Turek's
ORTHOPAEDICS
Principles and Their Application

Sixth Edition

Turek's
ORTHOPAEDICS
Principles and Their Application

Editors

Stuart L. Weinstein, MD

Ignacio V. Ponseti Chair and Professor
Department of Orthopaedics and Rehabilitation
University of Iowa Roy and Lucille Carver College of Medicine
University of Iowa Hospitals and Clinics
Iowa City, Iowa

Joseph A. Buckwalter, MD

Arthur Steindler Chair of Orthopaedic Surgery
Professor and Head of the Department of Orthopaedics
and Rehabilitation
University of Iowa Roy and Lucille Carver College of Medicine
University of Iowa Hospitals and Clinics
Iowa City, Iowa

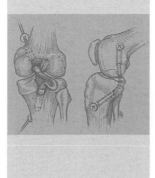

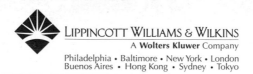

LIPPINCOTT WILLIAMS & WILKINS
A **Wolters Kluwer** Company
Philadelphia • Baltimore • New York • London
Buenos Aires • Hong Kong • Sydney • Tokyo

Acquisitions Editor: Robert Hurley
Developmental Editor: Tanya Lazar / Nancy Winter
Project Manager: David Murphy
Manufacturing Manager: Benjamin Rivera
Marketing Manager: Sharon Zinner
Production Services: Schawk, Inc.; Publishing Solutions for Retail, Book, and Catalog
Printer: Edward Brothers

Fifth Edition
Fourth Edition
Third Edition
Second Edition
First Edition

530 Walnut Street
Philadelphia, Pennsylvania 19106 USA
351 West Camden Street
Baltimore, Maryland 21201-2436 USA

Printed in the United States of America

Library of Congress Cataloging-in-Publication Data

Library of Congress Cataloging-in-Publication Data

Turek's orthopaedics : principles and their application / editors, Stuart L. Weinstein, Joseph A. Buckwalter.— 6th ed.
     p. ; cm.
   Includes bibliographical references and index.
   ISBN 0-7817-4298-6 (alk. paper)
   1. Orthopedics. I. Weinstein, Stuart L. II. Buckwalter, Joseph A. III. Title: Orthopaedics. [DNLM: 1. Orthopedics. WE 168 T9342 2005]
RD731.T8 2005
616.7—dc22
                              2005006236

10 9 8 7 6 5 4 3 2 1

Contributors

Robert F. Ashman, MD
Professor of Internal Medicine and Microbiology
Department of Internal Medicine: Rheumatology
University of Iowa Roy and Lucille Carver College
 of Medicine
VA Medical Center
Iowa City, Iowa

Joseph A. Buckwalter, MD
Professor and Head of the Department of
 Orthopaedics and Rehabilitation
University of Iowa Roy and Lucille Carver College
 of Medicine
University of Iowa Hospitals and Clinics
Iowa City, Iowa

Peter Devane, MBBhB, MSc, FRACS
Senior Lecturer in Orthopaedic Surgery
Wellington School of Medicine and Health Sciences
Wellington, New Zealand

Matthew B. Dobbs, MD
Assistant Professor
Department of Orthopaedic Surgery
Washington University School of Medicine
Children's Hospital
St. Louis, Missouri

Polly J. Ferguson, MD
Assistant Professor
Department of Pediatrics
University of Iowa Roy and Lucille Carver College
 of Medicine
University of Iowa Hospitals and Clinics
Iowa City, Iowa

Evan L. Flatow, MD
Bernard J. Lasker Professor of Orthopaedic Surgery
Department of Orthopaedics
Mount Sinai School of Medicine;

Chief of Shoulder Surgery
The Mount Sinai Hospital
New York, New York

John C. France, MD
Department of Orthopaedics
West Virginia University School of Medicine
Morgantown, West Virginia

Neil E. Green, MD
Department of Orthopaedics
Vanderbilt University Medical Center
Nashville, Tennessee

Gregory P. Guyton, MD
Greater Chesapeake Orthopaedic Associates
Union Memorial Hospital
Baltimore, Maryland

Geoffrey Horne, MBChB, FRCSc, FRACS
Professor of Surgery
Wellington School of Medicine and Health Sciences
Wellington, New Zealand

Jacob IJdo, MD, PhD
Assistant Professor
Department of Internal Medicine: Rheumatology
University of Iowa Roy and Lucille Carver College
 of Medicine
University of Iowa Hospitals and Clinics
Iowa City, Iowa

Eric T. Jones, MD, PhD
Professor, Orthopaedic Surgery
Department of Orthopaedics
West Virginia University School of Medicine
Morgantown, West Virginia

Kenton R. Kaufman, PhD, PE
Director
Motion Analysis Laboratory

Division of Orthopedic Research
Mayo Clinic Rochester
Rochester, Minnesota

Hyun Woo Kim, MD, PhD
Associate Professor
Department of Orthopaedic Surgery
Yonsei University College of Medicine
Severance Hospital
Seoul, Korea

Kenneth A. Krackow, MD
Professor
Department of Orthopaedics
State University of New York at Buffalo School of
  Medical and Biomedical Sciences;
Clinical Director of Orthopaedics
KALEIDA Health
Buffalo General Hospital
Buffalo, New York

Joseph M. Lane, MD
Department of Orthopedic Surgery
Hospital for Special Surgery and Weill Medical
  College of Cornell University;
Metabolic Bone Disease Service
Hospital for Special Surgery
New York, New York

George V. Lawry II, MD
Professor
Department of Internal Medicine: Rheumatology
University of Iowa Roy and Lucille Carver College
  of Medicine
University of Iowa Hospitals and Clinics
Iowa City, Iowa

Edward W. Lee, MD
Clinical Shoulder Fellow
Mount Sinai School of Medicine
Department of Orthopaedic Surgery
Mount Sinai Medical Center
New York, New York

Julie T. Lin, MD
Physiatry Department
Hospital for Special Surgery and Department of
  Rehabilitation Medicine
Weill Medical College of Cornell University;
Metabolic Bone Disease Service
Hospital for Special Surgery
New York, New York

Mary M. Moore, MD
Department of Pediatrics
University of Iowa Roy and Lucille Carver College
  of Medicine
University of Iowa Hospitals and Clinics
Iowa City, Iowa

José A. Morcuende, MD, PhD
Assistant Professor
Department of Orthopaedic Surgery and
  Rehabilitation
University of Iowa Roy and Lucille Carver College
  of Medicine
University of Iowa Hospitals and Clinics
Iowa City, Iowa

Sandeep Munjal, M.ch(orth), MD
Clinical Assistant Instructor
Department of Orthopaedics
State University of New York at Buffalo School of
  Medical and Biomedical Sciences
Buffalo, New York

Peter M. Murray, MD
Associate Professor
Division of Hand and Microvascular Surgery
Department of Orthopaedic Surgery
The Mayo Graduate School of Medicine
Rochester, Minnesota;
Senior Associate Consultant
The Mayo Clinic
Jacksonville, Florida

Joseph Jacob Nania, MD
Assistant Professor of Pediatric Infectious Disease
Department of Pediatrics
Vanderbilt University Medical Center
Nashville, Tennessee

Kenneth Noonan, MD
Associate Professor
Department of Orthopaedics and Rehabilitation
Department of Pediatrics
University of Wisconsin
Madison, Wisconsin

Hui Wan Park, MD
Professor
Department of Orthopaedic Surgery
Yonsei University College of Medicine
Yongdong Severance Hospital
Seoul, Korea

Paul M. Peloso, MD
Associate Professor of Internal Medicine and
  Epidemiology
Department of Internal Medicine: Rheumatology
University of Iowa Roy and Lucille Carver College
  of Medicine
University of Iowa Hospitals and Clinics
Iowa City, Iowa

Laura Prokuski, MD
Assistant Professor
Department of Orthopedics and Rehabilitation
University of Wisconsin Hospitals
Madison, Wisconsin

John W. Rachow, MD, PhD
Assistant Professor
Department of Internal Medicine
University of Iowa Roy and Lucille Carver College
of Medicine
University of Iowa Hospitals and Clinics
Iowa City, Iowa

Haraldine A. Stafford, MD, PhD
Associate Professor
Department of Internal Medicine: Rheumatology
University of Iowa Roy and Lucille Carver College
of Medicine
University of Iowa Hospitals and Clinics
Iowa City, Iowa

Rebecca S. Tuetken, MD, PhD
Assistant Professor
Department of Internal Medicine:
Rheumatology
University of Iowa Roy and Lucille Carver College
of Medicine
University of Iowa Hospitals and Clinics
Iowa City, Iowa

Scott A. Vogelgesang, MD
Associate Professor
Department of Internal Medicine: Rheumatology
University of Iowa Roy and Lucille Carver College
of Medicine
University of Iowa Hospitals and Clinics
Iowa City, Iowa

Anand M. Vora, MD
Illinois Bone & Joint Institute
Lake Forest, Illinois

Kristy L. Weber, MD
Johns Hopkins University
Department of Orthopaedic Surgery
Baltimore, Maryland

Stuart L. Weinstein, MD
Ignacio V. Ponseti Chair and Professor
Department of Orthopaedics and Rehabilitation
University of Iowa Roy and Lucille Carver College
of Medicine
University of Iowa Hospitals and Clinics
Iowa City, Iowa

Preface

In the fifth edition of this classic textbook, the entire format was revised to reflect the dramatic changes that had occurred in orthopaedic surgery since the previous edition. The text was condensed to one volume and structured to be concise enough for the resident and medical student to obtain a broad presentation of the specialty in a limited amount of time. The textbook maintained the broad approach to adult and pediatric orthopaedics, but eliminated the details of specific surgical treatment as technologic advances that dictate surgical alternatives require more in-depth presentations that are only appropriate for the advanced-level resident. In the sixth edition, we have added 16 new authors, all authorities in their fields, and have added a chapter on biomechanics and gait and one on the fundamentals of fracture repair and management.

The sixth edition of the textbook remains true to the original purpose of *orthopaedics*—to transmit knowledge that stimulates enthusiasm for the practice of orthopaedics and creates interest and curiosity that leads to further investigation that advances the specialty.

Stuart L. Weinstein, MD
Joseph A. Buckwalter, MD
Iowa City, Iowa 2005

Contents

III   *Regional Disorders of the Musculoskeletal System* 321

11   *The Neck* 323

Eric T. Jones
John C. France

I

Orthopaedics and the Musculoskeletal System

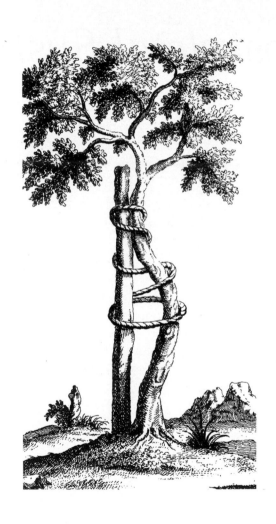

1

Joseph A. Buckwalter

Musculoskeletal Tissues and the Musculoskeletal System

The stability and mobility of the body depend on the tissues that form the musculoskeletal system: bone, cartilage, dense fibrous tissue, and muscle. These tissues differ in vascularity, innervation, mechanical and biological properties, and composition, but they share a common origin from mesenchymal cells. Understanding of diseases and injuries of the musculoskeletal system and their treatment depends on knowledge of these tissues. Failure to consider the biological and mechanical properties of the tissues, tissue changes caused by disease or injury, or the responses of the tissues to persistent changes in use can lead to misinterpretation of diagnostic information, suboptimal treatment decisions, and undesirable results of treatment. Furthermore, future advances in the diagnosis and treatment of musculoskeletal problems will depend on increased knowledge of the cell and matrix biology of the musculoskeletal tissues.

To provide the basis for understanding musculoskeletal diseases and injuries, this chapter reviews the structure and composition of the musculoskeletal tissues and the organization of the musculoskeletal system. The first section summarizes the distinctive characteristics of connective tissues including mesenchymal cells and the matrices they synthesize. The next sections review the structure, composition, and properties of bone; periosteum; the dense fibrous tissues (tendon, ligament, and joint capsule); tendon, ligament, and joint capsule insertions into bone; articular cartilage; growth cartilage; meniscus; synovium; muscle-tendon junction; and intervertebral disc. Although skeletal muscle is not a connective tissue, it is included in this chapter, because it forms a critical part of the musculoskeletal system. The last section discusses the formation and development of the musculoskeletal system.

CONNECTIVE TISSUE

The gross and microscopic studies of nineteenth-century histologists and pathologists led them to view connective tissue as a continuous basic tissue, or connecting substance, that extended throughout the body and assumed specialized forms including cartilage, periosteum, bone, tendon, fibrous septa, and fascia in different locations without altering the basic character of the tissue. The definition of basic connective tissue structure proposed by Virchow, "the greater part of the tissue is composed of intercellular substance, in which, at certain intervals cells are embedded," remains unchanged.

The role of connective tissue is most apparent in the musculoskeletal system, but all tissues and organ systems of multicellular organisms depend on connective tissue for mechanical support. The parenchymal cells of liver, kidney, and brain could not maintain the organization of these tissues or the tissue functions without their structural connective tissue framework. Normal function of the respiratory and cardiovascular systems depends on the repetitive mechanical performance of the connective tissues that form the airways and the blood vessels.

The group of specialized connective tissues that form the supporting structure and joints of the musculoskeletal system (bone, cartilage, dense fibrous tissue ligaments, tendons, and joint capsules) have primarily mechanical functions. Because of their obvious mechanical roles, and the prominence of their matrix component relative to their cellular component, these tissues are often regarded as homogeneous and inert. Yet, even in the mature skeleton they remain metabolically active, the cells and matrices are degraded and replaced, and the tissues respond to hormonal, metabolic, and mechanical stimuli.

Mesenchymal Tissues Versus Epithelial Tissues

During embryonic development two morphologic and functional classes of tissues appear: epithelium and mesenchyme. The skeletal connective tissues originate from a subdivision of the mesenchyme. Mesenchyme (Greek mesos, middle and enchyma, infusion) refers to the location of mesenchyme between the epithelial layers of endoderm and ectoderm. Epithelial tissues may develop from endoderm, ectoderm, and mesoderm, but mesenchyme appears to develop only from mesoderm.

The relationships of the cells to each other and the relationship of the cells to the matrix distinguish epithelia from mesenchyme. Epithelial cells form sheets or layers of cells. They establish close relationships with adjacent cells, frequently binding their membranes together with specialized cell junctions and devoting a large portion of their membranes to contact with other cells. Epithelial tissues generally have a sparse extracellular matrix, and a specialized form of matrix, basement membrane, that frequently serves as the bed for epithelial cells and separates them from mesenchymal tissue. Mesenchymal cells do not generally form sheets or layers. In the mesenchyme forming the skeletal connective tissues, cells rarely establish extensive contact with other cells and they surround themselves with an abundant extracellular matrix consisting of a macromolecular framework synthesized by the cells and water that fills the macromolecular framework. The cell membranes bind to specific macromolecules within the matrix, and although the cells may appear fixed in place by the surrounding matrix, they can migrate through the matrix.

Mesenchymal Cells

Undifferentiated mesenchymal cells not only can move through the tissue, they have the potential to divide rapidly and differentiate into specialized musculoskeletal tissue cells including the cells of cartilage, bone, dense fibrous tissues, and muscle. Systemic factors including nutrition and hormonal balance combined with local factors in the cell environment such as the composition of the matrix, concentrations of oxygen, cytokines and nutrients, pH, and mechanical forces influence mesenchymal cell proliferation and differentiation. These systemic and local factors interact with the genomic potential of the cell to determine the progression from undifferentiated stem cells to highly differentiated cells like chondrocytes and osteocytes.

The progressive differentiation proceeds through a series of stages with transition from one stage to the next dependent on signals from the local environment. The variety of forms these mesenchymal cells can assume include blood, fat, and muscle cells as well as the specialized connective tissue cells, fibroblasts, chondrocytes, osteoblasts, and osteocytes. Cell differentiation creates persistent, but not necessarily permanent changes in the cells. In general, the differentiated cell form persists through many generations of the cell. Some cells, like chondrocytes, rarely divide but maintain their differentiated form for their entire life. During cell differentiation, the cells not only change their form but also change the types of molecules they synthesize and thus the composition and organization of the matrix that surrounds them.

Even in the skeletally mature individual, undifferentiated mesenchymal cells persist. With increasing age they may lose some of their capacity for proliferation and differentiation, but they can still respond to appropriate signals by migrating, proliferating, and differentiating into the mature cells of bone, cartilage, and dense fibrous tissue including osteoblasts, osteocytes, chondrocytes, and fibroblasts.

Mesenchymal Matrices

The matrices of the musculoskeletal tissues consist of elaborate highly organized frameworks of organic macromolecules filled with water. Light microscopic examination of these matrices shows fibrils embedded in an amorphous ground substance. Biochemical examination shows that the fibrils consist of multiple types of collagen and elastin, the ground substance consists primarily of water and proteoglycans, and the matrix contains another class of macromolecules called noncollagenous proteins. In addition to an organic matrix, bone has an inorganic matrix that consists primarily of calcium phosphate.

Organic Matrix Macromolecules

COLLAGENS. Collagens give all connective tissues their basic form and tensile strength, but the tissues vary in collagen concentration and organization, and in the types of collagens that form part of their organic matrix. All collagens function as structural proteins in the extracellular matrix and a significant portion of each collagen molecule consists of a triple helix formed from three amino acid chains (Figure 1-1). This helical structure gives the molecules stiffness and strength.

More than 20 genes direct the synthesis of at least 16 different types of collagen. Differences in molecular topology and polymeric form divide the 13 known collagen types into three classes: class I (fibrillar collagens), class II (basement membrane collagens), and class III (short chain collagens). A specific type of collagen may vary slightly among tissues. For example, bone type I collagen, which normally mineralizes, appears to differ in structure and composition from tendon type I collagen, which does not mineralize under normal conditions.

Class I Collagens (Fibrillar Collagens). Class I collagens form the cross-banded fibrils seen by electron microscopy in all connective tissues. The five collagens in this group—types I, II, III, V, and XI—have triple helical domains consisting of about 1,000 amino acid residues in each of three polypeptide chains. Type I collagen forms the principal matrix macromolecule of skin, bone, meniscus, annulus fibrosis, tendon, ligament, joint capsule, and all other dense fibrous tissues. Figure 1-2 shows the assembly of type I collagen microfibrils. Type II collagen forms the banded fibrils found in hyaline cartilage, the nucleus pulposus of the intervertebral disc, and the vitreous humor of the eye. The "minor" fibrillar collagens, types V and XI, also contribute to the matrices of the connective tissues. Type V forms part of the matrix in tissues containing type I collagen, usually about 3% of the amount of type I. Type XI forms part of the type II collagen fibrils. Type III collagen occurs in association with type I collagen in most tissues other than bone and appears in repair tissue.

Class II Collagens (Basement Membrane Collagens). The class II collagens—types IV, VII and VIII—form critical parts of basement membranes. Type IV contributes the major structural component of basement membranes. Type VII acts as an anchoring filament in epithelial basement membranes, and type VIII forms part of endothelial basement membranes.

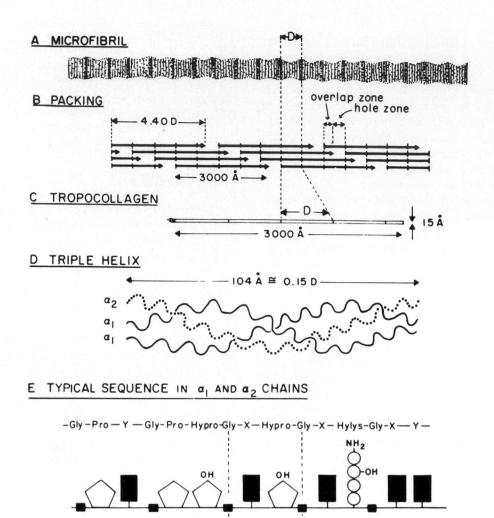

FIGURE 1-1. Type I collagen. **(A)** A stained microfibril of collagen exhibiting characteristic cross-striations with a regular repeat period (D) of approximately 680 Å. **(B)** A two-dimensional representation of the packing arrangement of tropocollagen macromolecules in the microfibril. **(C)** Each tropocollagen molecule has large numbers of darkly staining bands, and five of these, which are separated by a regular distance of 680 Å, account for the repeat period **(D)** in the microfibril. The H$_2$N-terminal and probably the HOOC-terminal ends of the molecule are atypical and nonhelical in structure and are called "telopeptides." **(D)** Each tropocollagen molecule consists of three polypeptides, two with identical amino acid sequences (α_1 chains) and one with a slightly different amino acid sequence (α_2 chain). Each α chain is coiled in a tight left-handed helix with a pitch of 9.5 Å, and the three chains are coiled around each other in a right-handed "super-helix" with a pitch of about 104 Å. **(E)** Gly occurs in every third position throughout most of the polypeptide chains, and large amounts of Pro and Hypro occur in the other two positions. X and Y represent any amino acid other than Gly, Pro, Hypro Lys, or Hys. (Grant ME, Prockop DJ. The biosynthesis of collagen. N Eng J Med 1972;286:194, 242, 291)

Class III Collagens (Short Chain Collagens). The forms and functions of class III collagens—types VI, IX and X—remain less understood than the forms and functions of the other classes of collagens. Type VI collagen appears in small amounts in many tissues. When examined by electron microscopy, it appears as filamentous banded aggregates. These aggregates often appear in the matrix immediately surrounding cells. Type IX collagen forms covalent bonds with type II collagen molecules and thus contributes to the extracellular matrix of hyaline cartilage. It may influence type II collagen fibril diameter

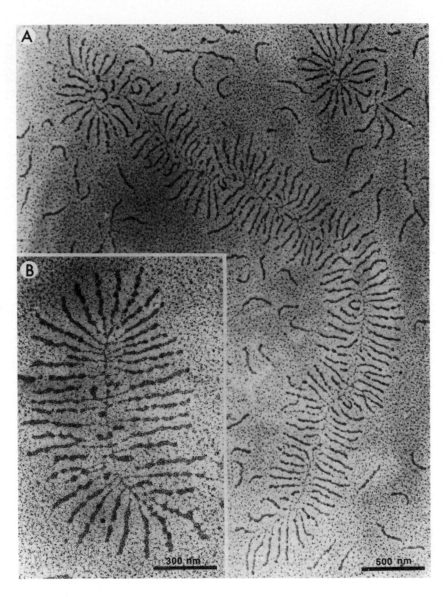

FIGURE 1-2. Electron micrographs showing the structure of proteoglycan aggregates. **(A)** A large aggregate. The central filament is hyaluronic acid and the projecting side arms are proteoglycan monomers. **(B)** A smaller proteoglycan aggregate.

and the organization of the hyaline cartilage matrix. Type X collagen occurs in the calcified cartilage region of the physis, articular cartilage, and bone fracture callus. Although its limited distribution suggests that it may have an important role in chondrocyte enlargement or cartilage mineralization, its functions remain unknown. The forms and functions of types XII and XIII collagens likewise remain unknown.

ELASTIN. Elastin, like collagen, forms protein fibrils, but elastin fibrils lack the cross-banding pattern seen in electron microscopic studies of fibrillar collagens (Figure 1-3) and differ from collagens in amino acid composition, confirmation of the amino acid chains, and mechanical properties. In addition,

elastin also forms lamellae or sheet-like structures. Unlike collagen, elastin can undergo some deformation without rupturing or tearing. Following deformation it returns to its original size and shape. Amino acid chains of elastin contain two amino acids not found in collagens (desmosine and isodesmosine), and the elastin amino acid chains form random coils, unlike the highly ordered triple helices of collagens. The random coil confirmation of the amino acid chains makes it possible for elastin fibers and sheets to undergo some deformation without molecular damage and then resume their original shape and size.

Elastin does not form part of the matrices of hyaline cartilage or bone, and it contributes only a small amount to the extracellular matrices most of

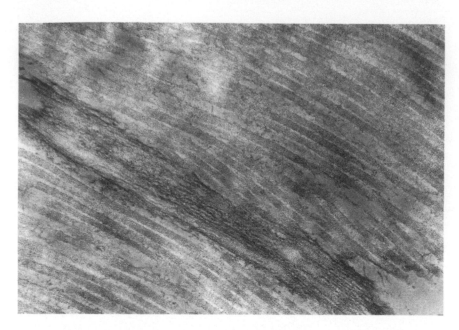

FIGURE 1-3. Electron micrograph showing cross-banded collagen fibrils lying parallel to an elastic fiber consisting of multiple dark microfibrils and regions of amorphous elastin.

other connective tissues. Trace amounts appear in the intervertebral disc and meniscus. Many ligaments also have some elastin, usually less than 5%, but a few ligaments, such as the nuchal ligament and the ligamentum flavum, have high elastin concentrations, up to 75%.

PROTEOGLYCANS. Proteoglycans form the major nonfibrillar macromolecule of the cartilage, intervertebral disc, dense fibrous tissue, bone, and muscle matrices. These musculoskeletal tissues vary considerably in the concentration and possibly the function of proteoglycans. The highest concentrations of proteoglycans occur in hyaline cartilages and nucleus pulposus. In these tissues the concentration of proteoglycans may approach 30 to 40% of the tissue dry weight, and these molecules significantly influence fluid flow through the matrix and help give the tissues stiffness to compression and resilience. They may have similar space-filling and mechanical roles in the other tissues, but the much lower concentrations in these tissues (in the dense fibrous tissues and bone, they contribute at most a few percent of the dry weight) make their effect on the tissue mechanical properties proportionately less. Muscle also contains specific types of proteoglycans, but they form only a small fraction of the tissue.

Proteoglycan aggrecan molecules (formerly called monomers), the basic units of proteoglycan molecules, consist of polysaccharide chains covalently bound to protein. Most types of proteoglycans contain relatively little protein, about 5% or less. Glycosaminoglycans, a special class of polysaccharide consisting of repeating disaccharide units containing a derivative of either glucosamine or galactosamine and carrying one or two negative charges, form the principal part of proteoglycan molecules (Figure 1-4). Connective tissue glycosaminoglycans include hyaluronic acid, chondroitin 4 sulfate, chondroitin 6 sulfate, dermatan sulfate, and keratan sulfate.

Aggrecans (proteoglycan monomers) and Proteoglycan Aggregates. Aggrecans consist of protein core filaments with multiple covalently bound oligosaccharides and longer chondroitin and keratan sulfate chains. Each glycosaminoglycan chain creates a string of negative charges that bind water and cations in solution. Because of this property, aggrecans can expand to fill a large domain in solution. In most musculoskeletal tissues, an intact collagen fibril network limits the swelling of the proteoglycans, but loss or degradation of the collagen fibril network will allow a tissue that contains a high concentration of large proteoglycans to swell, increasing the water concentration, and the permeability of the tissue.

Proteoglycan aggregates, consisting of a central hyaluronic acid filament with multiple attached aggrecans and link proteins, may reach a length of more than 10,000 nanometers with more than 300 aggrecans (Figure 1-2). Link proteins stabilize the association between monomers and hyaluronic acid and may have a role in directing the assembly of aggregates in the matrix. Aggregates appear to help

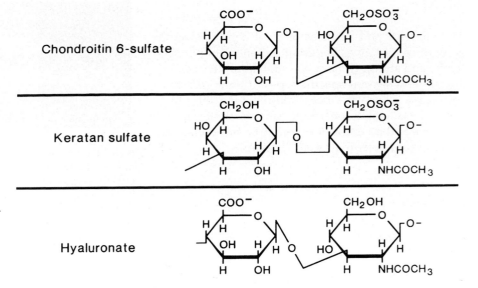

FIGURE 1-4. Diagrammatic representation of the structures of the glycosaminoglycans, chondroitin sulfate, keratan sulfate, and hyaluronate. Chondroitin sulfate has two negative charges per disaccharide and the others have one. (From Buckwalter JA, Cooper RR. The cells and matrices of skeletal connective tissues. Chapter 1. In: Albright JA, Brand RA, eds. The Scientific Basis of Orthopaedics. Norwalk, CT: Appleton & Lange, 1987:23)

anchor aggrecans within the matrix, preventing their displacement and thereby organizing and stabilizing the macromolecular framework. They also help determine the permeability of the matrix and thus the flow of water through the matrix.

Small Nonaggregating Proteoglycans. Small nonaggregating proteoglycans may contain chondroitin sulfate and dermatan sulfate. They consist of one or two glycosaminoglycan chains covalently bound to a protein core. They form specific associations with collagen fibrils and may influence matrix organization and the ability of cells to bind to the matrix collagen fibrils.

NONCOLLAGENOUS PROTEINS. Less is known about noncollagenous proteins and glycoproteins than about the collagens, elastin, or proteoglycans. Although they form part of the macromolecular framework of musculoskeletal tissues, few noncollagenous proteins have been identified and their functions have not been well defined. Most of them consist primarily of protein with small numbers of attached monosaccharides and oliosaccharides. They appear to have roles in the organization and maintenance of the macromolecular structure of the matrix and in establishing and maintaining the relationships between the cells and the other matrix macromolecules.

Examples of noncollagenous proteins found within the musculoskeletal tissue matrices include link protein, fibronectin, and tenascin. Link protein helps organize and stabilize the extracellular matrix through its effect on proteoglycan aggregation. Soluble fibronectin occurs in many body fluids including plasma, urine, amniotic fluid, and cerebral spinal fluid. Insoluble or cellular fibronectin appears in most musculoskeletal tissue matrices. Fibronectins examined by electron microscopy appear as fine filaments or granules. They may coat the surface of fibrillar collagens and associate with cell membranes. Tenascin, another matrix glycoprotein, occurs in perichondrium, periosteum, tendon, and muscle-tendon junction.

Inorganic Matrix

Normal function of the musculoskeletal tissues depends on rapid controlled mineralization (deposition of relatively insoluble mineral within the organic matrix) of some organic matrices and prevention of mineralization in others, yet the conditions that control and promote normal and pathologic mineralization of musculoskeletal tissues remain poorly understood. Bone, the growth plate cartilage longitudinal septa, and a thin zone of articular cartilage organic matrices all mineralize normally. The organic matrices of other cartilage regions and dense fibrous tissues mineralize in association with certain diseases including chondrocalcinosis, and muscle and some dense fibrous tissues mineralize following some injuries. The deposition of mineral in the organic matrix radically changes the properties of the tissue. It increases stiffness and compressive strength of bone, but pathologic mineralization of cartilage and dense fibrous tissue may accelerate or be associated with degenerative changes in these tissues.

BONE

The strength and stiffness of bone combined with its light weight gives vertebrates their mobility, dexterity, and strength. Bone has an elaborate vascular supply and several specific types of bone cells that form and resorb the bone matrix. Like the other musculoskeletal tissues, bone consists of mesenchymal cells and an extracellular matrix, but unlike the other tissues bone matrix mineralizes.

Structure

Gross Structure

BONE SHAPES. Bones assume a remarkable variety of shapes and sizes. They vary in size from the ear ossicles to the long bones of the leg. The variety of shapes allows them to be classified into three groups: long bones, short bones, and flat bones. Long bones like the femur, tibia, or humerus have an expanded metaphysis and epiphysis at either end with thick walled tubular diaphysis. The thick cortical walls of the diaphysis become thinner and increase in diameter as they form the metaphysis, and articular cartilage covers the epiphyses where they form synovial joints. The metacarpals, metatarsals, and phalanges, like the larger limb bones, have the form of long bones. Short bones, like the tarsals, carpals, and centra of the vertebrae, have approximately the same length in all directions. Flat or tabular bones have one dimension that is much shorter than the other two, like the scapula or wing of the ilium.

CORTICAL AND CANCELLOUS BONE. Examination of the cut surface of a bone shows that the tissue assumes two forms: the outer cortical or compact bone and the inner cancellous or trabecular bone (Figure 1-5). Cortical bone forms about 80% of the skeleton and surrounds the thin bars or plates of cancellous bone with compact lamellae. In long bones, dense cortical bone forms the cylindrical diaphysis that surrounds a marrow cavity containing little or no trabecular bone. In the metaphyses of long bones, the cortical bone thins and trabecular bone fills the medullary cavity. Short and flat bones usually have thinner cortices than the diaphyses of long bones and contain cancellous bone. Cancellous and cortical bone modify their structure in response to persistent changes in loading, hormonal influences, and other factors.

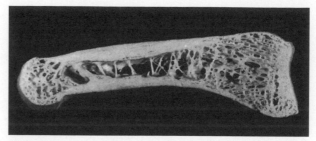

FIGURE 1-5. Longitudinal section of a human phalanx. Outer lamellae of cortical bone surround the inner cancellous bone. The metaphyses contain more cancellous bone than the diaphysis and the thick cortical bone of the diaphysis becomes thinner in the metaphysis. Larger bones like the femur follow the same structural pattern. (From Buckwalter JA, Cooper RR. Bone structure and function. In: AAOS Instructional Course Lectures, XXXVI, Park Ridge, IL: American Academy of Orthopaedic Surgeons, 1987:27–48)

Because of their differences in density and organization, equal size blocks of cortical and cancellous bone have different mechanical properties. The two types of bone have the same composition, but cortical bone has much greater density. Because the compression strength of bone is proportional to the square of the density, cortical bone has compressive strength that may be in order of magnitude greater than that of cancellous bone. Differences in the organization and orientation of cortical and cancellous bone matrices may also make a difference in their mechanical properties.

Microscopic Structure

MINERALIZED AND UNMINERALIZED BONE MATRIX. During skeletal growth and bone remodeling, osteoblasts form seams of unmineralized bone organic matrix, called osteoid, on the surface of mineralized bone matrix. Normally, osteoid mineralizes soon after it appears. Therefore, normal bone contains only small amounts of unmineralized matrix.

Osteoid lacks the stiffness of mineralized bone matrix. For this reason, failure to mineralize bone matrix during growth or during normal turnover of bone matrix in mature individuals produces weaker bone. Individuals with impaired mineralization of bone matrix may develop skeletal deformities or fractures. In children, the clinical condition associated with impaired mineralization, rickets, predisposes the patient to skeletal deformity. In adults, the clinical condition associated with impaired mineralization, osteomalacia, predisposes the patient to fractures.

WOVEN AND LAMELLAR BONE. Mineralized bone exists in two forms: woven (immature, fiber, or primary) bone and lamellar (mature, secondary) bone. Woven bone forms the embryonic skeleton and the new bone formed in the metaphyseal parts of growth plates. Mature bone replaces this woven bone as the skeleton develops and during skeletal growth. Small amounts of woven bone may persist after skeletal maturity as part of tendon and ligament insertions, the suture margins of cranial bones, and the ear ossicles. With these exceptions, woven bone rarely appears in the normal human skeleton after 4 or 5 years of age, although it is the first bone formed in many healing fractures at any age and it also appears during the rapid turnover and formation of bone associated with metabolic, neoplastic, and infectious or inflammatory diseases.

Woven and mature bone differ in mechanical properties and the rate of bone formation. Cells rapidly form the irregular, almost random, collagen fibril matrix of woven bone. The appearance of the irregular arrangement of collagen fibrils gives woven bone its name. It contains approximately four times as many osteocytes per unit volume of lamellar bone, and they vary in size, orientation, and distribution. The mineralization of the woven bone matrix also follows an irregular pattern with mineral deposits varying in size and their relationship to collagen fibrils. In contrast, cells form lamellar bone more slowly and the cell density is less. The collagen fibrils of lamellar bone vary less in diameter and lie in tightly aligned parallel sheets forming distinct lamellae 4 to 12 microns thick with an almost uniform distribution of mineral throughout the matrix.

Because of the lack of collagen fibril orientation, the high cell and water content, and the irregular mineralization, the mechanical properties of woven bone differ from those of lamellar bone. It is more flexible, more easily deformed, and weaker than mature lamellar bone. For this reason, the immature skeleton and healing fractures have less stiffness and strength than the mature skeleton or a fracture remodeled with lamellar bone.

Composition

Cells

The formation and maintenance of bone depends on the coordinated actions of different types of bone cells. The morphology, function, and characteristics of bone cells separate them into four groups: undifferentiated or osteoprogenitor cells, osteoblasts, osteocytes, and osteoclasts.

UNDIFFERENTIATED OR OSTEOPROGENITOR CELLS. Undifferentiated or osteoprogenitor cells, small cells with single nuclei, few organelles, and irregular forms, remain in an undifferentiated state until stimulated to proliferate or differentiate into osteoblasts. They usually reside in the canals of bone, the endosteum, and the periosteum, although cells that can differentiate into osteoblasts also exist in tissues other than bone.

OSTEOBLASTS. Osteoblasts, cuboidal cells with a single, usually eccentric, nucleus, contain large volumes of synthetic organelles: endoplasmic reticulum and Golgi membranes (Figure 1-6). They lie on bone surfaces where, when stimulated, they form new bone organic matrix and participate in controlling matrix mineralization. When active, they assume a round, oval, or polyhedral form and a seam of new osteoid separates them from mineralized matrix. Their cytoplasmic processes extend through the osteoid to contact osteocytes within mineralized matrix. Once they are actively engaged in synthesizing new matrix, they can follow one of two courses. They can decrease their synthetic activity, remain on the bone surface, and assume the flatter form of a bone surface lining cell or they can surround themselves with matrix and become osteocytes.

OSTEOCYTES. Osteocytes contribute more than 90% of the cells of the mature skeleton. Combined with the periosteal and endosteal cells, they cover the bone matrix surfaces. Their long cytoplasmic processes extend from their oval- or lens-shaped bodies to contact other osteocytes within the bone matrix or the cell processes of osteoblasts, forming a network of cells that extends from the bone surfaces throughout the bone matrix (Figures 1-7 and 1-8). The cell membranes of the osteocytes and their cell processes cover more than 90% of the total surface area of mature bone matrix. This arrangement gives them access to almost all the mineralized matrix surface area and may be critical in the cell mediated exchange of mineral that takes place between bone fluid and the blood. In particular, they may help maintain the composition of bone fluid and the body's mineral balance.

OSTEOCLASTS. Osteoclasts, large irregular cells with multiple nuclei, fill much of their cytoplasm with mitochondria to supply the energy required for

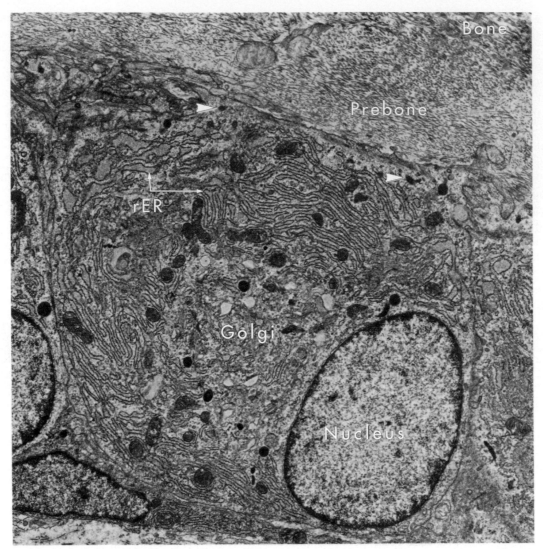

FIGURE 1-6. Electron micrograph of an osteoblast from demineralized rat alveolar bone showing the arrangement of the organelles. Numerous collagen fibrils, which these cells secrete, are present in the adjacent prebone or osteon and bone (*upper right*). The procollagen, which is the precursor of the collagen fibrils, is carried within secretory granules (*arrowheads*) originating from the Golgi saccules. Procollagen is released into the prebone by fusion of the secretory granule with the apical plasma membrane of the cell. (×12,000) (From Melvyn Weinstock; Ham AW, Cormack DH. Histology, 8th Ed. Philadelphia: JB Lippincott, 1979)

these cells to resorb bone. They usually lie directly against the bone matrix on endosteal, periosteal, and Haversian system bone surfaces (Figure 1-9), but unlike osteocytes, and presumably osteoblasts, they can move from one site of bone resorption to another. Osteoclasts appear to form by fusion of multiple bone-marrow-derived mononuclear cells. When they have finished their bone resorbing activity, they may divide to reform multiple mononuclear cells.

One of the most distinctive features of osteoclasts is the complex folding of their cytoplasmic membrane where it lies against the bone matrix at sites of bone resorption (Figure 1-10). This ruffled or brushed border appears to play a critical role in bone resorption, possibly by increasing the surface area of the cell relative to the bone and creating a sharply localized environment that rapidly degrades bone matrix. The fluid between the brush border and the bone matrix probably has a high concentration of hydrogen ions and proteolytic enzymes: the acidic environment could demineralize bone matrix, and the enzymes could degrade the

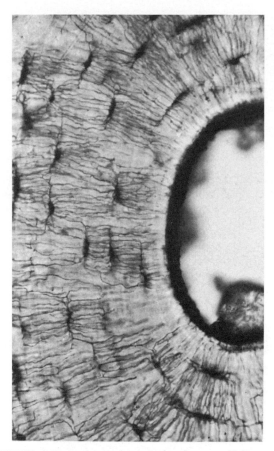

FIGURE 1-7. A photomicrograph of a ground bone section. The lacunae in which the osteocytes reside are dark flattened oval structures. The fine lines connecting these are canaliculi. The canaliculi extend to the empty canal on the right. In life this contained blood vessels that supplied tissue fluid to the canaliculi. (Preparation by H. Whittaker; Ham AW, Cormack DH. Histology, 8th Ed. Philadelphia: JB Lippincott, 1979)

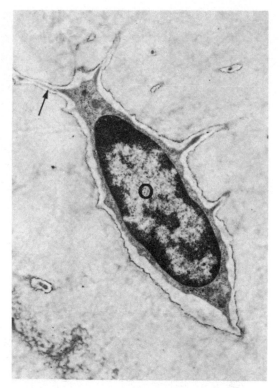

FIGURE 1-8. Low-power electron micrograph of an osteocyte and its processes in a section of decalcified bone. The nucleus (0) and an arrow point to a process in a canaliculus. Two processes in canaliculi cut in cross section can be seen one near the upper right corner and the other toward the lower left corner. (From S. C. Luk and G. T. Simon; Ham AW, Cormack DH. Histology, 8th Ed. Philadelphia: JB Lippincott, 1979)

organic bone matrix. In cancellous bone, osteoclasts resorbing the bone surface create a characteristic depression called a Howship's lacuna. In cortical bone, several osteoclasts lead the osteonal cutting cones that remodel dense cortical bone.

Bone Matrix

Bone matrix consists of the organic macromolecules, the inorganic mineral, and the matrix fluid. The inorganic matrix component contributes approximately 70% of wet bone weight, although it may contribute up to 80%. The organic macromolecules contribute about 20% of the bone wet weight and water contributes 8 to 10%. The organic matrix gives bone its form and provides its tensile strength; the mineral component gives bone strength in compression.

Removal of the bone mineral or digestion of the organic matrix show the contributions of the inorganic and organic matrix components to the mechanical properties of bone. Removal of either component leaves bone with its original form and shape, but demineralized bone, like a tendon or ligament, has great flexibility. A demineralized long bone, such as the fibula, can be twisted or bent without fracture. In contrast, removal of the organic matrix makes bone brittle. Only a slight deformation will crack the inorganic matrix and a sharp blow will shatter it.

ORGANIC MATRIX. The organic matrix of bone resembles that of dense fibrous tissues like tendon, ligament, annulus fibrosis, meniscus, and joint capsule. Type I collagen contributes over 90% of the organic matrix. The other 10% includes small

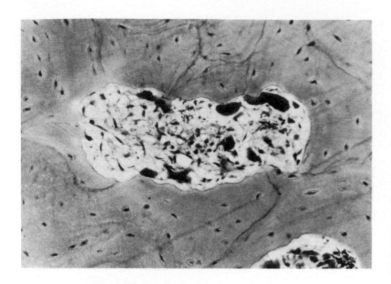

FIGURE 1-9. Photomicrograph of a cross section of the shaft of a bone showing a resorption cavity in cross or somewhat oblique section. The large dark cells are osteoclasts; their activity explains the etched-out borders of the cavity. (Ham AW, Cormack DH. Histology, 8th Ed. Philadelphia: JB Lippincott, 1979)

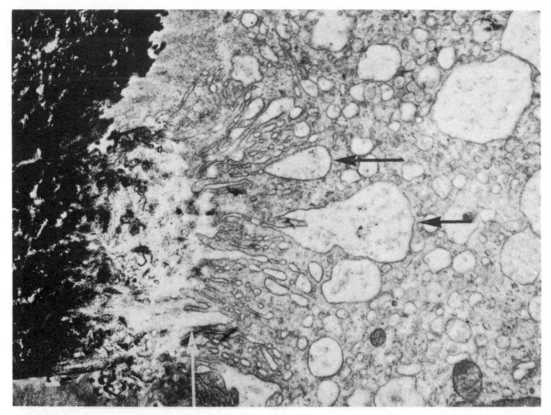

FIGURE 1-10. Electron micrograph of a section of a bone surface undergoing resorption. Calcified bone appears black at the left. The main part of the picture is occupied by the cytoplasm of an osteoclast. Extending from the top to the bottom, in the middle of the picture, is the ruffled border of the osteoclast; this consists of complex folds and projections that abut on the bone at the left. Between the ruffled border of the osteoclast and the heavily calcified bone is an area where the calcium content is much less, which suggests that the osteoclast is dissolving or otherwise removing mineral from this area. Black granules of mineral can be seen in some of the large vesicles that are indicated by horizontal arrows, and that probably form because of the bottom of crypts being pinched off. In the original print a collagenic microfibril showing typical periodicity could be seen at this site indicated by the vertical arrow. (×20,000) (From B. Boothroyd and N. M. Hancox; Ham AW, Cormack DH. Histology, 8th Ed. Philadelphia: JB Lippincott, 1979)

proteoglycans, many of noncollagenous proteins including osteonectin and small amounts of type V collagen and possibly other collagens.

Mineralization changes and stabilizes the composition of the bone organic matrix. Compared to bone organic matrix, osteoid contains more noncollagenous macromolecules and water. Once mineralization occurs, the organic matrix remains stable until resorbed. Abnormalities of the organic matrix can weaken bone. For example, many patients with osteogenesis imperfecta have disturbances of synthesis, secretion, or assembly of the collagen component of the bone organic matrix that increase bone fragility.

INORGANIC MATRIX. The mechanisms that initiate and control the transformation of osteoid into mineralized bone matrix remain unclear, but morphologic studies show that soon after osteoblasts produce osteoid, mineral appears within the bone type I collagen fibrils and then extends through the matrix without altering the organization of the collagen fibrils (Figure 1-11) or affecting osteocytes within the mineralized matrix. Mineralization of the bone matrix not only increases the stiffness and strength of bone, it provides a reservoir for minerals needed for normal function of other tissues and organ systems.

The bone matrix contains about 99% of the body's calcium, 80% of the phosphate, and large proportions of the sodium, magnesium, and carbonate.

Newly mineralized bone matrix contains a variety of calcium phosphate species that range from relatively soluble complexes to insoluble crystalline hydroxyapatite. As bone matures, the inorganic matrix becomes primarily crystalline hydroxyapatite, although sodium, magnesium, citrate, and fluoride may also be present. Because the degree of mineralization increases with maturation, the material properties of bone change as well. In particular, with increasing mineralization, bone stiffness increases. This change helps explain why children's and adult's bones may differ in their patterns of fracture. When subjected to excessive load, normal adult bone usually breaks rather than deforming permanently. In contrast, children's bones may bow or buckle rather than break.

Control of Bone Cell Activity

Throughout life, osteoclasts remove bone matrix and osteoblasts replace it. The reason for this physiologic turnover of bone tissue has not been established, but

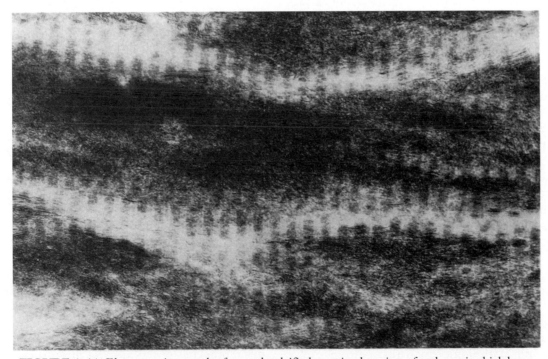

FIGURE 1-11. Electron micrograph of an undecalcified unstained section of embryonic chick bone. The ordered disposition of the dense mineral phase along the axial direction of the collagen fibrils is evident. Note also that the mineral phase is in lateral register as well. (×110,000) (Glimcher MJ. A basic architectural principle in the organization of mineralized tissues. Clin Orthop 1968:61:16)

it may have a role in maintaining the structural integrity of the bone tissue. To preserve normal bone mass and mechanical properties, osteoblastic bone formation must balance osteoclastic bone resorption. A variety of stimuli can alter this balance. For example, repetitive loading of the skeleton can increase bone formation relative to bone resorption and thereby increase bone mass and strength. Immobilization decreases bone formation relative to bone resorption, thereby decreasing bone mass and strength.

Bone mass normally changes with age. It increases to a maximum value about 10 years after completion of skeletal growth, remains stable for a variable period, and then begins to decrease, progressively weakening the skeleton. The reasons for the age-related loss of bone mass and the mechanisms that normally coordinate and control bone cell function remain poorly understood, but investigations of bone turnover show that both systemic and local factors help control osteoclast and osteoblast function.

Systemic Factors

Systemic factors that influence the balance between bone resorption and bone formation include nutrition, exercise, and hormonal activity, especially parathyroid hormone. Additional factors include Vitamin D and its metabolites, thyroid hormone, growth hormone, insulin, estrogens, testosterone, and calcitonin. Dietary abnormalities, lack of physical activity, and some disturbances of hormone balance are the most common known causes of clinically significant systemic increases in bone resorption relative to bone formation. Protein deficiency impairs bone formation during bone growth and remodeling. Prolonged lack of exercise will decrease bone mass. Vitamin D deficiency and abnormalities of Vitamin D metabolism produce rickets or osteomalacia. Excessive parathyroid hormone increases bone turnover and decreases bone mass; excessive thyroid hormones can have similar effects. Exogenous corticosteroids decrease the synthetic activity of osteoblasts and may interfere with the ability of undifferentiated cells to assume the form of osteoblasts and adversely affect calcium balance. As a result, patients receiving corticosteroids for prolonged periods may develop severe osteopenia and multiple pathologic fractures. Estrogen also influences bone cell function. In many women, bone mass begins to decrease rapidly after menopause and then continues to decrease rapidly for 5 to 10 years. Estrogen replacement can slow or reverse this rapid loss.

Local Factors

In addition to systemic factors, local factors including oxygen tension, pH, local ion concentrations, interactions between cells, local concentrations of nutrients and metabolites, mechanical and electrical signals, and interaction between cells and matrix molecules can influence the balance between bone loss and bone formation. Localized mechanical loading of bone has particular significance. Immobilization or decreased loading of a limb causes a relatively rapid loss of bone mass whereas repetitive increased loading can increase bone density.

Recent work suggests that cytokines, small protein molecules that influence multiple cell functions, can influence bone cell function and may help couple bone resorption and formation. Cytokines produced by neoplasms may increase bone formation or, more frequently, increase bone resorption. Interleukin-1, a cytokine produced by monocytes, stimulates osteoclast formation and osteoclastic bone resorption. It may contribute to the loss of bone in conditions like rheumatoid arthritis. Transforming growth factor β, a cytokine present in bone matrix, may be one of the factors that balances bone resorption and bone formation. Osteoclastic resorption of bone matrix may release or activate transforming growth factor β. Activated transforming growth factor β then may inhibit osteoclastic activity and stimulate osteoblasts to form bone.

Blood Supply

An elaborate system of vessels extends throughout bone, penetrating even the densest cortical bone (Figure 1-12). No cell lies more than 300 microns from a blood vessel.

Long bone diaphyses and metaphyses have three sources of blood supply: nutrient arteries, epiphyseal and metaphyseal penetrating arteries, and periosteal arteries (Figure 1-13). The nutrient arteries pass through the diaphyseal cortex and branch proximally and distally forming the medullary arterial system that supplies the diaphysis. The proximal and distal branches of the nutrient arteries join multiple fine branches of periosteal and metaphyseal arteries that contribute to the medullary vascular system.

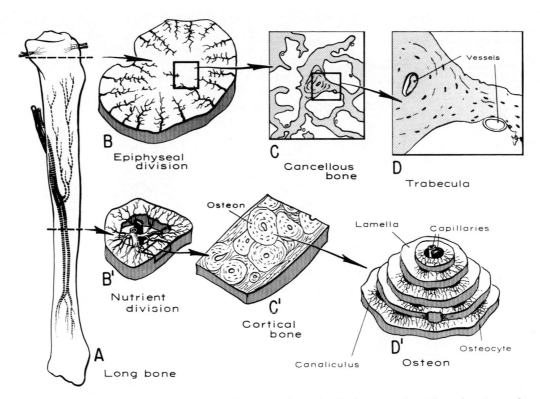

FIGURE 1-12. Distribution of nutrient blood supply to the diaphyseal and epiphyseal regions of a long bone. **(A)** Basic pattern of nutrient circulation to a long bone (human tibia). **(B)** Pattern of circulation in epiphyseal–metaphyseal region. Arteries perforate thin cortical shell to enter cancellous bone. **(C)** Structure of cancellous bone. **(D)** A trabeculae of bone. Capillaries abut against thin trabecula. In thicker trabecula, an osteon can be seen. **(B′)** Cross section of mid diaphysis. Here there is a single nutrient artery and vein. Lateral branches arise from the artery to supply the cortical bone. **(C′)** Cortical bone. Osteons and interstitial bone between osteons. **(D′)** Diagrammatic concept of a single osteon canaliculi of the osteocytes are canals in which the processes of the osteocytes are located. It is by way of these canaliculi that nutrition if derived from the vessels in the Haversian canal (Kelly PJ, Peterson LFA. The blood supply of bone. Heart Bull 1963;12:96)

Under normal circumstances this medullary vascular system supplies most of periosteum covered bone, therefore the primary direction of blood flow through the cortex is centrifugal. In regions of dense fascial insertions into bone, such as muscle insertions or interosseous membrane insertions, periosteal or insertion site vessels usually supply the outer third of the bone cortex.

Before closure of the physis, medullary vessels rarely cross the growth plate, and epiphyses depend on penetrating epiphyseal vessels for their blood supply. With closure of the physis, interosseous anastomoses develop between the penetrating epiphyseal arteries and the medullary arteries, but these anastomoses rarely provide sufficient blood flow to support the epiphyseal bone cells without the contribution of the epiphyseal vessels. For this reason, even after closure of the physis, the blood supply to many epiphyses is vulnerable to interruption. This is a particular problem in the region of the femoral head where a dislocation of the hip or damage to the epiphyseal penetrating vessels can cause necrosis and eventually collapse of the femoral head.

Nerve Supply

Nerve fibers have been identified within the medullary canals of bone and particularly in association with blood vessels. Presumably, these nerves have the primary function of controlling bone blood flow. Specialized complex nerve endings have not been described within bone tissue.

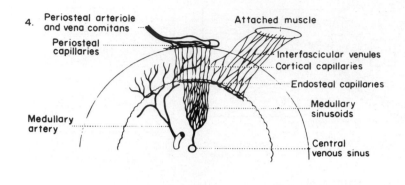

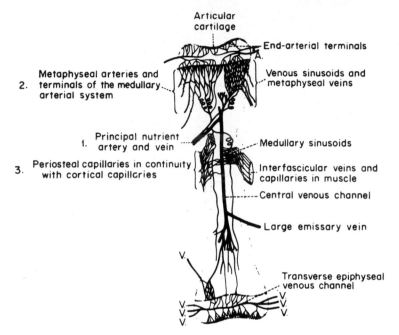

FIGURE 1-13. Blood supply of a long bone. Three basic blood supplies are shown: (1) nutrient; (2) metaphyseal, which anastomoses with epiphyseal after epiphyseal closure; and (3) periosteal. The numerous metaphyseal arteries arise from periarticular networks and anastomose with terminal branches of ascending and descending medullary arteries. Periosteal capillaries emerge from the cortex (efferent blood flow). (4) A periosteal arteriole feeds capillaries that provide afferent blood flow to a limited outer layer of cortex (Rhinelander FW. Circulation of bone. In: Bourne GH (ed). The Biochemistry and Physiology of Bone, 2nd Ed. New York: Academic Press, 1972: 2)

PERIOSTEUM

Except for the articular cartilage surfaces and the insertions of tendons, ligaments, joint capsules, and interosseous membranes, a tough thin membranous fibrous tissue, the periosteum, covers the external surface of bone. It allows some ligaments, tendons, and joint capsules to attach to bone and also provides a source of cells that can form new bone or cartilage.

Structure

Two tissue layers form the periosteum: an outer fibrous layer and an inner more cellular and vascular layer (Figure 1-14). The outer layer consists of a dense fibrous tissue matrix and fibroblast-like cells. Tendon, ligament, and joint capsule insertions that

do not penetrate directly into bone attach to this layer. In some regions, the dense fibrous tissue insertions form a continuous sheet or membrane of tissue with the periosteum. The inner osteogenic, or cambium, layer contains cells capable of forming cartilage and bone.

Periosteum changes with age. The thick cellular vascular periosteum of infants and children readily forms new bone. It shows this capacity when osteomyelitis or trauma destroys the diaphysis of a young individual's bone and the periosteum regenerates a new diaphysis. With increasing age periosteum becomes thinner and less vascular and its ability to form new bone declines. The cells of the deeper layer become flattened and quiescent, although they continue to form new bone that increases bone diameter and they still have the potential to form bone or cartilage in response to injury.

FIGURE 1-14. A longitudinal section of a rabbit's rib close to a fracture that had been healing for a short time. During this time the osteogenic cells of the periosteum have proliferated and some have differentiated into osteoblasts, which have laid down a layer of new bone on the original bone that was fractured. Three layers are labeled at the right: periosteum, new bone, and old bone. Within the periosteum the fibrous layer is labeled FIB.L., the osteogenic layer, OS.L., and the layer of osteoblasts, OB. Within the layer of new bone the intercellular substance is labeled I.S., and osteocyte in a lacuna is labeled O.S. in LAC., and the cementing line between the new bone and the old is labeled C.L. Within the old bone intercellular substance is labeled I.S., an osteocyte in a lacuna, O.S. in LAC., and a blood vessel in a canal is labeled B.V. (Ham AW, Cormack DH. Histology, 8th Ed. Philadelphia: JB Lippincott, 1979)

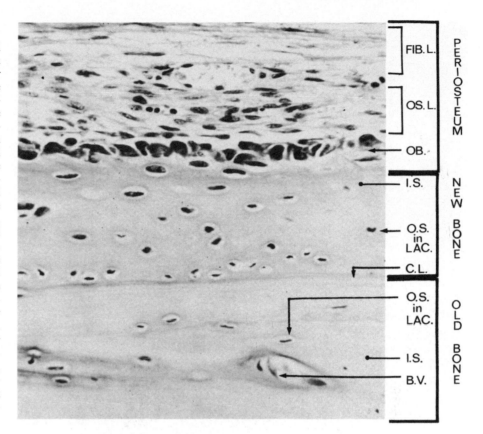

Blood Supply

In many areas a plexus of small vessels lies on the outer fibrous layer of the periosteum. At intervals these periosteal blood vessels anastomose with the vessels of the overlying muscle. Branches of the vessels on the surface of the periosteum penetrate the fibrous layer and contribute to the vascular system of the deeper layer of the periosteum and to the blood vessels that penetrate bone to join the medullary vascular system.

Nerve Supply

Nerve cell processes lie on the external periosteal surface and often accompany periosteal blood vessels. Presumably, they help regulate periosteal blood flow.

TENDON, LIGAMENT, AND JOINT CAPSULE

The specialized musculoskeletal dense fibrous tissues—tendon, ligament, and joint capsule—have a major role in providing the stability and mobility of the musculoskeletal system. These tissues differ in shape and location, and vary slightly in structure, composition, and function, but they have in common their insertion into bone and their ability to resist large tensile loads with minimal deformation. Tendons transmit the muscle forces to bone that produce joint movement; ligaments and joint capsules stabilize joints and the relationships between adjacent bones while allowing and guiding joint movement. Diseases or injuries that affect these tissues can destabilize joints or lead to loss of muscle function. Contractures of these tissues limit muscle and joint motion and contribute to skeletal deformity.

Structure

Tendons, ligaments, and joint capsules take the form of tough yet flexible and pliant fibrous sheets, bands, and cords that consist of highly oriented dense fibrous tissue. The high degree of matrix organization and density of the matrix (reflecting a high concentration of collagen) (Figure 1-15) distinguish these tissues from irregular dense fibrous tissues and loose fibrous tissues.

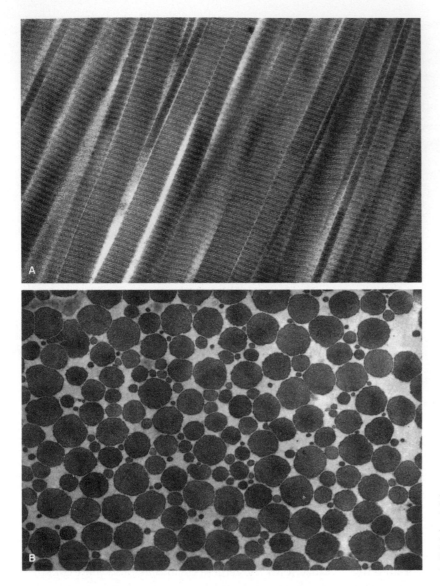

FIGURE 1-15. Electron micrographs of the type I collagen fibrils of ligament. **(A)** A longitudinal section shows the densely packed highly oriented collagen microfibrils. **(B)** A transverse section also shows the densely packed collagen microfibrils.

Tendon

Tendons vary in shape and size from the small fibrous strings that form the tendons of the lumbrical muscles to the large fibrous cords that form the Achilles tendons, but in any shape or size they unite muscle with bone and transmit the force of muscle contraction to bone. They consist of three parts: the substance of the tendon itself, the muscle-tendon junction, and the bone insertion (Figure 1-16). Connective tissues surrounding tendons allow low friction gliding and access for blood vessels to the tendon substance. Many tendons have a well-developed mesotendon, a structure that attaches the tendon to the surrounding connective tissue and consists of loose elastic connective tissue that can stretch and recoil with the tendon and provide a blood supply to the tendon substance. In certain locations, the surrounding connective tissue forms sheaths that enclose the tendon, and specialized pulleys of dense fibrous tissue that influence the line of tendon action.

TENDON SUBSTANCE. Multiple fascicles or bundles, consisting of fibroblasts and dense linear arrays of collagen fibrils, form the tendon substance and give tendons their fibrous appearance. The endotendon—a less dense connective tissue containing fibroblasts, blood vessels, nerves, and lymphatics—surrounds individual tendon fascicles. The separation of tendon fascicles by endotendon may allow small gliding movements between adjacent tendon bundles. The endotendon tissue continues to form the epitenon, a thin layer of connective

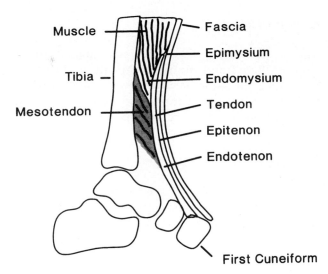

FIGURE 1-16. Diagrammatic representation of the tibialis anterior tendon showing the muscle-tendon junction, the tendon substance, and the bone insertion. The epimysium and endomysium of muscle and the epitenon and endotenon of tendon form continuous structures. The epimysium consists of a fibrous envelope that surrounds the muscle, and the endomysium consists of the fine sheaths that surround individual muscle fibers. Permysium refers to the fibrous sheath enveloping primary bundles of muscle fibers. Loose connective tissue surrounds the tendon proximally where it pursues a straight course, but a sheath forms distally where it changes direction. (From Buckwalter JA, Maynard JA, Vailis AC. Skeletal fibrous tissues: tendon, joint capsule, and ligament. Chapter 14. In: Albright JA, Brand RA, eds. The Scientific Basis of Orthopaedics. Norwalk, CT: Appleton & Lange, 1987:388)

tissue that covers the surface of the tendon. Where the tendon joins the muscle, the fibrous tissue of the epitenon continues as the thin fibrous covering of the attached muscle called the epimysium.

MUSCLE-TENDON JUNCTIONS. Muscle-tendon junctions must efficiently transmit the force of muscle contraction to the tendon. The attachment of muscle to tendon occurs through continuation of the collagen fibrils of the fibrous tissue layers of muscle (epimysium, perimysium, and endomysium) into the collagen fibrils of the tendon and through elaborate interdigitation of the muscle cell membrane with the collagen fibrils of the tendon. This interdigitation of muscle cell and tendon has the appearance of interlocking fingers when examined by electron microscopy, and provides a strong bond between the muscle cell and the tendon collagen. Collagen fibrils do not enter the muscle cells but lie next to their basement membranes. The muscle cell plasma membrane thickens at the muscle-tendon junction and muscle myofilaments extend directly to it.

PERITENDONOUS STRUCTURES. Normal tendon gliding, efficient transmission of muscle forces to move joints and tendon nutrition, depend on the peritendonous connective tissue structures sometimes called peritenon. These structures range from loose connective tissue to elaborate well-defined mesotendons, sheaths, and pulleys.

Where tendons follow a straight course, the surrounding tissue usually consists of loose areolar tissue. In some locations, this tissue must stretch several centimeters and then recoil without tearing or disrupting the tendon blood supply. It consists of an interlacing meshwork of thin collagen fibrils and elastic fibers filled with abundant soft, almost fluid ground substance.

Where tendons change course between their muscle attachment and their bone insertion, often as they cross or near a joint, the surrounding connective tissue may form a bursa or a discrete tendon sheath. These structures allow low friction movement between the tendon and adjacent bone, joint capsule, tendon, ligament, fibrous tissue retinacula, or fibrous tissue pulleys. Tendon bursae and sheaths consist of flattened synovial-lined sacks that usually cover only a portion of the tendon circumference. Tendon sheaths and bursae resemble synovial joints in that they consist of cavities lined with synovial-like cells, they contain synovial-like fluid, and they facilitate low friction gliding between two surfaces. Mesotenons generally attach to one surface of a tendon within a tendon sheath and provide the blood supply to this portion of the tendon.

Distinct dense fibrous tissue retinacula, pulleys, or fascial slings lie over the outer surface of some regions of tendon sheaths. These firm fibrous structures direct the line of tendon movement and prevent displacement or bowstringing of the tendon that would decrease the efficiency of the muscle-tendon unit. For example, the dense fibrous tissue (extensor tendon retinacula) of the wrist keep the wrist and digital extensor tendons from displacing dorsally when they extend the fingers and dorsiflex the wrist. The flexor tendons of the fingers and thumb pass through a more elaborate series of pulleys and sheaths that make efficient finger flexion possible.

Joint Capsule and Ligament

Joint capsules and ligaments have similar structures and functions, and in some regions ligament and capsule form a continuous structure. Like tendons, both of them consist primarily of high-oriented, densely packed collagen fibrils. Unlike tendons, they more often assume the form of layered sheets or lamellae. Both ligament and capsule attach to adjacent bones and cross synovial joints, yet allow at least some motion between the bones. Ligaments have the primary function of restraining abnormal motion between adjacent bones. Joint capsules also restrain abnormal joint motion or displacement of articular surfaces, but usually to a lesser extent. Both capsule and ligament consist of a proximal bone insertion, ligament, or capsular substance and a distal bone insertion, and both contain nerves that may sense joint motion and displacement.

JOINT CAPSULE. Joint capsules form fibrous tissue cuffs around synovial joints. A synovial membrane lines the interior of the joint capsule and loose areolar connective tissue covers the exterior. This loose tissue often contains plexes of small blood vessels that supply the capsule. Nerves and blood vessels from this loose connective tissue penetrate the fibrous capsule to supply the capsule and outer later of synovium. Each end of the capsule attaches in a continuous line around the articular surface of the bones forming the joint, usually near the periphery of the articular cartilage surface. Tendons and ligaments reinforce some regions of joint capsules. For example, the glenohumeral ligaments form part of the glenohumeral joint capsule and the expansion of the semimembranosus tendon contributes to the posterior oblique ligament of the knee and part of the knee joint capsule.

LIGAMENT. Surgeons and anatomists have named ligaments by their location and bony attachments (for example, the anterior glenohumeral ligament or the anterior talofibular ligament) or by their relationship to other ligaments (the medial collateral ligament of the knee or the posterior cruciate ligament of the knee). Unlike joint capsules, ligaments vary in their anatomic relationship to synovial joints. This variability separates ligaments into three types: intra-articular or intracapsular ligaments, articular or capsular ligaments, and extra-articular or extracapsular ligaments. Intra-articular ligaments, including the cruciate ligaments of the knee, have the form of distinct separate structures. In contrast, capsular ligaments, like the glenohumeral ligaments, appear as thickenings of joint capsules. Extra-articular ligaments, like the coracoacromial ligament, lie at a distance from a synovial joint. Despite these differences in relationship to joints, the function of the three ligament types remains that of stabilizing adjacent bones or restraining abnormal joint motion.

Composition

Individual tendons, ligaments, and capsules differ slightly in cell and matrix composition; but they all contain the same basic cell types, share similar patterns of vascular supply and innervation, and have the same primary matrix macromolecule, type I collagen.

Cells

Fibroblasts form the predominant cell of tendon, ligament, and joint capsule. The endothelial cells of blood vessels, and in some locations nerve cell processes, exist within tendon, ligament, and joint capsule, but they form only a small part of the tissue. The fibroblasts surround themselves with a dense fibrous tissue matrix and throughout life continue to maintain the matrix. They vary in shape, activity, and density among ligaments, tendons, and joint capsules and among regions of the same structure. Most dense fibrous tissue fibroblasts have long small diameter cell processes that extend between collagen fibrils throughout the matrix. Generally, younger tissues have a higher cell density and cells with a larger cytoplasmic volume and intracellular density of endoplasmic reticulum. With increasing age, the cell density usually decreases and the cells appear to become less active.

Matrix

Tissue fluid contributes 60% or more of the wet weight of most dense fibrous tissues, and the matrix macromolecules contribute the other 40%. Because most dense fibrous tissue cells lie at some distance from blood vessels, these cells must depend on diffusion of nutrients and metabolites through the tissue fluid. In addition, the interaction of the tissue fluid and the matrix macromolecules influences the mechanical properties of the tissue.

Collagens, elastin, proteoglycans, and noncollagenous proteins combine to form the macromolecular framework of the dense fibrous tissues. Collagens, the major component of the dense fibrous tissue molecular framework, contribute 70 to 80% of the dry weight of many dense fibrous tissues. Type I collagen commonly forms more than 90% of the tissue collagen. Type III collagen also occurs within the dense fibrous tissues; in some tissues it forms about 10% of the total collagen, and other collagen types may also be present in small amounts. Most dense fibrous tissues have some elastin, less than 5% of their dry weight, but some ligaments, in particular the nuchal ligament and ligamentum flavum, have much higher elastin concentrations, up to 75% of the tissue dry weight. Proteoglycans usually contribute less than 1% of the dry weight of dense fibrous tissues, but may have important roles in organizing the extracellular matrix and interacting with the tissue fluid. Most dense fibrous tissues appear to contain both large aggregating proteoglycans and small nonaggregating proteoglycans. The large proteoglycans presumably occupy the interfibrillar regions of the matrix and the small proteoglycans lie directly on or near the surface of collagen fibrils. Noncollagenous proteins also form a critical part of the dense fibrous tissue matrix even though they contribute only a few percent to the dry weight of most of the tissues. Fibronectin occurs in all dense fibrous tissues; other noncollagenous proteins also contribute to the structure of these tissues, but their composition, structure, and function have not been well defined.

Insertions into Bone

The bony insertions of tendons, ligaments, and joint capsules attach the flexible dense fibrous tissue securely to rigid bone, yet they allow motion between the bone and the dense fibrous tissue without damage to the dense fibrous tissue. Despite their small size, insertions have a more complex and variable structure than the substance of the tissue; and they have different mechanical properties. They vary in size, strength, and the angle of their collagen fiber bundles relative to the bone and in the proportion of their collagen fibers that penetrate directly into bone. Based on differences in the angle between the collagen fibers of the dense fibrous tissue structure and the bone and on the proportion of collagen fibrils that penetrate directly into bone, dense fibrous tissue insertions can be separated into two types: direct insertions (insertions where many of the collagen fibrils pass directly into bone) and indirect or periosteal insertion (insertions where only a few of the collagen fibrils pass directly into bone) (Figure 1-17).

Direct Insertions

Direct insertions, like the insertion of the medial collateral ligament of the knee into the femur, consist of sharply defined regions where the ligament joins the bone; only a thin layer of the substance of the ligament, tendon, or capsule joins the fibrous layer of the periosteum. Most of the collagen fibrils at the insertion pass directly from the substance of the tendon, ligament, or joint capsule into the bone cortex, usually entering at a right angle to the bone surface. These fibrils then mingle with the collagen fibrils of the organic matrix of bone creating a strong bond between the tendon, ligament, or capsule and the bone matrix. Where dense fibrous tissue structures approach the bone surface at oblique angles, the collagen fibrils may make a sharp turn to enter the bone at a right angle.

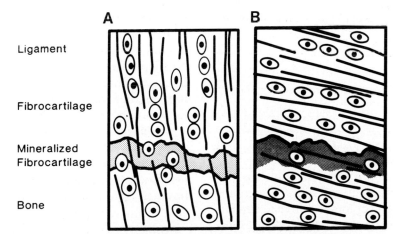

FIGURE 1-17. Diagrammatic representations of direct and indirect dense fibrous tissue insertions into bone. **(A)** In direct insertions, a high proportion of the collagen fibers pass directly into bone, and the fibrocartilage and mineralized fibrocartilage zones are well developed. **(B)** In indirect insertions, a high proportion of the collagen fibers pass into the periosteum and the fibrocartilage and mineralized fibrocartilage zones often are not well developed. (From Buckwalter JA, Maynard JA, Vailis AC. Skeletal fibrous tissues: tendon, joint capsule, and ligament. Chapter 14. In: Albright JA, Brand RA, eds. The Scientific Basis of Orthopaedics. Norwalk, CT: Appleton & Lange, 1987: 391)

The deeper collagen fibers that enter the bone pass through four zones of increasing stiffness: the substance of the dense fibrous tissue structure, fibrocartilage, mineralized fibrocartilage, and bone.

In the fibrocartilage zone, the cells are larger than the fibroblasts of the tendon, joint capsule, or ligament and more spherical. A sharp border of unmineralized matrix separates the zone of fibrocartilage from the mineralized fibrocartilage zone.

Indirect Insertions

The less common indirect insertions, like the insertion of the medial collateral ligament of the knee into the tibia, usually cover more bone surface area than direct insertions because a larger proportion of their collagen fibrils join the periosteum. Like direct insertions, indirect insertions have superficial and deep collagen fibrils, but most of their collagen fibrils form the superficial layer that joins the fibrous layer of the periosteum. The deep collagen fibrils enter the bone cortex, but they generally do not pass through sharply defined zones of mineralized and unmineralized fibrocartilage.

Blood Supply

Most dense fibrous tissues have well-developed networks of blood vessels extending throughout their substance. Generally, these vascular systems follow the longitudinal pattern of the collagenous matrix, but they may have multiple anastomoses between parallel vessels. Some blood vessels in tendon, ligament, and joint capsule insertions enter the bone.

Nerve Supply

In addition to nerve cell processes next to blood vessels, like those found in periosteum and bone, dense fibrous tissues have specialized nerve endings that lie on the surface or within the substance of the tissue. Presumably, the nerve fibers in the dense fibrous tissues function as pain receptors, vasomotor efferents, and mechanoreceptors sensitive to stretching or distortion. The mechanoreceptors presumably sense joint position, muscle tension, and loads applied to ligaments, capsules, and tendons. In tendons, they can adjust muscle tension. In ligaments and capsules, they may have a role in initiating protective reflexes that oppose potentially damaging joint movements.

MENISCI

Like articular cartilages, menisci perform important mechanical functions in synovial joints including load bearing, shock absorption, and participation in joint lubrication. They may also contribute to joint stability. Menisci and meniscus-like structures consist of dense fibrous tissue, or fibrocartilage, and project from the margins of synovial joints to interpose themselves between articular cartilage surfaces. They include the knee menisci (two C-shaped menisci that lie on the tibial plateaus and form part of the knee joint), the articular discs of the sternoclavicular and acromioclavicular joints, the triangular fibrocartilage that binds the distal ends of the ulna and radius together and forms part of the wrist joint, and the labra found in some joints like the hip and shoulder. Because the structures other than the knee menisci have not been extensively studied, this section refers only to the knee menisci.

Structure

Within the knee, menisci collagen fibril diameter and orientation and cell morphology vary from the surface to the deeper central regions. The superficial regions that lie against articular cartilage usually consist of a mesh of fine fibrils. Immediately deep to these fine fibrils, small diameter collagen fibrils with a radial orientation relative to the body of the meniscus form a thicker subsurface layer. The flattened ellipsoid shaped cells of this layer orient their maximum diameter roughly parallel to the articular surface. In the deeper central or middle region, the bulk of the meniscus is made up of large diameter collagen fibril bundles that surround larger cells with a more spherical shape. The deeper collagen fibril bundles follow the curve of the menisci and smaller radially oriented fibril bundles weave among the circumferential fibril bundles. The circumferential arrangement of the large collagen bundles gives the menisci great tensile strength for loads applied parallel to the orientation of the fibers. The radial fibers may resist the development and propagation of longitudinal tears between the larger circumferential collagen fiber bundles.

Composition

Cells

Meniscal cells, like many other types of mesenchymal cells, lack cell-to-cell contacts and attach their membranes to specific matrix macromolecules.

They have the primary function of maintaining the meniscal matrix. Most of them lie at a distance from blood vessels, so like chondrocytes, they rely on diffusion through the matrix for transport of nutrients and metabolites.

Matrix

Water contributes 60 to 75% of the total wet weight of meniscus. As in the other musculoskeletal tissues, the interactions between the matrix fluid and the macromolecular framework significantly influence the mechanical properties of menisci.

The macromolecular framework of meniscus contributes 25 to 40% of the meniscus wet weight and consists of collagens, noncollagenous proteins, proteoglycans, and elastin. The collagens give menisci their form and tensile strength and contribute approximately 75% of the dry weight of the tissue. Type I collagen makes up more than 90% of the total tissue collagen. Type II collagen, type V collagen, and type VI collagen each contribute 1 to 2% of the total tissue collagen. Noncollagenous proteins, including link protein, fibronectin, and other noncollagenous proteins, contribute 8 to 13% of the dry weight. Large aggregating proteoglycans and smaller nonaggregating proteoglycans together contribute about 2% of meniscal dry weight. Presumably they have functions like the proteoglycans found in other dense fibrous tissues. Elastin forms less than 1% of the tissue dry weight. This small amount of elastin probably does not significantly influence the organization of the matrix or the mechanical properties.

Blood Supply

Most menisci and meniscal-like structures have some blood supply, at least in their more peripheral regions. Branches from the geniculate arteries form a capillary plexus along the peripheral borders of the knee menisci. Small radial branches project from the circumferential parameniscal vessels into the meniscal substance. These vessels penetrate into 10 to 30% of the width of the medial meniscus and 10 to 25% of the width of the lateral meniscus, leaving the cells of the inner portions of the menisci dependent on diffusion of nutrients and metabolites.

Nerve Supply

Nerves lie on the peripheral surface of the knee menisci and other meniscal-like structures. Although these nerves enter the more superficial regions of some parts of the tissue, they generally do not penetrate into the central regions. The functions of these nerve endings have not been clearly defined, but they may contribute to joint proprioception.

SYNOVIUM

Synovium lines the nonarticular regions of synovial joints and the bursae and sheaths of tendons. In synovial joints, synovium attaches directly around the margins of the articular cartilage. It covers the inner surfaces of the joint capsule, bone surfaces, and intra-articular ligaments and tendons. Normally it does not extend over articular cartilage, intra-articular discs, or menisci. When examined from inside a joint, most of the synovial membrane has a smooth even surface, but some regions may have small projections or villi, and in others the synovium may form folds or fringes that project into the joint cavity. Fat lying outside the synovial membrane contributes to the ability of synovium to fill potential spaces in the joint cavity.

Structure

Synovial membranes consist of two layers: an inner intimal layer and a peripheral subintimal layer that lies on joint capsule or periarticular fat. Both layers vary in thickness among joints and among different regions of the same joint.

Intima

In most areas the intima consists of one or more layers of synovial cells in an amorphous matrix. The cells vary considerably in shape from flattened ellipsoids, to elongated cells, to polyhedral or spherical cells, and they may have cell processes. The synovial cells do not form a continuous layer; in some regions they leave gaps between cell membranes that fill with extracellular matrices. Unlike epithelial cells, the superficial synovial cells do not lie on a basement membrane.

Two types of synovial cells (A and B cells) have been identified. Type A cells have surface filopodia, plasma membrane invaginations, and vesicles. They contain mitochondria, lysosomes, cytoplasmic filaments, and Golgi membranes. B cells lack most of these characteristics, but contain a high concentration of endoplasmic reticulum. Some investigators have proposed that A and B cells have different primary functions: they suggest that A cells produce the hyaluronic acid that serves as part of the synovial fluid and have phagocytic capability, and that B cells synthesize proteins, including enzymes. Cells with features of both A and B cells appear commonly; and the two cell types may not represent distinct phenotypes, but morphologic variants of the same cell.

Subintima

The subintimal layer separates the intimal synovial cell layer from the joint capsule or the other synovial-covered tissues including bone, tendon, and ligament. The cells of the subintima include blood vessel endothelial cells, fibroblasts, macrophages, mast cells, and fat cells. The subintimal matrix may have a loose areolar form or a denser matrix with a higher concentration of collagen and elastin.

Blood Supply

The subintimal layer of synovium commonly has an extensive network of small blood vessels. The network forms from vessels that pass through the joint capsule. Where synovium covers bone, tendon, or ligament, the subintimal blood vessels form anastomoses with blood vessels from the underlying tissue.

HYALINE CARTILAGE

Like bone and dense fibrous tissues, cartilage consists of a sparse population of mesenchymal cells embedded within an abundant extracellular matrix. The cells contribute about 5% of the total tissue volume, and the matrix contributes approximately 95%. The roughly spherical shape of most cartilage cells, or chondrocytes; the unique composition of the matrix they synthesize, assemble, and maintain; and the lack of blood vessels and nerves distinguish cartilage from dense fibrous tissues and bone.

Differences in matrix composition, distribution within the body, mechanical properties, and gross and microscopic appearance differentiate three types of adult human cartilage: hyaline, fibrous, and elastic cartilage. Elastic cartilage forms the auricle of the external ear, a portion of the epiglottis, and some of the laryngeal or bronchiolar cartilages; it does not form part of the musculoskeletal system. Fibrous cartilage (also considered a form of dense

fibrous tissue) forms part of the intervertebral discs, pubic symphysis, and tendon, ligament, and joint capsule insertions. Menisci consist of a specialized form of fibrous cartilage. The most widespread form of cartilage, hyaline cartilage, forms most of the skeleton before it is removed and replaced by bone through the process of enchondral ossification. It also forms the physeal cartilages that produce longitudinal bone growth until skeletal growth ceases; in adults it persists as the nasal, laryngeal, bronchiolar, articular, and costal cartilages. This section discusses the structure of two specialized forms of hyaline cartilage that have important roles in the musculoskeletal system: articular cartilage and growth cartilage.

Structure

Articular Cartilage

Function of synovial joints, for example, the hip or the knee, depends on the unique mechanical properties of the articular cartilage that forms their bearing surfaces. It distributes loads, thereby minimizing stresses on subchondral bone. When loaded, it deforms and when unloaded, it regains it original shape. It provides a surface with almost unequalled gliding properties and has remarkable durability.

Although only a few millimeters thick at most, articular cartilage has an elaborate internal organization. This organization can be described by dividing articular cartilage into four successive zones beginning at the joint surface: the superficial or gliding zone, the intermediate, middle or transitional zone, the deep or radial zone, and the calcified cartilage zone (Figure 1-18 and Color Figure 1-1). Within zones, differences in matrix composition and organization distinguish three regions or compartments: the pericellular region, the territorial region, and the interterritorial region.

CARTILAGE ZONES. Cartilage zones differ in matrix composition, water concentration, collagen fibril orientation and cell alignment, and morphology.

Superficial Zone. The superficial or gliding zone, the smallest cartilage zone, forms the joint surface. A thin cell-free layer of matrix, containing primarily fine fibrils, lies directly next to the synovial cavity. Deep to this layer, elongated flattened chondrocytes surrounded by a larger volume of matrices per cell align their major axes parallel to

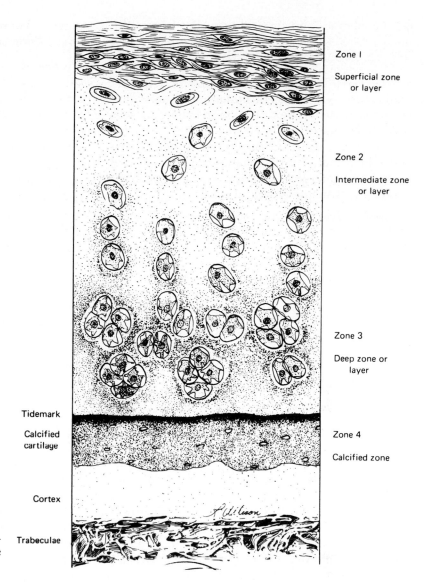

Zone 1
Superficial zone or layer

Zone 2
Intermediate zone or layer

Zone 3
Deep zone or layer

Tidemark

Calcified cartilage

Zone 4
Calcified zone

Cortex

Trabeculae

FIGURE 1-18. Diagrammatic representation of the organization of articular cartilage into zones.

the articular surface. The collagen fibrils of this zone lie roughly parallel to the articular surface.

Middle Zone. The middle or transition zone has several times the volume of the superficial zone. Its more spherical cells contain greater volumes of endoplasmic reticulum, Golgi membranes, mitochondria, and glycogen. The larger interterritorial matrix collagen fibrils of the transitional zone have a more random orientation than those of the gliding zone.

Deep Zone. The cells of the deep or radial zone resemble the spherical cells of the transitional zone but tend to align themselves in columns. This zone has the largest collagen fibrils, the highest proteoglycan content, and the lowest water content.

Calcified Cartilage Zone. The thin calcified cartilage zone separates the hyaline cartilage from the stiffer subchondral bone. Collagen fibrils penetrate from the deep zone of cartilage directly through calcified cartilage into bone, thereby anchoring articular cartilage to subchondral bone.

MATRIX REGIONS. Matrix regions differ in their proximity to chondrocytes, collagen content, collagen fibril diameter, collagen fibril orientation, and proteoglycan and noncollagenous protein content and organization.

Pericellular Matrix. The smallest matrix compartment, the pericellular matrix, consists of a thin layer of matrix containing little or no fibrillar collagen. It appears to attach directly to the chondrocyte cell membranes and probably contains noncollagenous proteins that help chondrocytes bind themselves to the matrix.

Territorial Matrix. An envelope of territorial matrix surrounds the pericellular matrix and sometimes pairs or clusters of chondrocytes and their pericellular matrices. Thin collagen fibrils in the territorial matrix near the cells appear to bind to the pericellular matrix. At a distance from the cell they spread and intersect at various angles, forming a basket like structure around the cells.

Interterritorial Matrix. The interterritorial matrix, the largest matrix compartment, has collagen fibrils of greater diameter than the territorial matrix. The organization and orientation of these interterritorial collagen matrix fibrils change as they pass from the articular surface to the deep region of the cartilage. In the most superficial zone they lie primarily parallel to the joint surface, in the transition zone they assume a more random orientation, and in the deep zone they tend to lie perpendicular to the joint surface.

Growth Cartilage

Bones elongate by growth of the cartilage forming the physes or growth plates (Figure 1-19). The complex structure of the physes (Figure 1-20) makes it possible for them to produce precisely directed longitudinal bone growth. The growth cartilages increase their volume and therefore bone length by synthesizing new matrices and by cell swelling. The organization of the growth cartilage matrix and the surrounding fibrous tissue directs the increasing volume of cells and matrices, so that it produces longitudinal bone growth. In the region of the growth cartilage nearest to the metaphysis, the longitudinal cartilage septae of the growth cartilage mineralize, and in the metaphysis, osteoblasts cover the mineralized cartilage bars with new woven bone. Osteoclasts then resorb the woven bone and calcified cartilage and osteoblasts form lamellar bone to complete the replacement of cartilage by mature bone.

Growth cartilages have a layered or zonal organization and a regional organization similar to that found in articular cartilage. The matrix regions, like those of articular cartilage, consist of the pericellular, territorial, and interterritorial compartments. The layered or zonal organization differs considerably from that of articular cartilage. The identified growth cartilage layers or zones consist of reserve or resting, proliferative, and hypertrophic or maturing zones.

Reserve or Resting Zone. Reserve zone cells, located in a thin layer at the epiphyseal pole of the growth plate, show relatively little evidence of metabolic activity. The functions of these small cells have not been clearly established, but they may serve as stem cells for the proliferative zone.

Proliferative Zone. In the proliferative zone, chondrocytes rapidly divide, synthesize a new matrix, and assume a highly oriented flattened disclike shape. In rapidly growing bones they create long columns of highly ordered cells that resemble stacks of plates.

Hypertrophic or Maturing Zone

Toward the bottom of the proliferative zone, the proliferative cells begin to enlarge, creating the hypertrophic zone. From the proliferative zone to the last part of the hypertrophic zone they increase their volume fivefold to tenfold, contributing significantly to bone growth, and assume a spherical or polygonal shape. As the cells enlarge, their matrix changes: the territorial matrix volume per cell increases significantly as its collagen concentration decreases and mineral appears in the interterritorial matrix.

The orientation of the interterritorial matrix collagen fibrils of the growth cartilage changes among zones. In the reserve zone and upper region of the proliferative zone, the fibrils have little apparent orientation, but in the middle and lower regions of the proliferative zone and throughout the hypertrophic zone, these interterritorial matrix collagen fibrils lie parallel to the long axis of the bone forming longitudinal columns or septae that surround the chondrocyte columns and their territorial and pericellular matrices.

In the last part of the hypertrophic zone, the zone of provisional calcification, the longitudinal septae mineralize. The enlarged chondrocytes condense and metaphyseal capillary sprouts penetrate the territorial matrix and cell lacunae, bringing osteoblasts that begin to form new bone on the calcified cartilage septae.

Composition

Chondrocytes

Unlike the other musculoskeletal tissues, cartilage contains only one cell type, the chondrocyte

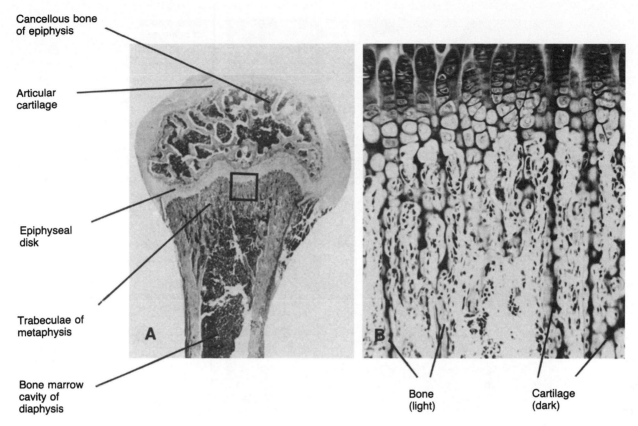

Cancellous bone of epiphysis

Articular cartilage

Epiphyseal disk

Trabeculae of metaphysis

Bone marrow cavity of diaphysis

Bone (light)   Cartilage (dark)

FIGURE 1-19. Micrographs showing the structure of a long bone physis. **(A)** A low-power photomicrograph of a longitudinal section cut through the end of a long bone of a growing rat. At this stage of development osteogenesis has spread out from the epiphyseal center of ossification so that only the articular cartilage above and the epiphyseal plate below remain cartilaginous. On the diaphyseal side of the epiphyseal plate are the metaphyseal trabeculae, which **(B)** consist of cartilage cores on which bone has been deposited. (Ham AW, Cormack DH. Histology, 8th Ed. Philadelphia: JB Lippincott, 1979)

(Figures 1-21 and 1-22), and no nerve cell processes or blood vessels. Like many other mesenchymal cells, chondrocytes surround themselves with the matrix they synthesize, attach themselves to the matrix macromolecules, and do not form contacts with other cells.

The relationship between chondrocytes and their matrix does not end with the synthesis and assembly of the matrix. The normal degradation of matrix macromolecules, especially proteoglycans, forces the cells to synthesize new matrix components to preserve the tissue. In addition, the matrix acts as a mechanical signal transducer for the chondrocytes. Deformation of the matrix generates signals, transmitted through the matrix, that cause the cells to alter their synthetic activity. For example, absence of joint loading and motion causes deterioration of the articular cartilage matrix, possibly because of the lack of mechanical signals to stimulate normal chondrocyte function.

Matrix

Tissue fluid forms the largest component of cartilage. Depending on the type of cartilage and its age, water contributes 60 to 80% of the wet weight of cartilage. The volume concentration, organization, and behavior of the tissue fluid depend on its interaction with the structural macromolecules. These molecules contribute 20 to 40% of the wet weight of cartilage and include collagens, proteoglycans, and noncollagenous proteins. Hyaline cartilage does not contain elastin. In most hyaline cartilages, collagens contribute about 50% of the tissue dry weight, proteoglycans contribute 30 to 35%,

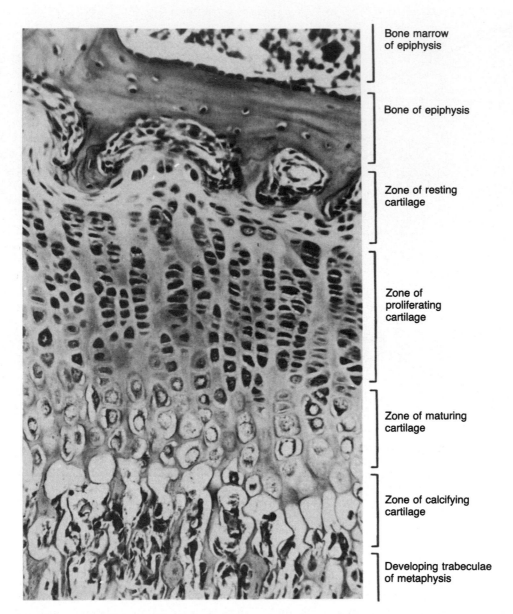

Bone marrow
of epiphysis

Bone of epiphysis

Zone of resting
cartilage

Zone of
proliferating
cartilage

Zone of maturing
cartilage

Zone of calcifying
cartilage

Developing trabeculae
of metaphysis

FIGURE 1-20. High-power photomicrograph of longitudinal section cut through upper end of tibia of a guinea pig. Note different zones of cells in the epiphyseal plate. (Ham AW, Cormack DH. Histology, 8th Ed. Philadelphia: JB Lippincott, 1979)

and noncollagenous proteins contribute about 15 to 20%. The collagens form the fibrillar meshwork that gives cartilage its tensile strength and form. The proteoglycans and noncollagenous proteins bind to the collagen network or become mechanically entrapped within it, and the chondrocytes attach themselves to the matrix macromolecules.

Type II collagen fibrils form the cross-banded fibrils identified by electron microscopy and account for 90 to 95% of total hyaline cartilage collagen. Hyaline cartilage also contains at least two other collagens, types IX and XI, and may contain trace amounts of other collagens. The mineralizing regions of articular cartilage and growth plate cartilage also contain small amounts of type X collagen.

Proteoglycans form a much larger portion of the matrix structure in hyaline cartilage than in any

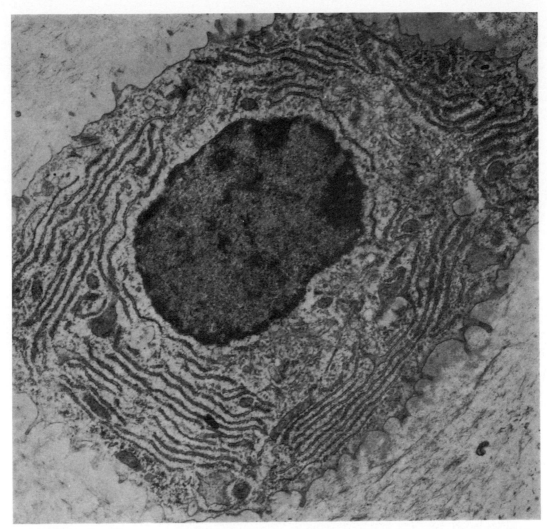

FIGURE 1-21. Ultrastructural characteristics of a chondrocyte. The cytoplasm reveals well-developed rough-surfaced vesicles of endoplasmic reticulum and a well-developed Golgi apparatus. The cytoplasmic processes extend off into the intercellular substance (cytoplasmic footlets). As the chondrocyte becomes older and synthesis of protein is less, the rough-surfaced vesicles and Golgi apparatus become less prominent, and glycogen and lipid material accumulate in the cytoplasm. (Ham AW. Histology, 7th Ed. Philadelphia: JB Lippincott, 1974)

other musculoskeletal tissue except for the nucleus pulposus. Hyaline cartilage has a high concentration of large aggregating proteoglycans that give the tissue its unique material properties in compression. It also contains smaller nonaggregating proteoglycans like those found in dense fibrous tissues. The large aggregates help control the fluid flow through the matrix.

Noncollagenous proteins also have an important role in hyaline cartilage. Link proteins stabilize and increase the size of proteoglycan aggregates. Chondronectin and anchorin CII may have a role in matrix organization and in establishing and maintaining the relationships between the chondrocytes and the matrix macromolecules.

INTERVERTEBRAL DISC

Normal function of the spine depends greatly on the mechanical properties of the intervertebral discs. These 23 specialized connective tissue structures unite adjacent vertebral bodies from the second and third cervical vertebrae to the fifth lumbar

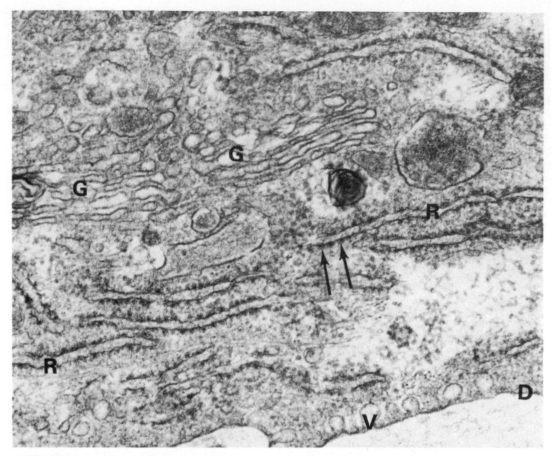

FIGURE 1-22. Part of a chondrocyte showing paired membranes of rough endoplasmic reticulum (R) with ribosome granules (*arrows*). The rough endoplasmic reticulum (R) with ribosome granules (*arrows*). The rough endoplasmic reticulum contrasts with the smooth membranes of the Golgi apparatus (G). Micropinocytotic vesicles (V). Limiting cell membrane (D). Transmission electron micrograph ×37,500. Glutaraldehyde. (Meachim G. The matrix. In Freeman MA. Adult Articular Cartilage, 2nd Ed. London: Pitman, 1973:1)

vertebrae and sacrum. They vary in size from the small diameter thin discs in the cervical region to the large diameter thick discs of the lower lumbar region. Throughout the spine they contribute to stability while allowing movement between vertebrae and absorbing compressive loads. With age the gross and microscopic appearance, cell content and matrix composition of disc tissues change more than any other tissues.

Structure

Human intervertebral discs consist of four tissues: hyaline cartilage endplate, annulus fibrosis, transition zone, and nucleus pulposus. These tissues vary in structure, composition, cell populations, and mechanical properties.

Cartilage Endplate

Hyaline cartilage endplates cover the superior and inferior surfaces of each disc and separate the other disc tissues from the vertebral bone. Grossly and microscopically they closely resemble other hyaline cartilages. The dense collagen fibers of the annulus fibrosis pass through the outer edges of the endplates into the vertebral bodies. With age the cartilage plates mineralize and eventually cannot be identified as distinct structures.

Annulus Fibrosis

Annulus fibrosis consists primarily of densely packed collagen fibers formed into two components: the outer circumferential rings of collagen lamellae or layers (Figure 1-23) and an inner larger fibrocartilaginous component. The collagen

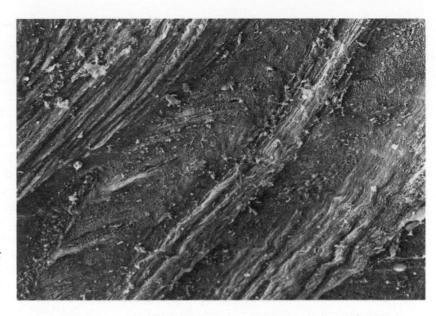

FIGURE 1-23. Electron micrograph of the cut surface of a human annulus fibrosus. Notice the dense layers of collagen fibers.

lamellae that form the outer concentric rings of the annulus have a high degree of orientation: collagen fibrils within a layer lie parallel to each other; collagen fibrils within adjacent layers lie at 40 to 70° angles to the collagen fibers within layers on either side. In the fibrocartilaginous component of the annulus, collagen fibrils run concentrically and vertically but lack the high degree of orientation found in the outer concentric rings.

Transition Zone

When the intervertebral disc first forms, the nucleus pulposus and annulus fibrosus have a sharp boundary where the gelatinous nucleus pulposus lies directly against the fibrous annulus. With growth, a transition zone appears that lies between the fibrocartilaginous component of the annulus fibrosis and the nucleus pulposus.

Nucleus Pulposus

In newborns and young individuals the soft gelatinous nucleus pulposus tissue has a translucent appearance. It contains relatively few collagen fibers, and they lack any apparent orientation (Figure 1-24). With age, the nucleus pulposus becomes more fibrous making it increasingly difficult to separate

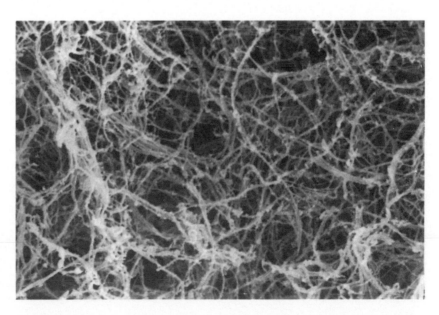

FIGURE 1-24. Electron micrograph showing the collagen fibers of a human nucleus pulposus. Notice loose arrangement of the fibers compared with the annulus fibrosus.

the nucleus pulposus from the transition zone and the fibrocartilaginous part of the annulus fibrosus.

Composition

Intervertebral disc tissues consist of water, cells, and matrix macromolecules. The composition of the hyaline cartilage plates has not been extensively studied, but it appears to resemble other hyaline cartilages. The annulus, like other dense fibrous tissues, has water concentration of 60 to 70% throughout life. In contrast, the water concentration of the nucleus pulposus declines from about 80 to 90% at birth to about 70% in adults.

Cells

Intervertebral discs contain two principal cell types: notochordal cells and connective tissue cells. Notochordal cells form the nucleus pulposus in the fetus. With growth, development, and aging they gradually disappear, and the cells found in the nucleus of older individuals have the appearance of connective tissue cells, often resembling chondrocytes. The connective tissue cells of the outer annulus have the appearance of fibroblasts, like those found in other dense fibrous tissues. The connective tissue cells of the inner regions of the annulus and other disc components have a more spherical form, like chondrocytes. The cells of the cartilage endplate tissue have the shape and organelles of hyaline cartilage chondrocytes.

Notochordal Cells

Clusters and cords of large irregular notochordal cells populate the nucleus pulposus of the newborn human intervertebral disc (Figure 1-25). These cells contain endoplasmic reticulum, Golgi membranes, mitochondria, glycogen, and bundles of microfilaments. Unlike mesenchymal cells, notochordal cells form multiple specialized junctions with other cells and their membranes form elaborate interdigitations with those of other cells. During skeletal growth, the notochordal cell clusters or cords disappear and the glycogen content of the cells declines. In some regions they retain cell-to-cell contact by elongated cell processes. With aging, the density of notochordal cells declines further, and definite notochordal cells have not been identified in the human nucleus pulposus after age 32.

CONNECTIVE TISSUE CELLS. In the outer annulus the fibroblasts lie with their long axes parallel to the collagen fibrils. In the inner fibrocartilaginous region of the annulus more of the cells assume a spherical form like those seen in other fibrocartilages (Figure 1-26). In the nucleus pulposus connective tissue cells have oval nuclei and slightly elongated form, but most have a more spherical shape. The proportion of viable nucleus pulposus cells declines with age, but even in discs from elderly people some viable connective tissue cells survive.

Matrix

The matrix macromolecular framework of the human intervertebral disc forms from collagens,

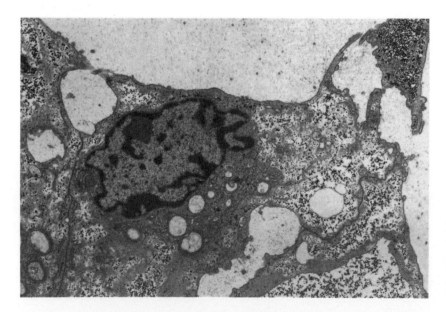

FIGURE 1-25. Electron micrograph of a human nucleus pulposus notochordal cells. Notice that, unlike connective tissue cells, the membranes of notochordal cells bind to the membranes of adjacent cells.

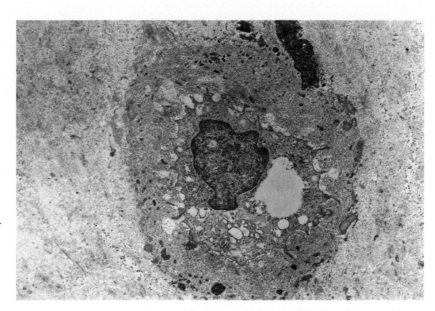

FIGURE 1-26. Electron micrograph of a human connective tissue cell from the inner region of the annulus fibrosus. Notice that this cell lacks any contact with other cells and has formed a distinct pericellular matrix.

elastin, proteoglycans, and noncollagenous proteins. The concentrations and specific types of these molecules vary among the disc tissues.

The collagens, including fibrillar and short chain collagens, give the disc its form and tensile strength. The concentration of collagen decreases progressively from the outer annulus to the most central portion of the nucleus. In the adult disc the contribution of collagen to the tissue dry weight declines from 60 to 70% in the outer rim of the annulus to 10 to 20% in the most central part of the nucleus.

The annulus fibrosus contains fibrillar and short chain collagens. The fibrillar collagens found in the annulus fibrosus include type I, type II, type III, and type V. The concentration of type I collagen declines from about 80% of the total collagen in the outer rim of the annulus to 0 in the transition zone and nucleus. The concentration of type II collagen follows the opposite pattern. It increases from 0 to 80% of the total collagen from the outer rim of the annulus to the transition zone and nucleus. Type III collagen occurs in trace amounts and type V collagen contributes about 3% of the total collagen of the annulus fibrosus. The short chain collagens found in annulus fibrosus include type VI and IX. Type IX collagen forms only about 1% of annulus fibrosus collagen, but type VI occurs in unusually high concentrations; it forms about 10% of total annulus fibrosus collagen.

Fibrillar and short chain collagens also form part of the matrix of the nucleus pulposus. It contains at least three fibril-forming collagens: type II, type III, and type XI. Type II is the predominant collagen contributing about 80% of the total nucleus pulposus collagen. Type III occurs in trace amounts, and type XI contributes about 3% of the total collagen of the nucleus. Nucleus pulposus short chain collagens include type VI and type IX. As in the annulus fibrosus type IX forms only about 1% of the total collagen, but type VI contributes even more to the nucleus than to the annulus, forming about 14 to 20% of the total collagen. The reason for the unusually high concentration of type VI collagen in the annulus and nucleus remains unknown. This short chain collagen forms banded fibrillar aggregates of longitudinal fibrils about 5 nm in diameter with alternating transverse bands consisting of two 15 nm wide dark bands separated by a 15 nm wide lucent strip. These fibrillar aggregates occur most frequently in the matrix immediately surrounding cells. They may have a role in resisting tensile loads on the matrix or may provide a loose fibrillar network that helps organize other matrix molecules.

Aggregating and nonaggregating proteoglycans form a significant part of the disc macromolecular framework and help give disc stiffness to compression and resiliency. Their concentration increases from the periphery of the disc to the center. They contribute about 10 to 20% of the dry weight of the outer annulus and as much as 50% of the dry weight of the central nucleus.

Annulus fibrosus and nucleus pulposus proteoglycans differ from those found in hyaline cartilages like the disc cartilage endplates, articular cartilage, or epiphyseal or growth plate cartilage.

The proteoglycan populations found in annulus fibrosus and nucleus pulposus include fewer aggregates, smaller aggregates, and smaller more variable aggrecans. Many disc proteoglycan aggregates consist of star-shaped clusters of monomers rather than long aggregates. Aggregated and nonaggregated disc proteoglycan monomers have shorter protein core filaments, vary more in size, and have less chondroitin sulfate and more keratan sulfate than those found in hyaline cartilages. The high concentration of these small variable monomers in the nucleus pulposus suggests that fragments of degraded proteoglycans accumulate in the central regions of the disc.

Elastin occurs in trace amounts in annulus fibrosis and nucleus pulposus. In the annulus, elastin appears as fusiform or cylindrical fibers lying parallel to the collagen fibrils. In the nucleus, elastin assumes irregular lobular shapes without apparent relationship to collagen fibrils. The contribution of elastin to disc mechanical properties remains unclear.

As in other musculoskeletal tissues, noncollagenous proteins appear to help organize and stabilize the extracellular matrix of intervertebral disc and may facilitate adhesion of cell membranes to other matrix macromolecules. The concentration of disc noncollagenous proteins increases with age. In the annulus, the proportion of tissue dry weight contributed by noncollagenous proteins increases from 5 to 25% with increasing age and in the nucleus it increases from 20% of the dry weight to 45% of the dry weight. Some of the increasing concentration of noncollagenous proteins may be due to accumulation of degraded molecules. Electron microscopic studies have identified dense granular sheaths around disc collagen fibers. These sheaths increase in volume with increasing age, suggesting that they represent collections of noncollagenous proteins.

Blood Supply

Small blood vessels and plexes of vessels lie on the surface on the annulus fibrosus, and occasional small vessels penetrate a short distance into the outer layers of the annulus. The intraosseous blood vessels of the vertebrae contact but do not penetrate the cartilage endplates. This arrangement of blood vessels leaves the central disc as the largest avascular structure in the body. The cells must rely on diffusion of nutrients and metabolites through a large volume of matrix. Mineralization of the endplates with increasing age may further compromise diffusion of nutrients to the central regions of the disc.

Nerve Supply

Perivascular and free nerve endings lie on the outer surface of the annulus and some of these nerve cell processes penetrate the outer most collagen lamellae. Despite multiple investigations of disc innervation, no nerves have been identified deep to the outer annular layers. The cartilage plates also have perivascular nerves.

Age-Related Changes in Disc Tissues

Growth, maturation, and aging dramatically alter disc tissues, especially the nucleus pulposus. The four tissue components of the disc are easily identified in the newborn. A clear gelatinous nucleus fills almost half the disc and consists almost entirely of notochordal tissue. A narrow transition zone and larger ring of annulus fibrocartilage surround the nucleus. The outermost layers of the annulus encircle the annular fibrocartilage. As the disc grows and matures during childhood the nucleus gradually becomes opaque. The decreasing water concentration makes it dense, firm, and difficult to separate from the fibrocartilage and transition zones. The annular fibrocartilage ring increases in size as the proportion of the disc occupied by the nucleus decreases. In the elderly, the components of the disc inside the outer annular layers consist almost entirely of fibrocartilage, and clefts and fissures appear in the central parts of the disc.

The disc cells also change with age. Viable notochordal cells fill most of the fetal nucleus pulposus. With growth and maturation, their numerical density progressively decreases and cells with the morphologic features of connective tissue cells appear in the nucleus pulposus. In adults, few if any notochordal cells remain and the percent of necrotic cells in the nucleus increases from about 2% in the fetus to about 50% in adults. In adults and the elderly a dense pericellular matrix forms around most cells in the nucleus pulposus and the inner annulus fibrosus, possibly because of accumulation of cell products and metabolites. In the elderly less than 20% of the nucleus cells remain viable. The causes of these age changes remain unclear. They may result from decreased nutrition of central disc cells due to increased disc volume, decreased diffusion of nutrients into the disc following mineralization of the cartilage endplates, and accumulation of cell products and metabolites in the matrix.

MUSCLE

The ability of muscle cell contraction to produce joint motion or stabilize joints against resistance depends not only on the composition and structure of the muscle cells, but on the muscle nerves and blood vessels, the organization of the tissue, and the attachment of muscle cells to tendons. Unlike the musculoskeletal connective tissues, muscle consists primarily of cells contained within a small volume of highly organized matrix (Figure 1-27). The matrix contains collagens, elastin, proteoglycans, and noncollagenous proteins that maintain the structure of the tissue including the muscle nerves and blood vessels.

Structure

Muscle cells (myofibers or muscle fibers) cluster into bundles called fascicles. Aggregates of fascicles combined with their extracellular matrix form named muscles. Although the extracellular matrix makes up only a small fraction of muscle volume (Figure 1-28), it is critical for normal muscle function, maintenance of muscle structure, and healing. A basal lamina containing collagens, noncollagenous proteins, and muscle-specific proteoglycans surrounds each myofiber. The basal lamina together with the surrounding irregularly arranged fine collagen fibers form the endomysium. A thicker matrix sheath composed primarily of collagen fibers and elastic fibers (the perimysium) covers muscle fasciculi. The epimysium, a denser peripheral sheath of connective tissue, covers the entire muscle and usually joins with the fascia overlying the muscle and with the muscle-tendon junction.

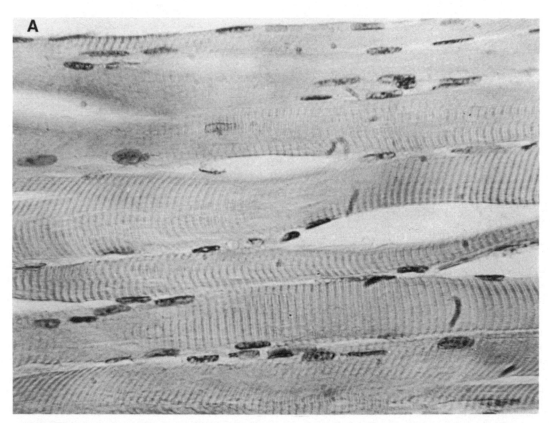

FIGURE 1-27. (A) Skeletal muscle, longitudinal section. Note that the fibers do not branch or anastomose. Each fiber has many flattened, slender sarcolemmal nuclei lying peripherally beneath the membrane and oriented parallel with the long axis of the fiber. In muscle disease these nuclei come to occupy a central position. Large numbers of axially disposed myofibrils are contained within the fiber. (×670) **(B)** Striated muscle, cross section. An enlargement of a muscle fiber is depicted. The myofibrils are separated by sarcoplasm. The matrix consists of the endomysium, perimysium, and epimysium.

continued

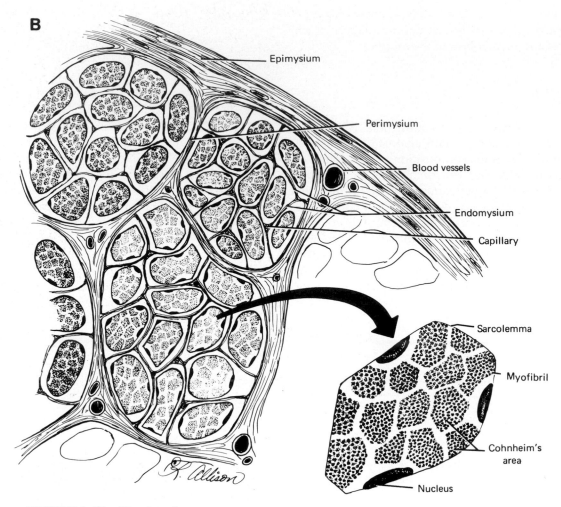

FIGURE 1-27. *(Continued)*

Composition

Cells

Muscles contain connective tissue cells, endothelial cells of blood vessels, and nerve cell processes, but most of the tissue consists of large highly differentiated muscle cells. Each muscle cell, or myofiber, contains multiple nuclei, a unique form of endoplasmic reticulum called the sacroplasmic reticulum and contractile protein filaments (actin and myosin) organized into cylindrical organelles called myofibrils (Figure 1-28). When viewed by the electron microscope, actin filaments appear as thin filaments and myosin filaments appear as thick filaments (Figures 1-29 and 1-30). Each myofibril consists of regular repeating units, consisting primarily of actin and myosin, called sarcomeres. These myofibrils often extend through the entire length of the

cell and fill most of the cell volume. Flattened vesicles of sarcoplasmic reticulum surround the myofibrils and a series of invaginations of the cell membrane, called transverse tubules, extend from the cell surface to lie next to each myofibril and the membranes of the sarcoplasmic reticulum (Figure 1-31). The interfibrillar sarcoplasm contains mitochondria, lysosomes, and ribosomes.

Myofibers form by fusion of multiple small mesenchymal cells called myoblasts. Myofibers cannot proliferate; therefore, increase in muscle mass occurs through cell growth. The myofibers can grow in length by fusion with myoblasts, thereby increasing the number of nuclei. They can grow in diameter by increasing the size and number of myofibers. In mature individuals, some myoblasts survive. They remain next to mature myofibers, and following muscle injury they can proliferate and fuse to form new muscle cells.

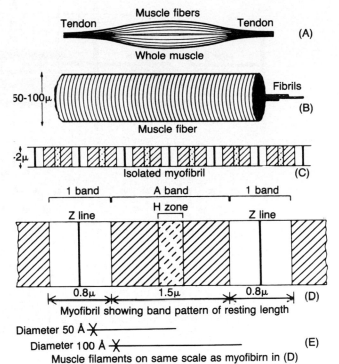

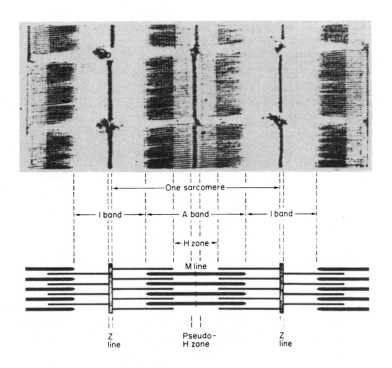

FIGURE 1-28. The dimensions and arrangement of the myofibrils in a muscle. The whole muscle **(A)** is made up of fibers **(B)** that contain cross-striated myofibrils **(C, D)**. Myofibrils consist primarily of actin and myosin filaments **(E)** that overlap and interdigitate in a stereospecific manner. (Huxley HE. The molecular basis of contraction. In: Bourne GH, ed. The Structure and Function of Muscle. New York: Academic Press, 1972)

FIGURE 1-29. Longitudinal section of frog sartorius muscle (*top*) together with a diagram showing the overlap of filaments that gives rise to the band pattern. The A band is most dense in its lateral zones where the thick and thin filaments overlap. The central zone of the A band (the H zone) is less dense, since it contains thick filaments only. The I bands are less dense still because they contain only thin filaments. The sarcomere length here is about 2.5 u. (Huxley HE. The molecular basis of contraction. In: Bourne GH, ed. The Structure and Function of Muscle. New York: Academic Press, 1972)

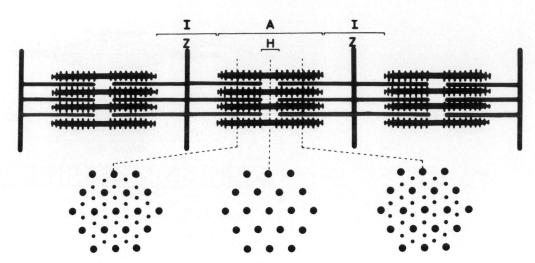

FIGURE 1-30. Structure of striated muscle, showing overlapping arrays of actin- and myosin-containing filaments, the latter with projecting cross-bridges on them. To facilitate showing the relationships, the diagram is drawn with considerable longitudinal foreshortening, with filament diameters and side-spacings as shown. The filament lengths should be about five times the lengths shown. (Huxley HE. The molecular basis of contraction. In: Bourne GH, ed. The Structure and Function of Muscle. New York: Academic Press, 1971)

Matrix

Because of difficulties in extracting, purifying, and studying the small volume of matrix found in muscle, the composition and organization of the muscle matrix remains poorly understood. The muscle basal lamina contain laminin (a noncollagenous protein that forms part of basement membranes), types IV and V collagen, and heparin sulfate proteoglycan. The outer connective tissue envelopes of muscle consist primarily of type I collagen fibrils.

Blood Supply

Large numbers of blood vessels penetrate the epimysium passing between muscle fasciculi within the muscle tissue matrix. They then enter the muscle fascicles to form rich capillary networks around individual myofibrils.

Innervation

Initiation, coordination, and control of muscle contraction require elaborate innervation. Nerves that sense muscle tension terminate on intrafusal fibers and Golgi tendon organs. Three types of motor neurons supply myofibers: (1) α motor neurons innervating extrafusal myofibers, (2) β motor neurons innervating both extrafusal and intrafusal myofibers, and (3) γ motor neurons innervating intrafusal myofibers.

One motor neuron innervates each myofiber, but each motor neuron generally innervates more than one myofiber. A motor unit consists of the motor neuron and the muscle fibers it innervates. Motor nerves attach to myofibers through neuromuscular junctions that transmit signals from the motor nerve terminas to limited regions of the myofibers. Neuromuscular junctions consist of five principal parts: (1) the nerve terminal filled with thousands of vesicles containing neurotransmitter, (2) a Schwann cell overlying the nerve terminal, (3) a synaptic space lined with basement membrane, (4) the postsynaptic membrane containing receptors for the neurotransmitter, and (5) postjunctional sarcoplasm necessary for the structural and metabolic support of the postsynaptic membrane. Release of neurotransmitter from the motor nerve terminal into the synaptic space creates an action potential in the muscle cell membrane. The action potential in the muscle cell membrane extends into folds in the cell membrane to the sarcoplasmic reticulum. The sarcoplasmic reticulum releases calcium ions, and the rapid increase in intracellular calcium triggers simultaneous contraction of myofibers throughout the cell.

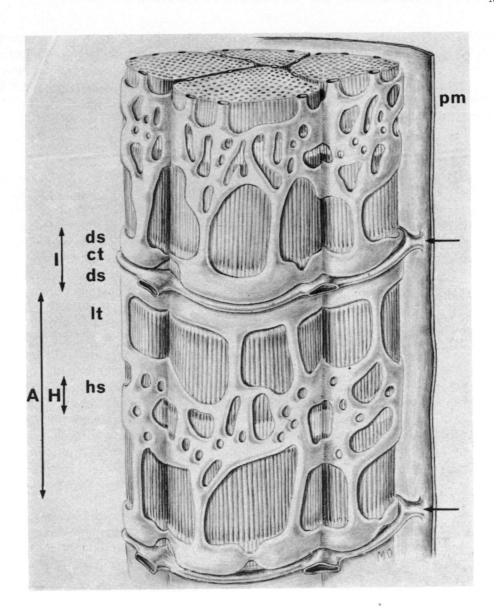

FIGURE 1-31. Three-dimensional drawing of parts of four myofibrils to illustrate (1) the sarcolemma (labeled pm on the right), (2) the transverse tubules that extend into the substance of the fiber from the sarcolemma (from points indicated by arrows on the right), and (3) the sarcoplasmic reticulum, which is interposed, and so lies between myofibrils, over their I, A, and H portions (labels for the latter on left). The transverse tubules are delicate tubules that are invaginations of the sarcolemma; hence their walls are composed of cell membrane, and their lumens open onto the outer surface of the sarcolemma. Transverse tubules (in the frog) enter the fiber at the level of Z line (indicated by arrows on right side), and each one branches as it extends across the fiber so as to surround myofibrils whose Z lines are in register with the site where it entered, as is shown by following the two tubules in this illustration, from right to left. The sarcoplasmic reticulum consists of cisternae and channels of smooth-surfaced endoplasmic reticulum that lie between and so surround myofibrils. In the region of the I band, the extent of which is indicated at the left of the illustration, the cisternae, known as terminal cisternae, are large and flattened, but they may be more or less distended (ds); they lie to either side of the transverse tubule (ct). The cisternae, by means of channels that run longitudinally (lt) over the A band to the region of the H zone, connect with a network of more or less flattened sacs called the H sacs (hs). The site of the H zone in the A band is indicated at the left of the illustration. (From C. P. Leblond; Ham AW. Histology, 7th Ed. Philadelphia: JB Lippincott, 1974)

FORMATION AND DEVELOPMENT OF THE MUSCULOSKELETAL SYSTEM

Normal structure and function of the musculoskeletal system depend on the formation and growth of the specific skeletal connective tissues and muscle, and the integration of these tissues into the system that provides the stability and mobility of the body. Cartilage, muscle, bone, and dense fibrous tissue form, grow, and become organized into the musculoskeletal system during early prenatal life so that by 6 months the final form of the musculoskeletal system is easily recognized (Figure 1-32). Disturbances of these processes cause congenital abnormalities including failure of segmentation of vertebrae, congenital dislocations of the hip, clubfeet, and absence of part or all of a limb. Following birth the musculoskeletal system continues to grow and modify its form until the physes close.

Cartilage, Muscle, and Bone

Within the first few weeks of intrauterine life, the embryo takes shape, developing the head, the trunk, and protrusions called limb buds. Between the ectoderm and the entoderm lies the diffuse, loose, cellular mesenchyme, which differentiates into the musculoskeletal connective tissues and skeletal muscle. The first recognizable musculoskeletal structures appear as dense concentrations of mesenchymal cells that take the shape of the bones.

As early as the fifth embryonic week, mesenchymal cells enlarge, become more compact, and differentiate into a sheet of cells recognized as pre-cartilage. Then, matrix is laid down between the cells (Figures 1-33 and 1-34). Cartilage increases in thickness by growth, both internally and externally (Figure 1-35). Internal growth occurs by multiplication of cartilage cells and production of new matrix. Peripheral growth occurs from the investing sheath (the perichondrium), whose inner cells are transformed into chondrocytes. Figure 1-33 shows the development of cartilage and skeletal muscle from mesenchyme.

Bone first appears after the seventh embryonic week. It forms either from mesenchymal membranes (e.g., facial and cranial bones) or from cartilage (e.g., the long bones of the limbs). Although the bone is identical in each instance, in the latter type the cartilage must first be removed before bone can be laid down.

Intramembranous Bone Formation

The mesenchymal or connective tissue membrane first forms the original model of the facial and the cranial bones. At one or more central points of the membrane, intramembranous ossification begins (Figure 1-36). These ossification centers are characterized by the appearance of osteoblasts that lay down a meshwork of bony trabeculae spread radially in all directions. The mesenchyme at the periphery differentiates into a fibrous sheath (the periosteum), the undersurface of which differentiates into osteoblasts, which in turn deposit parallel plates of compact bone (the lamellae). This is periosteal ossification, by which

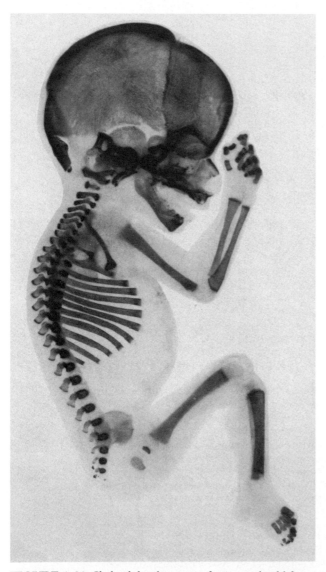

FIGURE 1-32. Skeletal development of a 6-month-old fetus.

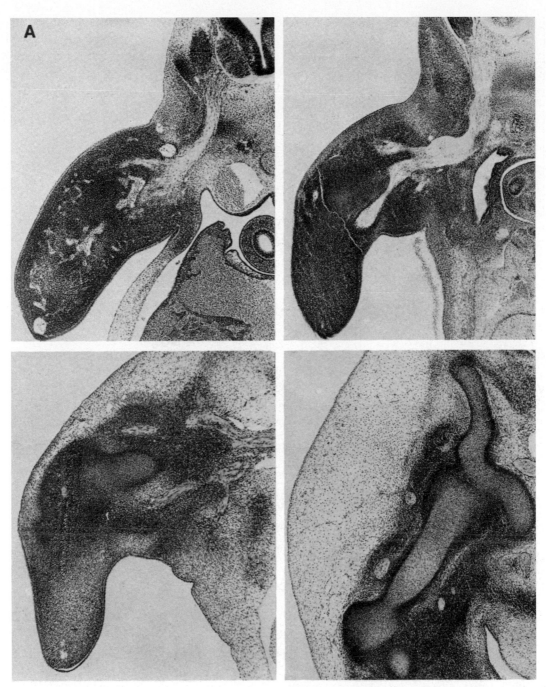

FIGURE 1-33. (A) Origin of a limb bud. Development of the upper limb bud and histogenesis of the humerus are shown. The limb bud originates as a small elevation of the body wall and at first consists of a condensed mass of proliferating mesoblastic cells. Within a few days, a central condensation of mesoblasts occurs. This is the skeletomuscle condensation, so-called because separate muscle and skeleton cannot be identified. At the same time, a broad sheet of branching nerve trunks from the cord and the spinal ganglia stream into the base of the arm bud (*top, left*). A few days later, muscular and skeletal condensations become distinct, and massive nerve trunks enter the center of the muscle condensations (*top, right*). In the next section, definite muscle groups can be identified (*bottom, left*) containing conspicuous nerve trunks, and major branches of the brachial plexus are obvious. At the same time, the central part of the skeletal condensation is being transformed into cartilage (this tissue appears lighter in color). The cartilage of different bones is deposited separately in the last section (*bottom, right*) so that these central cartilaginous cores within the skeletal bed acquire the shape of the bones of which they are forerunners. These sections represent developmental periods of about 2 days each. **(B)** These diagram drawings correspond to these sections in A. (From the Carnegie Institution of Washington, Streeter GL. Developmental horizons in human embryos (Pub 583), Contrib Embryol 1949;33:149.)

continued

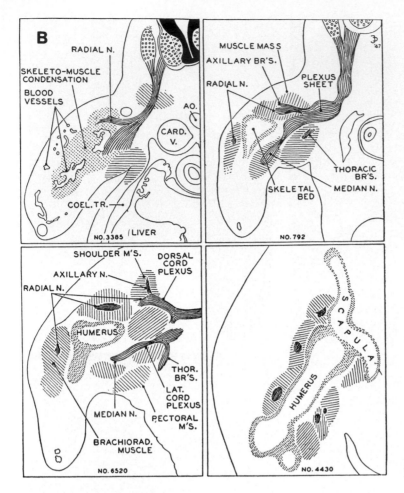

FIGURE   1-33. *(Continued)*

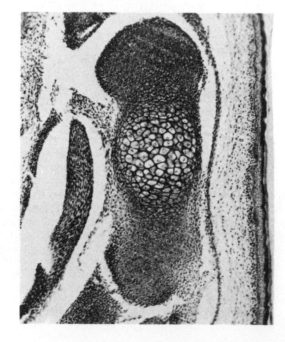

FIGURE 1-34. Early fetal anlage of a long bone. It is composed of mesenchyme at the center of which the cells become rounded and assume the appearance of chondrocytes. Later, the peripheral mesenchyme will give rise to vascular tissue that will invade the calcified cartilage and replace the latter with bone.

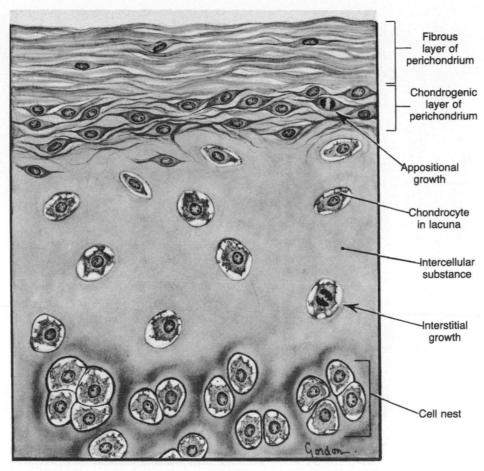

FIGURE 1-35. Appositional and interstitial cartilage growth. Cartilage grows from the perichondrium when fibroblast-like cells enlarge into chondroblasts and become encapsulated. They multiply, form groups, and synthesize new matrix producing appositional growth. Cells within the tissue also proliferate and synthesize matrix producing interstitial growth. (Ham AW. Histology, 7th Ed. Philadelphia: JB Lippincott, 1974)

the inner and the outer tables of the skull are formed. Trabeculae are arranged mainly along lines of greatest stress.

Enchondral Bone Formation

A cartilaginous model of the structure precedes destruction of cartilage and its replacement by bone. Two processes are involved: ossification centrally within the cartilage, or endochondral ossification, and ossification peripherally beneath the perichondrium (or periosteum), or perichondrial or periosteal ossification.

In the center of the cartilaginous precursor, the cells enlarge and become arranged radially as the matrix mineralizes. Invading from blood vessels the perichondrium (Figures 1-37 and 1-38) bring

osteoblasts that deposit new bone that replaces the cartilage.

As the central bone formation occurs, the cells of the inner layer of perichondrium (now more appropriately named the periosteum) lay down parallel layers of compact bone. The cartilaginous physes form at the end of each long bone and produce enchondral bone throughout skeletal growth. Periosteal ossification contributes to growth thickness of the structure.

Joints

Two types of joints develop between bones: synarthorses, which allow little movement, and diarthroses, which allow low friction movement.

The synarthorses form by the differentiation of mesenchyme into a uniting layer of connective tissue

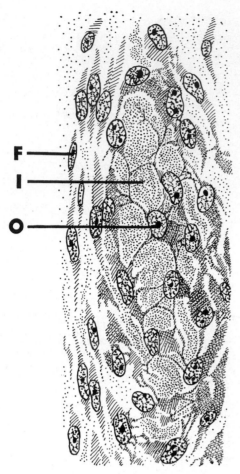

FIGURE 1-36. Intramembranous bone formation. Fibroblasts (F). Homogeneous interstitial bone substance (I), collagenous fibrils no longer visible. Connective tissue cells (O) that have developed processes to become osteoblasts and later osteocytes.

(the suture or syndesmosis), cartilage (the synchondrosis), or bone (the synostosis).

Diarthroses have joint cavities that arise from a cleft in the mesenchyme. The joint capsule and ligaments form from the dense external tissue, which is continuous with the periosteum. The cells on the inner surface of the capsule flatten into the synovial membrane. Menisci and meniscus-like structures form from mesenchyme that projects into the joint cavity.

The Axial Skeleton

The notochord is the primitive axial support for the body. Mesenchymal tissue (designated as sclerotomes) migrate toward the notochord and come

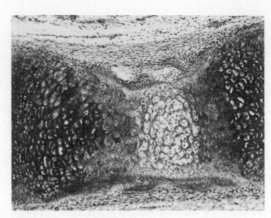

FIGURE 1-37. Ossification of a fetal cartilaginous long bone. The cartilage cells at the center of the calcified cartilage have become enlarged, and the matrix is sparse. A bone collar has formed about this level and is gradually replacing the cartilage.

to lie in paired segmental masses alongside the notochord. Intersegmental arteries separate each sclerotomic mesenchymal mass from similar masses before and behind. Each sclerotome then differentiates into a caudal compact portion and a cranial less dense half. The denser caudal half then unites with the looser cranial half of the succeeding sclerotome to form the substance of the vertebra (Figure 1-39). Both the condensed and the looser portions grow about the notochord to form the body of the vertebra. From the denser (now cranial) half, dorsal extensions pass around the neural tube to form the vertebral arch, and paired ventrolateral outgrowths form the costal processes or forerunners of the ribs. The mesenchymal tissue in the intervertebral fissure gives rise to the intervertebral disc. The nucleus pulposus in the disc constitutes the remnant of the notochord. The two parts of sclerotomes, in joining, enclose the intersegmental artery, which therefore passes through the center of the vertebral body. In the seventh embryonic week, centers of chondrification appear, two in the vertebral body and one in each half of the vertebral arch. These four centers enlarge and fuse into a complete cartilaginous vertebra. Vertebral ossification starts in the tenth week. A single center in the body and one in each half of the arch appears, but union is not completed until several years after birth (Figure 1-40).

Continued growth in length of the body occurs by enchondral ossification at the cephalad and the caudad epiphyseal plates. About the rim of the superior and the inferior surfaces, a prominent ring of

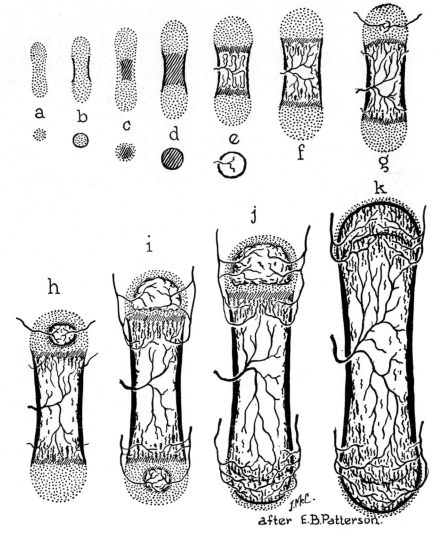

FIGURE 1-38. Development of a typical long bone. **(a)** Cartilage model. **(b)** Periosteal bone collar appears. **(c)** Center of calcifying cartilage. **(d)** Further development of calcified cartilage. **(e)** Vascular mesenchyme enters, resorbs calcified cartilage, and new bone is laid down toward either extremity of the model. **(f)** Endochondral ossification is further advanced, bone increased in length. **(g)** Blood vessels and mesenchyme enter upper epiphyseal cartilage. **(h)** Development of epiphyseal ossification center. **(i)** Ossification center develops in lower epiphysis. **(j and k)** The lower and then the upper epiphyseal cartilage plates disappear, bone ceases to grow in length, a continuous bone marrow cavity traverses the entire length of the bone, and blood vessels of diaphysis, metaphysis, and epiphysis intercommunicate. (Redrawn from Maximow AA, Bloom W. A Textbook of Histology. Philadelphia: WB Saunders, 1968)

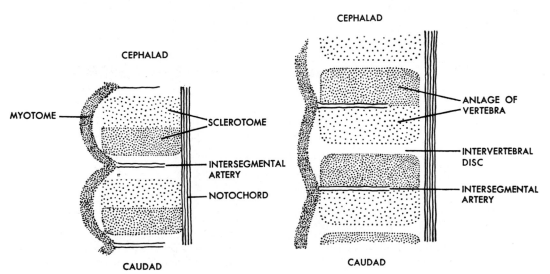

FIGURE 1-39. Early stages of differentiation of vertebrae. (Redrawn from Arey LB. Developmental Anatomy. Philadelphia: WB Saunders, 1974)

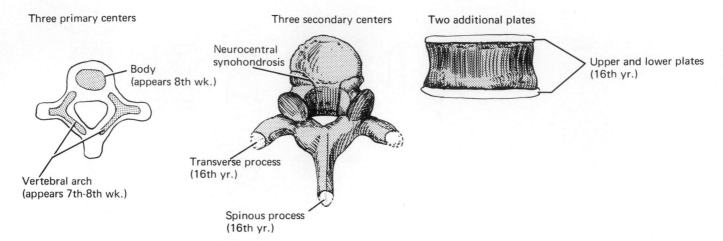

FIGURE 1-40. Development of vertebra. Three primary ossification centers develop in utero; three secondary centers appear during the growth period and, with epiphyseal plates, become completely ossified as growth is completed. (After Goss CM. Gray's Anatomy, 28th Ed. Philadelphia: Lea and Febiger, 1966)

cartilage exists to which is attached the fibers of the longitudinal ligament of the spine (Figure 1-41). It does not participate in growth. Gradually, it develops secondary ossification centers that are triangular in cross section but actually skirt the rim of the body. Eventually, this center appears as a line parallel with the upper and the lower surfaces of the body and resembles a plate (Figure 1-42). The term *plate* is reserved for the growth cartilage that intervenes

between the ring and the main body of bone. The secondary centers fuse with the main body by the age of 17. The central artery can be seen up to 6 years of age, after which it is obliterated (Figure 1-43). It may persist beyond this time in certain conditions (e.g., Scheuermann's disease).

An exception in the development of the vertebra occurs in the atlas. The body differentiates typically but soon is taken over by the axis serving as a

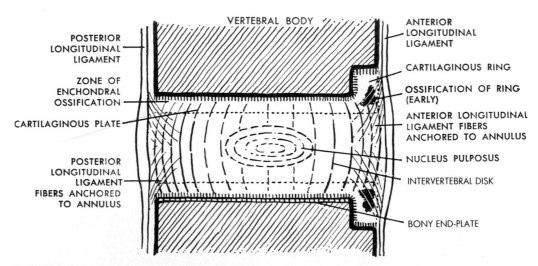

FIGURE 1-41. Sagittal section through adjacent vertebral bodies during ossification of the cartilaginous ring. (Redrawn from Schmid P. Zur Entstehung der Adolezentenkyphose. Dtsch Med Wochenschr 1949;74:798)

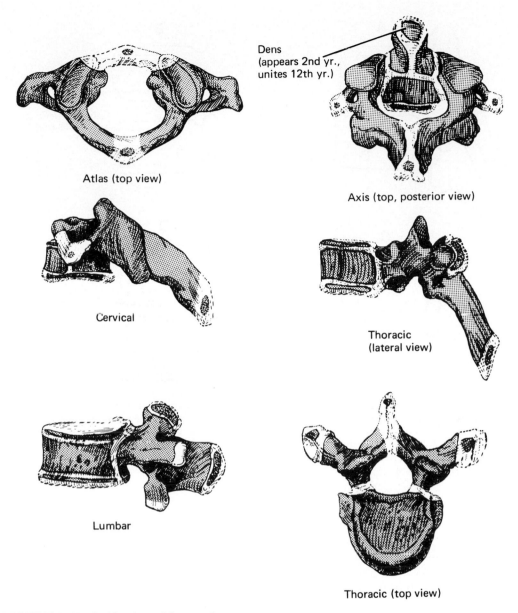

Atlas (top view)

Dens (appears 2nd yr., unites 12th yr.)

Axis (top, posterior view)

Cervical

Thoracic (lateral view)

Lumbar

Thoracic (top view)

FIGURE 1-42. Ossification of the vertebrae.

peg-like extension (dens) of the latter, about which the atlas rotates. The atlas is left as a ring. The sacral and the coccygeal vertebrae represent vertebra with reduced vertebral arches. The sacral vertebrae eventually fuse into a single mass. The coccygeal vertebrae exist as rudimentary structures. The entire spine at birth displays one continuous curve convex posteriorly. As the erect posture is assumed after the first year, secondary forward curves develop the cervical and the lumbar regions.

Finally, the lordosis in the cervical and the dorsal regions is balanced by the kyphosis in the thoracic and the sacral regions.

The original union of the costal process with the vertebra is replaced by a joint for the head of the rib. The center of ossification appears at the tangle of the rib. However, the distal ends of the long ribs always remain cartilaginous. In the neck the ribs are represented by their tubercles, which are fused with the transverse processes and their heads fused with

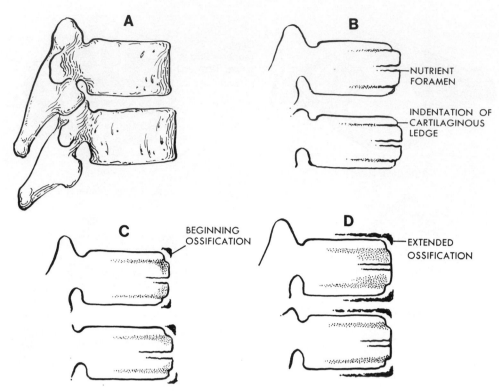

FIGURE 1-43. The appearance of normal thoracic vertebrae in children at various ages. **(A)** Normal thoracic vertebrae, fully developed, lateral view. **(B)** Lateral roentgenographic view of vertebral bodies in children under 6 years of age. **(C)** Lateral view in children, 6 to 9 years of age. Ossification starting in the cartilaginous ring is most visible anteriorly. **(D)** At 9 to 15 years of age. Ossification is more extensive in the ring and progresses posteriorly. The nutrient foramen normally is obliterated after 6 years of age.

the bodies; between these processes is an interval, the transverse foramen, through which the vertebral arteries course. When the costal processes are overdeveloped in the cervical region, a supernumerary rib is formed, which may lead to compression of nerve structures.

The sternum originates from the junction of two bars of ventrolaterally placed mesenchyme, which initially have no connection with the ribs or which each other.

At birth, the posterior bony arch is separated from the anterior bony centrum by cartilaginous bridges. The bony arch is completed by the second year. Junction between arch and body occurs between the third and sixth years.

The Appendicular Skeleton

The appendicular skeleton is derived directly from the unsegmented somatic mesenchyme. Definite masses are formed at the sites of the future pectoral and pelvic girdles and limb buds. The sequence of bone development through cartilaginous and osseous stages follows.

The clavicle is the first bone of the skeleton to ossify. Before ossification, a peculiar tissue resembling both membranous and cartilaginous tissue makes it difficult to classify the origin. Two primary centers of ossification appear.

The scapula is a single plate with two chief centers of ossification and several epiphyseal centers that appear later. An early primary center forms the body and the spine. The other, after birth, gives rise to the coracoid process.

The humerus, the radius, and the ulna all ossify from a single primary center in the diaphysis and an epiphyseal center at each end. Additional epiphyseal centers are constant at the lower end of the humerus. Each carpal bone ossifies from a single center. The metacarpals ossify from a single primary center and an epiphyseal center (Figures 1-44 and 1-45).

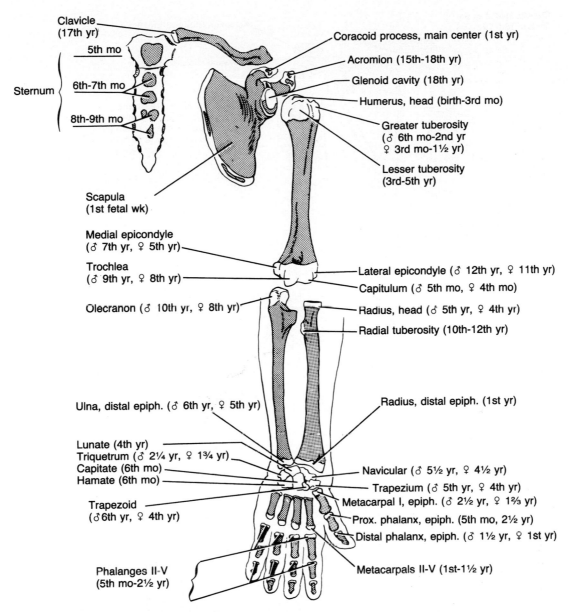

FIGURE 1-44. The appearance at birth of the upper extremity. The ages at which the ossification of the epiphyses appear are shown with the differentiation between male and female indicated.

At first, the cartilaginous plate of the pelvis lies perpendicular to the vertebral column. Later, it rotates to a position parallel with the vertebral column and in relation to the first three sacral vertebrae. Three main centers of ossification appear for the ilium, the ischium, and the pubis. The three elements join at a cup-shaped depression, the acetabulum, the articulation for the head of the femur.

The development of the femur, the tibia, the fibula, the tarsus, the metatarsals, and the phalanges corresponds to that of the bones of the upper extremity (Figures 1-46 and 1-47).

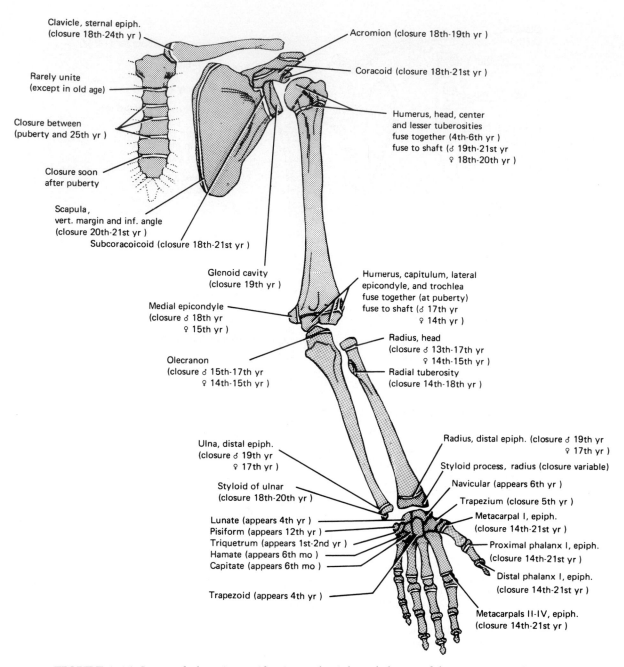

FIGURE 1-45. Stages of advancing ossification and epiphyseal closure of the upper extremity.

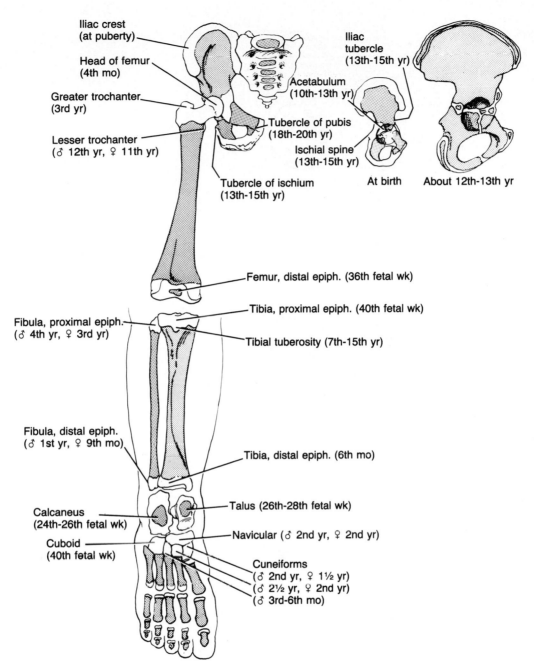

FIGURE 1-46. The appearance at birth of the lower extremity. The ages at which ossification of the epiphyses appear are shown with the differentiation between male and female indicated.

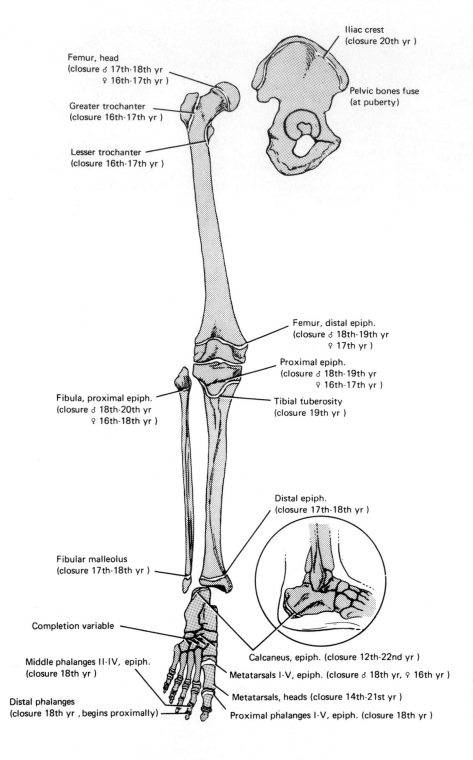

Iliac crest
(closure 20th yr)

Pelvic bones fuse
(at puberty)

Femur, head
(closure ♂ 17th-18th yr
♀ 16th-17th yr)

Greater trochanter
(closure 16th-17th yr)

Lesser trochanter
(closure 16th-17th yr)

Femur, distal epiph.
(closure ♂ 18th-19th yr
♀ 17th yr)

Proximal epiph.
(closure ♂ 18th-19th yr
♀ 16th-17th yr)

Fibula, proximal epiph.
(closure ♂ 18th-20th yr
♀ 16th-18th yr)

Tibial tuberosity
(closure 19th yr)

Distal epiph.
(closure 17th-18th yr)

Fibular malleolus
(closure 17th-18th yr)

Completion variable

Middle phalanges II-IV, epiph.
(closure 18th yr)

Distal phalanges
(closure 18th yr , begins proximally)

Calcaneus, epiph. (closure 12th-22nd yr)

Metatarsals I-V, epiph. (closure ♂ 18th yr, ♀ 16th yr)

Metatarsals, heads (closure 14th-21st yr)

Proximal phalanges I-V, epiph. (closure 18th yr)

FIGURE 1-47. The stage of advancing ossification and epiphyseal closure of the lower extremity.

SUMMARY

The musculoskeletal system consists of skeletal connective tissues (bone, cartilage, and dense fibrous tissues) and muscle formed into functional units that make possible movements that vary from the finely controlled motions of the upper limbs necessary to play musical instruments, to the powerful motions of all four extremities and the spine necessary to lift a heavy weights from the ground, to the rapid coordinated repetitive motions required for success in many sports. Mesenchymal cells form all musculoskeletal tissues, but specific tissues differ in structure, composition, mechanical properties, innervation, and blood supply. The skeletal connective tissues (bone, cartilage, and dense fibrous tissue) consist of sparsely distributed cells surrounded by a large volume of extracellular organic matrix synthesized by the cells. Their matrix molecular frameworks consist of collagens, proteoglycans, and noncollagenous proteins. Each tissue has a unique combination of these three classes of macromolecules, and in some tissues, like meniscus, intervertebral disc, and ligament, elastin also forms part of the organic matrix. In addition to their organic matrix, bone and some cartilage regions have an inorganic matrix consisting of relatively insoluble mineral deposited within the organic matrix. These differences in matrix composition give the skeletal connective tissues different mechanical properties. Hyaline cartilage has the stiffness in compression, the ability to distribute loads and the durability to form the low friction gliding surfaces of synovial joints. The dense fibrous tissues have the tensile strength and flexibility to serve as tendons and ligaments, and bone has the stiffness and strength to provide the rigid support necessary for normal function of the other tissues. Hyaline cartilage lacks nerves. Bone contains perivascular nerves and some regions of the dense fibrous tissues have nerves that may sense tissue deformation as well as perivascular nerves, but none of the connective tissue cells have direct innervation. Hyaline cartilage, the intervertebral disc (except for the outermost layers of the annulus fibrosus), and some regions of dense fibrous tissue lack blood vessels. Unlike the skeletal connective tissues, skeletal muscle consists primarily of cells with only a small volume of extracellular matrices, the tissue has a network of blood vessels that reaches every cell, a motor nerve innervates each muscle cell, and the cells generate the force necessary to produce movement.

Although knowledge of the tissues provides the basis for understanding orthopaedic diseases, musculoskeletal function and dysfunction cannot be understood in terms of individual tissues alone. The mobility, strength, and stability of the body depend on the organization and integration of these tissues into functional units. Voluntary movement requires skeletal muscle contraction, but the mechanisms by which muscle contraction produces joint motion, or the failure of muscle contraction to produce joint motion, cannot be understood by considering muscle cells alone. Muscles move or stabilize synovial joints and the spine by transmitting the force generated by individual muscle cells to tendons through elaborate muscle-tendon junctions. Many tendons pass through sheaths and retinacula that make it possible to effectively transmit the force generated by muscle to bone through distinct insertions into bone or periosteum. The force then acts on synovial joints consisting of articular cartilage, menisci, bone, joint capsule, synovium and ligaments, or the spine. The spine includes these tissues with the addition of the intervertebral disc. Ultimately muscle contraction causes joint motion or stabilizes joints against resistance, but synovial joint or spine function can only be understood by considering how the multiple musculoskeletal tissues perform simultaneously as parts of a functional unit. Likewise understanding orthopaedic diseases depends on considering how disturbances in the structure or function of one or more tissues alters musculoskeletal function measured in terms of motion, strength, and stability.

Annotated Bibliography

Arnoczky SP, McDevitt CA. The Meniscus: structure, function, repair and replacement. In: Buckwalter JA, Einhorn T, Simon S, eds. Orthopaedic Basic Science—Biology and Biomechanics of the Musculoskeletal System. Rosemont, IL: American Academy of Orthopaedic Surgeons, 2000:531–545.
This book chapter provides an overview of meniscal structure, composition, and function.

Bostrom MPG, Boskey A, Kaufman JJ, Einhorn TA. Form and function of bone. In: Buckwalter JA, Einhorn T, Simon S, eds. Orthopaedic Basic Science—Biology and Biomechanics of the Musculoskeletal System. Rosemont, IL: American Academy of Orthopaedic Surgeons, 2000:319–370.
This book chapter discusses current understanding of bone structure and function.

Buckwalter JA, Boden SD, Eyre DR, Mow VC, Weidenbaum M. Intervertebral disc structure, composition and function. In: Buckwalter JA, Einhorn T, Simon S, eds. Orthopaedic Basic Science—Biology and Biomechanics of the Musculoskeletal System. Rosemont, IL: American Academy of Orthopaedic Surgeons, 2000:547–556.
This book chapter provides a detailed overview of human intervertebral disc structure, composition, and function.

Buckwalter JA, Ehrlich MG, Sandell LJ, Trippel SB (eds). Skeletal Growth and Development: Clinical Issues and Basic Science Advances. Rosemont, IL: American Academy of Orthopaedic Surgeons, 1998.
This book discusses current understanding of skeletal growth and development, including the clinical presentation of selected disorders of skeletal growth and development.

Buckwalter JA, Glimcher MJ, Cooper RR, Recker R. Bone biology. part I. structure, blood supply, cells, matrix and mineralization. J Bone Joint Surg 1995;77A:1256–1275.

Buckwalter JA, Glimcher MJ, Cooper RR, Recker R. Bone biology. part II. formation, form, modeling and remodeling. J Bone Joint Surg 1995;77A:1276–1289.
These two articles discuss the structure, composition, and biology of bone.

Buckwalter JA, Mankin HJ. Articular cartilage I. Tissue design and chondrocyte-matrix interactions. J Bone Joint Surg 1997;79A:600–611.
This article presents an overview of articular cartilage structure and biology.

Garrett WE, Best TM. Anatomy, physiology and mechanics of skeletal muscle. In: Buckwalter JA, Einhorn T, Simon S, eds. Orthopaedic Basic Science—Biology and Biomechanics of the Musculoskeletal System. Rosemont, IL: American Academy of Orthopaedic Surgeons, 2000:683–716.
This chapter provides a review of skeletal muscle structure and function.

Iannotti JP, Goldstein S, Kuhn J, Lipiello L, Kaplan FS, Zaleske DJ. The Formation and growth of skeletal tissue. In: Buckwalter JA, Einhorn T, Simon S, eds. Orthopaedic Basic Science—The Biology and Biomechanics of the Musculoskeletal System. Rosemont, IL: American Academy of Orthopaedic Surgeons, 2000:77–109.
A book chapter that reviews the formation, growth, remodeling, and maturation of skeletal tissues.

Mankin HJ, Mow VC, Buckwalter JA. Articular cartilage structure, composition and function. In: Buckwalter JA, Einhorn T, Simon S, eds. Orthopaedic Basic Science—Biology and Biomechanics of the Musculoskeletal System. Rosemont, IL: American Academy of Orthopaedic Surgeons, 2000:443–470.
This book chapter discusses articular cartilage structure and biology.

Woo SL-Y, An KN, Frank CB, Livesay GA, Ma CB, Zeminski J, Wayne JS, Meyers BS. Anatomy, biology and biomechanics of tendon and ligament. In: Buckwalter JA, Einhorn T, Simon S. eds. Orthopaedic Basic Science—Biology and Biomechanics of the Musculoskeletal System. Rosemont, IL: American Academy of Orthopaedic Surgeons, 2000:581–616.
This book chapter reviews the structure, function, and biology of tendons and ligaments.

2

Joseph A. Buckwalter

Musculoskeletal Tissue Healing

Recovery from musculoskeletal injuries or success in the operative treatment of many musculoskeletal diseases and deformities depends on healing the musculoskeletal tissues: that is, restoration of tissue structure and function following injury. Healing occurs by repair, replacement of damaged or lost tissue by fibrous or fibrocartilaginous tissue that fails to duplicate the normal tissue structure and function, or by regeneration, replacement of damaged or lost tissue by tissue that duplicates the normal tissue structure and function. Most isolated muscle lacerations heal by repair with scar; bone fractures heal by regeneration of bone. Over the last two decades orthopaedic surgeons have dramatically advanced their ability to promote healing of damaged bones and joints. Using new methods of internal fixation, external fixation, and rehabilitation, they now successfully treat even the most severe fractures and many severe joint injuries.

Patients with injuries of dense fibrous tissue structures (tendon, ligament, joint capsule, and meniscus) or skeletal muscle present problems as difficult as patients with bone or articular cartilage injuries. Furthermore, injuries to these latter tissues may leave patients with more significant disability than fractures. For these reasons optimal treatment of musculoskeletal injuries and diseases requires understanding of the responses of the musculoskeletal tissues to injury and the healing of these tissues.

BONE HEALING

Fractures, acute disruptions of bone tissue, result from applications of forces to the skeleton that exceed the strength of the tissue. The intensity of the applied force determines the severity of the injury as measured by the extent of bone and soft tissue damage. A fracture initiates a sequence of inflammation, repair, and remodeling that can restore the injured bone to its original state. Inflammation begins immediately after injury and is followed

rapidly by repair. After repair has replaced the lost and damaged cells and matrix, a prolonged remodeling phase begins that commonly restores normal bone structure and function.

Inflammation and Repair

An injury that fractures bone not only damages the cells, blood vessels, and bone matrix (Figure 2-1), but also the surrounding soft tissues, including the periosteum and muscle. A hematoma accumulates within the medullary canal, between the fracture ends and beneath elevated periosteum. The damage to the bone blood vessels deprives osteocytes of their nutrition, and they die as far back as the junction of collateral channels, leaving the immediate ends of the fracture without living cells (see Figure 2-2). Severely damaged periosteum and marrow, as well as other surrounding muscle, may also contribute necrotic material to the fracture site.

Inflammatory mediators released from platelets and from dead and injured cells cause blood vessels to

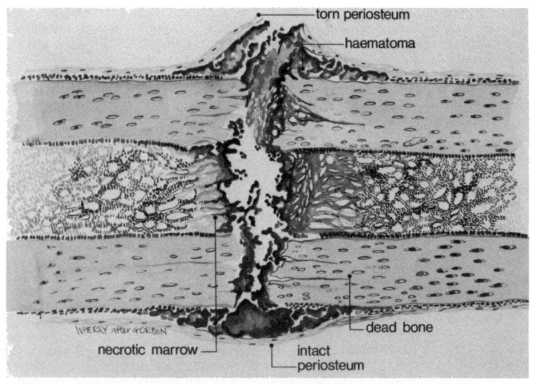

FIGURE 2-1. Initial events following fracture of a long bone diaphysis. **(A)** Drawing showing that the periosteum is torn opposite the point of impact, and may remain intact on the other side. A hematoma accumulates beneath the periosteum and between the fracture ends. There is necrotic marrow and cortical bone close to the fracture line. **(B)** A photomicrograph of a fractured rat femur 3 days after injury showing the proliferation of the periosteal repair tissue.

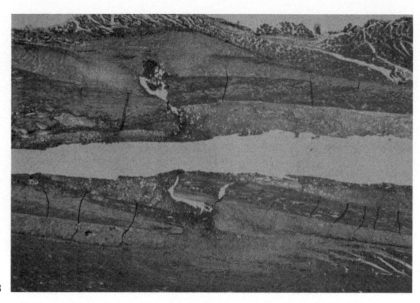

FIGURE 2-1. *(Continued)* **B**

dilate and exude plasma leading to the acute edema seen in the region of a fresh fracture. Inflammatory cells migrate to the region, including polymorphonuclear leukocytes followed by macrophages and lymphocytes. These cells also release cytokines that stimulate angiogenesis. As the inflammatory response subsides, necrotic tissue and exudate are resorbed, and fibroblasts and chondrocytes appear

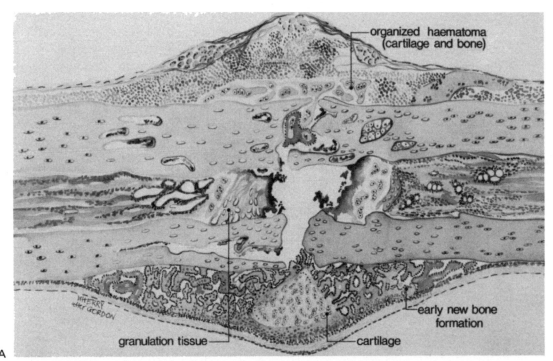

FIGURE 2-2. Early repair of a diaphyseal fracture of a long bone. **(A)** Drawing showing organization of the hematoma, early woven bone formation in the subperiosteal regions, and cartilage formation in other areas. Periosteal cells contribute to healing this type of injury. If the fracture is rigidly immobilized or if it occurs primarily through cancellous bone and the cancellous surfaces lie in close apposition, there will be little evidence of fracture callus. **(B)** Photomicrograph of a fractured rat femur 9 days after injury showing cartilage and bone formation in the subperiosteal regions. (Reprinted from Clin Ortho Rel Res with permission [5])

continued

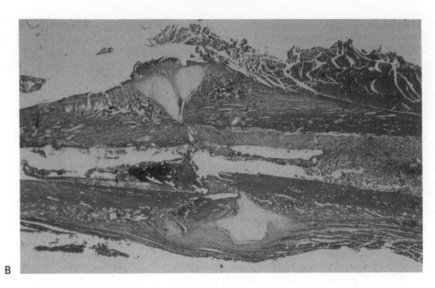

B

FIGURE 2-2. *(Continued)*

and start producing a new matrix, the fracture callus (Figures 2-2 and 2-3).

The mechanical stability of the fracture site influences the repair process. The summaries of fracture repair and remodeling that follow immediately below first describe healing of closed fractures that are not rigidly stabilized; that is, fractures where repair proceeds in the presence of motion at the fracture site (Figure 2-4). A closed clavicle fracture that is not treated by internal fixation provides an example of repair and remodeling of an unstable fracture. The second summary describes healing of stable fractures; that is, fractures where repair proceeds at a rigidly stable fracture site with the fracture surfaces held in contact. Transverse diaphyseal fractures of the radius and ulna treated by open anatomic reduction and rigid internal fixation provide examples of the repair and remodeling of stabile fractures.

Repair and Remodeling of Unstable Fractures

Disruption of blood vessels in the bone, marrow, periosteum, and surrounding tissue at the time of injury results in the extravasation of blood at the fracture site and the formation of a hematoma. Organization of this hematoma is usually recognized as the first step in fracture repair (Figure 2-2). Loss of the hematoma impairs or slows fracture healing suggesting that the hematoma and an intact surrounding periosteal soft tissue envelope that contains the hematoma may facilitate the initial stages of repair.

Although the volume of the vascular bed of an extremity increases shortly after fracture, presumably because of vasodilation, vascular proliferation also occurs in the region of the fracture. It appears that, under ordinary circumstances, the periosteal vessels contribute the majority of capillary buds early in normal bone healing, with the nutrient medullary artery becoming more important later in the process. Growth factors may be important mediators of the angiogenesis in fracture healing, but the exact stimuli responsible for vascular invasion and endothelial cell proliferation have not been defined.

The bone ends at the fracture site, deprived of their blood supply, become necrotic and are resorbed. In some fractures this may create a radiographically apparent gap at the fracture site several weeks or more after the fracture. The cells responsible for this function, the osteoclasts, come from a different cell line than the cells responsible for bone formation. They are derived from circulating monocytes in the blood and monocytic precursor cells from the bone marrow, whereas the osteoblasts develop from the undifferentiated mesenchymal cells that migrate into the fracture site.

Pluripotential mesenchymal cells, probably of common origin, form fibrous tissue, cartilage, and eventually bone at the fracture site. Some of these cells originate in the injured tissues, while others migrate to the injury site with the blood vessels. Cells from the cambium layer of the periosteum form the earliest bone (Figure 2-1A). Osteoblasts from the endosteal surface also participate in bone formation, but surviving osteocytes do not appear to form repair tissue. The majority of cells responsible for osteogenesis during fracture healing appear in the fracture site with the granulation tissue that replaces the hematoma.

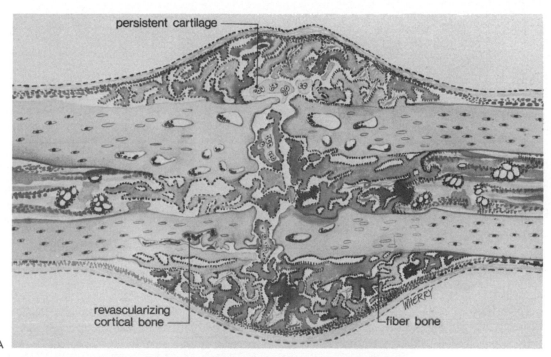

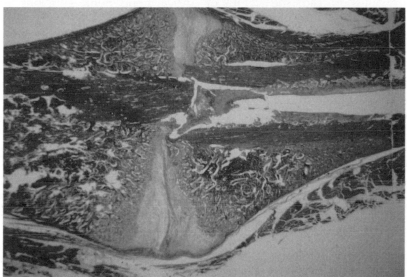

FIGURE 2-3. Progressive fracture healing by fracture callus. **(A)** Drawing showing woven or fiber bone bridging the fracture gap and uniting the fracture fragments. Cartilage remains in the regions most distant from ingrowing capillary buds. In many instances, the capillaries are surrounded by new bone. Vessels revascularize the cortical bone at the fracture site. **(B)** Photomicrograph of a fractured rat femur 21 days after injury showing fracture callus united the fracture fragments. (Reprinted from Clin Ortho Rel Res with permission [5])

The mesenchymal cells at the fracture site proliferate, differentiate, and produce the *fracture callus* consisting of fibrous tissue, cartilage, and woven bone (Figure 2-3). The fracture callus fills and surrounds the fracture site, and in the early stages of healing can be divided into the hard or bony callus and the softer fibrous and cartilaginous callus. The

bone formed initially at the periphery of the callus by intramembranous bone formation is the *hard callus*. The *soft callus* forms in the central regions and consists primarily of cartilage and fibrous tissue. Bone gradually replaces the cartilage through the process of endochondral ossification, enlarging the hard callus and increasing the stability of the fracture

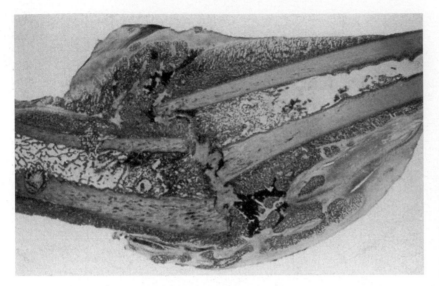

FIGURE 2-4. Light micrograph showing healing of a diaphyseal fracture under conditions of loading and motion. This femur fracture occurred in a pig that continued to use the limb for 3 weeks. Even though the fracture was not stabilized, it is healing. A large fracture callus consisting primarily of woven bone surrounds and unites the two fracture fragments. As the callus matures, it progressively stabilizes the fracture. Notice that the fracture callus contains areas of mineralized and unmineralized cartilage.

fragments (see Figure 2-4). This process continues until new bone bridges the fracture site, reestablishing continuity between the cortical bone ends.

As mineralization of fracture callus proceeds, the bone ends gradually become enveloped in a fusiform mass of callus containing increasing amounts of woven bone. The increasing mineral content is closely associated with increasing stiffness of the fracture callus. Stability of the fracture fragments progressively increases because of the internal and external callus formation, and eventually *clinical union* occurs—that is, the fracture site becomes stable and pain-free. *Radiographic union* occurs when plain radiographs show bone trabeculae or cortical bone crossing the fracture site and often occurs later than clinical union. However, even at this stage healing is not complete. The immature fracture callus is weaker than normal bone, and it only gains full strength during remodeling.

During the final stages of repair, remodeling of the repair tissue begins with replacement of woven bone by lamellar bone and resorption of unneeded callus. Although fracture callus remodeling results from an elaborate sequence of cellular and matrix changes, the important functional result for the patient is an increase in mechanical stability.

Repair and Remodeling of Stabilized Fractures (Primary Bone Healing)

As described above, when motion occurs within certain limits at a fracture site, fracture callus progressively stabilizes the bone fragments, and re-modeling of the fracture callus eventually produces

lamellar bone. However, when the fracture surfaces are rigidly held in contact, fracture healing can occur without grossly visible callus in either cancellous or cortical bone. Some surgeons refer to this type of fracture healing as *primary bone healing*, indicating that it occurs without the formation and replacement of visible fracture callus.

In most fractures that are rigidly stabilized with the bone ends directly apposed, the bone ends are in contact in some regions of the fracture line and other areas where there are small gaps. Where between bone ends contact, lamellar bone can form directly across the fracture line by extension of osteons. A cluster of osteoclasts cuts across the fracture line, osteoblasts following the osteoclasts deposit new bone, and blood vessels follow the osteoblasts. The new bone matrix, enclosed osteocytes, and blood vessels form new haversian systems. Where gaps exist that prevent direct extension of osteons across the fracture site, osteoblasts fill the defects with woven bone. After the gap fills with woven bone, haversian remodeling begins, reestablishing normal cortical bone structure. Cutting cones consisting of osteoclasts followed by osteoblasts and blood vessels traverse the woven bone in the fracture gap, depositing lamellar bone and reestablishing the cortical bone blood supply across the fracture site without grossly visible fracture callus. If a segment of cortical bone is necrotic, gap healing by direct extension of osteons still can occur, but at a slower rate, and areas of necrotic cortical bone remain unremodeled for a prolonged period.

Many impacted epiphyseal, metaphyseal, and vertebral body fractures where cancellous and in some regions cortical bone surfaces interlock have sufficient stability to permit primary bone healing at sites where bone surfaces make direct contact. The same type of cancellous bone healing can occur at osteotomies through metaphyseal bone, rigidly stabilized intra-articular fractures, and surgical arthrodesis treated with rigid stabilization. Most diaphyseal osteotomies, acute diaphyseal fractures of long bones, and unstable metaphyseal fractures require use of devices that compress and rigidly stabilize the fracture site to allow primary healing.

Failure of Fracture Healing

Despite optimal treatment, some fractures heal slowly or fail to heal. It is difficult to set the time when a given fracture should be united, but when healing progresses more slowly than average, the slow progress is referred to as *delayed union*. This indolent fracture healing may be related to the severity of the injury, poor blood supply, the age and nutritional status of the patient, or other factors. Failure of bone healing, or *nonunion*, results from an arrest of the healing process. A nonunion that occurs despite the formation of a large volume of callus around the fracture site is referred to as a *hypertrophic nonunion* (Figure 2-5), in contrast to an *atrophic nonunion* (Figure 2-6) where little or no callus

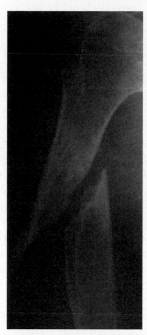

FIGURE 2-6. Atrophic nonunion of a humeral shaft fracture 18 months after fracture. Note the absence of callus.

forms and bone resorption occurs at the fracture site. In some nonunions, cartilaginous tissue forms over the fracture surfaces and the cavity between the surfaces fills with a clear fluid resembling normal joint or bursal fluid creating a *pseudoarthrosis*, or false joint. Pseudoarthroses may or may not be painful, but they almost uniformly remain unstable indefinitely. In other nonunions the gap between the bone ends fills with fibrous or fibrocartilaginous tissue. Occasionally dense fibrous and cartilaginous tissue firmly stabilizes a fracture creating a *fibrous union*. Although fibrous unions may be painless and unite the fracture fragments, they fail to restore the normal strength of the bone.

ARTICULAR CARTILAGE HEALING

Articular cartilage forms the bearing surfaces of synovial joints. It may be injured by mechanical forces that disrupt the articular cartilage alone or the articular cartilage and the underlying bone. Visible disruptions of articular cartilage are referred to as *osteochondral or intra-articular fractures* when they involve both the articular cartilage and subchondral bone; when they involve only the cartilage, they are referred to as *chondral fractures*. In addition to direct mechanical injury, articular cartilage can sustain damage by disruption of the synovial membrane

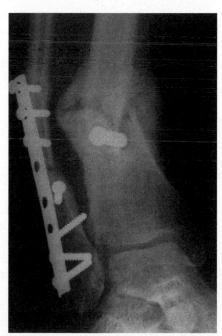

FIGURE 2-5. Hypertrophic delayed union of a distal tibial fracture 5 months after injury. Note the abundant callus but incomplete bridging of the fracture gap.

leading to exposure of the articular cartilage to air. Because of these special features, acute traumatic injuries to synovial joints can be separated into the following categories: disruption of the soft tissues of the synovial joint without direct mechanical cartilage injury and mechanical injury of articular cartilage. Because cartilage lacks blood vessels, it cannot respond to cell damage with inflammation. However, injuries that disrupt subchondral bone as well as the overlying cartilage initiate the fracture healing process, and the repair tissue from bone will fill an articular cartilage defect. Cartilage healing then follows the sequence of inflammation, repair, and remodeling like that seen in bone or dense fibrous tissue. Unlike these tissues, the repair tissue that fills cartilage defects from subchondral bone initially differentiates toward articular cartilage rather than toward dense fibrous tissue or bone.

Healing Following Disruption of Synovial Joint Soft Tissues

Exposure of cartilage to air by disruption of the joint capsule and synovial membrane can alter cartilage matrix composition by stimulating degradation of proteoglycans or suppressing synthesis of proteoglycans. A decrease in matrix proteoglycan concentration decreases cartilage stiffness and may make the tissue more vulnerable to damage from impact loading. Prompt restoration of the synovial environment by closure of the synovial membrane allows chondrocytes to repair the damage to the macromolecular framework of the matrix, and the tissue may regain its normal composition and function. However, prolonged exposure of the articular surface to air can desiccate the tissue and kill chondrocytes.

Healing Following Damage to the Articular Surface

Osteochondral fractures mechanically disrupt cartilage and bone tissue at the fracture site, but in addition, osteochondral fractures may be associated with blunt trauma limited to cartilage, abrasions of the articular surface, or chondral fractures. Alternatively, blunt trauma to a synovial joint may occur without an associated bone or cartilage fracture. Therefore, acute articular cartilage injuries can be separated into those caused by blunt trauma that does not disrupt or fracture tissue and those caused by blunt trauma that mechanically disrupts the tissue. Injuries that fracture or disrupt cartilage can be further divided into those limited to articular cartilage and those affecting both cartilage and subchondral bone.

BLUNT TRAUMA WITHOUT ARTICULAR CARTILAGE DISRUPTION

Acute blunt trauma may damage articular cartilage even when there is no grossly apparent tissue disruption; and these injuries may lead to later degeneration of the articular surface. Physiologic levels of impact loading have not been demonstrated to produce cartilage injury, and clinical experience suggests that acute impact loading considerably greater than physiologic loading, but less than that necessary to produce detectable fractures, rarely causes significant articular cartilage injury. However, acute impact loading less than that necessary to produce visible tissue disruption may cause cartilage swelling and alter the relationships between collagen fibrils and proteoglycans. This observation suggests that blunt trauma may disrupt the macromolecular framework of the cartilage matrix and possibly injure cells without producing detectable fracture of the cartilage or bone. Presumably this tissue damage makes cartilage more vulnerable to subsequent injury and progressive deterioration if the cells do not rapidly restore the matrix. This type of injury may help explain the development of articular cartilage degeneration following joint dislocations or other types of acute joint trauma that do not cause visible damage to the articular surface.

TRAUMA THAT DISRUPTS ARTICULAR CARTILAGE

Injuries Limited to Articular Cartilage

Lacerations, traumatically induced splits of articular cartilage perpendicular to the surface, or chondral fractures kill chondrocytes at the site of the injury and disrupt the matrix. Viable chondrocytes near the injury may proliferate, form clusters of new cells, and synthesize new matrix. They do not migrate to the site of the injury, and the matrix they synthesize does not fill the defect. A hematoma does not form, and inflammatory cells and fibroblasts do not migrate to the site of injury. This minimal response may be due to the inability of chondrocytes to respond effectively to injury, the inability of undifferentiated mesenchymal cells to invade the tissue defect, and the lack of a clot that attracts cells and gives them a temporary matrix to adhere to and replace with more permanent tissue. Although the response of chondrocytes to injury will not heal a clinically significant cartilage defect, most traumatic defects limited to small areas of articular cartilage do not progress.

Osteochondral Injuries

An articular cartilage injury that also damages subchondral bone stimulates bone fracture healing including inflammation, repair, and remodeling. Blood from ruptured bone blood vessels fills the injury site with a hematoma that extends from the bony injury into the chondral defect. The clot may fill a small chondral defect, generally one less than several millimeters wide, but it usually does not completely fill larger defects. Inflammatory cells migrate through the clot followed by fibroblasts that begin to synthesize a collagenous matrix. In the bone defect and the chondral defect some of the mesenchymal cells assume a rounded shape and begin to synthesize a matrix that closely resembles the matrix of articular cartilage.

Within weeks of injury the repair tissue forming in the chondral portion of the defect and the tissue forming in the bony portion of the defect begin to differ. Tissue in the chondral defect has a higher proportion of repair cells and matrix which resemble hyaline cartilage (Figure 2-7), while the repair tissue in the bone defect has started to form new bone. Within 6 weeks of injury repair tissue in the two locations is distinguished by the new bone formed in the bone defect, the absence of bone in the chondral defect, and the higher proportion of hyaline cartilage repair tissue in the chondral defect.

While the initial repair of an osteochondral injury usually follows a predictable course, subsequent changes in the cartilage repair tissue vary considerably among similar defects. In some chondral defects the production of a cartilaginous matrix continues, and the cells may retain the appearance and some of the functions of chondrocytes, including production of type II collagen and proteoglycans. They rarely, if ever, restore the matrix to the original state, but they may succeed in producing fibrocartilaginous tissue that maintains the integrity of the articular surface and provides clinically satisfactory joint function for years. Unfortunately, in many other injuries the cartilage repair tissue deteriorates rather than remodels.

It becomes progressively more fibrillar, and the cells lose the appearance of chondrocytes and appear to become more fibroblastic. The fibrous matrix may begin to fibrillate and fragment, eventually leaving exposed bone (Figure 2-7). The reasons why healing of some osteochondral injuries results in formation of fibrocartilage that may provide at least temporary joint function, while others fail to repair, have not been well defined.

Failure of Articular Cartilage Healing

When the healing response fails to restore a functional articular surface, or the cartilaginous repair tissue deteriorates, the joint loses its ability to provide pain-free motion. It becomes stiff and frequently becomes painful, a condition called posttraumatic osteoarthritis. The risk of posttraumatic osteoarthritis increases with the severity of the joint injury as measured by the degree of disruption of the articular surface and with the age of the patient. Residual joint articular surface incongruity and joint instability increase the risk of degeneration of remaining normal articular cartilage, and thereby increase the risk of posttraumatic osteoarthritis.

DENSE FIBROUS TISSUE HEALING

In general, acute soft tissue injuries can be identified as blunt, tearing, or penetrating injuries or combinations of these types of injury. *Blunt injuries* compress and crush tissue and range from mild contusion to severe crushing. *Tearing injuries* can range from minimal elongation or stretching to rupture, avulsion, or tearing away of tissue. *Penetrating injuries* vary in depth and the extent to which they cleanly lacerate tissue or cause combinations of blunt and tearing injuries. Generally the extent of tissue damage from penetrating injuries can be relatively easily determined. It is more difficult to define the extent of cell and matrix injury from blunt or tearing trauma.

Like bone, the response of vascularized dense fibrous tissue to acute injury includes inflammation, repair, and remodeling, and the repair tissue matrix consists primarily of type I collagen. Although the repair tissue formed following injury to dense fibrous tissue can replace damaged or lost tissue, it rarely duplicates the structure and properties of the uninjured tissue. The specialized forms of dense fibrous tissue follow the same general pattern

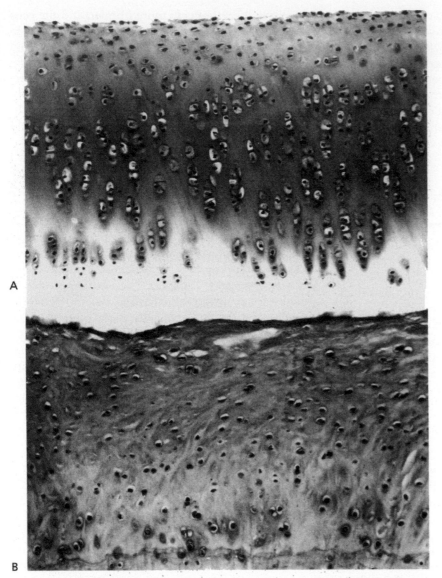

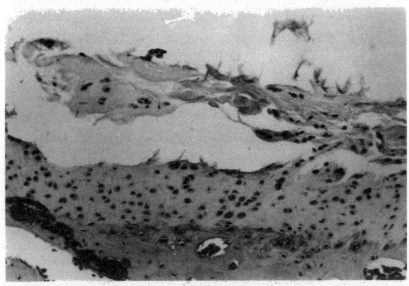

FIGURE 2-7. (A) Normal rabbit articular cartilage showing the homogenous extracellular matrix. The chondrocytes near the articular surface are relatively small and flattened, whereas those in the middle and deeper zones of the articular cartilage have a more spherical shape. **(B)** Well-formed fibrocartilaginous repair cartilage. Notice that the extracellular matrix is more fibrillar and the chondrocytes do not show the same organization as normal articular cartilage. Nonetheless, this repair cartilage does fill the defect in the articular surface. In most instances after osteochondral injury, this type of tissue forms within 6 to 8 weeks. **(C)** Photomicrograph showing fibrillation and fragmentation of fibrocartilaginous repair tissue. Because fibrocartilaginous repair tissue lacks the mechanical properties of normal articular cartilage, it often degenerates over time. (Reprinted from Buckwalter JA, Mow VC. Cartilage repair and osteoarthritis. In: Moskowitz RW, Howell DS, Goldberg VM, et al., eds. Osteoarthritis Diagnosis and Medical/Surgical Management, 2nd Ed. Philadelphia: WB Saunders, 1992:86–87, with permission)

of healing, but because of the differences in their structure and function, tendon, ligament, and joint capsule and meniscus healing present different clinical problems.

Tendon

All three tendon components, tendon substance, tendon insertions, and muscle-tendon junctions, may suffer acute traumatic injuries. Complete disruption of any part of the muscle-tendon unit allows the muscle to retract, increasing the gap at the injury site. If the injury is left untreated, scar tissue may eventually fill the gap between the tendon ends, but it will leave the muscle-tendon unit longer than before injury and may bind the tendon to the surrounding tissues. Without restoration of normal tendon length and gliding, the function of the muscle-tendon unit will be compromised. Furthermore, even when tendons are repaired, gaps at the repair site may prevent healing tendons from gaining strength and stiffness at the same rate as repaired tendons with gaps. The decreased strength increases the risk of tendon rupture. For these reasons restoration of muscle-tendon unit function following a complete disruption usually requires a surgical repair that reestablishes normal muscle-tendon unit length and has sufficient strength to allow immediate motion of the tendon relative to the surrounding tissues.

Injuries to Tendon Substance

The specialized structure of tendons makes it possible for them to transmit the force of muscle contraction to bone, thereby producing joint motion. Some tendons pass through well-defined synovial-lined sheaths and dense fibrous tissue pulleys. Achieving healing of lacerated digital flexor tendons within these tendon sheaths while preserving the pulleys and the tendon motion presents a unique problem in the treatment of musculoskeletal injuries. The cut tendon ends can be sutured and will heal, but if the repair tissue scars the tendon to the sheath or the pulleys, tendon motion will be restricted and may cause joint contracture. Tendons without sheaths do not usually present this problem because scarring of their repair tissue to surrounding loose areolar tissue often will not severely restrict motion.

Tendon healing begins with inflammatory cell and fibroblast migration into the site of injury.

Granulation tissue proliferates around the injury site and between the ends of the sutured tendons and deposits randomly-oriented collagen fibrils (Figure 2-8). The density of fibroblasts increases up to 3 weeks after injury when granulation tissue fills and surrounds the repaired area. If the tendon has been sutured, the suture material holds the tendon ends together until the fibroblasts have produced sufficient collagen to form a "tendon callus." The tensile strength of the repaired tendon depends on the collagen concentration and the orientation of the collagen fibrils. The collagen fibrils become longitudinally oriented by about 4 weeks, and during the next 2 to 3 months the repair tissue remodels until it resembles normal tendon (Figure 2-8). The amount and density of the scar tissue adhesions between the tendon injury site and surrounding tissues depend on the intensity, extent, and duration of the inflammatory and repair phases of healing and the mobility of the tendon during repair.

Early controlled mobilization of a repaired tendon can reduce scar adhesions between the tendon injury site and the surrounding tissue and facilitate healing, but excessive loading may disrupt the repair tissue and create gaps at tendon repair sites. Thus, optimal tendon healing depends on surgical apposition and mechanical stabilization of the tendon ends without excessive soft tissue damage and on creating the optimal mechanical environment for healing. This mechanical environment includes sufficient tendon mobility to prevent adhesions and sufficient loading to stimulate remodeling of the repair tissue matrix along the lines of stress, but loads applied to the tendon must not exceed the strength of the surgical repair.

Injuries to Tendon Insertions

Disruption of tendon insertions into bone often involves a fracture or avulsion of a bone fragment at the site of injury. These injuries usually can be treated by surgically reducing and stabilizing the fracture or reinserting the tendon into the bone and stabilizing the insertion. Healing occurs either by bony union or by union of the bone to the tendon substance.

Injuries to Muscle-Tendon Junctions

Partial muscle-tendon junction injuries usually will heal successfully if further injury can be prevented, but complete or nearly complete avulsions or tears

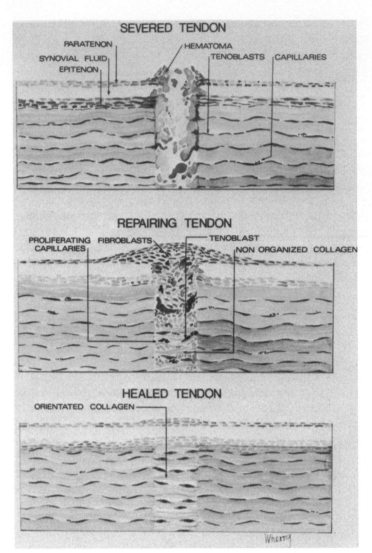

FIGURE 2-8. The sequence of events following a tendon laceration. A hematoma forms between the tendon ends. Inflammatory cells, undifferentiated mesenchymal cells, fibroblasts and blood vessels grow into the gap between the tendon ends. The fibroblasts repair the tendon defect by proliferating and synthesizing a new matrix. This repair tissue remodels until it closely resembles the uninjured tendon tissue.

can present difficult problems because attempts to suture muscle tissue consisting primarily of muscle cells to tendon is unlikely to restore the structure and function of the muscle-tendon junction. Optimal healing of these injuries depends on approximation of the avulsed tendon and any remnants of the tendon remaining attached to the muscle or, when available, muscle fascia. Although it may appear that muscles attach to tendons over a small area, in many muscles thin extensions of their tendons penetrate long distances within the muscle bellies. Identification of these thin bands of tendon within muscle may make it possible to suture them to an avulsed or partially avulsed tendon in the proximal and distal thirds of many muscles and as far as the middle third of some muscles.

LIGAMENT AND JOINT CAPSULE

Ligament and joint capsule substance healing follows the sequence described for healing of tendon substance by extrinsic cells (Figure 2-8). Also, as in tendon healing, early motion and loading of injured ligaments can stimulate healing. Because controlled normal motion of a joint does not necessarily cause large forces in the ligaments and joint capsule, limited joint motion will not necessarily disrupt the repair of the tissue.

If ligament or capsular tears heal with a significant gap or fail to heal, the resultant joint instability may increase the probability of subsequent joint injury and degenerative joint disease. For this reason, restoration or maintenance of near-normal ligament and capsule length and maintenance of normal joint motion should be the objectives of treatment. The most favorable condition for healing divided ligaments and joint capsules is direct apposition of the divided surfaces. Apposition and stabilization of the injury site decreases the volume of repair tissue required to heal the injury, minimizes scarring, and may help provide near-normal tissue length. A sutured ligament can heal with a minimal gap. When tested under tension, sutured ligaments are stronger than those that heal with a significant length of scar tissue, and ligaments that heal with a gap between the cut ends may have a decreased ability to stabilize the adjacent joint. However, many ligament and joint capsule tears heal without surgical repair and function as well or better than surgically repaired ligaments and capsules if the torn ends do not retract and the tear occurs through tissue with an adequate blood supply.

Meniscus

The response of meniscal tissue to tears depends on whether the tear occurs through a vascular or an avascular portion of the meniscus. The vascular regions respond to injury like other vascularized dense fibrous tissues. This response can heal a meniscal injury and restore the tissue structure and function if the torn edges remain apposed and if the repair tissue is not disrupted in the early stages of healing. Providing these conditions frequently requires surgical repair of meniscal tears or tears of meniscal attachments. The avascular regions of meniscal tissue, like articular cartilage, do not repair significant tissue defects. Cells in the region of the injury, like chondrocytes in the region of the injury limited to articular cartilage, may proliferate and synthesize new matrix but there is no evidence that the cells migrate into the defect site or produce new matrix that can fill the defect site.

Failure of Dense Fibrous Tissue Healing

Injuries to tendons, ligaments, joint capsules, and menisci may fail to heal despite treatment. Instead of a firm scar aligned along the lines of stress, the injury site contains filmy loose connective tissue, myxoid tissue, or granulation tissue. The reasons for failure of healing are unclear in some instances, but identifiable causes include a large gap at the injury site, extensive damage to the surrounding tissue including loss of vascular supply, excessive

early loading and motion of the repair tissue, and injury-related necrosis of the tissue. Surgical treatment may also contribute to poor healing. Extensive dissection can devascularize traumatized tissue, and inappropriate suture technique may also damage the blood supply to the injury site or place excessive tension on a sutured tissue.

SKELETAL MUSCLE HEALING

The same mechanisms of acute trauma that damage dense fibrous tissue structures (i.e., blunt trauma, lacerations, and tearing injuries) also injure muscle.

Types of Muscle Tissue Injury

Acute muscle injuries can be grouped into three types that differ in their potential for healing based on the components of the muscle left intact (Table 2-1).

A *type I muscle injury* damages muscle fibers but leaves the extracellular matrix, blood vessels, and nerve supply intact. Blunt trauma, including surgical trauma, mild stretching injuries, and temporary ischemia can cause a type I injury. The muscle fibers will be damaged but the basal lamina and other components of the extracellular matrix, the blood supply, and the nerve supply remain intact. These injuries occur frequently and can heal through spontaneous muscle fiber regeneration that restores the original structure, composition, and function of the muscle.

A *type II muscle injury* damages the nerve supply and may include damage to the myofibers, but leaves the extracellular matrix and blood supply intact. Type II injuries may result from isolated peripheral nerve damage, blunt trauma, or stretching of nerve and muscle. Because the matrix maintains the muscle structure, if regenerating nerve fibers reach intact neuromuscular junctions, the potential for restoration of function exists.

A *type III muscle injury* causes loss or necrosis of all muscle tissue components, including myofibers and extracellular matrix and/or prolonged loss of blood and nerve supply. Type III injuries result from severe blunt trauma, tearing, or penetrating trauma. If the vascular supply remains intact, the inflammatory response can remove the necrotic tissue, but some type III injuries compromise the blood supply, and the necrotic muscle is not removed and must be surgically debrided. If the necrotic tissue is removed, repair can begin. Cells capable of differentiating into

TABLE 2-1.
Acute Skeletal Muscle Injuries

Injury Type	Description	Tissue Response	Potential for Healing
I	Damage to muscle fibers without significant disruption of their extracellular matrix, blood vessels and nerves. (These injuries result from blunt trauma, including surgical trauma, mild stretching injuries, and temporary ischemia.)	Organized muscle fiber regeneration Formation of fibrous tissue after an inflammatory response	A significant inflammatory response may lead to some scar formation, but most of these injuries result in normal structure and function.
II	Damage to nerves that leaves the muscle extracellular matrix and blood supply intact but may include damage to the myofibers. (These injuries may result from isolated peripheral nerve damage, blunt trauma, or stretching of nerve and muscle.)	Organized nerve fiber and muscle fiber regeneration Formation of fibrous tissue after an inflammatory response	If regenerating nerve fibers reach intact neuromuscular junctions, the potential for restoration of function exists.
III	Loss or necrosis of all muscle tissue components, including myofibers and extracellular matrix. (These injuries result from prolonged ischemia and loss of innervation and from severe blunt trauma, tearing, or penetrating trauma.)	Disorganized muscle fiber regeneration Formation of fibrous tissue	Scar formation with scattered myoblasts result in loss of function in the injured region. The scar may allow function of adjacent intact or less severely injured muscle.

Data from Caplan A, Carlson B, Faulkner J. et al. Skeletal muscle. In: Woo SL-Y, Buckwalter JA, eds. Injury and Repair of the Musculoskeletal Soft Tissues. *Park Ridge, Illinois: American Academy of Orthopaedic Surgeons, 1988:213–291; and Carlson BM, Faulkner JA. The regeneration of skeletal muscle fibers following injury: a review* Med Sci Sports Excer *1983; 15:187–198, with permission.*

myoblasts survive even severe injuries or migrate into the injury site. However, the lack of an extracellular matrix to guide regeneration of myofibers usually prevents formation of organized muscle tissue. Even if such tissue forms, lack of guidance for reinnervation prevents regenerated myofibers from regaining function. For these reasons, the usual result of a type III muscle injury is healing by scar formation with scattered myoblasts attempting to form myofibers.

Blunt trauma to skeletal muscle occurs frequently as an isolated injury or in association with fractures. The results vary from type I to type III muscle injuries. Mild blunt trauma to skeletal muscle damages myofibers without disruption of extracellular matrix, nerves, or vessels—a type I muscle tissue injury. A slightly more severe injury ruptures blood vessels as well as myofibers, causing hemorrhage and inflammation. Healing of these injuries generally results in restoration of normal function. At the other extreme, blunt trauma can crush all components of skeletal muscle resulting in a type III muscle tissue injury that heals with scar tissue or that may not heal. If the area of the crushing injury is relatively small, muscle function may not be noticeably altered. However, following an extensive crushing injury, the cells replace large areas of the muscle with

noncontractile regenerating myofibers and scar, permanently decreasing muscle strength.

Most penetrating injuries of muscle result from lacerations or combinations of blunt trauma and lacerations. Because lacerations necessarily damage myofibrils, extracellular matrix, nerves, and blood vessels, they are type III tissue injuries. Following complete laceration and suture repair the separated muscle fragments heal primarily by scar, with a small number of regenerated myotubes within the scar. True regeneration of functional muscle tissue and nerves across complete lacerations has not been demonstrated, and muscle fragments separated from their nerve supply show the changes of denervation. Transected myofibers may form buds, but these buds fail to restore normal tissue across the laceration.

Muscle healing, like healing of the other vascularized tissues, proceeds through inflammation, repair, and remodeling.

Inflammation

Damage to myofibers initiates inflammation, which includes migration of inflammatory cells into the injured muscle and, in most injuries, hemorrhage and formation of a hematoma. In addition to hematoma formation, and the other events seen following injury to vascularized tissues, an important part of the inflammatory process in skeletal muscle is the removal of damaged muscle fibers by phagocytic inflammatory cells that penetrate and fragment necrotic myofibers. After they enter damaged muscle fibers, these cells phagocytize bundles of contractile filaments and other cytoplasmic debris. This macrophage activity not only removes damaged cell organelles, it may have an important role in stimulating regeneration of myofibers.

Repair

As macrophages remove damaged or necrotic myofibers, spindle-shaped myogenic cells appear and begin to proliferate and fuse with one another to form long syncytial myotubes with chains of central nuclei. Frequently, several of these early regenerating myotubes form within the basement membrane tube of a single necrotic muscle fiber. As they enlarge, the myotubes construct their sarcoplasmic reticulum and begin to assemble organized bundles of contractile filaments. The central chains of nuclei break up and migrate to the periphery of the myotube, completing the transition of the myotube into a muscle fiber. Contractile proteins continue to accumulate and form myofibrils. To become functional, a regenerating muscle fiber must be innervated, including formation of a neuromuscular junction.

At the same time myotubes are regenerating, fibroblasts are producing granulation tissue necessary to repair the matrix of the muscle. However, this granulation tissue can interfere with the orderly regeneration of the myofibers producing a disorganized mass of scar and partially regenerated myofibers. This type of tissue may restore the continuity of the muscle, but not its contractile function. Therefore, the optimal results of muscle healing require a balance between myofiber regeneration and synthesis of new matrix and appropriate organization and orientation of these two components of the healing muscle.

Remodeling

Once muscle fibers have appeared, the extracellular matrix continues to remodel. If excessive scar formation can be avoided and the muscle cells are innervated, controlled muscle contraction and loading increases the strength of the injured muscle.

Failure of Skeletal Muscle Healing

Muscle trauma that destroys myofibers and their extracellular matrix heals with scar. In some instances, the scar joins remaining intact muscle to either tendon or adjacent intact muscle. If the remaining muscle hypertrophies it can restore at least some normal function. Blunt trauma to muscle may also stimulate bone formation, myositis ossificans. The new bone can be contiguous with periosteum or lie entirely within muscle, free of any connection with underlying bone. Extensive myositis ossificans may weaken the muscle and restrict joint motion.

SUMMARY

The primary tissues that form bones and joints and bone and articular cartilage differ in their composition, structure, and capacity for healing. Bone fractures initiate a response that begins with inflammation (the cellular and vascular response to injury), proceeds through repair (the replacement of damaged or lost cells and matrices with new cells and matrices), and ends with remodeling (removal, replacement, and reorganization of the repair tissue, usually along the lines of mechanical stress). Injury to articular cartilage does not trigger an inflammatory response, but the cells respond to injury with an effort at cell proliferation and synthesis of new matrix. This effort rarely, if ever, restores a normal articular surface. When injuries extend through articular cartilage into bone, the repair tissue that forms in the bone extends into the region of the chondral injury and produces a fibrocartilaginous tissue that in some instances restores a functional articular surface. The principles of treating acute bone and joint injuries include preventing further tissue damage, avoiding treatments that compromise the natural healing process, and creating the optimal mechanical and biological conditions for healing. This treatment may include removing necrotic tissue, preventing infection, rapidly restoring blood and nerve supply when necessary, and in some circumstances providing apposition, alignment, and stabilization of injured tissue. The ideal result of healing—restoration of the original structure, function, and composition of the tissue—may occur following certain dense fibrous tissue injuries and some skeletal muscle injuries. Achieving ideal results is most likely to occur following fibrous tissue injuries in tissues with an excellent blood supply and injuries that do not cause segmental tissue loss. Following type I and type II injuries, skeletal muscle can regain normal structure and function. Dense fibrous tissue injuries that lead to segmental tissue loss and type III muscle injuries heal by formation of scar consisting primarily of a dense collagenous matrix containing primarily type I collagen and fibroblasts. Scar tissue may restore clinically acceptable function of injured tissue, especially in some tendon and ligament injuries and lacerations of skeletal muscle. As with bone and joint injuries, the principles of treating acute musculoskeletal soft tissue injuries include preventing further tissue damage, avoiding treatments that compromise the natural healing process, and creating the optimal mechanical and biological conditions for healing. Treatment includes removing necrotic tissue, preventing infection, rapidly restoring blood and nerve supply when necessary, and in some circumstances providing apposition, alignment, and stabilization of injured tissue. Early controlled loading and motion of the repair and remodeling tissues improves healing of many injuries, but uncontrolled

or excessive loading can adversely affect or even prevent healing.

Annotated Bibliography

Buckwalter JA. Tendon, Ligament, Meniscus and Skeletal Muscle Healing. In: Green DP, Bucholz RW, Heckman JD, eds. Fractures. 5th Ed. Philadelphia: JB Lippincott, 2001:273–284.
This book chapter reviews in detail the healing of tendon, ligament, meniscus, and skeletal muscle.

Buckwalter JA, Einhorn TA, Marsh JL. Bone and Joint Healing. In: Green DP, Bucholz RW, Heckman JD, eds. Fractures. 5th Ed. Philadelphia: JB Lippincott, 2001:245–271.
This book chapter reviews bone healing in detail.

Day SM, Ostrum RF, Chao EYS, Rubin CT, Aro HT, Einhorn TA. Bone Injury, Regeneration and Repair. In: Buckwalter JA, Einhorn T, Simon S, eds. Orthopaedic Basic Science—The Biology and Biomechanics of the Musculoskeletal System. Rosemont, IL: American Academy of Orthopaedic Surgeons, 2000:371–400.
This book chapter discusses bone regeneration and repair.

Woo SL-Y, Buckwalter JA, eds. Injury and Repair of the Musculoskeletal Soft Tissues. Park Ridge, IL: American Academy of Orthopaedic Surgeons, 1988.
This book reviews the structure, composition, function, and response to injury of the musculoskeletal soft tissues: tendon, ligament, tendon and ligament insertions into bone, muscle-tendon junctions, skeletal muscle, peripheral nerve, peripheral blood vessel, articular cartilage, and meniscus.

3

Kenton R. Kaufman

Gait Analysis

Human locomotion is a complex task. Because of inherent differences in anatomical structure, motor control patterns, and pathological or chronological changes, each person's gait pattern is unique. However, because everyone has the same basic anatomic and physiological makeup, human locomotion occurs in a similar manner for everyone. The cyclical and highly automated movement pattern during human locomotion involves rhythmic, alternating motions of the trunk and extremities. This movement pattern provides a unique characteristic of limb movement that can be studied with a high degree of accuracy. This specific branch of biomechanics is defined as gait analysis—a quantitative description of human locomotion.

Human motion analysis has widespread applications spanning many disciplines. In the field of medicine, motion analysis studies are fundamental to understanding the mechanics of normal and pathological movement. This information is useful for the diagnosis and treatment of patients with motor deficiencies. Others in the field of medicine use human models for the development of functional electrical stimulation protocols to restore mobility to paralyzed individuals. Sports medicine physicians also use motion analysis to test strategies for optimizing various sports movements. Clearly motion analysis techniques have widespread applications in medicine.

Motion analysis laboratories provide quantitative information that can be used as a basis for appropriate therapeutic intervention, as well as to objectively evaluate the effectiveness and efficacy of treatment methods. Clinical gait analysis is used to quantify the mechanics of walking and to identify deviations in normal movement. The causes of abnormal movement can then be distinguished from compensations in order to provide appropriate treatment recommendations. The ability to objectively quantify movement patterns is critical for prescribing specific treatment modalities. The focus of this chapter is on the methods for objective assessment of human movement. This chapter discusses available measurement technology and application of this technology for clinical treatment planning and assessment.

HISTORICAL PERSPECTIVE

The concept of depicting and recording human motion began during the Renaissance period. Giovanni Alfonso Borelli, a student of Galileo, was among the first scientists to analyze motion while developing his theory of muscle action based on mechanical principles. The quantitative study of human locomotion began in the nineteenth century. Duchenne conducted the first scientific systematic evaluation of muscle function. His findings were published in the monumental work, *Physiologie des Mouvements*, published in 1867. Leland Stanford, governor of California and horse breeder, hired Eadweard Muybridge in 1872 to determine whether a trotting horse had all four feet off the ground at any instant in time. Muybridge placed cameras at regular intervals along a race track. Thin threads stretched across the track triggered the shutters. The horse's hooves triggered cameras in order, and a series of photographs clearly depicted the gait sequence. Muybridge subsequently compiled a detailed photographic expose of human and animal locomotion, which was published in three volumes (original work published in 1887).

At the turn of the twentieth century in Germany, Braune and Fischer (1895) became interested in measuring the motion of human body segments. They placed Geissler tubes, containing a rarified nitrogen gas, on various limb segments of a human subject dressed in black. Electrical circuits connected to the tubes created incandescence, and cameras recorded the illuminated tubes as the subject walked. Experiments were carried out at night because there was no means to darken the room in which studies were performed. It took 10 to 12 hours to put this apparatus on the subject, whereas data collection was completed in minutes using four cameras. The images were digitized using a precision optical device. Coordinate geometry was used to extract three-dimensional coordinates. Equations needed to calculate resultant forces and moments at the joints of a 12-segment rigid body model were formulated. Their quantitative results were published in 1895 and are still valid today.

Inman and colleagues combined rudimentary motion recordings with electromyography (EMG) in the mid-1900s. Their pioneering work in limb prosthetic research laid the foundation for modern gait analysis. Their accumulated experience was published in 1981 as a textbook, *Human Walking,* which represents the seminal textbook in the field.

Since this pioneering work, much effort has been put into developing the needed technology for human movement analysis. Automated movement tracking systems have replaced hand digitization. Advances in the aerospace industry have been utilized for the development of force plates for kinetic analysis. Computerized electromyography systems have replaced hand palpation. Currently, the technology and knowledge for gait analysis has advanced to a level that permits rapid analysis. Gait analysis laboratories now exist in many different centers, and gait analysis is used for orthopedic surgery, clinical rehabilitation, sports medicine, and industrial ergonomics.

EQUIPMENT AND METHODS

Observation

The simplest form of gait analysis is observational gait analysis. A systematic approach for observational gait analysis was developed at the Rancho Los Amigos Medical Center in Downey, California. An experienced observer can detect many gait deviations during both stance and swing phases. However, an obvious limitation of observation in gait analysis is the difficulty of observing multiple events and multiple body segments interacting concurrently. Further, it is not possible to visualize the location of force vectors in space or electromyographic activity of muscles. Events happening faster than $\frac{1}{12}$ of a second (83 ms) cannot be perceived by the human eye. More consistent observations are obtained when motion videotapes are reviewed in slow motion. Three expert observers rated video footage of 15 children who had lower limb disability and wore braces. Pearson's correlation coefficient was 0.6 within observers and less between observers. Thus, observational gait analysis is a convenient, but only moderately reliable technique. Saleh and Murdoch (1985) utilized experienced observers to study the gait of transtibial amputees. The prosthetic limbs of the amputees were intentionally misaligned in the sagittal plane. The agreement of experienced observers with a biomechanical model was 22%. In a similar study, 54 licensed physical therapists with varying amounts of clinical experience rated three patients with rheumatoid arthritis. Generalized Kappa coefficients ranged from 0.11 to 0.52 indicating that clinician assessments are only slightly to moderately reliable. Thus, it is easy to see that limitations in observational gait analysis can lead to misinterpretation of the patient's locomotion capabilities. Hence, it is important to utilize advances in gait analysis techniques to more precisely quantify the patient's functional status. Extensive instrumentation has been developed for recording the various parameters used to describe gait.

Movement Measurement

In the biomechanical analysis of motion, skeletal segments are studied as rigid links moving through space. These rigid links are assumed to be interconnected through a series of frictionless joints. Measurement systems that are aimed at capturing the spatial trajectories of body segments usually involve a camera system or an electromagnetic system that tracks a series of body-fixed markers.

External markers are used to define orthogonal coordinate systems affixed to each body segment, whose axes define the position of these body segments. With a camera-based system, either passively reflective or actively illuminated markers are used (Figure 3-1A). These markers are commonly attached to the subjects as either discrete points or rigid clusters with multiple markers on each cluster. Placement of these external markers on the surface of the body segments are aligned with particular bony landmarks. As the patient walks along a marked walkway, the cameras track and record the marker trajectories. Using stereophotogrammetric principles, the planar projections of markers viewed by each camera are used to reconstruct the three-dimensional instantaneous position of the markers relative to an inertially fixed laboratory coordinate

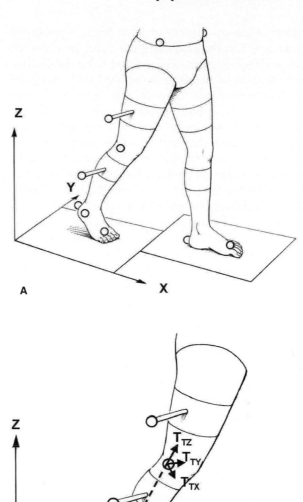

FIGURE 3-1. Body-fixed reflective markers used for establishing anatomical coordinate systems. **(A)** Video camera motion measurement systems calculate the location of external markers placed on the body segments and aligned with specific bony landmarks. **(B)** A body-fixed external coordinate system is then computed from three or more markers on each body segment. **(C)** Subsequently, a subject calibration relates the external coordinate system with an anatomical coordinate system through the identification of anatomical landmarks, for example, the medial and lateral femoral condyles and medial lateral malleoli. *continued*

system. If the position of at least three noncolinear points fixed to the body segment can be obtained (and the body segment is assumed to be rigid), then the 6 degrees of freedom associated with the position and orientation of each segment can be obtained. Initially, a body-fixed coordinate system is computed for each body segment (Figure 3-1B). For instance, consider the markers on the shank at an instant in time. A vector, S_{TZ}, can be formed from the lateral malleolus (B) to the lateral knee marker (A). Another vector can be formed from the lateral malleolus to the marker on the shank wand (C). The vector cross-product of these two vectors is a vector S_{TX}, which is perpendicular to the plane containing all three markers. The unit vector, S_{TY}, may be determined as the vector cross-product of S_{TZ} and S_{TX}. Thus, the vectors S_{TX}, S_{TY}, and S_{TZ} form an orthogonal body fixed coordinate system, called a technical coordinate system. In a similar manner, the marker based or technical coordinate system may be calculated for the thigh, that is, T_{TX}, T_{TY}, and T_{TZ}. These segments are linked and thus lack independence of movement. Hence, their points of attachment, that is, the joints, are the points of principal kinematic significance. Once the position of adjacent limb segments has been determined, it is possible to determine the relative angle between adjacent limb segments in three dimensions. This assumes that the technical coordinate systems reasonably approximate the anatomical axes of the body segments, for example, T_{TZ} approximates along axis of the thigh and S_{TZ} approximates along the axis of the shank. A more rigorous approach adapts a subject calibration procedure to relate the technical coordinate systems with pertinent anatomical landmarks. Additional data can be collected that relates the technical coordinate system to the underlying anatomical coordinate system. The subject calibration is performed as a static trial with the subject standing. Additional markers are typically added to the medial femoral condyle and the medial malleolli during the static calibration trial. These markers serve as anatomical references for the knee axis and ankle axis. The hip center location is estimated from markers placed on the pelvis. The technical coordinate system is then transformed into alignment with the anatomical coordinate system for each limb segment, for example, S_{AX}, S_{AY}, S_{AZ} (Figure 3-1C). The marker system is coupled to a biomechanical model. Once the position of adjacent limb segments has been determined (and each body segment is assumed to be rigid), it is possible to determine the relative angles between adjacent limb segments in

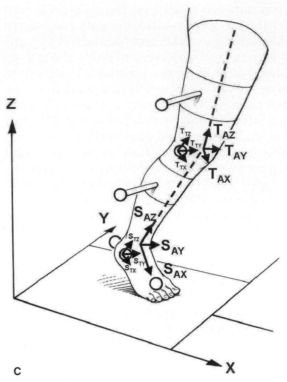

c

FIGURE 3-1C. *(Continued)*

three dimensions. Motion measurements are made in reference to the joint centers. The Euler/Cardan system is the most commonly used method for describing three-dimensional motion (Figure 3-2). It describes angular motion as a sequence of ordered

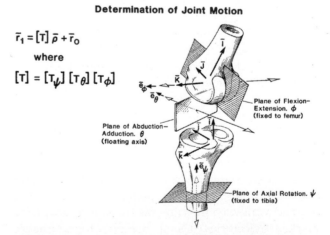

Determination of Joint Motion

$$\bar{r}_1 = [T]\,\bar{p} + \bar{r}_0$$

where

$$[T] = [T_\psi]\,[T_\theta]\,[T_\phi]$$

FIGURE 3-2. Description of knee joint motion using Eulerian angle system. An axis fixed to the distal femur defines flexion–extension motion, Φ. An axis fixed to proximal tibia along its anatomical axis defines internal–external rotation, Ψ. A floating axis is orthogonal to the other two axes and used to measure abduction-adduction, Θ. (Reproduced with permission from Chao, 1980)

rotations about the axes of the Cartesian coordinate system. Although the rotations are sequence dependent, the Cardan angle description defines relative joint motion in a manner that is physically meaningful and clinically relevant.

Recently, advances have been made in the animation industry that will have future applications in the biomechanics field. Computerized motion analysis systems have been developed that provide marker trajectory data in real time. These systems are now available for applications in biomechanics. These applications make it possible to obtain results of gait analysis studies much faster and will make gait analysis much more clinically available.

Another recent development to be used for quantifying human motion is an electromagnetic tracking system. Electromagnetic systems detect the motion of sensors placed on each segment using an electromagnetic field. A three-axis magnet dipole source and a three-axis magnetic sensor are used (Figure 3-3). The excitation of the source and the resulting sensor output are represented as vectors. The source excitation pattern is composed of three sequential excitation states, each of which produces an excitation vector that is linearly independent of the other two. The sensor is connected to a system controller through a cable. The sensor outputs are pre-amplified, multiplexed, and transmitted to a system electronics unit. The resultant set of three sensor output vectors contains information sufficient to determine both the position and orientation of the sensor relative to the source. Thus, these systems can provide real-time 6 degree-of-freedom movement data. The use of this equipment is growing in areas of human motion analysis. The instrumentation is simple to use and is insensitive to limb interference. The limitations are the sampling frequency and the sensitivity to magnetic interference from nearby ferromagnetic metallic structures such as a total joint replacement. Nonetheless, as these electromagnetic system capabilities increase, it is expected that these devices will be used more frequently for movement analysis.

Force Measurement

Gait analysis is also concerned with the forces that cause the observed movement and the assessment of their effect on locomotion (kinetic analysis). Kinetics is the branch of mechanics focusing on the forces and moments transmitted across the joints of the body. Forces acting on the human body can be divided into internal and external forces. The external forces represent all physical interactions between

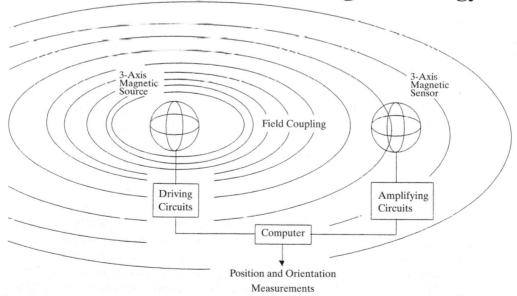

Electromagnetic Tracking Technology

FIGURE 3-3. System block diagram of an electromagnetic tracking system. The 3-axis magnetic source emits three sequential excitation states that are picked up by the 3-axis magnetic sensor. The resultant set of sensor excitation vectors is used to calculate the position and orientation of the sensor relative to the source.

the body and the environment. These forces include gravitational, ground reaction forces, and inertial forces. The internal forces are those transmitted by body tissues that include muscular forces, ligament forces, and forces transmitted through joint contact.

While the motion capture system records the body segment movements, force plates simultaneously measure the force generated by the interaction of the foot with the ground. This resultant force is referred to as the ground reaction force (GRF). Current force plates typically use strain gauge or piezoelectric transducers. These devices are embedded in the walkway of the laboratory and measure the magnitude and direction of the resultant GRF applied to the foot by the ground (Figure 3-4). The GRF vector is three dimensional and consists of a vertical component plus two shear components acting along the force plate surface. The shear forces are applied parallel to the ground and require friction. These shear forces are usually resolved in the anterior-posterior and medial-lateral directions. An additional variable, the center of pressure, is needed to define the location of this GRF vector. The center of pressure is defined as the point about which the distributed force has zero moment when applied to the foot. It is found by determining the line of action of the forces measured by the platform and calculating where that line intersects the surface of the force platform.

This force data is combined with kinematic data using Newton's second law to calculate the intersegmental forces and moments causing motion

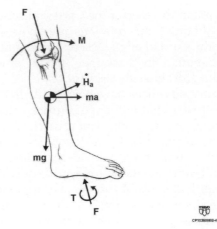

FIGURE 3-5. The joint dynamics, which include the intersegmental forces and moments, are computed through the use of Newtonian mechanics. The computation accounts for the external loads applied at the foot, for example, the ground reaction forces, F and T, the weight of the limb segment, mg, and the inertial loads, ma and H_a, in order to calculate the intersegmental force, F, and moment, M.

(Figure 3-5). The process of proceeding from known kinematic data and external forces to obtain intersegmental joint forces and moments is called the inverse dynamics approach. The gravitational forces acting on each body segment are determined from the relevant mass and location of the center of mass for each segment. These quantities are calculated along with the segmental mass moments of inertia using prediction techniques from anthropometric dimensions. The inertial forces are obtained from calculations of angular and linear position, as well as velocity and acceleration of the body segments with respect to either a fixed laboratory coordinate system or referenced to another body segment using kinematic data. This information is then combined to solve the inverse dynamics problem (Figure 3-6). Joint power may also be calculated. This data provides an understanding of the subtle musculoskeletal adaptations, which are utilized by patients to maintain dynamic balance during gait. Kinetic data is available at the hip, knee, and ankle joint. When the position of this force line with respect to joint center has been established by combining force and movement data, the extrinsic joint moment, which is the product of lever arm and the ground reaction force, plus gravity and inertia is calculated. This moment is of great importance because the lower extremity muscles act during load bearing. Thus, the external moment defines the requirements for intrinsic (muscle) force. For example, when the force line falls behind the knee joint center, quadriceps muscle

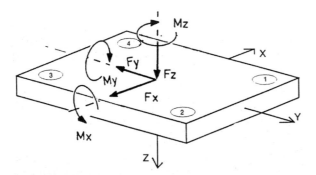

FIGURE 3-4. A force plate is used to measure the location and magnitude of the ground reaction force. Transducers are located in the four corners of the plate. The ground reaction force is divided into three force (F_x, F_y, F_z) and three moment (M_x, M_y, M_z) components. F_x and F_y are shear forces. F_z is the vertical force. Some force plates only measure the moment around the vertical axis, that is, M_z. This assumes that no tensile forces are imposed on the force plate; that is, the foot does not stick to the plate. Under this assumption, the other moments are zero.

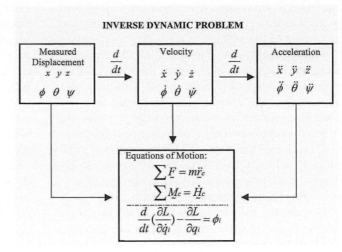

INVERSE DYNAMIC PROBLEM

FIGURE 3-6. Solution process for inverse dynamics problem. Displacement information must be differentiated twice to yield acceleration. Either Newtonian or Lagranian formulations can be used to formulate the equations of motion.

action is required to prevent knee collapse, and when the force line falls in front of the knee, extensor muscle force is not needed. When surgical intervention or nonsurgical treatment such as an orthoses is prescribed for a patient, the kinetic parameters offer insight into the treatment effectiveness.

At each joint, a state of equilibrium exists where the external joint forces are balanced by the internal joint forces. The measurement of internal forces requires sophisticated techniques that are invasive. Analytical procedures have been developed for estimating internal joint forces. These analytical approaches use classical mechanics and mathematical optimization routines. These analytical approaches require the use of simplifying assumptions about the mechanical structure and knowledge of muscle physiology principles. Thus, the accuracy of the analytical predictions depends not only on the quality of the input data but also on the validity of the assumptions. In general, it is necessary to evaluate the estimated quantities by comparing them with experimental observations. Typically, electromyographic data is obtained to provide information regarding muscle activation patterns.

Electromyography

Electromyography (EMG) is the recording of electrical activity during muscle contraction. Neuromuscular coordination is required to adjust the varying muscular and ligamentous forces interacting with the abundant degrees of freedom in the joints and other parts of passive locomotive system to obtain dynamic balance during gait. Electromyographic

data is useful to provide information about the timing of muscle activity and the relative intensity of muscle contraction. Both surface and fine-wire electrodes have been used for gait kinesiologica EMG. Each type of electrode has its advantages and disadvantages. Surface electrodes are convenient, easy to apply to the skin, and do not cause irritation or discomfort to the subject. However, they pick up signals from other active muscles in the general area of application. This feature makes surface electrodes the ideal choice for analysis of global activity in superficial muscles or muscle groups. In addition, surface electrodes are sensitive to movement of the skin under the electrodes and have poor specificity. They are influenced by significant muscle "cross-talk," in which the electrode signals of one muscle interfere with the signals from another. Thus, the activity of adjacent muscle groups can interfere and lead to false results. However, a double differential technique has been shown to reduce cross-talk in surface EMGs. The major advantage of fine-wire electrodes is selectivity to measure the activity of specific muscles. The influence of electrical activity of nearby muscles is greatly reduced. Nonetheless, a number of disadvantages are associated with fine-wire electrodes. Patient discomfort on insertion, the difficulty of accurate placement, wire movement with muscle contraction, and the need for licensure to utilize wire electrodes are some of the drawbacks. Electrical stimuli is usually given to confirm the accuracy of fine-wire placement. Furthermore, subjects with in-dwelling electrodes walk more slowly after insertion of the electrodes. Because needle electrodes are inserted transcutaneously, they must be sterilized and sufficiently strong to resist breakage. Commonsense considerations, such as time, expense, discomfort experienced, the tolerance of the subject to multiple needle insertions, and the influence of in-dwelling electrodes on walking, necessitate a selection of the muscles most relevant to the specific movement abnormalities. Large muscles near the surface can be studied well with surface electrodes, whereas small muscles and those surrounded by other muscles require insertion of fine-wire electrodes. EMG systems are available in either hardwired or telemetry versions. The hardwired versions now send multiple signals on a single cable. These systems are reliable and less expensive than telemetry. Telemetry systems do not encumber the subject with cables but are susceptible to electromagnetic interference.

Once the EMG data is acquired, it must be processed further to provide information about the timing of muscle activity and the relative intensity of the muscle activity. The EMG data is recorded throughout the gait cycle. The gait cycle is indicated either with synchronization of the kinematic data, foot-switch information, or force plate data to indicate each foot strike and toe-off. Analysis of the EMG is done by a phase–time plot of the activity of the muscle against events of the gait cycle. The raw EMG signal can be analyzed or processed further. The most common methods of EMG signal processing are full wave rectification, linear envelope, and integration of the rectified EMG. The linear envelope is created by low-pass filtering the full wave rectified signal. Integrated processing of the rectified signal is usually performed over short duration, that is, 2% gait cycle, and then the integration is reset and accumulated again. Normalization schemes may also be used to aid in analysis. Normalization may be based on the maximum manual muscle test or maximum EMG signal obtained during gait. The muscle is considered to be activated when at least 5% of the maximum electrical activity obtained during a manual muscle test is present for 5% of the gait cycle.

The electromyogram provides a means for studying muscle activity. The signals that result from action potentials and muscle fibers are stochastic and nonstationary, adding to uncertainty in interpretation. While the ultimate source of locomotor activity is muscle force, no study has established that electromyographic signals represent muscle force. The EMG signal is a measure of the bioelectric events that occur in conjunction with contraction of the muscle fibers. Thus, it is a phenomenon related to the initiation of muscle contraction rather than an effect of the muscles mechanical action. There are many difficulties in correlating the EMG signal amplitude with muscle force magnitude. Both linear and nonlinear relationships between the force level of skeletal muscles and the EMG signal have been reported. Consequently, the EMG is commonly used in clinical gait analysis to determine phasic patterns for individual muscles or muscle groups. It is possible to examine simple on/off patterns, or the EMG can be processed to find a graduation of signal level, after which EMG patterns are examined as defined by the level of activity over the gait cycle. In the latter process, it is common to normalize the signal as a percentage of voluntary maximum muscle contraction. The process of detecting when a muscle is "turned on or off" is usually one of testing whether the average level of the signal is above some predefined limit. This limit is often defined as a percentage of the maximum voluntary muscle contraction. The determination of on/off time is often done by calculating the EMG level and then testing for occasions when the level exceeds some threshold value. EMG on/off times are generally more variable from step to step than either kinematic or kinetic gait measurements.

Intramuscular Pressure

Problems occur in dynamic situations when using electromyographic activity as a measure of muscle functional capability. A dynamic force produced by a muscle is not proportional to the degree of muscular activity. Other factors may affect the muscle force, such as a change of the muscle length, change of the contraction velocity, the rate and type of muscle contraction, joint position, and muscle fatigue. It is desirable to find an alternative measurable mechanical parameter related to muscle force. The electromyographic signal does not assess the tension produced by a muscle, because the tension reflects the sum of both the active contraction and the passive stretch. A technique that may provide information about muscle force is measurement of intramuscular pressure. A new microsensor has been developed for measuring intramuscular pressure. The pressure microsensor has a 360 μm diameter (Figure 3-7). It has an accuracy, repeatability, and linearity better than 2% full scale output (FSO) and the hysteresis of 4.5% FSO.

Intramuscular pressure (IMP) is a mechanical variable that is proportional to muscle tension. The relationship between IMP and active and passive

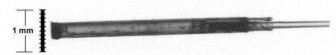

FIGURE 3-7. Microscopic view of a pressure microsensor for measuring intramuscular pressure.

muscle tension has been quantified. The fiber length–isometric tension curve was characterized by an "ascending limb" at a length less than muscle optimum length (L_0) and a "descending limb" at lengths greater that L_0 (Figure 3-8A). The shape of this curve presumably represents a scaled and distorted version of a sarcomere length–tension curve previously published. Passive muscle tension increased in a fairly exponential fashion at lengths $>L_0$. The length–pressure relationship generally mimics the shape of the length–tension curve with an ascending limb at lengths less than L_0 and descending limb at length greater that L_0 (Figure 3-8B). A positive linear relationship has been found between IMP and muscle stress for both the ascending and descending limbs. Further, the IMP accurately reflects the muscle passive tension. These data indicate that IMP measurement provides an accurate index of muscle tension under both active and passive conditions.

It is possible to obtain IMP measurements during gait and relate these measurements to the timing and intensity of muscle contraction. IMP increased at the beginning of single-limb stance (opposite toe-off) (Figure 3-9). The increase on IMP corresponded with the increase in electromyographic activity of the gastrocnemius. The greatest muscle activity in the plantar flexors was required near the end of single-limb stance to meet the high intrinsic plantarflexion moment occurring at the

ankle joint (Figure 3-10B) and to reverse the direction of ankle movement (Figure 3-10A). It should be noted that the IMP reading continued briefly after cessation of the EMG. Furthermore, it can be noted that lower levels of IMP are recorded during the swing phase of gait. During the stance phase of gait, the peak IMP recording corresponds to the time when the ankle moment is at a maximum (opposite foot strike) (Figure 3-10B). Furthermore, during the swing phase of gait, the peak of IMP corresponds to the point of time when the ankle is at peak dorsiflexion (Figure 3-10A). Thus, the peaks in IMP during gait can be correlated with the peaks of active contraction and passive stretch of the gastrocnemius.

INTERPRETATION OF GAIT DATA

Once the data that describes the biomechanics of the patient's gait has been collected, the most crucial step of interpreting the data remains to be performed. Gait analysis produces a large number of measurements. The data must be synthesized and integrated in order to supply clinically relevant information. Human locomotion is very complex and multifaceted. The clinical interpretation of pathological gait disorders involves holding in human memory a large number of graphs, numbers, and clinical tests from data presented on hard copy, chart radiographs, video, and computer generated three-dimensional graphics from multiple trials of a subject walking. Further, comparisons must be made to data from an able-bodied normal population in order to identify the potential movement problems for a given individual. The referring clinician, who may not be an expert in gait analysis, is

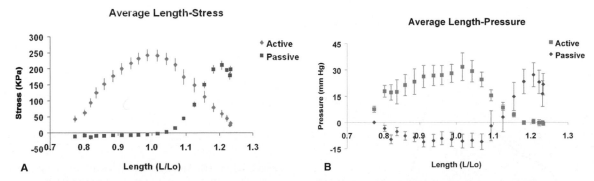

FIGURE 3-8. Relationship between relative muscle length (L/L_0) and **(A)** isometric force, or **(B)** intramuscular pressure. The intramuscular pressure reflects both the active and passive tension characteristics of muscle. (Reproduced with permission from Davis, Kaufman, and Lieber, 2003)

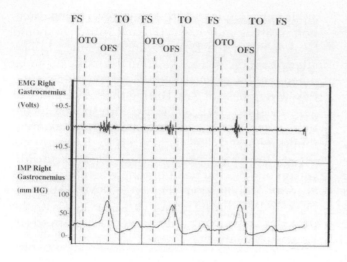

FIGURE 3-9. Raw data for a single subject during gait. Both EMG and intramuscular pressure are being recorded from the gastrocnemius muscle. The stance phase of gait occurs from FS to TO. The swing phase of gait occurs from TO to FS. Single-limb stance occurs from OTO to OFS. Peaks in intramuscular pressure during gait can be correlated with peaks of active contraction and passive stretch of the gastrocnemius. (Reproduced with permission from Kaufman and Sutherland, 1995)

overwhelmed by the magnitude of the number of measurements included in a typical gait report. The person interpreting the data must integrate this information. While data collection techniques for gait analysis have continually evolved over the last 50 years, the method of data presentation has not changed over this time. The data is still reported in two-dimensional charts with the abscissa usually defined as a percentage of the gait cycle and the ordinate displaying the gait parameter.

Recent developments in computer animation may make it possible to apply advanced methods to visualize human movements. The large volume of variables currently found in a typical clinical report

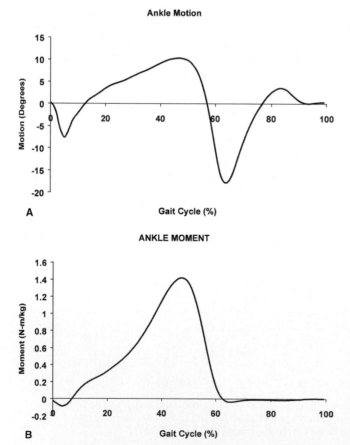

FIGURE 3-10. Ankle motion **(A)** and moment **(B)** during gait. The gait cycle is defined as the events that occur between successive footsteps of the same foot. The gait cycle begins with foot strike, continues through stance and swing phases, and ends with foot strike of the same foot.

could be replaced with a few graphic images that succinctly provided the needed information. It is difficult to fully appreciate and understand the relationships between motion dynamics and biomechanical variables without scientific graphic visualization. Presently, computer software packages have advanced to the stage where it is possible to provide a gait analysis report using animation of fully three-dimensional, realistic graphical depictions of human locomotion. The format used for reporting test results is a matter of considerable importance. The data must be presented in an accurate, clear, and concise format. If the results are not communicated in an effective format, they will be of little use to the clinician regardless of quality.

TREATMENT PLANNING

Clinical gait analysis is useful for assessing abnormal gait patterns, disease progression, and treatment effectiveness. Pathological gait results from a number of different clinical conditions. There are four main causes of pathological gait: (1) structural (i.e., skeletal deformities or lower limb amputation); (2) joint and soft tissue pathology (i.e., arthritis or ligament deficiency); (3) myopathic disorders (i.e., muscular dystrophy); and (4) neurologic disorders (i.e., progressive or nonprogressive pathology of the peripheral or central nervous system).

For each of these categories, gait analysis can be used to measure the dynamic functional limitations of the patient. Careful assessment of this data provides objective selection criteria for different management options. For example, gait analysis can be used to determine if an orthoses is providing functional support for a patient. Similarly, an equinovarus foot deformity can result from several distinct dynamic patterns, for example, overactivity of the tibialis anterior or tibialis posterior, which can be differentiated with gait analysis and dynamic EMG. For patients with myopathic disorders, gait analysis can identify transitional stages of disease progression and provide objective evidence of quadriceps insufficiency requiring long-leg bracing. In chronic neurological impairment, gait analysis can be used to differentiate fixed contracture, that is, static deformity, from muscular overactivity, or, dynamic deformity. Thus, gait analysis is useful for determining the appropriate treatment intervention.

When treatment is being planned, the main objective is to differentiate between the primary causes and compensations for the patient's functional problems.

If the treatment is directed at compensation, the patient will lose their ability to compensate and their movement problems will worsen. A patient may display adaptations in their gait pattern due to their pain, injury, deformity, instability, and/or inappropriate muscle activation patterns. The ramifications of these problems cannot be fully assessed without an instrumented gait study. Patients can undergo dynamic adaptation related to the biomechanics of walking, which must be factored into the treatment algorithm. For example, it has been shown that when planning corrective osteotomy knee surgery, patients with the same bony deformity will have differing knee loading due to dynamic adaptations. These dynamic adaptations will have a direct effect on surgical outcome. The patients who dynamically compensated for their malalignment had a better long-term outcome. For patients with progressive disorders, these dynamic adaptations will also change with time as the disease progresses. It is possible to use motion analysis studies to quantify these dynamic changes in locomotor patterns.

RATIONALE

In this era of government reimbursement for medical services, the ability to document the need and effectiveness of a particular treatment will assume an increasingly important role. Managed care will require validation for many types of therapeutic interventions. Pre- and posttreatment measurement will become mandatory. Outcomes will have to be compared. Practitioners and facilities will be rated on their outcomes. Maximizing anticipated outcomes will be required to document that a treatment plan is worthwhile. Objective gait analysis is an essential tool to meet these demands. The technology is at a level where it is both feasible and affordable to provide an objective form of patient assessment.

In all areas of medical care, a need exists for instrumentation and procedures to aid in a differential diagnosis and treatment of patients. Further, information is required to objectively document patient response to treatment. The ability to diagnose, prescribe treatment, and document results is common to all areas of medical care. However, the technology available in different medical specialties varies widely. This is particularly evident when the current medical technology for treating patients with cardiovascular conditions is compared to the technology for treating patients with neuromuscular

TABLE 3-1.
Current Medical Technology

| Level | Exam | Test Modality | |
		Cardiovascular Patients	Neuromuscular patients
I	Static	ECG	X-ray
		EBCT	CT
		MRI	MRI
		PET	Nuclear Imaging
		Ultrasound	
		Nuclear imaging	
II	Dynamic	Stress Test	Motion Analysis
		Echocardiography	
III	Invasive	Angiography	Diagnostic EMG
			Kinesiological EMG

conditions (Table 3-1). For both types of patients the technology can be divided into three levels: static examinations, dynamic examinations, and invasive procedures. Typically, the approach is to utilize the technology available at the lowest level that will meet the requirements for aiding in differential diagnosis and treatment planning. When a patient reports to a physician that he or she is experiencing chest pain and the risk factors for a myocardial infarction exist, the patient is monitored with an electrocardiogram. In some centers, a computed tomography (CT) scan is obtained to assess the amount of arteriosclerosis in the vessels of the heart muscle. These tests are obtained while the patient is either sitting or lying down. Hence, these constitute static exams. Other static modalities include MRI, PET, ultrasound, and nuclear imaging. If the physician has a high index of suspicion, dynamic tests may be undertaken. These tests include a stress test or echocardiography. Finally, angiography may be utilized as an invasive procedure to further examine the heart.

Conversely, for a patient with neuromuscular dysfunction, most of the modalities utilized are static modalities. Current modalities include radiograph, CT, MRI, and nuclear imaging. It is also common to obtain diagnostic electromyography (EMG) to further elucidate the neuromuscular status of the patient. However, during all these examinations, the patient is static and non–weight bearing. Dynamic assessment of patients with neuromuscular dysfunction can only be obtained using motion analysis techniques along with acquisition of kinesiological EMG.

An objection sometimes raised is that these studies are too costly. However, this objection is unfounded. In terms of cost–benefit ratio, the most compelling consideration is the high cost of inappropriate treatment. It is important to remember that unsuccessful treatment results in unfavorable changes in function and may require subsequent procedures to deal with the original problem. There is, of course, no assurance that gait studies performed prior to treatment planning ensures favorable outcome, but careful planning, based on objective data, provides a solid foundation for decision making. Posttreatment studies give the information required for objective evaluation of treatment results. The rate at which gait analysis technologies become more common depend on the market, the manufacturers, and managed care requirement. Objective patient assessment using gait analysis techniques facilitates the identification of optimal treatment regimens and provides a solid foundation for clinical decision making.

SUMMARY

Human function cannot be fully understood without studies of movement. The modern motion analysis laboratory that has evolved with technological advances has the potential for opening new opportunities for progress in the treatment of patients. Current gait analysis laboratories offer sophisticated automatic tracking systems, force platforms, and electromyographic activity measurements. When coupled with a biomechanical model, this analysis technique is able to provide a complete, three-dimensional, dynamic description of the patient's gait along with information on the timing and intensity of muscle activity. The function of a motion analysis laboratory is to objectively measure the dynamic aspects of an individual patient's performance that cannot be assessed in the clinical setting. Gait dysfunction is, most often, multifactorial in etiology. This quantitative data can facilitate the differentiation of functional deficits from compensations for the deficits. Appropriate intervention requires a thorough understanding of the pathophysiology of the gait deviations along with the appropriate treatment options. Interpretation of this data makes it possible to integrate morphology and functional adaptations. Sound clinical judgment is also indispensable for the management of gait dysfunction. The clinician and gait specialist form an essential team for elucidating the factors contributing to pathological gait and the selection of effective treatment options.

ACKNOWLEDGMENT

This chapter was supported in part by National Institutes of Health Grant R01 HD31476. Appreciation is also expressed to Barb Iverson-Literski for her careful assistance with manuscript preparation.

Annotated Bibliography

An KN, Jacobsen MC, Berglund LJ, et al. Application of a magnetic tracking device to kinesiologic studies. J Biomech, 1988;21(7):613–620.
This is the first article to describe the use of a magnetic tracking device for application in biomechanical research.

Bell AL, Pedersen DR, and Brand RA. Prediction of hip joint centre location from external landmarks. Hum Movement Sci 1989;8:3–16.
This article provides a method to locate the hip center based on measurements from the ASIS and PSIS landmarks.

Bogey RA, Barnes LA, and Perry J. Computer algorithms to characterize individual subject EMG profiles during gait. Arch Phys Med Rehabil 1992;73(9):835–841.
This article describes a computer program for automated analysis of electromyographic signals during gait.

Borelli GA. De motur animalium. Batavis: Lugduni, 1685.
This is the classic work that forms the initial concepts for analyzing the biomechanical effects of muscle action.

Braune W, and Fischer O. Der Gang des Menschen [The Human Gait]. Leipzig: BG Teubner. 1895:25.
This is the first objective measurement of human walking.

Cappozzo A, Catani F, Croce UD, et al. Position and orientation in space of bones during movement: anatomical frame definition and determination. Clin Biomech 1995;10(4):171–178.
This article describes a method for converting technical coordinate systems to anatomical coordinate systems using a subject calibration procedure.

Chao EYS. Determination of applied forces in linking systems with known displacements: with special application to biomechanics. Iowa City: University of Iowa, 1971.
The first description of the inverse dynamics techniques for use in biomechanics.

Chao, EYS. Justification of triaxial goniometer for the measurement of joint rotation. J Biomech 1980;13:989–1006.
This article contains a detailed description on the use of Eulerian angles for human movement analysis.

Davis J, Kaufman KR, and Lieber RL. Correlation between active and passive isometric force and intramuscular pressure in the isolated rabbit tibialis anterior muscle. J Biomech 2003;36(4):505–512.
This article demonstrates that intramuscular pressure reflects both active and passive muscle tension.

Duchenne, GBA. Physiologie des mouvements démontrée a l'aide de l'expérimentation électrique et de l'observation clinique et applicable a l'étude des paralysies et des déformations, J.B. Bailliere ed. Paris, 1867.
This classic article describes how muscles function during gait.

Eastlack, ME, Arvidson J, Snyder-Mackler L, et al. Interrater reliability of videotaped observational gait-analysis assessments. Phys Ther 1991;71(6):465–472.
This article demonstrates that the inter-rater reliability of videotaped observational gait analysis assessments are only slightly to moderately reliable.

Gage JR, and Ounpuu S. Gait analysis in clinical practice. Sem Orthop 1989;2:72–87.
This article presents examples of how gait analysis is used in current clinical practice.

Gordon AM, Huxley AF, and Julian FJ. The variation in isometric tension with sarcomere length in vertebrate muscle fibres. J Phys (Lond) 1966;184:170–192.
This classic article describes the sarcomere length–tension relationship.

Grood ES, and Suntay WJ. A joint coordinate system for the clinical description of three-dimensional motions: application to the knee. J Biomech Eng 1983;105(2):136–144.
This article is often quoted to describe the Eulerian angle system.

Inman, VT, Ralston HJ, and Todd F. Human Walking. Baltimore: Williams & Wilkins, 1981.
This is the classic textbook on clinical applications of the engineering analysis of human walking.

Kadaba, MP, Ramakrishnan HK, and Wootten ME. Measurement of lower extremity kinematics during level walking. J Orthop Res 1990;8(3):383–392.
This article describes a biomechanical model that is commonly used in gait analysis, the so-called Helen Hayes marker set.

Kaufman KR, and Sutherland DH. Dynamic intramuscular pressure measurement during gait. Oper Tech in Sports Med 1995;3(4):250–255.
This article demonstrates that intramuscular pressure reflects both active and passive muscle tension in vivo.

Kaufman KR, An KN, and Chao EY. A comparison of intersegmental joint dynamics to isokinetic dynamometer measurements. J Biomech 1995;28(10):1243–1256.
This article contains a rigorous mathematic description of inverse dynamics.

Kaufman KR, An KW, Litchy WJ, et al. Physiological prediction of muscle forces—I. Theoretical formulation. Neuroscience 1991;40(3):781–792.
A rigorous description of the optimization technique for predicting muscle and joint forces.

Kaufman KR, Wavering T, Morrow D, et al. Performance characteristics of a pressure microsensor. J Biomech 2003;36(2):283–287.
A description of the smallest pressure sensor currently available for measuring biological pressure signals.

Koh TJ, and Grabiner MD. Cross talk in surface electromyograms of human hamstring muscles. J Orthop Res 1992;10(5):701–709.
A description of an instrumentation technique used to reduce crosstalk in electromyographic measurements.

Komi PV. Relationship between muscle tension, EMG, and velocity of contraction under concentric and eccentric work. New Developments in Clinical Neurophysiology. J.E. Desmet, ed. Basel, Switzerland: Karger, 1973.
This article illustrates that EMG is not a direct measure of muscle force. The EMG varies for the same muscle force during dynamic muscle contraction.

Krebs DE, Edelstein JE, and Fishman S. Reliability of observational kinematic gait analysis. Phys Ther 1985;65(7):1027–1033.
This study presents the within-rater and between-rater reliability of observational gait analysis in a pediatric sample of patients wearing ankle–foot orthoses.

Muybridge E. Human and Animal Locomotion. Vols. 1–3. New York: Dover, 1979. (Original work published in 1887).
This three volume set provides the first photographic documentation of human and animal movement.

Perry J, Easterday CS, Antonelli DJ. Surface versus intramuscular electrodes for electromyography of superficial and deep muscles. Phys Ther 1981;61(1):7–15.
The relative selectivity of surface electrodes was compared to fine-wire electrodes. The EMG values obtained with surface electrodes reflect a composite of electrical activity from the target muscle and muscles in proximity to the target muscle, that is, cross-talk.

Perry J. Gait Analysis: Normal and Pathological Function. Thorofare, NJ: Slack, 1992.
This textbook is a must read for individuals interested in normal and pathological gait.

Prodromos CC, Andriacchi TP, and Galante JO. A relationship between gait and clinical changes following high tibial osteotomy. J Bone Joint Surg Am 1985;67(8):1188–1194.
This article demonstrates that patients can have the same anatomical alignment and can have different clinical outcomes because they alter their dynamic knee joint loading during gait.

Raab FH, Blood EB, Steiner TO, et al. Magnetic position and orientation tracking system. IEEE Transactions on Aerospace and Electronic Systems 1979;AES-15(5):709–718.
This article describes the mathematical principles of a magnetic tracking system.

Rack PMH, and Westbury DR. The effects of length and stimulus rate on tension in the isometric cat soleus muscle. J Physiol (Lond) 1969;204:443–460.
The classic article describes the length–tension relationship in whole muscle.

Saleh M, and Murdoch G. In defence of gait analysis. Observation and measurement in gait assessment. J Bone Joint Surg [Br] 1985;67(2):237–241.
This report demonstrates the inadequacy of visual observation as a diagnostic method. It emphasizes the need for objective measurements.

Sutherland DH, Olshen R, Cooper L, et al. The pathomechanics of gait in Duchenne muscular dystrophy. Dev Med Child Neurol 1981;23(1):3–22.
This classic article classifies patients with Duchenne muscular dystrophy into three groups: early, transitional, and late, based on their gait characteristics. It describes changes in gait patterns of these subjects during disease progression.

Sutherland DH, Olshen RA, Biden EN, et al. The development of mature walking. Oxford, England: Mac Keith,1988.
This classic text explains the electromyographic pattern changes during the development of gait in normal children.

Wang JW, Kuo KN, Andriacchi TP, et al. The influence of walking mechanics and time on the results of proximal tibial osteotomy. J Bone Joint Surg 1990;72(6):905–909.
This is a follow-up to the Prodromos et al. (1985) study. The article describes the relationship between the magnitude of a knee adduction moment during walking and the outcome of proximal tibial osteotomy. The patients with a low adduction moment have less recurrence of varus deformity over a greater period of time.

Waters RL, Frazier J, Garland DE, et al. Electromyographic gait analysis before and after operative treatment for hemiplegic equinus and equinovarus deformity. J Bone Joint Surg 1982;64(2):284–288.
This article demonstrates that it is necessary to obtain dynamic EMG in order to differentiate between the action of tibialis anterior and tibialis posterior contributing to equinovarus foot deformity.

Winter DA. Biomechanics and Motor Control of Human Movement, 2nd Ed. New York: Wiley & Sons,1990.
A classic textbook on the biomechanics of human movement with emphasis on kinetic analysis.

Woods JJ, and Bigland-Ritchie B. Linear and nonlinear surface EMG/force relationships in human muscles. Amer J Phys Med Rehab 1983;62(6):287–299.
This article reports how it is possible to have both linear and nonlinear relationships between EMG and muscle force.

Wooten, ME, Kadaba MP, and Cochran GUVB. Dynamic electromyography. II. Normal patterns during gait. J Orthop Res 1990;8:259–265.
A description of the mathematical technique for analyzing changes in electromyographic activity level during gait.

Young CC, Rose SE, Biden EN, et al. The effect of surface and internal electrodes on the gait of children with cerebral palsy, spastic diplegic type. J Orthop Res, 1989;7(5):732–737.
This study demonstrates that the addition of electromyographic recording apparatus causes a change in the gait of subjects being studied.

Laura Prokuski

Principles of Fractures

Bone has various roles. Bones are responsible for the shape and structure of the body. Bone provides origin and insertion sites for muscles and tendons, and is critical for locomotion. Bones such as the skull, sternum, and ribs protect vital organs. Finally, bone is a reservoir for minerals, and plays a role in mineral homeostasis.

Bone is a unique, dynamic, well-organized tissue. The cells and matrix that comprise bone are constantly remodeling in response to changes in loading. Bone is unique in that it is a self-repairing tissue. As microdamage is accumulated, an infinitely complex and well-orchestrated cascade of cellular events works to repair it. Bone can alter its properties and geometry in response to changes in mechanical load and metabolic demand. Bone is capable restoring the structural and functional roles of the tissue even after a catastrophic failure (fracture).

BONE BIOMECHANICS

Bone is a dynamic tissue that responds to specific stimuli. The mechanical environment around the bone can induce changes in structure. Bone responds to increased loads by increasing the amount and density of tissue, and by changing shape in order to optimally withstand applied forces. Similarly, disuse results in osteopenia. With less force applied to bone, the quantity and density of bone will diminish to match the perceived demand. Bone structure and quality is also sensitive to the complex biochemical cascades that accompany certain metabolic disorders, aging, and exposure to drugs such as glucocorticoids and bisphosphonates.

The strength of bone is related to the quality and amount of collagen, mineral content, and overall density. Bone is like a two-phase material consisting of a collagenous matrix and a mineralized crystalline lattice. The collagen matrix is stronger in tension than in compression. The mineral phase of orderly apatite crystals is stronger in compression than tension.

Bone is anisotropic. The mechanical properties are different when load is applied in different directions. The tensile strength of bone is greater when it is loaded along its longitudinal axis, compared to when it is loaded perpendicular to the longitudinal axis. Therefore, cortical bone is weak in tension and shear, but tough under compression. For weight-bearing bones, this appears to be adaptive.

Bone is viscoelastic. The mechanical properties are different when load is applied at different rates. More energy can be absorbed by bone at higher loading rates than lower loading rates. Therefore, the more strenuous the activity, the stronger the bone. The elastic component defines maximum deformity that is achieved prior to failure. The viscous component determines the time taken to reach the maximum deformity.

The amount of deformation a material demonstrates prior to failure is a reflection of ductility or brittleness. Ductile substances can undergo a large amount of deformation prior to failure. Brittle substances have ultimate strains similar to yield strains. Failure occurs under very small deformations. Cortical bone is ductile in loading under compression. Cortical bone exhibits a ductile to brittle transition as the strain rate increases.

Trabecular bone material properties are very sensitive to density. Density can vary greatly from area to area. Bone can easily regulate its strength and stiffness by adjusting density. Subtle changes in density result in large changes in strength.

FRACTURE BIOMECHANICS

A fracture is the structural failure of bone. Energy absorbed by bone during loading is released within the bone as it fractures. Extrinsic and intrinsic factors affect bone failure. The extrinsic factors are the external forces applied to the bone. The magnitude and area of force distribution, as well as the rate at which the bone is loaded are important factors in fracture occurrence and pattern.

Bone fails under applied compression, tension, rotation, shear, or a combination of forces. Because bone has particular mechanical characteristics, specific loads applied at specific directions and rates will produce predictable patterns of failure. A pure tensile force will produce a transverse fracture. An uneven bending force results in an oblique fracture. The cortex under compression breaks before the transverse tension failure is complete. This results in comminution or a butterfly fragment at the site of compression. Spiral patterns of fracture are result of torsional load. With torsion, some bending force coexists, which limits endless propagation of the spiral. Pure compressive forces result in uniform impaction. Four-point bending produces two sites of tension, and a segmental fracture results (Figure 4-1).

The intrinsic factors are related to the structure's biomechanical characteristics, or how much energy the bone can absorb prior to failure (toughness). Because bone is anisotropic, it absorbs more energy prior to failure if the load is applied in the longitudinal axis of the bone. Conversely, it takes less energy to fracture if the bone is loaded perpendicular to the longitudinal axis. Because bone is viscoelastic, the rate of loading affects the amount of energy the bone can absorb. With higher loading speeds, more energy is absorbed, and failure results in more damage to the bone structure, reflected in the degree of comminution of the fracture pattern. Lower loading speeds allow less energy to be absorbed prior to failure, resulting in a simpler fracture pattern.

BONE FATIGUE

Microstructural fatigue failure can be summarized in three phases: crack initiation, crack propagation, and complete structural failure. Repetitive loading over long periods results in the development of microcracks. Irregularities in the microstructure, such as Haversian canals, lacunae, or canaliculi act as stress risers and are the sites of crack initiation. The repair response to accumulated microdamage is termed adaptation. Adaptation is targeted at the repair of microdamage. If the repair response is insufficient, crack propagation will proceed, resulting in a slow

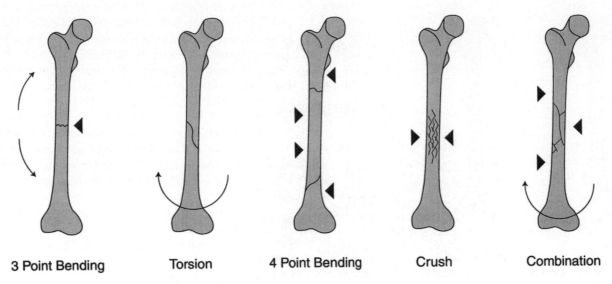

3 Point Bending   Torsion   4 Point Bending   Crush   Combination

FIGURE 4-1. Bone fails differently under different loading conditions.

but steady decrease in strength and stiffness of the bone. As microcracks propagate, larger cracks form in interfaces such as cement lines between osteons. If crack propagation continues, cracks become larger and coalesce (Figure 4-2). The mechanical properties of the bone cannot support additional load and a fracture occurs. Areas of the bone experiencing tension forces have more microdamage than areas under compression. Fatigue damage increases with increasing strain rate.

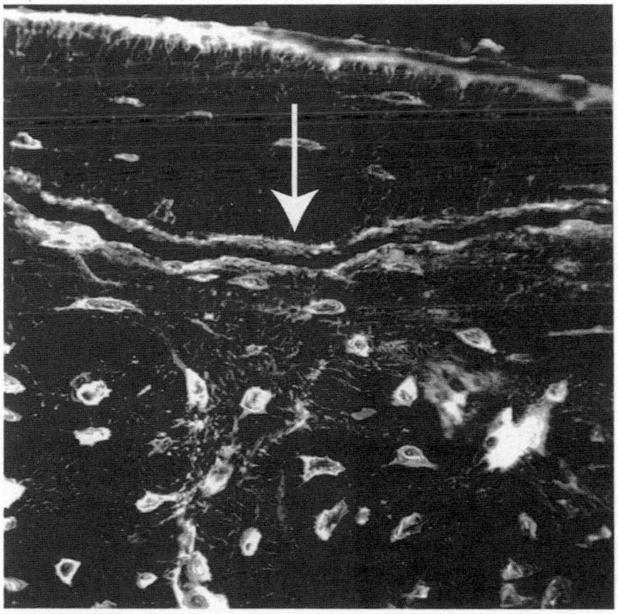

Fatigue fracture can occur in normal bone with repeated application of strain. Fatigue fracture can also occur with fewer cycles or less strain in pathologic bone. Fatigue fractures are often not associated with a specific traumatic event and occur in previously adapted bone. Alterations to peak strain, number of loading cycles, the quantity of microdamage within bone, and the adaptive response are key variables that influence the risk of fatigue fracture.

FRACTURE CLASSIFICATION

The nomenclature of fractures first starts with the name of the bone that is injured. Further descriptive terms can be used that describe the anatomic location injured, such as diaphyseal or metaphyseal (Figure 4-3). The morphology of the fracture can be described. Common terms include, but are not limited to, transverse, oblique, spiral, or comminuted (Figure 4-4). A fracture can be described as intra-articular if it involves a joint surface. An impacted fracture occurs when the diaphysis is driven into metaphyseal trabecular bone. A greenstick fracture indicates an incomplete or bending fracture. A compression fracture of the metaphyseal region with cortical buckling in a child is a torus fracture.

The failure of bone does not occur in isolation. Injury to overlying soft tissue always occurs. Rupture

FIGURE 4-2. Confocal microscopic image of cortical bone after subcatastrophic fatigue loading. Osteocytes and their canalicular networks are outlined in white. The arrow demonstrates a microcrack.

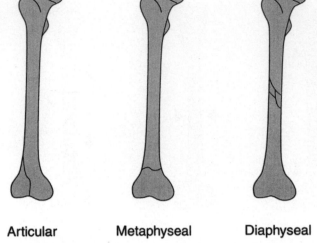

Articular   Metaphyseal   Diaphyseal

FIGURE 4-3. The anatomic location of a fracture.

of the periosteum, local blood vessels, and muscle always accompany a fractured bone. Occasionally the soft tissue injury includes major named arteries or nerves, subcutaneous tissue, and skin. When the skin is violated, the fracture is termed an open fracture (Figure 4-5).

When bone ends move away from each other, changing the alignment, they are displaced. Displacement is described by the position of the distal fragment relative to the proximal fragment. Alternatively, displacement with angulation can be described by the direction of the apex of the fracture (Figure 4-6).

Fractures can be classified in many ways. Classification systems have been created to organize almost

every type of fracture. The intent of creating a classification system is to highlight particular variations in a specific type of fracture. These variations are used either to select a treatment algorithm or assist in predicting outcome. Several comprehensive fracture classification schemes have been created to compartmentalize all fractures. The two most frequently used are the AO/ASIF and Orthopaedic Trauma Association (OTA) classification systems. These systems are used primarily as research tools and, to a lesser extent, to communicate between medical professionals. More often, descriptive terms are used.

Traumatic fractures occur when the force applied to a normal bone exceeds its capacity to absorb energy. An example is the fracture of a humerus in a motor vehicle crash (Figure 4-7).

Pathologic fractures are the result of normal physiologic forces on abnormal bone. The bone in a pathologic fracture is weakened by a neoplastic process. Both primary bone tumors and metastases can cause destruction of the bone structure and impairment of the adaptation response, rendering it vulnerable to failure under normal loads (Figure 4-8). Pathologic fractures have also been associated with osteopenia from abnormal bone metabolism; these are also referred to as insufficiency fractures (Figure 4-9).

Fatigue or stress fractures are common in military recruits and athletes. Repetitive physiologic load can produce microcracks that propagate to nondisplaced fractures before significant repair can occur. It has been theorized that muscle fatigue plays a role in this mechanism of injury. Skeletal muscle normally diverts some stress from the bone,

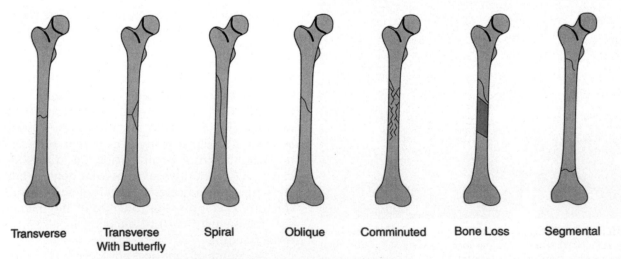

Transverse   Transverse   Spiral   Oblique   Comminuted   Bone Loss   Segmental
**   With Butterfly**

FIGURE 4-4. The pattern of the fracture.

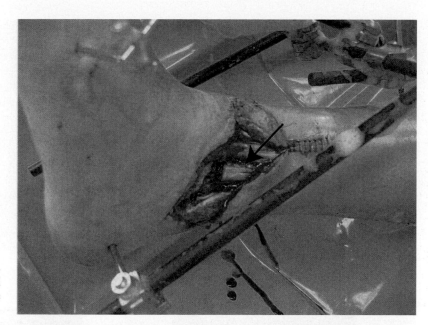

FIGURE 4-5. The photograph demonstrates an open ankle fracture stabilized with a bridging external fixator. Note the exposed fibula in the wound (*arrow*).

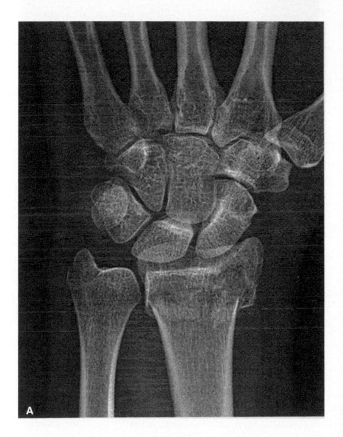

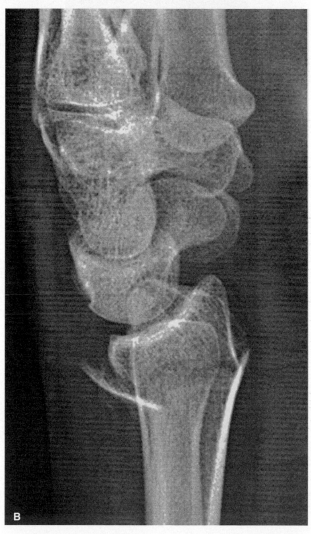

FIGURE 4-6. Posteroanterior **(A)** and lateral **(B)** radiographs of the wrist demonstrate a displaced distal radius fracture. The displacement is posterior, or dorsal. The displacement can also be described as apex anterior angulation.

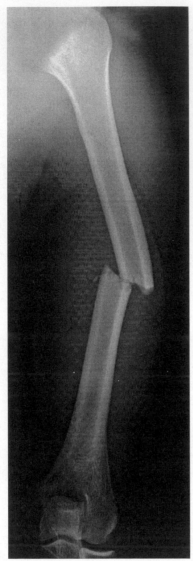

FIGURE 4-7. Anterioposterior radiograph of the humerus demonstrates a traumatic fracture.

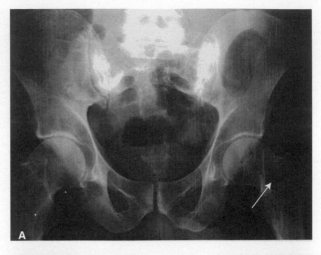

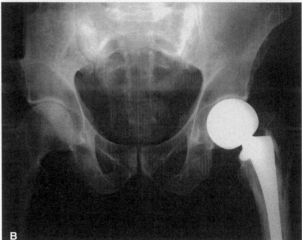

FIGURE 4-8. (A) Anterioposterior radiograph of the pelvis demonstrates multiple myeloma in the femoral neck (*arrow*). There is a nondisplaced pathological fracture of the basicervical region. (B) This fracture was treated by curettage and cemented hemiarthroplasty. Immediate weight bearing was allowed.

but with muscle fatigue, this protective maneuver is lost (Figure 4-10).

Fractures can be classified by the mechanism that caused them. A single application of force sufficient to cause a fracture can be applied directly or indirectly. Direct trauma such as the application of blunt, crush, or penetrating force to the body will cause soft tissue injury and fracture at the site the force was applied (Figure 4-11). Indirect trauma includes tension, angulation, rotation, compression, and a combination of forces applied at an area remote to the fracture. Transmission of forces through muscle contractions results in a fracture. An example of an indirect force causing fracture is the strong

contraction of the triceps with a fixed forearm, resulting in an olecranon fracture (Figure 4-12).

EFFECTS OF FRACTURES

A fracture is a mechanical failure, but the process triggers a biologic response that starts the repair process. Bleeding occurs from the ruptured periosteum and surrounding muscle. Bone marrow contents are released into the vicinity of the fracture and can be distributed systemically. Inflammatory mediators such as prostaglandins and leukotrienes are released.

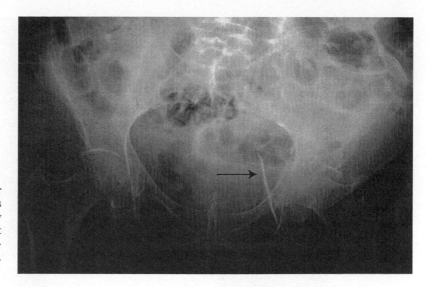

FIGURE 4-9. An anterior-posterior radiograph of the pelvis demonstrates profound osteopenia in an elderly woman. A fall from a standing height produced a displaced acetabular fracture and central hip dislocation (*arrow*). This is an insufficiency fracture.

Clinically, a fracture is suspected when an appropriate force has been applied that would cause failure of the bone. A supraphysiologic load applied to a normal bone, for example during a motor vehicle accident, is appropriate to cause a tibial shaft fracture. Passive range of motion of the knee is not an appropriate force to cause a tibial shaft fracture in a normal ambulatory person, but is an appropriate mechanism for a paraplegic with severe disuse osteopenia and spasticity. The absence of an appropriate mechanism of injury should warrant a search for abnormal bone. Neoplastic conditions, metabolic disorders of bone, and the clandestine use of drugs that adversely affect bone metabolism (glucocorticoids) may be diagnosed by a fracture. An inappropriate mechanism of injury may also suggest a situation of abuse and should be suspected in those with few defense mechanisms (children, women, elderly, disabled.)

Clinical signs of fracture vary with the age of the patient and the area of the body injured. General signs include pain, swelling, deformity, abnormal mobility, and loss of function. Pain is caused by bleeding, swelling, abnormal motion on surrounding soft tissues, and release of inflammatory mediators. Deformity and abnormal mobility are due to lack of structural support that the bone provides. Altered function of a limb is a function of pain and lack of normal structural integrity. Inability to walk or painful ambulation is a reliable sign of spine or lower extremity fracture in those with poor communication capacity, such as children and the elderly. Radiographs confirm the clinical suspicion.

Fractures can result in some form of alteration of function, both temporarily and permanently. With the diminished ability to use a limb, the patient experiences functional losses. The injured patient's role in the family and society is often altered. The capacity to earn a living is compromised, and medical bills can be significant, leading to emotional concerns and financial strains. Patients often have problems adjusting to their disability and suffer psychological sequelae related to change in body image and function. Laborers with fractures that lead to permanent disability often need to retrain and find more sedentary vocations.

SINGLE VERSUS MULTIPLE FRACTURES

Patients with an isolated fracture should be differentiated from multiply injured patients. The effect of multiple fractures on the systemic physiology is not the same as the sum of the individual fractures. Bleeding from multiple fractures can produce shock. Pelvic fractures with displaced sacroiliac dislocations, sacral fractures, and symphyseal disruptions can be associated with life-threatening hemorrhage from ruptured pelvic veins. Injuries to named arteries can also occur with pelvic and acetabular fractures, and can produce rapid and profound hemorrhage. Fractures with associated arterial injuries can also be a source of shock. For example, scapulothoracic dissociation is associated with injury to the subclavian vessels and can lead to

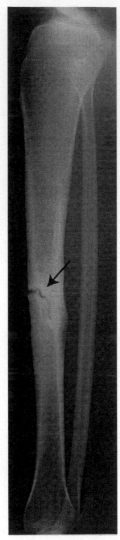

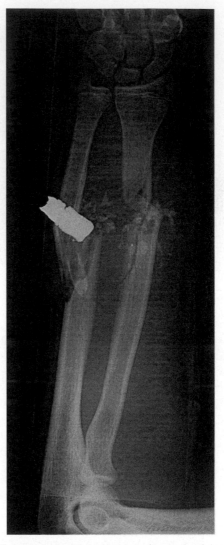

FIGURE 4-10. Lateral radiograph of the tibia demonstrates a subacute stress fracture of the tibial diaphysis (*arrow*). Note the sclerosis surrounding the fracture cleft.

FIGURE 4-11. Anterior-posterior radiograph of the forearm demonstrates an injury from direct penetrating trauma. Massive comminution reflects the high energy nature of the injury.

rapid and significant blood loss. Thighs with broken femurs can accommodate one liter of blood. Multiple open fractures can be a source of significant external blood loss. Multiple skeletal injuries in combination with visceral injuries can produce significant bleeding and consumption of platelets and coagulation factors.

The release of marrow elements into the general circulation is increased with multiple fractures. Although this occurs to some degree with every fracture, certain patients react with a clinical syndrome known as fat embolism syndrome. Respiratory insufficiency is the primary clinical sign, ranging from increased oxygen demands to full-blown acute

respiratory distress syndrome (ARDS), which can be fatal. Other clinical manifestations include petechiae, anemia, thrombocytopenia, and central nervous system dysfunction. The cause not completely understood, but hypotheses include microcirculatory occlusive phenomenon, generalized inflammation, and cell membrane dysfunction. It is also not understood what factors make some susceptible to develop fat embolism syndrome, while the same clinical situation does not produce the syndrome in others.

Multiple areas of injury increase the occurrence of venous thromboembolism and pulmonary embolus. The factors important in thrombogenesis are

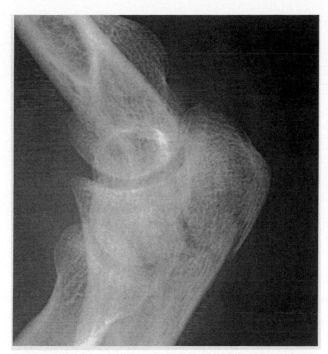

FIGURE 4-12. Lateral radiograph of the elbow demonstrates an injury from an indirect source. A nondisplaced fracture of the olecranon was caused by strong contraction of the triceps with a fixed forearm.

venous endothelial injury, venous stasis, and activated coagulation. A fracture results in diffuse intimal damage in the vessels in the zone of injury. With immobilization of an injured limb, the forceful muscle contractions that facilitate venous return to the heart are minimized, and stasis occurs in the veins. Prolonged recumbency from multiple injuries increases the risk of venous stasis exponentially. Without prophylaxis, venous thromboembolism occurs in the majority of injured patients. Pulmonary embolism is the leading cause of death in those who survive the initial injury.

Patients with multiple fractures often require prolonged periods in the recumbent position to manage the skeletal instability and pain. Multiple adverse affects of this position have been observed. Pulmonary function is compromised due to suboptimal ventilation. Pain results in poor inspiratory effort and positioning leads to atelectasis, dependent edema, and aspiration. Narcotic pain medications decrease the respiratory rate. The sum of these factors leads to hypoxia and pneumonia. Nutrition is compromised due to the adverse effects narcotic medication has on gastrointestinal function and difficulty eating in an atypical position. With pain and decreased mobility, urinary catheters are needed, which ultimately lead to urinary tract infections.

Immobility leads to skin breakdown and deep venous thrombosis. In this patient population, early surgical treatment of multiple fractures, especially pelvic and femur fractures, reduces time in bed, and greatly improves outcomes.

INITIAL MANAGEMENT OF FRACTURES

Realignment

The preferred initial treatment for a fracture is realignment and splinting. Realignment of a grossly angulated limb will improve arterial flow and venous drainage distal to the injury. Bleeding will diminish as the volume around the fracture is reduced, and tamponade can occur. Nerve function improves when anatomically aligned.

Realignment can be performed with several simple techniques. Simple manipulation of an angulated limb into a more anatomic position is recommended. Longitudinal traction is the simplest way to reduce a fracture. Generally, the segment that can be controlled manually is realigned to the less mobile segment. More challenging techniques include reduction maneuvers where the deformity is accentuated, then corrected. The maintenance of alignment after the latter technique depends on an intact soft tissue hinge around the fracture. Impediments to realignment include interposed soft tissue between the fracture ends and lack of soft tissue hinge around the fracture, making the reduction difficult to maintain.

Displaced open fractures should be realigned prior to splinting. Gross contamination can be removed, but formal irrigation in the emergency department is not recommended. Reintroduction of a contaminated bone end into the wound is tolerated. The entire wound will be subsequently debrided in the operating room. A sterile dressing should be applied over the wound and maintained until the patient is in the operating room.

Splinting

A splint is a noncircumferential device that maintains alignment of a limb with a fracture and decreases motion at the fracture site. Limitation of excessive fracture motion may prevent additional injury to vulnerable soft tissues. There is always concern that an unsplinted closed fracture may be converted into an open fracture from the motion of sharp bone ends. Splinting reduces bleeding and release of marrow elements from the fracture site, and thus may contribute to resuscitation. By reducing pain, patient transport and evaluation are facilitated.

A variety of splinting techniques can be used in a variety of fractures. In a hospital, simple materials can be effective splints. Sheets folded to a swathe or commercially available slings can help reduce pain for clavicle, scapula, or proximal humerus fractures. Padded fiberglass or plaster slabs can be customized to splint fractures of the humerus, forearm, wrist, and hand, as well as fractures distal to the knee. Prefabricated adjustable knee immobilizers are helpful in splinting injuries around the knee. A circumferential sheet can be tied around the pelvis and thighs to reduce the pelvic volume in an open book pelvic ring injury. Pillows or sandbags can be used to reduce the motion of a fractured femur. Philadelphia collars or sandbags can immobilize a cervical spine fracture. A long rigid board is the method of choice for spine splinting.

DEFINITIVE TREATMENT OF FRACTURES

Evaluation of the Patient

Definitive treatment of fractures is performed when the general condition of the patient is optimized, and the patient will tolerate the process of treatment. The goals of treating the injured patient are to save life first, then save limb, and limit disability. The goals of fracture treatment are to obtain stability of the injured limb, facilitate healing, and accelerate rehabilitation.

Characteristics of the patient and the fracture are important to consider when deciding on a definitive treatment plan. The overall condition of the patient is of utmost concern. For multiply injured patients, resuscitation is necessary. Multiple fractures, as well as visceral injuries, can cause significant hemorrhage. Suboptimal perfusion of organs can occur from this hemorrhage and is referred to as shock. Shock can be manifested by tachycardia, hypotension, changes in mental status, peripheral vasoconstriction, poor urine output, and ultimately death. Laboratory findings involving shock can include anemia, thrombocytopenia, and elevated clotting times, which represent bleeding and consumption of coagulation factors. As perfusion decreases, cellular metabolism turns from aerobic to anaerobic, liberating the waste product lactic acid. Lactic acid production results in metabolic acidosis.

Reversal of shock is termed resuscitation. Resuscitation principles are to stop ongoing hemorrhage and replenish lost circulating volume . This is accomplished with infusions of lactated Ringer's or normal saline solution, or blood products, if hemorrhage has been significant. Transfusion of red blood cells, platelets, and plasma (containing coagulation factors) may be required to replace lost circulating volume and replenish consumed factors and cells. Surgical intervention may be necessary to stop hemorrhage. Surgical removal of an irreparable bleeding organ (spleen) or ligation of bleeding arteries may be a necessary component of resuscitation. Restoration and maintenance of pelvic volume with external devices may be necessary to promote tamponade of bleeding pelvic vessels after injury. Alternatively, in some cases, angiographic identification and intravascular embolization of major bleeding vessels is also in the algorithm used to control hemorrhage.

Treatment of fractures should be delayed until the patient is hemodynamically stable. Fracture surgery will result in additional blood loss to an already compromised patient and may contribute to the patient's demise. Open fractures can be temporized in a hemodynamically unstable patient with removal of gross contamination, limited irrigation of exposed bone, placement of a sterile dressing, and splinting. Definitive debridement and skeletal stabilization can be performed when the patient's condition is compatible with surgery. Although this step may increase the rate of infection at the fracture site, it may be a necessary precaution. Fracture surgery can be considered when the patient's blood pressure and heart rate have stabilized, and when end organ perfusion is judged adequate. No active hemorrhage should be ongoing, and hematologic parameters should be in a reasonable range. General guidelines are a hematocrit around 30%, INR < 1.4, and platelets > 80,000/mm^3.

Associated injuries may preclude immediate operative treatment of fractures. For patients with a head injury, secondary brain injury is associated with hypotension and hypoxia. Operative treatment of fractures in a poorly resuscitated patient may result in a secondary brain injury. A severe pulmonary injury is a controversial contraindication to early definitive fracture care.

Elderly patients require particular consideration. Older patients are limited functionally by poor eyesight, diminished hearing, and limited mobility from other medical conditions. Nonoperative treatment of some fractures requires immobilization in a cast or brace. Casts or braces limit an elderly person's mobility and functioning more than similar restrictions in a younger adult. Weight-bearing restrictions and the introduction of crutches or a walker can significantly diminish an elderly patient's mobility and may contribute to subsequent falls and injuries. Lack of ability to comply with weight-bearing restrictions has led to loss of reduction and fixation. Additional problems seen with external immobilization include skin breakdown, often contributed to by poor sensation, delicate skin, and other comorbid conditions such as diabetic neuropathy and vasculopathy. Access to medical care may be limited, or patients may not want to complain, leading to delayed diagnosis of pressure areas. After operative treatment of fractures, mobilization of an elderly patient is much slower than in a young adult. Irreversible loss of function also happens more frequently in elderly patients. After hip fractures, only one-third returns to preinjury function. Perioperative complications and death are more common due to multiple medical problems and lack of physiologic reserve. Malnutrition is common in the elderly, which delays wound and fracture healing.

Elderly patients and others with significant medical problems require comprehensive evaluation prior to definitive treatment of the fracture. The presence or treatment of chronic medical problems can lead to injuries. Syncope from a new antihypertensive medication or existing arrhythmia can cause a fall in an elderly patient, producing a hip fracture. New medical problems can also cause injuries. An acute myocardial infarction sustained while driving can lead to a crash. Optimization of the patient's medical condition prior to surgery is warranted. Any reversible problems such as dehydration, hypertension, infections (urinary tract infection, pneumonia) and renal insufficiency should be reversed. Any anticoagulation requires reversal, as well.

For patients with delicate constitutions and multiple medical problems, extensive preoperative evaluation is often necessary to understand the patient's risk for significant perioperative complications. With this information, a realistic discussion with the patient and family of the risk–benefit ratio of surgery can be performed. Chronic renal failure, congestive heart failure, chronic obstructive pulmonary disease, hip fracture, and an age greater than 70 years have been identified as critical risk factors for inpatient mortality. Postoperative complications associated with significant increases in mortality include myocardial infarction, acute renal failure, pulmonary embolus, pneumonia, and cerebrovascular accident. Perioperative testing can also provide information that may modify the perioperative plan. Those with significant pulmonary compromise may elect to have regional instead of a general anesthesia to prevent prolonged intubation and ventilation postoperatively. Decisions can be made about the perioperative management of medical problems, including the need for postoperative monitoring.

For elderly patients with multiple injuries or multiple medical problems, fractures usually treated operatively may be treated nonoperatively if the patient's overall condition is not favorable. Often there is a good salvage procedure if the patient has pain or functional limitations with a malunion. A good example is an elderly woman in a motor vehicle accident with a depressed tibial plateau fracture. In isolation, the fracture would require surgical treatment to correct limb axis deviation and knee instability. However, the patient also suffered a blunt chest injury and has a pericardial effusion, which has produced a new arrhythmia. The risks of immediate surgery may be greater than the risks of reconstructive surgery done at a later date, with an accepted salvage technique.

The patient's functional status and demands are important to consider. An elderly nonambulatory patient would not necessarily need operative treatment for a hip fracture if pain were well controlled. A dentist would not be able to tolerate nonoperative treatment for a mallet fracture. The splint required for successful nonoperative treatment would not be tolerated with frequent hand washing required by the occupation. A displaced intra-articular lower extremity fracture in a paraplegic patient would not require operative reduction and fixation, as it would in an ambulatory patient. However, an upper extremity injury in a paraplegic patient may be treated operatively to maximize function and limit disability, when it may be treated nonoperatively in an ambulatory patient.

Evaluation of the Limb

The condition of the limb should be assessed. Particular attention should be made to the skin condition, vascular inflow, and innervation. Skin condition is important to observe, for it is a source of morbidity with either nonoperative or operative fracture treatment. Acute changes in the skin from the injury include wounds, hematomas, degloving injuries, ecchymoses, and blisters. Any wound in proximity to a fracture should be considered an open fracture until proven otherwise in the operating room. Degloving injuries are common with crush or shear mechanisms of injury. The zone of internal injury is often greatly underestimated by the external appearance of the limb. The skin and subcutaneous tissue are separated from the underlying fascia in an open wound, or without break in the skin. Degloved areas may lead to infected seromas or hematomas. Incisions through a degloved area are often ill advised. A degloving injury associated with an acetabular fracture, referred to as a Morel-Lavallee lesion, is associated with increased rates of surgical wound infection. It is generally recommended that the degloving injury be treated and healed before an incision is made in the area to treat the fracture. Areas of poor skin quality from previous injuries, surgery, burns, grafts, or ulcers, must be noted. Poor skin quality may affect the decision to treat operatively, if the tissues can't tolerate the incisions needed, or nonoperatively, if the tissues can't tolerate an immobilization device.

The vascular supply to a limb is a critical consideration in treatment decision making. Changes in arterial inflow of a limb are seen with acute injuries. An injury with an associated fracture can cause diffuse vascular damage to the bone, periosteum, and muscle. Fractures with injuries to major named arteries can occur with penetrating trauma. Injuries to proximal arteries often, but not always, result in limb ischemia. Injuries to more peripheral arteries rarely produce ischemia due to the extensive anastamotic system present between the vessels.

Acute interstitial swelling can proceed to the point where capillary pressure is overcome. Diffusion of red blood cells and delivery of oxygen at the cellular level is diminished. This physiologic process is known as compartment syndrome. Left untreated, the tissues in the limb become ischemic.

Ischemia can lead to a variety of problems in the limb. Skeletal muscle can tolerate approximately 6 hours of ischemia before widespread irreversible myonecrosis occurs. Nerves are also particularly sensitive to ischemia, although absolute tolerances are not known. Prolonged ischemia may affect fracture treatment decisions. Previously treatable fractures in a limb with prolonged ischemia may be more amenable to amputation.

Peripheral vascular disease or diffuse diabetic small vessel can diminish vascular inflow to the point where wound and fracture healing are impaired. Poor wound healing may increase the chance of infection. Clinical signs of poor arterial inflow include lack of hair on the ischemic segments, lack of palpable pulses, poor sensation, and ulcers. Ankle/brachial index is a simple noninvasive test that can quantify the adequacy of peripheral circulation in the lower extremities. In patients with suspected vascular disease, a vascular surgery consultation should be obtained to assess the adequacy of blood flow to the limb. Reversible forms of ischemia can be addressed, which may reduce the complications of the fracture treatment. For those with irreversible ischemia, significant counseling with the patient and family is necessary to understand the dire situation. Often, the results of fracture treatment are poor and the complication rate is high, whether operative or nonoperative treatment is pursued.

Chronic venous stasis disease can complicate both operative and nonoperative treatment methods. An incision through tortuous dilated veins leads to difficulty in hemostasis, bleeding, hematoma formation, and occasionally difficulty with wound healing. Varicosities predispose to venous stasis, especially in an immobilized limb. The risk of venous thrombosis and pulmonary embolism are increased.

Sensibility and motor strength should be assessed. Acute changes in sensibility or motor strength are attributed to the injury. Fractures can be associated with neuropraxia, axonotmesis, or neurotmesis of named peripheral nerves. Loss of sensation in certain areas of the body can be functionally debilitating. Loss of sensation in the fingers from an injury to the radial, median, or ulnar nerves can have adverse effects on dexterity. Loss of sensation to the plantar aspect of the foot is important in making limb salvage treatment decisions. Acute changes in strength in the setting of injury can be attributed to direct musculotendinous injury or associated nerve injury. These associated injuries will influence treatment decision making.

Many patients have sensory deficits prior to injury. The most common cause of chronic sensory loss is diabetes mellitus, which results in a diffuse peripheral neuropathy. Other common causes include hereditary motor and sensory neuropathies, acquired compressive neuropathy, radiculopathy, spinal cord pathology, peripheral vascular disease, and medications. These conditions can also cause chronic motor weakness. It is important to ask about any preexisting neurovascular conditions, to fully appreciate the effect of the injury.

The overall bone quality is important to observe and may affect treatment plan. As aging occurs, there is a diminution in the bone mineral density. Osteopenia is also seen in patients with malnutrition, metabolic disorders, and chronic glucocorticoid use (transplant recipients, systemic inflammatory disease). Cortical diameters become larger to optimize the toughness of less dense bone. Trabecular lines become thinner. Remodeling of accumulated microdamage is diminished. This remodeling offers particular problems with treatment decision making. Operative treatment of osteopenic fractures is fraught with problems. Poor purchase of standard implants is becoming more of a recognized problem. Poor fixation leads to loss of reduction, resulting in a suboptimal outcome or the need for revision surgery. Solutions to this problem include using different fixation strategies in osteopenic bone and modifying existing implants to strengthen the bone-implant construct. For example, for a patient with an osteopenic hip fracture, intramedullary hip screws are supplanting the use of dynamic hip screws. The intramedullary hip

screw has the mass closer to the axis of the bone, creating a stronger construct. New implants have been developed that are ideally suited for fixation in osteopenic bone. The traditional plate and screw construct has been modified so that the threaded screw head engages a complementary threaded screw hole. This modification creates a fixed angle construct. Placing several locked screws in the plate creates multiple fixed angle devices (Figure 4-13). This device fails differently than traditional screw/plate constructs. Instead of sequential loosening or breaking of screws, the locked construct fails by catastrophic pullout of the entire device. This type of failure is rare, even in osteopenic bone. These new implants have improved the ability to maintain a reduction in osteopenic bone until the fracture heals.

Finally, the fracture characteristics should be assessed. Fractures in different bones often require different treatment plans. For example, metatarsal fractures are most commonly treated nonoperatively because they heal well with minimal intervention. Femoral neck fractures are more likely to

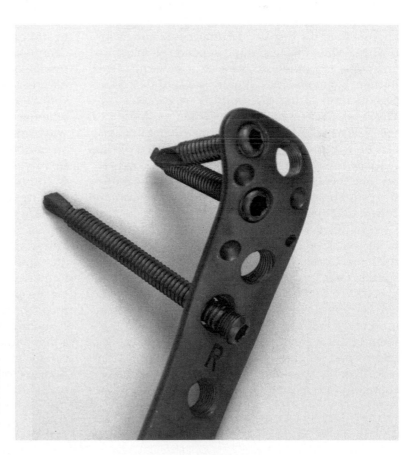

FIGURE 4-13. The photograph demonstrates a locking plate and screws. Note the threaded heads of the screws, which engage complementary threads in the plate hole. Multiple fixed angle devices are created, which drastically improves fixation in osteopenic bone.

be treated operatively to restore weight bearing immediately. The location within the bone, pattern of fracture, and the amount of displacement should be observed. In some bones, the amount of displacement and the area in which the bone is fractured determines whether the injury is treated operatively or nonoperatively. A nondisplaced diaphyseal tibia fracture can be treated nonoperatively, where a displaced proximal metaphyseal fracture in the same bone usually requires operative treatment.

Nonoperative Treatment

Nonoperative treatment of fractures consists of obtaining adequate alignment, and maintaining the alignment in an external immobilization device. For nondisplaced fractures, no change in alignment is necessary, and this step is skipped. For displaced fractures, closed reduction improves alignment. Reduction can be obtained by techniques such as the application of gentle axial traction. The intact soft tissue hinge guides the fracture to the correct alignment. The simplest example is having a patient with a humeral shaft fracture sit up. Gravity provides longitudinal traction on the arm, and the alignment of the displaced humerus fracture is improved. When this technique depends on intact ligamentous attachments around a fracture, it is termed ligamentotaxis (Figure 4-14). Other times accentuation of the deformity is necessary to unkink a soft tissue hinge before manipulation into the desired alignment is performed. Fractures that can be reduced, and reductions maintained in an external immobilization device are considered stable. Fractures that cannot be reduced, or lose reduction in an external immobilization device, are considered unstable.

Devices used to maintain the reduction supplement the stability achieved with the reduction of the bone. Common immobilization devices include splints, casts, and braces. The external immobilization device contributes a little to the stability of the fracture by increasing the hydrostatic pressure around the fracture. They will not prevent displacement of an unstable fracture. They immobilize the injured part for pain relief and to prevent further injury. They also position the limb in a way to prevent common contractures.

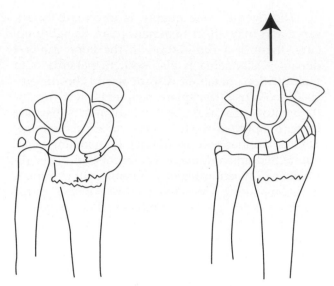

FIGURE 4-14. This schematic demonstrates reduction of a displaced distal radius fracture. Longitudinal traction on bone fragments with ligamentous attachments leads to fracture reduction via ligamentotaxis.

Splints and Casts

Splints are thoughtfully constructed slabs of plaster molded around a limb to provide immobilization of a fracture, without circumferential compression. They are commonly used as the first treatment of a fracture. The noncircumferential nature accommodates swelling. Lower extremity splints are either short or long leg, depending on whether the knee is immobilized. The ankle is always immobilized in a neutral position to prevent an equinus contracture (Figure 4-15). Upper extremity splints are more varied. A long arm splint is commonly used to immobilize a radial head fracture, where a short arm splint is used on a distal radius fracture. Specialized upper extremity splints include the coaptation, sugar tong, and gutter splints. A coaptation splint is used to immobilize a proximal or shaft fracture of the humerus. It consists of a U-shaped slab of padded plaster molded from the axilla, around the elbow, then up the lateral arm and around the shoulder. A sugar tong splint is a device used to immobilize a distal radius fracture. It controls the flexion and extension of the wrist as well as forearm rotation. A sugar tong splint involves a long slab of plaster placed from the dorsal metacarpophalangeal joints,

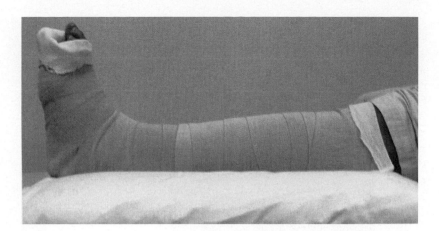

FIGURE 4-15. A padded posterior plaster slab has been used to form a short leg splint. Ace wraps accommodate swelling. The foot is kept in a neutral position to prevent an equinus contracture.

along the dorsum of the forearm, around the elbow, and to the metacarpophalangeal joints on the anterior side. Full, unrestricted metacarpophalangeal motion should be allowed (Figure 4-16). A gutter splint is applied to the radial or ulnar border of the hand, and is commonly used to immobilize metacarpal fractures. The metacarpophalangeal joints are immobilized in 70° to 90° of flexion, to prevent contractures of the collateral ligaments (Figure 4-17). Splints are wrapped with ace wraps or other expandable covering to accommodate swelling.

Casts can be made from plaster or synthetic material. Plaster casts are moldable and can be shaped to fit the limb. Plaster casts are applied over a few layers of cotton padding. The plaster rolls are applied snugly and tucked where free ends are created. The plaster is molded to the shape of the limb. The forearm and arm are molded into flattened cylinders. The thigh is molded into a square shape, and the leg into a triangle. Careful contouring over anatomical structures such as the concavity of the palm and malleoli is performed to fit the cast accurately to the complex geometry of the limb. Three-point pressure can be applied to the cast while it is drying to create a construct that supports the reduction. If angular alignment of the fracture in the cast is suboptimal, wedging can be performed to change the reduction a small degree. Wedging cannot be used to change malreductions of length or rotation. Casts made of synthetic materials cannot be molded as well as plaster. Casts made of

synthetic materials should be used when simple immobilization of a stable fracture is desired, and no maintenance of a reduction is required (Figure 4-18). Synthetic casts are also useful in preventing common contractures after injury.

Patient education on cast and splint care is critical to their success. Patients should be instructed that their splints should be left on. Many, not knowing this restriction, will remove the splint if it becomes uncomfortable, and jeopardize the reduction. The patient's reapplication of the splint is usually not correct, leading to pressure necrosis and contractures. Initially after the injury, volume changes with dependency of the injured limb will manifest with throbbing pain, tightness, and color change. Patients must be educated to react to these sensations with elevation of the extremity, preferably above the heart. Active movement of fingers or toes is also encouraged to promote venous and lymphatic drainage, and prevent stiffness of these joints. Pain or the sensation of unrelenting constriction after a period of elevation should result in the patient's seeking medical attention to loosen or replace a too tight splint or cast. Any complaints of rubbing or burning of the skin should be investigated immediately for soft tissue injury. Patients should be instructed not to stick anything into the cast, for it can cause skin abrasion, laceration, or pressure necrosis. Casts and splints must be kept clean and dry. Wet cast padding will cause maceration of the skin and breakdown. Special synthetic liners are available that dry easily, but are not used routinely.

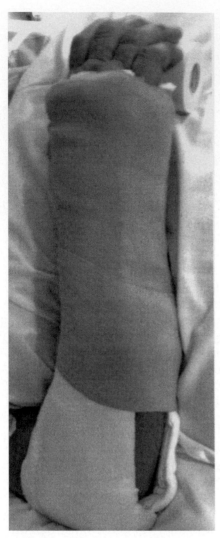

FIGURE 4-16. A padded plaster slab is fashioned around the elbow and forearm to form a sugar tong splint for a forearm fracture. The metacarpophalangeal joints have unrestricted motion.

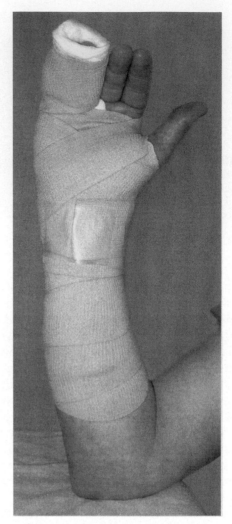

FIGURE 4-17. A padded plaster slab is used as an ulnar gutter splints to immobilize a metacarpal neck fracture. The fingers are included with the metacarpophalangeal joints at 70° of flexion and the interphalangeal joints in full extension. This "safe position" prevents contractures.

The most common complication of splints and casts is skin breakdown. Focal pressure over a bony prominence or an inadvertent depressed area caused by the surgeon's ill-placed fingers may cause skin and soft tissue pressure necrosis. Areas at risk are those with little soft tissue covering, such as the ulnar styloid, heel, and malleoli. Careful attention to padding and cast application will minimize these problems. Patients' attempts to soothe itching and irritation under the casts with the insertion of long and often sharp objects can also be the source of skin lacerations and abrasions. All complaints of pain under a splint or cast should be investigated by its removal and a thorough physical examination. A lost reduction can always be regained, but an area of pressure necrosis can threaten the viability of a limb. Extreme caution should be exercised when placing a splint on a patient that cannot communicate the presence of discomfort. Circumferential casts should be avoided in this patient population. Diligent skin checks are required.

A circumferential compressive device such as a cast can contribute to increased pressure in the compartments of the injured extremity. Because casts are nonyielding, swelling in the underlying compartments can result in compartment pressures high enough to cause ischemia to the limb.

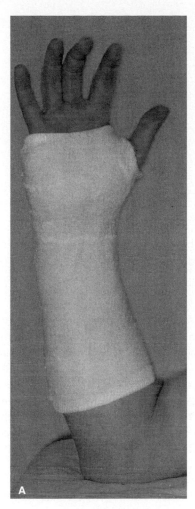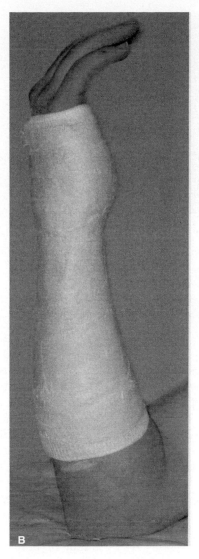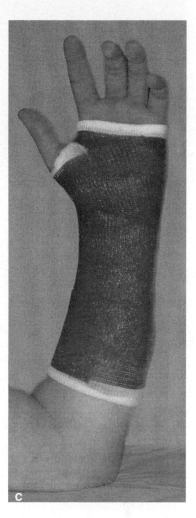

FIGURE 4-18. (A and B) A short arm plaster cast is demonstrated. Note the molding of the cast to resemble the shape of the palm. The forearm is molded into a cylinder. **(C)** A fiberglass short arm cast is shown. Much less molding is allowed with this material.

All complaints of unrelenting compression should be investigated. A cast can be bivalved, and one half removed at a time to inspect the limb. A reduction maintained by the cast, if lost by removing the cast, can always be regained. The sequelae of compartment syndrome are irreversible. Other complications of immobilization devices include joint stiffness, peripheral nerve palsy, and regional pain syndrome.

Traction

Traction is a type of splint. Traction will improve alignment and plays some role in reducing fracture motion by restoring soft tissue tension. Traction can be applied to the skin or through the skeleton. Skin traction is used in pediatric patients with femur fractures. Skeletal traction involves placing a transfixion pin through the distal femur, proximal tibia, or calcaneus. The pin is tensioned with a bow, and weights applied (Figure 4-19). The pull of the weights should be executed in line with the femur if traction is used for pelvic or femoral fractures, and in line with the longitudinal axis of the tibia if used for tibial fractures. Complex balanced suspension systems have been erected to suspend the limb; however, a pillow under the leg is often all that is required to keep pressure off the heel. Skeletal traction is useful in restoring pelvic morphology when there is superior migration of a hemipelvis after fracture. It is also used as a temporizing device in patients with lower extremity

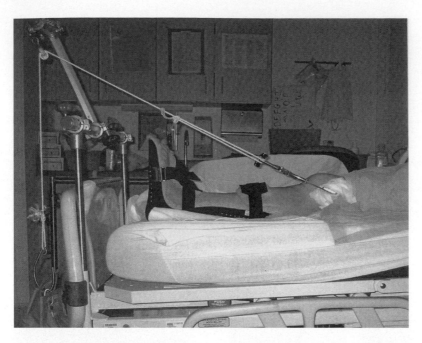

FIGURE 4-19. A temporary skeletal traction set up is demonstrated in this photograph. A pin is placed in the distal femur. A prefabricated padded splint with heel relief is placed on the foot to prevent equinus contracture and to protect against pressure necrosis.

fractures when the patient or the limb is not ready for definitive operative treatment. In a patient with severe head injury, elevated intracranial pressures, and a femur fracture, definitive treatment of the femur fracture may result in secondary brain injury. Length and alignment of the femur fracture can be maintained in traction until the brain injury improves. Distal tibia fractures are often accompanied by major soft tissue swelling and blistering. With the foot elevated on a Braun-Bohler frame, calcaneal traction can maintain limb length and alignment until the skin is ready for operative treatment.

Skeletal traction is rarely used for definitive treatment. If a patient with a fracture can't tolerate surgery, or if the fracture cannot be treated with the resources available, traction can be used for definitive treatment. This technique is fraught with complications associated with prolonged bed rest including global deconditioning and muscular atrophy, skin breakdown, venous thromboembolism, urinary tract infections, pneumonia, malnutrition, and the development of psychiatric disorders.

Operative Treatment

The priorities in treating the injured patient are to first save life, then limb, joints, and finally to restore function. Operative treatment of fractures does have

a role in resuscitation and can prevent mortality. Operative reduction of an anterior-posterior compression type pelvic ring injury with external fixation can reduce pelvic volume and facilitate tamponade. Judicious early stabilization of pelvic and femur fractures has been shown to reduce mortality. However, early definitive operative treatment of all fractures may not be warranted. For a selected group of severely injured patients, definitive stabilization of long bone fractures may be detrimental. A more limited surgical approach with external fixation of pelvic and long bone fractures to restore length and alignment, or "damage control orthopedics," may be a safer approach until the patient's overall condition improves. Limb salvage priorities involve debridement of open fractures to reduce the risk of infection, vascular repair for ischemic limbs, and soft tissue reconstructive procedures. Joint salvage involves reconstruction of articular injuries, ligament reconstruction, and implementation of a rehabilitation exercise program.

Benefits of operative treatment of a fracture include stabilization of the injured limb, which reduces pain, facilitates mobility and rehabilitation, and shortens hospital stay. Operative restoration of correct limb alignment and articular congruity maximizes the chances of long-term successful rehabilitation. These benefits are noted; however, there are risks associated with operative treatment of fractures. Bleeding may occur that requires transfusion. Risks associated with transfusion include transfusion reaction, and the transmission of bloodborne pathogens. HIV and hepatitis have been transmitted by transfusion. Donor testing has reduced the risk of transmitting HIV and hepatitis, but has not eliminated it. Other bloodborne pathogens likely exist but are currently not identified. Mutations in currently existing nonpathogens may yield new pathogens. In addition, transient immunosuppression is seen with blood transfusions.

Infection is a risk of any surgical procedure. Risk factors for surgical site infections in orthopedic patients are related to increasing age, additional nosocomial infections, wound contamination, and number of operations. Open fractures have higher rates of surgical site infections than closed fractures. The infection rate in open fractures is even higher in the host with an immune deficiency.

Postoperative wound infections are a significant source of morbidity and mortality in the United States. The number of antimicrobial-resistant pathogens infecting wounds is on the rise. Wound infections almost always require rehospitalization and further surgery. Surgical debridements carry the risks of additional surgery. Antibiotic therapy often involves an indwelling central venous catheter and months of antibiotics. Antibiotics are potentially toxic to bone marrow, liver, hearing, and kidneys.

With the use of correct antibiotic prophylaxis, the rate of wound infections can be diminished but not eliminated. Factors in correct prophylactic antibiotic usage include using the correct antibiotic and redosing after two half-lives during the procedure. Antibiotics should be infused prior to the start of the procedure, up to 1 hour before. Prophylaxis should be stopped 24 hours after the procedure, to prevent the development of antimicrobial-resistant organisms.

Surgical treatment of fractures requires a complete knowledge of the surrounding anatomy. Injuries to nerves, arteries, and veins have been reported with operative treatment of almost every fracture. Nerve injuries can include neuropraxia or neurotomesis. Surgery about the spine runs the risk of spinal cord or nerve root injury. Vascular injuries can result in significant hemorrhage, and/or limb ischemia, and often require an intraoperative vascular surgery consultation. Tendon or ligament injury has also inadvertently occurred during surgery.

Other events that can occur in the perioperative period include myocardial infarction, cerebral vascular accident, pulmonary embolus, anesthesia complications, and nerve palsies and soft tissue breakdown from positioning and unrelieved pressure. Death can occur after fracture surgery. The rate of acute mortality after inpatient orthopedic surgical procedures is approximately 1% for all patients, and 3.1% for those having surgery for hip fractures.

Problems with delayed healing and nonunion occur with surgical treatment. Some patient factors contribute to delayed healing. Protein malnutrition, smoking, and use of nonsteroidal anti-inflammatory agents all prolong healing times and may predispose to nonunions. Surgeon-controlled factors include the degree of soft tissue stripping around the fracture. Every surgical move has its biological consequence. With every incision, the blood supply to the fracture is diminished. Careful consideration should be made to minimize iatrogenic ischemia to the fracture. Diminished blood supply from aggressive soft tissue stripping leads to longer healing times and higher infection rates.

Other problems that can arise with surgical treatment include loss of fixation, loss of reduction, regional pain syndrome, uncosmetic scarring, and stiff joints.

Despite these risks, there are indications for operative treatment of fractures. If acceptable alignment cannot be obtained, or if the alignment cannot be maintained by nonoperative means, then operative treatment is required. In some cases immobilization of a fracture is morbid to the patient or to the limb. Operative treatment of certain fractures is required to restore immediate weight bearing. The vast majority of hip fractures fall into this category (Figure 4-20). Irreducible fracture dislocations require operative reduction and internal fixation (Figure 4-21). Some fractures have so much displacement, healing without open reduction is unlikely (Figure 4-22). Open fractures are always treated operatively. Debridement of contamination and devitalized tissue reduces the rate of infection. Fractures associated with arterial injuries are treated operatively, to restore perfusion. Skeletal stabilization prevents disruption of the reestablished blood flow. Fractures with compartment

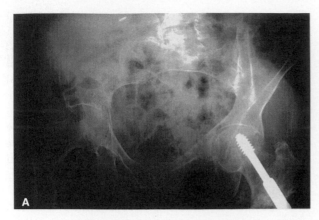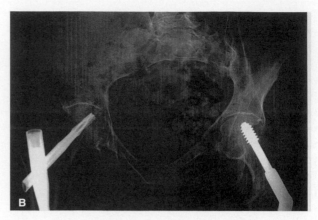

FIGURE 4-20. (A) Anterior-posterior radiograph of the pelvis of an elderly woman demonstrates a right intertrochanteric femur fracture with subtrochanteric extension (*arrow*). Note the previous left hip fracture treated with internal fixation. **(B)** The right proximal femur fracture was treated with an intramedullary hip screw. Weight bearing may start immediately postoperatively.

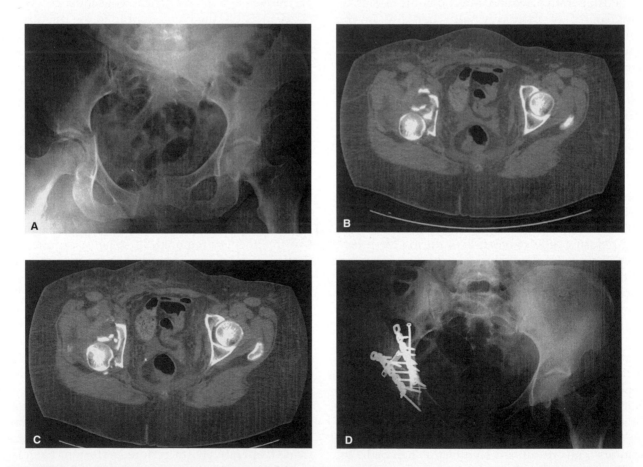

FIGURE 4-21. (A) Anterior-posterior radiograph of the pelvis demonstrates a symphysis pubis diastasis and a fracture dislocation of the right hip. Reduction of the hip is impossible due to osteochondral fragments in the acetabulum. **(B and C)** Axial computerized tomography images further demonstrate the posterior dislocation of the hip and intra-articular blocks to reduction. Operative reduction and internal fixation of the fracture were required. **(D)** Postoperative anterior-posterior radiograph demonstrates a reduced hip and internal fixation of the acetabular fracture.

syndrome are treated with fasciotomy and bony stabilization. Stabilization of the fracture prevents further soft tissue injury. Fractures caused by pathological processes invading and weakening the bone are treated operatively (Figure 4-8). Displaced articular fractures are thought to have the best outcome with anatomic reduction and internal fixation (Figure 4-23). Finally, patients who are multiply injured mobilize better with their fractures stabilized and have lower rates of morbidity and mortality. Fractures that, if occurred in isolation, are treated nonoperatively, such as humeral shaft fractures, can be treated operatively in multiply injured patients. Certain areas of the body require immediate mobility of the adjacent joints to prevent stiffness and diminished function. The upper extremity is extremely sensitive to prolonged immobilization. Fractures about the elbow and fingers are often treated operatively, so enough stability can be obtained that immediate range of motion exercises can be performed in the surrounding joints.

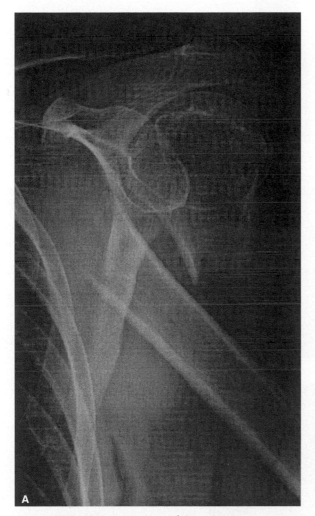
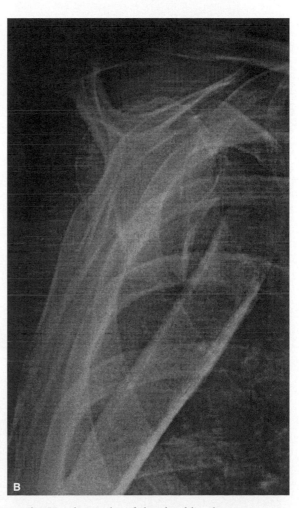

FIGURE 4-22. (A and B) Anterior-posterior and scapular Y radiographs of the shoulder demonstrate a widely displaced humeral neck fracture. Healing is unlikely with this degree of displacement, and operative reduction and fixation are indicated. **(C and D)** Neer anterior-posterior and axillary views of the shoulder postoperatively demonstrate better reduction of the fracture and internal fixation with a locked plate.

continued

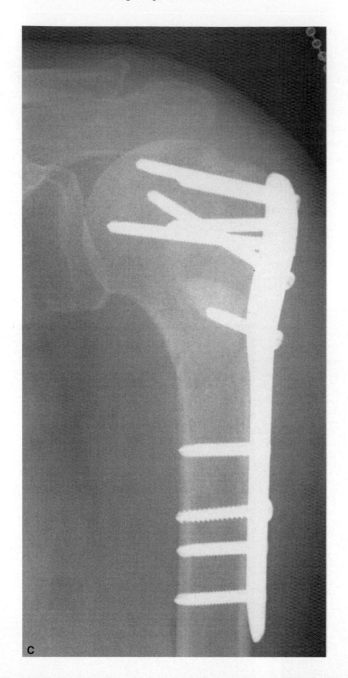

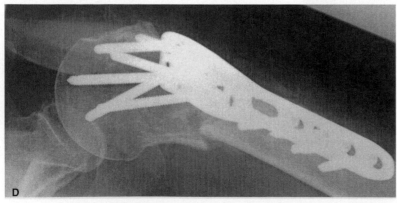

FIGURE 4-22. *(Continued)*

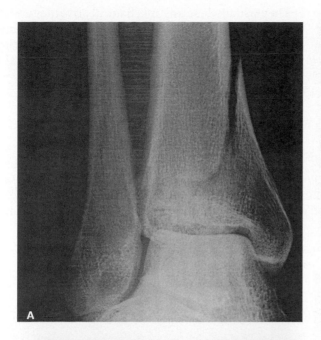

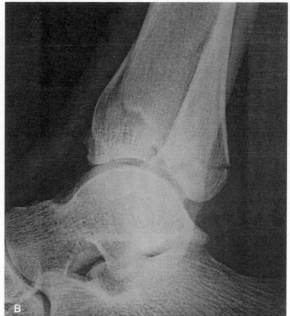

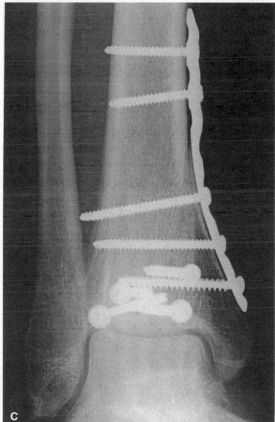

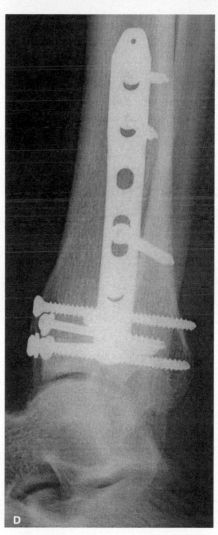

FIGURE 4-23. (A and B) Mortise and lateral views of the ankle demonstrate a distal tibia fracture with intra-articular extension. Gap and step-off of articular fragments creates an irregular joint surface. **(C and D)** Postoperative mortise and lateral radiographs reveal reduction of the articular surface maintained by plates and screws.

OPERATIVE TECHNIQUES FOR FRACTURE REDUCTION AND STABILIZATION

Closed Reduction and Percutaneous Pinning

Percutaneously placed Kirschner wires can supplement stability of a closed reduction. The small diameter wires have some purchase on both cortices, which supplements the stability of the construct (Figure 4-24). They have definite limitations in their ability to hold a reduction in unstable fractures.

They usually lose any mechanical advantage within several weeks. Percutaneously placed pins almost always require supplemental stabilization with a splint, cast, or external fixator (Figure 4-25C and D).

External Fixation

An external fixation system consists of threaded pins placed bicortically in bone, coupled to external bars and clamps. This technique provides relative stability. External fixation has several advantages. It can be quickly applied and is completely modular.

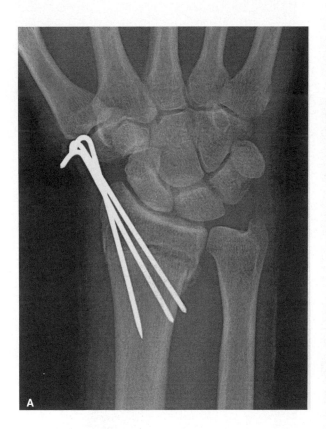

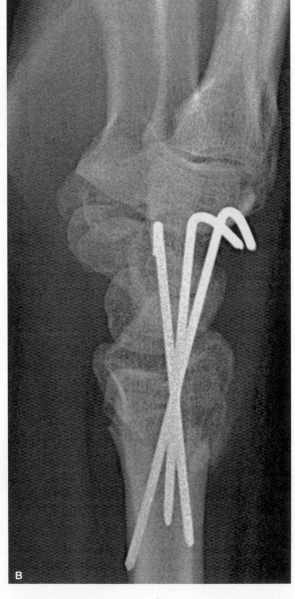

FIGURE 4-24. Posterior-anterior **(A)** and lateral **(B)** radiographs of the wrist demonstrate a distal radius fracture. Three Kirschner wires help maintain the reduction.

Pins can be placed at the surgeon's discretion, and the frame can be custom built. The fixation construct can also be modified at will. External fixation is the only fixation method where the surgeon has direct control over the construct stability. Stability is increased with anatomic fracture reduction, increased size of pins, increased pin spread within a fragment, decreased distance of bars to bone, increased number of bars, and a multiplanar frame. Conversely, the frame can be destabilized to decrease the stability. It is a good way to maintain proper length and rotation of the extremity. This is commonly referred to as "traveling traction." The technique is tissue friendly. Pins can be placed around wounds or marginal

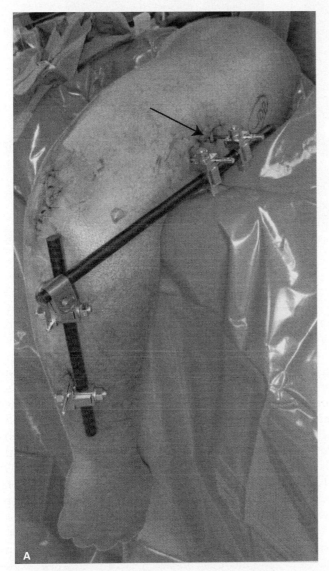

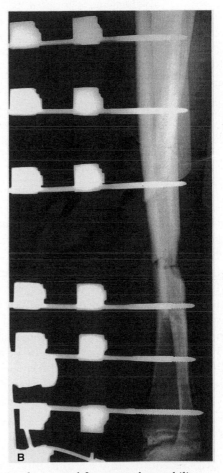

FIGURE 4-25. (A) This clinical photograph demonstrates a simple external fixator used to stabilize an open distal humerus fracture. A generous incision was created to insert the humeral pins in an effort to avoid injury to the radial nerve. **(B)** Lateral radiograph of the tibia demonstrates a diaphyseal fracture with posterior bone loss. The reduction is maintained with an external fixator. Two sets of pin-to-bar clamps are seen anterior to the tibia. As the bone heals, the frame can be destabilized by gradually disassembling the construct. **(C and D)** External fixation is useful for definitive treatment of distal radius fractures. Anterior-posterior and lateral radiographs of the wrist demonstrate this application. The traction provided by the external fixator maintains the metaphyseal reduction with the assistance of Kirschner wires.

continued

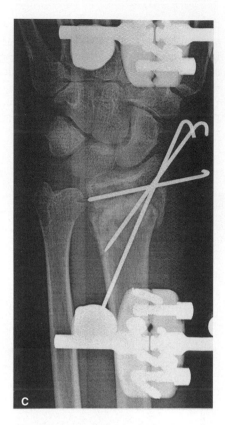
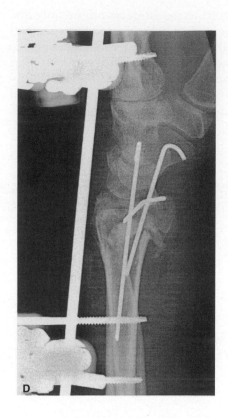

FIGURE 4-25. *(Continued)*

quality skin. The technique can also be used for reconstructive tasks such as deformity correction or distraction osteogenesis.

Different types of external fixators exist. Inserted into the bone are large threaded pins or small tensioned wires. Pins can be cylindrical or tapered. The pins are generally coupled to bars and clamps, and thin wires are tensioned and connected to rings. External fixation systems can be completely modular, or consist of prefabricated frames with use directed toward specific regions (wrist, ankle). New hinged external fixators are used to hold the reduction of an unstable knee or elbow, while allowing range of motion of the joint.

Pins are usually inserted through stab incisions in the lower extremity. In the femur, pins are placed into the anterolateral quadrant. Tibial pins are inserted from the medial border. Talar and calcaneal pins are inserted from medial to lateral, avoiding the medial neurovascular bundle. In the upper extremity, pins are inserted through a generous incision and dissection to avoid nerve injury (Figure 4-25A). A thorough knowledge of cross-sectional anatomy is required before placing small transfixion pins. At least two pins or wires should be inserted into each fragment.

Pin failure is the limitation of the technique. Pin failure is the result of infection and loosening. Pin tract infection is nearly universal. The incidence of infection varies by site. Fleshy areas such as the arm, pelvis, and thigh have more pin site infections than areas with less tissue, such as the tibia. Slight purulent drainage or localized cellulitis is treated with increased local care and oral antibiotics. If this fails, or cellulitis becomes regional, systemic antibiotics are required. With advanced infection, osteolysis occurs around the pin and can be visualized on radiographs. With the pins loose, they must be removed, and the tract curetted. Osteomyelitis or a sequestrum can develop from infected pins. Additional pins in noninfected area may need to be placed to accommodate for the lost stability of the construct.

Despite the ubiquitous problem of pin tract infections, no standard pin care system has been recommended. Physicians vary in their recommendations from half strength peroxide, peroxide, Betadine, soap and water, chlorhexidine solution, and dilute bleach. The pins should be covered to prevent external contamination. Fleshy areas should be compressed with the dressings to prevent pistoning of tissue on the skin, which contributes to tissue necrosis and infection. Pins should have complete release of the surrounding soft tissue. Tenting of the skin causes necrosis, which predisposes the tract to infection. The threaded portion of the screw should stay below the skin surface. Pin tract infections will definitely affect future stabilization options. In the tibia, a pin tract infection is considered a contraindication for subsequent intramedullary nailing. This scenario is tolerated somewhat better in the femur.

Taking steps to preserve the pin-bone interface can minimize pin loosening. Mechanical and thermal damage to the bone from drilling and pin insertion can cause osteonecrosis, which weakens the critical interface and predisposes to infection. Drills should be sharp and irrigation cooled, and pins inserted under manual power. As the rigidity of the construct increases, less strain on the pins occurs. This also helps preserve the critical interface. Weight bearing on an unstable fracture should be avoided. Stress overload at the pin-bone interface puts pin at risk for failure. The bone-pin interface is stronger in cortical than cancellous bone. Hydroxyapatite coating on the pins improves osteointegration and the strength of the bone-pin interface, and prevents loosening. This corresponds to a reduction in infection of pin tract.

With time, almost all pin-bone interfaces will become loose, and the frame will become ineffective in maintaining alignment of the bone. This is why external fixation often leads to nonunion or malunion when prolonged stabilization is required. Open tibia fractures, which have long healing times, develop more malunions with external fixation compared to intramedullary nailing. Hydroxyapatite-coated pins have been shown to reduce malalignment with external fixation systems left on for long periods of time, such as for tibial lengthening.

External fixation may be used as a temporizing technique until the patient or limb is ready for definitive stabilization. Care must be taken with subsequent intramedullary nailing in the tibia, for infection rates are higher. External fixation can also be used as definitive treatment.

External fixation is a good method of definitive treatment for fractures that have an articular injury and metaphyseal comminution. Distal radius and distal tibial fractures are common fractures that fit this description. These injuries require precise articular reduction with maintenance of correct length through the comminuted metaphyseal segment. External fixation is usually applied to preserve length of the limb, and articular reduction is performed through small, directed incisions. Fixation in the metaphyseal and diaphyseal sections are not required, they will heal with callus (Figure 4-25C and D).

External fixation is suited to fractures that require a dynamic mechanical environment. The modularity of the frame of an external fixator allows the surgeon to slowly destabilize the frame as the fracture heals, gradually applying more load to the bone and less to the fixator (Figure 4-25B).

In cases with large bony defects, external fixation may play a role in reconstruction. With large areas of bone loss, the external fixator will allow acute shortening of the limb, followed by gradual lengthening via distraction osteogenesis. This technique may obliviate the need for formal soft tissue coverage with local or rotational muscle flaps.

Intramedullary Nailing

The term *intramedullary nail* can be used to describe a variety of devices that are inserted into the medullary canal of a long bone. These implants are used to stabilize fractures, osteotomies, impending pathological fractures, and new regenerate bone after lengthening.

Intramedullary nails may be classified by some of their physical characteristics. Flexible nails have small diameters and uniform curvatures. Fixation is achieved by stacking several into the medullary canal, or by placing the curved nail to achieve three-point fixation. Larger diameter rigid nails are solid or hollow. Hollow or cannulated nails may be inserted over a guide wire. Hollow nails can be open section (slotted) or closed sectioned. Rigid nails may have interlocking capabilities. Proximal and distal perforations through the nail allow placement of screws that pass through bone and nail. Dynamic locking of the nail is with interlocking screws in one end. This locking allows some compression and micromotion at the fracture site. This treatment should be used only with axially stable fractures. Static locking uses interlocking screws in both fragments and is the best technique to control length and rotation. Nails are inserted with or without reaming. Reaming is the process where the intramedullary canal is enlarged by a motorized rotary curette. This method allows for the placement of a larger, stronger implant.

Nails are preferably inserted with closed technique, not exposing the fracture. Traction, manipulation, and fluoroscopy are required to achieve and maintain reduction. In open nailing, the fracture site is exposed. Currently, the preference is to avoid open nailing, except in certain subtrochanteric fractures where closed reduction almost always fails. By default open fractures are nailed with an open technique.

Many different styles of intramedullary nails have evolved over the past decades. Currently two types are used. Small diameter flexible nails are curved to achieve three-point fixation in the medullary canal of the bone. Multiple nails are used in the same bone to achieve many points of contact and interference fit between each other. These devices hold angulatory alignment well, but are less proficient in maintaining length and rotation. They are often used in children's fractures (Figure 4-26C). Adult femur and tibia fractures are treated with a cannulated interlocking nail. The cannulated design allows the use of a smaller guide wire to obtain the reduction. Reaming and nail insertion are performed over the guide wire (Figure 4-26A and B). Static interlocking is generally performed.

The nail and the bone form a composite material. The nail acts as a splint. Nail contact with the bone occurs at the insertion site, diaphysis, and interlocking screws. There is some motion at the

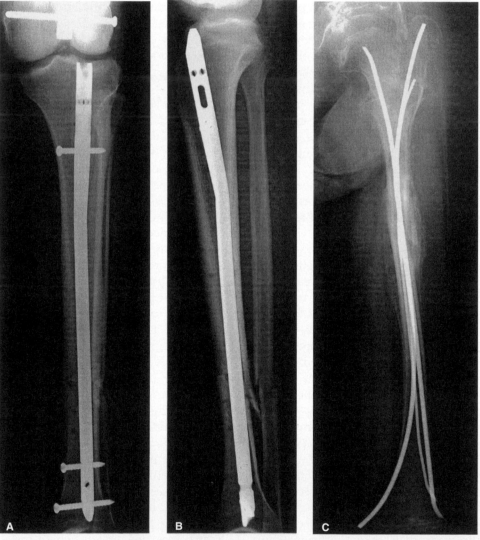

FIGURE 4-26. (A and B) Anterior-posterior and lateral radiographs of the tibia demonstrate a statically locked intramedullary nail placed to stabilize a diaphyseal tibia fracture. Note the intramedullary nail in the femur as well. **(C)** Anterior-posterior radiograph of the femur in a child demonstrates multiple small flexible nails stabilizing a femoral shaft fracture.

fracture site. This promotes callus formation. As the bone heals, it gradually assumes more of the load and less stress is seen by the implant. Ideally, the bone-nail composite has enough fatigue resistance to allow fracture healing to occur, yet is not overly rigid to impair the physiologic stimulus for healing. One advantage of this technique is that the implant is load sharing, and the construct is strong enough to allow immediate weight bearing.

Advantages of intramedullary fixation include providing good fracture stability through a minimally invasive technique of insertion. The soft tissue envelope around the fracture is preserved, minimizing surgical devascularization of the injured bone. The implant is central in the bone, close to the mechanical axis of the limb, which is optimally positioned to reduce bending forces. Proximal and distal locking control length and rotation. Early weight bearing, even in comminuted fractures, is allowed with this configuration.

Reamed statically locked nails is the method of choice for fractures of the diaphyseal femur and tibia. New nail designs with more peripheral and variable angle interlocking screws, and with techniques such as blocking screws, can be used for fractures in the metaphyseal area. Nailing is not always the best treatment method for all long bones. Intramedullary nailing of humerus fractures results in more complications, and more secondary surgery. Intramedullary nails have also been developed for the fibula and forearm, but have limited indications.

Disadvantages of intramedullary nailing are few. Loss of fixation, loss of reduction, and malunion occur, but are usually due to poor patient selection or poor implant selection. The fracture is usually too peripheral for the interlocking screws to hold the reduction, and an alternative fixation scheme may provide more stable fixation. Another source of healing problems is hardware failure. Smaller interlocking screws used with smaller nails in tibia fractures tend to break more often, however, hardware failure is not always associated with nonunion or malunion.

The timing of fracture fixation in the multiply injured patient, particularly the timing of femoral nailing, is often controversial. For the vast majority of patients, fixation of long bone (particularly femur fractures) within the first 1 to 2 days is beneficial. Shorter duration of ventilator dependence, shortened length of stay in the hospital, and lower rates of acute respiratory distress syndrome, pneumonia, and other pulmonary problems has been reported.

It is thought that some multiply injured patients cannot tolerate early intramedullary nailing of the femur or tibia. It has been proposed that those patients with significant pulmonary injuries have higher rates of adult respiratory distress syndrome and mortality after this procedure, but others have disputed this conclusion.

There is also concern about early intramedullary nailing of femur fractures in patients with closed head injuries and elevated intracranial pressures. The fear is that the femur stabilization will cause secondary brain injury. Factors associated with secondary brain injury are hypotension, hypoxia, and subsequent decreased cerebral blood flow. Cerebral perfusion pressure has been found to decrease intraoperatively during reamed intramedullary nailing of the femur. Early fixation of femur fractures in patients with head injury is thought to be safe; however there is no clear-cut guidance from the literature and treatment should be tailored to the individual patient.

Open Reduction and Internal Fixation

Open reduction and internal fixation is indicated for fractures with unacceptable alignment after closed reduction and immobilization, lower extremity limb malalignment, and articular incongruity. In some cases open reduction and internal fixation is warranted to allow immediate weight bearing, or because the patient's outcome will be better than nonoperative treatment.

In general, for some fractures the quality of reduction is very important. Articular fractures are thought to require perfect anatomic reduction for best outcome. Gaps or step-offs in the articular surface produce areas of stress concentration, which is thought to lead to posttraumatic arthrosis. However, not all joints require perfect articular reduction for good results. The outcome of acetabular fractures is dependent on the quality of reduction. However, there is little proof that accurate articular reduction of tibial plateau fractures is important for a good clinical outcome. The results in intra-articular fractures about the proximal interphalangeal joint depend more on maintaining joint reduction than articular reduction. Other factors such as age and infection also affect the outcome after articular fracture.

Reduction in nonarticular fractures can have a significant affect on function. The radius morphology must be anatomically reduced to allow full forearm rotation (Figure 4-27). Metacarpal and phalangeal fractures must have no malrotation or the fingers will not be parallel, which is functionally disabling. Apex anterior angulation of a metatarsal neck fracture will lead to plantar prominence of the metatarsal head, producing a painful prominence with weight bearing.

In fractures of the lower extremity, restoration of correct axial alignment of the limb is just as important as the quality of articular reduction. If a fracture malreduction leads to varus or valgus alignment of the knee or ankle relative to the floor, ambulation becomes awkward and painful, deformity results with subsequent degenerative changes in the affected joints. For the femur and tibia, varus and valgus tolerances approach 5°. Malrotation in the lower extremities is poorly tolerated if the difference between limbs exceeds 10°. Shortening of

the lower limb greater than 1 cm results in symptomatic leg length discrepancy, and often requires orthotic management.

A variety of implants are used in internal fixation. Different fractures require different types of stability. Screws are usually considered to be cortical or cancellous. Cancellous screws have a larger outer diameter, a deeper thread, and a larger pitch than cortical screws. Screws used to obtain compression across a fracture site are termed lag screws. Compression occurs between the screw head on one cortex, and thread purchase on the far cortex. Screws are also used to secure a plate to the bone. Locked screws have threaded heads that fit into a corresponding thread on the plate hole, creating a fixed angle device (Figures 4-13, 4-28). Screws range in size from 1.1 mm to 7.3 mm. Screws can be solid or cannulated. Cannulated screws are placed over a smaller

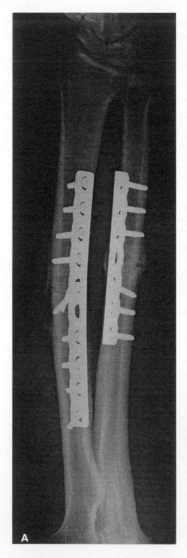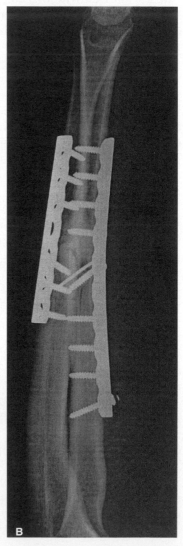

FIGURE 4-27. Anterior-posterior **(A)** and lateral **(B)** radiographs of the forearm demonstrate anatomic reduction of the radius and ulna. The reduction is maintained by 3.5 mm low contact dynamic compression plates and cortical screws. Perfect reduction of the radius is critical in restoring full forearm rotation.

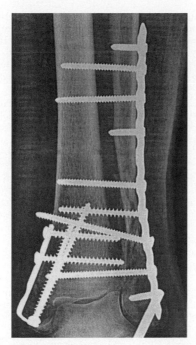

FIGURE 4-28. Anterior-posterior radiograph of the ankle in an elderly woman. Note the profound osteopenia. This difficult fracture is stabilized using a locking fibular plate. Several screws are passed from the fibula into the tibia to improve purchase of the implants.

guide wire, which may improve the accuracy of implant placement in critical areas.

Implants are broken into categories in the AO system. Minifragment implants include cortical screws from 1.1 mm to 2.7 mm. Small fragment screws are 3.5 mm cortical screws and 4.0 mm cancellous screws. Large fragment implants use 4.5 mm cortical and 6.5 mm cancellous screws. Cannulated 7.3 mm cancellous screws are available as a separate set. The size of the screw needed depends on the size of the bone, size of the fragment, and surgeon preference.

Plates vary in size and shape. The characteristics of a plate affect the plate's strength and contourability. Plates vary from 1.5 mm wafers in the minifragment set to stout, broad 4.5 mm dynamic compression plates. Tubular plates are thin, moldable, and placed in areas with little subcutaneous tissue. Dynamic compression plates allow variable placement of screws in the holes. With eccentric screw placement, compression can be achieved indirectly across the fracture. Limited contact dynamic compression plates have a lesser footprint to lessen the deleterious effect plates have on the underlying cortical circulation. Reconstruction plates have deep grooves between holes to allow more

complex contouring. Periarticular plates are designed to fit on a certain portion of a certain bone. The plate shape and type transitions as the needs differ in various areas of the bone.

A plate should be used to perform a specific task. Lag screws provide compression across a fracture site, but the lever arm is too limited to resist functional loading. Lag screws are often supplemented with a plate that resists these forces. This is a neutralization plate. A plate functions as a tension band when applied to the tension side of a fracture. Compression plating can be performed to compress a fracture without lag screws. A buttress plate has a supporting role. A locked plate acts as an internal external fixator, stabilizing the fracture with multiple fixed angle devices.

Internal fixation can produce absolute or relative stability. Absolute stability is achieved with lag screws and a neutralization plate. Motion is reduced to such an extent at the fracture site that primary bone healing occurs. Relative stability confers that all motion is not eliminated, but enough stability exists to allow bone healing and rehabilitation. A bridge plate is an example of relative stability. The screws couple the plate to the bone proximal and distal to the fracture, leaving this area alone.

Internal fixation implants maintain the desired alignment of the bone until the fracture heals. Unlike intramedullary nails, these implants are less load sharing, and weight bearing is usually not allowed until the bone heals.

REHABILITATION

An injury results in decreased physical activity for the patient. When the fracture is fresh or unstable, pain limits activity. Problems with limited activity include global deconditioning, muscle atrophy, joint stiffness, and disuse osteopenia. However, as the fracture heals, pain lessens, and activity level should slowly increase. Treatment modalities such as casts or braces will immobilize joints, producing stiffness. Immobilization also decreases cartilage nutrition, further insulting the joint. Some lower extremity fractures require physician-imposed restrictions on weight bearing, which makes locomotion with a walker or crutches unnatural and cumbersome.

The goal of treatment of a fracture is to return the patient to his or her vocational and recreational activities. Every injury is different, but each patient can tolerate some exercise. Patients should be encouraged to participate in joint range of motion exercises and muscle strengthening or maintenance exercises. An exercise program for all limbs should be established. For example, upper extremity strengthening exercises will improve crutch-walking endurance in the patient with a lower extremity injury.

When healing has progressed, gait training may be helpful as the patient transitions from wheelchair to independent ambulation. Balance and proprioception training are important factors in regaining normal function. Water exercise may be beneficial in maintaining strength and endurance in those who have restrictions on weight bearing, or are not quite comfortable exercising on land.

A licensed physical therapist may be helpful in providing instruction and feedback to the patient. The therapist also monitors the patient's progress, alerting the physician if no improvement or regression occurs. It should be made clear, however, that it is the patient's responsibility to perform all exercises as instructed, every day. Exercise should not be limited to physical therapy sessions only. The consequences of noncompliance should be emphasized.

Rehabilitation from upper extremity injuries can also be difficult. The emphasis in the upper extremity is early joint range of motion to prevent stiffness. Again, a licensed physical or hand therapist is part of the methodology, but should not be the sole source of exercise for the injured patient.

There are many facets to recovery. The rehabilitation team consists of not only physicians, nurses, and therapists, but also dieticians, social workers, and vocational counselors. The psychological impact of injury tends to be under-recognized by the medical team. The inclusion of a health psychologist to the team may benefit the injured patient. Considerable psychological distress has been identified in patients up to 2 years after severe lower extremity injury, and few get any mental health services.

Annotated Bibliography

Bone and Fracture Biomechanics

Bostrom MPG, Boskey A, Kaufman JK, et al. Form and Function of Bone. In: Buckwalter JA, Einhorn TA, Simon SA, eds. Orthopaedic Basic Science. 2nd Ed. Aurora, IL American Academy of Orthopedic Surgeons, 2000: 320–369.
This comprehensive chapter reviews the structure and function of bone. Topics covered include bone morphology, cellular mechanisms of bone remodeling, bone matrix composition, bone blood flow, biomechanics of bone, material properties of bone, bone metabolism and mineral homeostasis, age-related changes in bone mass and morphology, and metabolic bone disease.

Burr DB. Targeted and nontargeted remodeling. Bone 2002;30:2–4.
This is a review of the current understanding of bone microdamage and repair mechanisms.

Day SM, Ostrum RF, Chao EYS, et al. Bone injury, regeneration, and repair. In: Buckwalter JA, Einhorn TA, Simon SA, eds. Orthopaedic Basic Science. 2nd Ed. Aurora IL American Academy of Orthopedic Surgeons, 2000:371–400.
This comprehensive chapter is a definitive source of information on all aspects of bone injury and repair. The effects of bone repair after surgical intervention are well presented.

Harkess JW, Ramsey WC, Harkess JW. Principles of fractures and dislocations. In: Rockwood CA, Green DP, Bucholz RW, et al., eds. Rockwood and Green's Fractures in Adults. 4th Ed. Philadelphia: Lippincott-Raven, 1996:3–120.
This chapter in this classic fracture textbook provides a comprehensive review of important concepts related to fractures and dislocations.

Perren SM, Claes L. Biology and biomechanics in fracture management. In: Ruedi TP and Murphy WM, eds. AO Principles of Fracture Management. New York: Thieme, 2000:7–32.
This chapter is a well-illustrated and succinct summary of the biology of fracture healing, and how the process is altered by surgical stabilization.

Fractures in Multiply Injured Patients

Advanced Trauma Life Support Instructor Course Manual. Shock. 6th Ed. Chicago: American College of Surgeons, 1997.
This chapter summarizes the physiology, clinical manifestations, and treatment of hemorrhagic shock.

Geerts WH, Code KI, Jay RM, et al. A prospective study of venous thromboembolism after major trauma. N Engl J Med 1994;331:1601–1606.
This study reported the prevalence of thromboembolic disease in injured patients with no prophylaxis. Fifty-eight percent of patients had deep venous thrombosis (DVT), detected by screening venography and impedance plethysmography. Three of the 716 patients died of pulmonary embolism prior to screening. Five independent risk factors were determined for the development of DVT: older age, blood transfusion, surgery, fracture of femur or tibia, and spinal cord injury.

Pape HC, Giannoudis P, Krettek C. The timing of fracture treatment in polytrauma patients: relevance of damage control orthopedic surgery. Am J Surg 2002;183:622–629.
A historical overview of treatment philosophies for multiply injured patients with fractures is presented. The authors favor a "damage control orthopedics" philosophy when treating those multiply injured patients at high risk of developing systemic complications. This involves temporary stabilization, followed by definitive treatment when the patient's condition allows.

Initial Management of Fractures

Bottlang M, Krieg JC. Introducing the pelvic sling: pelvic fracture stabilization made simple. J Emerg Med Serv 2003;28:84–93.
Significant and rapid reduction in pelvic volume can be achieved in patients with pelvic ring injuries using simple methods of external compression.

Evaluation of the Limb

Hak DJ, Olson SA, Matta JM. Diagnosis and management of closed internal degloving injuries associated with pelvic and acetabular fractures: the Morel-Lavallee lesion. J Trauma 1997;42:1046–1051.
This is a review of the authors' experience with 34 patients with closed degloving injuries. Positive cultures were obtained in 46% of the patients and were related to time from injury to debridement. The authors recommend early debridement of the degloving injury, either before or at the time of fracture fixation, and leaving the wound open.

McQueen MM, and Court-Brown CM. Compartment monitoring in tibial fractures. The pressure threshold for decompression. J Bone Joint Surg Br 1996;78-B:99–104.

The authors determined the differential pressure measurement (diastolic pressure—compartment pressure) of 30 mm Hg to be a reliable threshold for fasciotomy. Using this criterion led to no missed cases of compartment syndrome in this group.

Complications of Operative Fracture Treatment

Bhattacharyya T, Iorio R, Healy WL. Rate of and risk factors for acute inpatient mortality after orthopaedic surgery. J Bone Joint Surg Am 2002;84-A:562–572.
Overall mortality for inpatient orthopedic procedures was 0.92%. The mortality rate was 3.1% for patients with hip fractures, and 0.5% for patients without hip fractures. Five critical risk factors were identified as most helpful in identifying patients at risk for death: chronic renal failure, congestive heart failure, chronic obstructive pulmonary disease, hip fracture, and age of greater than 70 years. A linear increase in mortality was seen with increasing numbers of critical risk factors.

deBoer AS, Mintjes-de Groot AJ, Severijnen AJ, et al. Risk assessment for surgical-site infections in orthopedic patients. Infect Control Hosp Epidemiol 1999;20:402–407.
Age, additional nocosomial infections, wound contamination class, preoperative stay, and numbers of operations were identified as important risk factors for orthopedic surgical-site infections in Dutch patients.

Farouk O, Krettek C, Miclau T, et al. Minimally invasive plate osteosynthesis: does percutaneous plating disrupt femoral blood supply less than the traditional technique? J Orthop Trauma 1999;13:401–406.
A cadaver vascular injection study demonstrated that a percutaneous submuscular plating technique preserved more blood supply to the bone than traditional open methods of plate application.

Giannoudis PV, MacDonald DA, Matthews SJ, et al. Nonunion of the femoral diaphysis: the influence of reaming and nonsteroidal anti-inflammatory drugs. J Bone Joint Surg Br 2000; 82-B:655–658.
A group of patients with femoral nonunions was compared to a group of patients with healed femur fractures. Fewer nonunions were noted in comminuted femoral fractures and in patients allowed early weight bearing. Nonsteroidal anti-inflammatory use after injury was significantly associated with femoral nonunion.

Harvey EJ, Agel J, Selznick HS, et al. Deleterious effect of smoking on healing of open tibia shaft fractures. Am J Orthop 2002;31: 518–521.
A retrospective review of tibial fractures treated with either external fixation or intramedullary nailing demonstrated patients who smoked had decreased rates of union, slowed healing, and increased complications.

Paiement GD, Hymes RA, LaDouceur MS, et al. Postoperative infections in asymptomatic HIV-seropositive orthopedic trauma patients. J Trauma 1994;37:545–550.
A retrospective review of patients with orthopedic injuries demonstrated a higher infection rate among asymptomatic HIV seropositive patients (16.7%) compared to HIV seronegative patients (5.4%). Differences in infection rate after open fractures were also significant, and became more significant as the severity of the open fracture increased.

Pinney SJ, Keating JF, Meek RN. Fat embolism syndrome in isolated femoral fractures: does timing of nailing influence incidence? Injury 1998;29:131–133.
The incidence of fat embolism syndrome was reviewed in a consecutive series of 274 patients with isolated femur fractures. No fat embolism syndrome was seen in patients older than 35 years. In those <35, if nailing of femoral fracture was performed early (<10 hours from injury), no fat embolism syndrome was observed. If femoral fracture stabilization was delayed, a 10% incidence of fat embolism syndrome was observed.

Raymond DP, Kuehnert MJ, Sawyer RG. CDC/SIS Position Paper. Preventing antimicrobial-resistant bacterial infections in surgical patients. Surg Infect (Larchmt) 2002;3:375–385.
The authors developed a multistep approach to help surgeons prevent antibiotic-resistant bacterial infections in their patients. The

focus of the recommendations includes steps to prevent infection, diagnose and treat infection effectively, use antibiotics appropriately, and prevent transmission of organisms.

Simon AM, Manigrasso MP, O'Connor JP. Cyclo-oxygenase-2 function is essential for bone fracture healing. J Bone Miner Res 2002;17:963–976.
Fracture healing failed in rats given COX-2 inhibitors and in COX-2 knockout mice. COX-2 is required for normal endochondral ossification.

External Fixation

Behrens F, and Johnson W. Unilateral external fixation: methods to increase and reduce frame stiffness. Clin Orthop 1989;241: 48–56.
This is a review of the mechanical properties of different external fixator constructs.

Moroni A, Vannini F, Mosca M, et al. State of the art review: techniques to avoid pin loosening and infection in external fixation. J Orthop Trauma 2002;16:189–195.
Hydroxyapatite coating of external fixator pins was the most effective technique to improve bone-pin interface. The effect was most evident with the use of tapered pins.

Tornetta P III, Bergman M, Watnik N, et al: Treatment of grade-IIIb open tibial fractures: a prospective randomised comparison of external fixation and non-reamed locked nailing. J Bone Joint Surg Br 1994;76-B:13–19.
This study demonstrated no advantage of external fixation in treating severe open tibia fractures. The rate of malunion was less in the group treated with intramedullary nailing. The authors feel the soft tissue management was improved with stabilization by intramedullary nails.

Intramedullary Nailing

Anglen JO, Luber, K, Park T. The effect of femoral nailing on cerebral perfusion pressure in head-injured patients. J Trauma 2003;54:1166–1170.
Seventeen patients with an intracranial pressure monitor underwent femoral nailing. A decrease in the cerebral perfusion pressure occurs nearly universally intraoperatively. The authors suggest careful management of the mean arterial pressure intraoperatively is critical to maintain cerebral perfusion pressure.

Bone LB, Johnson KD, Weigelt J, et al. Early versus delayed stabilization of femoral fractures: a prospective randomized study. J Bone Joint Surg Am 1989;71-A:336–340.
This prospective randomized study found that delayed stabilization of femur fractures in multiply injured patients resulted in increased rates of pulmonary complications and longer hospital stays.

Bone LB, Sucato D, Stegemann PM, et al. Displaced isolated fractures of the tibial shaft treated with either a cast or intramedullary nailing: an outcome analysis of matched pairs of patients. J Bone Joint Surg Am 1997;79-A:1336–1341.
This study examined the outcomes of operative versus nonoperative treatment of displaced tibial shaft fractures. Those treated with intramedullary nailing had shorter times to union. This group also had better knee, ankle, and SF-36 scores.

Bosse MJ, MacKenzie EJ, Riemer BL, et al. Adult respiratory distress syndrome, pneumonia, and mortality following thoracic injury and a femoral fracture treated either with intramedullary nailing with reaming or with a plate. J Bone Joint Surg Am 1997;79-A:799–809.
Patients with femoral fractures were treated with early reamed intramedullary nailing or plating, depending on the institution they were at. Groups included those with and without a significant chest injury. For patients without a chest injury, no difference in the rates of ARDS, pneumonia, pulmonary embolus, multi-organ failure, or death was seen between the two groups. Similarly, no differences in these complications were seen between the groups with a chest injury, when the two

stabilization techniques were compared. The authors concluded the use of reamed intramedullary nailing for acute stabilization of femur fractures in multiply injured patients who have a thoracic injury does not increase the occurrence of pulmonary complications or death.

Brumback RJ, Toal TR Jr., Murphy-Zane MS, et al. Immediate weight-bearing after treatment of a comminuted fracture of the femoral shaft with a statically locked intramedullary nail. J Bone Joint Surg 1999;81:1538–1544.
In patients with femur fractures treated with reamed statically locked intramedullary nails, immediate weight bearing is safe, even if the fracture is comminuted.

Charash WE, Fabian TC, Croce MA. Delayed surgical fixation of femur fractures is a risk factor for pulmonary failure independent of thoracic trauma. J Trauma 1994;37:667–672.
This duplication of Pape's study yielded different results. Delayed surgical fixation was associated with higher pulmonary complication rates, independent of the severity of thoracic injury.

Fakhry SM, Rutledge R, Dahners LE, et al. Incidence, management, and outcome of femoral shaft fracture: a statewide population-based analysis of 2,805 adult patients in a rural state. J Trauma 1994;37:255–261.
Nonsurgical treatment of femoral shaft fractures resulted in increased mortality. For multiply injured patients (ISS > 15) skeletal stabilization at 2 to 4 days was associated with the lowest mortality. In this group a trend toward higher mortality was observed with stabilization in the first day. The authors suggest further study warranted in the multiply injured patients, and an individualized approach is warranted.

Giannoudis PV, Veysi VT, Pape HC, et al. When should we operate on major fractures in patients with severe head injuries? Am J Surg 2002;183:261–267.
This review determines the available literature does not give definite guidance in the management of patients with fractures associated with brain injuries. The authors feel that treatment of the skeletal injuries should be tailored to the individual patient.

Johnson KD, Cadambi A, Seibert GB. Incidence of adult respiratory distress syndrome in patients with multiple musculoskeletal injuries: effect of early operative stabilization of fractures. J Trauma 1985;25:375–384.
This retrospective study demonstrated a significant increase in ARDS associated with a delay (>24 hours) in operative stabilization of major fractures in multiply injured patients. This was more apparent with the more severely injured patients (Injury Severity Scores > 40).

Keating JF, O'Brien PJ, Blachut PA, et al. Locking intramedullary nailing with and without reaming for open fractures of the tibial shaft: a prospective randomized study. J Bone Joint Surg Am 1997;79-A:334–341.
This study compared the outcomes of nails inserted with and without reaming in open tibial fractures. Equivalent outcomes were observed, with a higher rate of hardware failure in the unreamed group. Reamed intramedullary nailing is safe for open tibia fractures.

Pape HC, Auf'm'Kolk M, Paffrath T, et al. Primary intramedullary femur fixation in multiple trauma patients with associated lung contusion—a cause of post traumatic ARDS? J Trauma 1993;34:540–548.
In the presence of significant pulmonary injury, early intramedullary nailing causes additional pulmonary damage and may trigger ARDS. In the absence of chest trauma, early definitive stabilization of femoral fractures is beneficial to the patient.

Blachut PA, O'Brien PJ, Meck RN et al. Interlocking intramedullary nailing with and without reaming for the treatment of closed fractures of the tibial shaft. J Bone Joint Surg Am 1997;79-A:640–646.
This study compared the outcomes of nails with and without reaming in closed tibia fractures. Increased rates of delayed union and hardware failure were seen in the unreamed group.

Scalea TM, Scott JD, Brumback RJ, et al. Early fracture fixation may be "just fine" after head injury: No difference in central nervous system outcomes. J Trauma 1999;46:839–846.
A review of patients with head injuries and associated pelvic or lower extremity injuries was performed looking for differences between early versus delayed skeletal fixation. Early fracture fixation was not found to negatively influence brain injury outcome or mortality.

Open Reduction and Internal Fixation

Matta JM. Fractures of the acetabulum: accuracy of reduction and clinical results in patients managed operatively within three weeks after the injury. J Bone Joint Surg Am 1996;78-A: 1632–1645.
This review of operative treatment of acetabular fractures demonstrated the quality of reduction was related to the postoperative clinical results. Anatomic reduction and avoidance of complications resulted in the best clinical results.

Marsh JL, Buckwalter J, Gelberman R, et al. Articular fractures: does an anatomic reduction really change the result? J Bone Joint Surg Am 2002;84-A:1259–1271.
The authors review the data available on articular reduction and patient outcome. Topics covered include the effects of articular injury, articular step-off, accuracy of the measurement of articular displacement, and the effects on the accuracy of reduction on outcomes of specific fractures.

McCormack RG, Brien D, Buckley RE, et al. Fixation of fractures of the shaft of the humerus by dynamic compression plate or intramedullary nail: A prospective, randomised trial. J Bone Joint Surg Br 2000;82-B:336–339.
A prospective randomized trial of intramedullary nailing versus dynamic compression plating for unstable humerus fractures demonstrated higher rate of complications with the use of intramedullary nails. The authors feel that intramedullary nails may have specific indications, but dynamic compression plating is the standard of care.

Perren SM, Frigg R, Hehli M, et al. Lag Screw. In: Ruedi TP and Murphy WM, eds. AO Principles of Fracture Management. New York: Thieme, 157–168.
This well-illustrated chapter provides a concise review of the mechanics and applications of lag screws.

Wittner B, and Holz U. Plates. In: Ruedi TP and Murphy WM, eds. AO Principles of Fracture Management. New York: Thieme, 2000:169–186.
This well-illustrated chapter provides a concise review of the mechanics and use of different types of plates in fracture surgery.

Rehabilitation

Eastwood EA, Magaziner J, Wang J, et al. Patients with hip fracture: subgroups and their outcomes. J Am Geriatric Soc 2002;50:1240–1249.
In this review of 571 patients with hip fractures, 33 to 37% returned to prior levels of function 6 months after fracture. Only 25% were independent ambulators at that time. The authors developed five subgroups with 6 month outcomes that clinicians may use to predict functional recovery for patients.

McCarthy ML, MacKenzie EJ, Edwin D, et al. Psychological distress associated with severe lower-limb injury. J Bone Joint Surg Am 2003;85-A:1689–1697.
Two years after severe lower extremity injury, almost one-fifth of patients had severe phobic anxiety and/or depression (versus 2 to 3% rate in general population). Factors associated with psychological disorders in these patients include poorer physical function, younger age, nonwhite race, poverty, a likely drinking problem, neuroticism, poor sense of self-efficacy, and limited social support.

II

General Disorders of the Musculoskeletal System

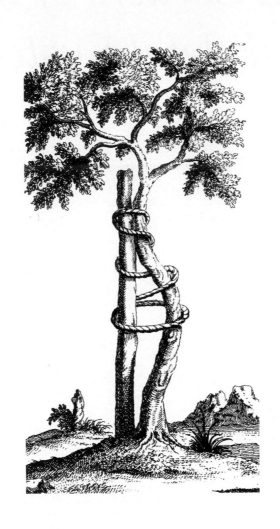

Neil E. Green
Joseph Jacob Nania

Bone and Joint Infections in Children

This chapter discusses the diagnosis and treatment of different forms of acute and subacute osteomyelitis and septic arthritis. The treatment of these bone and joint infections has evolved. We currently recommend a short course of IV antibiotics for almost all types of bone and joint infections followed by oral therapy. Surgical debridement is necessary for infections with documented abscesses and where there has been bone destruction. The debridement of the infected bone enhances antibiotic penetration and thereby shortens the course of IV antibiotics. Antibiotic therapy alone is sufficient if the bone infection is diagnosed early, and there is no abscess found or bone destruction seen radiographically. The need for arthrotomy for the drainage of acute septic arthritis of the hip has become controversial. Nevertheless, most authors and pediatric orthopaedic surgeons feel that anterior arthrotomy of the hip is the safest and most secure means of drainage of the infected hip. Other forms of bone and joint infection are discussed thoroughly.

DIAGNOSIS AND TREATMENT OF OSTEOMYELITIS AND SEPTIC ARTHRITIS

The treatment of bone and joint infections in children has continued to evolve since the development of antibiotics in the early 1940s. We have witnessed the development of penicillin resistance by staphylococci and the subsequent development of the semisynthetic penicillins and cephalosporins, which eradicate these penicillin-resistant staphylococci. Because of the risk of chronic bone infection, acute hematogenous osteomyelitis was traditionally treated with 6 weeks of intravenous (IV) antibiotics in the hospital. However, a short course (5 to 10 days) of IV antibiotics in the hospital followed by a longer course of oral therapy has been shown to be effective in eradicating these infections. The incidence of acute bone and joint infections in children has declined. The reason for the decline is unclear; however, numerous articles in the literature have documented this reduced incidence of these infections.

ACUTE HEMATOGENOUS OSTEOMYELITIS

Classification

Osteomyelitis in children may be classified in various ways. The age of the child at the onset of the infection determines the type of infection that develops. Acute hematogenous osteomyelitis behaves differently in neonates from the way it does in children. Because of the existence of blood vessels that cross the growth plate in neonates and infants younger than age 18 months, the bone infection that develops in that age group will likely cross the physis; however, in older children, acute infections rarely cross the growth plate (Figure 5-1).

Osteomyelitis may also be classified according to the severity of the infection and the rapidity with which it develops. Acute hematogenous osteomyelitis has a rapid onset, and children with this illness are usually seen within one to several days from the onset of the infection. Another form of bone infection is subacute hematogenous osteomyelitis, which resembles the acute form; however, the children are less ill, and the infection causes fewer systemic findings (Table 5-1). Chronic osteomyelitis is usually present for months before either detection or treatment. It may also result from inadequate treatment of an acute bone infection. It more commonly

is the result of an infection that is secondary to an open fracture of a long bone.

Osteomyelitis may result from hematogenous spread of the infecting organism, which is the most common means of production of osteomyelitis in the child. Bone may also become infected secondarily from the spread of a contiguous area of infection, although this is uncommon. A bone infection may also result from direct inoculation of bacteria. If infection occurs, it is usually the result of an open fracture of a long bone or penetration of a bone such as is seen after nail punctures of the foot. Lastly, bone infections may be classified according to the type of infectious agent. Both pyogenic and granulomatous organisms may infect bone. We discuss only pyogenic infections in this chapter.

Pathogenesis

The metaphyses of long bones is where acute hematogenous osteomyelitis begins. The nutrient artery of the long bone divides within the medullary canal of the bone, ending in small arterioles that ascend toward the physis. Just beneath the physis, these arterioles bend away from the physis and empty into venous lakes that drain into the medullary cavity. It is here, in the bend of these arterioles, that the infection begins. Bacteria injected into the osseous circulation are phagocytosed in the medullary cavity of the bone; phagocytosis, however, seems to be less active in the metaphysis. This differential in phagocytosis may explain the predilection of the metaphysis for the development of acute hematogenous osteomyelitis. A lack of reticuloendothelial cells in the metaphysis often exists, so bacteria that lodge there are more likely to multiply and establish an infection. The bacteria may also lodge in the metaphysis because of a decrease in the rate of circulation at the bend of the terminal arterioles before they empty into the venous lakes. Nade has shown with the use of electron microscopy that the new metaphyseal vessels that are growing as the physis itself grows have a lack of an endothelial lining. Therefore, the blood that circulates in these vessels is in direct contact with the recently ossified metaphyseal bone. Not only would the red blood cells be in direct contact with the osteocytes, but any circulating bacteria would also directly contact the metaphyseal bone. This fact is the most likely reason for the nearly universal localization of acute hematogenous osteomyelitis in the metaphysis of long bones.

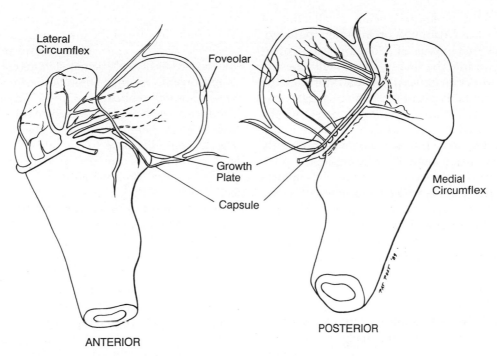

FIGURE 5-1. Views of the hip in a neonate. The intraosseous circulation in the femoral head of a neonate is different from that in a child older than 12 to 18 months. Blood vessels are seen crossing the growth plate in the femoral neck and head of a neonate.

Trauma may be associated with the establishment of a bone infection in a certain location. Children with acute hematogenous osteomyelitis frequently complain of trauma as an inciting incident. It is well known that the trauma may simply bring the child's attention to a preexisting lesion. It has been shown, however, that rabbits in whom a bone is traumatized develop an infection more frequently in the traumatized bone than in nontraumatized areas after the production of a bacteremia. Clinical evaluations of patients with acute hematogenous osteomyelitis frequently reveal a history of blunt trauma to the affected bone. This may well be an accurate cause and effect, but the association of trauma is always considered by anyone who has a painful extremity whether or not trauma is the cause.

Once established, the infection produces an exudate, and if the infection remains untreated, pus is produced. The fluid formed seeks the path of least resistance for egress from the metaphysis. The fluid can spread in one of three ways. It can spread from the metaphysis into the diaphysis; it can spread into the epiphysis across the physis; or it can exit

TABLE 5-1.
Comparison of Acute and Subacute Hematogenous Ostemyelitis

	Acute	Subacute
White blood cell count	Frequently elevated	Frequently normal
Erythrocyte sedimentation rate	Frequently elevated	Frequently elevated
Blood cultures	50% positive	Rarely positive
Bone cultures	90% positive	60% positive
Localization	Metaphysis	Diaphysis, metaphysis, epiphysis, cross physis
Pain	Severe	Mild to moderate
Systemic illness	Fever, malaise	No
Loss of function	Marked	No or minimal
Prior antibiotics	Occasional	30%–40%
Initial radiograph	Bone normal	Frequently abnormal

the cortex of the bone, producing a collection of subperiosteal pus. Although an infection that commences in the metaphysis of a long bone may occasionally spread into the diaphysis, it rarely does so. Instead, the infection generally spreads through the cortex of the metaphysis of the bone of a child. It is important to this discussion to understand the anatomy of a human bone at different ages to appreciate how the same infection behaves differently in patients of various ages. For example, the presence of transphyseal vessels in the neonate allows an infection that begins in the metaphysis of a long bone to easily spread into the epiphysis through these vessels (see Figure 5-1).

In the child older than 1 year to 18 months, an osteomyelitis that begins in the metaphysis of a long bone usually spreads through the cortex of the metaphysis. The metaphyseal cortex of the infant is porous, thereby providing easy access for the egress of an exudate or pus. As the fluid exits the bone cortex, it elevates the periosteum, which in the child is loosely adherent to the cortex of the bone. The periosteum is, however, thick and therefore not easily penetrated, so the pus remains subperiosteal until there is enough periosteal destruction to allow the development of a soft tissue abscess. The periosteum of the adult is more thickly adherent to the bone cortex, but it is also much thinner and easily torn.

If an osteomyelitis progresses in a child, the infection that begins in the metaphysis produces loss of the endosteal blood supply of the involved bone because of thrombosis of the venous and arterial blood supply. Once pus escapes through the metaphyseal cortex, it elevates the periosteum, thereby depriving the bone of its remaining vascular supply. The portion of the bone that has become avascular is termed *a sequestrum*. The elevated periosteum remains viable because its blood supply, which is derived from the overlying muscle, is undisturbed. The cambium layer of the periosteum continues to produce bone; however, this bone is produced at a distance from the bone cortex because the periosteum has been elevated. This new periosteal bone is termed the *involucrum*.

Acute hematogenous osteomyelitis begins with a "cellulitis" phase in which no obvious pus has been produced. The patient will exhibit at the signs of a bone infection, but there will be no obvious pus formation. If this infection is left unchecked, an abscess will form. The pus then escapes through the cortex of the metaphysis of the long bone, producing a subperiosteal abscess. This concept of an initial cellulitis of bone is important because it is during this stage that medical treatment alone usually results in cure of the infection.

Staphylococcus aureus—the organism that causes the most cases of acute hematogenous osteomyelitis—is responsible for more than 90% of cases in otherwise normal children. Other organisms may produce acute hematogenous osteomyelitis, such as bacteroides, pneumococcus, *Kingella kingae*, and *Haemophilus influenzae*. In neonates, *Staphylococcus* is still common, as are group B *Streptococcus* and Gram-negative organisms. In patients with sickle cell disease, both *Staphylococcus* and *Salmonella* are known to cause acute hematogenous osteomyelitis. Group-A β-hemolytic *streptococcus* is the most common organism in patients with bone, joint, and soft tissue infections (necrosing fasciitis), which occur as a complication of varicella. This organism may also be seen in children who have not been infected with varicella. They tend to be very young (preschool age), have a very high temperature, and have a high leucocytosis.

Diagnosis

The diagnosis of acute hematogenous osteomyelitis depends on a high index of suspicion. Children with acute bone pain and systemic signs of sepsis should be considered to have acute hematogenous osteomyelitis until proved otherwise. Unfortunately, not all children with osteomyelitis have the characteristic findings typically associate with this disease, so the diagnosis is not always easily made. It is important, however, to make the diagnosis of acute hematogenous osteomyelitis early in the course of the disease, because both the course of the disease and its ultimate prognosis depend on the rapidity and adequacy of treatment.

For those instances in which an absolute diagnosis has not been established, the diagnosis of acute hematogenous osteomyelitis may be established if a patient fulfills two of the following criteria: (1) bone aspiration yields pus; (2) bacterial culture of bone or blood is positive; (3) presence of the classical signs and symptoms of acute osteomyelitis exists; and (4) radiographic changes typical for osteomyelitis occur. It is important to have diagnostic criteria for acute hematogenous osteomyelitis; these criteria should include the typical patient history and physical findings because occasionally the cultures of bone may be negative. Even with negative cultures one may make the presumptive diagnosis of acute hematogenous osteomyelitis if other criteria have been established. Most of the time, however, the diagnosis of acute hematogenous osteomyelitis may result from the typical history and physical findings combined with positive bone and blood cultures. Not all patients with acute hematogenous osteomyelitis will have positive bone or blood cultures; therefore, the other above criteria may have to be used to confirm the diagnosis. Interestingly, it has been shown that culture negative patients have a less severe disease than do culture positive patients with acute hematogenous osteomyelitis. They are less likely to have antecedent trauma, overlying skin changes, and less duration of pain.

History and Physical Examination

Children with acute hematogenous osteomyelitis usually present with a history of bone pain of one to several days' duration. The pain may be well localized if the child is old enough to cooperate. The pain may be poorly localized if the child is young or if the area of involvement produces confusing findings, such as might be seen in patients with osteomyelitis of the pelvis. The pain usually is severe enough to seriously limit or completely restrict the use of the involved extremity. The child usually is febrile and relates a history of generalized malaise consistent with the generalized sepsis. Some children, however, present without generalized sepsis and therefore do not exhibit all of these complaints. Thus, do not exclude the diagnosis of acute hematogenous osteomyelitis simply on the basis of a lack of sepsis, because this disease may be more or less virulent depending on the organism involved and the host resistance.

The physical examination of these children is extremely important to establish the correct diagnosis. The examination may be difficult to perform because these children are frightened and experience considerable pain. Approach the child slowly and carefully, gaining the child's confidence before beginning the examination. This usually takes a few extra minutes, but the time is well spent. First attempt to establish which limb is involved before the examination begins and also have an idea where in the limb the pain is localized. The examiner begins by palpating the uninvolved areas of the extremity after the rest of the child has been examined. The final portion of the examination focuses on the area of involvement.

Children with acute hematogenous osteomyelitis usually have swelling of the involved extremity. The swelling is localized to the area of the infection unless the infection has spread to involve much of the soft tissues of the extremity. Early in the course of the disease, the swelling is localized to the metaphysis of the involved long bone, which is warm. The overlying skin, however, is not red unless the bone involved is subcutaneous or unless the infection has spread and a subcutaneous abscess has developed.

Laboratory Data

It is important to obtain laboratory studies in every child suspected of having osteomyelitis; however, acute bone and joint infections are diagnosed by clinical means, and laboratory studies are used only as confirmatory evidence and never to make a diagnosis.

A complete blood count and an erythrocyte sedimentation rate should be obtained, both of which are usually elevated. In addition, the differential count of the white blood cells frequently shift left. Although these blood studies are usually abnormal in children with acute hematogenous osteomyelitis, never dismiss the diagnosis of acute hematogenous osteomyelitis simply because the white blood cell (WBC) count or the sedimentation rate is normal. Neonates frequently have no signs of infection; which makes the diagnosis of osteomyelitis more difficult in them.

Radiographic Findings

Radiographs of the involved extremity should be obtained; however, the bone changes that are characteristic of osteomyelitis are not seen for at least 10 to 14 days after the onset of the infection. Soft tissue swelling with loss of the normal soft tissue planes is seen before bone changes become apparent. The radiographic finding of soft tissue swelling, however, simply confirms the findings of a good physical exam that has established the existence of the swelling and determined its location (Figure 5-2). Magnetic resonance imaging (MRI) has not been shown to be of greater benefit for the evaluation of suspected osteomyelitis than have other more conventional modalities, but in some instances MRI may be useful in the evaluation. Gadolinium-enhanced MRI has the advantage of excellent delineation of fluid collections and soft tissue. It is, therefore, helpful in identifying medullary edema

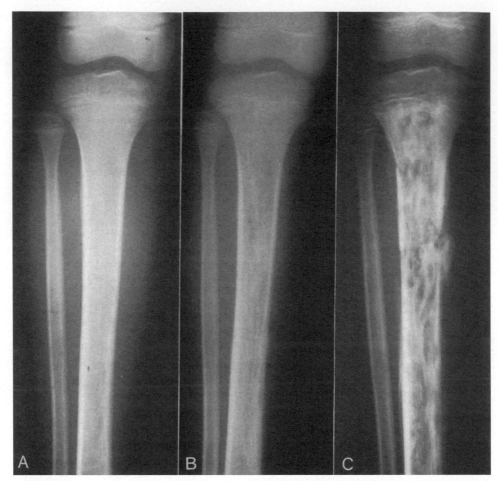

FIGURE 5-2. Radiographs of a child with progressive radiographic changes as the result of acute hematogenous osteomyelitis of the tibia. **(A)** AP radiographs of the tibia that demonstrate soft tissue swelling with loss of the normal tissue planes. **(B)** Radiographs of the same leg taken 2 weeks after the one in A. Note the early mottled appearance of the tibia with a small amount of periosteal new bone seen on the medial cortex of the tibia. **(C)** Five weeks after presentation this AP radiograph of the tibia shows progressive destruction of the entire diaphysis and proximal metaphysis of the tibia. (Courtesy of Dr. R.H. Hensinger)

consistent with osteomyelitis in cases where the diagnosis is unclear and in identifying subperiosteal or adjacent soft tissue abscess that may require drainage. Additionally, MRI has been used to differentiate osteomyelitis from acute medullary bone infarct in patients with sickle cell disease and systemic lupus erythematosus. Cost and need for sedation in young children are the main disadvantages of MRI in comparison to other imaging techniques.

Bone Scan

Bone scanning has become a popular method for the evaluation of children with suspected osteomyelitis. With the advent of technetium-99m (^{99m}Tc) bone scanning, the evaluation of the abnormal bone in the child became possible. The low radiation dose of this radioisotope and its affinity for bone make it ideal for the evaluation of the skeleton. The ^{99m}Tc is taken up in areas of rapid bone formation or in areas of increased blood flow. Thus, one would expect that there would be increased uptake of ^{99m}Tc in areas of acute hematogenous osteomyelitis, but this is not always the case. The bone scan has been shown to have an accuracy rate as low as 80% in patients with acute hematogenous osteomyelitis. In some children, especially those in whom the infection is fulminant, the involved bone may have become avascular by the time of the scan, producing a cold scan. The reason for the cold scan is the loss of the endosteal circulation as a result of occlusion of the nutrient artery along with the loss of the periosteal circulation resulting from the elevation of the periosteum by a subperiosteal abscess. •This cold scan should alert one that the infection of the bone demands immediate drainage.

The bone scan may be used to help confirm the diagnosis of osteomyelitis much as one would use the sedimentation rate or the WBC count; however, treatment must never be delayed while awaiting the results of a bone scan. It is important to note that needle aspiration of a bone does not alter the bone scan. Thus, bone aspiration itself will not cause a bone scan to be positive.

Bone scanning may be helpful when the exact localization of an acute infection is in doubt, such as in infections of the spine or the pelvis. Bone scanning may be of use in neonates, in whom multiple sites of infection are common, and it may also be helpful in the case of bone pain in children with sickle cell disease, for whom the differential diagnosis of acute hematogenous osteomyelitis from acute bone infarction is difficult.

Gallium scanning has been advocated by some authors, because radioactive gallium localizes in white blood cells and would seem to be more specific for osteomyelitis than is ^{99m}Tc. Gallium scanning may be more specific than technetium scanning, but it is not more sensitive. If a ^{99m}Tc scan is negative, a gallium scan is likely to be negative also. In addition, the gallium scan requires at least 24 to 36 hours for an adequate study. Some authors have advocated the use of gallium scanning for the differentiation of bone infarction from osteomyelitis in patients with sickle cell disease.

MRI may help with the diagnosis of subperiosteal or soft tissue abscess, especially if there is an inadequate response to antibiotic therapy.

Bone Aspiration

Once a clinical diagnosis of acute hematogenous osteomyelitis is established, a bacteriologic diagnosis is made by culturing the involved bone. Bone aspiration is mandatory not only to establish an accurate bacteriologic diagnosis but also to determine whether an abscess is present. Aspiration of the bone should be performed immediately after completion of the physical evaluation so that treatment may be started.

The bone should be aspirated at the point of maximum swelling and pain, which is usually at the metaphyseal end of a long bone. Use a large bore needle such as a 16- or 18-gauge spinal needle

with an inner stylet. The stylet is necessary to prevent plugging the end of the needle with bone. The needle is inserted just to the outer cortex of the bone, and the subperiosteal space is aspirated. If an abscess is encountered, the pus is cultured and a Gram's stain is performed. In this instance, the diagnosis has been firmly established, and the need for drainage of the abscess has been determined. If no abscess is encountered, the needle is advanced into the bone through the cortex, which can be accomplished with ease in the metaphysis. The needle is gently twisted as it is advanced into the bone. Once the needle is through the cortex and is in the medullary cavity of the bone, the marrow is aspirated. Usually one obtains only marrow, but this must be cultured because almost invariably the cultures are positive. If no pus is found, the infection is in an early cellulitis stage (i.e., before an abscess has developed). If an abscess is encountered, it should be cultured and surgically drained.

In addition to obtaining cultures of the involved bone, obtain cultures of any and all lesions that could potentially have been the source of a bacteremia. Blood cultures should be obtained, too, but they should not be relied on to make a bacterial diagnosis because only 50% of patients with acute hematogenous osteomyelitis have positive blood cultures. We have studied a large group of patients with confirmed acute hematogenous osteomyelitis to evaluate the rate and location of bacterial recovery. We found that there were about 50% of blood cultures positive as has previously been reported. In addition, about 60% of the bone aspirations were positive for bacteria. When we combined both bone and blood culture the bacterial recovery rate was 70%, therefore, the likelihood of obtaining a bacteriologic diagnosis is enhanced if cultures of all possible sources plus the blood have been obtained. Isolating an etiologic organism for susceptibility testing has become even more important in recent years as rates of colonization and infection with methicillin-resistant *S. aureus* (MRSA) continue to rise in pediatric patients. MRSA is found not only in patients with identifiable risk factors (i.e., health care acquired), but also increasingly in those lacking traditional risk factors (i.e., community acquired).

Treatment

To effectively treat acute hematogenous osteomyelitis, sufficient antibiotic must be delivered to the site of the infection for an adequate period to sterilize the bone and eradicate the infection. Controversy occasionally arises between pediatrician and orthopaedist concerning the appropriate form of treatment. The pediatrician may recommend only parenteral antibiotic therapy, whereas the orthopaedic surgeon may recommend both surgical drainage and antibiotic treatment. This controversy will not arise if acute hematogenous osteomyelitis is considered an infectious disease rather than either a surgical or a medical disease. Principles of the treatment of infection then become evident. It is well established that sequestered abscesses require surgical drainage, but areas of simple inflammation without abscess formation respond to antibiotics alone. Therefore, bone aspiration is important in determining the future course of therapy for the child with an osteomyelitis. If an abscess is encountered either under the periosteum or within the bone itself, surgical drainage of the abscess is required. If no abscess is found, antibiotics alone should suffice in eradicating the infection, because treatment begins during the cellulitis stage of the infection, before the formation of an abscess.

Surgical drainage should also be considered when the patient does not respond to appropriate antibiotic therapy after a negative bone aspiration. In that instance, an abscess may have developed that requires drainage. If a child with acute hematogenous osteomyelitis does not show symptomatic improvement with decrease in swelling and tenderness after 36 to 48 hours of appropriate antibiotic treatment, the bone should be aspirated again and surgical drainage considered. The fever should also begin to decline, although it may remain elevated for several more days.

If surgical treatment is necessary, the bone involved should be approached directly over the area of involvement. A subperiosteal abscess should be thoroughly drained and debrided. Whether or not the bone should be opened is subject to debate. Some authors think that if a subperiosteal abscess is found, an intraosseous abscess is not likely because it would have spontaneously drained itself into the subperiosteal space through the porous metaphyseal cortex. Conversely, if no abscess is found under the periosteum, the intraosseous abscess will not have drained itself into the subperiosteal space, and the bone must be opened. Although we and others have not found pus under pressure within the bone cortex at the time of drainage of a subperiosteal abscess, it is probably wise to drill the metaphyseal cortex to be certain that no abscess is sequestered within the bone. It is probably not necessary to widely open the bone to curette it unless pus is discovered at the time of drilling of the bone cortex.

Surgical treatment, if needed, should not create more tissue damage than has already been created by the infection itself. If pus escapes through the metaphyseal cortex, the periosteum is elevated and the periosteal blood supply is compromised, leaving the bone cortex avascular. When draining an abscess, do not elevate the periosteum more than it has already been elevated, so as to avoid creating further sequestration of the bone.

Once the abscess is adequately debrided, the wound may be closed over a drain. It is not necessary nor recommended to leave the wound open, unless dealing with a chronic, long-standing osteomyelitis. A suction drain or a Penrose drain may be used and removed in 2 to 4 days. Closed suction-irrigation is not necessary and introduces a significant risk of superinfection with Gram-negative organisms.

Antibiotics

Antibiotics are begun immediately after all cultures are obtained, whether or not surgical drainage is necessary. The initial choice of antibiotic is made on a best-guess basis. At least 90% of the cases of acute hematogenous osteomyelitis in otherwise normal children are caused by coagulase-positive staphylococci. Thus, the antibiotic chosen should be one that effectively treats this organism. For patients who are not allergic to penicillin, a semisynthetic penicillin that is β-lactamase resistant should be chosen. The antibiotic of choice is either oxacillin or nafcillin. Methicillin is also effective, but this antibiotic carries a higher risk of interstitial nephritis than do the others. These agents remain the most rapidly bactericidal drugs for susceptible strains of staphylococci, have a desirably narrow spectrum of activity, and demonstrate a proven track record in the treatment of acute osteomyelitis. In choosing nafcillin, be careful with peripheral needle sites for the administration of the drug IV, because nafcillin may cause significant sloughing of the skin and subcutaneous tissues if infiltration of the IV solution occurs (Table 5-2). Cefazolin is an acceptable alternative, at a dosage of 150 mg/kg/24 hr, in place of the semisynthetic penicillin. In patients with identifiable risk factors for MRSA, empiric use of vancomycin should be considered while awaiting culture and susceptibility data. In places where a significant percentage of community-acquired staphylococcal isolates are

TABLE 5-2.
Doses of Antibiotics Used in Osteomyelitis

Medication	Daily Dose in mg/kg (adult maximum)	Interval in Hours
Intravenous		
Nafcillin or Oxacillin	150–200 (12 g)	6
Cefazolin	100-150 (6 g)	8
Clindamycin	40 (2.7 g)	6–8
Vancomycin	60 (4 g)	6–8
Foot Puncture Wounds:		
Ceftazidime	150 (6 g)	8
Cefepime	150 (4 g)	8
Piperacillin	200-300 (18 g)	4–6
Ticarcillin (+/- Clavulanate)	200–300 (24 g)	6
Tobramycin	5-7.5 (5 mg)	8
Oral		
Dicloxacillin	100 (2 g)	6
Cephalexin	150 (4 g)	6
Cefadroxil	50 (2 g)	12
Clindamycin	20 (1.8 g)	6–8
Rifampin	20 (600 mg)	12
(not appropriate for monotherapy)		
Foot Puncture Wounds:		
Ciprofloxacin	30 (1.5 g)	12
(see text for comment on use in children)		

methicillin resistant, local susceptibility patterns of such isolates should guide empiric antibiotic choice. Clindamycin has generally been effective in treating community-acquired MRSA infections in children, including acute osteomyelitis, and this is a particularly attractive option in patients who are allergic to penicillin. Regardless of risk factors or local rates of resistance, it is recommended that patients with life-threatening infections likely to be staphylococcal be treated empirically with both vancomycin and a semisynthetic penicillin such as oxacillin or nafcillin.

The recommended dosage of oxacillin is 150 to 200 mg/kg administered in divided doses over 24 hours. The appropriate length of therapy has been a subject of debate for many years. In the past, children with acute hematogenous osteomyelitis were treated for 6 weeks with IV antibiotics in the hospital. It became apparent that this was excessive, and a regimen of 3 weeks of IV antibiotics followed by 3 weeks of oral therapy was adopted. Because studies have shown that adequate blood levels of antibiotic may be achieved with oral administration, the current mode of therapy involves a shorter period of initial IV therapy, given a good response by the patient, followed by oral therapy.

Combined IV and oral antibiotic therapy has now become accepted as the standard treatment for acute hematogenous osteomyelitis. This mode of therapy is more complicated than the simple treatment of the child with IV antibiotics for the entire course, because it requires the complete cooperation of the family and the child. In addition, the antibiotic must be adequately absorbed from the gastrointestinal tract, providing sufficient blood levels of the drug.

The current regimen is to begin treatment of the patient with IV antibiotics. If the patient responds quickly to this form of therapy, consider switching the child to oral antibiotics (Table 5-2). To do this, the patient must meet certain requirements (Table 5-3).

Antistaphylococcal antibiotic therapy is started while awaiting the culture results. Once the organism is identified, the antibiotic is adjusted if necessary. It is important to retain the bacteria so that the laboratory may test it against the antibiotic being used to be certain that adequate blood levels can be obtained. If the child responds quickly to the initial therapy with IV antibiotics, consider beginning oral therapy. The IV antibiotics are continued for at least 5 days, although some physicians prefer to treat with IV antibiotics for a longer period before beginning oral therapy. Oral therapy is begun 5 to 7 days after the initiation of IV therapy if the child shows a good clinical response to the initial treatment.

Oral therapy is begun in the hospital to be certain of compliance and patient tolerance of the drug. If the patient is reliable, he or she may be discharged

TABLE 5-3.
Contraindications to Oral Antibiotic Therapy

- Inability to swallow or retain the prescribed medicine
- Questionable or unreliable gastrointestinal absorption of antibiotics (e.g., short bowel syndrome, Crohn's disease, neonates)
- Inadequate response to intravenous therapy
- Response to intravenous antibiotic for which there is no oral equivalent (e.g., vancomycin) and etiologic agent not established
- Infection with organism for which there is no effective and acceptable oral antibiotic (e.g., multidrug resistant staphylococci)
- Parents' and patient's strict compliance with prescribed oral regimen in doubt

from the hospital and followed as an outpatient once all studies have been completed. Treatment should continue for a total of 4 to 6 weeks, which includes the time of IV and oral therapy combined (Table 5-3).

If there is adequate response to the IV therapy, oral dicloxacillin may be started at a dosage of 100 mg/kg/24 hr. As an alternative, cephalexin may be administered at a dosage of 150 mg/kg/24 hr. The oral suspension form of dicloxacillin is not palatable, and parents may find it difficult to persuade young children to swallow it. For that reason, cephalexin may be preferred, as the oral suspension of this antibiotic is more palatable. Cephalexin may also be used as the IV drug, at a dosage of 150 mg/kg/24 hr, in place of the semisynthetic penicillin. The oral dosage of clindamycin is 30 mg/kg/24 hr IV, followed by 50 mg/kg/24 hr by mouth. This is particularly attractive in patients who are allergic to penicillin. Clindamycin has excellent oral bioavailability, but as with dicloxacillin, the oral suspension has an unpleasant taste that may contribute to therapeutic noncompliance

Unfortunately methicillin resistant *S. aureus* (MRSA) has become a more common pathogen in bone and joint infections in children. This organism used to be thought of as hospital acquired, however, community-acquired MRSA is now seen very frequently. Accurate culture of bone and joint infections is necessary to document the organism because of the prevalence of MRSA. Any child who does not respond appropriately to adequate therapy should be considered to have infection caused by MRSA.

For methicillin-resistant staphylococcal organisms one should use vancomycin, 50 mg/kg/24 hr IV, combined with rifampin, 15 mg/kg/24 hr orally as covered earlier.

Neonatal Osteomyelitis

Osteomyelitis in the neonate is a different disease from that seen in children because of the variety of organisms involved, the frequency of multiple sites of infection, and the presence of transphyseal vessels

until age 12 to 18 months, which leads to infection on both sides of the physis. As a result, the infection destroys the center of ossification of the epiphysis and the physis itself, producing complete growth arrest (Figure 5-3). This is most likely to occur in the proximal femur, where the result is destruction of the head of the femur. The infection frequently spreads out of the involved epiphysis into the joint, producing a septic arthritis.

Osteomyelitis in the neonate frequently produces fewer clinical and laboratory signs than in the child. Although *Staphylococcus* may be the etiologic agent of the osteomyelitis, Gram-negative organisms and group B *Streptococcus* are also common; therefore, antibiotics that cover all of the organisms must be given while awaiting the results of cultures. Neonates with acute hematogenous osteomyelitis frequently have multiple sites of involvement—as often as 40% of the time. Infants with multiple sites of osteomyelitis are usually sick before the onset of

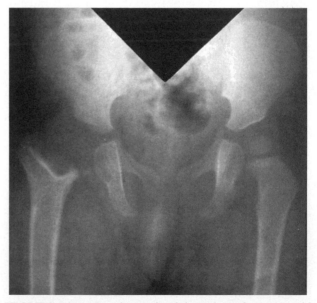

FIGURE 5-3. AP radiograph of the pelvis of a 1-year-old girl who had an osteomyelitis of the proximal femur and a septic arthritis of the hip as a neonate. These infections resulted in destruction of the physis and the epiphysis.

the infection, and most have an umbilical catheter. Infants with single sites of osteomyelitis have a milder disease and are generally less ill than those with multiple sites of infection.

Special Sites of Infection

Acute hematogenous osteomyelitis of the pelvis may be difficult to diagnose, requiring a high index of suspicion establish the correct diagnosis. Children with acute infection of the pelvis often are initially thought to have infection of the hip joint because the pain is frequently intense and often limits motion of the hip joint. The correct diagnosis can be established by performing a careful examination. Carefully moving the hip joint usually demonstrates a free, painless range of movement, whereas palpation of the pelvis establishes the area of maximum tenderness. Septic arthritis of the sacroiliac joint is also frequently confused with osteomyelitis of the pelvis. In this disease, tests specific for pain in the sacroiliac joint—such as the figure 4 test (one leg is placed across on top of the other leg with the knee bent to 90°, as in the number 4, and the pelvis is then rocked using the crossed leg as a lever arm) and pelvic compression—are positive. Plain radiographs of the pelvis are normal in the early stages of pelvic osteomyelitis and in septic arthritis of the sacroiliac joint. Bone scintigraphy usually is positive. As in acute osteomyelitis of other bones, however, a certain percentage of these infections have false-negative bone scans. Bacterial confirmation of the diagnosis is established by bone aspiration.

An abscess may develop in patients with acute hematogenous osteomyelitis of the pelvis. If this occurs, surgical drainage of the abscess is necessary. A child with acute hematogenous osteomyelitis of the pelvis should be evaluated in the same manner as the child with an infection of a long bone, with an appropriate history and physical examination. In addition, laboratory data should be obtained. Bone aspiration should also be performed, and antibiotics should be started once all cultures have been obtained. Because of the possibility of developing an intrapelvic abscess that is not detectable either on physical examination or through needle aspiration, CT or MRI scanning of the pelvis should be performed. If an abscess is seen, it should be drained through an appropriate surgical approach and the child treated with antibiotics to sterilize the bone (Figure 5-4).

Osteomyelitis of the spine in children and infants is rare, but does occur. As in osteomyelitis in other locations, *S. aureus* is the most common cause with a number of other organisms reported. Among the others, *Bartonella henselae* seems to have some predilection for infecting the vertebrae in an atypical manifestation of cat scratch disease. Also, *Salmonella spp.* have been reported as a cause of vertebral osteomyelitis in children without sickle cell disease. A much more common presentation of infection of the spinal column is the disc space infection, which is discussed in the subacute hematogenous osteomyelitis section. The mean age of patients with vertebral osteomyelitis is significantly higher than those with disc space infection. The latter is more commonly a disease of school-aged children (mean of 7 to 8 years), whereas the mean age for disc space infection is 2 to 3 years. True osteomyelitis of the spine produces significant bone destruction. Neonates with osteomyelitis of the spine develop abnormalities of the spine that resemble congenital defects.

Sickle Cell Disease

Acute hematogenous osteomyelitis in patients with sickle cell disease differs from osteomyelitis in otherwise normal patients. The two major differences in the two forms of osteomyelitis are that the infection in patients with sickle cell disease is usually located in the diaphysis of long bones rather than in the metaphysis. In addition, the organism responsible for the infection is frequently salmonella, although *S. aureus* is also common in patients with sickle cell disease. The salmonella bacteria enter the blood stream through microinfarcts in the gut lining, producing a bacteremia. The bacteria may then produce bone infection at the site of an acute bone infarction.

Patients with sickle cell disease and acute bone pain present a difficult diagnostic problem, because acute bone infarcts are painful and produce clinical findings often identical to those of patients with osteomyelitis. Thus, it is frequently difficult to differentiate between an area of acute bone infarction and one of acute osteomyelitis. The infarction and the infection are usually located in the diaphysis of a long bone, and both are associated with severe pain and restricted use of the involved extremity. Patients with acute osteomyelitis usually have a higher and more persistent fever than those with infarction. The sedimentation rate and peripheral WBC count may be elevated in both but are usually higher in patients with infection.

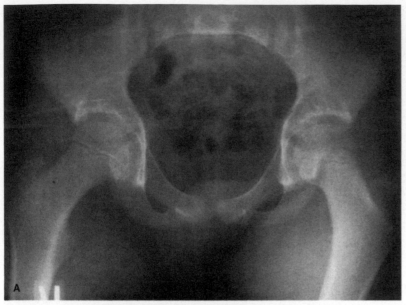

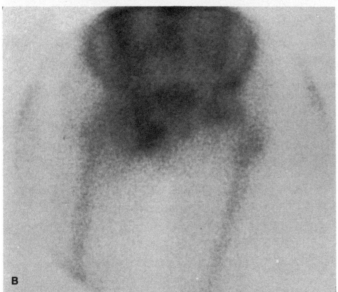

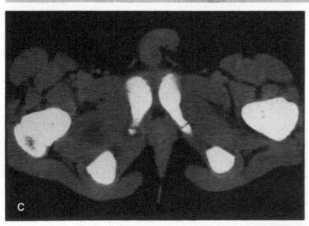

FIGURE 5-4. Eight-year-old boy with osteomyelitis of the pubis and a pelvic abscess. **(A)** AP radiograph of the pelvis of this child demonstrating no bony abnormalities. **(B)** Technetium-99m bone scan demonstrating increased uptake of the isotope in the region of the right pubis. **(C)** CT scan through the obturator region of the pelvis demonstrating an abscess in the obturator region of the right hemipelvis.

The diagnosis of acute osteomyelitis in these children may be difficult. As mentioned earlier, children with infection exhibit somewhat severer clinical findings. Bone scanning maybe helpful in these patients. Skaggs et al. (2001) have recently shown that one may be able to differentiate bone infarct from osteomyelitis with the use of both bone marrow and bone scans. They found that if the patient with bone pain has decreased uptake on a bone marrow scan and abnormal bone scan at the site of pain, the diagnosis of bone infarct could accurately be confirmed. If, on the other hand, there is normal uptake on bone marrow scan and abnormal uptake on bone scan, the diagnosis is suggestive of osteomyelitis. They also found that if both the bone marrow and bone scans were normal, the diagnosis was neither bone infarct nor osteomyelitis. One study with a relatively small number of patients, found gadolinium-enhanced MRI useful in distinguishing between bone infarct and osteomyelitis. Even with the findings on scanning that suggest the diagnosis of osteomyelitis, cultures of the patient's stool culture of the bone by bone aspiration should be performed to obtain bacteriological diagnosis.

SUBACUTE HEMATOGENOUS OSTEOMYELITIS

Subacute hematogenous osteomyelitis differs from acute osteomyelitis in the severity of the clinical signs. The systemic signs seen in patients with subacute forms of the disease are either absent or much less severe than those seen in patients with the acute form of the disease. In addition, the location of the subacute form of the disease may differ from that seen with acute osteomyelitis (see Table 5-1).

Classification

Some authors have classified subacute osteomyelitis according to the location and radiographic appearance of the lesion. This, however, does not consider the differences in clinical presentation of these different forms of subacute osteomyelitis. The classification based on radiographic appearance was first described by Gledhill and subsequently modified by others. In this classification, the type 1 lesion is a central metaphyseal lesion. The type 2 lesion is also metaphyseal, but it is eccentrically placed with cortical erosion present. The type 3 lesion is an abscess in

the cortex of the diaphysis, and the type 4 lesion is a medullary abscess in the diaphysis without cortical destruction but with periosteal reaction present. The type 5 lesion is primary epiphyseal osteomyelitis. The type 6 lesion is a subacute infection that crosses the physis (Figure 5-5).

This classification system excludes the subacute osteomyelitis that begins in the metaphysis and crosses the physis to involve the epiphysis. Acute hematogenous osteomyelitis in the child older than age 18 months rarely crosses the physis; however, subacute osteomyelitis frequently does. The lesion may be primarily metaphyseal with only a small portion of the physis and epiphysis involved (Figure 5-6). Conversely, much of the physis may be involved (Figure 5-7). In the neonate with acute hematogenous osteomyelitis that crosses the physis to involve the epiphysis, the physis is frequently destroyed as is the growth center of the epiphysis (see Figure 5-3). Conversely, the subacute infection that crosses the physis rarely causes permanent damage to the growth plate.

One may also subclassify subacute hematogenous osteomyelitis into two types according to the

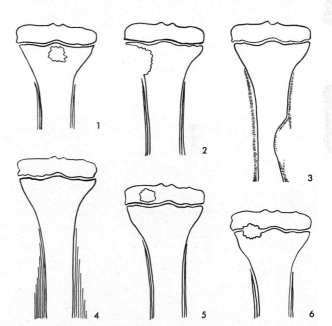

FIGURE 5-5. Classification of subacute osteomyelitis type 1 is a central metaphyseal lesion. Type 2 is an eccentric metaphyseal lesion with erosion of cortex. Type 3 is a lesion of cortex of diaphysis. The type 4 lesion of the diaphysis demonstrates periosteal new bone formation but without a definite bone lesion. Type 5 is primary subacute epiphyseal osteomyelitis, and type 6 represents subacute osteomyelitis that crosses physis involving both the metaphysis and epiphysis.

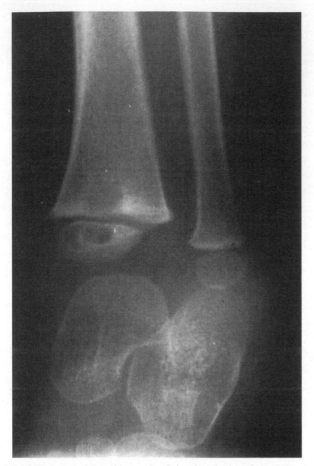

FIGURE 5-6. AP radiograph of the distal tibia demonstrating an area of subacute osteomyelitis that involves the metaphysis, physis, and the epiphysis.

rapidity of onset and severity of presenting symptoms. One type has a fairly acute presentation, and children with this type of infection usually present within a week or two of the onset of symptoms. Radiographic changes may be present at the time of presentation; however, the infection is usually diaphyseal. This type of infection thus encompasses types 3 and 4 of the Gledhill classification system. This diaphyseal infection could easily be confused with Ewing sarcoma, and a biopsy may be necessary to exclude this diagnosis. Frequently, however, the clinical and radiographic picture is characteristic enough to make a presumptive diagnosis of infection. Children with this type of subacute infection may have a fever, although it will not be as elevated in acute hematogenous osteomyelitis. In addition, children with this type of infection usually continue to walk even if the femur, the most commonly involved bone, is infected. They will, however, limp and complain of pain. The peripheral WBC count and the sedimentation rate may be elevated, although the sedimentation rate is more commonly elevated (Figure 5-8). The second type of subacute infection encompasses types 1, 2, 5, and 6. Children with this type of infection have minimal symptoms, but the complaints are frequently of longer duration. There are no systemic signs, and the peripheral WBC count and the sedimentation rate usually are normal. Radiographic changes are present at the time of presentation and may be described as a lucency located anywhere within a bone.

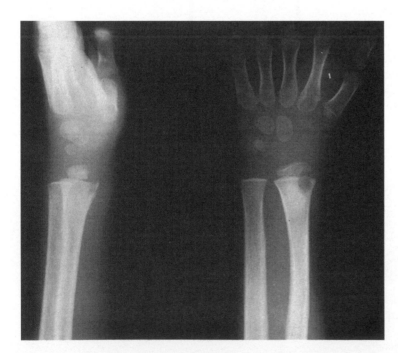

FIGURE 5-7. AP and lateral radiographs of a distal radius of a child with subacute osteomyelitis that crosses the physis. The AP radiograph demonstrates that the lesion involves both the metaphysis and the epiphysis. On the lateral radiograph, significant erosion of the epiphysis is seen.

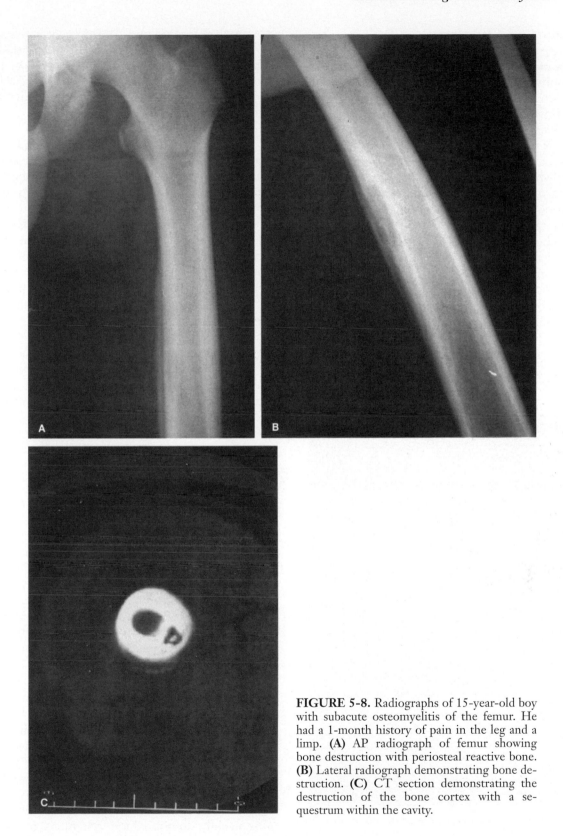

FIGURE 5-8. Radiographs of 15-year-old boy with subacute osteomyelitis of the femur. He had a 1-month history of pain in the leg and a limp. **(A)** AP radiograph of femur showing bone destruction with periosteal reactive bone. **(B)** Lateral radiograph demonstrating bone destruction. **(C)** CT section demonstrating the destruction of the bone cortex with a sequestrum within the cavity.

Diagnosis and Treatment

The diagnosis in patients with subacute infection of the diaphysis of a long bone is confirmed by bone aspiration for bacterial culture. The cultures usually are positive for S. *aureus*. The treatment of this diaphyseal lesion depends on several factors. If the diagnosis is in question, open biopsy may be required, at which time debridement is carried out if infection is established. If a sequestrum is present, sequestrectomy is required for eradication of the infection. Most commonly, however, the patient presents with minimal radiographic bone changes, and simple antibiotic therapy alone usually results in eradication of the infection, because no abscess is present.

Lesions of subacute osteomyelitis, of the metaphysis and epiphysis, can usually be diagnosed as subacute osteomyelitis radiographically; however, in some instances the diagnosis is in question. When the diagnosis is not clear radiographically, open biopsy is required in making the diagnosis (Figure 5-9). In addition, because there is a radiographic lesion, an

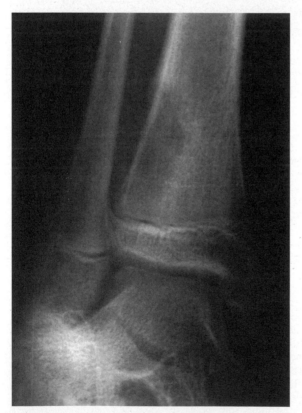

FIGURE 5-9. Oblique radiograph of the distal tibia of an 11-year-old girl with a 1-month history of pain, swelling, and redness of the ankle. A metaphyseal lesion of the distal tibia resembles subacute osteomyelitis; however, the biopsy revealed that the lesion was an osteogenic sarcoma.

abscess has formed and debridement is usually required, although some authors have reported healing without debridement. Frequently no pus is evident at exploration; however, one may find granulation tissue within the cavity that should be debrided. Cultures may be sterile, but *Staphylococcus aureus* and *Staphylococcus epidermidis* are the most common organisms. Some have suggested that debriding these lesions is not required. These lesions will heal with adequate antibiotic treatment. It has been recommended that patients be treated with antibiotics for at least 4 weeks or until significant healing is seen radiographically (Cole 1982; Ezra et al. 2002). Therefore, if one is comfortable with the radiographic diagnosis of subacute osteomyelitis, then antibiotic treatment alone without biopsy is appropriate. If there is inadequate response, as judged by the clinical course and radiographic healing, then biopsy is required.

The treatment of subacute osteomyelitis should be similar to that of acute osteomyelitis. Begin with IV antibiotics and switch to oral antibiotics if there are no contraindications. As mentioned earlier, debridement is usually necessary for subacute osteomyelitis with a radiographic lesion or if a sequestrum has formed or if the patient has not responded adequately to antibiotics.

CHRONIC RECURRENT MULTIFOCAL OSTEOMYELITIS

Chronic osteomyelitis may be defined as osteomyelitis presenting with symptoms that have been present for months or longer. Also included in the diagnosis of chronic osteomyelitis is any recurrent osteomyelitis. This chapter does not deal with the chronic osteomyelitis that results from a recurrence of a previously treated infection or from an open wound such as an open fracture. The only exception is the special circumstance of nail puncture wound infections of the foot, which are covered in the next section.

The cause of chronic multifocal osteomyelitis is unknown at the present time, but it is presumed to be due to an infectious agent. The disease produces vague bone pain in multiple sites. Frequently the symptoms seem to be unilateral, despite the fact that lesions occur bilaterally. Children with this disease usually do not exhibit systemic signs of infection such as an elevated temperature. Although the peripheral WBC count is normal, the sedimentation rate is frequently elevated.

Multiple lytic lesions that have little surrounding bone reaction and are generally located in the metaphyses of the long bones are seen radiographically (Figure 5-10). The medial end of the clavicle seems to be the bone that is most frequently involved, followed by the distal tibia and then the distal femur.

Based on clinical and radiographic findings, an infectious agent is thought to cause these lesions. The histology of these lesions is typical of osteomyelitis; however, the agent responsible has not as yet been identified with certainty. The treatment is symptomatic. The natural history of this disease usually involves spontaneous resolution of the lesions and the clinical signs and symptoms, which may take anywhere from 1 to 15 years.

Most authors have felt that this disease is an inflammatory disease that should be treated with nonsteroidal inflammatory drugs (NSAID). We have cultured *Mycoplasma* from three patients with this

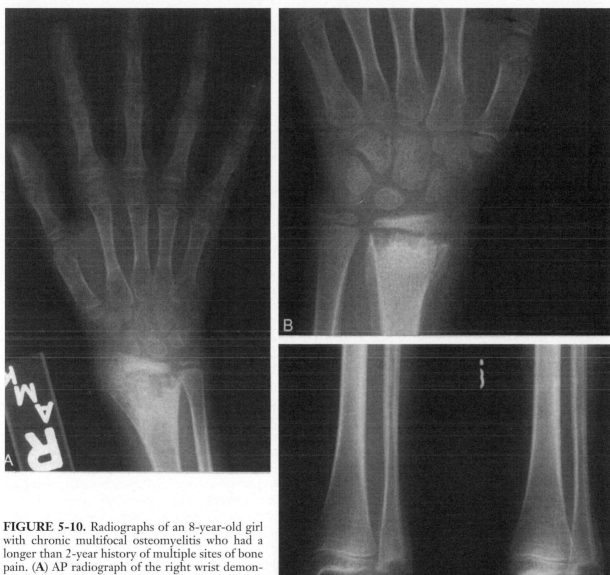

FIGURE 5-10. Radiographs of an 8-year-old girl with chronic multifocal osteomyelitis who had a longer than 2-year history of multiple sites of bone pain. (**A**) AP radiograph of the right wrist demonstrating bone destruction of the metaphysis, physis, and epiphysis. (**B**) AP radiograph of the left wrist demonstrating bone destruction in the metaphysis with periosteal reactive bone. (**C**) Radiographs of the left ankle demonstrating metaphyseal and physeal destruction of the distal fibula with periosteal reactive bone.

disease and have subsequently treated all of our patients with antibiotics that would be useful for *Mycoplasma*. All of our patients responded dramatically with resolution of their symptoms very shortly after beginning therapy. In addition, the sedimentation rate has shown a rapid decline to normal in all patients. As a result of these findings, we feel that this disease is infectious, likely the result of *Mycoplasma* infection, and believe that very long-term antibiotics such as doxycycline or clindamycin is appropriate for the treatment of this disease.

DISC SPACE INFECTION

Etiology

Controversy has arisen as to the cause of disc space infections, resulting in the term *diskitis*. This disease is usually regarded, however, as an osteomyelitis of the vertebral endplates that secondarily invades the disc without producing an acute osteomyelitis of the vertebral body. The organism that produces the infection in children is usually *S. aureus,* although other organisms are common in older patients, especially drug abusers and in debilitated patients.

Clinical Findings

Although disc space infection may occur at any age, it is most common in younger children, who may present with an inability to walk as the primary presenting feature, although the most common complaint is back pain. Unfortunately, in infants and toddlers diagnosing back pain may be difficult. Some children present with abdominal pain as the primary complaint. Frequently, the infant is irritable without other definite complaints.

The physical findings in these patients are characteristic, and the diagnosis can usually be established on the basis of the physical examination alone. Because the disc space infection usually occurs in the lumbar spine, the child splints the spine, refusing to flex it. Although the child may be able to bend at the waist, no flexion occurs in the spine itself. Some children are adept at compensating for the pain and may function relatively normally. They will, however, exhibit complete restriction of motion of the spine on examination.

This disease entity differs from osteomyelitis of the spine in that there are usually few, if any, systemic signs in patients with disc space infection. The patient's body temperature is usually normal as is the peripheral WBC count. The sedimentation rate is frequently, although not invariably, elevated.

Radiographic Findings

The radiographic findings depend on the delay in diagnosis. The disease characteristically produces narrowing of the disc space with irregularity of the adjacent vertebral endplates. This may be difficult to see radiographically, especially in a young child early in the course of the disease. Lateral tomography of the involved area of the spine is helpful in demonstrating the disc space and bone abnormality. These radiographs help eliminate the overlying gas that frequently obscures the spine in the lumbar region.

Bone scanning has been a popular method of diagnosing disc space infections. The bone scan usually demonstrates an area of increased uptake in the infected disc space, but some scans will be false-negative. Therefore, the diagnosis of disc space infection should not be excluded because of a normal bone scan. MRI has been shown to be able to accurately demonstrate an abnormal disc space, and we have recently demonstrated that the MRI is abnormal before the bone scan is positive and before radiographic changes are evident (Figure 5-11).

Diagnosis

The diagnosis of disc space infection is usually made on clinical grounds because of the characteristic physical findings. The clinical diagnosis is confirmed with radiographs that show the characteristic disc space narrowing and erosion of the vertebral endplates. Normally with a bone infection, a tissue or bacteriologic confirmation of the diagnosis would be necessary; however, because of the morbidity of needle aspiration of the spine, this procedure is usually not justified for the child exhibiting the characteristic findings of a disc space infection. The infecting organism is usually *S. aureus.* Aspiration biopsy of the spine should be reserved for the child who does not respond to initial treatment with antistaphylococcal antibiotics. One should also perform a biopsy of the disc space when the disease is unusual in any respect. If the infection involves an older child such as a teenager, or if drug abuse is

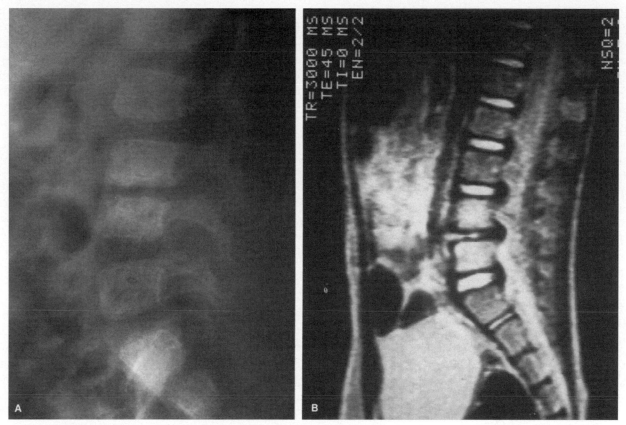

FIGURE 5-11. MRI of the spine demonstrating an abnormal L4-L5 disc. Note the loss of height and the change in the density of the disc. The bone scan, the plain radiographs, and the lateral tomograms of this patient were normal. The lateral radiograph of the spine subsequently demonstrated the typical changes seen in disc space infections.

suspected, a biopsy should be performed because of the possibility of a Gram-negative organism being the etiologic agent.

Treatment

Some authors, in the past, have advocated the use of spinal immobilization for children with disc space infection. They have shown that many patients respond to immobilization alone and consequently reserve antibiotics for the child who does not respond to immobilization alone. Currently most authors, however, favor the use of antibiotics as for any other bone infection. These children should, therefore, be started on oxacillin or cephazolin in doses that would be used for osteomyelitis. Treatment should be continued for 3 to 7 days with IV antibiotics, followed by oral antibiotics for another 4 weeks. The length of IV antibiotic therapy is determined by the patient's clinical response. One may also wish to use the C-reactive protein as a guide for treatment, because it falls more quickly than does the sedimentation rate during the treatment of osteomyelitis. We generally treat these children with IV antibiotics for several days only and then they are switched to oral antibiotics that are continued on an outpatient basis for a minimum of a total of 4 weeks of total antibiotic therapy.

Immobilization of the spine has been a mainstay of the treatment of disc space infection. However, most children with disc space infection usually respond quickly to IV antibiotics. Therefore, immobilization is used only in those patients who do not exhibit a rapid and dramatic response to the IV antibiotic treatment and need immobilization for comfort. One should also immobilize children with osteomyelitis of the spine because of the bony destruction that occurs.

PSEUDOMONAS: INFECTIONS OF THE FOOT FOLLOWING PUNCTURE WOUNDS

Clinical Presentation

Puncture wounds of the foot are relatively common injuries. The exact number of infectious complications of these injuries is not known, although rates up to 15% have been reported. Although the majority of infections are limited to the soft tissue, bone and joint infections occur in approximately 2% of puncture wounds of the foot.

The presentation of the infectious complications of nail punctures is characteristic. Typically, the patient is a child with tennis shoes who steps on a nail, sustaining a puncture of the foot that invariably either enters a bone or joint or punctures the plantar fascia. These children experience pain from the initial puncture wound, but this pain usually diminishes quickly. Children who develop a pseudomonal infection experience increasing pain in the foot 2 to 4 days after the initial trauma. These symptoms worsen so that within a day or so the child is not able to bear weight.

At presentation there is pain and swelling about the area of the puncture wound and throughout the area of the bone or joint infection, with signs of inflammation, including redness of the skin. Careful examination of the foot reveals pain and tenderness on the dorsum of the foot over the involved bone or joint.

Despite the fact that this is a foot infection, there frequently are no or few systemic signs of infection. The child's temperature usually is normal, as is the WBC count. Unfortunately, these findings have prompted many to underestimate the seriousness of this infection.

Treatment

The infection of the foot following puncture wounds is almost always caused by *Pseudomonas aeruginosa*, which has been grown from cultures taken from within the sole of tennis shoes. This infection requires thorough surgical debridement and antibiotic treatment. Antibiotic coverage alone does not eradicate the infection and only allows the infection to destroy more tissue. Once the diagnosis is made, a thorough debridement is performed. Prior aspiration of the area of infection may be performed but is not necessary because the signs and symptoms of this infection are so typical that culture of the tissues at the time of debridement is sufficient. However, do not give antibiotics until obtaining adequate cultures of the area of infection. Superficial cultures from the area of the puncture wound are not sufficient; it is necessary to obtain cultures from the bone or joint involved. *P. aeruginosa* rarely produces the thick pus typical of other infections. Rather, one finds a thin, watery, serosanguineous fluid typical of early *P. aeruginosa* infections.

The surgical approach to the area of infection depends on the area of involvement. If one is dealing with a septic arthritis of the metacarpophalangeal joint, the joint may be drained through a dorsal incision rather than through the puncture wound itself. If infection exists only within the sole of the foot under the plantar fascia, a plantar incision is necessary. If one of the bones of the foot is extensively infected, debridement may be required, using both dorsal and plantar incisions.

After thorough debridement and culture, IV antibiotics are required. Because the involved organism is usually *P. aeruginosa*, empiric antibiotics should have antipseudomonal activity. Additionally, the presence of cellulitis suggests infection with Gram-positive organisms (often in addition to *P. aeruginosa*) and should prompt empiric coverage that includes *S. aureus*. Local resistance rates of *P. aeruginosa* and *S. aureus* should dictate the empiric choice of antibiotics. For a bone infection alone, cefepime, ceftazidime, piperacillin, ticarcillin, or tobramycin are reasonable choices as single agents for empiric antipseudomonal therapy. If cellulitis accompanies the osteochondritis, the addition of an antistaphylococcal penicillin (i.e., nafcillin or oxacillin) to ceftazidime or tobramycin or the addition of a β-lactamase inhibitor to one of the antipseudomonal penicillins (i.e., piperacillin/tazobactam or ticarcillin/clavulanate) is warranted on an empiric basis. Cefepime has activity against both *S. aureus* and *P. aeruginosa* that is adequate for empiric therapy. If rates of methicillin resistance are high among local *S. aureus* isolates, the use of vancomycin for staphylococcal coverage may be warranted on an empiric basis. Antibiotic susceptibility data from the cultures collected during debridement should guide definitive antibiotic therapy.

The length of treatment depends on the patient's response, the extent of the infection, and the thoroughness of the debridement. The sedimentation rate may be used as a guide to the length of therapy, with the recommendation that antibiotics be discontinued when the sedimentation rate falls to normal. In general, the more thorough the debridement, the shorter the length of antibiotic treatment necessary. However, the largest available study in children suggests that an intravenous antibiotic course of 7 days following thorough surgical debridement is effective. In adult patients, a small study demonstrated the efficacy of oral ciprofloxacin for 7 to 14 days after surgery for pseudomonal osteomyelitis or septic arthritis of the foot. The use of fluoroquinolones in pediatric patients remains controversial. Due to cartilage damage in multiple juvenile animal models with therapeutic doses, fluoroquinolones are generally contraindicated, according to their FDA-approved labeling. There is not a single report of ciprofloxacin causing arthropathy in children, and the American Academy of Pediatrics Committee on Infectious Diseases states that the use of oral ciprofloxacin can be justified in certain cases. One such situation is when no other oral agent is available, necessitating an alternative drug be given parenterally. After the risks and benefits are explained to the parents, oral ciprofloxacin can be considered for pseudomonal osteomyelitis when the patient is well enough to be discharged from the hospital.

The sequelae of this infection depend on the interval between the puncture wound and the onset of appropriate treatment. The longer the delay before debridement of the foot and the commencement of aminoglycoside therapy, the worse the sequelae. To minimize sequelae, it is important to quickly establish the correct diagnosis and to perform the surgical debridement.

SEPTIC ARTHRITIS

Pathogenesis

Acute septic arthritis is a relatively uncommon disease. It may be associated with acute osteomyelitis, especially in the proximal femur, where bacteria escape the cortex of the metaphysis and invade the adjacent joint, producing a joint infection. In other cases, the joint infection is simply the result of hematogenous infection of the synovium or synovial fluid without prior bone infection. This isolated joint infection may be treated differently from the bone infection, which requires longer antibiotic therapy because of the possible presence of necrotic bone within the area of the infection. With a pure septic arthritis, bone sequestration does not occur. In addition, antibiotics are delivered across the synovium into the joint in high concentrations.

Organisms

Different organisms prevail as the most common infecting organisms depending on the age of the patient. *S. aureus* is the most common organism over all age groups. In the neonate, as we have seen in bone infections, group B *Streptococcus* is common, as are Gram-negative organisms. In the child between the age of 6 months to 5 years, type B *H. influenzae* was common, and in some series was the most common agent in septic arthritis in this age group; however, we have shown that since the advent of the H. Flu vaccine, the incidence of H. Flu septic arthritis has declined to near zero. In the older child *S. aureus* is the most common organism. Recently joint infections caused by *Kingella kingae* have been diagnosed relatively commonly, and in one recent report this organism has been seen more frequently than staph. This organism is present in the nasopharynx of normal children and may spread to produce joint infections via the bloodstream. In the teenager, however, *Neisseria gonorrhoeae* is common and may be the most common cause of septic arthritis. It is certainly the most common cause of polyarthritis in that age group.

Diagnosis

Children with septic arthritis usually exhibit all the clinical signs of sepsis, with elevated temperature, malaise, and local signs of inflammation. The exception is seen in children with acute septic arthritis secondary to *Kingella kingae* who frequently are not febrile at the time of diagnosis and may not have all of the signs of hip sepsis. The onset of septic arthritis is frequently more acute than is the onset of osteomyelitis. The child, especially the neonate, may present with pseudoparalysis of the extremity. The older child will protect the extremity, and if a joint of the lower extremity is involved, the child will usually refuse to walk.

The physical examination reveals an irritable child with a painful joint. Few other diseases produce such exquisite joint pain. The differential diagnosis includes acute rheumatic fever or acute juvenile arthritis, both of which may produce acute joint inflammation that is as painful as that produced by septic arthritis. In both of these diseases, the joint effusion also is significant, and the WBC count in the synovial fluid may occasionally be as high as 100,000 cells. The diagnosis usually can be made by other laboratory means, although the diagnosis occasionally is made retrospectively after treating a child for an infection.

Inspection of the child reveals a warm and painful joint with an effusion. The child will resist movement, splinting the joint in the position of greatest comfort. Laboratory data may be helpful. The peripheral WBC count is usually elevated, as is the sedimentation rate, although the diagnosis of septic arthritis should not be excluded simply on the basis of normal values for these two studies. Radiographs may demonstrate the joint swelling, although they are of little benefit early in the course of the disease except to exclude other problems.

Joint aspiration is mandatory for fluid analysis and culture of the synovial fluid. The joint fluid should be inspected visually. The fluid in patients with an infection of the joint varies in color from cloudy yellow to creamy white or gray, especially if the infection has been present for a period or if the organism is particularly virulent. Thus, the earlier the infection is diagnosed and the joint aspirated, the clearer the fluid. The fluid should be analyzed for cell count with a differential count of the WBCs. In most septic joints, the WBC count is greater than 50,000, and usually greater than 100,000. The one exception is in gonococcal arthritis, in which the WBC count is frequently lower than 50,000 cells. The differential count of polymorphonuclear leukocytes demonstrates that they constitute over 90%, and usually over 95%, of the total WBCs in the fluid.

A Gram's stain and culture of the synovial fluid is obviously important and provides the basis for the definitive diagnosis of septic arthritis. The fluid should be transported immediately to the laboratory and plated on the appropriate medium. Laboratory personnel must be informed that the fluid is from a joint and should also know what the physician suspects, which enables the technician to perform the appropriate cultures. Some special circumstances require special techniques for organism retrieval. *H. influenzae* is difficult to culture, and the plates must be incubated under a carbon dioxide environment. *Kingella kingae* is fastidious organism, and its recovery in the microbiology laboratory is increased significantly by direct inoculation of synovial fluid into automated blood culture system bottles. Despite meticulous culture techniques, a percentage of septic joints yield negative cultures. In some series, the percentage of organism retrieval was only 70%. Therefore, blood cultures should also be performed. Despite this, the diagnosis of septic arthritis may have to be made on clinical grounds in some patients because of negative bacterial cultures.

Because of the possibility of negative joint fluid cultures, one should also perform glucose determination on the joint fluid. In addition, lactic acid determination of the joint fluid and counter immunoelectrophoresis may be helpful for the detection of *H. influenzae*.

Treatment

The principles of treatment of septic arthritis do not differ from those of the treatment of infections in other areas of the body. The infection should be considered an abscess that requires drainage. In addition, the infection requires appropriate antibiotic therapy to sterilize the joint. The joint infection differs from other infections, in that it occurs in a closed space with easy access for needle aspiration and irrigation. In addition, antibiotics readily cross the synovial barrier and are concentrated in the synovial fluid.

Thorough debridement of the joint is required to completely eradicate the infection of the joint. In some instances, eradication may be accomplished with aspiration and irrigation of the joint without surgical debridement. Most reports of aspiration and irrigation technique of joint debridement of infection have reported good results. The requirements for this technique are specific. The major contraindication to aspiration irrigation technique for the treatment of joint infections is the hip joint being the site of infection. This joint must always be surgically drained in the face of an acute infection because the vascular supply of the hip joint is intracapsular, and therefore these vessels are easily obliterated if the pressure within the hip joint is elevated. In the case of acute septic arthritis of the hip joint, the joint must be surgically drained as an emergency. Recently, articles have been published that document satisfactory medical treatment of septic arthritis of the hip without surgical drainage. They state that the diagnosis must be made very early in the course of the disease and that there should be immediate response to treatment. They do make the diagnosis of septic arthritis of the hip with joint aspiration and then begin antibiotic treatment. It is probably safer to conservatively surgically drain the septic hip until adequate literature confirms the efficacy and safety of medical-only treatment.

The technique of aspiration irrigation of infected joints requires that the joint be easily accessible for aspiration. Because of its accessibility, the knee joint is most frequently treated with this technique. The ankle joint is also relatively accessible. The other joints of the body are less accessible and therefore more difficult to adequately debride through a needle.

Joint aspiration must be performed sterilely with the use of a large-bore needle. The fluid is fully drained from the joint and sent for appropriate studies. Without removing the needle, the joint is irrigated with sterile IV saline until the fluid that is returned is clear. The joint should be splinted, and the patient started on antibiotics while awaiting the culture results. If the WBC count of the fluid is low (i.e., below 80,000 to 100,000), and there is no particulate matter in the aspirate, this aspiration-irrigation may be the only mechanical treatment needed. The joint should be inspected the following day, and if the fluid has reaccumulated, a second aspiration-irrigation should be performed. If the reaccumulation of fluid is significant, and if the patient is still febrile, consider performing surgical drainage. If, in addition, the WBC count of the aspirated fluid is not significantly lower on the second day than that seen in the initial aspirate, surgical debridement should be strongly considered. If a second aspiration is performed and the fluid reaccumulates significantly on the third day, surgical drainage should be performed. Parenteral antibiotics enter the inflamed joint so readily that there is no need for direct joint instillation of antibiotics.

Initial arthrotomy of the joint should be performed when the fluid is thick (i.e., with a WBC count over 100,000), and when particulate matter is seen in the aspirate. This particulate matter is precipitated fibrin that must be removed to eradicate the infection. The arthrotomy of the knee joint should be performed through a small lateral parapatellar incision that allows inspection of the joint. A medial parapatellar incision is not performed because release of the medial retinaculum might lead to patellar subluxation. The joint may be closed over a small drain such as a Penrose drain. Suction drainage may be used; however, a suction-irrigation system should not be employed because of the possibility of superinfection with Gram-negative organisms. Arthroscopy has become a popular tool for the inspection of the joint and has been proposed for the debridement of the infected joint. Proponents state that one can effectively debride the joint and that the fibrinous material may be removed with the debridement tools available to the arthroscopist.

IV antibiotics should be started immediately after the joint fluid and blood have been cultured and the other studies such as Gram's staining and WBC count have been performed. The diagnosis may have to be confirmed on a presumptive basis; however, it is important to begin treatment as long as the criteria for making the diagnosis of septic arthritis have been met. In all age groups, most acute septic arthritis is caused by *S. aureus*. In children 6 months to 5 years, *H. influenzae* is a common cause in unvaccinated children. In the neonate, group B *Streptococcus* and Gram-negative organisms are common etiologic organisms. While awaiting the culture results, appropriate antibiotics should be started to cover the most likely organisms. Because *S. aureus* is ubiquitous, all acute septic joints are treated initially with an antistaphylococcal drug. The antibiotics are then modified when the culture and sensitivity results are known.

The dosages of the antibiotics are the same as for the patient with acute hematogenous osteomyelitis. The duration of antibiotic treatment, however, is not as long as in osteomyelitis because antibiotics reach the infected joint readily and in high concentration. In addition, one does not have to deal with necrotic bone in a septic arthritis as in a patient with osteomyelitis. Treatment of the septic joint should be started with IV antibiotics for 3 to 5 days. The patient may then be switched to oral antibiotics if the patient responded well to the treatment, which should include no fever for 24 hours and excellent clinical response. The total length of treatment is generally 2 to 4 weeks.

Hip Joint

An infection of the hip joint must be treated as an emergency because of the potential for the development of avascular necrosis of the femoral head. The initial evaluation of the hip joint is performed in the same manner used for any other joint. However, because the hip joint is deep and may be difficult to aspirate accurately, it must be aspirated using fluoroscopy. The needle may be directed from the anterior or medial approach. The anterior approach is used if the child is able to extend the hip. If, because of pain, the hip is in a position of abduction, flexion, and external rotation, a medial approach to the hip is easier. The exact needle entry point through the skin is easily determined by placing the needle on the skin and positioning the needle point using fluoroscopy. After skin penetration, the needle is directed toward the femoral neck at about the level of the junction of the head and the neck. If no fluid is collected from the joint, contrast medium is injected into the joint and an arthrogram obtained, which will reveal whether the hip joint has been entered.

Once the diagnosis of septic arthritis of the hip joint has been confirmed, the joint must be surgically drained as mentioned earlier. However, recent articles have documented excellent response to medical therapy alone in children with acute septic arthritis of the hip. These reports require critical evaluating before making a decision about the need for surgical drainage based on multiple factors. One need not await culture reports before draining the infected hip. Strong presumptive evidence is sufficient. Therefore, a positive Gram's stain or WBC count of the joint fluid of more than 90,000 to 100,000 cells is sufficient evidence if seen in combination with the characteristic history and physical findings.

The hip joint should never be treated with aspiration and irrigation because of the danger of avascular necrosis developing as a result of increased joint fluid pressure from the infection. The hip may be drained from either an anterior or a posterior approach. Each approach has its proponents. The posterior approach is generally easier and less damaging to the muscles of the hip. In addition, it allows for dependent drainage. If the femoral neck must be opened because of an intraosseous abscess, this cannot be performed posteriorly because the blood supply to the femoral head would be damaged. Thus, if the femoral neck should be windowed, the hip should be approached anteriorly. This approach allows one to drill the femoral neck in every patient (Figure 5-12). It is wise to always drain the infected hip joint from an anterior approach. This method allows easy access to the femoral neck for drilling if necessary.

The joint should be immobilized for several days to allow for a decrease in the acute inflammation. The hip may be placed in split Russell traction and the other joints splinted. Once the acute inflammation has subsided, motion should be instituted. Continuous passive motion has been advocated, and it may be used in children of adequate size. Joint motion helps prevent fibrosis and assists in cartilage nutrition.

Sacroiliac Joint

Septic arthritis of the sacroiliac joint is somewhat unusual because of its symptomatology and treatment, and therefore deserves separate discussion.

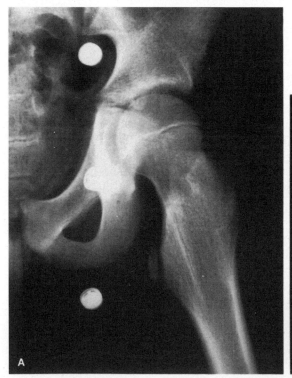
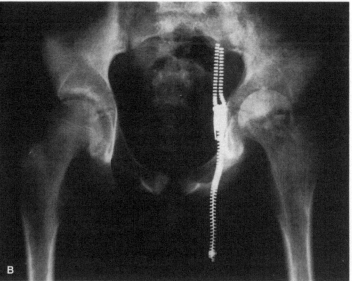

FIGURE 5-12. A 14-year-old boy with septic arthritis of his left hip. **(A)** AP radiograph of the left hip at the time of presentation. The hip was drained posteriorly, but the femoral neck was not drained. **(B)** AP radiograph of the left hip taken 6 weeks later demonstrating chondrolysis, avascular necrosis of the femoral head, and chronic osteomyelitis of the femoral neck with sequestrum within the femoral neck.

Sacroiliac (SI) joint infection may be difficult to diagnose unless one is familiar with its signs and symptoms and considers it in patients with pain about the pelvis and hip. Frequently, children with this disease are referred with abdominal or hip pain. Occasionally, they may be thought to have back pain. A careful history and examination, however, reveal that the pain is localized to the posterior pelvis. Pelvic compression is positive and usually produces exquisite pain in the region of the SI joint. The figure 4 test or Fabre test produces exquisite pain in the region of the SI joint.

The child usually is febrile, with signs of a systemic infection. The initial radiographs of the pelvis are usually normal, although tomograms of the SI joint may show some erosion of the margins of the joint if the infection has remained untreated for a sufficiently long period. Usually, however, all radiographs are normal. The ^{99m}Tc bone scanning may be positive; however, false-negative bone scans are seen in 25% or more of patients with acute infections. The diagnosis, therefore, depends on a careful history and examination, combined with confirmatory laboratory studies.

As in any other infection, joint aspiration is necessary to determine the bacteriologic cause of the infection; however, the SI joint is difficult to aspirate. Several descriptions of SI joint aspiration technique have been published, but even with this assistance the technique is demanding. Children with SI joint infection experience considerable pain and are usually distraught, making aspiration even more difficult. The SI joint is best aspirated using an approach with CT assistance. This approach allows for direct access to the joint. In our experience, little if any material is aspirated, however, whatever is obtained is submitted for Gram's stain and culture. Appropriate antibiotics are immediately begun while awaiting culture results. The infecting organism seen most commonly in non–drug-abusing children is *S. aureus*. Surgical drainage is not required unless the infection does not respond to IV antibiotics.

Gonococcal Arthritis

Septic arthritis secondary to infection with *N. gonorrhoeae* is probably the most common form of septic arthritis in the sexually active population. The typical syndrome of disseminated gonococcal infection frequently consists of three stages, although all patients with gonococcal septic arthritis do not go through all of these stages. The first stage is a septic stage that is similar to a septicemia caused by any other bacteria. The second stage is a transition stage, and the final stage is the septic joint stage. Eighty percent of patients with gonococcal arthritis complain of a migratory polyarthralgia, which is most commonly seen on the dorsum of the hands, wrists, ankles, and feet. This history is so characteristic that the diagnosis of gonococcal arthritis may be made on the basis of the history of migratory polyarthralgia combined with the typical joint findings.

About 60% of patients with gonococcal arthritis have more than one involved joint. The joints of the upper extremity, especially those of the fingers and wrist, are more commonly involved than are the joints of the lower extremity.

Joint aspiration is mandatory for culture and fluid analysis. Typically, the WBC count of the fluid is much lower than one would see in the fluid of a joint infected with another organism. In a series of teenagers with gonococcal arthritis, the average WBC of the synovial fluid was 48,000, with a range of 3,800 to 152,000. The organism is difficult to culture in the laboratory, and joint fluid cultures of septic joints are positive only half of the time. Therefore, it is necessary to culture all orifices in patients suspected of having gonococcal arthritis. Additionally, it is imperative that all patients with gonococcal infections be tested for other sexually transmitted infections (syphilis, hepatitis B, HIV) and treated presumptively for *Chlamydia trachomatis*.

Surgical drainage of the infected joints is usually not required because the organism is so easily eradicated with appropriate antibiotic therapy. In addition, the organism usually does not destroy the involved joint until late in the course of an infection; therefore, if an infection is treated promptly, no joint destruction should be expected. Penicillin and tetracycline resistance among *N. gonorrhoeae* isolates from the United States is common; therefore, penicillin is no longer an appropriate empiric choice for suspected gonococcal infection. In treating patients with gonococcal arthritis, one should follow the Centers for Disease Control and Prevention recommendations, which are to treat with ceftriaxone 50 mg/kg (up to 1g) as a single IV or IM dose for 7 days. Options for the cephalosporin allergic patient or in cases of proven cephalosporin resistant gonnococcal infection are spectinomycin or a fluoroquinolone, such as ciprofloxacin. Consider using a fluoroquinolone in patients under the age of 18 as discussed above in the section "*Pseudomonas*: Infections of the Foot Following Puncture Wounds." Presumptive treatment for

concomitant *C. trachomatis* infection is a single oral
dose of azithromycin 20 mg/kg (up to 1g). Additionally, evaluation and treatment of the patient's sexual
partners is important in preventing reinfection.

Annotated Bibliography

Abuamara S, Louis JS, Barbier-Frebourg N, et al. Kingella kingae
osteoarticular infections in children. A report of a series of
eight new cases. Arch Pediatr 2000;7(9):927–932.
*Kingella kingae is a Gram-negative bacillus that belongs to the
Neisseriaceae family, which is usually present in the nasopharynx. It has been recognized as the cause of bone and especially joint
infections. It is difficult to culture in the laboratory, and it is necessary to use blood culture bottles for inoculation. This organism
produces an infection that is usually less severe than seen with
staph. In this series only 75% of patients had a fever at the time of
diagnosis.*

Bowerman SG, Green NE, Mencio GA. Decline of bone and joint
infections attributable to haemophilus influenza type b. Clin
Orthop 1997;341:128–133.
*The authors demonstrate that H. Flu has virtually been eliminated
as a cause of bone and joint infections since the onset of widespread
inoculation with the H. Flu vaccine. Therefore, coverage for H. Flu
is not needed in patients who have been vaccinated.*

Blythe MJ, Kincaid R, Craigen MA, et al. The changing epidemiology of acute and subacute haematogenous osteomyelitis in
children. J Bone Joint Surg Br 2001;83(1):99–102.
*This article documents the decreasing incidence of both acute and
subacute osteomyelitis; however, the decrease in the incidence of acute
osteomyelitis was significantly greater than in the subacute form.*

Canale ST, Harkness RM, Thomas PA, et al. Does aspiration of
bones and joints affect results of later bone scanning? J Pediatr Orthop 1985;5(1):23–26.
*The authors demonstrate that bone aspiration with a needle does not
alter the bone scan. They emphasize that if bone scanning is to be
done in acute hematogenous osteomyelitis, it should not delay a
bone aspiration and treatment. Treatment should be carried out immediately, and if a bone scan is necessary, it may be done without
fear of altering the results after needle aspiration.*

Chen CE, Ko JY, Li CC, et al. Acute septic arthritis of the hip in
children. Arch Orthop Trauma Surg 2001;121(9):521–526.
*This study documents satisfactory results of septic arthritis of the
hip with arthrocentesis and antibiotic treatment without arthrotomy. They did have 4 of 7 with poor results, and all of those were
associated with osteomyelitis of the proximal femur. One should not
automatically assume this method of treatment without long-term
documentation of larger series of patients with septic arthritis of the
hip treated without arthrotomy.*

Cole WG, Dalziel RE, Leitl S. Treatment of acute osteomyelitis in
childhood. J Bone Joint Surg Br 1982;64(2):218–223.
*The authors present a review of 55 children with acute hematogenous
osteomyelitis. Ninety-two percent were cured if diagnosed early, and
their cure was effected with a single course of antibiotics without operation. The patients were kept in the hospital for less than 1 week.
The authors quickly switched to oral antibiotics as soon as the patient
had responded to the IV antibiotics with excellent results.*

Crosby LA, Powell DA. The potential value of the sedimentation
rate in monitoring treatment outcome in puncture wound–
related *Pseudomonas* osteomyelitis. Clin Orthop 1984;188:
168–172.
*The authors used the sedimentation rate for determining the course
of antibiotic treatment for pseudomonal osteomyelitis of the foot
after puncture wounds. They found that once the sedimentation
rate had returned to normal, the antibiotic therapy could be stopped.*

Early SD, Kay RM, Tolo, VT. Childhood diskitis. J Am Acad Orthop Surg 2003;11(6):413–420.
*Good review article demonstrating the etiology and appropriate
treatment of disc space infection in children. The authors confirm a
bacteriological etiology and advocate antibiotic therapy. Response to
treatment is rapid and permanent.*

Ezra E, Cohen N, Segev E, et al. Primary subacute epiphyseal osteomyelitis: role of conservative treatment. J Pediatr Orthop.
2002;22(3):333–337.
*The authors present a series of patients with subacute epiphyseal
and combined metaphyseal-epiphyseal osteomyelitis that were successfully treated with antibiotics alone. They recommend conservative, nonoperative treatment of subacute osteomyelitis.*

Floyed RL, Steele, RW. Culture negative osteomyelitis. Pediatr
Infect Dis J. 2003;22(8):731–736.
*The authors have studied children with culture negative os-
teomyelitis and have found that they are less likely to have had
antecedent trauma. In addition, their symptoms and clinical
presentation are less severe than children with culture positive
osteomyelitis.*

Gillespie WJ, Mayo KM. The management of acute hematogenous osteomyelitis in the antibiotic era. J Bone Joint Surg Br
1981;63-B(1):126–131.
*The authors review the treatment of acute hematogenous os-
teomyelitis seen in children between 1947 and 1976. They had a
high failure rate of 20% and found that failure was more common in
surgically treated patients. Their results are worse than one would
expect today. The organism recovered was S. aureus in more than
90%, but they isolated the organism in only 55% of patients who
were treated successfully.*

Green NE. *Pseudomonas* infections of the foot following puncture
wounds. AAOS Instruct Course Lect 1983;32:43.
*The author identifies the cause of pseudomonal infections of the foot
after puncture wounds. These require debridement in all cases and
prolonged antibiotic therapy.*

Green NE, Beauchamp RD, Griffin PP. Primary subacute epiphyseal osteomyelitis. J Bone Joint Surg Am 1981;63-A:107–114.
*The authors identify lesions of the epiphysis as representing pri-
mary subacute epiphyseal osteomyelitis. The lesions are characteristic with well-circumscribed borders. The treatment is debridement
and antibiotic therapy.*

Griffin PP, Green WT Sr. Hip joint infections in infants and children. Orthop Clin North Am 1978;9(1):123–134.
*The authors outline the appropriate treatment for acute septic
arthritis. They emphasize that early treatment of the infection is
mandatory and that poor results are more likely to be seen in infants
and young children than in older children and that poor results are
more common in children with a delay in the diagnosis and treatment. They also point out that associated osteomyelitis of the
femoral neck is more likely to result in a poor outcome.*

Gutman LT. Acute, subacute, and chronic osteomyelitis and pyogenic arthritis in children. Curr Probl Pediatr 1985;15(12):1–72.
*This is a good review of the diagnosis and treatment of osteomyelitis
in children. All forms of osteomyelitis are discussed, and the means
of diagnosis and treatment are outlined.*

Gwynne-Jones DP, Stott NS. Community-acquired methicillin-
resistant Staphylococcus aureus: a cause of musculoskeletal
sepsis in children. J Pediatr Orthop 1999;19(3):413–416.
*Methicillin-resistant staph aureus bone and joint infections have
become more commonplace. They documented a 20% incidence of
MRSA in community-acquired bone and joint infections in children. As a result one should be aware of and consider MRSA as the
potential cause of a bone or joint infection.*

Ibia EO, Imoisili M, Pikis A. Group A β-hemolytic streptococcal
osteomyelitis in children. Pediatrics 2003;112(1):22–26.
*The authors discuss the prevalence of GABHS in bone and joint
infections, especially in children who have concurrent varicella
infection.*

Jacobs RF, McCarthy RE, Elser JM. *Pseudomonas* osteochondritis complicating puncture wounds of the foot in children: a 10-year evaluation. J Infect Dis 1989;160(4):657–661.
They reviewed their patients with pseudomonas infections of the foot after nail puncture. Of 77 patients, 70 were wearing tennis shoes. They discovered that after aggressive surgical debridement a shorter course of antibiotics (7 days) was effective in obtaining a cure for the infection.

Jackson MA, Nelson JD. Etiology and medical management of acute suppurative bone and joint infections in pediatric patients. J Pediatr Orthop 1982;2(3):313–323.
The authors review the etiology and management of acute bone and joint infections and outline oral therapy of acute hematogenous osteomyelitis.

Johanson PH. *Pseudomonas* infection in the foot following puncture wounds. J Am Med Assoc 1968;204:262–264.
The author was the first to identify Pseudomonas *as the primary cause for infections of the bones of the foot after nail puncture wounds. These infections should be treated aggressively.*

Meller Y, Yagupsky P, Elitsur Y, et al. Chronic multifocal symmetrical osteomyelitis. Am J Dis Child 1984;138:349–351.
The authors identify the syndrome of chronic multifocal osteomyelitis. This is an unusual disease with no known cause as of yet. It seems to run a self-contained course that may last as long as 15 years.

Morrissy RT. Bone and joint sepsis in children. AAOS Instruct Course Lect 1982;31:49–61.
The author presents a good review of the cause, diagnosis, and treatment of bone and joint infections in children. He emphasizes the need for aspiration of the bone and joint for diagnosis and treatment.

Nelson JD, Bucholz RW, Kusmiesz H, et al. Benefits and risks of sequential parenteral-oral cephalosporin therapy for suppurative bone and joint infections. J Pediatr Orthop 1982;2:255–262.
The authors outline the sequential IV–oral treatment of acute bone and joint infections in children. They emphasize the need for high-dose antibiotics both in the IV and oral routes. They stress that the oral antibiotics should not be given unless the child has had an excellent response to the IV antibiotics.

Norden C, Gillespie J, Nade S. Infections in bones and joints. Blackwell Scientific Publications, 1994.
The authors review their findings of the origin of bone and joint infections and present good scientific evidence to demonstrate why acute hematogenous osteomyelitis begins in the metaphysis of long bones.

Roberts JM, Drummond DS, Breed AL, et al. Subacute hematogenous osteomyelitis in children: A retrospective study. J Pediatr Orthop 1982;2:249–254.
The authors outline the diagnosis of subacute hematogenous osteomyelitis in children. This disease does not produce systemic symptoms but does produce local findings. Treatment is debridement and antibiotic therapy.

Schreck P, Schreck P, Bradley J, et al. Musculoskeletal complications of varicella. J Bone Joint Surg 1996;78-A:1713–1719.
There is a 6% incidence of bone, joint, and soft tissue infections in patients with varicella, which included osteomyelitis, septic arthritis, and necrotizing fasciitis. Eighty-four percent of those infections were caused by group-A β-hemolytic streptococcus.

Scoles P, Quinn T. Intervertebral discitis in children and adolescents. Clin Orthop 1982;162:31–36.
The authors identify the syndrome of intervertebral diskitis in children. This is an infection of the disc space that should be treated aggressively.

Skaggs DL, Kim SK, Greene NW, et al. Differentiation between bone infarction and acute osteomyelitis in children with sickle-cell disease with the use of sequential radionuclide bone marrow and bone scans. J Bone Joint Surg Am 2001;83-A: 1810–1813.
The authors point out the efficacy of differentiating between bone infarction and osteomyelitis in patients with sickle cell disease with the use of sequential bone marrow and bone scans.

Sullivan JA, Vasileff T, Leonard JC. An evaluation of nuclear scanning in orthopaedic infections. J Pediatr Orthop 1981;1:73–79.
The authors demonstrate that bone scanning is less than 100% accurate in patients with acute hematogenous osteomyelitis. As a matter of fact, they find in their series only 80% of the children with acute hematogenous osteomyelitis had a positive bone scan. Therefore, the diagnosis of acute hematogenous osteomyelitis should not depend on bone scanning.

Szalay E, Green NE, Heller R, et al. MRI disc space infection. J Pediatr Orthop 1987;7:164.
The authors believe that MRI is the most sensitive means of early diagnosis of disc space infection in children.

Trueta J. The three types of acute hematogenous osteomyelitis: A clinical and vascular study. J Bone Joint Surg 1959;41-B: 671–680.
The author describes the three types of osteomyelitis—neonatal, childhood, and adult—and demonstrates the difference in blood supply that forms the basis for this classification system.

Umans H, Haramati N, Flusser G. The diagnostic role of gadolinium enhanced MRI in distinguishing between acute medullary bone infarct and osteomyelitis. Magn Reson Imaging 2000;18: 255–262.
The authors were able to distinguish between bone infarct and osteomyelitis in patients with sickle cell disease with the use of gadolinium-enhanced MRI. In acute infarcts, one saw thin linear rim enhancements on MRI while in osteomyelitis there was a more geographic and irregular marrow enhancement.

Wenger DR, Bobechko WP, Gilday DL. The spectrum of intervertebral disc-space infection in children. J Bone Joint Surg Am 1978;60-A:100–108.
The authors elucidate the cause, diagnosis, and treatment of disc space infection in children. They emphasize the infectious nature of this disease.

Robert F. Ashman
Polly J. Ferguson
Jacob W. IJdo
George V. Lawry II
Mary M. Moore
Paul M. Peloso

John W. Rachow
Haraldine A. Stafford
Rebecca S. Tuetken
Scott A. Vogelgesang

6

Rheumatic Diseases: Diagnosis and Management

The Normal Synovium
Robert F. Ashman

Characteristics of Normal Synovial Fluid

The structure of the *synovium*, or *synovial membrane* is discussed in Chapter 2.

Synovial fluid is a plasma transudate from synovial capillaries, modified by the secretory activities of the type B synovial lining cells. They secrete the hyaluronic acid-protein complex (mucin) that gives synovial fluid its viscosity and lubricating properties. Glucose and electrolytes are in equilibrium between synovial fluid and serum. The nutrition of hyaline cartilage depends on synovial fluid exchanged by diffusion plus compression and decompression of the cartilage during motion and weight bearing.

Normal fluid is clear, pale yellow, and sufficiently viscous that droplets expelled from a needle tip fall in a long string. Normal synovial fluid does not clot because it lacks fibrinogen. The normal volume of fluid in the largest synovial cavity, the knee, is 0.2 to 4 mL. Thus, aspiration of the normal joint may yield only enough fluid to wet the needle.

Laboratory analysis of normal fluid shows (1) sterile culture; (2) less than 100 leukocytes per cubic millimeter, mostly lymphocytes and monocytes; (3) specific gravity of 1.008 to 1.015; (4) protein content of 20 to 200 mg/mL, with an albumin/globulin ratio of 1.5:1; (5) mucin content that varies widely and is the main determinant of the high viscosity; (6) glucose that is normally more than 75% of the concentration in serum; and (7) no crystals.

Examination of Synovial Fluid

Aspiration of synovial fluid is a helpful diagnostic maneuver whenever the cause of arthritis is in doubt but especially when the inflammation is concentrated in a single joint or has an acute onset. Ruling out infection or crystal deposition as a cause of arthritis is the strongest indication for synovial fluid analysis because the treatment of these disorders is substantially different from that of other causes of joint inflammation. In the case of bacterial infection, the results of misdiagnosis can be catastrophic.

Routine analysis of synovial fluid includes (1) inspection for color, transparency, and viscosity; (2) cell count; (3) crystal examination; (4) bacterial culture; and, if bacterial infection is suspected clinically, (5) Gram's stain. Samples for both cell count and crystals can be collected in sodium heparin (green-top) tubes. All of these tests are most reliable when performed on fresh specimens. Culture of the fastidious gonococcus requires employing specialized culture techniques within a few minutes of collection.

Additional tests sometimes performed, which add little to the above information, include glucose, protein, and complement levels.

Crystal Examination

Crystal examination is the only known means of making the diagnosis of gout, pseudogout, and basic calcium phosphate (BCP) crystal disease. Examination of fresh synovial fluid on a polarizing microscope with a first-order red compensating filter permits the recognition of birefringence in addition to crystal morphology. *Sodium urate* crystals are thin, pointed, and strongly negatively birefringent (yellow if their axis is parallel to that of the compensator). *Calcium pyrophosphate dihydrate* (CPPD) crystals are short, thick, and weakly positively birefringent. Diagnosis is more certain if crystals are seen within phagocytes. BCP (including hydroxyapatite) crystals may sometimes be identified under ordinary light microscopy as small, chunky Alizarin red-staining crystals in clumps.

Crystal artifacts occasionally encountered include steroid crystals (flat parallelograms occurring in joints recently injected with depot steroid preparations).

Table 6-1 summarizes the results of synovial fluid analysis, with usual diagnostic implications. Typical cell counts and fluid characteristics overlap among the classifications, and only in the case of a positive crystal examination or culture can a definitive diagnosis be made from fluid alone. Because septic joints (especially if partially treated) may have low leukocyte counts, culture should be performed regardless of the fluid's appearance.

TABLE 6-1.
Results of Synovial Fluid Analysis

Group	Appearance	Cell Count/μL	Neutrophils (%)	Typical Diagnosis
Normal	Clear, colorless to straw colored, good string, low volume	< 100	< 25	None
I (Noninflammatory)	Clear, straw colored, good string	200–2,000	< 25	Degenerative arthritis, internal derangement, trauma, aseptic necrosis
IIA (Mild inflammatory)	Faintly cloudy, moderate string	1,000–10,000	25–50	Systemic lupus erythematosus and other immune complex arthritides, mild rheumatoid arthritis, spondyloarthropathies
IIB (Severe inflammatory)	Translucent but cloudy, yellow, drops like water	2,000–75,000	50–75	Moderate to severe rheumatoid arthritis, gout, pseudogout, tuberculosis
III (Septic)	Creamy, opaque, poor string	>50,000	> 80	Acute gout, bacterial infection

Furthermore, more than one diagnosis may be present, as in the gout patient with a septic joint.

A frankly bloody fluid may mean tumor, trauma, or hemophilia. A dark brown fluid full of hemosiderin is seen in hemophilia and pigmented villonodular synovitis. Fat floating on a bloody fluid indicates fracture or tumor exposing the marrow cavity to the synovial space. Floating fragments resembling ground pepper represent pigmented cartilage fragments in ochronosis. Small white clots ("rice bodies") represent fibrin bits seen in some inflammatory fluids. Phagocytic mononuclear cells with vacuoles may appear in rheumatoid arthritis (RA) and in reactive arthritis.

Synovial Biopsy

The indications for synovial biopsy are rare, because fluid analysis, direct visualization by arthroscopy, or arthrography usually provides most of the information required for diagnosis. The suspicion of tumor, pigmented villonodular synovitis, tuberculous or fungal arthritis, sarcoidosis, amyloidosis, or synovial chondromatosis may be confirmed by synovial biopsy.

Biopsy is most commonly obtained by arthroscopy. Biopsy tissue is usually formalin fixed for hematoxylin and eosin staining, but preservation of urate crystals requires absolute ethanol, and cultures require unfixed sterile samples. The yield of positive cultures from synovium in tuberculous and fungal arthritis is superior to that of fluid cultures. Other special staining procedures include iron stains for hemosiderin in pigmented villonodular synovitis or hemochromatosis and Congo red stains for amyloid.

Histologic findings of diagnostic import include the cartilage metaplasia of synovial chondromatosis, malignant synovial sarcoma and chondrosarcoma, metastatic tumors or leukemias, caseating granulomas (tuberculosis), noncaseating granulomas (sarcoidosis), the histiocytes and giant cells of multicentric reticulohistiocytosis, and the periodic acid Schiff-positive macrophages of Whipple disease. Of course, inflammation is a far more common finding, but unfortunately, the histology of inflamed synovium is similar in the major rheumatic diseases. Early in inflammatory arthritis, the synovial lining cells accumulate, capillaries proliferate, and then mononuclear cells (mostly monocytes and T lymphocytes) infiltrate the tissue. Finally, in the chronic phase, complete germinal centers resembling those of lymph nodes may appear. The exuberant thickening of this hypercellular synovium resembles granulation tissue and forms long villous fronds.

Osteoarthritis
Rebecca S. Tuetken

Pathogenesis and Clinical Manifestations

Osteoarthritis (OA), the most common joint disease, is age related, affecting more than 80% of people over the age of 55. It is more common in women, especially after menopause. OA in weight-bearing joints is strongly linked to body mass index. As life expectancy increases, and the rate of obesity reaches epidemic proportions, it is no surprise that OA is increasingly common. OA pathogenesis involves an imbalance between normal cartilage degradative and repair mechanisms, which results in net loss of cartilage, hypertrophy of bone, and generation of osseous outgrowths called osteophytes. OA has a predilection for finger joints, knees, hips, shoulders, and the spine. Occurrence in an atypical joint, such as an elbow, can usually be traced to prior trauma, a congenital joint abnormality, underlying systemic disease, or a chronic crystalline arthropathy. The heterogeneity of OA arises from the many factors that can contribute to cartilage damage.

Patients will typically report pain that is increased with activity, and relieved by rest, though rest pain occurs in advanced disease. "Gelling"—stiffness that occurs after any period of rest—is also common. Morning stiffness, when present, rarely lasts more than 30 minutes. Symptom severity ranges from asymptomatic disease diagnosed radiographically to significant pain with functional limitation. Physical exam findings of the affected joints include tenderness on palpation, crepitus (palpable friction) with movement, bony enlargement, abnormal alignment, decreased range of motion, and sometimes joint effusion.

Regional Variations and Radiographic Features

The characteristic radiographic features of OA are osteophytes, asymmetric joint space narrowing, subchondral bone sclerosis, and subchondral cysts. The severity of OA can be scored based on these four common features (Table 6-2). *Osteophytes,* commonly called "bone spurs," are osseous outgrowths that most commonly arise at the joint margins, and are the single most common feature of OA. *Joint space narrowing* results from loss of hyaline cartilage and should be present to some degree in all joints that exhibit osteophytes. Because cartilage loss is

TABLE 6-2.
Radiographic Classification of Degenerative Joint Disease

Grade	Description
KNEES	
0	Normal
1	Doubtful narrowing of joint space and possible osteophytic lipping
2	Definite osteophytes and possible narrowing of joint space
3	Moderate multiple osteophytes, definite narrowing of joint space, some sclerosis, and possible deformity of bone ends
4	Large osteophytes, marked narrowing of joint space, severe sclerosis, and definite deformity of bone ends. Subchondral cysts may be present.
HIPS	
0	Normal
1	Possible narrowing of joint space medially and possible osteophytes around the femoral head
2	Definite narrowing of joint space inferiorly, definite osteophytes, and slight sclerosis
3	Marked narrowing of joint space, slight osteophytes, some sclerosis and cyst formation, and deformity of femoral head and acetabulum
4	Gross loss of joint space with sclerosis and cysts, marked deformity of femoral head and acetabulum, and large osteophytes

(Adapted from the Council for International Organization of Medical Sciences, 1963)

greatest where the stress on the joint is greatest, radiographic joint space narrowing in OA is usually asymmetric, in contrast to the more uniform pattern that occurs in chronic inflammatory arthritides such as rheumatoid arthritis. *Subchondral bony sclerosis* also occurs in the most stressed areas of the joint, where cartilage is most thin. Once cartilage is lost, the bone surfaces rub and polish each other, a process termed *eburnation*. Eventually, in severe disease, cysts may form in the subchondral bone beneath eburnated or sclerotic surfaces.

Hands and Wrists

The most commonly affected hand joints are the distal interphalangeal (DIP), proximal interphalangeal (PIP), and the first carpometacarpal (CMC) joints. Osteophytes of the DIP joints (called *Heberden's nodes*), and of the PIP joints (called *Bouchard's nodes*) may be prominent and are sometimes tender (Figure 6-1). In severe cases, angular deformity, dislocation, or ankylosis may occur. OA of the first CMC (trapeziometacarpal) joint causes pain with grasping or pinching and crepitus on movement. Occasionally, the metacarpophalangeal (MCP) joints are involved but never without concomitant disease in the DIP and PIP joints. Isolated MCP degeneration is usually secondary to some other disease process, such as a recurrent crystal arthritis. Radiographs of the hand and wrist joints will show uniform or nonuniform joint space narrowing, osteophytes at the joint margin, bony sclerosis, and sometimes subchondral cysts. At the DIP and PIP joints, osteophytes have been described as "seagull wings" because the pattern of the marginal osteophytes with irregular joint space narrowing resembles a seagull flying (Figure 6-2). *Erosive osteoarthritis* of the DIP and PIP joints is a particularly painful disease primarily of middle-aged and older women, characterized by degenerative changes plus inflammation. Bone erosions occur centrally, but can also extend laterally along the joint margin, and coupled with marginal osteophytes, give a scalloped appearance to the joint on plain radiographs.

Knees

OA of the knees is common, and risk is strongly linked to body mass index. Symptoms include pain with walking, standing up from a chair, climbing or descending stairs; and stiffness after periods of rest. Exam findings may include joint effusion, crepitus with movement, and with more advanced disease, loss of full knee extension and a palpable osteophytic

ridge. Because it bears the most weight, the medial aspect of the joint tends to degenerate more rapidly than the lateral aspect, resulting in varus ("bow-legged") angulation of the knee, and asymmetric joint space narrowing on weight-bearing radiographs (Figure 6-3). Although less common, the opposite pattern of lateral joint space loss and valgus ("knock-kneed") deformity does occur. Plain films also typically reveal sclerosis, with or without subchoncral bone cysts, and osteophytes arising from the tibial spines, intercondylar notch, and from the joint margins of the tibia and femur. In patellofemoral disease, merchant and lateral radiographs of the knees will reveal narrowing of the patellofemoral space, often with the patellae displaced laterally, and osteophytes at the superior and inferior poles of the patella. Uniform tri-compartmental (medial, patellar, and lateral) joint space narrowing without osteophytes usually indicates the aftermath of an inflammatory arthritis, such as rheumatoid arthritis.

Hips

Symptoms of hip OA vary. Patients may report groin or buttock pain with walking, but sometimes experience pain that radiates toward the knees. The exam may reveal decreased range of motion, particularly internal hip rotation, sometimes with pain at the limit of rotation. Radiographs of early disease show changes concentrated in the superolateral aspect of the joint, the area under most mechanical stress. Joint space narrowing is followed by osteophyte formation, sclerosis, and cyst formation. Remodeling of the medial and lateral femoral head occurs and can lead to its collapse and flattening. The medial acetabulum space fills in with osteophytes, resulting in gradual superolateral migration of the femoral head (Figure 6-4). The cortex may thicken with new bone formation along the medial aspect of the femoral head (*buttressing*). In contrast, chronic inflammatory arthritis, such as rheumatoid arthritis, will typically lead to diffuse loss of joint space and medial migration along the axis of the femoral head, or *protrusio acetabuli*.

Spine

OA may affect any level of the spine, but most commonly occurs at C5, T8, and L3, the areas of greatest spinal flexibility. Joints of the spine include cartilaginous joints, *nucleus pulposus of the intervertebral discs;* synovial lined *apophyseal joints;* cervical pseudoarthroses called *uncovertebral joints;* and fibrous articulation, the *annulus fibrosus of the*

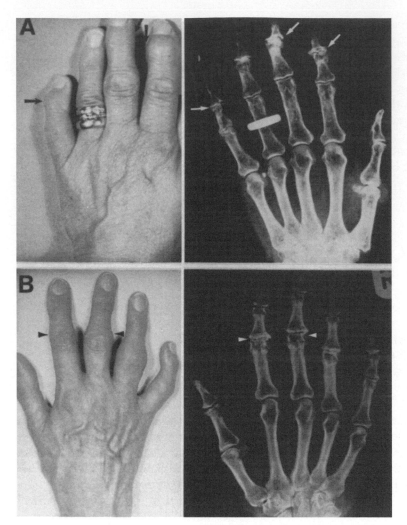

FIGURE 6-1. (A and B) Heberden's and Bouchard's nodes. **(A)** Enlargement of the distal interphalangeal joint (*arrow*) due to joint osteophytes is called a Heberden's node; **(B)** similar enlargement at the proximal interphalangeal joint is called a Bouchard's node (*arrowhead*).

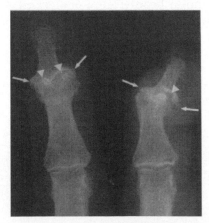

FIGURE 6-2. Osteoarthritis of the DIP joint: the combination of osteophytes at the margin (*arrow*) and irregular joint space narrowing (*arrowhead*) resembles a seagull flying.

intervertebral discs (Figure 6-5). OA will typically affect all spinal joints in the same area, but features of disease at each joint type are described separately for clarity.

Intervertebral (osteo)chondrosis is primary degeneration of the nucleus pulposus of the intervertebral discs. Radiographs reveal progressive uniform or nonuniform narrowing of the disc space and reactive subchondral sclerosis at the vertebral endplate with osteophytes extending from the anterolateral vertebral margins. Progressive desiccation or rupture of the disc will sometimes allow gas to appear in the disc substance, which on radiographs will appear as a thin linear lucency within the disc (*vacuum sign*) seen on extension and often disappearing on flexion (Figure 6-6, A and B). The vacuum sign

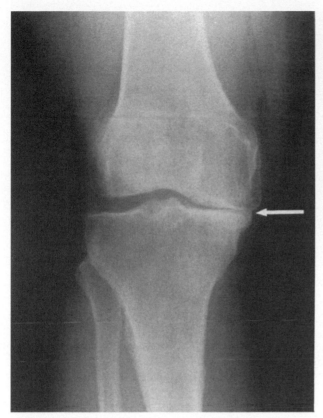

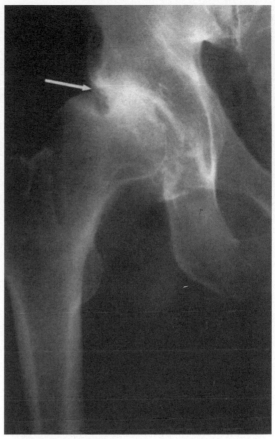

FIGURE 6-3. Degenerative joint disease of the knee is manifested by asymmetric joint space narrowing. The medial compartment (*arrow*) that bears the most weight is more affected than the lateral compartment.

FIGURE 6-4. Osteoarthritis of the hip. An AP radiograph of the hip joint illustrates superolateral migration of the femoral head (*arrow*) with asymmetric joint space narrowing.

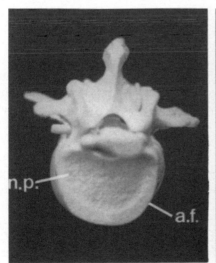
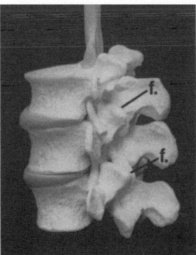
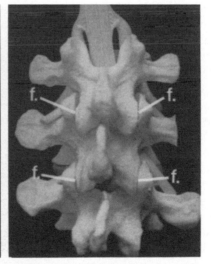

FIGURE 6-5. The vertebral bodies and intervertebral discs contain three structures that degenerate in OA. The intervertebral facet joints (f) show classic features of osteoarthritis. The intervertebral disc is composed of the central nucleus pulposus (n.p.), where disease is termed intervertebral osteochondrosis, surrounded by the annulus fibrosis (a.f.), where disease is termed spondylosis deformans.

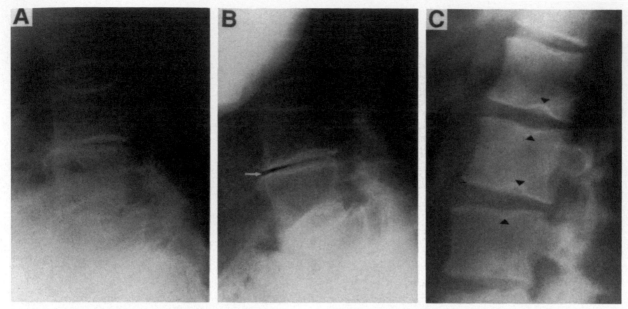

FIGURE 6-6. Lateral views of the lumbosacral spine show a horizontal linear lucency (*arrow*), called a vacuum sign, created when gas forms in the degenerated disc due to negative pressure. It is seen in extension (**B**) when disc pressure is lowest, and vanishes in flexion (**A**), which increases disc pressure. (**C**) A Schmorl node (*arrowhead*) forms when the nucleus pulposus herniates into an adjacent vertebral body.

helps to exclude infection as a cause of disc space loss. *Discogenic* low back pain caused by ruptured discs is typically worsened by flexing the spine, which increases pressure on the disc, and likewise decreased by extension of the spine, or by lying supine. The degenerating disc may herniate into the adjacent vertebral body, producing a *Schmorl node* (Figure 6-6C), or impinge on the spinal cord, causing spinal stenosis.

OA of the synovial apophyseal, or facet joints, is characterized by joint space narrowing, marginal osteophytes, and bony sclerosis. Lumbar facet disease may produce central low back pain that worsens on extension, which loads the facet joints and decreases with flexion. Osteophytes and hypertrophy of the joint capsule may cause spinal stenosis by encroaching onto the spinal cord or the nerve roots at the intervertebral foramina. Pain due to stenosis may radiate below the knee, worsen with exertion and extension, and resolve with rest or by bending forward, a pattern known as *neurogenic claudication* or *pseudoclaudication*. Concurrent intervertebral disc degeneration worsens intersegmental instability and increases the load on the lumbar facet joints, which can lead to subluxation of the joints, allowing the forward movement of one vertebral body over another (*spondylolisthesis*).

In the cervical spine, the posterior margins of the vertebral bodies project slightly beyond the disc to form pseudoarthroses called uncovertebral joints.

Osteophytes at both the uncovertebral and facet joints can cause cervical spinal stenosis.

Spondylosis deformans refers to degenerative disease of the annulus fibrosus of the intervertebral disc and is characterized by formation of large osteophytes along the anterior and lateral aspects of the spine. Osteophytes of axial OA are oriented horizontal to their point of origin, which distinguishes them from the fine, vertically oriented *syndesmophytes* of the inflammatory spondyloarthropathies (Figure 6-7). Axial osteophytes of OA also differ from the *paravertebral hyperostoses* of *diffuse idiopathic skeletal hyperostosis* or DISH. In DISH, there is ossification of the paravertebral ligaments, particularly at the anterolateral aspects of the vertebral bodies, producing upward or downward pointing hyperostoses, which are sometimes bridging, appearing to flow like candle wax from one vertebra to the next.

In general, anteroposterior (AP), lateral, and lumbosacral spot radiographs are adequate to diagnose OA of the spine, and oblique views of the lumbar spine to show the facet joints are not usually necessary. Magnetic resonance imaging (MRI), or alternatively, computed axial tomography (CT), are necessary to diagnose herniated vertebral discs and/or lumbar spinal stenosis. It is important to make a specific diagnosis when these problems are suspected, as physical therapy designed to alleviate one disorder may aggravate the other.

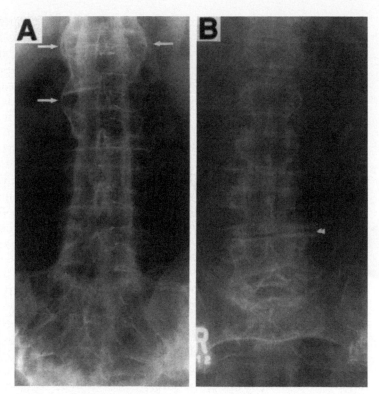

FIGURE 6-7. Osteophytes versus syndesmophytes. Syndesmophytes of spondyloarthropathy are fine, project vertically, and seem to flow from one vertebral body to the next (*arrows* in **A**), whereas osteophytes of OA are course and project more horizontally (*arrowheads* in **B**).

Sacroiliac Joints

OA of the sacroiliac joint occurs frequently in older individuals and presents on radiographs as asymmetric joint space narrowing, osteophytes at the inferior aspect of the joint, and distinct sclerotic joint margins. The finding of pseudowidened joint spaces, indistinct joint margins, and erosions or fusion of the joint, particularly in a young person, suggests the presence or aftermath of an inflammatory sacroiliitis, rather than OA.

Foot and Ankle

The metatarsophalangeal (MTP) joint of the great toe is prone to develop OA, with the usual radiographic findings of joint space narrowing, osteophyte formation, sclerosis, and subchondral cysts. It often presents with pain on walking, and limited dorsiflexion or plantar flexion of the MTP, or *hallux rigidus*. Asymmetric degeneration may lead to abduction of the great toe with lateral angulation of the joint, or *hallux valgus* (bunion) deformity.

Subtalar joint degeneration can lead to pain with inversion and eversion of the foot. Tibiotalar joint degeneration rarely occurs without prior trauma or an inciting anatomic abnormality. Rapid and destructive degeneration of the foot and ankle joints usually indicates a *neuroarthropathy* (Charcot joint), in which loss of sensation and proprioception leads to improper joint loading and repetitive trauma. The neuropathy associated with diabetes mellitus is the most common cause.

Laboratory Features

No laboratory studies are specific for degenerative arthritis, and none are needed to confirm the diagnosis. Studies are sometimes done, however, to rule out diseases that can be associated with or mimic OA. Assessment of serum creatinine and liver transaminases may be necessary in order to safely prescribe analgesics for pain. Analysis of synovial fluid from joints with OA typically reveals normal to mildly decreased viscosity and a cell count that is frequently less than 100 cells/μL, and rarely higher than 8,000 cells/μL. Cell counts at the high end of this range are more common in long-standing joint disease, and very high cell counts should prompt further investigation for infection, crystal arthritis, or other superimposed inflammatory joint disease. When new joint effusions occur, fluid should also be analyzed by polarized light microscopy for calcium pyrophosphate dihydrate (CPPD) crystals, as the incidence of CPPD is increased in degenerative arthritis. Basic calcium phosphate crystals are also increased in degenerative arthritis, but are too small to detect by light microscopy.

Medical Management

The goal of medical management of OA is not merely to reduce pain, but to slow or prevent further decline in functional status. The natural history of OA may be one of slow, chronic progression, or of stable periods with intermittent worsening. With new or increased pain there is a natural tendency to reduce activity. As activity decreases over time, so, too, does muscle bulk and strength, which may lead to decreased joint stability, worsening of joint degeneration, and further decline in functional status. Even though OA is not a systemic disease, the related decline in functional status can have major systemic consequences, affecting cardiovascular health, emotional health, and sense of well-being. Breaking this cycle may require a team approach targeted toward educating the patient and family, evaluating and sometimes altering the patient's lifestyle, offering assistive devices, and prescribing both physical and pharmacotherapy.

Nonpharmacologic Therapy

Patient education is vital, especially in early disease where intervention is most likely to be effective. Obesity is the number one *modifiable* risk factor for OA. Therefore, obese patients should be counseled by dietitians and be continually encouraged by their physicians to adhere to a diet program that *safely* promotes and maintains weight loss. Patients may alter the course of their disease and improve their level of safety and functioning, simply by losing weight and increasing or at least maintaining muscle strength. They need to understand the benefits and limitations of their medications, which are prescribed to alleviate pain and reduce inflammation, but by themselves may not alter the disease process or slow its progression.

Periodic rest of affected joints is appropriate, especially in acute disease exacerbations, but excessive rest or reduction in activity will begin the cycle of atrophy, weakness, and further functional decline, which may actually worsen pain over time. Exercise is required to strengthen muscles, and many studies have shown that regular, moderate exercise can both reduce pain, and improve the functional status of patients with mild to moderate OA.

Finally, exercise is often required, in addition to dietary modifications, for effective weight loss. The type and intensity of exercise should be tailored to the individual needs of the patient. For instance, for patients with OA of the knees who have not yet developed significantly abnormal joint angulation, a twice daily set of supine 10-second isometric quadriceps contractions can improve strength, reduce pain, and reduce the risk of falling. This exercise is generally well tolerated even by patients with moderately severe knee pain. In general, low impact exercise, such as walking, is preferred to high impact exercise, such as running or jogging. Exercise in water, which helps to unload the weight-bearing joints, can be especially beneficial when weight-bearing pain in the knees, back, or hips limits tolerance for land exercise.

The need for exercise guidance is just one of many reasons that physical therapy is an integral part of the management of OA. Physical therapists can instruct patients on the proper use of canes and walkers, to decrease weight-bearing stress on knees and hips, reduce the risk of injurious falls, and reduce the fear of falling that by itself can greatly limit patient mobility. Therapists can also instruct patients on the proper use of transcutaneous electrical nerve stimulation (TENS) units to reduce pain in specific areas. Insoles, braces, and orthopaedic shoes can benefit OA of the knees, ankles, and feet. Lateral wedged shoe inserts can sometimes reduce pain of medial knee joint OA by shifting weight to the less affected lateral compartment. Medial patellar taping may reduce the lateral compartment pain of patellofemoral syndrome. Patients with chronic back pain due to lumbar spinal stenosis will benefit from education about appropriate spinal biomechanics used in daily activities and about those positions of the spine that exacerbate back and leg pain.

Occupational therapy can be very beneficial for patients with hand and wrist OA. Therapists can fit patients with finger or first CMC splints to stabilize affected joints, and instruct them on how to reduce joint stress during daily activities. Small sleeves of silicone can pad tender Heberden's and Bouchard's nodes. Careful use of heat or cold may also alleviate pain. Paraffin baths are particularly soothing for the pain of erosive OA.

Pharmacotherapy

Pharmacotherapy for OA can be divided into topical (rubifacient) therapies, intra-articular therapies, oral analgesic therapies, and dietary supplements.

Rubifacients include counterirritant agents, which can have a transient, soothing effect on joint pain, and are generally safe. Topical capsaicin, if applied frequently and consistently to a region, can selectively reduce pain sensation in that region by depleting substance P from type C unmyelinated pain neurons. However, not everyone can tolerate the initial burning sensation caused by capsaicin, and patients must be well informed in order to use this agent properly.

Intra-articular corticosteroid injections are particularly helpful for OA of the knees, especially when there is inflammation and joint effusion, and can be safely repeated up to four times per year. The injection may work best if the knee joint is first aspirated to remove excess synovial fluid. If the fluid appears at all turbid, it should be sent for cell counts and for culture, and the corticosteroid injection should be postponed until it is clear that the joint is not infected. Epidural corticosteroid injections, performed under fluoroscopic guidance, can sometimes reduce pain of lumbar stenosis. *Viscosupplementation*, intra-articular injection of hyaluronic acid derivatives, may also be beneficial for mild to moderate OA of the knee, particularly for patients who cannot take analgesics, or who are not candidates for joint replacement.

Oral analgesics are still a mainstay in the management of OA pain, but choice of agent must be guided by knowledge of the patient's other medical conditions and concurrent treatment. Oral analgesics include acetaminophen, nonsteroidal anti-inflammatory drugs (NSAIDs), selective cyclooxygenase-2 (COX-2) inhibitors, nonacetylated salicylates, synthetic opioid agonists, and narcotics.

Acetaminophen is inexpensive, widely used, and for many patients will provide adequate pain relief when used at a full dose of 1 g three to four times per day. Though long thought to be very safe, a recent meta-analysis suggests that acetaminophen may cause more gastrointestinal and renal toxicity then originally believed, especially when used chronically. Impaired liver function is a contraindication for high dose acetaminophen.

For some patients, an oral NSAID or selective COX-2 inhibitor will be more effective than acetaminophen for relieving OA-related pain. However, the benefit of added pain relief must be balanced with the potential for significant toxicity, especially in the elderly, who are the majority of patients needing analgesics for OA. NSAIDs inhibit gastric COX-1, thus blocking production of gastroprotective prostaglandins, and are known to cause significant

gastrointestinal (GI) side effects and toxicity, including pain, acid reflux, gastric ulcers, and erosive esophagitis. Therefore, many patients who require chronic use of NSAIDs will also require concurrent use of gastroprotective agents such as misoprostal, or proton-pump, inhibitors. Selective COX-2 inhibitors are as effective as NSAIDs for relieving OA-related pain, and cause fewer GI side effects and ulcers, however, they may be associated with an increased risk of heart attack and stroke. Both NSAIDs and COX-2 inhibitors can reduce glomerular filtration, and thus increase sodium and fluid retention. Therefore, patients who have uncontrolled hypertension, renal insufficiency, or congestive heart failure should, in most cases, avoid these agents altogether and should certainly be monitored very closely when these agents are prescribed. The nonacetylated salicylates, which do not inhibit COX-1 or COX-2, may be safer choices for elderly patients with hypertension or mild renal insufficiency. However, ototoxicity and CNS side effects may limit tolerance to these medications.

Judicious use of narcotics or the synthetic opioid agonist, tramadol, has a role in management of OA-related pain. Short-term use for acute exacerbation of pain is safe and effective in most circumstances. Chronic use should generally be avoided, but may be appropriate in selective cases where pain and functional limitation are significant, surgery is not possible, and other medical conditions prohibit use of NSAIDs or COX-2 inhibitors. Narcotics and tramadol are often prescribed as combination pills containing acetaminophen, which may improve efficacy but also creates a risk for acetaminophen overdose if additional acetaminophen is taken along with them. Patients must be educated to avoid acetaminophen overdose.

Almost all oral analgesics have some potential for hepatic toxicity and should be used with caution in patients with liver disease. Physicians should obtain baseline creatinine and liver transaminases, and later repeat these tests, in all patients who are starting a course of chronic analgesic use for OA.

Dietary supplements, such as glucosamine sulfate, have gained great popularity and are now widely used. Studies in animal models suggest that glucosamine may slow cartilage breakdown. Human studies do show at least a modest benefit of reduced pain, or reduced need for other oral analgesics, such as acetaminophen. Human studies have also purported to show that glucosamine use reduces loss of knee cartilage, by showing differences in radiographic joint space between glucosamine versus placebo users. However, these studies have been criticized for not accounting for the possibility that pain reduction in the glucosamine users may have altered their stance and thus increased the measured joint space. Glucosamine is generally safe, but should be avoided by patients who are allergic to shellfish. Many glucosamine preparations also contain chondroitin sulfate, and small controlled trials suggest that this agent may also reduce pain of OA. However, chondroitin is derived from animal cartilage, which raises issues of safety, and there is little evidence that chondroitin will provide any additional benefit beyond that derived from glucosamine alone. The American College of Rheumatology Subcommittee on Osteoarthritis Guidelines does not recommend use of these agents at this time.

Surgical Management

Surgical intervention is considered for intractable pain or deformity that limits function and is discussed separately elsewhere. It does not obviate the need for continued medical management.

Rheumatoid Arthritis

Paul M. Peloso

Rheumatoid arthritis is a disease of chronic polyarticular inflammation that leads to joint swelling, joint deformity, loss of joint function, and early death. Advances in the underlying immunobiology, earlier diagnostic possibilities, and major therapeutic approaches could well limit the previous inexorable decline in function. RA occurs in 1 to 3% of the white adult population, but prevalence varies depending on age, race, and classification criteria used. Women are slightly more affected than men (3:2), but the disease is seen in all races, teenagers, and the elderly, and has a worldwide distribution.

Pathogenesis

Products of the HLA region or class II genes of the major histocompatibility complex control both immune responses and susceptibility to rheumatoid arthritis (Color Figure 6-1). People who are HLA DRB4 positive are more likely to develop erosive, disabling disease, but only one-third of RA patients are DRB4 positive. Infection is suspected to play a role in RA onset, although no specific bacterial or viral causes have been proven. Perhaps RA is a final common pathway for several infections.

In the early stages, edema, microvascular proliferation, and T-lymphocyte infiltration occur in the subsynovial tissue, followed by synovial lining cell proliferation. Increased cellularity includes synovial infiltration by B-cells, macrophages, and fibroblasts. B-cells develop into plasma cells and reside in the synovium chronically, producing rheumatoid factor (an immunoglobulin), leading to complement activation. Fibroblasts migrate to the synovial surface, with granulation tissue development, entailing further proliferation of fibroblasts, synovial lining cells, and enhanced vascular infiltration. Responding to chemotactic factors including complement byproducts, granulocytes migrate through capillary walls and synovial tissue into the joint space. These cells then permanently reside in the joint space and discharge enzymes. These hydrolases, DNAase, proteinases (elastase and collagenase) accumulate in the synovial fluid, articular cartilage, and bone-destroying structural proteins and other cells. Soluble pro-inflammatory substances produced by activated lymphocytes, monocytes, and macrophages (TNF-α, interleukin 1 and other cytokines, E series prostaglandins, leukotriene B4) are generated in the joint. These increase vascular permeability and further activate granulocytes, lymphocytes, and monocyte-derived macrophages, synovial cells, osteoclasts, and fibroblasts. Soluble mediators augment and perpetuate the inflammatory response.

In chronic RA, this proliferative granulation tissue, called pannus, advances across the joint surface, destroying marginal articular cartilage and invading subchondral bone. Pannus attached to the joint capsule, ligament, and tendons results in joint deformity. Active inflammation is accompanied by attempted repair, and collagen production may become dominant, leading to fibrosis and joint contractures.

Clinical Features

As in all inflammatory arthritis conditions, patients with RA are stiff and sore in the morning, lasting 1 to or more hours, improving with low-grade activity.

Visible joint swelling, especially that observed by an experienced health care provider, is highly specific for an inflammatory arthritis. Rheumatoid arthritis has a predilection for small joints of the hands (PIP and MCP), the wrists, the knees and the feet. Population-based studies suggest pain elicited by squeezing the MTPs or the MCPs in the presence of two or more swollen joints is highly specific for RA. Symmetrical involvement is typical of RA, and it can be associated with fatigue, malaise, fever, weight loss, and lymphadenopathy. Nodules may occur, typically along the olecranon border, Achilles tendon, or extensor surfaces of the hands and feet, but are often a later finding.

The onset may be explosive, or an additive, progressive polyarthritis. MRI reveals bone edema and cartilage degradation within weeks of symptom onset. In time almost all synovial joints may become involved, including TMJ, shoulders, elbows, wrists, MCP, PIP, knees, ankles, feet, and cervical spine. The hips may be spared early. Involvement of the DIPs of the hands and inflammatory spinal involvement are extremely rare. Tenosynovitis is common, especially in the hands and feet and can lead to nerve root entrapment (carpal and tarsal tunnel) and tendon rupture. Documentable joint inflammation is detected as palpable synovial swelling or joint tenderness. Although swelling is often visible and palpable, joint tenderness is elicited by applying direct pressure to the joint or at the end range of passive joint motion. Tenosynovitis is diagnosed as swelling along the tendon, pain with passive stretching of the tendon, and pain on resisted movement.

Diagnosis, Differential Diagnosis, and Prognosis

The American College of Rheumatology has developed diagnostic criteria, which require the presence of four or more of the following seven items:
   Morning stiffness for at least one hour and present for at least 6 weeks
   Swelling of three or more joints for at least 6 weeks
   Swelling of wrist, PIP, or MCP joints for at least 6 weeks
   Symmetrical joint swelling
   Hand radiograph changes typical of RA, including erosions or unequivocal bony periarticular decalcification
   Subcutaneous nodules
   Rheumatoid factor

The differential diagnosis of RA includes an acute viral polyarthritis, such as rubella or parvovirus, SLE, Sjögren's syndrome, sarcoidosis, systemic immune complex reactions, reactive arthritis, psoriatic arthritis, polyarticular CPPD (pseudogout), and erosive osteoarthritis involving mainly the PIPs. All can have polyarthritis, but historical features of infection, cutaneous abnormalities, and patterns of joint involvement all suggest these alternate diagnoses.

Spontaneous remission can occur and last months or years, in as many as 10% of patients. Risk factors for progression include rheumatoid factor positivity, DRB4 positivity, nodules, persistent elevation of the CRP, and a progressive, additive onset. Intermittent disease flares with increased systemic symptoms and increased numbers of swollen joints is the rule. Joint damage correlates with persistent joint inflammation.

Laboratory Features

Positive rheumatoid factor occurs in 60% of patients at 6 months and in 80% over time. Other conditions with positive rheumatoid factors include cryoglobulinemia, parvovirus 19 infection, hepatitis C, Sjögren's syndrome, SLE and occurs in 5% of normal, healthy individuals. A positive ANA occurs in 40%. The recently described anti–citrullinated cyclic peptide (anti-CCP) antibody can be positive early in RA when the rheumatoid factor is negative. It appears to have prognostic importance. Persistent elevation of the ESR or CRP and anemia of chronic disease are common in undertreated RA.

Radiographic erosions and joint space loss commonly affects the MCP, PIP, MTP, and ulnar-carpal joints, and are present in up to 30% of patients in the first year with 90% having erosions after 2 years. MRI is a far more sensitive test for erosions than is plain radiography.

Rheumatoid Deformities

Chronic unchecked inflammation leads to characteristic deformities. Rotation of the carpometacarpal complex on the radius, and volar subluxation of the carpus on the radius leads to reduced grip. Disruption of the distal radio-ulnar ligament leads to dorsal subluxation of the distal ulna, appreciated clinically as the "piano key sign." Damage to the joint capsule and collateral ligaments of the MCP joints combined with rotational deformity of the metacarpal complex leads to ulnar deviation of the fingers, often accompanied by volar or ulnar subluxation of the PIP joints. Swan neck deformity is fixed hyperextension of the PIP joint and accompanying flexion of the DIP joint. Boutonniere deformity is flexion contracture of the PIP joint with hyperextension of the DIP, resulting from damage to the central portion of the extensor tendon overlying the PIP joint. A Baker's cyst develops in the popliteal space from increased intra-articular pressure and a gradual weakening of the posterior capsule. Baker's cysts are prone to rupture, with acute pain, swelling, and heat in the calf, mimicking deep venous thrombosis or cellulitis. Ultrasonography can differentiate a cyst from venous thrombosis. Forefoot involvement includes widening of the forefoot, hallux valgus, hallux rigidus, and cock-up toe deformities. Atrophy of the soft tissue pads on the plantar surface of MTP results in weight-bearing pain and ulceration. Hindfoot involvement includes contracture of the subtalar joints or excessive laxity associated with abduction and pronation of the midfoot and forefoot.

RA frequently involves the cervical spine, paralleling hand involvement. Particularly concerning is weakening of ligaments attaching the odontoid process to C2 and to the lateral masses of C1. Anterior subluxation of C1 relative to C2 and the odontoid process leads to atlanto-axial subluxation. Progressive subluxation in concert with degenerative and inflammatory changes at levels below C2 may lead to neurological impingement and motor deficits. Cranial settling results when erosion of the occipital condyles or the lateral masses of C1 cause settling of the skull relative to the odontoid process. The odontoid may protrude into the foramen magnum where it compresses the medulla or pons.

Extra-Articular Manifestations

RA is a systemic disease and may entail nodules, serositis, and vasculitis. Nodules occur in 25% of patients and are often a late feature. They have a central area of fibrinoid necrosis surrounded by histiocytes and inflammatory cells. Common locations are elbows, hands, feet, although they can occur in all locations including internal organs. Repeated pressure may encourage their development. Sjögren's syndrome occurs in 10% of RA patients,

involving chronic inflammation of exocrine glands, most commonly the lacrimal and salivary glands. Clinically it presents as dryness of the eyes and mouth, leading to corneal ulceration and accelerated dental carries. Serositis is relatively uncommon and presents with recurring, moderate-sized exudative pleural effusions with a low glucose. Diffuse interstitial pulmonary fibrosis is bilateral, principally affecting the lower lung zones. Felty's syndrome is the co-occurrence of RA, splenomegaly, cytopenias (white cells or platelets), and leg ulcers. Systemic vasculitis can lead to ischemia of the skin (purpura), vasa nervorum (peripheral neuropathies), and rarely internal viscera. Small 1 to 2 mm hemorrhagic cutaneous infarcts in the periungal region of the digits are the result of an obliterative vasculopathy and do not indicate a systemic vasculitis.

Management of Rheumatoid Arthritis

The three major goals of rheumatoid arthritis management include reducing pain, reducing inflammation, and preventing disability (Figure 6-8). Other goals include minimizing drug toxicity and management of extra-articular features. These goals are best prioritized through careful history taking, physical examination, and selected laboratory and radiographic studies. Several well-validated patient-completed questionnaires of disability, such as the health assessment questionnaire (HAQ), predict short- and long-term functioning and should be a routine component of RA care.

Pain management is not equivalent to inflammation control, although they may be performed in concert. Analgesia with acetaminophen, nonsteroidal anti-inflammatory drugs, weak opiates (codeine and tramadol), use of local depot steroid injections, physical therapy, joint splinting, and education (Arthritis Foundation) are appropriate for pain management. NSAIDs and injections have only a minor role in inflammation management. Pain can result from several causes including inflammation, but also from joint and tendon damage, muscle pain, and fatigue and should not be assumed to be inflammation related. Joint inflammation is diagnosed by asking about inflammatory symptoms (morning stiffness and improvement with activity) and the presence of joint swelling. Laboratory tests (ESR/CRP) can be a helpful adjunct to the history and examination.

Pain Management	Inflammation Management	Disability Management	Management of Extra-Articular Disease Features
Analgesia with acetaminophen, NSAIDs, weak opiates. Physical therapy, occupational therapy, education. Injections. Total joint arthroplasty.	Corticosteroid injections. Short courses of oral corticosteroids (prednisone 10–25 milligrams for one to two weeks). Hydroxychloroquine, sulfasalazine, monocycline (low potency, low toxicity DMARDs). Methotrexate, azathioprine, leflunomide (antimetabolites with bone marrow and liver toxicity). Combinations of DMARDs. TNF alpha antagonists. (infection risks).	Control of inflammation (DMARDs). Management of comorbidities (depression and anxiety). Job site factor assessments (job physical capacity). Help from social workers, physical therapists and occupational therapists.	Sicca—eye drops, oral lozenges, pilocarpine. Nodules—injections and surgery rarely. Entrapment neuropathy—surgical release. Cervical Spine instability—peri-operative assessment and careful clinical follow-up. Vasculitis—intensive medical management.

FIGURE 6-8. Managing rheumatoid arthritis.

Inflammation is best managed with immuno-modulators, which do not have immediate onset. While oral corticosteroids (prednisone) and joint injections may provide temporary relief, their long-term toxicity and the availability of more effective drugs argue against their long-term use. Corticosteroids should be used temporarily, for 1 or 2 weeks with acute flares and while waiting for long-term inflammation control with disease-modifying agents. Low potency, low toxicity DMARDs include hydroxychloroquine, sulfasalazine, and minocycline. These drugs should be used early in patients with mild disease, and in combinations with more potent DMARDs as disease progresses. One of these drugs should be started as soon as the RA diagnosis is suspected.

Methotrexate, an antimetabolite, has been the mainstay of inflammatory control for the last 20 years, with two other antimetabolites, azathioprine and leflunomide, as alternatives. For persistent uncontrolled inflammation, research has shown that combinations of DMARDs (two or three of the above listed agents) or the addition of TNF-α inhibitors are required. Recent large, long-term, randomized controlled trials with TNF-α inhibitors have shown improvements in joint inflammation and joint damage, with prevention of radiographic erosions. Use of antimetabolites and TNF-α inhibitors require expert rheumatologist advice. The antimetabolites have important toxicity in the liver and bone marrow and are associated with infection risk. Recent data shows methotrexate does not impair wound healing. The TNF-α antagonists also have increased infection risk and should be stopped 2 to 4 weeks before surgery.

Prevention of disability may be the most challenging goal and requires optimal pain control, control of joint inflammation, and attention to personal, social and occupational factors that contribute to disability burden. Depression, anxiety, low educational attainment, a physically demanding job, and persistent unchecked inflammation all predict job loss. Involvement of the primary care provider, social workers, physical therapists, occupational therapists, and the work site may be required to match job requirements with the patient's abilities.

Extra-articular features require individualized management. Sicca complex (Sjögren's syndrome) may be improved with eyedrops, oral lozenges, and oral pilocarpine or oral cholinergic agonists. Nodules are best left alone unless they are causing pain and functional loss. Local corticosteroid injection may cause nodules to regress. They often recur after surgical removal. Entrapment neuropathies require surgical release. Tendon ruptures (especially wrist and finger extensors) require surgical repair. Recurrent Baker's cysts may respond to surgical excision.

Cord compression symptoms are the usual justification for surgical stabilization. Cervical instability requires cooperation between the orthopedist and the rheumatologist. Advanced degenerative disease responds well to total joint replacement, particularly knees and hips, although shoulder, wrist, MCP, and PIP arthroplasty may all be appropriate in some instances. The need for surgical intervention is evidence of unchecked inflammation in the past, and surgery is not an alternative to optimal medical management.

Felty's syndrome, rheumatoid lung, vasculitis, cytopenias, and drug toxicity mandate consultation with a rheumatologist and other appropriate medical specialists, with a rheumatologist coordinating care.

Advances in medical and surgical management can fundamentally alter the natural history and subsequent disability associated with rheumatoid arthritis. RA need not be a progressive, disabling condition, when expertly managed.

Systemic Lupus Erythematosus
Haraldine A. Stafford

Definition

Systemic lupus erythematosus (SLE) is a multisystemic chronic autoimmune disease that is distinguished by characteristic organ manifestations. It most commonly involves the musculoskeletal, cutaneous, and renal systems. Its cause is unknown but likely involves hereditary and environmental susceptibility factors. Autoantibodies are the hallmark of this condition and are directed primarily to cell nuclei and their constituents, for example, antinuclear antibodies (ANA), and anti–double stranded DNA (anti-dsDNA). They mediate tissue injury by forming immune complexes, which promote inflammation. They also promote cell destruction by the reticuloendothelial system and perhaps exert direct toxic effects on cell function.

SLE is primarily a disease affecting young women with a peak incidence in the reproductive years. It affects individuals of all races and ethnicities with a prevalence of 15 to 52 cases/100,000 persons. Diagnosis is made on the basis of characteristic clinical and laboratory features (for formal criteria used in making the diagnosis, see Tan 1982). The course is variable, and is related to race, type, and severity of organ involvement. Prognosis has improved dramatically over the last 50 years secondary to earlier recognition and more effective management.

Clinical Features

Patients with SLE may present with a variety of symptoms due to the multitude of clinical manifestations. Moreover, these clinical manifestations may change over time. Joint and skin complaints followed by constitutional symptoms (fever, fatigue, malaise, weight loss) are the most common presenting complaints. The majority of patients have arthralgias (95%), arthritis (90%), fever (90%), fatigue (81%), skin rashes (malar rash, discoid lupus, photosensitivity, 74%), or glomerulonephritis (50%) at some time in their illness. Myalgias and myositis occur less frequently. Other clinical features used in making the diagnosis of SLE include serositis, seizures, psychosis, and oral ulcers. The classic presentation of a butterfly (malar) rash (erythema over the cheekbones and nose) with simultaneous arthritis occurs in a minority of patients.

Joint complaints include pain (arthralgias), stiffness, and swelling (arthritis). Symptoms are inflammatory in nature, and may be evanescent and migratory, persistent, or progressive. Any peripheral joint may be involved, although the metacarpophalangeal and proximal interphalangeal joints of the hands, wrists, and knees are most frequently affected. Symmetric polyarthritis affecting the hands and wrists is the most common arthritis presentation. Pain and palpable tenderness is often more prominent than swelling. This joint distribution resembles the pattern in rheumatoid arthritis (RA), and often, patients are initially diagnosed with RA. The diagnosis of SLE becomes obvious when other characteristic clinical and laboratory features develop. Usually the joint complaints in SLE are milder than in RA, and destruction of cartilage and bone does not occur. Deformities of the joints can occur in SLE, and in the hand include ulnar deviation and subluxation, swan neck deformities, and hyperextension of the thumb interphalangeal joints. This usually reducible subluxation is called

Jaccoud's arthropathy, and occurs in 5 to 40% of patients. It results from stretching and laxity of ligaments and tendons rather than from destructive changes typical of RA. Jaccoud's arthropathy can occur in other joints as well. Symptomatic axial skeleton involvement is unusual, although radiographic evidence of sacroiliitis is frequently present.

Patients on glucocorticoids or immunosuppressive drugs are susceptible to a variety of musculoskeletal complications. Steroid myopathy can cause progressive weakness. Glucocorticoid-induced osteoporotic compression fractures are a potential cause of acute back pain. Stress fractures near a joint can cause joint pain and swelling, and should also be considered in those patients on chronic corticosteroids. Septic arthritis and osteonecrosis are other potential causes of joint pain. Immunosuppressives, glucocorticoids, and intrinsic susceptibility to infection predispose these patients to septic arthritis. Clinically apparent osteonecrosis occurs in 4 to 15% of these patients. It affects the humeral head in 80% of cases, followed by the knees and shoulders. Multiple joint osteonecrosis is common. Pain may be mild to severe and develops insidiously to abruptly. Thus, acute mono- or oligoarthritis needs to be further evaluated with arthrocentesis and MRI to eliminate septic arthritis and osteonecrosis, respectively.

Tendon involvement is common and includes changes resulting in Jaccoud's arthropathy, tenosynovitis, and tendon rupture. Tenosynovitis often involves the extensor tendons of the fingers and toes. Tendon rupture frequently affects the patellar tendons, long head of the biceps and triceps, and extensor tendons of the hands. Trauma and corticosteroid use are associated risk factors.

Pathologic and Radiologic Features

Histologic synovial changes in SLE arthritis resemble those observed in RA although they are milder in intensity. Typical features include perivascular inflammation, synovial cell proliferation, and fibrin deposition at the synovial membrane. Bone and cartilage destruction rarely occur, in contrast to what is observed in RA. Histologic examination of ruptured tendons may show inflammatory changes.

Radiographs of arthritic joints are often normal, but up to 50% of patients may have mild abnormalities. These abnormalities include soft tissue swelling, periarticular osteopenia, osteoporosis, and subluxation. Joint space narrowing and marginal erosions,

which are common in RA, are rarely if ever observed in SLE.

Laboratory Features

SLE patients with joint complaints usually have laboratory evidence of SLE. ANAs are present in greater than 98% of patients with SLE. However, the specificity of a positive ANA is low. Positive ANAs are observed frequently in other autoimmune diseases, as well as in healthy individuals and particularly in the elderly. Consequently, their utility is the greatest when used to support the clinical and laboratory impression of SLE. Anti-dsDNA and anti-Sm autoantibodies are more specific for SLE. Unexplained leukopenia, lymphopenia, hemolytic anemia, and thrombocytopenia are hematologic manifestations of SLE. Proteinuria, hematuria, and red blood cell casts suggest renal involvement by SLE.

Synovial fluid in SLE arthritis is usually mildly inflammatory. Fluid is clear with normal viscosity. White cell counts typically range from 2,000 to 15,000, although values up to 40,000 have been detected. There is often a lymphocyte predominance.

Management

Appropriate medical therapy for SLE is determined by the pattern and severity of organ involvement. If musculoskeletal complaints are accompanied by major organ involvement (kidneys, central nervous system, blood cells), then aggressive therapy with high dose glucocorticoids with or without immunosuppressive therapy is used. Cyclophosphamide, mycophenolate mofetil, and azathioprine are commonly used immunosuppressive agents. If musculoskeletal complaints accompany minor organ involvement (skin, oral mucosa, pleura), then antimalarials are often used. Isolated mild musculoskeletal complaints are initially treated with NSAIDs. If they are refractory or more severe, antimalarials are added. Methotrexate is used for arthritis that has failed antimalarial treatment. Low dose glucocorticoids (usually ≤ 10 mg prednisone each day) are used in arthritis that fails to respond to NSAIDs while waiting for antimalarials and/or methotrexate to become effective. More aggressive therapy of SLE arthritis with combination immunosuppressive therapy, such as that used for RA, is rarely indicated. TNF-α blocking agents are not used in SLE, and may worsen it.

Nonpharmacologic therapy is also indicated for SLE musculoskeletal complaints. Physical and occupational therapy are important adjuncts to pharmacologic therapy. Splints may be effective in limiting deformities and, with appropriate exercise, may preserve function. Surgical interventions may be necessary to correct deformities, restore joint function, and manage tendon rupture and osteonecrosis.

Spondyloarthropathies
George V. (Geordie) Lawry II

The spondyloarthropathies are an interrelated group of disorders which include ankylosing spondylitis, inflammatory bowel disease arthritis, reactive arthritis (Reiter's syndrome), and psoriatic arthritis. They are clinically, radiographically, pathologically and genetically related to ankylosing spondylitis. The absence of rheumatoid factor (leading to the name "seronegative" spondyloarthropathy) is not an essential diagnostic feature. The predilection of these disorders to axial, spinal inflammation is the dominant clinical feature leading to the preferred term *spondyloarthropathy*. A number of clinical distinctions permit differentiation from rheumatoid arthritis, including important differences in articular and extra-articular features as well as management and prognosis.

Clinical Hallmarks

The most distinctive feature of the spondyloarthropathies is the presence of "enthesopathy." An enthesis is the insertion point of tendons, ligaments, or joint capsule on bone and the term enthesopathy refers to a physical alteration at the site of such attachments. *Inflammatory enthesitis* is the clinical hallmark of all the spondyloarthropathies and is an important feature shared by all the members of this family. The presence of widespread enthesitis leads to multiple spinal and peripheral manifestations so characteristic of these disorders (Figure 6-9).

A second important hallmark is the presence of *axial (spinal) involvement.* Inflammatory synovitis and capsular enthesitis at the sacroiliac joints leads to sacroiliitis (Figure 6-9A). Inflammation of spinal entheses at paraspinous ligaments leads to spondylitis (inflammatory involvement of the spine). Inflammation at axial cartilaginous joints contributes to the arthritis at the SI joints, intervertebral discs, symphysis pubis, manubriosternal joint, and sternoclavicular joints.

The third hallmark of the spondyloarthropathies is the particular pattern of *peripheral joint involvement.* Axial "root" joint synovitis in shoulders and hips is most commonly seen in ankylosing spondylitis. An asymmetric lower extremity oligoarthritis (2 to 4 joints), especially involving the knee and ankle joints, is seen in patients with inflammatory bowel disease arthritis. A similar, predominantly large joint lower extremity oligoarthritis may be seen in reactive arthritis or Reiter's syndrome with the addition of small joint synovitis, particularly with distal interphalangeal (DIP) involvement of toes and fingers (DIP involvement is not usually seen clinically in RA). In addition, a particularly distinctive feature of the spondyloarthropathies (especially seen in reactive and psoriatic arthritis) is the presence of "sausage digits" (Figure 6-9D). This distinctive pattern of swelling represents the combination of synovitis of small synovial joints combined with enthesitis of tendon sheaths, tendon insertions, joint capsules and supporting ligaments, giving rise to sausage-like swelling of the entire digit. A spectrum of progressively increasing peripheral joint involvement is seen when comparing ankylosing spondylitis (least peripheral) to inflammatory bowel disease arthritis to reactive arthritis to psoriatic arthritis (most peripheral).

The fourth clinical hallmark of the spondyloarthropathies is the notable *extra-articular features* frequently present in this family of disorders: ocular (conjunctivitis and uveitis), GU (urethritis), GI (diarrhea and dysentery), and cutaneous (psoriasis) manifestations.

Ankylosing Spondylitis

Ankylosing spondylitis is estimated to occur in 0.5 to 1% of the population. It begins most frequently before age 40, usually in the third or fourth decades of life. Symptoms and signs of inflammatory spinal disease predominate. Inflammatory back pain, suggesting sacroiliitis and spondylitis, has five important historical features that help to

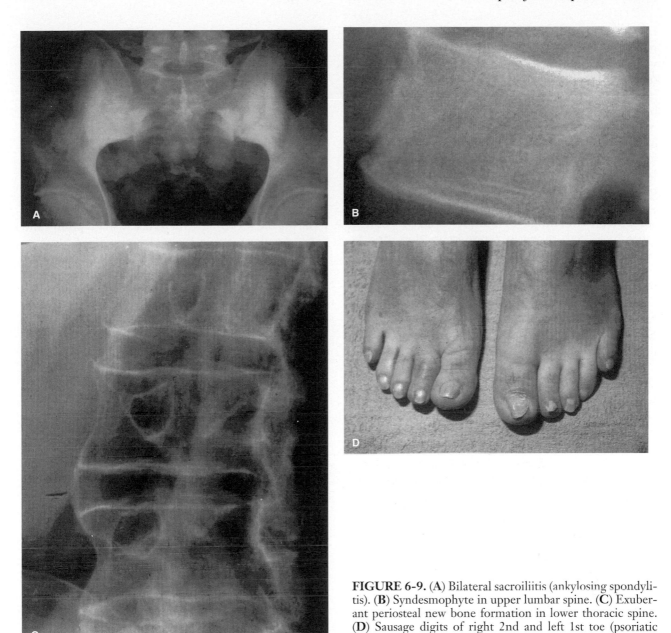

FIGURE 6-9. (A) Bilateral sacroiliitis (ankylosing spondylitis). (B) Syndesmophyte in upper lumbar spine. (C) Exuberant periosteal new bone formation in lower thoracic spine. (D) Sausage digits of right 2nd and left 1st toe (psoriatic arthritis).

distinguish it from more common mechanical low back pain: age less than 40, insidious onset, duration of less than 3 months, significant morning stiffness, and improvement with exercise. Patients with inflammatory back pain give a history that frequently sounds quite vague, the significance of which can easily be missed. Discriminating questions focusing on sleep, mornings, and the effect of rest and exercise can be extremely helpful in suspecting the correct diagnosis. Family histories of

patients with ankylosing spondylitis frequently reveal other individuals with early onset low back pain, uveitis or iritis, inflammatory bowel disease, or psoriasis.

Physical examination centers on evaluation of the spine. Sacroiliac joints may be tender to direct percussion. Specific maneuvers applying mechanical stress to the pelvis frequently result in discomfort felt directly at the SI joint (upper, inner buttock region). Visual inspection of the lumbar spine during flexion is very important. Due to extensive inflammation in spinal entheses, the lumbar lordotic curvature frequently does not reverse (as it should) during spinal flexion. Chest expansion may also be limited due to inflammatory changes at costovertebral joints in the thoracic spine. The cervical spine may also be involved, demonstrating restriction in all planes of motion (especially extension). Early loss of spinal range of motion in patients with ankylosing spondylitis may be due to inflammatory pseudofusion of spinal ligaments, and may be reversible with aggressive anti-inflammatory therapy combined with range of motion exercises. Later, more fixed reductions in range of motion, due to bony fusion, are not reversible.

Radiographic findings in ankylosing spondylitis reveal symmetric sacroiliitis characterized by sclerosis, articular erosions, and the later development of bony fusion across the joint. A single AP pelvis radiograph (Ferguson view) is the most helpful to confirm suspected sacroiliitis. Additional radiographic features of ankylosing spondylitis include progressive vertebral squaring and marginal sclerosis due to remodeling of the vertebral bodies and new bone formation. Syndesmophytes (bony bridging across the annulus of the intervertebral discs) may develop and, years later, result in the development of a bamboo" spine (multiple symmetrical syndesmophytes giving the radiographic appearance of bamboo).

Inflammatory Bowel Disease Arthritis

Arthritis may develop in 7 to 20% of patients with Crohn's disease or ulcerative colitis, and may involve either the sacroiliac joints or peripheral joints of the lower extremities.

Inflammatory back pain in such patients may be secondary to sacroiliitis with spondylitic symptoms characteristic of ankylosing spondylitis. Radiographically, these patients have symmetric sacroiliitis indistinguishable from ankylosing spondylitis. Inflammatory spondylitis may precede, occur simultaneously with, or follow inflammatory bowel disease (IBD). The clinical course of spondylitis is independent of the clinical activity of the bowel inflammation.

Peripheral arthritis in IBD tends to be a lower extremity, large joint oligoarthritis predominantly involving knees and ankles. The course of the peripheral arthritis tends to be episodic, but parallels the activity of the bowel disease.

Reactive Arthritis (Reiter's Syndrome)

Reactive arthritis describes the clinical syndrome of arthritis and extra-articular features sometimes seen in susceptible individuals following a genitourinary or gastrointestinal infection. Such patients characteristically have a seronegative (rheumatoid factor negative) arthritis lasting greater than 1 month associated with mucocutaneous, ocular, gastrointestinal (GI) or genitourinary (GU) manifestations. Mucocutaneous features include painless oral ulcers, balanitis (scaly rash on the glans penis), and keratoderma blennorrhagicum (scaly rash on palms and soles). Ocular features include conjunctivitis (which may be completely asymptomatic) or uveitis with ocular redness and photophobia. GI involvement is typically a dysenteric or diarrheal illness. GU involvement consists of urethritis or cervicitis.

The term *Reiter's syndrome* describes the classic triad of arthritis, urethritis and conjunctivitis. *Reactive arthritis* is a broader term that doesn't necessarily require all three features.

Infectious agents most commonly associated with GU or GI symptoms include *Chlamydia*, *Salmonella*, and *Shigella* species. These agents have not been cultured from synovial tissues despite the presence of significant joint swelling and synovitis, hence the term *reactive* arthritis.

Like patients with IBD arthritis, peripheral joint involvement in reactive arthritis is usually an asymmetric lower extremity oligoarthritis. However, small joint involvement is also seen in toes and fingers, particularly with the presence of sausage digits. Furthermore, the arthritis and extra-articular manifestations may occur at different times.

Symptomatic or radiographic sacroiliitis and spondylitis are seen in only a minority of patients.

Psoriatic Arthritis

Cutaneous psoriasis (psoriasis vulgaris) is a problem affecting at least 2% of the population. Psoriatic arthritis, however, develops in only about 5% of patients with cutaneous psoriasis. Psoriatic arthritis usually begins in young adulthood but may occur at any age. A number of patterns of clinical involvement can be seen with psoriatic arthritis, but the predominant peripheral expression of arthritis is an asymmetric oligoarthritis, so typical of the spondyloarthropathies. Approximately 50% of patients with psoriatic arthritis have a lower–upper extremity oligoarticularthritis. Approximately 30% will have an asymmetric to nearly symmetric polyarthritis, which may resemble rheumatoid arthritis. However, careful examination revealing persistent asymmetry, DIP joint involvement, sausage digits, and peripheral enthesopathy (Achilles tendonitis or plantar fasciitis) strongly suggests a spondyloarthropathy rather than rheumatoid arthritis. Less commonly, patients with psoriatic arthritis have sacroiliitis and spinal inflammation (approximately 20%), exclusive DIP involvement in hands and feet (approximately 10%) and, rarely, severe destruction of the finger joints called arthritis mutilans (uncommonly seen today). Sausage digits are frequently seen in psoriatic arthritis and may be very symptomatic or completely asymptomatic (thus, easily missed if both shoes and socks are not removed for a careful joint exam).

Extra-articular features of psoriatic arthritis are essentially confined to the skin and nails. The five most common site of cutaneous involvement include the elbows, knees, temporoparietal scalp, umbilicus, and intergluteal cleft (these last three sites can easily be missed if not inspected carefully).

Radiographic features of psoriatic arthritis include the development of fluffy periosteal new bone at sites of entheseal inflammation, very characteristic of the spondyloarthropathies. Extensive and aggressive inflammation at the distal interphalangeal joints may result in a classic "pencil in cup" deformity at the DIP joints of the hands or the IP joint of the great toe (a favorite site of inflammation in psoriatic arthritis).

Undifferentiated Spondyloarthropathy

Although four members of the spondyloarthropathy family are clearly recognized and distinguished, patients may present with clinical features suggesting a spondyloarthropathy (seronegative oligoarthritis and peripheral enthesitis) without additional abnormalities allowing a proper name diagnosis. Patients with such findings are best diagnosed as having an undifferentiated spondyloarthropathy, with treatment focused on dominant clinical features.

Principles of Management

Spinal Inflammation

Spinal inflammation involving sacroiliitis and spinal enthesitis is best managed with a combination of patient education (increasing understanding and reducing fear), nonsteroidal anti-inflammatory drugs (NSAIDs) to reduce pain and stiffness, development of a lifelong daily exercise program (to reduce the tendency toward spinal fusion) and, more recently, the addition of anti–tumor necrosis factor (anti-TNF) therapy including etanercept, infliximab and adalimumab, and others.

Peripheral Inflammation

Peripheral inflammation at entheses (Achilles tendon and plantar fascia and other sites) can best be managed through patient education, NSAIDs, and orthotics (heel cushions, arch supports, and splints to reduce physical stress on inflamed entheses). Selective, local corticosteroid injections may be helpful at reducing inflammation at painful entheses (with the exception of the Achilles tendon and its insertion, which should not be injected because of the danger of rupture).

Peripheral inflammation in synovial joints is best managed with patient education, NSAIDs, joint aspiration, and corticosteroid injection, and the addition of systemic medication to reduce the inflammatory process throughout the body. Sulfasalazine (enteric-coated preparations) can be an especially helpful for patients with peripheral arthritis. Methotrexate is perhaps the most widely used, potent anti-inflammatory and is usually given in weekly oral or parenteral pulses. More recently, anti-TNF therapy (etanercept, infliximab, and adalimumab) has been used in patients with spondyloarthropathy and severe axial and peripheral inflammation with significant disease-modifying effects. Long-term follow-up of patients given these newer biologic therapies (anti-TNF and other anticytokine therapy) will be required to firmly establish both their efficacy and toxicity. At present, the potential for serious infections appears to be the most significant adverse effect of these agents.

Extra-articular Features

Treatment of extra-articular features in patients with the spondyloarthropathies should be directed at the organs involved. Ocular involvement with uveitis frequently responds to topical and systemic corticosteroids. GI involvement with inflammatory bowel disease requires treatment of the underlying Crohn's disease or ulcerative colitis. GU involvement with urethritis may be treated with a tetracycline or erythromycin during acute episodes of reactive arthritis (which appears to have no beneficial effect on the duration and severity of subsequent arthritis). Cutaneous psoriasis frequently responds to topical preparations and especially well to weekly pulse methotrexate.

Juvenile Idiopathic Arthitis (a.k.a. Juvenile Rheumatoid Arthritis)

Mary M. Moore and Polly J. Ferguson

The term *juvenile idiopathic arthritis (JIA)* collectively refers to a heterogeneous group of diseases that occur in childhood with unknown etiology. The term *JIA* has recently replaced the American term juvenile rheumatoid arthritis (JRA) and European term juvenile chronic arthritis (JCA). Although the nomenclature continues to evolve, the rationale for new ILAR (International League of Associations for Rheumatology) classification is to recognize subgroups with enhanced homogeneity and to provide internationally standardized terminology in order to facilitate basic and clinical research.

The ILAR classification of JIA includes eight groups: systemic arthritis, oligoarthritis, extended oligoarthritis, polyarthritis (RF negative), polyarthritis (RF positive), psoriatic arthritis, enthesitis related arthritis, and an "other" arthritis category. It is important to correctly classify the subtype of arthritis as the pertinent differential diagnoses, the prognoses, and the complications vary with the mode of JIA onset. Common to all forms of JIA are the challenges involved in therapy of a chronic inflammatory condition occurring in growing, developing individuals. A multidisciplinary approach, including physical therapist, occupational therapist, medical social worker, orthopaedist, ophthalmologist, and rheumatologist, is necessary to ensure the best possible outcome.

The cause and pathogenesis of the JIA subgroups remain unknown. However, evidence suggests that both genetics and environment likely play a role. The strongest evidence is for linkage with certain HLA alleles, but increasing evidence shows non-HLA genes may be important as well.

Differential Diagnosis

Chronic arthritis in children (and many other conditions that present with arthralgia or apparent arthritis) have multiple causes. Essential to the diagnosis of JIA is the presence of chronic arthritis (longer than 6 weeks duration), onset before the 16th birthday and the exclusion of other conditions by history, physical examination, and appropriate laboratory testing. The possibility of malignancy must always be considered in the evaluation of a child with joint pain and ruled out with appropriate

studies prior to instituting therapy for the arthritis. Pain out of proportion to physical findings, cytopenia, elevated acute phase response with a normal or low platelet count, elevations in uric acid and/or LDH, and abnormalities on radiographs are all clues that malignancy may be the underlying cause of the joint symptoms. Giving corticosteroids to a child with occult malignancy can dramatically worsen outcome and should absolutely be avoided. Neuroblastoma and lymphoid malignancies are the most common neoplasms that present as arthritis in children.

Infection must also be considered in a child with arthralgia or arthritis. Analysis of synovial fluid is mandatory in cases in which septic arthritis is a diagnostic possibility. Other infectious causes of arthritis include Lyme disease and tuberculosis. Beyond malignancy and infection, the differential diagnosis is still extensive, including trauma, reactive arthritis, acute rheumatic fever, transient synovitis of the hip, hemophilia, inflammatory bowel disease, bacterial endocarditis, viral infections, serum sickness, lupus, dermatomyositis, metabolic disorders, among others. Growing pains, or benign limb pains, are common in school-aged children. These poorly localized pains usually occur in the lower extremities in the evening or at night and normally last a few days to weeks. Severe pain, altered gait, morning stiffness, and abnormalities on physical examination such as joint swelling suggest consideration of alternative diagnoses, including JIA.

Clinical Characteristics

Several features distinguish JIA from adult RA. Inflammatory arthritis in children (particularly younger children) is much less likely to present with complaints of pain, even when there is easily demonstrable inflammatory arthritis on examination. Like adults, children with chronic arthritis may develop destructive bony changes and soft tissue flexion contractures. Children, however, are much more prone to develop ankylosis of peripheral joints and the cervical spine. Growth disturbances can result from suppression of linear growth by inflammatory disease and premature epiphyseal closure. Alternatively, chronic inflammation can cause boney overgrowth due to enhanced blood supply to an open epiphysis. Only a minority of JIA patients are RF positive, and virtually all of these have polyarticular involvement at presentation.

Persistent Oligoarthritis and Extended Oligoarthritis

Oligoarthritis (also known as pauciarticular JRA) is the most common form of JIA. This designation is utilized for children with up to four joints affected within the first 6 months of disease onset. Typically, the large joints are affected. In about half of patients, the disease is limited to a single joint, most often the knee. Elbows and ankles are also commonly involved. This presentation often afflicts young girls, with a peak age of onset at about 2 years of age. These girls have a high incidence of concomitant inflammatory eye disease (uveitis) as well as serum ANA. Uveitis is typically asymptomatic in oligoarthritis.

Joint symptoms in pauciarticular disease are often mild and of insidious onset. The patient may present to the pediatrician for evaluation of abnormal gait or a reluctance to walk or play. These patients do not appear systemically ill. Undiagnosed or untreated disease may result in (and present with) muscular atrophy and joint contractures, particularly of the knee. As with other subtypes of JIA, growth disturbances of variable degree occur, depending on severity of disease, age of affliction, and duration of joint inflammation. Most patients persist with an oligoarticular course and are classified as "persistent oligoarthritis." However, a subset may go on to develop additional joint involvement over time. Those patients that develop a polyarticular course after the initial 6 months of oligoarthritis are classified as "extended oligoarthritis."

Polyarthritis (Rheumatoid Factor Negative)

Children have five or more joints involved during the first 6 months of their illness and do not have circulating serum rheumatoid factor. Patients often present with a gradual onset of symptoms: decreased activity, morning stiffness, joint swelling, and occasionally joint pain. Girls are most commonly affected. Both large and small joint involvement may be seen. Systemic symptoms occur, but are generally mild. Low-grade fever, fatigue, and poor appetite may occur for weeks or months before diagnosis. Examination reveals proliferative synovitis and effusions and often loss of range of motion. Mild adenopathy or hepatosplenomegaly is sometimes present. Chronic uveitis occurs less frequently than in the oligoarthritis category. JIA polyarthritis patients demonstrate a striking tendency for ankylosis of joints, particularly of the cervical spine.

Polyarthritis (Rheumatoid Factor Positive)

Patients may also present with a gradual onset of symptoms but many present with acute polyarthritis. Girls are most commonly affected, and both large and small joint involvement may be seen. Low-grade fever, fatigue, and poor appetite are often present. Examination reveals proliferative synovitis and joint effusions often with decreased range of motion. Mild adenopathy or hepatosplenomegaly may be present. Chronic uveitis is rare. These patients often have a persistent destructive arthropathy and associated subcutaneous rheumatoid nodules. This small group of patients represents the onset in childhood of classic adult RA.

Systemic Arthritis

Systemic onset of JIA (Still's disease) occurs in approximately 10% of cases. This diagnosis can be quite difficult to make, as the inflammatory arthritis is not always present on initial evaluation. These children present with high fever, malaise, and rash. The fever pattern in Still's disease is classically quotidian, with one or more daily spikes to the 38.8°C to 40.5°C (102°F to 105°F) range, followed by a return to normal or occasionally subnormal temperatures. The rash is often present only during fever spikes or after a hot bath, when it transiently appears as a fine, salmon-colored, macular eruption of the trunk, proximal extremities, and skin overlying affected joints. Most patients have adenopathy and hepatosplenomegaly and are found to have moderate to severe anemia and a striking neutrophilic leukocytosis. Other manifestations of systemic onset disease may include pericarditis, myocarditis, pleural effusion, and interstitial lung disease. Renal disease is rare. Other important considerations in the differential diagnosis include infections (particularly osteomyelitis and abdominal abscesses), inflammatory bowel disease, and malignancy. RF and ANA are usually absent, and diagnosis is made on the basis of clinical findings.

Psoriatic Arthritis

Children with psoriatic arthritis may have either psoriasis and arthritis, or arthritis plus two of the following: dactylitis, nail changes (pitting or onycholysis), or dermatologist-confirmed psoriasis in a first-degree relative. Generally, there are no associated systemic symptoms and the number of joints involved is variable. Rheumatoid factor is absent by definition. Psoriatic arthritis has a variable course but can be quite destructive.

Enthesitis-Related Arthritis

These patients are generally boys, who are older than 9 years and often have a family history of HLA-B27 spondyloarthropathy in a 1st or 2nd degree relative.

For diagnosis, patients have both enthesitis and arthritis. Or alternatively, they have only arthritis or only enthesitis plus two of the following: sacroiliac joint tenderness, presence of HLA-B27, a close relative with a spondyloarthropathy, symptomatic anterior uveitis, or, if male, onset of arthritis before 8 years.

Other Arthritis

Patients not fitting the seven categories or with features of two or more of the categories, make precise classification impossible. Future revisions of the ILAR criteria and further advances in establishing etiology will likely occur.

Course, Complications, and Prognosis

Considerable variability is found in the severity, prognosis, and the responsiveness to therapy of JIA. Patients with oligoarthritis (pauciarticular disease) generally have milder synovitis and a better prognosis. However, 10 to 15% of patients with oligoarthritis later progress to polyarticular disease. Children with oligoarthritis may develop significant disability due to joint contractures and muscular atrophy, even with control of inflammatory arthritis activity. One cannot overemphasize the importance of physical therapy in the management of these patients.

Polyarticular disease has a variable prognosis. Patients with RF often develop progressive disease extending into the adult years, and develop significant disability in the absence of effective therapy. New anticytokine therapies have brightened the long-term outcome for patients with polyarticular (both RF positive and RF negative) disease.

Patients with systemic onset generally recover from the acute systemic illness without major sequelae, but synovitis with either oligoarticular or polyarticular pattern may then persist. A subset develop persistent treatment-resistant arthritis. Mortality from JIA is rare but does occur. The vast majority of the deaths occur in children with systemic onset disease. Macrophage activation syndrome (MAS) is a rare form of the hemophagocytic lymphohistiocytosis syndrome, and when it occurs it is a life-threatening complication of the disease. Viral infections and drugs have been implicated in the onset of MAS. These children become rapidly ill with fever, worsening adenopathy, organomegaly, petechiae, and bleeding. ESR rapidly falls and pancytopenia is present. The ferritin level is often markedly elevated. This complication needs prompt recognition and treatment.

Ocular Complications

Eye involvement occurs in nearly a quarter of children with JIA and is typically asymptomatic at onset. This is most common in oligoarthritis patients but may be seen in up to 10% of rheumatoid factor negative polyarthritis patients, and rarely in systemic-onset patients. A chronic anterior uveitis occurs most commonly in young girls who are ANA positive. Insidiously progressive disease may result in posterior synechiae with resultant pupillary abnormalities. Occasionally band keratopathy may be seen. Loss of vision results from the development of secondary glaucoma, cataracts, and keratopathy. Early detection and treatment are essential to improving the outcome of JIA-associated uveitis. The eye disease is usually asymptomatic at onset. Patients with oligoarthritis should be seen by an ophthalmologist at least every 3 months during the first 2 to 3 years of disease, and then every 6 months for several more years. There is no correlation between the severity of arthritis and risk for development of uveitis. In addition, children with enthesitis-related arthritis may develop anterior uveitis, but it is typically symptomatic, presenting as a red, painful eye with or without photophobia.

Growth Disturbances

Children with chronic inflammatory disease of any type may have generalized inhibition of growth and subsequent short stature. Occasionally, periarticular hyperemia results in premature epiphyseal fusion with resultant shortening of the affected extremity. Prolonged hyperemia may at times cause accelerated bone growth. Leg length discrepancies are the most common orthopaedic sequelae of JIA and can be severe. Temporomandibular Joint (TMJ) involvement may result in a shortened mandible and micrognathia. This may result in disturbances of speech and chewing, in addition to the cosmetic alteration. Surgery may be complicated by difficulties with endotracheal intubation particularly in patients with associated cervical spine fusion.

Hip disease is unusual at onset of JIA, but is commonly seen later in patients with polyarticular disease. Muscle spasm and disuse may result in flexion contracture. Hip involvement in early childhood may contribute to valgus deformity of the femoral neck, persistent femoral anteversion, and dysplasia of both femoral head and acetabulum. Postoperative ectopic bone formation occasionally complicates surgical management of severe disease. Nonetheless, joint replacement can be successful in patients with disabling, end-stage disease. Knee involvement typically results in flexion contracture. Associated leg length discrepancy and hip disease may also contribute to development of contracture as well as genu valgus. Secondary scoliosis may occur. In the hand and wrist, deformities similar to adult rheumatoid arthritis are seen, although ulnar deviation at the wrist and radial deviation at the MCP joints is common. Additionally, some patients develop extensive fusion of carpal bones. Ankles and feet are similarly prone to fusion, particularly at the subtalar joint. Complex foot deformities may be seen as a result of soft tissue damage and growth disturbances.

Management

Essential to optimal outcome in JIA is the early diagnosis and prompt institution of treatment. As our arsenal of therapeutic agents grows and is utilized appropriately, we are likely to see long-term outcomes continue to improve.

NSAIDs are the most commonly used drugs in the treatment of JIA. They control pain, swelling, and stiffness, but have no effect on the long-term outcome. NSAIDs approved by the U.S. Food and Drug Administration for use in childhood include aspirin, ibuprofen, naproxen, and tolmetin sodium. Other NSAIDs are used for patients who cannot tolerate the FDA-approved NSAIDs. Ibuprofen, naproxen, and several salicylate preparations are available in liquid form. Aspirin has a long historical record of use in JIA but its use has decreased markedly due to the risk (albeit very slight) of Reye syndrome, the potential for drug toxicity, and the availability of other effective drugs. Salicylates (if used) should be promptly discontinued in JIA patients with concomitant influenza or varicella infections. Most children with JIA do not do well on an NSAID alone and require additional therapeutic intervention for maximum control of their disease.

In oligoarticular disease, intra-articular corticosteroids and/or anti-malarial drugs are frequently utilized along with regular physical therapy. Systemic corticosteroids are reserved for refractory cases of JIA and are particularly useful in the treatment of severe systemic JIA. The lowest possible dose should be used.

Methotrexate is commonly used in children with multiple joints involved. Increasingly, biologic agents are being utilized that block a particular pro-inflammatory cytokine. Children with severe polyarticular arthritis who fail or have an incomplete response to methotrexate are candidates for treatment with this class of agents. These drugs must still be used with caution, as their long-term safety has not yet been demonstrated.

Up to 10% of children with JIA seen in a pediatric rheumatology center require surgical intervention, and the specific procedures used are reviewed more extensively in the references. Children with severe JIA have significant osteoporosis and can experience spontaneous fractures. JIA patients require surgical intervention when medical and physical therapy (e.g., splinting, casting) are not sufficient to control pain, improve contracture, or correct deformity. The most common procedure in JIA patients is soft tissue release, particularly of the knee or hip. Occasionally, synovial biopsy may be necessary for diagnostic reasons. Synovectomy can be helpful for the child with severe pain or loss of function and is most commonly required for the knee in oligoarthritis patients. Arthroscopy can be performed, but the presence of severe pericapsular contracture may decrease distensibility and visibility of the joint. Severe bone ankylosis may require a corrective osteotomy to improve joint position. Joint replacement is a well-established treatment of end-stage JIA. Children with severe JIA are often smaller and lighter than other children of the same age, and the joint prosthesis may need to be custom made.

Careful preoperative medical and anesthetic evaluation is necessary in all children. Children on systemic corticosteroid therapy need intravenous stress corticosteroid coverage and are at greater risk of infection. Involvement of the cervical spine, TMJs, and cricoarytenoid joints can make airway management difficult.

Infectious Arthritis

Jacob W. IJdo

Infectious agents have been demonstrated to play an etiologic role in the initiation and propagation of some acute and chronic arthritides. Symptoms suggesting a possible infectious arthritis need to be evaluated promptly and treated appropriately, because failure to recognize infectious arthritis may result in avoidable catastrophic joint destruction. However, in reactive arthritis, the interaction of a genetic susceptible background, especially HLA-B27, with certain infectious agents (e.g., Campylobacter, Chlamydia, Clostridium, Salmonella, Shigella, or Yersinia) may result in inflammatory reactive arthritis. In these instances bacterial DNA may be found in joint fluid or tissue using PCR, but cultures remain negative. This section discusses infectious arthritis based on the different causes: bacterial, fungal, and viral.

Acute Septic Arthritis

Risk Factors

Nongonococcal bacterial arthritis can quickly progress to a destructive acute arthritis. Direct invasion of the joint by pyogenic bacteria may occur through inoculation, or by contiguous spread from soft tissue infection or from osteomyelitis. In the primary care setting, the majority of cases arise from hematogenous spread to the joint. Common predisposing factors include injection drug use, in-dwelling catheters, and underlying immuno-compromised states such as HIV infection, alcoholism, diabetes mellitus, malignancy, allogeneic transplants, chronic inflammatory arthritis, or concomitant use of immunosuppressive medications. Immuno-compromised patients may display few symptoms of infection, making the clinical diagnosis of septic arthritis difficult. Orthopedic surgeons are more likely to be confronted with joint infections as a result of trauma or surgical procedures. Examples include penetrating injury, introduction of a foreign body into a joint, arthroplasties, or total joint replacements. Late infections of prosthetic joints, albeit rare, may be the result of contamination at the time of surgery, or due to bacterial seeding during a bacteremic episode.

Microbiology

The major pathogens of nongonococcal septic arthritis of native joints are Gram-positive cocci (in 75% of all cases), whereas Gram-negative organisms are the second most common (15 to 20%). *Staphylococcus aureus* is the most common cause, both in native and prosthetic joints. Streptococci, including pneumococci, are the second most common Gram-positive bacteria isolated. *Staphylococcus epidermidis* is commonly encountered in prosthetic joints but rarely seen in native joint infections. In intravenous drug abusers or patients with comorbidities, such as in the elderly, Gram-negative organisms including *Escherichia coli*, *Proteus* spp., and *Serratia* spp., may be more commonly encountered.

Clinical Features

Acute septic arthritis is a medical emergency. Delay in initiating therapy may lead to joint destruction. Acute septic arthritis usually presents with joint swelling, warmth, pain, erythema, and loss of function. Although usually a single joint is affected (in about 80% of the cases), multiple joints can be infected, especially in immuno-compromised patients. Sudden onset of monoarticular arthritis should be considered septic until proven otherwise. The large weight-bearing joints, especially the knees, are most commonly involved. Ankles, shoulders, elbows, and wrists are other commonly affected sites. In a patient with known inflammatory polyarthritis, such as rheumatoid arthritis, the sudden worsening of a single joint out of proportion to disease activity in the other joints should suggest the possibility of septic arthritis. Nonarticular infection, such as cellulitis, pneumonia, dental abscess, or urinary tract infections, are often the distant source for bacterial seeding of joints.

Constitutional signs and symptoms, when present, are helpful in suggesting an infection but in themselves are nonspecific, as are general laboratory studies. An elevated ESR is common. Leukocytosis occurs in up to two-thirds of patients. Plain radiographs are usually normal early in infectious arthritis, except perhaps for evidence of soft tissue swelling or joint effusion. Nevertheless, joints with suspected infection should be radiographed at presentation, since a baseline study is useful in interpretation of subsequent examinations. Periarticular osteopenia may be seen but is nonspecific. Joint space narrowing due to cartilage destruction may occur in days to weeks without appropriate treatment. Subchondral bone destruction is a late finding. Contiguous osteomyelitis is a late but grave complication. Radionuclide imaging techniques, such as technetium gallium, or indium scans, may aid diagnosis of septic arthritis in joints difficult to aspirate, such as intervertebral, sacroiliac, or hip joints.

Laboratory Findings

The diagnosis of acute septic arthritis must be confirmed by arthrocentesis with synovial fluid analysis and culture. Synovial fluid is usually purulent, with greater than 50,000 cells/mm^3 and over 80% polymorphonuclear leukocytes. Initial leukocyte counts, however, may be only minimally elevated. In immuno-compromised hosts, leukocyte counts in synovial fluid may remain low or even normal. In cases with low or normal leukocyte counts, repeat arthrocentesis in 12 to 24 hours may demonstrate rising counts. A high leukocyte count in itself is not pathognomonic, since high counts may be seen in nonseptic inflammatory arthritis, especially crystal-induced arthritis or Reiter's syndrome. Identification of crystals, however, does not rule out septic arthritis, because both entities may occur simultaneously. The definitive diagnosis requires demonstration of the causative bacteria on Gram's stain, by culture, or both. The main reason for false-negative culture results are prior use of antibiotics and the special growth requirements of some fastidious microorganisms. In those cases the use of PCR may be extremely helpful. Although the utility of this sensitive technique is still being defined, DNA detection of *Neisseria gonorrhoeae* and *Mycoplasma* spp. has been shown to be useful when cultures remained negative.

Treatment

Prompt treatment will eradicate the infection, speed recovery, and reduce morbidity. Antibiotic treatment based on a presumptive diagnosis of septic arthritis should be initiated after arthrocentesis and collection of samples for microbiologic studies. The choice of antibiotic is guided by the history, clinical presentation, and results of the Gram's stain. If the Gram's stain of the synovial fluid reveals Gram-positive cocci, cefazolin or vancomycin are preferred choices. If there are Gram-negative organisms, a third generation cephalosporin is indicated. If *Pseudomonas aeruginosa* is suspected (in patients with injection drug use), ceftazidime with an aminoglycoside is the first choice. If a young, otherwise healthy, sexually active person presents with tenosynovitis and migratory joint pain, without any visible bacteria on Gram's stain, therapy against presumptive gonococcal infection may be appropriate (see next section).

Frequent drainage of the infected joint space will hasten eradication of the infection. Surgical drainage may be indicated if repeated aspirations are technically difficult. Although antimicrobial therapy needs to be tailored to the individual patient, typically, intravenous antibiotic therapy is given for 2 to 4 weeks followed by oral therapy for a total course of treatment of 4 to 6 weeks, depending on the severity of the infection. In prosthetic joints, therapy may be even more protracted.

Gonococcal Arthritis

In contrast to nongonococcal septic arthritis, the typical patient who develops gonococcal arthritis is frequently young and healthy. Infectious arthritis due to *N. gonorrhoeae* follows dissemination from a primary site, such as urethra, cervix, rectum, or pharynx. The clinical course is classically biphasic. The first stage is characterized by migratory polyarthralgias, polyarthritis, or tenosynovitis. Multiple vesiculopustular skin lesions that develop necrotic centers may be seen. Cultures from these skin lesions and from blood are often positive for *N. gonorrhoeae* during this stage. Untreated, the patient may develop the second stage, in which infection settles into one or a few joints, which become purulent. Cultures from purulent joints are positive only one-quarter of the time because *N. gonorrhoeae* is a fastidious organism and difficult to grow. Patients with suspected gonococcal infection should have all possible sites examined and cultured, including pharynx, rectum, blood, cervix in women, and urethra in men. Special transport media should be used if samples will be delayed in reaching the microbiology laboratory.

Treatment consists of ceftriaxone IV or IM until resolution of symptoms followed by a 2 weeks of oral cefuroxime or a quinolone. However, quinolone-resistant strains are common in Asia and the Pacific and are also increasingly noted in Hawaii and California, so quinolones are no longer appropriate in these areas. Concurrent treatment for *Chlamydia trachomatis* with doxycycline for 7 days is mandatory. Sexual partners should be traced and offered treatment as well.

Mycobacterial Arthritis

Mycobacterium Tuberculosis

Tuberculous arthritis should be considered in the differential diagnosis of chronic monoarticular and pauciarticular arthritis at any age. The arthritis is frequently insidious in onset. It tends to appear "cold," lacking the usual signs of active inflammation, especially erythema and heat. Pott's disease, tuberculous involvement of the spine, classically involves the thoracolumbar junction. Anterior destruction of vertebral bodies and disks eventually leads to angulation of the spine and kyphosis (gibbous deformity). Although constitutional signs of tuberculosis (e.g., fever, malaise, and weight loss) may be present, active pulmonary tuberculosis is rare. A history of past infection may be absent. A positive skin test for tuberculosis is helpful, although a negative test in the presence of anergy does not rule out the diagnosis. Diagnosis is based on finding acid-fast bacilli in synovium or synovial fluid or caseating granulomas in biopsied synovium. A CT-guided biopsy of inaccessible sites may be required. Synovial fluid or tissue cultures are positive 90% of the time. Tuberculosis and its complications should be considered in patients with AIDS or with a history of immigration from an endemic area. In addition, reactivation of latent tuberculosis may occur as a result of treatment with corticosteroids or tumor necrosis factor-α (TNF-α) antagonists. Tuberculous arthritis is usually due to hematogenous spread, and thus active disease elsewhere needs to be investigated. Poncet's disease is defined as reactive arthritis during active tuberculosis, most commonly seen as polyarticular arthritis of the hands and feet, while cultures of synovial fluid remain negative. Improvement ensues with antituberculous medication. Antimicrobial treatment of tuberculous arthritis or osteomyelitis is the same as for pulmonary tuberculosis.

Nontuberculous Mycobacteria

Atypical mycobacterial joint infection can mimic tuberculous arthritis. The most common strains include *M. marinum*, *M. kansasii*, and *M. avium intracellulare*. Infections are indolent. Diagnosis is made by the demonstration of the organism in the synovial fluid or tissue. Delay of diagnosis up to a year or more is not uncommon. Most nontuberculous mycobacterial joint infections are due to local trauma, surgery or intra-articular injection. Treatment may require surgical debridement for both diagnosis and therapy, especially for the closed spaces of the hand and the wrist and for infections of long bones, in addition to specific drug therapy.

Mycobacterium Leprae

Of all cases of leprosy diagnosed in the United States, more than 85% of patients are immigrants. The six countries with the highest incidence of leprosy include Brazil, India, Madagascar, Mozambique, Myanmar, and Nepal. Lepromatous leprosy may present with polyarthralgia or polyarthritis. Erythema nodosum leprosum is an associated finding and consists of nodules on the legs, arms, or trunk. Malaise and fever may occur. Swollen hands syndrome is another presentation of leprosy. Thickening of peripheral nerves and typical skin changes suggest the diagnosis. Chronic erosive arthritis may resemble rheumatoid arthritis and improves with treatment of the leprosy. A classic finding in the late stages of leprosy is the Charcot joint as a result of sensory neuropathy with repeated minor trauma. The diagnosis is made by identifying *M. leprae* in aspirates of skin lesions or biopsy specimens. *M. leprae* may be found in synovial and periarticular tissues. Combination therapy of several drugs with activity against *M. leprae* has replaced monotherapy with dapsone.

Syphilis

Although rare as a cause of arthritis, secondary syphilis can cause inflammatory polyarthritis that can be confused with many other joint diseases such as rheumatoid arthritis, SLE, and sarcoidosis. Syphilis is suspected if there is a concomitant maculopapular rash on the palms and soles. Other characteristics may include a systemic illness with fever, lymphadenopathy, sore throat, and mucosal ulcers. The arthritis is symmetric and involves predominantly the lower extremities. *Treponema pallidum* spirochetes cannot be grown from human specimens *in vitro*, and hence cultures of joint fluid are negative. The diagnosis relies on serology (RPR or VDRL) and a confirmatory FTA-ABS.

"Saber shins" are a classic manifestation of congenital syphilis. The congenital form of syphilis is a severe, disabling, and often life-threatening condition, and occurs when the mother is infected and transmits the pathogen to her unborn infant. Perinatal mortality is high. Infants develop early stage and late-stage symptoms of syphilis if not treated. Early stage symptoms include irritability, failure to thrive, and fever. Bony abnormalities include osteochondritis, osteomyelitis, osteitis, and periosteitis. In older children, painless effusions, especially of the knees, may occur. In acquired primary syphilis, transient bone pain of a boring nature may be prominent. The tibia, humerus, and cranium are most frequently involved, but radiographs are normal.

In secondary syphilis, pain and tenderness with overlying soft tissue swelling may be seen in superficial bones, such as anterior tibia, sternum, ribs, and skull. Symptoms and signs are variable but characteristically worse at night. Proliferative periosteitis is the most common radiographic change. It is associated with new bone formation that may be extensive, resulting in marked cortical thickening. The tibia, sternum, ribs, and skull are most significantly involved, but changes may also be seen in the femur, fibula, clavicle, hands, and feet. Periosteitis in the adult that involves both clavicles or tibiae is frequently syphilitic. Destructive bony lesions suggest syphilitic osteomyelitis or osteitis, but these are less common than periosteitis. Areas of lysis may be seen.

Tertiary syphilis may be complicated by gummatous osseous lesions. The lesion pathologically resembles a tubercle with necrosis of adjacent bone. Lytic and sclerotic areas of bone may reach large size and may be associated with pathologic fracture. Periosteitis adjacent to gummatous lesions is frequent. Nongummatous osseous lesions that consist of periosteitis, osteitis, or osteomyelitis may occur in conjunction with or in the absence of gummatous bony lesions. Charcot joints, characteristically of the knees, result from loss of proprioception due to tabes dorsalis in tertiary syphilis. Hip, ankle, shoulder, elbow, spine, and other joints may be affected as well in tabes dorsalis.

Lyme Disease

Lyme disease is a systemic illness caused by the spirochete *Borrelia burgdorferi*. The geographic distribution of Lyme disease is dictated by the presence of the vector. In the Northeast and upper Midwest, transmission occurs by the tick *Ixodes scapularis* or deer tick. Although Lyme disease has been reported in most states, more than 90% of all cases in the Unites States are seen in only eight states: Massachusetts, Rhode Island, Connecticut, New York, New Jersey, Pennsylvania, Minnesota, and Wisconsin. Transmission in western states occurs by *Ixodes pacificus* (black-legged tick), while *Ixodes ricinus* is responsible for transmission in Europe. Normally ticks require up to 4 to 5 days to feed to completion and transmission of the organism occurs most efficiently after 48 hours. Ticks removed within 24 hours of attachment will not have transmitted the spirochete. Discovery and removal of an engorged tick on the day following outdoor activities in an endemic area is sufficient to prevent Lyme disease in most cases, provided that a "total body tick check" is performed. Less than 50% of patients ever recall a tick bite.

Clinical manifestations of Lyme disease include early localized, early disseminated, and late disease. *Early localized disease* includes the typical erythema migrans, or bull's eye rash, which occurs in about 80% of Lyme disease patients and within one month of the tick bite. The rash (usually more than 3 to 5 cm) should not be confused with the small local reaction (just a few mm), which occurs at the site of any bite. The diagnosis of this stage is made by the combination of the typical history and the rash.

The *early disseminated phase* occurs in several weeks to a few months and is characterized by disseminated skin lesions at sites other than the tick bite, cardiac disease, and neurologic involvement. This phase represents systemic infection. Spirochetes may be present in the skin, in cardiac tissue (leading to conduction block), and central nervous system (Bell's palsy).

Late disease is seen months after the initial infection. Most frequently it consists of a monoarthritis of the knee, but other large joints can be involved. Patients with Lyme arthritis are usually strongly seropositive. Episodes of joint inflammation may recur several times with disease-free intervals, but the ultimate outcome is favorable with eventual resolution of the inflammation over the course of several years. Late neurologic symptoms are designated as tertiary neuroborreliosis in analogy with tertiary neurosyphilis. Patients with neuroborreliosis are strongly seropositive. Features include encephalopathy, neurocognitive dysfunction, and peripheral neuropathy. Neuroborreliosis is relatively rare, especially because most patients are now correctly diagnosed and treated early within the disease course.

Laboratory confirmation of a clinical suspicion of Lyme disease is obtained by ELISA. Positive or equivocal ELISA results are confirmed by immunoblot, because significant false positive ELISA results are due to other (spirochetal) infections (i.e., relapsing fever, syphilis, Epstein-Barr virus) and other autoimmune diseases (i.e., rheumatoid arthritis and SLE). A positive Lyme test includes a positive

ELISA and a positive immunoblot consisting of at least two of three bands for IgM (23, 39 and 41 kD), or five of ten bands for IgG (18, 21, 28, 30, 39, 41, 45, 58, 68, 93 kD). Note that a positive IgM immunoblot can only be used to support the diagnosis within 4 weeks of onset of clinical disease. Laboratory testing in the setting of early disease is not recommended because of a high rate of false-negative results, but treatment should be initiated promptly.

Treatment of early localized Lyme disease consists of 3 weeks of 100 mg orally 2 times a day doxycycline, or amoxicillin 500 mg 4 times a day. Early disseminated or late Lyme disease requires 3 weeks of a third generation cephalosporin intravenously.

Brucella Arthritis

The organism of brucellosis is transmitted to humans from infected animals or through the ingestion of untreated milk or milk products; raw meat and bone marrow have also been implicated. Other portes d'entrée include skin abrasions and conjunctiva or by inhalation during contact with animals, especially by slaughterhouse workers, farmers, and veterinarians. Aerosolized *B. melitensis* is considered an agent of biological warfare.

Most countries of mainland Europe and Japan are free of brucellosis. However, it is suggested that even in developed nations, the true incidence of brucellosis may be up to twentyfold higher than official incidence numbers. In the United States, about 200 new cases are reported every year, but only a fraction of cases are recognized and reported. Consumption of imported cheese, travel abroad, and occupational exposures are the most frequently identified sources of infection. Brucellosis has many synonyms depending on geographical area (e.g., Mediterranean fever, Malta fever, etc). Four species can cause human brucellosis: *Brucella melitensis* (the most common cause of brucellosis) and is acquired primarily from goats and sheep; *B. abortus* from cattle; *B. suis* from hogs; and *B. canis* from dogs.

The clinical features of brucellosis are those of an acute febrile illness and are not specific for brucellosis. Acute infection is associated with bacteremia, fever, myalgias, polyarthralgia, headache, and general malaise. Most commonly, brucella arthritis is monoarticular and involves the large weight-bearing joints of the lower extremities. However, 30 to 40% of patients have reactive asymmetric polyarthritis involving the knees, hips, shoulders, and sacroiliac and sternoclavicular joints. Infection with brucella organisms commonly causes osteomyelitis of the lumbar vertebrae, starting at the superior endplate and occasionally progressing to involve the entire vertebra, disc space, and adjacent vertebrae. Extraspinal brucella osteomyelitis is rare. In brucella septic arthritis and osteomyelitis, the peripheral white cell count is typically normal, while the erythrocyte sedimentation rate may be either normal or elevated. Diagnosis is based on a positive culture or on a rising or high brucella antibody titer. Cultures of synovial fluid are positive in about 50% of cases. Radiologic investigations aimed at detecting skeletal involvement include plain radiography, bone scintigraphy, CT, and MRI. Bone scintigraphy is more sensitive than conventional radiography in detecting areas of spinal and extraspinal involvement, particularly in the early stage of infection. Plain lateral radiography of the spine may reveal bone sclerosis, with destruction and erosion of the superior end plate anteriorly. As the disease progresses, healing with osteophyte formation and reduction of disc space may take place.

Monotherapy for brucellosis has now been replaced by combination therapy because of the high rates of failure and relapse and the potential development of antibiotic resistance. Combination therapy lasting less than 8 weeks has also been associated with high rates of relapse. The combination of doxycycline and an aminoglycoside for 4 weeks followed by the combination of doxycycline and rifampin for 4 to 8 weeks is the most effective regimen.

Fungal Arthritis

Most fungal joint infections are insidious in onset, have an indolent course, and are associated with mild inflammation. Diagnosis is often delayed and frequently the only laboratory finding is a positive culture. Septic arthritis caused by *Candida albicans* is rare and is usually due to direct inoculation or hematogenous spread. *C. albicans* is a rare cause of infection in prosthetic joints (< 1%). In adults disseminated candida infections are usually related to IV drug abuse or severe illness requiring intensive care and the use of multiple broad-spectrum antibiotics, or associated with chemotherapy or immunosuppressive medication. Treatment includes amphotericin B, ketoconazole, and fluconazole.

Primary pulmonary infection with *Blastomycosis dermatitidis* can lead to hematogenous spread and skeletal infection, including osteomyelitis and arthritis. Osteomyelitis has a predilection for vertebral sites and ribs, and can mimic tuberculous infection. Large joint arthritis such as the knee can be acute, usually in the setting of pulmonary disease or cutaneous infections. Diagnosis is confirmed by culture and treatment options include amphotericin B, ketoconazole, and itraconazole.

Coccidioidomycosis occurs in the southwestern United States and is caused by *Coccidioides immitis*. It may present with erythema nodosum, periarthritis, and bihilar lymphadenopathy. This triad is also seen in sarcoidosis (known as Lofgren syndrome), and therefore, the two entities must be differentiated. In coccidioidomycosis, the triad is a hypersensitivity reaction to primary infection and resolves spontaneously within weeks. Persistent arthritis is uncommon, resulting from hematogenous spread or extension from contiguous osteomyelitis. The most commonly involved joints are knee, wrist and hand, ankle, elbow, and foot, in order of decreasing frequency. Arthritis progression is slow and indolent. Diagnosis is by synovial biopsy and culture.

Sporotrichosis due to *Sporothrix schenckii* typically occurs in agricultural or mine workers or in gardeners after minor skin trauma. Disease usually presents as a painful erythematous cutaneous nodule and spreads by local extension and via the lymphatic system. Indolent arthritis occurs rarely and involves the knee, hand, wrist, or ankle, in order of decreasing frequency. About half the patients have a monoarthritis. Alcoholism or myeloproliferative disease predisposes to infection. Diagnosis is by synovial histology and culture.

Cryptococcus neoformans spreads hematogenously and may seed the central nervous system and can result in bone and joint infection similar to blastomycosis. Demonstration of the organisms in joint fluid or biopsy specimens confirms the diagnosis.

Traditionally, treatment of fungal infections has been with amphotericin B but renal toxicity has been a major limitation. Newer agents including liposomal amphotericin and caspofungin seem to have less toxicity.

Viral Arthritis

The association of acute arthritis with certain viral infections has long been recognized. Viral arthritis characteristically is polyarticular and usually develops at the time of the rash or shortly thereafter. In most cases pathogenesis seems to be due to immune-complex deposition. It is important to remember that the arthritis associated with viral infections never leads to joint destruction or chronic joint inflammation.

Parvovirus B19 infections may be responsible for as many as 12% of patients presenting with recent onset of polyarthralgia or polyarthritis. B19, first described in 1975, is very common, and causes the common childhood exanthem erythema infectiosum, or fifth disease, characterized by "slapped cheeks" and a rash of the torso and extremities. A majority of adults have serologic evidence of past infection. About 10% of children with fifth disease have arthralgias, and 5% have arthritis, usually short-lived. In contrast, 60% of infected adults have arthralgias or frank polyarticular arthritis, in a distribution that resembles rheumatoid arthritis. In fact, the history of a viral syndrome and a B19 seroconversion may help differentiate viral polyarthritis from rheumatoid arthritis in an early stage. B19 can also cause transient aplastic anemia in patients with underlying hematologic disorders, and thus B19 infection may resemble SLE. A recent B19 infection is confirmed if a B19 IgM is detected, which is only present for several weeks (occasionally up to 2 to 3 months) after infection. IgG persists for years and is not helpful unless a seroconversion between paired samples is detected. Detection of B19 DNA by PCR is useful but can remain positive for months after the initial infection. The long-term outcome is good, though a few patients have recurrent episodes of arthralgias over several years.

Hepatitis B infection, clinically silent or icteric, is usually self-limiting, followed by the appearance of hepatitis B surface antibodies. However, 5 to 10 % of patients may develop a chronic infection, with continued antigen production (i.e., HBeAg, HBcAg, HBsAg). In the prodromal phase, which may precede clinical jaundice circulating immune complexes may cause symptoms ranging from arthralgias to a sudden and severe polyarthritis. Symptoms usually last several weeks, but in patients with chronic active hepatitis, arthralgias and arthritis may be prolonged. Because patients may not be icteric in chronic active hepatitis, laboratory testing for hepatitis may be an essential to the diagnosis. Polyarteritis nodosa (PAN) is frequently associated with chronic HBV viremia. PAN is characterized by inflammation of small and medium-sized arteries and is a multisystem disease: arteries in skin, kidneys, peripheral nerves (vasa nervorum), intestines, and muscles can be affected.

Hepatitis C has become a major cause of chronic hepatitis and cirrhosis. Mixed cryoglobulinemia is most frequently associated with HCV, although a number of other viruses and bacteria have also been implicated. Other disorders such as lymphoma and myeloma can also cause cryoglobulinemia. Clinical features of mixed cryoglobulinemia include palpable purpura, hepatitis, arthralgias/arthritis, renal involvement, Raynaud's and peripheral neuropathy. The cutaneous vasculitis and glomerulonephritis is immune-complex mediated, and a similar pathogenesis has been suggested for the arthritis. Treatment consists of interferon 2b, preferably the pegylated form, combined with ribavirin, with the objective of clearing the HCV. Glucocorticoids and immunosuppressive agents such as methotrexate have been used, but should probably be reserved for severe vasculitis due to the cryoglobulinemia, because these drugs may increase viral replication, and hence perpetuate the problem.

Rubella virus infection is characterized by a maculopapular rash, lymphadenopathy, and arthralgias or arthritis. The joint symptoms are usually self-limited. Vaccination with live attenuated strains can cause joint symptoms in up to 25% of vaccinated individuals.

Alphavirus infections have been responsible for viral epidemics with associated polyarthritis, but to date, these have been all outside North America.

The viruses include Sindbis, Mayaro, Ross River, Chikungunya, and O'nyong-nyong viruses, all of which are mosquitoborne. The recent emergence of West Nile virus in the United States demonstrates the potential that these viruses may be encountered in this country in the future. The arthritis is polyarticular with a preference for the small joint of the hands, wrists, elbows, knees, and ankles. Most cases resolve within a week, although joint symptoms persisting for up to a year have been reported.

Patients with HIV may be affected by several musculoskeletal syndromes, only a few of which are specifically related to HIV. Reiter's syndrome, without eye inflammation, has probably an increased frequency in HIV patients in the study populations. However, extra-articular manifestations such as eye inflammation may be absent. HIV increases the frequency of psoriatic arthritis in patients with psoriasis. Diffuse infiltrative lymphocytosis syndrome (DILS) and HIV-associated arthritis are seen specifically in HIV. These syndromes occur in the setting of significant immunosuppression. Treatment with combination antiviral therapy seems to reduce the incidence, suggesting that HIV may be involved directly or indirectly in the pathogenesis.

Crystal-Induced Arthritis

Scott A. Vogelgesang
John W. Rachow

Gout "is usually sudden, occurring in the night, and is of short duration." "The cause of this disease is an immoderate use of stimulating food and drinks. Plethoric persons are its most frequent victims."

R.V. Pierce, M.D., The People's Common
Sense Medical Advisor 1887

Gout

Few clinical presentations are as distinct and dramatic as an acute gout attack. With its clinical description rooted in antiquity, gout can be considered the prototypic acute monoarthritis as well as crystal-induced arthritis. Gout is due to the presence of monosodium urate (MSU) crystals in articular tissues.

Pathogenesis

Prolonged hyperuricemia at concentrations yielding supersaturation (generally, serum uric acid > 7.0 mg/dL) leads to precipitation of MSU crystals in soft tissues. When sufficient MSU accumulates within joints, several factors, such as trauma, abrupt dietary changes, acute illness, surgery, dehydration, and administration of serum urate-lowering medications, probably induce acute MSU crystal precipitation within joints or shedding of crystals from deposits in synovium into synovial fluid. MSU crystals recovered from joints are coated with a variety of serum proteins, notably immunoglobulins, which attract and enhance phagocytosis by polymorphonuclear (PMN) leukocytes. Crystal contact with leukocytes results in generation of mediators of inflammation and chemoattractants, including interleukin-1 and a specific PMN-derived, crystal-induced chemotactic factor. A massive influx of PMN into the joints ensues. Partially due to the membranolytic properties of the MSU crystals, PMN lysis occurs, releasing lysosomal contents that further intensify the inflammatory response. Simultaneous influx of serum factors into the joint, including lipoproteins and proteolytic enzyme inhibitors, help make gout attacks self-limited.

Epidemiology

Gout occurs after prolonged periods of sustained hyperuricemia. Consequently, the epidemiology of gout closely parallels the epidemiology of hyperuricemia. Because lower levels of serum uric acid are found in the normal population of prepubertal men and premenopausal women, gout develops mostly in postpubertal men or postmenopausal women. Other factors that result in sustained elevations of serum uric acid above the solubility product of MSU can lead to increased total-body urate and predispose to gout. Such factors can be divided into those that involve either uric acid underexcretion or overproduction.

Clinical Features

The classic gout attack is characterized by the rapid onset (usually over a few hours) of extreme pain, swelling, and erythema in one joint. The inflammatory response is so intense that patients describe an inability to tolerate anything touching the joint. The first metatarsophalangeal (MTP) joint is the most frequently affected joint (podagra). Other joints commonly affected early include the mid-foot (tarsalmetatarsal joints) and the ankle. The attacks are usually self-limited and resolve completely in 1 to 2 weeks without therapy. Recurrent episodes are common. The period of complete symptom relief between episodes of intense joint inflammation, termed the intercritical period, is a hallmark of crystal-induced arthritis.

With time, the intensity of attacks lessens and the intercritical period shortens leading to chronic polyarticular arthritis. Polyarticular gout can affect knees, wrists, elbows, metacarpophalangeal (MCP) joints and proximal interphalangeal (PIP) joints. Hips, shoulders and the axial spine are rarely affected.

Aggregates of MSU crystals can deposit into nodules called tophi that can be seen in cartilage, tendons and soft tissues. Extensor surfaces of the extremities and the Achilles tendon are common sites of deposition, but tophi can be seen on the ear, on the skin, and around the small joints of the fingers and toes. Tophi may drain spontaneously and may be confused with draining abscesses. The drainage from tophi usually includes particles of white, chalky material and may even have an appearance suggestive of toothpaste. Patients who have undergone organ transplant may develop gout that behaves differently than idiopathic gout. These patients may present initially with polyarticular, tophaceous gout.

Examination of the patient who presents with a monoarthritis should exclude cellulitis, bursitis, or tendonitis, which can all be associated with warmth, pain, and swelling. Demonstration of a joint effusion or pain on slight movement of the affected joint helps to confirm true joint involvement. The finding of redness over a joint with exquisite tenderness requires arthrocentesis to exclude an infected joint. MSU crystals can be demonstrated under polarized microscopy after aspirating a tophus or by touching a microscope slide to the tophaceous drainage.

The diagnosis of gout relies on the demonstration of MSU crystals within synovial fluid of an affected joint. Compensated, polarized light microscopy will reveal negatively birefringent, needle-shaped crystals found within PMNs. Other tests on synovial fluid are of limited use in acute, crystal-induced arthritis. Synovial fluid leukocyte counts should be clearly inflammatory, often in the 20,000 to 50,000 cells/µL range. In acute gout, synovial fluid leukocyte counts can be as high as those seen in septic arthritis or higher. Coexistent gout and septic arthritis is rare but can occur. If clinical suspicion of a septic joint persists, even after crystals are identified, synovial fluid Gram's stain and culture should be obtained.

Serum uric acid levels are often misused in evaluating patients with suspected acute gout. Although a gout attack is preceded by many months of sustained hyperuricemia, at the time of an acute gout attack, serum uric acid may be low, normal or high. Serum uric acid levels are not helpful in diagnosing acute gout; however, levels are useful in guiding uric acid-lowering therapy, later. Further laboratory investigation to characterize the hyperuricemia may be indicated when the acute gout attack resolves. In most cases, hyperuricemia is due to renal underexcretion of uric acid. If the onset of gout occurs in a man before the age of 20 years, in a menstruating woman, or in a patient without an obvious reason for renal underexcretion, it is appropriate to determine whether urate accumulation is a result of overproduction or underexcretion. This is accomplished by measuring 24-hour urine uric acid excretion. An excretion of greater than 800 mg of uric acid, on an unrestricted diet is evidence of uric acid overproduction. In the presence of normal renal function, a 24-hour urinary uric acid of less than 800 mg in a hyperuricemic patient indicates underexcretion.

Radiology

Radiographs of a joint undergoing an acute gout attack may only show nonspecific soft tissue swelling. With long-standing disease and a history of several attacks, asymmetric periarticular swelling suggestive of a soft tissue mass may indicate the existence of a tophus. Tophi may also develop inside juxta-articular bone and appear on radiographs as subchondral, cystic lucencies. Still later, bone erosions may be seen that are either intra-articular or extra-articular (proximal to the point of confluence of synovium, cartilage, and subchondral bone). These erosions may exhibit a characteristic appearance in which overhanging edges of the disrupted bone cortex are seen.

Treatment

The treatment of choice for acute gout is oral administration of a nonsteroidal anti-inflammatory drug (NSAID). An example of an effective regimen is indomethacin, 50 mg taken every 6 hours for 1 to 2 days then tapered to 50 mg taken every 8 hours for 1 to 2 days then tapered to 25 mg every 8 hours until the attack abates. There is little difference in efficacy among the NSAIDs and an inexpensive, short-acting choice may be the most appropriate. Caution should be exercised when using NSAIDs. Gastrointestinal ulceration is a major problem with chronic use. Worsening renal insufficiency or congestive heart failure can also occur. Decreased doses of NSAID and more frequent monitoring of serum creatinine is indicated in a high-risk patient. NSAIDs that inhibit cyclooxygenase 2 have a lower incidence of gastrointestinal toxicity but are no more effective, have the same potential renal toxicity and are more expensive. Concerns about cardiovascular morbidity may limit the use of these agents. Aspirin, other salicylates, allopurinol, and the uricosurics should be avoided in gout attacks, because they are likely to alter serum uric acid levels and lead to prolongation of the attack.

Colchicine has also been used for the treatment of acute gout. The traditional oral regimen is 0.6 mg every 1 to 2 hours until (1) improvement in the attack is seen; or (2) until the development of nausea, vomiting, or diarrhea; or (3) until a maximum of 10 doses (<6 mg in a 24-hour period) have been taken. Intravenous colchicine is rarely used because of the potential for severe bone marrow toxicity. The dose of colchicine should be reduced in those with impaired renal or hepatic function and in the elderly.

A short course of oral corticosteroids (e.g., prednisone 20 mg daily for 3 days, 15 mg daily for 3 days, 10 mg daily for 3 days, 5 mg daily for 3 days, then stop) is frequently efficacious and well tolerated. Intra-articular corticosteroids can also be ben-

eficial provided one is sure the joint is not infected. Intramuscular ACTH has been shown to be effective. Finally, in a patient with multiple comorbidities that limit therapy, simply controlling the pain while the self-limited attack abates may the most appropriate course.

Long-term management must be individualized. Some patients may suffer only a small number of gout attacks in their lifetime and never develop detectable tophi or joint damage. Intermittent use of NSAIDs in this case may be the most appropriate course. Repeated attacks, the development of tophi, joint damage, or renal damage may necessitate serum urate-lowering therapy. Allopurinol inhibits the enzyme xanthine oxidase and prevents the formation of uric acid. A usual dose is 300 mg orally, once a day. Smaller doses (i.e., 100 mg) may be appropriate in the elderly or in a patient with renal insufficiency. The dose is adjusted upward until a serum uric acid level of ≤5 mg/dL is achieved. Patients should be instructed to immediately discontinue allopurinol if they develop a new rash. The development of allopurinol hypersensitivity can rarely be associated with fatal toxic epidermal necrolysis. The indications for using allopurinol include three or more attacks in a year *and* one of the following: renal insufficiency, nephrolithiasis, or tophi.

Initiation of allopurinol therapy is associated with an increased frequency of gout attacks. Consequently, prophylaxis against acute attacks is usually administered for a week before the initiation of allopurinol and continued for 1 to 12 months in the form of oral colchicine 0.6 mg once or twice daily. Small doses of NSAID (i.e., ibuprofen 400 mg once or twice daily) may be substituted if the risk for NSAID associated toxicity is low.

Uricosuric drugs, which can lower serum uric acid, seem a rational choice in patients with uric acid underexcretion. There are some limitations to this approach: (1) normal renal function is required for the uricosuric drugs to be effective; (2) increased concentration of urine uric acid can result in acute stone formation—uricosuric drugs should not be used in patients with a history of stones; (3) serum uric acid reductions are likely to be modest compared with reductions achievable with allopurinol; (4) uricosuric drugs have a short half-life and must be given four times a day. Probenecid and sulfinpyrazone are both uricosuric drugs used in the long-term management of gout. Probenecid is usually begun at 500 mg/day and increased to 2000 to 3000 mg/day in four divided doses as needed to lower the serum uric acid. Sulfinpyrazone can be initiated at 100 mg/day and increased as needed to 800 mg/day in four divided doses. Increased fluid intake is recommended to lessen the risk of acute urinary stone formation. Just as with allopurinol, acute lowering of serum uric acid with uricosuric drugs can precipitate acute gout attacks, prophylaxis should be used.

Calcium Pyrophosphate Dihydrate (CPPD) Deposition Disease

In the early 1960s, patients with acute arthritis thought to have gout were found to have crystals in synovial fluid that were not MSU. Radiographs showed abnormal calcifications and later the crystals in synovial fluid were identified as calcium pyrophosphate dihydrate (CPPD).

Pathogenesis

Metabolic abnormalities that allow CPPD crystals to form intra-articular deposits are not well understood. There does not appear to be an increased whole-body load of inorganic pyrophosphate (PPi). Plasma, serum, and urinary levels of PPi are no different in most patients with CPPD crystal deposition than normal. Synovial fluid PPi concentrations are higher than plasma in many arthropathies but are highest in patients with CPPD crystal deposition. Accumulated evidence suggests that elevated intra-articular PPi concentrations are more likely due to excess production of PPi by cartilage than to impaired PPi clearance mechanisms. Impaired PPi hydrolysis may be an important factor in some cases. Breakdown of PPi *in vitro* by inorganic pyrophosphatases, which are widely distributed in human tissue, is inhibited by high calcium and low magnesium. This may partially explain the association of CPPD deposition with hyperparathyroidism and hypomagnesemia.

Epidemiology

CPPD crystal deposition occurs only in adults and uncommonly before the sixth decade. The incidence of chondrocalcinosis on radiographs steadily rises and may exceed 30% of the asymptomatic population over 85 years old. CPPD deposition also occurs more frequently in certain metabolic diseases such as hypothyroidism, hyperparathyroidism, hemochromatosis, hypomagnesemic states, and hypophosphatasia.

Clinical Features

CPPD can present in several different manners. Acute attacks of inflammatory arthritis (monoarthritis, often termed pseudogout, or oligoarticular arthritis) commonly occur first in the knees. However, the wrist, elbows, ankles, and shoulders are often involved. Involvement of the first MTP occurs, but is uncommon. Acute attacks are usually self-limited, lasting several days to weeks. Acute attacks may occur in a postoperative patient and, like in gout, may uncommonly coexist with a septic joint.

CPPD can also present as a polyarticular, inflammatory arthritis, commonly involving the knees, wrists, and elbows. Involvement of the small joints of the hands and feet can be seen but is uncommon. Low-grade, chronic joint pain and swelling can be seen in some with evidence of degenerative joint disease. Some patients will present with what appears to be a disintegrating, neuropathic joint as a result of CPPD crystal deposition. Finally, many have no clinical symptoms but chondrocalcinosis can be demonstrated on radiographs.

The diagnosis of CPPD relies on the demonstration of calcium pyrophosphate crystals within the synovial fluid of an affected joint. Compensated, polarized light microscopy will reveal positively birefringent, rhomboid-shaped crystals found within PMNs. Other tests on synovial fluid are of limited use. Synovial fluid leukocyte counts are similar to those seen in gout.

Radiology

The radiologic hallmark of CPPD is chondrocalcinosis: calcification of the fibrocartilage and hyaline cartilage of involved joints. The most commonly calcified fibrocartilage includes the knee, the pubic symphysis, and the triangular fibrocartilage of the wrist. Hyaline cartilage calcification tends to be more linear and parallels the subchondral bone. Joint space narrowing, subchondral sclerosis, and subchondral cysts can also be seen. Isolated patellofemoral joint space narrowing with osteophytes suggests the diagnosis of CPPD.

Treatment

The therapy for acute CPPD arthropathy is similar to that used for gout and includes NSAIDs, corticosteroids, colchicine, and intra-articular corticosteroids (if infection is excluded). Urate-lowering therapy is ineffective in CPPD.

BASIC CALCIUM PHOSPHATE. Calcium hydroxyapatite crystals (among other basic calcium phosphate crystals) can deposit into articular tissue and cause an acute, subacute, or chronic arthritis as well as a periarthritis (bursitis, tendonitis). The periarthritis may be associated with radiographic calcifications at the sites of inflammation. Commonly affected areas include the shoulder, the greater trochanter, the epicondyles, and tendinous attachments about the wrist and knee. The "Milwaukee shoulder" is the term applied to a progressive, erosive arthritis of the shoulder seen in older women. Calcium hydroxyapatite crystals are difficult to identify on polarized microscopy due in part to their small size. NSAIDs, colchicine, and oral and intra-articular corticosteroids have been used successfully in therapy.

Systemic Sclerosis
Rebecca S. Tuetken

Classification and Pathogenesis

The thickened, sclerotic skin lesion of *scleroderma*, which literally means "hard skin," is the key feature linking a heterogeneous group of conditions, commonly referred to by the same name. Scleroderma can be subclassified into disease of the skin only, or *localized scleroderma*, versus disease with internal organ involvement, or *systemic sclerosis*. Systemic sclerosis (SSc) is further classified by the extent of skin disease into *diffuse cutaneous systemic sclerosis* (dcSSc), versus *limited cutaneous systemic sclerosis* (lcSSc) (Table 6-3). By definition, limited skin involvement means the face, neck, feet, and upper extremity involvement that is most often distal to the wrist and virtually always distal to the elbow, whereas diffuse skin involvement includes the trunk and proximal extremities. This classification system is clinically useful because the pattern and extent of skin disease, coupled with the specific type of autoantibodies detected, correlates well with the pattern of organ involvement and overall disease mortality and morbidity. In rare cases SSc can occur without significant skin disease, or systemic sclerosis *sine scleroderma*. It may also occur as part of an overlap syndrome with other autoimmune diseases such as systemic lupus erythematosus, dermatomyositis, rheumatoid arthritis, and Sjögren's syndrome. The combination of Raynaud's phenomenon, with either abnormal nailfold capillaries or SSc-specific serologic markers is so predictive of underlying SSc, that it is often referred to as "pre-scleroderma."

SSc is a rare disease, with an estimated prevalence in the United States of about 240 per million, and an incidence of about 20 per million per year. It is more common in women than men by a ratio of about 4:1. The cause is unknown, but it most likely involves an interaction between genetic and environmental factors. The pathogenesis can best be viewed as an interacting triad of pathological immune system activation (as evidenced by autoantibodies to nuclear antigens), endothelial cell dysfunction (with resulting small vessel vasculopathy and tissue ischemia), and fibroblast dysfunction (with increased synthesis and deposition of extracellular matrix), all culminating in end organ damage, fibrosis, and atrophy.

Clinical Presentation

SSc affects multiple organ systems, including vascular, skin, musculoskeletal, pulmonary, renal, cardiac, and gastrointestinal systems. Organ-specific manifestations will be discussed first, followed by a discussion of characteristics that distinguish lcSSc and dcSSc.

Vascular

Vascular manifestations are particularly prominent, especially Raynaud's phenomenon (RP), which is often the first sign of SSc. RP is an exaggerated vasoconstrictive response of terminal arteries to stimuli such as cold or emotional stress, most noticeable in the digits, and manifested by coldness, ischemic pain, and striking color changes: pallor (white), followed by acrocyanosis (blue), then hyperemia (red) on reperfusion. In SSc-associated RP, vessel wall morphology is abnormal. Small and medium arteries show abnormal smooth muscle cell activation, with markedly increased $\alpha 2c$ adrenergic reactivity. Over time progressive intimal hyperplasia and fibrosis reduces the effective vessel lumen and limits dilatation, leading to chronic tissue ischemia, ulceration, and infarction.

TABLE 6-3.
Classification of Scleroderma and Subtype Associations

LOCALIZED SCLERODERMA

Linear (including en coup de sabre)
Morphea
   localized (circumscribed)
   generalized

SYSTEMIC SCLEROSIS

Pre-Scleroderma
   Raynaud's phenomenon, plus *either*
     • abnormal nailfold capillaries, *or*
     • anticentromere or anti-Scl-70 antibodies
Limited cutaneous systemic sclerosis (lcSSc)
   Cutaneous disease limited to the distal extremities, face, and neck
   CREST syndrome and anticentromere antibodies
   Severe Raynaud's phenomenon with digital ulceration, without nailfold capillary drop out
   Slow disease progression
   Generally less severe internal organ involvement
   Pulmonary arterial hypertension or interstitial lung disease
Diffuse cutaneous systemic sclerosis (dcSSc)
   Cutaneous disease includes trunk and proximal extremities
   ANA and anti-Scl-70 (topoisomerase) antibodies
   Mild Raynaud's phenomenon, with nailfold capillary drop out
   Rapid disease progression
   High incidence of significant internal organ involvement
     • interstitial lung disease
     • renal crisis
     • diffuse GI disease
Systemic sclerosis *sine* scleroderma
   Organ disease of SSc
   Absence of skin disease
   Raynaud's
Overlap syndromes with scleroderma
   Features of SSc, plus another autoimmune rheumatic disease, e.g., systemic lupus erythematosus, rheumatoid arthritis, dermatomyositis, or Sjögren's syndrome.

An ophthalmoscope set at 40 diopters can be used to examine capillary loops proximal to the fingernail cuticle (nailfold). In SSc this exam will reveal abnormally dilated and tortuous capillary loops, sometimes with areas of vessel loss. When RP is accompanied by this finding, even in the absence of autoantibodies, it is strong evidence for an underlying autoimmune disease. *Telangectasias* are dilated venules and capillaries, which form small (2 to 7 mm) polygonal macules on the hands, face, lips, oral, and intestinal mucosa.

Vascular disease is the direct cause of many organ system manifestations, including some of the pulmonary, gastrointestinal, and renal manifestations discussed in the following sections.

Skin and Musculoskeletal

Cutaneous sclerosis will often begin on the hands, which in early stages become diffusely edematous or "puffy" in appearance. As the swelling subsides, the skin becomes thickened and tough, and eventually "hidebound" to the deeper tissues. The normally plump finger tuft atrophies, causing the distal phalanx to shrink behind the fingernail. The face and neck may also be involved. Perioral skin may take on a puckered appearance with radial folds, and the oral aperture, measured as the inter-incisor distance, decreases. Skin will feel tight and sometimes pruritic. Scleroderma of the fingers is called *sclerodactyly*. When the hands are involved proximal to the fingers, but the trunk is spared, this is termed *acrosclerosis*. The hands and face are involved in both major disease subtypes, but rapid progression to involve the trunk and proximal extremities indicates the diffuse cutaneous form of SSc.

Calcinosis is the abnormal tissue deposition of basic calcium phosphate. Usually a late manifestation, it eventually occurs in up to a third of patients. Lesions can persist for years, and can occur anywhere, but are most often found in the distal finger tufts, near the proximal interphalangeal joints, along extensor surfaces, or near other bony prominences, such as the elbows and knees. Calcinoses may be painful, especially when they occur in highly innervated locations such as the fingertip. They will sometimes ulcerate and leak a whitish material, and secondary infection is a common complication.

About 20 to 30% of patients complain of joint pain, and as many as 20% will have arthritis, mainly affecting the finger joints. Synovial biopsy reveals fibrosis rather than synovitis. Radiographs will sometimes show joint erosions, or the virtual disappearance of the distal phalanx, termed *acro-osteolysis*. Flexion contractures of the finger joints result from tightening of the periarticular skin, fascia, and tendons. Tendon friction rubs—a palpable or audible crepitus with movement of the tendon—occur in over 50% of patients with dcSSc, and occasionally in those with lcSSc.

Disuse atrophy is the most common muscle manifestation. However, a true primary myopathy with proximal muscle weakness and mild elevation of creatinine kinase has been reported. Muscle biopsies reveal interstitial fibrosis and fiber atrophy, without much evidence of inflammatory cell infiltration.

Gastrointestinal

The gastrointestinal (GI) tract is affected in the vast majority of patients, and at least half are symptomatic. Though any level of the tract may be involved, the most common symptoms arise from the esophagus. Esophageal hypomotility and incompetence of the distal sphincter lead to recurrent acid reflux, which in turn can cause erosive esophagitis, Barrett's esophagus, and stricture formation. Patients report dysphagia, acid reflux, or regurgitation. Gastric or intestinal disease results in loss of normal peristalsis, bacterial overgrowth, malabsorption, and resulting malnutrition. Patients report prolonged satiety or loss of appetite, weight loss, bloating, constipation, and diarrhea. Telangectasias in the gut will sometimes bleed and cause anemia.

Pulmonary

Pulmonary involvement is now the single leading cause of disease-related death in SSc, and over 70% patients have some form of lung involvement. There are two main types: interstitial lung disease (ILD) (also called fibrosing alveolitis or pulmonary fibrosis); and vascular disease of the lung leading to pulmonary arterial hypertension (PAH). Other pulmonary complications include aspiration pneumonia due to severe esophageal reflux, pleural fibrosis, bronchiectasis, and spontaneous pneumothorax.

ILD most frequently occurs with dcSSc, but can also occur in lcSSc, and usually presents as dyspnea on exertion and cough. Examination will reveal bilateral basal lung crepitations. The 8-year survival of patients with dcSSc and ILD is about 50%.

PAH is almost always associated with lcSSc, occurring in about 10% of these patients, and is associated with high mortality. Life expectancy is less than 1 year once gas exchange drops to 25% of the normal value. Patients report an insidious onset of dyspnea on exertion. Lower extremity edema and hepatic congestion will occur with advancing disease.

Renal

Renal disease, sometimes called "scleroderma renal crisis," is much more common in dcSSc than in lcSSc, and is actually another manifestation of SSc vasculopathy, so it is not surprising that it often begins during cold weather. As renal arterioles become narrowed, afferent renal blood flow decreases, activating the renin-angiotensin system, resulting in hypertension, which, if untreated, can quickly progress to malignant hypertension and renal failure. Patients may present with ophthalmic evidence of hypertensive retinopathy (hemorrhages, cotton wool exudates, and papilledema).

Cardiac

Although up to 80% of autopsies reveal myocardial fibrosis, clinically significant myocardial dysfunction is uncommon. Radionuclide-exercise studies may reveal fixed thallium perfusion abnormalities, even when angiography is normal, indicating that the lesion is due to small vessel disease. Clinically significant pericardial disease may occur in up to 10% of patients, but frank tamponade or hemodynamically significant effusions are very rare.

Other

Fibrosis of the thyroid gland may cause hypothyroidism in up to 25% of patients. Dry mouth and eye symptoms may occur with fibrosis of exocrine tear and salivary glands. SSc spares the central nervous system, but peripheral nerve entrapment syndromes, such as carpal tunnel syndrome or facial nerve palsies, sometimes occur secondary to fibrosis and sclerosis of surrounding tissue. Osteoporosis may occur, usually as a consequence of malabsorption and malnutrition from GI disease.

Disease Variation by Classification

The majority of SSc patients will eventually be classified as lcSSc, where skin disease spares the trunk and proximal extremities, and is frequently limited to the hands or fingers. LcSSc is sometimes referred to as the CREST syndrome, an acronym for the most common disease manifestations: *c*alcinosis cutis, *R*aynaud's phenomenon (RP), *e*sophageal dysmotility, *s*clerodactyly, and *t*elangectasias. LcSSc tends to have a longer and more indolent disease course than dcSSc, with lower overall disease mortality and generally later onset of significant internal organ disease. RP may be present for years before other signs of disease appear. However, RP tends to be more severe in lcSSc, with a higher incidence of digital ulcers and necrosis. About 10% of patients will develop significant PAH, and this group will have a very poor prognosis. ILD can occur, but is less common than in dcSSc. Renal crisis is rare.

About one-third of SSc patients will develop the extensive skin involvement that defines dcSSc. Early clues that a patient will develop this pattern include appearance of skin disease before or within one year of onset of RP, dilated capillary loops *with dropout* at the nailfold, tendon friction rubs, and early onset of ILD, renal crisis, or diffuse GI disease. ILD occurs frequently, and mortality can be high. However, in some patients the disease course is one of initial worsening, followed by a plateau, and then some improvement or stabilization thereafter. Diagnosis and organ-specific treatment early in the disease may significantly improve the prognosis.

DcSSc and lcSSc are also characterized by distinct serologic markers, which are discussed in the following section.

Diagnostic Evaluation

A thorough history and physical examination are essential for diagnosing early SSc. A complete review of systems is key, as patients seeking evaluation for puffy hands may not spontaneously report mild dyspnea, or new nocturnal heartburn. Patients with dcSSc, should be taught to monitor their own blood pressure frequently, and report any consistent elevation. Assessment of skin tightness, and use of a standard scoring system, can help to detect rapidly progressive disease. The most commonly used system involves measurement at 17 sites, scoring each site on a scale of 0 (normal) to 3 (hidebound skin). Skin biopsy is rarely needed to confirm scleroderma and should generally be avoided as healing may be impaired. Radiographs of the hands may detect acro-osteolysis, calcifications, or joint erosions, but will have little impact on the overall disease management.

The majority of patients with SSc will have detectable antinuclear antibodies (ANA), and the pattern detected on immunofluorescence is very important (Table 6-4). An anticentromere pattern (ACA) is detected in 70 to 80% of patients with lcSSc, but is unusual in patients with dcSSc. ACA correlates positively with PAH and *negatively* with ILD or renal disease. A speckled ANA pattern may indicate antibodies to topoisomerase-1 called anti-Scl-70, which can be measured directly in a separate assay. Anti-Scl-70 antibodies are found in about 30% of

TABLE 6-4.
Common Serum Autoantibody Associations in Systemic Sclerosis

Autoantibody(antigen)	SSc Classification (% positive)	Positive Disease Association	*Negative* Disease Association
anticentromere antibodies (centromere kinotochore)	lcSSc (70–80%)	pulmonary hypertension	*interstitial lung disease, renal crisis*
anti-Scl-70 (topoisomerase)	dcSSc (30%) few lcSSc	interstitial lung disease	*pulmonary hypertension*
ANA, speckled or nucleolar (RNA polymerase I and III)	SSc (20%) more dcSSc than lcSSc	pulmonary hypertension, muscle disease	

[Note: italics in fourth column only, to emphasize that the association is negative]

patients with dcSSC but fewer patients with lcSSc, and correlate positively with ILD and *negatively* with PAH. Autoantibodies to several other nuclear antigens have been linked with SSc. As many as 20% of patients with dcSSc will have an antinucleolar or speckled ANA pattern due to antibodies to RNA polymerase I and III, a finding that correlates with renal disease. The false-positive rates for detection of ACA and anti-Scl-70 among disease-free controls are both very low, giving these tests a high degree of specificity for SSc. However, negative antibody tests, including ANA, do not rule out SSc.

Beyond establishing a diagnosis, a variety of laboratory, functional, and imaging studies are useful to detect and monitor disease in each affected organ system. Serum creatinine should be checked periodically in patients with dcSSc to monitor renal function. Oxygen saturation or arterial blood gas profile, pulmonary function tests including DLCO, and chest radiographs, should be obtained at diagnosis of SSc, and repeated with any new respiratory symptoms to detect onset of ILD or PAH. Additional studies may include high-resolution chest CT to confirm fibrosis, and/or echocardiography with Doppler to estimate pulmonary artery pressure. Invasive studies such as bronchoscopy for bronchoalveolar lavage, or right-heart catheterization to directly measure pulmonary artery pressure, may be needed to confirm a diagnosis before beginning treatment with high-risk medications. Gastrointestinal disease can be detected and monitored with radiographic studies such as barium swallow, gastric emptying tests, or abdominal CT. Esophageal manometry, upper endoscopy, or colonoscopy may also be needed.

Treatment

No single agent has been identified as disease-modifying for all SSc manifestations. Disease management is therefore primarily organ based. Search is under way, however, for treatments that will prevent tissue fibrosis, and thus reduce the risk of end organ failure.

Patient education is very important for management of SSc. Occupational therapists can help to educate patients on how to keep warm, protect their fingers while performing activities of daily living, and maintain flexibility. Because nicotine will worsen RP, and smokers have a significantly higher risk for finger ulcers and digital necrosis, patients must be advised that smoking cessation is absolutely necessary. Medications that trigger vasospasm must be avoided. Hypothyroidism will worsen Raynaud's, so hypothyroid patients must be on adequate replacement hormone. Some antihypertensives, such as β-blockers, may worsen RP, or at least limit use of other antihypertensives that will more effectively treat RP.

Long-acting calcium channel blockers are the drugs used most frequently to treat RP, and efficacy is well established. Use may be limited, however, by intolerable side effects such as postural hypotension, dependent edema, and significant gastroesophageal reflux, especially in those who already have an incompetent esophageal sphincter. ACE inhibitors and angiotensin receptor blockers have been used with mixed success. They are generally well tolerated, and do not worsen esophageal function. Platelet serotonin may play a role in the pathogenesis of RP. The selective serotonin-reuptake inhibitor, fluoxetine, has been reported to be beneficial, and was superior to nifedipine in one small trial. Most authors recommend daily aspirin (81 to 325 mg) to prevent formation of microthrombi, though actual benefit is unproven. Anecdotal reports support use of pentoxifylline, which may improve microcirculation. There are promising reports that the phosphodiesterase inhibitor, sildenafil, is effective and well tolerated for short-term management of severe Raynaud's, but controlled trials are needed to prove efficacy in SSc-associated RP.

Aggressive therapy is sometimes needed to prevent or treat impending digital infarction. Topical nitroglycerine may improve circulation to the affected digit, but intolerance may limit its use. Several synthetic prostacyclins have been used for this indication, but the need for constant IV infusion limits use to the hospital setting, and there may be rebound worsening once infusion is stopped.

To some extent, PAH may be thought of as "Raynaud's of the lungs." Unfortunately, it does not respond adequately to most of the oral medications used to treat Raynaud's. The endothelin receptor blocker, bosentan, has been shown to help stabilize pulmonary function in patients with significant PAH. Controlled trials showed slight functional improvement (as measured by 6 minute walking distance) in bosentan-treated SSc patients, while untreated control patients showed significant continuing decline. Bosentan may also be effective for severe digit-threatening Raynaud's, but cost will likely limit any off-label indication. Intravenous prostaclycin analogues are effective in PAH but costly. Administration by continuous subcutaneous infusion, or by inhalation, is showing promise in clinical trials. Sildenafil and other oral phosphodiesterase inhibitors may also have a role in management of PAH, either alone or in combination with the synthetic prostacyclins.

Early diagnosis is key to the successful management of SSc-related ILD. The goal is to treat the disease with aggressive immunosuppression in the early inflammatory phase and thereby reduce the risk of progressive fibrosis and decline in function that may follow. Retrospective data supports this approach but prospective studies are needed to confirm this strategy. Cyclophosphamide, either by daily oral dose or pulse IV dosing, is the current drug of choice for treatment of ILD. Some recommend adding daily low dose prednisone, but there is limited evidence that this is helpful.

An ACE inhibitor is recommended for any patient with hypertension and SSc. Renal crisis was once the major cause of death in SSc, but ACE inhibitors have proven to be very effective at controlling hypertension and reducing the rate of subsequent renal failure. Studies have shown long-term benefit, even if creatinine levels increase after starting an ACE inhibitor.

Proton pump inhibitors are useful for treating severe gastroesophageal reflux, and to reduce the risk for esophagitis and recurrent aspiration. Prokinetic agents such as metoclopromide may help patients with delayed gastric emptying and poor appetite. Cyclic oral antibiotics are used to treat bacterial overgrowth in advanced disease. Dieticians may be needed to guide the use of oral supplements when malabsorption leads to malnutrition. Some patients do eventually require total parenteral nutrition.

Skin disease has proven difficult to treat with any degree of efficacy. The fact that sclerosed skin may spontaneously start to soften many years after disease onset complicates interpretation of long-term studies. Many agents reported to be beneficial in small open trials have not shown benefit when studied in large double-blind studies. D-Penicillamine has shown promise in some trials but not in others. Studies on methotrexate have shown benefit or at least a trend favoring treatment, but further studies are needed. Minocycline inhibits cation-dependent matrix metaloproteases,

which have been implicated in the tissue damage that follows inflammation in SSc. Minocycline 100 mg twice/day did seem to soften the skin of several patients with advanced dcSSc in one small open-label trial, but this needs to be repeated in a larger trial. Corticosteroids play no role in managing the skin disease of SSc and topical steroids are contraindicated.

Surgery in Systemic Sclerosis

In view of the significant microvascular disease of SSc and resulting poor healing of wounds, surgical procedures are relatively contraindicated. Circumstances will arise, however, which necessitate surgery, such as severe esophageal strictures, and small or large bowel obstructions.

Hand surgery may be of benefit in selective circumstances. Patients with severe carpal tunnel syndrome may benefit from surgical release. When sclerodactyly leads to severe (> 90°) contracture of the PIP joints, arthrodeses or joint replacements may be of benefit. Debridement and amputation of ischemic digits will occasionally be indicated to address secondary infection, but should be done conservatively, to allow the maximum possibility of spontaneous healing. In general, this should follow aggressive medical therapy with a parenteral prostacyclin and possibly a trial of bosentan.

Cervical sympathectomies have been tried for upper extremity RP, and can now be performed thorascopically, but they rarely provide long-lasting benefit, probably due to accessory sympathetic pathways and the upregulation of sympathetic receptors on vascular smooth muscle following denervation. Lumbar sympathectomies, by contrast, have proven very effective for Raynaud's of the feet with lasting benefits.

Microarteriolysis (digital sympathectomy) has been shown to relieve pain and ulceration of severe RP, including cases secondary to SSc. Yee and colleagues (1998) report very favorable outcomes in their series of 13 procedures in 9 patients. They conclude that adventitial stripping of the arteriole both denervates and decompresses the vessel, which is why their procedure was effective even in patients who showed no discernable response to sympathetic blockade prior to surgery. This procedure should be considered when medical management fails or is contraindicated by other medical conditions.

Fibromyalgia
Robert F. Ashman

Definition

Fibromyalgia is a clinical syndrome of diffuse pain (present at rest but exacerbated by activity), fatigue, and sleep disturbance. The American College of Rheumatology defined two criteria for diagnosing fibromyalgia in 1990: (1) a history of widespread pain and (2) pain in at least 11 of 18 defined tender point sites on digital palpation with a force of 4 dynes/cm^2 (Figure 6-10).

Clinical Features

Symptoms

"Hurting all over" is the usual chief complaint, although pain may be concentrated in the neck and shoulder girdle area, in the buttocks and thighs, or in an area previously injured. Typically the patient cannot point to an exact location for the pain, nor can it be localized anatomically to particular muscles, particular joints, or to the area of distribution of particular nerves. Stiffness may be present, but it is not relieved by heat or gentle activity, and thus differs from the morning stiffness characteristic of inflammatory disorders such as rheumatoid arthritis or polymyalgia rheumatica. Usually there is a clear trend toward diminishing motor activity over months or years, and patients may feel disabled by their pain.

Patients usually complain of severe fatigue with dozing off during the daytime. On prompting, they describe disordered sleep hygiene of long duration: difficulty falling asleep, shallow sleep with frequent awakening, and arising unrefreshed.

Other common features are (1) numbness and tingling of hands and/or feet—because the whole hand or limb is involved in fibromyalgia, it can be distinguished from nerve entrapment syndromes where the numbness conforms to the area served by a particular nerve; (2) irritable bowel syndrome, characterized by alternating diarrhea and constipation; (3) dysuria with normal urinalysis; and (4) a history of having taken many different pain medications without relief. Periods of more intense symptoms typically follow events that force reduced motor activity (e.g., hospitalization for surgery), intensified sleep

disturbance (e.g., assuming care of an elderly parent), a painful injury (e.g., a motor vehicle accident), or a period of increased stress or muscle tension (e.g., combat duty lawsuit). This is how susceptible patients with rheumatoid or osteoarthritis can develop superimposed fibromyalgia symptoms.

Signs

The only characteristic finding on physical exam is the presence of the nine pairs of tender points (Figure 6-10). Fingertip pressure on these sites, which would be judged mildly unpleasant by a normal subject, produces an aversive reaction and is

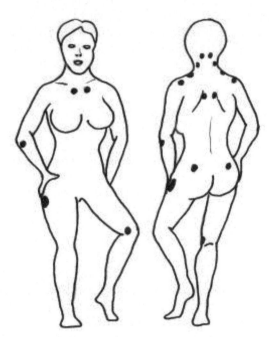

FIGURE 6-10. Fibromyalgia tender points. The ACR published clinical criteria for fibromyalgia in 1990, emphasizing the characteristic nine pairs of tender points: insertion of cervical paraspinals on the occipital condyles, cleidomastoid muscle over lateral transverse processes of C5-7, belly of trapezius, supraspinatus, wrist extensor insertion on lateral epicondyle, pectoralis insertions on 2nd rib near sternum, upper outer buttock, gluteus insertion on greater trochanter, and insertion of vastus medialis on medial condyle of the femur. The diagram also shows a common tenth tender point over the rhomboids. *Control points:* middle of forehead; volar aspect of midforearm; thumbnail; muscles of anterior thigh.

perceived as painful by fibromyalgia patients. While the ACR criterion of 11 of 18 tender points is a useful general guide for diagnosing fibromyalgia, strict conformance with this criterion is not necessary in the clinic. Some patients have palpable tender knots representing localized areas of muscle spasm. Trigger points, where local pressure produces referred pain over an entire region, is unusual in fibromyalgia. Joint and neurologic exams are normal. So is muscle strength, although "breakaway weakness" due to pain may be observed. In especially severe cases, the tenderness may be generalized to the point that control points or even gentle pinching of skin are also painful, a condition called allodynia.

Epidemiology

More than 90% of fibromyalgia patients are female. All ages are susceptible, but the pain pattern often begins in the teens. Community surveys, confirmed with tender point examinations, have estimated that pain thresholds tend to be stable over time in a given individual, and that females whose pain threshold falls in the lower 5% tend to develop fibromyalgia symptoms when they encounter a prolonged reduction in motor activity or a prolonged deprivation of deep sleep. Family histories positive for fibromyalgia are common.

Pathogenesis

PET scans of the brain of fibromyalgia patients show that peripheral stimulation of muscle pressure receptors produces activation of thalamic regions typical of pain rather than touch. Impulses interpreted centrally as pain are carried by peripheral myelinated or unmyelinated nerve fibers in fibromyalgia, whereas in normals they are confined to unmyelinated fibers. In fibromyalgia, as in other chronic pain states, there is progressive failure of inhibitory neurons in the spinal cord to focus afferent sensory impulses appropriately, leading to "central sensitization," which widens the range of sensory impulses perceived as pain, and also enlarges the area of pain, making it difficult for the patient to localize pain. Research in progress focuses on the role in central sensitization of endorphins (regenerated by exercise and deep sleep), serotonin, and other neurotransmitters in the central nervous system.

An abundant literature on histologic, physiologic, and biochemical changes in fibromyalgia muscles can be summarized as showing many abnormalities typical of fatigued incompletely relaxed muscle, but no *primary* physiologic abnormalities of muscle have been proven.

The controversial relationship of fibromyalgia to psychiatric conditions has recently been clarified. In general, psychological profiles of fibromyalgia patient resemble those of other chronic pain patients. The only psychiatric diagnoses more frequent in fibromyalgia patients than in controls are mood and anxiety disorders. Furthermore, in community-based surveys, this association only occurs among the subset (about one-third) of persons with fibromyalgia who seek medical intervention for their symptoms, and does not apply to the others who learn from experience how to control their own symptoms. One symptom characteristic of inadequately treated depression is an inability to initiate and carry out a treatment program, which may make it especially difficult for such a patient to control their fibromyalgia symptoms. Patients with anxiety disorders have difficulty tolerating the short-term muscle pain experienced during exercise, fearing that they will damage themselves. Thus, the psychiatric associations with fibromyalgia have less to do with primary pathology than with the probability of treatment success.

Radiologic and Laboratory Features

There are no typical radiologic or laboratory features of fibromyalgia other than normal values. The initial workup should focus on ruling out fibromyalgia mimics or exacerbating conditions such as hypothyroidism (TSH), diabetes (Hemoglobin A1c) or inflammatory conditions (ESR and CRP). If muscle spasm is prominent, creatinine, electrolytes, calcium, and magnesium may be useful. Anemia should be ruled out as a cause of fatigue. Rheumatoid factor and ANA are meaningless in the absence of specific clinical features of those diseases. Males should be tested for hypogonadism (free and bound testosterone).

Medical Management

Many patients expect that when they get sick, they will visit the physician, get treated with a medicine, and recover. This paradigm does not apply in fibromyalgia, where the success or failure of treatment depends on the patient, who must faithfully carry out his or her own treatment program on a daily basis over many weeks to alleviate his or her pain. The physician's role is to rule out alternative diagnoses, educate the patient, and arrange the first meeting with the physical therapist who will act as "coach."

The management strategy encompasses three main aspects: (1) patient education; (2) therapeutic exercise; and (3) achievement of stage 3 sleep. Analgesic drugs have little impact on fibromyalgia symptoms, and thus play a minor role, especially when the patient is severely symptomatic.

Education

Even today, patients may have been told that fibromyalgia is psychosomatic, and many are reassured to learn that it is a recognized medical disorder with a physiologic basis. The two key points are the relationship of symptoms to deprivation of sleep and reduced physical activity. The essential message is that by following the treatment plan the patient will learn how to control his or her symptoms, but that this control is won slowly over weeks or months. Patients should be taught to identify and avoid the exacerbating circumstances in their own lives. Examples include stress causing muscle spasm or sleep interruption or occupations entailing tonic muscle tension (orchestra conductors, keyboard operators, bus drivers). They must learn that chronic pain does not have the protective warning function we all associate with acute pain, and that it is not harmful to engage in painful exercises today in order to decrease the pain you will experience next month.

A therapist experienced in fibromyalgia should be able not only to apply the standard treatments, but also to direct appropriate patients to second line treatments such as ultrasound, biofeedback (for muscle relaxation), and acupuncture. Such a therapist should also be able to individualize the exercise program for each patient and make adjustments when other health events occur (e.g., abdominal surgery, because of the prolonged inactivity, usually requires returning to an earlier stage of the treatment protocol).

Physical Therapy

Three elements comprise the standard fibromyalgia treatment protocol: (1) gentle stretching, (2) graduated conditioning, and (3) transcutaneous nerve stimulation.

1. The patient begins with muscles that are incompletely relaxed, which will hurt if contracted too vigorously. Tai Chi-style slow-motion stretching toward the limit of each motion promotes relaxation and produces short-term pain relief, which can be applied several times per day. Contrasting activities to be avoided in the early stages of treatment are quick forceful contractions. An athlete needs to warm up before running a dash to avoid painful muscle spasm, whereas the fibromyalgia patient needs to warm up in order to perform normal daily activity.

2. The conditioning program begins with a low level of gentle exercise, designed to accelerate breathing and heart rate, and cause less than an hour of delayed pain. Swimming or moving limbs through a full range of motion in a swimming pool three times per week is ideal, but walking and other gentle land-based exercises are an effective second choice. A gradual increase in the intensity and duration of exercise occurs until pain is controlled. Exercises designed to build strength are especially painful and may be counterproductive in the early stages of treatment. Normal daily activities are encouraged, but do not substitute for therapeutic exercise.

3. Transcutaneous nerve stimulators (TENS) help to relax thin muscles lying close to the skin, so they work much better in the neck and shoulder region than in the low back and buttocks. A brief trial with the therapist will usually show whether TENS will work in a particular patient, who can then rent a unit on prescription and use it at home or at work.

The goal of therapy is a patient trained to carry out a well-designed program on his or her own; prolonged "hands on" treatment by a therapist is generally unnecessary, whereas periodic reassessments for advancing the program are helpful. The most common reason for failure of a treatment program is that the patient has not been doing the exercise. Reassessment for undertreated depression should be considered in such a patient. Fibromyalgia patients should be strongly encouraged to seek accommodations in their work environment (such as short breaks for stretching) so they can remain productive. Social security disability from fibromyalgia is unusual.

Drug Treatment

The only drugs with well-documented efficacy in fibromyalgia are the tricyclics, such as amitriptyline, trazodone, nortriptyline, desipramine, or cyclobenzaprine. A dose given 2 hours before bedtime should increase the proportion of stage 3 sleep. Intolerable morning grogginess may necessitate cutting the dose in half or taking it earlier. Lack of effect over several nights means a higher dose is needed. Lack of effect plus morning grogginess means a different tricyclic should be selected. Usually the beneficial effects of a regimen become evident between 2 weeks and 3 months. Sleep apnea may need to be ruled out by polysomnography, and treated if present for progress to be made.

Failure to respond to opioids and other analgesics is so typical of severe fibromyalgia that it is considered to have diagnostic importance. As the patient's pain responds to exercise and treatment, the response to conventional analgesics (such as ibuprofen, Tylenol, or tramadol) reemerges. Opioids may be partially effective in some patients. However, breakthrough pain increases with time, leading to dose escalation. Also narcotics can impair deep sleep. Narcotic rebound pain can be difficult to distinguish from fibromyalgia. For these reasons, opioids are not recommended in fibromyalgia.

Annotated Bibliography

Osteoarthritis

American College of Rheumatology Subcommittee on Osteoarthritis Guidelines. Recommendations for the Medical Management of Osteoarthritis of the Hip and Knee. Arthritis Rheum 2000 update;43:1905–1915. *Also available at:* http://www.rheumatology.org/publications/guidelines/oa-mgmt/oa-mgmt.asp
Following the principles of evidence-based medicine, the ACR subcommittee provides a detailed review of current knowledge regarding many modes of treatment for OA of the hip and knee, both pharmacologic and nonpharmacologic, and provides a consensus recommendation for the nonsurgical management of OA in the hip and knee. The most current version of these guidelines can be found at the above web address.

Felson DT, Zhang Y, Hannan MT et al. Risk factors for incident radiographic knee osteoarthritis in the elderly. The Framingham Study. Arthritis Rheum 1997;40:728–733.
An excellent study demonstrating the correlation between weight and incident radiographic knee OA in an elderly population.

Kraus VB. Pathogenesis and treatment of osteoarthritis. Med Clin North Am 1997;81:85–112.
This article provides an authoritative review of normal joint tissue physiology, and the epidemiology, genetics, and pathology of osteoarthritis. Kraus also reviews the clinical features of OA, and discusses treatment in terms of both primary and secondary intervention, including the concept of chondroprotection.

Minor MA. Exercise in the treatment of osteoarthritis. Rheum Dis Clin North Am 1999;25:397–415.
Minor makes a strong argument that exercise is integral to the successful management of OA. This article includes exercise recommendations and safety considerations.

Rheumatoid Arthritis

Choy EHS, Panayi GS. Cytokine pathways and joint inflammation in rheumatoid arthritis. N Engl J Med 2001;344:907–916.
This article reviews the latest science on the role of cytokines in the pathogenesis of RA and describes several potential therapeutic targets with the use of anticytokine therapy.

Harris ED Jr., Schur PH. Risk factors for and possible causes of rheumatoid arthritis. In: Rose, BD, ed. UpToDate, Wellesley, MA, 2003.
This article reviews the epidemiology of rheumatoid arthritis as well as the pathogenesis.

Harris ED Jr., Schur PH. Overview of the systemic and nonarticular manifestations of rheumatoid arthritis. In: Rose, BD, ed. UpToDate, Wellesley, MA, 2003.
This article reviews the complications of the disease as well as the drugs used to treat RA (such as steroid induced osteoporosis, entrapment syndromes, etc.)

Venables PJW, Maini RW. Clinical features of rheumatoid arthritis. In: Rose, BD, ed. UpToDate, Wellesley, MA, 2003.
This article reviews the clinical features of RA including extra-articular features, as well as discussing factors leading to a poorer outcome.

Venables PJW, Maini RW. Diagnosis and differential diagnosis of rheumatoid arthritis. In: Rose, BD, ed. UpToDate, Wellesley, MA, 2003.
This article reviews the diagnostic features of RA, including laboratory testing, the other forms of arthritis that may present similarly to RA and discusses a rationale approach to making the diagnosis

Systemic Lupus Erythematosus

Egol KA, Jazrawi LM, DeWal H et al. Orthopaedic manifestations of systemic lupus erythematosus. Bull Hosp Jt Dis 2001;60:29–34.
This review summarizes the common musculoskeletal manifestations of SLE from an orthopaedic viewpoint, and gives an overview of surgical interventions commonly used.

Mont MA, Jones LC. Management of osteonecrosis in systemic lupus erythematosus. Rheum Dis Clin North Am 2000;26:279–309.
This excellent review summarizes the epidemiology, diagnosis, and medical and surgical management of osteonecrosis in SLE patients.

Nalebuff EA. Surgery of systemic lupus erythematosus arthritis of the hand. Hand Clin 1996;12:591–602.
This review describes the features of lupus arthritis of the hands and wrists and the conservative and surgical approaches to its sequelae.

Pisetsky DS, Gilkeson G, St Clair, EW. Systemic lupus erythematosus: diagnosis and treatment. Med Clin North Am 1997;81:113–128.
This review details the clinical and laboratory diagnostic criteria for SLE, and summarizes the medical therapeutic approach for SLE by organ involvement.

Tan EM, Cohen AS, Fries JF et al. Revised criteria for the classification of systemic lupus erythematosus. Arthritis Rheum 1982;25:1271–1277.
This paper describes the 11 clinical and laboratory features that are used in the diagnosis of patients with SLE. These diagnostic criteria were developed for the standardization of subjects for research studies, but are now used frequently in substantiating the diagnosis of SLE.

Spondyloarthropathies

Dougados M, van der Linden S, Juhlin R et al. The European Spondyloarthropathy Study Group preliminary criteria for the classification of spondyloarthropathy. Arthritis Rheum 1991;34:1218–1227.
A very comprehensive helpful presentation of the wide spectrum of clinical features within the family of spondyloarthropathies.

Khan MA. Update on spondyloarthropathies. Ann Intern Med 2002;136:896–907.
A well-written, comprehensive, and extensively referenced review of the spondyloarthropathies.

McGonagle D, Conaghan PG, Emery P. Psoriatic arthritis: a unified concept twenty years on. Arthritis Rheum 1999; 42:1080–1086.
An excellent discussion of the clinical features and centrality of entheseal inflammation in psoriatic arthritis.

Mease PJ. Disease-modifying antirheumatic drug therapy for spondyloarthropathies: advances in treatment. Curr Opin Rheumatol 2003;15:205–212.
A review of recent progress in disease-modifying therapy for spondyloarthropathy, including the newer biologic agents.

Juvenile Idiopathic Arthritis

Cassidy JT, Petty RE. Textbook of Pediatric Rheumatology, 2nd Ed. New York: Churchill Livingstone, 1990.
This is an excellent comprehensive general reference.

Petty RE, Southwood TR, Baum J et al. Revision of the proposed classification criteria for juvenile idiopathic arthritis: Durban, 1997. J Rheumatol 1998; 25(10):1991–1994.
This article describes revisions of the International League of Associations for Rheumatology (ILAR) criteria for JIA.

Schneider R, Passo MH. Juvenile rheumatoid arthritis. Rheum Dis Clin North Am 2002; 28:503–530.
This article presents an overview of JRA utilizing the new JIA classifications. It offers a review of the genetics, prognosis, special aspects of the disease, and treatment in JIA.

Web sites with current information about JIA:

Arthritis Foundation: http://www.arthritis.org

American College of Rheumatology: http://www.rheumatology.org

Infectious Arthritis

Garcia-De La Torre I. Advances in the management of septic arthritis. Rheum Dis Clin N Am 2003;29:61–75.
A compact up-to-date review of the current treatment of septic arthritis.

Klippel JH, Crofford LJ, Stone JH et al. Primer on Rheumatic Diseases, 12th Ed. Atlanta: Arthritis Foundation, 2001.
This textbook is popular with medical students and residents interested in learning more about rheumatic diseases. The succinct book provides sufficient detail, without being overwhelming.

Mody GM. Infection and arthritis. Best Practice Research Clin Rheumatol 2003;17;183–363.
This issue reviews specific topics of joint infections.

Reveille JD. The changing spectrum of rheumatic disease in human immunodeficiency virus infection. Semin Arthritis Rheum 2000;30:147–166.
This book reviews rheumatic disease related to HIV.

West SG. Rheumatology Secrets, 2nd Ed. Philadelphia: Hanley and Belfus, 2002.
This concise book is extremely helpful to find answers quickly to virtually all questions on rounds, in the clinic, and on exams. It is a favorite with residents and fellows.

Crystal-Induced Arthritis

Conaghan PG, Day RO. Risks and benefits of drugs used in the management and prevention of gout. Drug Safety 1994;11: 252–258.
Conaghan and Day review the quantity and quality of evidence supporting therapeutic options in gout.

Halverson PB, Carrera GF, McCarty DJ. Milwaukee shoulder syndrome: fifteen additional cases. Arch Intern Med 1990; 150:677–682.
Halverson, Carrera, and McCarty review an additional 15 cases of Milwaukee shoulder syndrome describing common clinical features and discuss potential predisposing factors.

McGill NW. Gout and other crystal-associated arthropathies. Baillieres Best Pract Res Clin Rheumatol 2000;14:445–460.
McGill provides a thorough review of gout, calcium pyrophosphate deposition (CPPD), and basic calcium phosphate crystalline disease.

Rott KT, Agudelo CA. Gout. J Am Med Assoc 2003;289:2857–2860.
Rott and Agudelo provide a more concise review of the pathogenesis and treatment of gout.

Terkeltaub RA. Gout. N Engl J Med 2003;349:1647–1655.
Terkeltaub briefly reviews the clinical presentation of gout, followed by a more in-depth discussion of the therapy of gout with supporting references.

Systemic Sclerosis

Hummers LK, Wigley FM. Management of Raynaud's phenomenon and digital ischemic lesions in scleroderma. Rheum Dis Clin North Am 2003;29:293–313.
The authors review the quantity and quality of evidence supporting both common and less common treatments for Raynaud's, and lay out a practical approach for disease management.

Lin AT, Clements PJ, Furst DE. Update on disease-modifying antirheumatic drugs in the treatment of systemic sclerosis. Rheum Dis Clin North Am 2003;29:409–426.
The author reviews existing data for and against a series of agents used for the long-term management of SSc.

Medsger TA. Natural history of systemic sclerosis and the assessment of disease activity, severity, functional status, and psychologic well-being. Rheum Dis Clin North Am 2003;29:255–273.
Medsger summarizes data from several large case series to define the frequency of different disease manifestations in early versus late disease, and in lcSSc versus dcSSC; and also discusses the tools used to measure disease activity.

Pope JE. Musculoskeletal involvement in scleroderma. Rheum Dis Clin North Am 2003;29:391–408.
Pope provides a thorough review of the joint, tendon, muscle, and other connective tissue lesions of systemic sclerosis.

Yee AM, Hotchkiss RN, Paget SA. Adventitial stripping: a digit saving procedure in refractory Raynaud's phenomenon. J Rheumatol 1998;25:269–276.
The authors describe their generally favorable experience with digital microsurgery for severe Raynaud's in patients with systemic disease and conclude that efficacy is due to both denervation and decompression of the ischemic vessel.

Fibromyalgia

Bennett RM. Emerging concepts in the neurobiology of chronic pain: evidence of abnormal sensory processing in fibromyalgia. Mayo Clin Proc 1999;74:385–398.
This is a clearly written summary of the neurophysiology of fibromyalgia and its relationship to other chronic pain syndromes.

Carette S, Bell MJ, Reynolds WJ et al. Comparison of amitriptyline, cyclobenzaprine, and placebo in the treatment of fibromyalgia. Arthritis Rheum 1994; 37:32–40.
This article describes randomized double-blind placebo-controlled trial of two tricyclics in fibromyalgia.

Kennedy M, Felson DT. A prospective long-term study of fibromyalgia syndrome. Arthritis Rheum 1996; 39:682–685.
Prospective study of fibromyalgia patients showed 66% were "a little or a lot better" and 55% said they "felt well" after 10 years, but most still had some symptoms.

Wolfe F, Smythe HA, Yunus MB et al. The American College of Rheumatology 1990 criteria for the classification of fibromyalgia: report of the Multicenter Criteria Committee. Arthritis Rheum 1990;33:160–172.
This article reviews different criteria and proposes standard criteria to diagnose fibromyalgia. It underscores the difficulties one encounters in diagnosing these patients.

Wolfe F, Ross K, Anderson J et al. The prevalence and characteristics of fibromyalgia in the general population. Arthritis Rheum 1995; 38:19–28.
This article describes a population-based study of fibromyalgia prevalence.

7

Julie T. Lin
Joseph M. Lane

Metabolic Bone Disease

BONE GROWTH AND DEVELOPMENT

Bone is a living organ that is made primarily of type I collagen. It provides structural and mechanical support and plays a central role in mineral homeostasis. Its roles include protecting vital organs and housing bone marrow—as a site for muscle attachments and as the primary reservoir for calcium and phosphate.

Bone is comprised of cells and extracellular matrices. It is a dynamic entity regulated by osteoblasts, which are responsible for bone formation, and osteoclasts, which are responsible for bone resorption. Pluripotent mesenchymal cells give rise to marrow stromal-cell progenitors that can proliferate and differentiate into osteoblasts. Peak bone mass is established between 20 and 30 years of age. Multiple factors influence peak bone mass including race, genetics, nutrition, exercise, and in women, regular menstrual cycles. Bone strength is related to bone mass, distribution of the mass, microarchitectural structure, and quality of the bone.

Nutrition

Poor nutritional states such as anorexia nervosa, especially prevalent in adolescents, disrupt the hypothalamic-pituitary-gonadal axis, resulting in disturbance of menstrual cycles. Eating disorders such as anorexia nervosa are increasingly prevalent, with prevalence rates estimated at 0.5 to 1% among adolescents and young adults. Certain variables may identify those patients with anorexia nervosa at highest risk for low bone density. Lean body mass and low body mass index have been strongly correlated with amenorrhea and may be even more important than variables such as participation in physical exercise. Length of amenorrhea in patients with anorexia nervosa has been inversely correlated with bone density in the lumbar spine and hip. Additional important variables include greater than 12 months since onset of weight loss, calcium intake less than 600 mg/day, and body mass index less than 15. Regional bone loss may be predicted on the basis of low body weight.

Prevention of osteoporosis during adolescence in all patients includes a combination of adequate calcium intake and exercise, which together may represent the most significant factors. Adolescent women are at particularly high risk of poor nutrition and limited caloric intake. One study showed that half of adolescent females skipped one meal per day, more than half were trying to lose weight, and almost three-fourths were trying to keep from gaining weight.

The female athlete triad of disordered eating, amenorrhea, and osteoporosis, also commonly seen in adolescents, represents a complex interplay of poor nutrition and disrupted menstrual cycles leading to osteopenia and osteoporosis. This triad may be particularly prevalent in sports that place high emphasis on appearance, such as gymnastics and figure skating. Additional nutritional conditions contributing to osteoporosis include alcoholism, especially in men. Low bone density in alcoholics appears to be multifactorial in origin, with hormonal factors, malabsorption, and liver disease all possible contributors.

Poor intake of calcium, vitamin D, and total protein directly impact bone density. Poor nutritional states such as protein and calorie malnutrition stimulate bone resorption and impair bone formation secondary to reduced serum insulin-like growth factor-I. Gastrointestinal disorders such as malabsorption syndromes secondary to celiac sprue, ulcerative colitis, and Crohn's disease; primary biliary cirrhosis; chronic obstructive jaundice; and hepatitis are associated with bone loss. Specifically, the cytokines that are involved in inflammatory bowel disease and possibly celiac sprue stimulate bone resorption.

Menstrual Cycles

Regular menstrual cycles in women are exceedingly important for bone health. Hypoestrogenism is a well recognized cause of osteoporosis. In young women, the early diagnosis of primary amenorrhea is of paramount importance because it strongly correlates with osteopenia. Eating disorders, hyperandrogenism, and exercise-induced amenorrhea are all associated with amenorrhea and oligomenorrhea.

The regulation of menstrual cycles is extremely important and oral contraceptive pills are usually utilized to regulate cycles. The composition of the pills appears to be an important factor; it has been suggested that the use of the progestin-only contraceptive pills, as well as the depot medroxyprogesterone acetate may have deleterious effects on bone accretion. Therefore, special care may need to be taken when prescribing oral contraception for the regulation of menstrual cycles.

Hypogonadism

Hypoestrogenism in women and low testosterone levels in men are associated with low bone density. Men who receive treatments for conditions like prostate cancer with luteinizing hormone-releasing hormone (LHRH) agonist analogues are at increased risk for low bone density. The sex steroids are important in men, both during peak bone formation as well as for the maintenance of bone strength in adults.

Calcium and Vitamin D

Adequate calcium intake is essential during adolescence and has been shown to increase bone mineral density. It may be most beneficial to those adolescent girls who are greater than 2 years after menarche. Vitamin D deficiency has been correlated with low bone mineral density in adolescent girls, particularly in the lumbar spine.

In adults, adequate calcium and vitamin D intake remains a priority, with recommended minimum daily intakes of 1200 mg and 400 IU, respectively.

Elderly postmenopausal patients may benefit from higher doses of calcium and vitamin D. The use of calcium and vitamin D in the elderly can result in gains in bone mineral density in the spine and hip ranging from 1% to 3%.

Vitamin D is mainly produced in the skin with the activation of sunlight. It is photoconverted from 7-dehydrocholesterol in the skin to cholecalciferol (vitamin D3) by UV radiation from sunlight and in the diet is supplied as either vitamin D3 or from the plant sterol ergosterol as vitamin D2 (ergocalciferol). Vitamin D is hydroxylated at the 25 position in the liver and is then hydroxylated by the 1 α-hydroxylase enzyme in the kidney to the active metabolite 1,25 (OH) 2D.

Vitamin D is needed to maintain calcium homeostasis as it increases intestinal absorption of dietary calcium. With low dietary calcium intake, osteoblasts signal osteoclast precursors to mature and dissolve the calcium stored in bone. Vitamin D is metabolized in the liver and then the kidney under parathyroid hormone control to 1, 25-dihydroxyvitamin D. 1, 25-dihydroxyvitamin D receptors are present in many organs, including the intestine, bone, brain, heart, stomach, and pancreas.

In the elderly, the most common cause of increased bone resorption is calcium deficiency. Both calcium and vitamin D deficiency are very common in the elderly and can be attributed to poor diet, lack of sunlight, malabsorption syndromes, and various drugs that are degraded by the liver enzymes. Postmenopausal patients supplemented with calcium and vitamin D have shown preservation of bone mineral density and a reduction in osteoporotic fractures. Vitamin D deficiency appears to be widely underdiagnosed and undertreated. Nonambulatory elderly housebound adults are at particularly high risk of vitamin D deficiency. Exposure to sunlight can increase bone mineral density in elderly osteoporotic patients through elevation of 25-hydroxyvitamin D levels. Vitamin D is an essential vitamin that helps to regulate serum calcium. Vitamin D deficiency is associated with poorer function and increased hip fracture prevalence. Women with vitamin D deficiency can present with normal levels of calcium, increased serum PTH, and hypocalciuria. Vitamin D and calcium supplementation are associated with a decreased risk of hip fractures (< 25%) and are shown to be cost effective.

Calcium and vitamin D may be ingested in foods naturally containing these nutrients as well as with foods supplemented with the nutrients. Calcium occurs naturally in dairy products and broccoli. Foods fortified with calcium including orange juice and cereals can help to increase dietary intake of calcium. Vitamin D occurs naturally in foods such as salmon and mackerel and in fish oils including cod liver oil. Cereals, bread products, and milk fortified with vitamin D are good supplemental sources of vitamin D.

Exercise

Physical activity during childhood and adolescence, the peak bone forming years, is essential. Peak bone mass accretion during childhood and adolescence may be as important as bone loss, which occurs during adulthood. Weight-bearing exercise throughout the life cycle has been shown to be beneficial and appears to be especially important in adolescence. In combination with calcium supplementation, weight-bearing exercise has been shown to increase bone mineral density in adolescent women. High impact weight-bearing exercises may be particularly effective in premenarchal girls. In mature women, exercise will not increase bone mass but will improve the quality of bone and decrease fracture risk.

Weight bearing is essential, while lack of weight bearing has deleterious effects on bone mineral density. Prolonged immobilization, secondary to conditions such as spinal cord injury or coma, as well as prolonged space flight are known to have deleterious effects on bone density.

Accumulation of Peak Bone Mass

Peak bone mass is accrued during childhood and adolescence, with almost half of peak adult bone mass acquired during adolescence. Failure to achieve peak bone mass can contribute to osteopenia and osteoporosis. Numerous factors contribute to peak bone mass formation during this time period. These factors include gender, heredity, nutrition, exercise, and the presence of endocrinopathies. The role of nutrition, exercise, and presence of endocrinopathies is discussed elsewhere in this chapter.

Menopause

During the perimenopausal years, bone resorption is increased and bone loss accelerated. This is more marked in the trabecular than in cortical bone because of the trabecular bone's greater surface area. In estrogen deficient states, remodeling increases: more bone is remodeled on its endosteal surface and within these sites even more bone is lost as more bone is resorbed while less is replaced, accelerating architectural delay. The bone loss that occurs during menopause is associated with increased periosteal apposition, which partially preserves bone strength. Areas of the skeleton with primarily trabecular bone, such as the distal forearm and vertebrae, are particularly susceptible to fracture during this time.

Osteoporosis: Scope of Problem

Osteoporosis is the most common metabolic bone disease and affects 200 million worldwide and 25 million in the United States. It is a disease that is often underlooked and undertreated—likely in part because it is a clinically silent disease until it manifests in the form of fracture. Osteoporosis has significant physical, psychosocial, and financial consequences.

Osteoporosis Definition

Osteopenia and osteoporosis are determined on the basis of bone mineral density readings. Osteoporosis is a condition in which bone mineral density decreases and the fragility of bone leads to increased susceptibility to fracture. The World Health Organization has defined osteopenia as a T-score of –1 to –2.5 standard deviations below peak bone mass in controls and osteoporosis as a T-score of –2.5 standard deviations or greater below peak bone mass in controls.

Risk Factors for Osteoporosis

Low bone density represents the main risk factor for osteoporosis. Major primary risk factors include personal history of fracture as an adult, history of fragility fracture in a first degree relative, low body weight (less than 127 lbs), and current smoking. Additional risk factors include Caucasian race, advanced age, female sex, dementia, estrogen deficiency (early menopause, bilateral ovariectomy; prolonged premenopausal amenorrhea (> 1 year), low lifelong calcium intake, alcoholism, impaired eyesight despite correction, inadequate physical activity, and poor health/frailty. Numerous medical conditions and

medications are associated with low bone density. These conditions include hyperparathyroidism, hyperthyroidism, osteomalacia/rickets, malabsorption syndromes, inflammatory bowel disease, and multiple myeloma. Medications associated with increased risk include prolonged heparin use, anticonvulsants, cytotoxic drugs, and tamoxifen.

Bone Mineral Density Testing

Bone mineral density testing may be performed using dual energy x-ray absorptiometry (DEXA), quantitative CT, or other modalities, but DEXA is considered the gold standard. DEXA represents the areal bone density. Sites of measurement are the spine, the hip, and the wrists. Precision between tests approximates 2%. The National Osteoporosis Foundation recommends that bone mineral density should be measured in the following groups of patients:

1. All women 65 years and older regardless of risk factors.
2. All postmenopausal women under age 65 years with one or more risk factors for osteoporosis (other than being white, postmenopausal, and female).
3. Postmenopausal women who are considering therapy for osteoporosis, if bone mineral density testing would facilitate the decision.
4. Postmenopausal women who present with fractures (to confirm diagnosis and determine disease severity).

Medicare coverage for bone mineral density testing is as follows:

1. Estrogen deficient women at clinical risk for osteoporosis.
2. Individuals with vertebral abnormalities.
3. Individuals receiving, or planning to receive, long-term corticosteroid therapy.
4. Individuals with primary hyperparathyroidism.
5. Individuals being monitored to assess the response or efficacy of an approved osteoporosis drug therapy.

Fracture Determinants

Osteoporotic fractures typically occur in regions with large volumes of cancellous bone. The ability of a structure like cancellous bone to carry loads depends on several factors including bone quantity or tissue volume, architecture or tissue geometry, and material or tissue composition.

Falls

Falls or applied loads are implicated in the development of osteoporotic fractures, especially hip fractures. Falls are exceedingly common in community dwellers and in the nursing home setting. Hip fractures are most often associated with falls directly onto the hip. Determinants of fracture risk in the setting of falls include hard impact surfaces, quantity of soft tissue covering the hip region, and low bone density. Causes of falls are multifactorial and include medications, underlying medical conditions such as peripheral neuropathy, neuromuscular deficits including weakness, decreased visual acuity, cognitive impairment, and poor general physical health. Screening for falls risk should include neuromuscular examination, watching the patient ambulate and perform tandem gait and simple functional tests, including the get-up-and-go-test and 6-minute walk test. These simple tests may be performed in the physician's office or a physical therapy gym.

In 2003, the *Cochrane Review* assessed the effects of 62 trials involving 21,668 people using interventions designed to reduce falls risk in the elderly. The trials focused on falls and number of fallers. The *review* concluded that interventions likely to be beneficial in reducing falls included multidisciplinary, multifactorial, health and environmental risk factor screening; programs of muscle strengthening and balance retraining; home hazard assessments and modifications professionally prescribed for older people with a history of falling; withdrawal of psychotropic medication; cardiac pacing for fallers with cardioinhibitory carotid sinus hypersensitivity; and a 15-week Tai Chi group exercise intervention. The authors found that interventions of unknown effectiveness included nutritional supplementation, group-delievered interventions, vitamin D supplementation, pharmacological therapy, cognitive/behavioral interventions alone, amongst others. The authors concluded that there are interventions that are likely to reduce falls, but that further studies assessing prevention of injuries related to falls are needed.

DIFFERENTIAL DIAGNOSIS OF OSTEOPOROSIS

Secondary causes of osteoporosis should be considered in the differential diagnosis of osteoporosis and ruled out appropriately. In one review of 1,015 female patients, a secondary cause for osteoporosis was found in 8.6% of 384 osteoporotic patients. The most common secondary causes of osteoporosis included thyrotoxicosis and parathyroid adenoma. Additional conditions to be considered in the differential diagnosis of osteoporosis should include diseases of the bone marrow such as multiple myeloma, connective tissue diseases such as Ehlers-Danlos and osteogenesis imperfecta, other endocrinopathies such as type I diabetes mellitus, and Paget's disease. These conditions are outlined in the following sections.

Bone Marrow Diseases

Multiple Myeloma

Multiple myeloma is the most common primary neoplasm of the skeleton. In the United States, approximately 12,000 cases of multiple myeloma are diagnosed each year. Bone pain related to lytic lesions is the most common presentation of multiple myeloma. Additional presentations include systemic symptoms including weakness, infections, fever, or weight loss. Multiple myeloma should be ruled out with the use of serum and urine immunoelectrophoresis, serum and urine protein electrophoresis, complete metabolic panel, and complete blood count. In a review involving 1,027 patients diagnosed with multiple myeloma, anemia was present in 73% of patients, hypercalcemia in 13% of patients, and serum creatinine level of 2 mg/dL or more in 19%, β_2-microglobulin level was increased in 75%, serum protein electrophoresis revealed a localized band in 82% of patients, immunoelectrophoresis or immunofixation showed a monoclonal protein in 93%, and a monoclonal light chain was found in the urine in 78%.

Multiple myeloma may have two distinct presenting subtypes: presenting with bone lesions and a nodular growth pattern and the other presenting with anemia and infiltrative growth pattern.

Connective Tissue Disorders

Patients with connective tissue disorders including osteogenesis imperfecta, Ehlers-Danlos, and Marfan syndrome can present with low bone density. Patients with these disorders have clinical findings related to collagen defects. Patients with osteogenesis imperfecta can present with an array of physical findings including bone fragility, dentinogenesis, scoliosis, blue sclera, and hyperlaxity; Ehlers-Danlos patients have hypermobile joints and hyperelastic skin; and patients with Marfan syndrome have disorders of the musculoskeletal, cardiovascular, and ocular systems.

Endocrinopathies

Primary Hyperparathyroidism

Primary hyperparathyroidism occurs secondary to parathyroid gland adenoma in 85% of cases. Other causes include parathyroid gland hyperplasia or glandular adenocarcinoma. Primary hyperparathyroidism results in disturbances in serum calcium homeostasis, which are detected by the kidney. In response to primary hyperparathyroidism, the kidney increases tubular resorption of calcium, decreases resorption of phosphate and bicarbonate, and excretes excessive amounts of calcium in the urine.

Optimal localization imaging techniques include 99m Tc-sestamibi scintigraphy and ultrasonography. This combination helps to detect nodular goiter. In addition, a 24-hour urinary calcium excretion should be obtained in order to rule out familial hypocalciuric hypercalcemia.

Familial forms of hyperparathyroidism associated with MEN syndromes including MEN I and MEN II. MEN I is associated with hyperplasia of the parathyroid gland, with islet cell tumor and pituitary adenoma. MEN IIa is associated with medullary thyroid carcinoma with bilateral pheochromocytoma and hyperplasia of the parathyroid gland and MEN IIb has these findings with neurocutaneous manifestations without primary hyperparathyroidism.

In primary hyperparathyroidism serum levels of calcium are elevated and serum levels of phosphate are decreased. Patients present with weakness, urolithiasis, peptic ulcer disease, pancreatitis, and bone and joint pain and tenderness. In primary hyperparathyroidism, the excessive secretion of parathyroid hormone results in different effects in cortical and trabecular bone. In cortical bone, bone turnover increases, resulting in increased resorption at the endosteal envelope, increased cortical porosity, and thinned cortical bone. This condition is contrasted to cancellous bone, where there is reduced osteoclastic resorption and osteoblastic bone formation at individual bone multicellular units, resulting in diminished erosion depth, decreased bone formation, and decreased thickness of bone structural units.

Patients with mild primary hyperparathyroidism can be treated with bisphosphonates at doses similar to those administered in osteoporosis. In addition, surgical treatment has been very successful in situations where medical management is insufficient.

Secondary Hyperparathyroidism

Hypocalcemia stimulates parathyroid hormone secretion and chronic conditions stimulate parathyroid gland hyperplasia resulting from end-organ resistance to parathyroid hormone. This can be caused by several different mechanisms including intestinal causes, impaired PTH action, and loss of calcium from the extracellular compartment. It is most commonly caused by renal disease.

Intestinal causes of secondary hyperparathyroidism include impaired dietary calcium intake, impaired dietary calcium absorption, and vitamin D–deficient states. Impaired PTH action can result in renal failure, in impaired gut calcium absorption, impaired parathyroid calcium sensing, and in pseudohypoparathyroidism. Loss of calcium from the extracellular compartment can occur during bone growth, during recovery postlactation, in association with bisphosphonate treatment, during lactation, in cases of idiopathic hypercalciuria, in increased sodium excretion, with the use of loop diuretics, and in rhabdomyolysis and sepsis. Nutritional disorders, with resulting reduced calcium and vitamin D, can also cause secondary hyperparathyroidism.

Secondary hyperparathyroidism is commonly caused by chronic kidney disease which can lead to significant bone loss. It stems from disruptions in calcium, phosphorus, vitamin D, and parathyroid hormone metabolism. Early treatment for renal failure should include restricting dietary levels of protein and phosphorus as well as supplementation of calcium levels. In secondary hyperparathyroidism, bone is removed from a dwindling bone mass, with concurrent bone formation on the periosteal bone surface during aging that in part offsets bone loss and increases bone's cross sectional area.

Treatment of secondary hyperparathyroidism in end stage renal patients is critical. Important medications in these patients include noncalcemic vitamin D analogs including 22-oxacalcitriol (Maxacalcitriol), 19-nor-1a, 25(OH)2D2 (Paracalcitriol), and 1a (OH)2D2 (Doxercalciferol) and calcimimetic agents that bind parathyroid calcium sensing receptors and reduce PTH secretion.

Tertiary Hyperparathyroidism

Tertiary hyperparathyroidism that occurs in situations of long-standing secondary hyperparathyroidism is a condition in which the cause for secondary hyperparathyroidism has been corrected but the parathyroid glands function autonomously producing hormone despite a lack of calcium imbalance hormone synthesis.

Radiologic findings in hyperparathyroidism include demineralized and poorly defined bone and the presence of brown tumors. Rugger jersey spine describes ill-defined bands of increased bone density next to the vertebral endplates that can occur in any situation associated with hyperparathyroidism. A bone scan demonstrates generalized uptake in the skeleton with diminished soft-tissue activity, giving the "super scan" appearance. Uptake also may be increased in the long bones, periarticular regions, calvarium, mandible, a "tie" sternum, and "beading" of the costochondral junctions.

Diabetes Type I

Postteenage women with type I diabetes mellitus have lower bone mineral density than controls, and are at increased risk of osteoporosis. Diagnosis is made on the basis of elevated glucose levels.

Cushing's Syndrome

Cushing's syndrome, in which there is excessive endogenous glucocorticoid production, is associated with both osteopenia and osteoporosis. Diagnosis is made by measurement of urinary-free cortisol, with surgical treatment the preferred method of treatment. Iatrogenic Cushing's disease is common and occurs after treatment for asthma and polymyalgia rheumatica.

Hyperthyroidism

Thyroid hormone suppresses bone formation and patients with hyperthyroidism are noted to have low bone density. Thyroid hormone increases osteoclast activity to a greater extent than osteoblastic activity. Patients with thyrotoxicosis have increased fracture risk. Surface area of unmineralized matrices increase, with increased numbers of osteoclasts and resorption sites. Obese patients often use thyroid overdosage to control their weight.

Rickets and Osteomalacia

Vitamin D deficiency can result in rickets and osteomalacia in childhood and adulthood, respectively. Rickets is a disease in growing children or adolescents, and is characterized by failure or delayed mineralization of endochondral new bone at the growth plates. Osteomalacia is a failure of mineralization of newly formed osteoid at sites of bone turnover or periosteal or endosteal apposition in adults.

Cases of rickets and osteomalacia include lack of dietary absorption and diminished gut absorption of vitamin D or of calcium. This may be found in malabsorption syndromes such as Crohn's disease or small bowel resection and liver (biliary and hepatocellular) diseases that lead to problems with gut absorption of vitamin D and interference with 25-hydroxylation of vitamin D, respectively.

Rickets can be seen in patients with hereditary defects in vitamin D-signaling molecules, in disorders of phosphate metabolism, and in situations where there is extrarenal synthesis of 1,25-Hydroxyvitamin D such as in granulomatous disease. Renal diseases can interfere with 1-hydroxylation of 25-vitamin D. Renal tubular disorders (vitamin D–resistant rickets), such as x-linked hypophosphatemia and cystinosis, result in abnormally increased clearance of inorganic phosphorus (hypophosphatemia) with diminished ability to mineralize osteoid. Medications such as Dilantin and phenobarbital can interfere with vitamin D hydroxylation and function.

Clinical findings in patients with rickets and osteomalacia include painful limbs and muscle weakness, particularly in the elderly. Common laboratory abnormalities include low normal calcium, low phosphate, increased intact PTH, increased bone and total alkaline phosphatase, and low urinary calcium.

Irregular trabeculae may be visualized on radiologic imaging in both rickets and osteomalacia.

In rickets, there is undermineralization of osteoid at growth plates (metabolically active sites), particularly noted at sites of rapid bone growth such as proximal and distal femur, proximal tibia, proximal humerus, and distal radius. Therefore, findings include widened and irregularly shaped physeal lucencies, many times with flaring of metaphyses and rachitic rosary in ribs secondary to involvement at multiple costochondral junctions. Radiographic findings in osteomalacia include lucent, coarsened bones, due to a mixture of decreased bone density, and possibly radiographic density contributed by nonmineralized osteoid. Looser zones or pseudofracture, which are linear foci of undermineralized osteoid at sites of mechanical loading, are classically present, and often appear as linear lucencies perpendicularly oriented to the cortex of the bone with incomplete penetration of bony width, which usually occur along concave aspects of bone. These characteristics are commonly seen in the femoral neck, pubic rami, posterior part of ribs, and below the lesser femoral trochanter and less frequently in the lateral border of the scapulae, forearm, and wing of ilium. Bone scan can detect cortical infarctions, which are precursors to Looser's zones. Vertebral bodies can have a ground glass appearance.

Rickets and osteomalacia are both treated with high doses of vitamin D.

Paget's Disease of Bone

Paget's disease of bone is a progressive bone disease in which there is bone hypertrophy and disorganized bone remodeling. It is characterized by bone expansion, cortical bone thickening, and trabecular bone thickening. It is suspected that Paget's disease has an underlying viral cause. Osteoclasts and osteoclast precursors respond abnormally to 1,25 (OH)2 D3 and RANK ligand. Osteoclasts are activated with resultant osteolysis, followed by an osteoblastic response until a new equilibrium is established between bone production and bone lysis. Histologically, there is a mosaic-like appearance of osteoid secondary to rapid disordered bone resorption and production.

Clinical presentations of Paget's disease of the bone can include pain, osteoarthritis, deformities, unsteady gait, and hearing impairments. The three stages of Paget's disease include (1) lytic phase; (2) mixed lytic and blastic phase, which corresponds to onset of osteoblastic activation in response to osteoclastic bone resorption; and (3) sclerotic phase.

Laboratory values include normal serum phosphorus and calcium levels but elevated serum alkaline phosphatase, serum, and urine hydroxyproline. Radiographic imaging and bone scans are useful diagnostic imaging tools. Radiologic findings of Paget's disease include "osteoporosis circumscripta," which is acutely marginated bone demineralization during the lytic phase of disease in the skull, and the "blade of grass and flame-shaped margin," which describes acutely marginated demineralization of long bones. In addition, there are "picture frame vertebrae," which describes the mixed lytic and sclerotic phase in the spine, and "cotton wool" skull, which describes the mixed lytic and sclerotic phase in the skull.

Complications of Paget's disease include osteoarthritis, basilar skull invagination, insufficiency fractures, protrusio acetabuli, and proximal femoral varus deformity. Neurologic complications related to osseous expansion include sensorineural and conductional hearing loss and spinal stenosis. Osteosarcoma can rarely develop in these patients.

Treatment with bisphosphonates is the treatment of choice, and it addresses osteoclastic-mediated bone resorption. Calcitonin can also be used for treatment.

TREATMENT OF OSTEOPOROSIS

Medical

Calcium/Vitamin D

Patients with osteoporosis require between 1,200 and 1,500 mg of elemental calcium per day and between 400 and 800 IU of vitamin D per day. It is essential that calcium and vitamin D are taken together. Dairy products are a good source of calcium but most individuals require dietary supplementation with calcium carbonate or calcium citrate. Vitamin D is found in fish, such as salmon and mackerel; in fish liver oils, such as cod oil; and in fortified foods, such as orange juice and cereals.

Bisphosphonates

Bisphosphonates represent the most potent class of drug in the prevention and treatment of osteoporosis. This class of drugs are pyrophosphate analogs, which strongly bind to the hydroxyapatite of bone, inhibiting osteoclast activity. Alendronate (Fosamax) and risedronate (Actonel) are the two main oral bisphosphonates utilized for osteoporosis, with the intravenous bisphosphonates pamidronate (Aredia) and zolendronate (Zometa) used off label. Adverse effects for the oral bisphosphonates include gastrointestinal complications such as gastritis or esophagitis, abdominal pain, nausea, vomiting, diarrhea, and constipation, while adverse effects for the intravenous bisphosphonates include fevers and a flu-like syndrome. The administration of concurrent acetaminophen, antihistamine, and nonsteroidal anti-inflammatory medication helps to minimize these transient complications.

Alendronate has been proven to be effective in postmenopausal osteoporosis in increasing bone mineral density and decreasing the risk of fracture. A 5 mg daily dose of alendronate administered for 24 months, and then increased to 10 mg, results in fewer radiographic vertebral fractures in the treatment group versus placebo, with average increases in the lumbar spine BMD of about 5% after one year, and then 1.5% per year for the next 2 years. At the end of 3 years, BMD increases by about 6% in the femoral neck and about 7% in the trochanter.

Alendronate has demonstrated efficacy in men and individuals on steroids. A single weekly dose is as clinically effective as daily dosages. Alendronate decreases spinal and appendicular fractures by 50%.

Risedronate has also been shown to be effective in increasing BMD and in reducing fracture risk. Treatment with a 5 mg daily dose of risedronate reduces the risk of new vertebral fractures by 62% versus control and reduces new vertebral fractures by 90% versus control. A 5 mg oral daily dose of risedronate results in BMD increases after only 6 months of therapy, and at 24 months, lumbar spine BMD is increased from baseline by 4%, with increases of 1.3% and 2.7% seen in the femoral neck and femoral trochanter, respectively. A 35 mg once weekly dose of risedronate appears to be as effective as a 5 mg daily dose in reducing vertebral fracture risk. Like alendronate, risedronate also decreases hip fractures.

Parenteral pamidronate has also been used off label in the treatment of postmenopausal women with osteoporosis who are intolerant to oral bisphosphonates. It has been shown to be have comparable effects on bone mineral density when compared with alendronate. Fracture data are currently not available.

Parenteral zolendronate, also used off label, administered at intervals of one year, produced comparable effects on bone turnover and BMD to those seen with oral dosing with bisphosphonates. A randomized, double-blind, placebo-controlled trial documented bone mineral density increases in the treatment group that were 4.3 to 5.1% higher than those in the placebo group, with suppressed biochemical markers of bone formation.

Parathyroid Hormone

Parathyroid hormone is the anabolic agent approved for the treatment of osteoporosis. Approved by the U.S. Food and Drug Administration in November 2002, this subcutaneous daily medication has shown promising results in prospective studies.

The 20-mcg dose of 1-34 parathyroid hormone has been shown to both increase bone mineral density and decrease fracture risk, with fewer side effects than the 40-microgram dose. In a study involving 1,637 postmenopausal women with prior vertebral fractures, women who took a 20-mcg daily dose of 1-34 parathyroid hormone demonstrated a 0.35 relative risk of fracture compared to placebo and increases of 9% in the lumbar spine and 3% in the femoral neck.

The use of parathyroid hormone in the treatment logarithm of osteoporotic patients remains unclear. Clinical studies have suggested that the concomitant administration of parathyroid hormone with bisphosphonate medication may mitigate parathyroid hormone's effects. In a study involving 83 men with low bone density randomized to received alendronate, parathyroid hormone, or both, bone density in the lumbar spine and femoral neck increased significantly than in the other groups ($p < 0.001$). The combination therapy group had increased bone density in the lumbar spine and femoral neck compared to those in the alendronate group. Another study involving 238 postmenopausal women using 100 mg of daily parathyroid hormone (1-84), alendronate or both showed that the volumetric density of the trabecular bone at the spine in the parathyroid hormone group increased about twice that in either of the other groups after 12 months.

Calcitonin

Nasal calcitonin (Miacalcin) is helpful in the management of bony pain secondary to fracture and also works to increase bone mineral density and decrease fracture risk. Typically, analgesia for bone pain is achieved as early as the first to second week of use. The mechanism of activity is not well understood, though the endogenous opiate system may play a role in mediating the analgesic effects. A 5-year, double-blind, randomized, placebo-controlled study in 1,255 women with established osteoporosis demonstrated that the 200 IU dose reduces the risk of new vertebral factures by 33% compared to placebo, with gains of 1 to 1.5% in the lumbar spine bone mineral density in patients receiving 100, 200, and 400 IU of calcitonin daily. It has no protective action regarding hip fractures.

Estrogen/Selective Estrogen Receptor Modulators

Estrogen used for the alleviation of symptoms following menopause may increase bone density and decreases fractures by 35%, but is not used as a primary agent in the treatment of osteoporosis due to its many potential complications. Estrogen has been associated with increased incidence of coronary heart disease events, strokes, pulmonary embolisms, and invasive breast cancers in patients receiving conjugated equine estrogens plus progestin. Therefore, it has been concluded that the overall health risks from estrogen exceeds the benefits from use.

Selective estrogen receptor modulators such as raloxifene may increase bone mineral but are not considered primary agents in the treatment of osteoporosis. They decrease spine fracture by 35 to 40% but have no effect on hip fractures. Furthermore, they have been associated with venous thromboembolism and hot flashes.

Nonmedical Management of Osteoporosis

The nonmedical treatment of osteoporosis represents an extremely important, though often overlooked, facet of the appropriate management of osteoporotic individuals. Treatments, including physical therapy, the use of orthoses such as the posture training support and hip protectors, and the minimally invasive spine procedures vertebroplasty and kyphoplasty, are exceedingly important players in a comprehensive multidisciplinary management approach to osteoporosis.

Physical therapy and exercise programs should be specifically geared toward the patient with osteoporosis. Balance exercises and strengthening exercises of the bilateral lower extremities and weight-bearing exercises may help to decrease fall risks. In particular, Tai Chi has been shown to reduce falls risk almost by 50%. Back extensor strengthening exercises can decrease thoracic kyphosis and possibly prevent vertebral compression fractures. In addition, aerobics and weight-bearing and resistance exercises can increase bone mineral density in the spine, and walking can result in increased bone mineral density in the hip.

Hip protectors are orthoses comprised of padding placed in undergarments worn over the greater trochanter to help absorb impact on fall. They have been documented to significantly decrease hip fracture risk in elderly institutionalized patients. Poor patient compliance remains the main obstacle to their use. The posture training support, CASH (cruciform anterior spinal hyperextension) brace, and the Jewett brace can all be used in individuals with symptomatic vertebral compression fractures to minimize thoracolumbar flexion. The posture training support may minimize the symptoms accompanying painful vertebral compression fractures.

Vertebroplasty and kyphoplasty are two minimally invasive spine procedures utilized in the management of painful vertebral compression fractures that have demonstrated excellent results in alleviation of pain. Both procedures involve placement of polymethylmethacrylate into a symptomatic fractured vertebral body. Kyphoplasty provides excellent reduction of fracture, restoring vertebral body height and restoring function.

CONCLUSIONS

Bone is a dynamic organ that has many functions. Many factors, including nutritional status, hormonal status, calcium and vitamin D, and regular weight-bearing exercise, play a role in bone development.

Osteoporosis is a condition with decreased bone mineral density and resulting increased fragility. It is the most common metabolic bone disease but is often underdiagnosed and undertreated. Osteoporosis can be treated with medical management as well as a comprehensive multidisciplinary approach.

The differential diagnosis for osteoporosis includes other metabolic bone diseases, including hyperparathyroidism, rickets/osteomalacia, and Paget's disease, among others. These conditions should be ruled out appropriately.

Annotated Bibliography

Bone Growth/Development

Grados F, Brazier M, Kamel S et al. Effects on bone mineral density of calcium and vitamin D supplementation in elderly women with vitamin D deficiency. Joint Bone Spine 2003;70(3):203–208.
In this placebo-controlled, double-blind randomized study, elderly vitamin D–deficient women (defined as serum 25(OH)D ≤12ng/ml) in the study group were given calcium carbonate and vitamin D. Compared to controls, women in the study group had significantly improved bone mineral density in the lumbar spine, femur, trochanter, and whole body after 1 year.

Calcium supplementation on bone loss in postmenopausal women. Cochrane Database Syst Rev 2003;4:CD004526.
This review of 15 trials involving 1,806 participants found efficacy for calcium after 2 or more years of treatment on bone mineral density. Percentage increases range from 1.6% in the hip to 2.05% for the total body. Relative risk for fracture was 0.79 and 0.86 for the vertebrae and nonvertebral fractures, respectively.

Isaia G, Giorgino R, Rini GB et al. Prevalence of hypovitaminosis D in elderly women in Italy: clinical consequences and risk factors. Osteoporos Int 2003;14(7):577–582.
This multicenter study involving 700 elderly Italian women identified vitamin D deficiency in 76% of women, with severe vitamin D deficiency in 27% of women. Hypovitaminosis D was associated with diminished ability to perform activities of daily living and higher hip fracture prevalence.

Heinonen A, Sievanen H, Kannus P et al. High-impact exercise and bones of growing girls: a 9-month controlled trial. Osteoporos Int 2000;11(12):1010–1017.
This study involving 64 pre- and postmenarchal girls participating in a supervised 9-month step aerobic program found that more

significant gains in bone mineral acquisition could be achieved before menarche than following menarche.

Feskanich D, Willett W, Colditz G. Walking and leisure-time activity and risk of hip fracture in postmenopausal women. JAMA 2002;288(18):2300–2306.
This study involving 61,200 postmenopausal nurses found that moderate levels of exercise, such as walking, are correlated with lower risks of hip fracture. For each increase of 3 metabolic equivalent hours per week of activity, risk of hip fracture was lowered by 6%.

Seeman E. Invited review: pathogenesis of osteoporosis. J Appl Physiol 2003; 95(5):2142–2151.
This is a good review of the abnormal bone modeling and remodeling that takes place in osteoporosis.

Osteoporosis

Osteoporosis prevention, diagnosis, and therapy. NIH Consensus Statement 2000;17(1):1–45.
Summarizes the conclusions and recommendations of the NIH Consensus Development Conference on Osteoporosis Prevention, Diagnosis, and Therapy.

van der Meulen MC, Jepsen KJ, Mikic B. Understanding bone strength: size isn't everything. Bone 2001;29(2):101–104.
This is an excellent overview of the determinants of bone strength.

Greenspan SL, Myers ER, Kiel DP et al. Fall direction, bone mineral density, and function: risk factors for hip fracture in frail nursing home elderly. Am J Med 1998;104(6):539–545.
In this prospective, case-controlled study, a fall to the side, low hip bone density, and impairment in mobility were all identified as independent risk factors for hip fracture in frail, elderly nursing home fallers.

Tinetti ME. Clinical practice. Preventing falls in elderly persons. N Engl J Med 2003; 348(1):42–49.
This is a good review of fall management in the elderly, particularly useful for primary care physicians and other physicians caring for the elderly.

Gillespie L, Gillespie W, Robertson M et al. Interventions for preventing falls in elderly people. Cochrane Database Syst Rev 2003; 4:CD000340.
This is a comprehensive meta-analysis of the various interventions for preventing falls. This review included 62 trials with 21,668 participants. Effective measures include multidisciplinary health and environment risk factor screening and intervention programs, muscle strengthening and muscle retraining programs, home hazard assessment and modification, withdrawal of psychotropic medication, cardiac pacing, and Tai Chi.

Differential Diagnosis of Osteoporosis

Marx SJ. Hyperparathyroid and hypoparathyroid disorders. N Engl J Med 2000; 343(25):1863–1875.
This is a good review of hyperparathyroidism.

Treatment of Osteoporosis

Lin JT, Lane JM. Bisphosphonates. J Am Acad Orthop Surg 2003; 11(1):1–4.
This is a review of the current knowledge of the oral and intravenous bisphosphonate medications in various metabolic bone disorders relevant to orthopedists.

Black DM, Cummings SR, Karpf DB et al. Randomised trial of effect of alendronate on risk of fracture in women with existing vertebral fractures. Fracture Intervention Trial Research Group. Lancet 1996; 348(9041):1535–1541.
This study involved 2,027 women in the Fracture Intervention Trial, whose goal was to assess the effect of alendronate on the risk for morphometric and clinically evident fractures in postmenopausal women with low bone mass. The study concluded that women who received alendronate for 36 months had reduced frequency of morphometric and clinically apparent vertebral fracture compared to controls.

Gonnelli S, Cepollaro C, Montagnani A et al. Alendronate treatment in men with primary osteoporosis: a three-year longitudinal study. Calcif Tissue Int 2003; 73(2):133–139.
In this study involving 77 osteoporotic men, subjects who received alendronate plus calcium compared to calcium alone demonstrated significant improvements in bone mineral density.

Luckey MM, Gilchrist N, Bone HG et al. Therapeutic equivalence of alendronate 35 milligrams once weekly and 5 milligrams daily in the prevention of postmenopausal osteoporosis. Obstet Gynecol 2003;101(4):711–721.
This 1-year, double-blind study of postmenopausal women found that alendronate 35 mg weekly is therapeutically equivalent to alendronate 5 mg daily. Weekly alendronate is associated with greater dosing convenience and good tolerability.

Watts NB, Josse RG, Hamdy RC et al. Risedronate prevents new vertebral fractures in postmenopausal women at high risk. J Clin Endocrinol Metab 2003;88(2):542–549.
This study combined data form two randomized, double-blind studies and found that significant fracture risk is noted 1 year after treatment. There was a risk reduction of new vertebral fractures by 62% and reduction of multiple new vertebral fractures by 90%, compared to controls.

Fogelman I, Ribot C, Smith R et al. Risedronate reverses bone loss in postmenopausal women with low bone mass: results from a multinational, double-blind, placebo-controlled trial. BMD-MN Study Group. J Clin Endocrinol Metab 2000; 85(5):1895–1900.
This study found that postmenopausal women with low bone mass who received risedronate 5 mg daily demonstrated increases in bone mineral density as early as 6 months following treatment and had upper gastrointestinal adverse events that were similar to placebo.

Watts NB, Lindsay R, Li Z et al. Use of matched historical controls to evaluate the anti-fracture efficacy of once-a-week risedronate. Osteoporos Int 2003; 14(5):437–441.
Using matched historical control data from previous placebo-controlled trials, the authors found that risedronate 35 mg weekly appears to have similar efficacy to risedronate 5 mg daily in reducing the risk of new vertebral fractures in the first year of treatment.

Heijckmann AC, Juttmann JR, Wolffenbuttel BH. Intravenous pamidronate compared with oral alendronate for the treatment of postmenopausal osteoporosis. Neth J Med 2002; 60(8).315–319.
This retrospective study compared the efficacy of intravenously administered pamidronate with oral alendronate and found that monthly intravenous pamidronate is at least as good as oral alendronate in improving bone mineral density in women with postmenopausal osteoporosis.

Reid IR, Brown JP, Burckhardt P et al. Intravenous zoledronic acid in postmenopausal women with low bone mineral density. N Engl J Med 2002;346(9):653–661.
In this 1-year, randomized, double-blind, placebo-controlled trial, the authors found that intravenous zoledronic acid in postmenopausal women resulted in increased bone mineral density and suppressed biochemical markers of bone resorption as great as those achieved with oral daily dosing with bisphoshponates.

Neer RM, Arnaud CD, Zanchetta JR et al. Effect of parathyroid hormone (1-34) on fractures and bone mineral density in postmenopausal women with osteoporosis. N Engl J Med 2001;344(19):1434–1441.
This important randomized trial involving 1,637 postmenopausal women found that daily injections of parathyroid hormone in postmenopausal women with prior vertebral fractures resulted in decreased risk of vertebral and nonvertebral fractures and increased vertebral, femoral, and total-body bone mineral density.

Black DM, Greenspan SL, Ensrud KE et al. The effects of parathyroid hormone and alendronate alone or in combination in postmenopausal osteoporosis. N Engl J Med 2003; 349(13): 1207–1215.
This randomized, double-blind trial compared the effects of parathyroid hormone and alendronate alone or in combination and found that there was no evidence of synergistic effects of parathyroid hormone and alendronate. Instead, there was the suggestion that concurrent use of alendronate may reduce the anabolic effects of parathyroid hormone.

Finkelstein JS, Hayes A, Hunzelman JL. The effects of parathyroid hormone, alendronate, or both in men with osteoporosis. N Engl J Med 2003;349(13):1216–1226.
This randomized trial involved 83 men with low bone density and compared the effects of parathyroid hormone, alendronate, or both. The authors found that bone mineral density increased more in the lumbar spine and femoral neck than in the alendronate group, and bone mineral density increased more in the lumbar spine in the combination therapy group than in the alendronate group. The authors concluded that alendronate appears to limit the effects of parathyroid hormone on bone mineral density in the lumbar spine and femoral neck in men.

Chesnut CH III, Silverman S, Andriano K et al. A randomized trial of nasal spray salmon calcitonin in postmenopausal women with established osteoporosis: the prevent recurrence of osteoporotic fractures study. PROOF Study Group. Am J Med 2000;109(4):267–276.
This 5-year, randomized, double-blind, placebo-controlled trial involving 1,255 postmenopausal osteoporotic women found that salmon calcitonin nasal spray resulted in significant risk reductions of new vertebral fractures.

Rossouw JE, Anderson GL, Prentice RL et al. Risks and benefits of estrogen plus progestin in healthy postmenopausal women: principal results From the Women's Health Initiative randomized controlled trial. JAMA 2002;288(3):321–333.
This well-known trial reported the results of the risks and benefits of estrogen plus progestin in 16,608 healthy postmenopausal women after a mean of 5.2 years and determined that the overall health risks exceeded benefits. Risks included increased coronary heart disease, stroke, pulmonary embolus, and breast cancer.

Lin JT, Lane JM. Nonmedical management of osteoporosis. Curr Opin Rheumatol 2002;14(4):441–446.
This is a review of the nonmedical management of osteoporosis, including strengthening and weight-bearing exercise, Tai Chi, bracing, and hip protectors.

Wolf SL, Barnhart HX, Kutner NG et al. Reducing frailty and falls in older persons: an investigation of Tai Chi and computerized balance training. Atlanta FICSIT Group. Frailty and injuries: cooperative studies of intervention techniques. J Am Geriatr Soc 1996;44(5):489–497.
This prospective, randomized, controlled clinical trial involving 200 elderly participants with an intervention length of 15 weeks, found that Tai Chi can reduce the risk of multiple falls by 47.5%.

Bonaiuti D, Shea B, Iovine R et al. Exercise for preventing and treating osteoporosis in postmenopausal women. Cochrane Database Syst Rev 2002;(2):CD000333.
This meta-analysis included 18 randomized, controlled trials involving exercise for preventing and treating osteoporosis in elderly women and found that aerobic, weight-bearing, and resistance exercises all had positive effects on bone mineral density of the spine. However, the authors criticized the studies for having low quality reporting of the trials.

Parker MJ, Gillespie LD, Gillespie WJ. Hip protectors for preventing hip fractures in the elderly. Cochrane Database Syst Rev 2004;(3):CD001255.
This meta-analysis included 13 randomized trials involving the use of hip protectors for preventing hip fractures in the elderly. Data from the cluster randomized studies suggests that hip protectors reduce the incidence of hip fractures in patients with high risk of hip fractures living in institutionalized settings.

Deramond H, Mathis JM. Vertebroplasty in osteoporosis. Semin Musculoskelet Radiol 2002;6(3):263–268.
This is a good review of the use of vertebroplasty in osteoporotic patients.

Ledlie JT, Renfro M. Balloon kyphoplasty: one-year outcomes in vertebral body height restoration, chronic pain, and activity levels. J Neurosurg Spine 2003;98(1 Suppl):36–42.
This retrospective chart review followed the authors' first 96 patients with 133 fractures and reported that kyphoplasty increased vertebral body height, decreased back pain, and restored function.

8

Kenneth Noonan

Neuromuscular Diseases

T his chapter will cover the diagnosis and management of the most common neuromuscular disorders. These disorders present some of the most challenging problems in orthopaedics.

ORTHOPAEDIC MANIFESTATIONS OF CEREBRAL PALSY

Although the brain injury that results in the clinical picture of cerebral palsy (CP) is static, the orthopaedic manifestations are often evolving, due to the effects of abnormal muscle tone and movement disorders over the individual's lifetime. For instance, one of the first features of CP may be delay in the normal motor milestones of development. For example, some eventually spastic patients may first present with hypotonia and be considered a "floppy baby." Later the child will demonstrate retardation in normal motor development. In general, most children are able to sit independently by 6 months and the normal range of walking onset is from 9 to 18 months. Patients with CP will have delay in these milestones that is concordant to their level of brain injury. Hemiplegic patients may walk in the upper range of normal gait onset or have delays of several months. Diplegic patients may not walk until 2 to 3 years of age; severely involved diplegic patients or quadriplegic patients may never walk. Understandably, families are focused on the potential for ambulation for their children. Bleck has described a rating system based on retention of certain neonatal reflexes beyond one year of age; this system can be used to predict eventual walking. One point is given for the presence of asymmetric tonic neck reflex, neck-righting reflex, Moro reflex, an absent parachute reaction, an absent foot-placement reaction, and extensor thrust. If more than two are present the prognosis for ambulation is poor. In general, if a child is unable to sit unsupported by 4 years of age, the potential of independent ambulation is low.

Abnormal muscle forces and control may result in altered function and development of every aspect of the musculoskeletal system. In general, the more severe fixed skeletal deformities result in those individuals with spasticity. A child with significant components of movement disorders such as athetosis tends to not develop fixed contractures. These children will move their extremities about and tend to provide excellent range of motion therapy on their own. Results of orthopaedic treatment are less predictable in patients with movement disorders then in those with pure spasticity. The bulk of treatment options, which we will discuss, are directed toward those patients with spasticity as a major feature of their CP.

Musculoskeletal interventions for patients with CP are individualized for each patient and may consist of a variety of different modalities. Rehabilitative methods include physical and occupational therapy, casting or orthotic use, seating programs, and medical management to reduce spasticity (oral baclofen or valium) or injection of phenol around the motor nerves or botulinum A toxin injection. The later modality has revolutionized the care of spasticity in younger patients with cerebral palsy. Botulinum A toxin is a potent neurotoxin produced by clostridium botulinum that induces a prolonged, but reversible, paralysis of skeletal muscle. The toxin diffuses locally and prevents the release of acetylcholine at the neuromuscular junction. The effects on the neuromuscular junction are not permanent, but rather reversible, further suggesting the possibility for botulinum A toxin as a temporary agent. The effect of the toxin is related to the dose, the concentration of the dose injected, and the location within the muscles. With time, the temporary

blockade is reversed with new sprouting of nerve fibers, which then tend to retract once the original toxin effect at the neuromuscular blockade is reversed. In general, botulinum A toxin lasts for 3 to 4 months with better results seen in younger patients and patients with initial treatment. Efficacy tends to wane with repeated doses and increased age of the patients. Although commonly used to combat dynamic contractures (spasticity) in an attempt to avoid the morbidity from surgical release of muscle contractures, some clinicians have attempted to expand the indications of botulinum A toxin to individuals with muscle contractures. Unfortunately it is unknown whether the combination of chemical muscle relaxation (botulinum A toxin) and progressive stretch (serial casting) will actually make muscles longer.

Neurosurgical methods of spasticity control include selective dorsal root rhizotomy (SDR) and intrathecal baclofen (ITB) pump placement. Selective dorsal root rhizotomy (SDR) is useful in the 4- to 5-year-old diplegic patients with pure spasticity and no fixed joint contractures who are ambulatory. These children are usually a result of premature delivery and with a higher association of low birth weights. The indications for SDR have regional differences; some centers have broad experience while others tend to utilize orthopaedic surgery as the primary method to improve function. The primary benefit of SDR is to reduce spasticity and improve the quality and smoothness of gait. This translates into more efficient gait with less oxygen need. These individuals may still require orthopaedic surgery for bony abnormalities or residual contractures. Patients who undergo SDR should be admitted for intensive therapy for approximately one month. Potential complications include development of spinal deformity in 5 to 10% of patients, of which, very few require eventual spinal stabilization. Surgical treatment of muscle contractures or residual bony malalignment should be delayed for a year after SDR.

Intrathecal baclofen pump placement can also be used in patients with spasticity and may be more effective in patients who have movement disorders as a component of their involvement. Use of intrathecal baclofen was first described in 1984 and was shown to reduce spasticity in selected patients with spinal cord injury and multiple sclerosis. Long-term ITB was introduced several years later and is considered safe and effective in reducing spasticity in patients with CP. The advantages of ITB pump placement are its relative reversibility (it can be removed) and the ability to increase or decrease the effect of baclofen. The disadvantages include risks of infection, trunk weakness, spinal deformity, and the need to refill the pumps with baclofen. Although designed to reduce lower extremity spasticity, both SDR and ITB pump placement may concurrently decrease some upper extremity spasticity.

Orthopaedic treatment is tailored to the individual and his or her potential for ambulation, sitting, or other activities of daily living. For instance, a child who is severely involved usually has diminished function and the orthopaedist may contribute care that is designed to balance sitting and to prevent contractures that preclude comfortable sitting. Conversely, a mild hemiplegic patient may benefit from sophisticated tendon transfers, which may essentially normalize hand and foot function. In general, more severely involved patients will present with abnormalities of the entire skeletal system while more minimally involved individuals have fewer problems with the spine and hips and present with problems more distal in the extremities.

Spine Deformities

Spinal deformity is usually restricted to the most severely involved patients with cerebral palsy. In a recent survey, we documented an 87% incidence of scoliosis in 77 severely involved adult patients with CP. The incidence in hemiplegic patients is much less and approaches that seen in adolescent idiopathic scoliosis. Spinal deformity may also develop as a sequelae of ITB pump placement or SDR (Figure 8-1). The most common spinal deformity is thoracolumbar scoliosis with attendant pelvic obliquity. In the sagittal plane, these patients may also have fairly significant lordosis, which is due to concurrent hip flexion contractures and spasticity of the paraspinous muscles. The deformity differs from curves encountered in patients with idiopathic scoliosis. Cerebral palsy curves tend to be long C-shaped curves without compensatory curves. As such, patients tend have unbalanced sitting posture.

Treatment for scoliosis is individualized to the patient and his or her level of function. In general, sitting programs, bolsters, and orthoses have a minimal to no effect in slowing the evolution or eventual progression of scoliosis. They may have a role in preventing rapid progression and allow one to delay surgical treatment in immature patients. The decision to perform surgery is often difficult and

two important indications: (1) severe curves greater than 50° and sitting imbalance that may reduce sitting endurance and increase pain, and (2) the patient should be of sufficient health and function in order to gain maximal improvement. Surgery is recommended for those individuals with head control and some cognitive abilities such as caregiver or environmental recognition. Surgical treatment may not be needed in patients who are cognitively devastated and is contraindicated in patients with severe hip extension contractures. Such patients will not benefit from improved axial alignment as the hips preclude sitting balance.

The decision to perform such an invasive surgery is complex and involves a great deal of time discussing the benefits versus the risks of surgery. Families should be given the opportunity to decide if the risks outweigh the benefits, and each decision is individualized. In general, the main benefits are to prevent curve progression and to improve sitting balance. It could be argued that the latter doesn't directly improve the quality of life of severely involved patients. On the other hand, patients with severe scoliosis and sitting imbalance are often difficult to care for. If spine surgery improves the ability of these patients to sit, it is less likely that they will be bed bound as they age.

In general, fusion to the pelvis is performed to reduce pelvic obliquity. Rarely one will encounter less involved ambulatory patients with curves similar to those seen in idiopathic scoliosis; in these patients surgical stabilization that corrects the curve without necessary stabilization to the pelvis is recommended. Fixation is performed with rods, sublaminar wires, and judicious use of pedicle screws and hook fixation. Pelvic fixation may be performed with Galveston fixation or iliac and sacral screws. Many have found good results with the unit rod construct. Anterior release and interbody fusion is indicated in patients with severe curves that do not reduce on unbending or traction films (> 45°) or if pelvic obliquity is greater than 15° on preoperative traction films (Figure 8-2). In younger patients, anterior fusion may be indicated to prevent crankshaft phenomenon due to anterior growth. Others have demonstrated that posterior segmental fixation and fusion may prevent clinically significant spinal deformity as a result of continued anterior growth. Anterior release and interbody fusion is usually performed on the same day that the posterior surgery is performed. Spinal cord monitoring with somatosensory evoked potentials is utilized in nonambulatory patients with voluntary bowel and

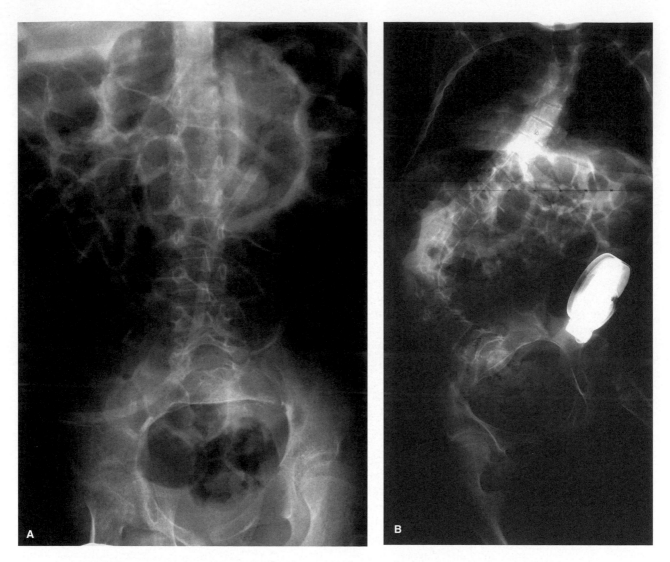

FIGURE 8-1. (A) AP radiograph of a 15-year-old male with severe spastic quadriplegia. Prior to placement of baclofen pump demonstrating a left thoracic curve with a Cobb angle of 10°. **(B)** AP radiograph 17 months after baclofen pump placement demonstrating a left thoracic curve with a Cobb angle of 76°.

bladder function. However, it is not used in severely involved nonambulatory individuals with no motor control, as the signals are often difficult to evaluate in those severely affected individuals. Practically speaking, improved spinal alignment is more beneficial even if the severely affected individual without any voluntary muscle control suffers some neural compromise.

The list of potential morbidities and complications from spinal surgery is long and includes risk of infection, blood loss and need for transfusion, and anesthetic complications such as aspiration

pneumonia. The complication rates, and especially rates of infection, seem to be higher in patients who are more severely involved and with poor nutritional status. Careful nutritional assessment is needed to optimize the nutritional status prior to surgery. Some patients begin central venous nutrition in the immediate postoperative period. Often these patients are chronically malnourished, and it is difficult to get adequate caloric and protein intake following large surgeries. Dying within 1 year of surgery may result from complications from surgery at a rate of about 1 to 3%; this is certainly more

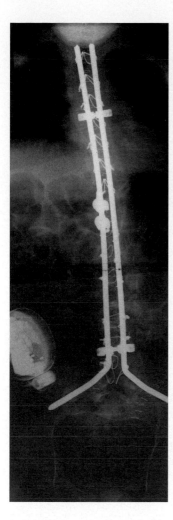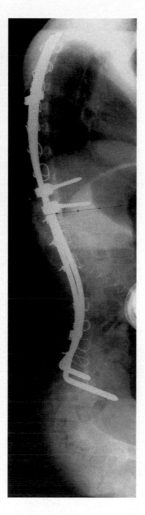

FIGURE 8-2. AP and lateral radiograph after anterior release and posterior instrumentation and fusion.

common in the more involved patients with CP spinal deformity. Other complications include pressure sores from new pelvic position and superior mesenteric artery syndrome. The later is a result of significant surgical correction and poor nutrition. These patients will present with vomiting, obstruction, and potentially fatal electrolyte abnormalities with prolonged vomiting. Treatment of obstruction is with hyperalimentation via a feeding tube placed past the obstruction.

Postsurgical pain control in patients with CP is among the most challenging to control. These patients will development muscle spasms in the lengthened tendons that result in increased pain in cut muscles leading to more spasm and pain. The use of epidural catheter placement and infusion with local anesthetics, narcotics or clonidine produces good results. Supplemental intravenous narcotics and benzodiazapenes are helpful to keep these patients comfortable in the challenging postoperative period.

Hip Dysplasia

Patients with CP are born with normally located hips; yet a broad spectrum of hip abnormalities may develop as a result of abnormal muscle forces. These abnormalities may range from hip contractures to hip dislocation. The development of hip deformity in spastic patients is thought to be secondary to asymmetric muscle forces produced across the hip by the hip adductors, iliopsoas, and hamstrings. Persistent femoral anteversion, coxa valga, acetabular dysplasia and pelvic obliquity often result from retained neonatal reflexes and abnormal muscle forces and have also been implicated in the evolution of hip subluxation. The increased muscle forces lead to hip migration in a posterior and superior direction. Hip migration leads to femoral head deformity and acetabular dysplasia. One percent of patients may have dislocation in an anterior direction as a result of overactive hip extensors (gluteus maximus and hamstring muscles) and hip abductors. It may be hard to recognize anterior instability on standard radiographs but is better documented on CT studies (Figure 8-3).

Hip subluxation and dislocation in individuals with CP may result in a serious problem for affected patients. The incidence of hip subluxation or dislocation in these patients varies from 2.6 to 75% seen in more severely involved patients with spastic quadriplegic patients. Uncorrected hip subluxation or dislocation may lead to later problems with pain, perineal care, and sitting balance. Patients with anterior dislocation may be more likely to have pain than posterior dislocations. Studies estimate the rates of eventual pain as a result of hip dislocation to be from 0 to 50%. In a recently completed study of severely involved adults with CP, 15% of hips were dislocated and radiographic arthritis was detected in 23% of hips.

Wide ranges of hip abnormalities are seen in children with CP and include contractures that hinder activities of daily living, acetabular or femoral dysplasia, and hip subluxation and hip dislocation with or without adaptive or degenerative changes in the pelvis and femur. As a result, surgical procedures are recommended in children with progressive hip displacement in an attempt to prevent progression and to treat the present state of dysplasia and possible hip dislocation. Surgery can be classified as *reconstruction* procedures where the hip is stabilized or reduced with a combination of soft tissue releases, femoral or pelvic osteotomy. *Salvage* procedures are used in patients

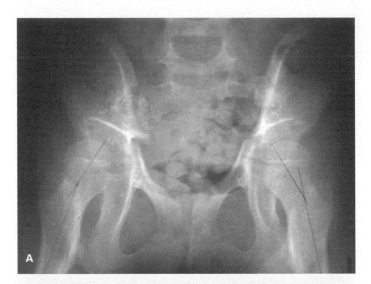

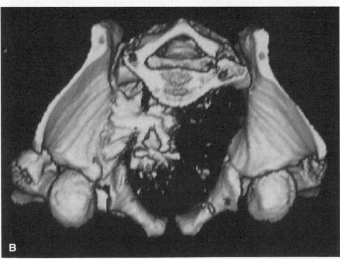

FIGURE 8-3. (A) AP radiograph of a 9-year-old girl with cerebral palsy. Radiograph demonstrates capacious acetabulum with deficient anterior coverage. **(B)** CT scan confirms anterior displacement of both femoral heads.

with long-standing and painful dislocation with or without arthrosis.

Reconstructive treatment for subluxation or dislocation in hips of CP patients varies depending on the degree of subluxation, patient age, range of motion, and presence of pain or arthrosis. Soft tissue releases such as adductor release or transfer, psoas release, and abductor advancement have been variably recommended for hips considered likely to progress to subluxation or dislocation. Adductor release is performed through a transverse groin incision; the adductor longus is sectioned at its origin once the gracilis has been identified. Lengthening of the gracilis follows and portions of the brevis may also be released in order to obtain 45 to 50° of hip abduction. If a hip flexion contracture greater then 20° exists, the iliopsoas muscle insertion may also be released off of the lesser trochanter through the interval of the pectineus and the adductor brevis. In ambulatory patients it's better to lengthen the psoas tendon more proximally. "Over the brim" isolated psoas lengthening provides better hip flexion power (retained iliacus function) as opposed to direct removal off of the lesser trochanter (loss of both psoas and iliacus). Finally, it's important to remember that the medial hamstrings are often hip adductors and may need to be concurrently lengthened. Following soft tissue releases use nighttime bracing for up to a year. Patients should be followed for several years as the contractures may recur and progressive hip subluxation may become evident.

Unfortunately, once a hip begins to subluxate, the success of stabilization with only soft tissue procedures rapidly decreases. The decision to perform femoral and acetabular procedures is dependent on the amount of femoral head coverage and age. Complete hip dislocation at any age will require bony surgery for stabilization. Stabilization of the hip is obtained via femoral osteotomy, acetabular osteotomy, or augmentation, or a combination of these procedures may be recommended. Femoral osteotomy is recommended for older patients (< 6 years of age) with greater than 50% uncovering of the femoral head. Concurrent pelvic osteotomy is recommened in older patients with greater than 50% uncovering. The goals of femoral osteotomy are to reduce the neck shaft angle by placing the head in varus, shortening of the femur and with external rotation of the distal shaft. The neck shaft angle is reoriented 95 to 105° in nonambulatory patients and 110 to 115° in ambulatory patients. A great deal of soft tissue and muscle tension can be obtained by removing a 2-cm wedge of bone. This may obviate the need for hamstring release. Derotation of the femur and reducing the persistent femoral anteversion may be of some benefit in patients with significant femoral internal torsion. In patients with asymmetric hip subluxation, one may perform bilateral femoral osteotomy, to reduce the displaced hip and shorten and equalize the less-dysplastic side. It may be wise to perform bilateral soft tissue releases if contractures occur in the contralateral hip. Contralateral hip subluxation can occur if one fails to recognize abnormal tone in the contralateral hip. A windswept hip appearance can occur by releasing muscles only in the more severed hip.

Pelvic osteotomies are performed in order to improve the coverage of the femoral head by correcting the dysplasia mentioned above. These patients tend to have capacious acetabuli with focal areas of deficiency. Pelvic osteotomies such as the Dega, Pemberton, and the San Diego osteotomy are effective at reducing the volume of the acetabulum and improving coverage. The Pemberton works well to improve anterior coverage occasionally seen in those patients with anterior dislocations. Triple innominate osteotomies are effective for extensive and congruent dysplasia.

The above *reconstructive* procedures are not recommended in patients with long-standing dislocations or with painful osteoarthritis. In these patients *salvage* procedures are chosen and include proximal femoral resection and interposition of muscle, valgus femoral osteotomy with or without femoral head resection, hip fusion, or hip replacement. Proximal femoral resections with muscle interposition have good reliability in reducing pain in nonambulatory patients but may not completely remove all of the discomfort. Resection and interposition arthroplasty is performed through an extended lateral position. Careful extraperiosteal dissection is performed; the proximal femur is resected at a level that is equal to a line drawn across the ischial tuberosities. More proximal resection of only the femoral head and without interposition of muscle will likely lead to proximal migration and continued preoperative pain levels. The vastus lateralis and rectus femoris is pulled over the proximal femoral shaft while the gluteus medius and psoas are sutured into the hip capsule. The patients will benefit from indomethacin or other anti-inflammatory medicines to reduce heterotopic bone. Alternatively a single treatment of 700 rads of radiotherapy is used. Patients that undergo proximal femoral resection may be stabilized in traction, with external fixation for several weeks in order to allow soft tissue healing. A pica cast application with two external fixation half pins in the distal femur is recommended.

Valgus osteotomy may also be indicated in non-ambulatory patients and is most useful in painful hips with severe adduction contractures. Hip replacement is most effective in marginal to better ambulatory patients who require the ability to position the hip in extension for ambulation and flexion for sitting. Hip fusions have less utility in these patients.

Lower Extremity Contractures

There is a continuum of muscle pathology in patients with CP. Muscle spasticity due to the abnormal stretch reflex is the primary problem. During physical examination, patients with only spasticity will have increased tone; however, the joints can be positioned adequately at near normal extremes of flexion and extension by prolonged and slow stretch. However, with time, muscle contracture results from the prolonged spasticity. For example, hamstring muscle contracture is detected when the knee cannot be fully extended with the hip flexed at 90°. Hamstring contracture without knee contracture is present if the knee can be fully extended with the hip extended. Finally prolonged muscle contracture may lead to fixed contracture of the joint. In our previous example, a knee contracture can develop from long-standing hamstring contracture. The evidence showed restricted knee motion despite placing the hip in any position of flexion or extension. In this instance, isolated hamstring lengthening would be expected to have minimal effect on intrinsic knee stiffness. Other procedures such as arthrotomy or extension osteotomy would be needed to fully extend the knee.

It is important to tailor surgical treatment for muscle spasticity and contractures according to each patient's functional levels. Ambulatory patients are classified as *community* ambulators if they are able to ambulate with minimal assistance in public. These individuals occasionally require the use of orthotics. *Household* ambulatory patients require wheelchairs for travel outside the home but can use walkers or crutches to be independent at home. *Functional* ambulators may stand to transfer and take a few short steps with maximal assist for balance and power. *Nonambulatory* patients require full assistance for transfer from the bed to chair and back. It is intuitive to consider that treatment is more beneficial in community and household ambulatory patients. Yet on the other hand, it is important to maintain as much standing as possible in functional ambulators. This is of paramount importance for parents who see that their ability to assist and care for the children would decrease with aging and the increase in size of the children. In these children it is of benefit for them to have standing abilities maintained by avoiding severe hip and knee flexion contractures.

The assessment of gait abnormalities in community or household ambulatory patients with CP is often challenging and treatment has traditionally been selected based on physical exam and observational gait analysis (OGA). In the early 1980s, methods of three-dimensional gait analysis (GA) became popular and have evolved into sophisticated measures of gait. Today, instrumented GA is performed in motion analysis laboratories and usually consists of physical exam, videotaping for OGA, and calculation of time–distance parameters. Kinematic assessment of joint motion and kinetic evaluation for powers and moments is obtained with the use of reflective markers, multiple recording cameras, and refined computer software and force plate data. Finally, surface or fine wire electrodes are often applied for electromyographic measurement of muscle activity.

Proponents of modern gait analysis cite an increased ability to document and quantify preoperative abnormalities in all planes. Such precise assessment theoretically enables the surgeon to detect all of the pathologic and compensatory components of gait and to plan and perform all of the procedures required for their correction during the same anesthetic session. When performed postoperatively, gait analysis generates objective data that allows for assessment of treatment and guides further treatment in similar patients. Detractors of modern gait analysis believe that past methods are perfectly adequate for assessment of gait abnormalities and possible treatment interventions. These physicians also cite cost (over $2,000 for each gait analysis) and the difficulty in reproducing similar data in the same patient.

It is currently recognized that certain muscles tend to be more problematic than others. For instance, diarthrodial muscles such as the psoas, hamstring, rectus femoris, and gastrocnemius muscles cause greater difficulty with ambulation. These muscles cross two joints and are more likely to invoke abnormal stretch reflexes due to their increased muscle excursion during gait. Common gait abnormalities as a result of contracture or spasticity include equinus gait or back-kneeing in stance (gastrocsoleus), crouch gait (hamstring and/or psoas), scissor gait (adductors), and stiff-kneed gait (rectus and hamstring). Selective lengthening or transfer (rectus femoris) of the pathologic muscles at one operative setting is reasonable once a child reaches 7 to 8 years of age. Earlier surgery tends to result in recurrence prior to maturity, and younger children tend to respond well to nonoperative modalities such as botulinum A toxin injections and casting or bracing.

In general it is better to try and correct all significant deforming muscles at the same time. A good example of this principle exists in a patient with tight tendoachilles and hamstrings and hip flexion contractures. If the tendoachilles was solely lengthened, the patient would lose knee extension moment and would tend to crouch more due to the persistent knee flexion deformity of the hamstrings. Conversely, release of the hamstrings only would lead to severe back-kneed gait. Further hamstring release in the face of severe hip flexion contracture would lead to increase in pelvic tilt.

It is important to lengthen only those muscles that are leading to deformity, such as in the patient with equinus in gait. This deformity may be treated via lengthening of the Achilles tendon (in effect, lengthening the soleus and the gastrocnemius) or just the gastrocnemius fascia. The first surgery is more appropriate when an equinus contracture exists whether the knee is in either full extension or in 90° of flexion. Isolated gastrocnemius lengthening by the Strayer or Vulpius method is better considered in that patient whose foot can only be dorsiflexed past neutral with the knee flexed. (By flexing the knee the gastrocnemius is relaxed and the test isolates the soleus muscle.) In general, medial hamstring contractures are treated in ambulatory patients by Z-lengthening of the semitendinosis and gracilis and a fascial lengthening of the semimembranosis. Consideration for transfer of the gracilis and semi tendinosis is reasonable in the face of weak hip extensors or marginal hip flexion contracture. Lengthening of the fascia of the biceps tendon is reasonable in patients with a concurrent knee flexion contracture or who are nonambulatory. In these later patients it is perfectly acceptable to simply cut the semi tendinosis and gracilis without Z-lengthening them.

In ambulatory patients, bony surgery is indicated in older patients with recurrent flexion deformities of the hip and knee (extension osteotomy) (Figure 8-4) or in patients with rotational malalignment (external rotational osteotomy of the femur or internal osteotomy of the tibia). In these individuals rotational abnormalities can be a hindrance to gait. For instance, excessive femoral anteversion can lead to significant knee valgus in stance phase as well as in toeing with the feet hitting in swing phase. External rotation deformity at the tibia will lead to lever arm dysfunction. In this scenario, the externally rotated foot presents a shorter moment arm, thus diminishing the knee extension moment in stance phase as the leg proceeds from the second to the third ankle rocker.

Foot Deformities

Foot deformities in patients with cerebral palsy usually involve an equinus component and may have a varus or valgus deformity of the hind foot. Varus or supination deformity tends to predominate in hemiplegic patients and some diplegic patients. This is due to various combinations of overactivity of the posterior tibialis or supination of the forefoot as a result of anterior tibialis spasticity. It can be difficult to determine which muscle is the deforming force. If the posterior tibialis is the deforming force, the foot seems to have more hind foot varus without foot supination that is seen when the anterior tibialis forces. Spastic posterior tibialis may be appreciated by palpating the taunt tendon behind the malleolus. Fine wire EMG can help determine whether the anterior tibialis or the posterior tibialis is the deforming force. In normal gait, the posterior tibialis is most active in stance phase and should be relatively quiescent in swing phase. The tibialis anterior dorsiflexes the foot at the start of swing phase due to concentric contraction. In addition, it also fires in the early stance phase, allowing eccentric lengthening and lowering of the foot to the floor. Deviations from these patterns on EMG will delineate the most likely cause of the foot inversion.

Surgical treatment of these deformities includes selective lengthening or transfer of all or part of the offending muscles. The most common treatment of equinovarus deformity includes lengthening of the gastrocsoleus (if the foot is in equinus irregardless of knee position) or the gastrocnemius (if no equinus exists when the knee is flexed). The two most common methods of correcting the foot inversion is via a split posterior tibialis transfer to the peroneus brevis or with a combination of posterior tibialis lengthening and split anterior tibialis transfer. In the latter procedure, the lateral half of the anterior

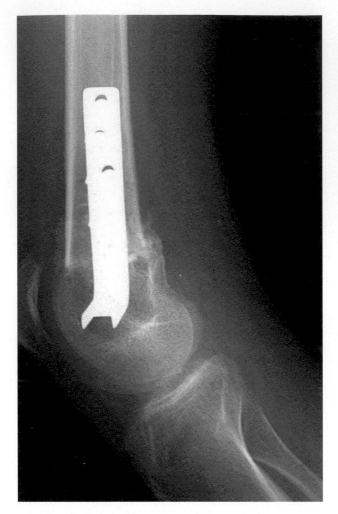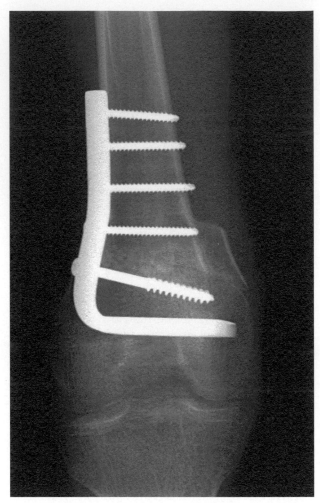

FIGURE 8-4. AP and lateral radiograph of distal femoral osteotomy for knee flexion contracture in an older patient with cerebral palsy.

tibialis is placed into the cuboid bone. Each procedure has their proponents but in general each case must be individualized as other methods including isolated posterior tibialis lengthening or transposition may be more appropriate. In general, patients should be treated with a postoperative ankle-foot orthosis (AFO) for at least 1 year. Although rare, severe equinovarus deformities may exist in the nonambulatory patients. Surgical treatment is indicated for lateral pressure sores or due to an inability to provide proper shoe wear. In these cases triple arthrodesis is a good method to insure a plantargrade foot with low recurrence rate.

Flat foot deformities are usually seen in nonambulatory quadriplegic patients; these deformities usually do not require treatment beyond an orthosis. Surgical treatment may be indicated in cases of

extreme deformity with foot sores and pain. Flat foot deformities may also be seen in ambulatory patients with spastic diplegia. In these cases, the equinus contracture will lead to collapse of the midfoot at Chopart's joints and an increase in forefoot abduction. The collapse causes a vertical positioning of the talus with potential for pressure sores; the abducted foot will contribute to lever arm dysfunction as the foot is externally rotated on the shank of the tibia. This inefficiency may hinder knee extension in the later stages of stance phase. Most patients tolerate the planovalgus foot deformities with little problems, and an accommodative ankle-foot-orthosis (AFO) is sufficient to prevent problems. Surgical treatment may be necessary in rare patients with skin breakdown or pain; treatment options usually require Achilles contracture release in addition to subtalar arthrodesis, sliding calcaneal osteotomy, or lengthening osteotomy of the calcaneus. In the later operation the calcaneus is cut between the anterior and medial facets with insertion of a block of bone. The lengthening of the lateral column of the foot induces reduction of the talonavicular joint. Long-term results for this operation are pending and early recurrences may be prevented when the lateral lengthening is combined with medial reefing of the posterior tibialis and talonavicular joint. The flat foot deformity is associated with excessive pronation of the first ray with the development of hallux valgus deformity. This deformity is rarely symptomatic; however, in rare cases metatarsal phalangeal joint arthrodesis may be needed. Standard hallux valgus operations are usually prone to failure and recurrence.

Upper Extremity Deformities

Most orthopaedists have concentrated in understanding, diagnosing and treating lower extremity problems in CP patients, yet an increased interest in hand and upper extremity function has concurrently developed. Patients with upper extremity spasticity yield a variety of deformities that may affect function as well as cosmesis and hygiene. The latter issues are of relevant importance in the more severely affected individuals. Severe muscle contractures lead to thumb-in-palm deformities and finger and wrist flexion deformities that may result in poor hygiene and skin maceration. Upper extremity function may be diminished in the more functional hemiplegic or diplegic patients at different levels. At the shoulder, patients can have spontaneous abduction when excited or running. At the elbow, patients usually have a dynamic flexion contracture with activities or when excited; the forearm can be pronated relative to the upper arm. The wrist is often flexed and ulnarly deviated due to increased activity in the flexor carpi ulnaris or other wrist flexors (Figure 8-5). Treatment is needed to correct functional problems such as elbow flexion deformity, diminished pronation, wrist flexion and ulnar deviation, extrinsic finger contractures, and intrinsic muscle imbalances. The latter may result in thumb adduction and finger swan necking.

Occupational therapy and splinting can help prevent fixed deformities. Botulinum A toxin may also benefit these patients. The latter is usually more successful in the upper than the lower extremity and is a result of the ability to place sufficient quantities

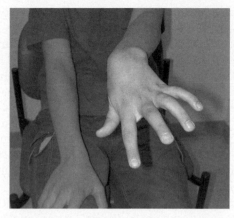

FIGURE 8-5. The flexed, pronated, and ulnarly deviated hand is commonly seen in patients with hemiplegia.

of toxin in the smaller muscles. Surgical treatment of contractures with lengthening or transfers of muscles and tendons improves hand function one to two levels. Less functional patients with severe or fixed deformities may be treated to improve hygiene and cosmesis with surgical release, transfer, or arthrodesis. Concurrent flexion deformities of the elbow, wrist, and fingers may be treated with a flexor–pronator slide. In this procedure the common flexor origin may retract a great deal when an extensive extraperiosteal release is performed with dissection of the neurovascular structures. The flexor pollicis longus may require an isolated lengthening in the face of severe flexion deformity. Wrist arthrodesis is useful in older patients or in patients with recurrent or severe flexion deformity. Through a dorsal approach, a proximal row carpectomy is performed and will functionally lengthen the wrist and finger flexors. Occasionally, a volar approach and Z-lengthening or release of the wrist flexors, profundus tendons, or the superficialis tendons may also be needed. A dorsal plate is placed across the distal radius, the capitate, and the third metacarpal and will provide stabilization while the morselized scaphoid, lunate, and triquitrium provides bone graft (Figure 8-6). Release of thumb adductors and intrinsic flexors improves the position of the thumb out from the palm. Augmentation of the thumb abductors prevents recurrence of thumb in palm deformity.

More sophisticated procedures may be performed in hemiplegic patients in order to improve function. Prior to surgical intervention, careful serial physical examinations with an experienced hand therapist helps identify the functional problems. Use of dual videotaping and EMG monitoring helps delineate which muscles are firing during specific activities. Prior to surgery, selective nerve blockade may simulate potential results of muscle transfer or release. In general, surgery should be delayed until the patient is able to cooperate with postoperative occupational therapy. In addition, there may be higher chances of recurrence or overcorrection in younger patients. Adolescent patients tend to be excellent candidates as they have the maturity to decide if treatment is in their best interest and, therefore, desire maximum improvement in function through postoperative occupational therapy.

Patients with dynamic flexion deformities of the elbow may be treated with fascial lengthening of the brachialis and Z-lengthening of the biceps tendon. Concomitant release of the lacertus fibrosis increases the ability of the biceps to improve supination. Pronation contracture is treated with isolated release of the pronator teres or pronator teres transfer. The latter is usually efficacious when the patient

has active pronation without fixed contracture. Transfer through the interosseous membrane to the dorsum of the radius converts the pronator into a supinator. Other tendon transfers, such as dorsal transfer of the flexor carpi ulnaris may also increase supination power.

Flexion deformity of the wrist is treated by weakening of the wrist flexors (simple lengthening of the flexor carpi radialis and ulnaris) or increasing the wrist extensor power via augmentation (central transfer of the extensor carpi ulnaris or brachioradialis). Dorsal transfer of flexor carpi ulnaris is indicated when a patient has weak wrist or finger extension in addition to overactive wrist flexion. Transfer to the finger extensors is indicated when the patient has weak release and to the extensor carpi radialis brevis when they have weak grasp. Care is needed to ensure that concurrent finger flexion contractures are not present and, if so, are treated with fractional lengthening.

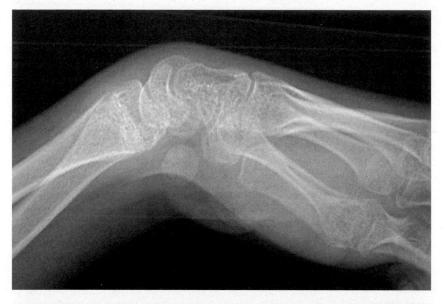
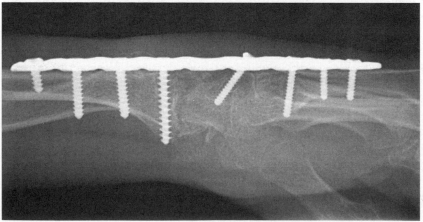

FIGURE 8-6. Preoperative and postoperative radiographs in a skeletally mature individual with severe cerebral palsy that underwent proximal row carpectomy and wrist arthrodesis.

Thumb deformities have been classified as simple thumb adduction (type 1), thumb adduction with MP joint contracture (type 2), thumb adduction with MP hyperextension (type 3), and thumb adduction with flexion deformity of both the MP and IP joints (type 4). Treatment of thumb deformity requires release of contracted tissues and augmentation of the weakened thumb abductors and extensors. Adduction is released with a 2- or 4-flap Z-plasty of the first web space and subsequent release of the adductor pollicis muscle and tendon as well as the first dorsal interosseus muscle off of the first metacarpal. If the IP joint of the thumb is contracted, Z-lengthening of the flexor pollicis longus is indicated. Hyperextension deformity of the MP is treatable with MP capsulodesis or MP arthrodesis. Alternatively, this deformity may stabilize after rebalancing of the thumb muscles. Tendon transfers to increase thumb abduction include exterior pollicis longus EPL re-routing through the first dorsal compartment, transfer of the extensor pollicis brevis to the abductor pollicis longus (APL) tendon, or transfer of the brachioradialis to the APL. Finger deformities such as flexion contracture may be treated with release of the flexor digitorum superficialis or fascial lengthening. Swan neck deformities are treated with lateral band transfer or flexor digitorum superficialis tenodesis.

ORTHOPAEDIC MANIFESTATIONS OF MYELODYSPLASIA

Several contrasts exist in CP patients in comparison to MMC patients. In general, deformities in MMC result from muscle imbalance due to paralysis of muscles. In CP, joint deformities are usually a result of asymmetric spasticity in addition to weakness. Furthermore, most patients with MMC have low to normal intelligence despite severe motor impairment and, therefore, are able to communicate effectively with the health care team. On the other hand, MMC patients tend to have comorbidities such as frequent urinary tract infections and therefore higher rate of opportunistic infections. These patients may have unrecognized hormone imbalances and the potential for obesity and increased energy consumption during ambulation. Patients usually require self-catheterization for urinary retention; spine fusions may make it impossible for female patients to perform this task. Fusions may predispose recurrent skin and joint problems as the inherent flexibility of

joints is sacrificed. As such, adjacent and insensate skin and joints must accommodate and are therefore predisposed to breakdown (skin sores and bony Charcot changes). Spine fusions may also predispose to decubitus ulcers due to stiffening of the spine and pelvis.

When born, parents of the affected children are very concerned about the potential for independent ambulation. A functional level of the third lumbar nerve root (medial hamstring function) is needed to have the possibility of some independent ambulation. Furthermore, the level of motor function is predictive for independent ambulation and for the different orthopaedic manifestations. For instance, patients with a motor level in the thoracic spine will never walk independently and will have hip instability with the potential for spinal deformity. Upper lumbar levels (L1 and L2) may have some ambulation in the early years but as they age and grow this is usually lost. Spinal deformity is less common but hip instability is more common than in thoracic-level deformities. Lower lumbar levels (L3 and L4) maintain ambulatory potential for longer periods of time and have a slightly lower rate of hip instability issues than in the upper lumbar level patients. Finally, L5 and sacral level patients have good ambulatory potential throughout life but are hampered by inefficient gait from weak hip extensors and abductors (L5 level) and foot deformities (sacral levels).

Ambulatory function in patients with myelomeningocele is not static; there is a tendency to undergo progressive degeneration. This is partially due to society's acceptance of people with special needs and the ease at which affected individuals are able to live. As patients age and their weight increases, it becomes increasingly more difficult to ambulate with crutches and braces and more acceptable to use wheelchairs. In addition, degeneration of the central nervous system may be present due to several possible causes. These causes include Arnold-Chiari malformations, tethered cord, shunt malfunctions and hydrocephalus, and syrinx development. The neurological deterioration can be sudden or very slow and insidious. It is extremely important that the orthopaedic surgeon carry out a detailed neurological evaluation at each visit. Any change in neurological function may be the first sign that there are problems. Also, any change in neurological function should generate referral to the neurosurgeon for appropriate evaluation.

The orthopaedic treatment of the MMC patient is complicated by multiple medical problems, which require treatment by other medical specialists (neurosurgeons, urologists, developmental pediatricians, and therapists). The mental development of the child, and the formation of parent–child bonding, may take precedence over the correction of skeletal deformity, especially during early infancy. Very few orthopaedic deformities cannot delay treatment until the child is one year old. Most of the problems of infancy such as shunt malfunction, feeding difficulties, respiratory problems, and developmental delay have been addressed. Orthopaedic treatment should be coordinated with the overall treatment plan for the child and also considered in light of orthopaedic deformities of the spine, hips, knees, and feet. For instance, severe congenital foot deformity in a patient with thoracic level paralysis (nonambulatory patient) takes precedence over the possible presence of a dislocated hip. On the other hand, severe kyphosis occasionally seen in thoracic level patients should be corrected prior to foot deformities. Correction of the spinal deformity provides more significant overall patient improvement. The following centers discussion on anatomic area of involvement in patients with myelodysplasia.

Spinal Deformity in Myelodysplasia

In myelodysplasia, the many unique patient aspects and anatomic features of the spine make treatment a challenge. Issues pertinent to the immature spine with myelomeningocele include failure of the neural arch to close, resulting in deficiency in the posterior elements. The lack of posterior elements increases the difficulty of obtaining surgical fixation and also decreases the bone available for fusion. As such, individuals with severe spinal deformity and myelomeningocele require anterior and posterior spine fusions to obtain the fusion and improve fixation. In addition, the open posterior canal increases the incidence of inadvertent injury to the thecal sac. Sagittal plane abnormalities tend to be more extreme in spina bifida than in idiopathic scoliosis with extreme lumbar lordosis and risk for increased kyphosis in the thoracic spine. The posterior musculature of the spinal erector muscles are anterior to the axis of the spine and may lead to further kyphosis. In addition, a higher incidence of congenital anomalies of the spine exists (hemivertebrae, unsegmented bars, diastematomyelia, lipomas, and dermoid cysts). Patients with myelomeningocele have high rates of urinary tract infections, which lead to a higher rate of secondary infection of the spine following surgery.

Scoliosis is prevalent in many patients with myelomeningocele. Most patients with thoracic level paraplegia have spinal deformity; the incidence falls to 50 to 60% in patients with low lumbar level paraplegia. In general, the curves tend to be greater at an earlier age, therefore, increasing the potential for significant curves with time. If the spinal deformity rapidly progresses, MRI scan is needed to rule out syrinx in the cervical and thoracic spine. The lumbar spine is also scanned for dermoid cysts, lipomas, and tethering of the cord.

Observation is recommended in patients with curves less than 30°. Bracing may be considered in selected individuals with curves greater than 30° who are less than 7 years of age. Unfortunately, bracing is not as efficacious as in idiopathic scoliosis, and progression of the spinal deformity can be expected. In addition, problems with skin sores and rib deformities may result from the use of bracing. Surgical stabilization is indicated in patients with progressive curves or curves greater than 45°. The goals of surgical treatment include obtaining a level pelvis, restoring normal sagittal and coronal balance, and preventing further deformity. In general, fusion levels are considered to extend from the neutral vertebral body proximally into the distal stable zone. If questions arise, it is more advisable to fuse longer than shorter. In general, instrumentation is planned to avoid ending the fusion in the middle of a sagittal curve.

Fusion to the pelvis is generally indicated in patients with pelvic obliquity greater than 15° or in patients with thoracic or upper lumbar level paraplegia. Unfortunately, fusion to the pelvis may increase secondary problems, such as pressure sore development. Importantly, female patients should be informed of the possibility of increased difficulty of self-catheterization due to stabilization of the lumbar spine. Anterior interbody fusion is needed to augment the fusion rates, particularly in the regions of deficient posterior elements. Fixation of the posterior elements is possible with the use of pedicle screws; sublaminar wires and cables are placed in the intact lamina proximally and transverse connectors will prevent collapse of the spine. Contoured rods may be placed over the ala of the sacrum, or into the first sacral foramen. Anterior rods and instrumentation may be used in patients with extreme deformity and increased stabilization can be expected. Anterior only instrumentation for isolated lumbar curves without posterior surgery may be considered; however, posterior instrumentation should be considered in addition to this technique in patients with larger curves or high level of thoracic deformity. Instrumentation should be low profile, due to the poor skin and problems that can result from deficient soft tissues in myelomeningocele.

As mentioned, congenital scoliosis is occasionally seen in patients with myelomeningocele and may be treated somewhat differently than in those patients with scoliosis without congenital anomalies. In general, anterior and posterior spine fusion over the apices of the deformity is needed to prevent further progression. Earlier surgery is indicated in those patients who have congenital anomalies that are prone to rapid progression, such as contralateral bars and hemivertebrae. Anterior fusion is done through an open anterior approach; however, transpedicular approaches can be used to obtain anterior fusion. Rarely, osteotomies are needed to correct significant deformities.

Young patients with spina bifida may present or develop severe kyphosis that merits treatment. Children with significant kyphosis will have difficulty with independent sitting without using their upper extremities for balancing. Cephalad displacement of the abdominal contents will restrict breathing, prevent normal nutrition, and may lead to failure to thrive for these individuals. Try to correct the kyphosis early in order to improve the ability of the child to sit independent without the necessary use of the upper extremities. Bracing is usually ineffectual. In general, kyphectomy is performed by decancellation of the vertebrae above and below the apical vertebrae and is done to avoid violation of the endplates and, therefore, the growth centers of this deformity. Instrumentation is placed extraperiosteally to allow for future growth. Usually a Luque rod is contoured and placed over the ala of the sacrum or into the first sacral foramen. Proximal fixation with pairs of sublaminar wires placed in an extraperiosteal fashion will allow for continued growth. At closure, the paraspinal muscles are closed posteriorly over the instrumentation, reducing them to an anatomic position and decreasing the propensity for progressive kyphosis. Rigid S-shaped kyphosis may be treated with cordectomy and resection of the vertebral bodies and fixation with segmental fixation.

Hip Dysplasia in Myelodysplasia

Individuals with myelomeningocele are more likely to have hip dislocation and dysplasia. The incidence of dislocation of the hip is 20% compared to 0.1% in the general population. This is presumably due to altered forces across the hip in utero and in the postnatal period. Thoracic level patients may have contractures of their hips due to positioning. Upper lumbar level patients will have actively firing hip adductors and hip flexors, but will be deficient in hip abductors and hip extensors. This muscle imbalance leads to higher rates of dislocation and dysplasia than in thoracic level patients. Compared to thoracic level and lower lumbar, sacral level patients will usually have stronger hip extensors and abductors, in addition to weight-bearing activities, which will prevent dislocations.

The goal of treatment in the thoracic level patients is to avoid hip contractures, which will preclude comfortable sitting, as well as standing. Thoracic level patients with dislocated hips or progressively dislocating hips should not undergo surgery to reduce the hips. Surgery is only performed in order to prevent significant hip contractures that preclude sitting or standing. All children who develop independent sitting by 18 to 24 months of age should be started on a prone standing program in order to improve their upper extremity function. Patients with the upper lumbar level function may be candidates for a reciprocating gate orthosis. In these patients, swaying of the hips in a side-by-side manner will allow for forward propulsion. Unfortunately, in order to use this orthosis, patients must be fairly contracture free.

The upper lumbar level patients will have higher rates of hip dislocation and dysplasia than in the thoracic level paraplegic patients. Historically, efforts have been made to maintain the hip position in these patients, including muscle transfers. Today, treatment in these patients is similar to those in the thoracic level paraplegic patients and surgery is only indicated to prevent muscle contractures. In the past, was recommended reduction of hips in lower lumbar patients with the addition of different tendon transfers designed to augment weak hip extension and abduction. These reductions include transfer of the psoas muscle to the greater trochanter; posterior transfer of the origins of the adductor longus, brevis and gracilis muscles; external oblique transfer to the greater trochanter; and posterior tensor fascia lata transfer to the gluteal muscle sling. Controversy surrounds whether these extensive muscle transfers prevent later dysplasia and improve the function and gait of these patients. Recently, surgeons have not been reducing dislocated hips in lumbar level patients, unless patients are experiencing ongoing pain. The function of these patients whether the hips are dislocated or located does not seem to vary; and they seem to function whether the hips are located or not.

Dislocated hips in patients with sacral level paralysis should undergo hip reduction and stabilization procedures. Standard open reduction through an anterior approach and femoral shortening in older patients may be indicated. If weakness of the hip abductors is noted, the transfer of the external oblique is probably appropriate.

Knee Problems in Myelodysplasia

The knee in patients with myelomeningocele can have several problems, including hyperextension deformity, flexion contracture, and valgus deformities of the knee. The important knee functions of motion and stability are to be reasonably maintained in patients in order to allow sitting, standing, and gait.

Hyperextension deformities of the knee are common in patients with L3 level of motor function. These patients have active quadriceps function with no hamstring function thus leading to hyperextension deformities. These deformities are usually treated well with physical therapy or casting in the early period. Surgery may be performed in cases with persistent dislocation of the knee and inability to obtain flexion. In these patients, the hamstring muscles can subluxate anteriorly and provide a deforming knee extensor moment verses the normal knee flexion. These patients are treated with an anterior VY quadriceps plasty, thus allowing the hamstring muscles to then drift posteriorly to the axis of the knee.

Flexion contractures may develop in ambulatory patients with myelodysplasia. Patients with deformities less than 20° may be treated with an anterior floor reaction AFO and progressive stretching. If contractures are greater than 30°, this degree of flexion will preclude efficient gait and may lead to anterior knee pain, due to increased stresses of the patellofemoral joint. Posterior release is indicated in patients with a significant flexion contracture. In this technique, the hamstring muscles are transferred proximally to the insertion of the gastrocnemius muscle. The gastrocnemius muscle can be released if it is a deforming force for flexion. Posterior capsulotomy and partial sectioning of the cruciate ligaments may be needed in order to obtain full extension. In the author's experience, posterior capsulotomy is a procedure that works better in younger patients. Older patients tend to have higher rates of recurrence. Therefore, distal femoral osteotomy with extension is more reproducible in older patients. It is important to ensure that the patient has active knee flexion greater than 100° of flexion, as distal femoral extension osteotomy will decrease the flexion arc. Anterior physeal stapling may be indicated in growing patients with knee flexion contracture, avoiding the morbidity of distal femoral osteotomy.

Some ambulatory myelomeningocele patients will develop progressive valgus deformities of the knee. This may be due to tightness of the iliotibial band and increased valgus moment of the knee as a result of the Trendelenburg gait. Patients with a valgus deformity of the knee can be treated with a knee-ankle-foot orthosis. Selective surgical procedures may include iliotibial band release, osteotomy of the distal femoral joint and medial distal femoral physeal stapling.

Foot Deformities in Myelodysplasia

In caring for the foot in spina bifida, the correction of foot pathology requires treatment of structural deformity and balance of the extrinsic and intrinsic foot muscles as well. The preservation, removal, or transfer of muscle activity must be carefully considered in relationship to the function of the foot during walking. For instance, a muscle that functions as a deforming force may not have the power to fully correct the structural deformity after transfer. Transfer of a tendon may result in muscle weakness and production of a secondary problem. In thoracic level and upper lumbar level patients, the feet should be kept contracture and deformity free to allow appropriate orthosis wear and prevention of foot sores. This is important for shoeing and to start standing protocols, which may promote future independence with activities of daily living. Lower level lumbar patients have good long-term ambulatory potential and may require removal of deforming forces in the foot to maximize ambulatory potential and to prevent areas of high pressure and subsequent pressure sores. The motion of the joints in the foot should be preserved as much as possible. This will allow preservation of the shock absorptive capacity of the foot, and lessen the possibility of ulceration and joint degeneration. Sacral level patients have at least moderate plantar flexion power in the triceps surae, yet intrinsic paralysis may lead to foot deformities consisting of hind foot and forefoot malalignment.

Clubfoot

Talipes equinovarus is the most common congenital foot abnormality and accounts for over 50%

of foot deformities. The clubfoot deformity is significantly stiffer and more resistant to manipulate in comparison to idiopathic clubfeet (Figure 8-7). As such, correction of the equinovarus deformity in MMC patients is rarely accomplished by nonoperative means. An attempt to manipulate and cast the deformity during the newborn period may be worthwhile in the extremely rare instance when the foot is supple and can be manipulated into a satisfactory position prior to the application of plaster. If the foot has not achieved satisfactory correction by the time the infant is 3 months old, make no further attempts at conservative treatment; surgical correction is recommended when the child is 1 year old. Performing the surgery at an age when the child is able to stand utilizes weight bearing as well as an orthosis to maintain correction.

Skin coverage of the posteromedial aspect of the foot presents a major potential problem during surgical correction of the severe hind foot deformity common in the MMC clubfoot. Many different incisions have been tried, but no approach is completely devoid of limitations. After skin incision, all 1 to 2 cm of the paralyzed and spastic tendons should be resected rather than lengthened. Additionally, in patients with L5 level paraplegia the functioning, anterior tibialis and the peroneal tendons will often result in a calcaneal valgus deformity.

In these cases, consider resection of these tendons, as it is better for the patient to have a flaccid braceable foot than a deformed foot due to muscle activity that is inappropriate for standing. Limited surgery rarely corrects the clubfoot. Complete circumferential subtalar release is necessary in order to allow the calcaneus to rotate sufficiently underneath the talus to reduce varus and align the axis of the foot with the axis of the ankle and knee. Postoperatively, the patient is placed into a long leg cast and the pins are removed at 6 weeks. The child is then fitted for a night splint and AFOs are worn during the day.

Recurrent clubfoot deformity is seen with a greater frequency in those patients with an MMC. The treatment of the recurrent deformity depends on several factors including the age of the patient, the functional level of the patient, as well as the previous treatment of the clubfoot. In toddlers treat recurrent clubfoot with a repeat posteromedial release. Recurrent clubfoot deformity may require talectomy; however, the resultant correction is rarely satisfactory due to possible recurrence. Less severe deformities may be managed with a combination of osteotomies such as a tarsal or metatarsal osteotomy to correct the midfoot deformity and a calcaneal osteotomy to correct the fixed varus deformity of the heel.

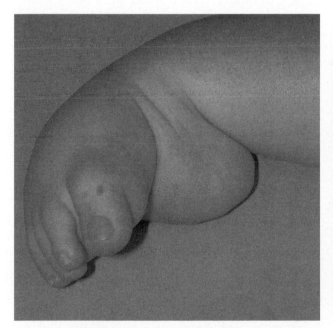
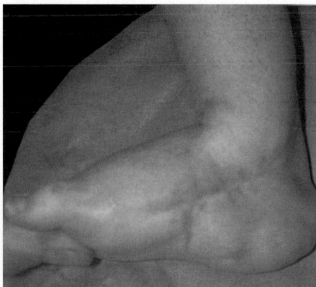

FIGURE 8-7. Preoperative and postoperative photographs from a child with severe clubfoot treated with extensive posterior medial and lateral release.

Calcaneal Deformity

These foot deformities are primarily due to the unopposed voluntary or spastic pull of the anterior tibialis muscle, the toe extensor muscles, or the peroneal muscles. With time, the calcaneus eventually becomes vertical underneath the talus, promoting excessive pressure under the calcaneus and preventing the forefoot from contacting the floor. Nonoperative treatment of calcaneal deformity is rarely successful in the long term. Simple resection of the offending tendons at an early age (in the child under 5 years of age) allows the foot to be brought into satisfactory position for bracing. However, in cases of more severe deformity with vertical alignment of the calcaneus, the anterior tibialis tendon is transferred through the interosseous membrane and attached to the os calcis. The remaining tight anterior structures are released so that the foot can be brought into a satisfactory plantarflexed position for bracing. The transferred tendon rarely provides enough power for braceless ambulation and is designed to make the foot braceable and ulcer free, not to eliminate brace use.

Congenital Vertical Talus

Congenital valgus deformities are usually due to contraction of the lateral musculature of the foot with equinus deformity of the calcaneus; severe cases present with lateral displacement of the calcaneus from beneath the talus. The deformity may be flexible or rigid; in the former, a trial of manipulation and cast treatment followed by an orthosis designed to hold the foot in the corrected position may be successful. In the rigid form of congenital vertical talus, an aggressive surgical approach is needed. As in 1-year-old patients, surgery consists of an extensive subtalar release, resection of deforming tendons, and postoperative ankle release. The anterior tibialis tendon can either be resected or transferred back to the neck of the talus. After postoperative cast immobilization, it is important to protect the foot and ankle with a rigid ankle foot orthosis to prevent neuropathic degeneration of the ankle joint.

Valgus Deformity

Valgus and external rotation of the foot is a common deformity seen in older children. The valgus deformity may occur in the subtalar joint, in the ankle, or in both sites. Ankle valgus is noted on radiographs when the fibular physis is above the level of the plafond, if there is wedging of the distal tibia epiphysis and if the longitudinal axis of the tibia is not perpendicular to the dome of the talus. In many cases, the deformity is mild and requires only custom inserts such as a UCBL. In rare cases, the ankle valgus deformity will be excessive and lead to decreased knee extension moment in stance phase. In such instances, correction may be obtained with a supramalleolar osteotomy that corrects both the valgus and rotation or, alternatively, a medial tibia epiphysiodesis may be used in cases of valgus deformity without external rotation of the ankle.

Failing to have radiographic evidence of ankle valgus implies that valgus is present in the subtalar joint. Several different options exist when the valgus is due to the subtalar joint. These options include medial calcaneal osteotomy, calcaneal lengthening or subtalar arthrodesis. The use of subtalar arthrodesis will usually restore normal hind foot alignment but does remove motion from the subtalar joint. This increases the risk of sores and Charcot-like changes in the ankle joint as the child matures.

Cavus

Cavus foot deformity is due to muscle imbalances and is most commonly seen in sacral level MMC. Muscle weakness leads to dropped first metatarsal and claw toes. The muscle imbalance (weak peroneals) and plantar flexed metatarsal leads the hind foot into varus. Children with a cavus deformity have sufficient sensation and voluntary muscle control to walk without an orthosis. Deformity will frequently be progressive, resulting in ulcerations on their toes and over their metatarsal heads. Failure of conservative treatment with severe calluses or ulcerations and ankle instability due to hind foot varus is an indication for surgical correction. Cavus is corrected via plantar fascia release and osteotomy of the metatarsals or midfoot. Balancing of muscles may include transfer of the IP joints, transfer at toe flexors to the extensors, and occasionally extensor hallucis longus recession will be used to increase foot dorsiflexion power. A calcaneal osteotomy is necessary when a dorsiflexion attitude of the calcaneus is present and accentuates the cavus deformity. Following osteotomy the calcaneus is moved backward and laterally as needed to correct cavus or cavovarus deformities.

Charcot Arthropathy

Neuropathic arthropathy is a progressive joint degeneration due to lack of protective sensation. This is primarily a problem in the ambulatory young adult who has decreased sensation of the knee, ankle, and foot. The L4–L5 patient appears to be the most vulnerable; however, patients with paralysis at the S-1 level of paraplegia may also have Charcot changes. The pathologic process follows a traumatic episode that may be quite mild. Progressive destruction results after the patient continues to walk leading to further microfractures and joint destruction. Following initial trauma there is usually a considerable amount of swelling and redness around the joint and the appearance of the foot resembles an infection and cellulitis. Because the initial radiographs are often unremarkable, the patient may be given antibiotics for the mistaken diagnosis of infection.

Appropriate treatment consists of complete joint protection following the initial episode and before additional injury occurs. Immobilization may be accomplished by splinting or casting and non weight bearing. Typically, the swelling and erythema will subside after 1 or 2 weeks and complete healing will take approximately 6 to 8 weeks. If the early treatment is successful, then radiographic changes may never be identified. If redness and swelling recurs after the onset of weight bearing, then protection must be resumed for a longer period of time. In some cases diagnosis and treatment are delayed and the radiograph becomes positive for joint deformity or degeneration. Prolonged immobilization and protection must be provided until the process has run its course. With this plan, joint instability and the development of bony prominences are hopefully avoided. Such treatment may take up to 6 to 8 months and joint protection should be maintained until there is radiographic evidence of healing of the joint, and all swelling and erythema has disappeared.

Fractures in Myelodysplasia

Myelomeningocele patients who are ambulatory can occasionally present with fractures of the lower extremity following minimal trauma. These fractures occur in patients who are between 3 and 7 years of age and typically occur in the distal femur and proximal tibia. Fractures occur at the epiphyseal plate or in the metaphysis. Presenting signs and symptoms include erythema, swelling, and fever; moderate elevations in sedimentation rate may be noted. Differential diagnosis includes the possibility of cellulitis and osteomyelitis. Fractures should be considered the primary cause, unless other signs and symptoms and positive cultures are consistent with infection. These fractures are

treated with a bulky soft dressing with splinting for 3 weeks until callus formation is noted and then progressive weight bearing is started to prevent further osteopenia.

In summary, patients with myelomeningocele have multiple problems and issues regarding the hip, knee, and foot. Treatment is indicated and individualized to the patient according to the general medical health of the child, the level of paraplegia and the functional deficits inherit to each patient.

SPINAL MUSCULAR ATROPHY

Spinal muscular atrophy is due to dysfunction in the anterior horn cells of the spinal cord, resulting in distal weakness. The inheritance is autosomal recessive in nature and consists of different clinical pictures, based on differences in severity. Spinal muscular atrophy is classified clinically into three types. Type I is termed Werdnig-Hoffmann disease. Type II is a chronic form of Werdnig-Hoffmann disease and Type III is the milder form of Spinal Muscular Atrophy, termed Kugelberg-Welander disease. No clear demarcation in the extent of disease, onset of disease and progression of deformity exists between the three types. However, patients are often classified into these three categories, even though clinical presentation may not distinctly place a child into each of the different groups. In general, the earlier onset of the disease results in more severe clinical effects and poor outcome.

Type I or acute Werdnig-Hoffmann disease is diagnosed prior to 6 months of age. These patients present with severe pulmonary restriction and complications resulting in early death. As such, orthopaedic treatment is rarely needed except occasionally to provide immobilization for pathologic fractures in the postnatal period. Type II or chronic Werdnig-Hoffmann disease is diagnosed after 6 months of age. These patients never become ambulatory and may live into the middle decades of life. Type III or Kugelberg-Welander disease is usually diagnosed after 2 years of age. These patients are ambulatory, with decreasing ambulation over time, as weakness increases. These patients have proximal muscle weakness and may have some similar physical exam features as those seen in muscular dystrophy.

Orthopaedic treatment needed in spinal muscular atrophy is needed for resultant muscle weakness, which leads to contractures of the soft tissues, hip instability, and progressive spinal deformity.

Due to the muscle weakness, muscle contractures become common, and muscle is replaced with fat and fibrosis. Decreased function and an inability to ambulate predispose individuals to develop hip and knee flexion contractures. Physical therapy and orthoses may be of some benefit in maintaining motion. As these individuals are usually wheelchair dependent, muscle contractures are rarely severe enough to require surgical intervention.

In order to prevent pelvic obliquity, difficult seating, and pain, it is desirable to maintain reduction of the hips, even in nonambulatory patients. Many patients have a life expectancy into the fourth and fifth decade. Treatment to prevent hip displacement includes surgical release of those muscle contractures that lead toward displacement. These treatments include surgical releases of the adductors and hamstrings. In patients with rapid subluxation, femoral osteotomy may be of benefit. In patients with dislocated hips, an open reduction, femoral osteotomy and pelvic acetabuloplasty osteotomy may be required. Salvage operations, such as Chiari and shelf operations will maintain posterior coverage, while increasing lateral coverage.

Spinal deformity is common in patients with spinal muscular atrophy. All type II patients will develop scoliosis within the first decade of life. Individuals with type III spinal muscular atrophy will have a more variable incidence of scoliosis. In general, scoliosis is characterized as a long, C-shaped scoliosis involving pelvic obliquity. Occasionally, isolated thoracic curves will be noted. It is expected that all type II patients and most type III patients will have progression of the deformity and will require surgical intervention. Be that as it may, it is a benefit to delay surgery as long as possible. Therefore, bracing with use of a TLSO, (Thoracic, Lumbar, Sacral, Orthosis) may be indicated in patients younger than 8 or 9 years with minor curves. Bracing will allow patients to have improved sitting balance. The main benefit allows increased spinal growth and obviates the need to consider anterior and posterior spinal fusion. Surgery is uniformly indicated in patients with curves over 40° and who maintain good pulmonary function. Pulmonary function is affected in response to weakness of the intercostal muscles. Pulmonary function may be further affected by cephalad displacement of the abdominal contents from severe scoliosis. Decreased complications and improved outcome can be anticipated in patients whose expected forced vital capacity is greater than 30 to 40%.

The benefits of surgery include an increase in sitting balance, an improvement in self-image, and cosmesis. Similar to spine fusion in other neuromuscular disorders, posterior spine fusion instrumentation improves the ability of the caregiver to provide for the patients. Posterior spine fusion may also decrease or remove the aching back pain that may occasionally be seen in individuals with severe deformity. Scoliosis is corrected with posterior spine fusion and instrumentation to the pelvis in order to reduce pelvic obliquity, if present. Pelvic fixation is obtained with Galveston instrumentation or multiple screw placements into the lower lumbar vertebra, sacrum, and the iliac wing. Due to the significant osteoporosis seen in these individuals, sublaminar wires at every level are preferred to segmental instrumentation via hooks. Anterior release and instrumentation is rarely indicated in these patients, due to the potential for exacerbating poor pulmonary function. Increased blood loss and need for transfusion is noted, as well as increased risk of infection, due to complexity and length of these procedures. Spinal cord monitoring is utilized. In general, spinal cord monitoring benefits patients with muscle disease in order to maintain any residual bowel and bladder function, as well as to maintain the protective sensation, thus preventing decubitus ulcers.

Postoperatively, these patients are managed with aggressive pulmonary toilet Continuous positive airway pressure (CPAP) is often beneficial in maintaining lung ventilation and decreases atelectasis. Epidural pain control is of further benefit in order to prevent the splinting of respiration as a result of postoperative pain.

FRIEDREICH'S ATAXIA

Friedreich's ataxia is considered one of several spinal cerebellar degenerative disorders and has an autosomal recessive inheritance. These individuals present with increased ataxia as the first presenting symptom. On physical exam, there is a loss of the knee and ankle reflexes, and a positive Babinski sign. In addition, there is a loss of proprioceptive and vibratory sense. The average age at clinical onset is from 7 to 15 years of age, with rare cases of delayed onset up to 25 years of age. Ataxia and symmetric weakness leads to progressive decrease in walking and patients often become wheelchair bound by the second to third decade. Weakness is usually symmetric, involving the proximal musculature (gluteus maximus), more than in the distal musculature. Premature death occurs in the fourth or fifth decade as a result of complications from cardiomyopathy or pulmonary dysfunction following complicating events, such as aspiration pneumonia. The orthopaedic manifestations of Friedreich's ataxia include foot disorders and spinal deformity.

Individuals with Friedreich's ataxia will occasionally have a cavovarus foot deformity as a presenting symptom. Ambulation becomes difficult as a result of the foot deformity, combined with ataxia. In order to produce a plantar grade foot, surgical treatment of the cavovarus deformity requires muscle rebalancing, bony osteotomies, or fusion. Soft tissue releases include plantar fascia release, tendoachilles lengthening, transfer of the posterior tibialis tendon, or lengthening and transfer of the anterior tibialis tendon. When a transfer of the anterior or posterior tendon in entertained, it is usually placed into the dorsum of the third cuneiform in the center of the foot. Residual skeletal deformity of the foot may be managed with calcaneal and midfoot osteotomies versus a triple arthrodesis.

Scoliosis develops in nearly all patients with Friedreich's ataxia. Several distinct differences in spinal deformity exist between patients with Friedreich's ataxia and patients with spinal deformity as a result of muscle weakness. Patients with Friedreich's ataxia develop scoliosis not as a function of muscle weakness, but as a result of abnormalities in balance. It is theorized that the spinal deformity in Friedreich's ataxia is a result of the perturbations in the proprioceptive and balance systems. This theory is similar to the theories for the cause of curves in patients with idiopathic scoliosis. Because of the similarities, the progression, curve pattern, and treatment are more similar to patients with adolescent idiopathic scoliosis. Curve onset may occur while individuals are walking, as opposed to those patients with muscular dystrophy. In the latter case, curve progression usually develops when patients become wheelchair dependent. Similar to idiopathic scoliosis, progression of scoliosis is age dependent; younger patients will have rapid progression and larger final magnitudes than patients with later onset of scoliosis. The curve pattern in Friedreich's ataxia is also similar to idiopathic scoliosis with greater incidences of double major curve patterns, single thoracic and thoracolumbar curves. This is in contrast to scoliosis from muscular dystrophy, which is characterized by long C-shaped curves and pelvic obliquity.

The treatment for scoliosis in Friedreich's ataxia is similar to that in patients with adolescent idiopathic scoliosis. Bracing may be utilized in younger, immature patients with mild to moderate curves.

Bracing may provide some decrease in progression of the curve; however, the use of the TLSO may limit the patient's ability to walk. Surgery is generally indicated in patients who have curves greater than 50°. Surgical planning and treatment is similar to adolescent idiopathic scoliosis, with the bulk of patients requiring posterior spine fusion with instrumentation. Because the curves rarely result in pelvic obliquity, fusion to the pelvis is not indicated in most cases. posterior instrumentation with segmental fixation from the upper thoracic to the low lumbar region, maintaining curve balance in both the sagittal and coronal planes is recommended. Unnecessary fusion to the sacrum with screw fixation or Galveston fixation in an ambulatory patient may significantly decrease their ability to walk. Anterior release is indicated in those curves with severe rigidity and with poor sitting balance.

ORTHOPAEDIC IMPLICATIONS OF DUCHENNE MUSCULAR DYSTROPHY (DMD)

Clinical onset is usually between 3 to 6 years of age with noted decreases in ambulation, often heralded with new onset of toe walking. On initial physical exam, patients have loss in reflexes and pseudohypertrophy of the calves. Delayed onset of toe walking due to DMD is uniquely different from that seen in idiopathic toe walking. These individuals walk on their toes from the very beginning of independent ambulation. Patients with DMD may also present with increased tripping, difficulty running, and climbing stairs. These patients have difficulties as a result of proximal muscle weakness in the shoulder and hip musculature. Weakness in the lower extremity begins in the gluteus maximus, quadriceps, and anterior tibialis muscle. In the upper extremity, weakness is noted in the deltoid, pectoralis, and trapezius muscles. Pelvic weakness results in an abnormal gait that is typical for muscular dystrophy. These individuals have weak hip extensors and, therefore, develop compensatory flexion of the hips and increased lordosis of the lumbar spine. Muscle contractures in the tensor fascia lata promote development of a wide-based gait. Static examination will further reveal contractures of the tensor fascia lata, with a positive Ober test. In addition, Trendelenburg lurch results from weak hip abductors. These patients have further difficulty compensating for the abnormal gait due to concurrent weakness in the upper extremity that precludes crutch use. They will present with a positive Gower's sign, which is decreased ability to rise from a sitting position without use of the upper extremities.

Treatment is based on maintaining ability to ambulate, prevention of contractures which preclude sitting in nonambulatory patients and prevention of significant spinal deformity. In ambulatory patients, judicious release of these contractures, in combination with aggressive physical therapy in the motivated patients can preserve an ambulatory ability for 2 to 3 more years. Such surgical procedures are minimally useful in wheelchair-dependent patients. Other treatment indications include pain from severe muscle contractures.

Limiting foot deformities in DMD include equinus and equinovarus foot deformities. The latter results from a combination of the hypertrophy of the gastrocnemius muscle weakness of the anterior tibialis and over-pull of the posterior tibialis muscle. These patients are treated with percutaneous tendoachilles Z-lengthening and posterior tibialis transfer through the interosseous membrane. Postoperative use of an AFO will prevent recurrence. Ambulatory patients with abduction contractures may benefit from selective release of the iliotibial band and the fascia lata. Nonambulatory individuals with DMD may also develop hip flexion contractures, which result in increased lordosis and occasional back pain. Selective release of the sartorius, rectus femoris, and tensor fascia lata may improve the hip flexion contractures in nonambulatory patients. Knee flexion contractures may occasionally be painful in nonambulatory patients and hamstring releases can reduce the pain and spasms.

Ninety-five percent of patients with DMD develop scoliosis. The onset of scoliosis is concurrent with loss of ambulation in most patients. Rapid progression of the curve can be expected as soon as a child becomes wheelchair dependent. Most spinal deformity is a long thoracolumbar curve, with concurrent pelvic obliquity. Nonoperative treatment for scoliosis may be indicated in selective patients who have poor sitting balance and who have contraindications for surgery. Use of an orthosis will not prevent curve progression in affected individuals, but may help sitting balance in those patients who are poor candidates for surgical treatment.

Posterior spine fusion with instrumentation is indicated for a child with a 25° curve. There is no benefit to waiting as relentless progression of scoliosis and concurrent decrease in lung function may be expected. Standard surgical technique includes posterior instrumentation from T2 to L5 or to the pelvis. Most utilize instrumentation to the pelvis, especially if the curves are greater than 40° with attendant pelvic obliquity. Posterior instrumentation with Luque wiring provides solid fixation. Fixation to the pelvis can be accomplished with pedicle or sacral screws into the sacrum or the ilium. Alternatively, a unit rod may be placed into the pelvis via the Galveston method. Spinal cord monitoring is used throughout surgery to detect spinal cord injury. Although patients are nonambulatory, maintenance of bowel and bladder function and protective sensation is important.

The risks of surgery are increased in DMD patients in comparison to those with idiopathic scoliosis. Patients with DMD may have cardiomyopathy; therefore, a preoperative cardiology evaluation is mandatory. All patients with DMD have a decrease in pulmonary function. Once the child becomes wheelchair dependant, further loss of pulmonary function is inevitable. Spinal fusion is reasonably safe in patients who have a forced vital capacity greater than 30 to 40% of the expected values. Increased complications from surgery may result when the forced vital capacity is lower than 30% of expected values. With aggressive postoperative pulmonary toilet, surgical intervention may still be possible in patients with forced vital capacity of 20%. However, families of these patients should be informed of the significant risk and need for postoperative intubation. Posterior spine fusion with instrumentation has also been noted to stabilize the loss of pulmonary function. As such, increased life expectancy can be expected as a result of posterior spine fusion in patients who have an uncomplicated postoperative course.

Other surgical risks include excessive blood loss and need for transfusion. Higher rates of infection are also present as a result of the long duration of surgery and as a result of the significant blood loss. Surgical complications such as hardware failure have also been reported. The benefit of surgical treatment for spinal deformity is a clear improvement in the quality of life for affected individuals by maintaining an erect sitting position and improving their self image and cosmesis. On the other hand, some patients may have increased difficulty in feeding, as it is harder to get food to their mouth with their posture restored to near normal.

BECKER TYPE MUSCULAR DYSTROPHY

Becker type muscular dystrophy is best considered as a mild form of DMD. Although the anatomic distribution and problems are similar to those seen in DMD, the onset of symptoms is later, at approximately 7 years of age or older. Fortunately, the severity of the problems and the extent of disability are much less and these patients can expect to be ambulatory into the teen and young adult years.

Anatomic deformities include equinus and equinovarus deformities, as well as a milder form of scoliosis (Figure 8-8). Treatment for these deformities is individualized, using some of the same surgical and nonoperative treatment strategies seen in DMD. For instance, AFO use may prevent contracture and improve ambulatory potential. If this fails, tendoachilles lengthening, plantar fascia release, and posterior tibialis transfer may be needed. Affected individuals with scoliosis need their treatment individualized according to the location of the curve and extent of the curve size.

EMERY-DREIFUSS MUSCULAR DYSTROPHY

Emery-Dreifuss muscular dystrophy is also a sex linked recessive muscular dystrophy. Clinical onset is noted by early muscle contractures, such as equinus contractures. Paraspinal weakness, spasm, and tightness of these muscles may lead to cervical spine contractures. Affected individuals will also have elbow flexion contractures. These patients can walk for many decades and treatment is individualized to release any formal contractures of the foot. In rare cases, patients with this disorder require stabilization of the spine when curves are greater than 40°.

FACIOSCAPULOHUMERAL MUSCULAR DYSTROPHY

The two variations of Facioscapulohumeral muscular dystrophy are differentiated according to differences in genetic pattern. Patients with infantile Facioscapulohumeral muscular dystrophy have an autosomal recessive inheritance. This is a very severe form of muscular dystrophy, with onset of facial weakness in the first decade of life. Patients become wheelchair dependent by the second decade and will develop pulmonary complications resulting in death in the second to third decade. Patients have very severe weakness of the hip extensors, resulting in extreme lumbar lordosis and hip flexion

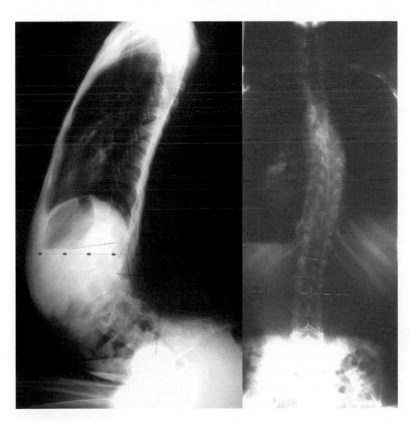

FIGURE 8-8. Lateral and AP of a 16-year-old boy with Becker muscular dystrophy. Extreme lordosis and minimal scoliosis is present.

contractures. In these patients, orthopaedic surgery is rarely helpful in improving function.

Compared to the infantile form, the autosomal dominant variety of Facioscapulohumeral muscular dystrophy has a variable expression with a less malignant course. The onset of clinical symptoms is in late childhood and early adolescence. Patients present with facial weakness and lack of facial mobility; decreased scapulothoracic motion, and scapular winging is noted. Following onset of facial abnormalities and scapulohumeral changes, weakness of the pelvic muscles and anterior tibialis is noted (Figure 8-9). Patients rarely present with scoliosis. The major orthopaedic problem is winging of the scapula, resulting in decreased shoulder flexion and

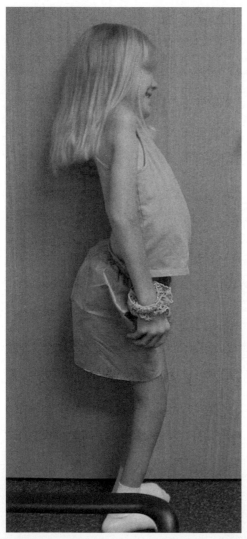

FIGURE 8-9. A 10-year-old female with fascioscapulohumeral muscular dystrophy. Note hyperlordosis and knee flexion secondary to weakness in the hip extensors and triceps surae.

abduction. In these patients, posterior stabilization of the scapula to the thorax may benefit by improving shoulder flexion and abduction. These surgical results are reliably maintained over time.

LIMB-GIRDLE MUSCULAR DYSTROPHY

Limb-girdle muscular dystrophy is a form of autosomal recessive muscular dystrophy. It is relatively benign in its clinical course in comparison to patients with Duchenne muscular dystrophy. The anatomic distribution is similar to that seen in Facioscapulohumeral muscular dystrophy, except no involvement of the face is noted. Clinical symptoms start in the second and third decade with weakness in hip extensors, hip flexors, and quadriceps. The clinical exam is similar to that seen in Becker and Duchenne muscular dystrophy, except more accentuated effects may be noted in the shoulder girdle region. Treatment is initiated in order to prevent and control muscle contractures, which are similar to those in Duchenne and Becker muscular dystrophy.

MYOTONIC DYSTROPHY

Myotonia is defined as an inability of the muscles to relax after spontaneous or reflexive muscle contracture; and it is this early feature of myotonic dystrophy that is noted on physical exam. Other clinical signs of myotonic dystrophy such as gradual atrophy of the muscle, frontal baldness, and cataracts may be present in older individuals. Cardiac problems such as arrhythmias or mitral valve prolapse may be common in patients with myotonic dystrophy. Myotonia tends to decrease with disease progression as a result of the muscle weakness. Myotonic dystrophy is inherited as an autosomal dominant disorder. Succeeding generations may have increased clinical effects than preceding generations. Clinical onset of functional muscle abnormalities begins in adolescence to early adulthood. As opposed to muscular dystrophies, myotonic dystrophy results in more marked abnormalities in the distal musculature. Early decreased function in the hands and decreased grip strength is followed by more proximal abnormalities. As the disease progresses, individuals will have impaired walking, due to weakness of the quadriceps, hamstring, and hip extensor muscles. Patients tend to lose their ability to ambulate within 15 to 20 years of disease onset. Very few orthopaedic deformities of myotonic dystrophy merit surgical treatment. Foot deformities, such as hind foot varus may be amenable to orthotic use.

HEREDITARY MOTOR SENSORY NEUROPATHIES (HMSN)

Hereditary motor sensory neuropathies (HMSN) are a diverse group of peripheral neuropathies, which have variable inheritance patterns. The first three HMSNs have a predominant onset in childhood and adolescence. Hereditary motor sensory neuropathies IV–VII, typically present in the adult population. Charcot-Marie-Tooth disease is considered the prototypical hereditary motor sensory neuropathy. Charcot-Marie-Tooth disease is classified as HMSN I if it is of the hypertrophic form. The less affected neuronal form of Charcot-Marie-Tooth disease is considered HMSN II.

The more severe form of HMSN I presents with decreased deep tendon reflexes and more weakness in the distal extremities, as opposed to the proximal muscle weakness. The more severe form of Charcot-Marie-Tooth disease has marked decreased nerve conduction velocity studies. The milder form of Charcot-Marie-Tooth disease (HMSN II) has clinically normal deep tendon reflexes with only mild aberrations noted in the nerve conduction velocities. These individuals have less weakness and, therefore, lead to later disease onset and less significant deformity. The diagnosis of HMSN can now be reliably made via genetic testing.

The orthopaedic problems of HMSN I and II result from muscle imbalances; usually resulting in cavovarus foot deformities, hip dysplasia, spinal deformity, and decreased upper extremity function. The predominant cavovarus foot deformity results from weakness of the peroneal muscles and relatively normal power of the posterior tibialis tendon. This deformity leads to foot inversion, abduction, and a varus hind foot. Cavus results from contracture of the plantar fascia and intrinsic muscle weakness. Preferential loss in strength in the peroneus brevis versus the peroneus longus will also contribute to a plantar flexed first ray and the cavus deformity. The cavus deformity and hind foot muscle imbalance (increased tone in the posterior tibialis tendon, compared to the peroneals) results in a varus hind foot deformity. This deformity is initially flexible, but may become fixed with time. Anterior tibialis weakness

results in over-activity of the extensor tendons to the toes. This weakness combined with intrinsic contracture leads to claw toe deformity.

Treatment options for these foot deformities include observation, orthotic use, and surgical treatment. The nonoperative methods are reasonable in patients with mild or nonprogressive deformities. Surgical indications include progressive deformity, ankle instability, and pain due to lateral column overload. Surgical treatment involves muscle balancing by removing or weakening the deforming forces and augmenting the deficient forces. The need for bony surgery in the hind foot is based on whether the hind foot varus is fixed or flexible. The Coleman Block Test is useful in determining whether the hind foot varus is fixed or flexible. With this maneuver, a $1\frac{1}{2}-\frac{3}{4}$-inch wooden block is placed under the lateral aspect of the foot and fifth metatarsal. Soft tissue only procedures would be appropriate if the hind foot can correct to a valgus or neutral position with this maneuver. Failure to correct the varus deformity implies a fixed skeletal deformity. In these cases, forefoot balancing procedures are combined with hind foot osteotomy or fusion.

The cavus deformity is treated with a plantar fascia release and in fixed deformities will require plantar based osteotomy, either through the metatarsals or the first cuneiform. The peroneus longus is usually transferred to the peroneus brevis tendon. Supination and hind foot varus is treated with anterior tibialis transfer to the third cuneiform if good power is present in the anterior tibialis tendon. If the anterior tibialis muscle is weak, posterior tibialis tendon transfer through the interosseous membrane will assist in balancing the foot. If the individual has weak dorsiflexion, a transfer of the extensor hallucis longus to the first metatarsal may increase dorsiflexion power with the added advantage of diminishing the tendency for clawing at the first ray. Fixed hind foot varus may be treated with calcaneal sliding osteotomy, closing wedge osteotomy, or hind foot triple arthrodesis. Tendoachilles release is rarely indicated as most of the equinus deformity is due to forefoot plantar flexion. Triple arthrodesis may be indicated in the severely deformed foot. However, complications with this operation include overcorrection, undercorrection, and pseudoarthrosis. Adjacent arthrosis in the ankle and midfoot may occur with longer term follow-up. Toe deformities in Charcot-Marie-Tooth disease may be treated with tenotomy of the long toe flexor in flexible deformities. Dorsal transfer of the long toe flexors may be indicated in more moderate deformities. The latter operation, however, has risks of complications to the neurovascular structure. Other treatment options for toe deformities include a resection arthroplasty of the Interphalangeal joints.

Hip displacement may be present in less than 10% of patients with hereditary sensory motor neuropathy type I and II; a higher incidence is noted in patients with more severe HMSN I. The spectrum of hip abnormalities may include dislocation at birth, as well as progressive acetabular dysplasia, coxa valga, or hip subluxation. In general, radiographic dysplasia is asymptomatic. On occasion, patients may present with hip pain and the above anatomic deformities are subsequently diagnosed. Treatment for progressive or symptomatic acetabular dysplasia and subluxation involve balancing of deforming muscle forces across the hip. Femoral and acetabular osteotomies may be utilized in the rare patients with progressive hip subluxation or dislocation.

The incidence of spinal deformity is also less than 10% of those in patients with HMSN I or II. Females seem to have a higher incidence than males, and the deformity is more likely in those individuals with more severe HMSN I. The spinal deformity is similar to that seen in adolescent idiopathic scoliosis with usual age of onset at 10 years of age and with development of similar curve patterns, to 0. In the unusual instance of large curves (35 to 40° in rapidly growing individuals) orthotic treatment with a brace may be indicated. Posterior spine fusion with segmental instrumentation and fusion is indicated in those rare patients with progressive deformities greater than 50 to 60°. Use of spinal cord monitoring during surgery may be limited due to the poor nerve conduction inherent to the demyelinization of the patients with hereditary sensory motor neuropathies.

Decrease sensory function and upper extremity deformities may be present in severely involved patients with HMSN I. These patients have intrinsic weakness, resulting in claw hands of the second through fifth digits (Figure 8-10). In addition, decrease in the intrinsic muscles will result in decrease pinch and opponens function of the thumb. Surgical treatment may be considered in those patients with severe clawing and would consist of flexor digitorum superficialis tenodesis.

ARTHROGRYPOSIS

Arthrogryposis is not a diagnosis per se, but a condition with joint contractures, atrophy of muscles noted on physical examination. In general, there are over 60 identifiable causes for arthrogryposis, and all patients have joint contractures detected at birth. No unifying theory as to the origin of these disorders is currently identified. Some may be due to in utero infection of some variety that affects the anterior horn cells; some may have a strong genetic component such as in Larsen's syndrome. Yet all have the characteristic of limited movement of the limb in utero that probably leads to the fibrosis and stiffness seen at birth. A diagnosis of arthrogryposis may be suspected in a fetus that has limited movement and with characteristic deformities such as clubfeet noted on ultrasound. Once delivered, these infants may have their arthrogryposis grossly classified according to distribution of the deformities. These contracture syndromes may involve all four extremities, as seen in patients with Larsen's syndrome or arthrogryposis multiplex congenita. Contractures may involve just the hands and feet and be considered distal arthrogryposis. Pterygium syndromes include those patients

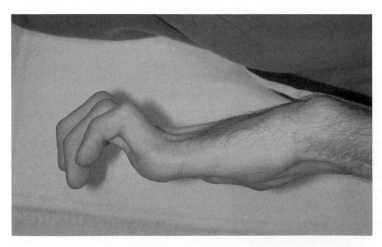

FIGURE 8-10. Intrinsic minus hand seen in a 20-year-old with HMSN I.

with severe pterygia of their major joints. Initial work-up involves consultations with a pediatric geneticist and neurologist and may require evaluation with MRI scans and skin or muscle biopsies.

Patients with arthrogryposis multiplex congenita have a characteristic appearance of the limbs. Limbs appear tubular without normal contours of the muscles and joints and the overlying skin is without wrinkles; however, there may be occasional dimples over joints or muscles. The shoulder is typically adducted and internally rotated; and the elbow is usually fixed in extension. At the wrist, the hand is invariably flexed and ulnarly deviated and there may be a thumb and palm deformity with severe finger flexion. More severe finger deformity is noted on the ulnar side of the hand as opposed to the radial side. Hips are usually flexed, abducted, and externally rotated; we have occasionally seen children with hips and knees in frank breech position. Knees may be fixed in the extension and the feet usually have severe, stiff clubfeet. In general, examination of the joints demonstrates a rigid block to motion with firm nonelastic endpoints.

Histologically, the muscles are very small and fibrotic with large amounts of fibrous and fatty deposition between the muscle fibers. Myopathic and neuropathic features can be noted in the muscles. The joints have severe ankylosis with dysplastic and contracted joint capsules with thickening and fibrosis of the ligaments and joint capsules. Intra-articular deposits of fibrocartilagenous material may accompany the contracted joint capsules and be a mechanical block to reduction in the hips (pulvinar) and the knees. As time progresses, joint motion is not likely to worsen. Eventually, 25% of patients will fail to develop ambulation due to stiffness of the joints and with variable weakness in the extremities.

Goals of treatment are identified in order to improve the lower limb alignment and allow ambulation. Upper extremity treatment may be geared with the goal to improve the ability of the hand to feed and assist with perineal care and with transfers. Physical therapy is important for increasing range of motion, which is started at an earlier age. Orthotics can be used to maintain a standing position and also to brace the upper and lower extremity into positions of functions. In general, surgical release of soft tissues is done at an earlier age in order to improve joint motion and correct deformity. It is not uncommon for initial surgical correction to be lost and then to require further surgical treatment to correct residual or recurrent deformity. However, bony operations such as osteotomy

or fusion are usually done at a later age to correct residual deformity.

Dislocation of the hip or dysplasia of the acetabulum may be noted in 60% of patients. In general, the goals of hip treatment are to improve motion and allow the hips to be in a functional position for standing and sitting. Maintaining a located hip based on radiographic presentation is less important; it is reasonable to accept bilaterally dislocated hips that are freely mobile without pain. On the other hand, patients with unilaterally dislocated hips generally do not function as well as in patients with bilaterally dislocated hips. Therefore, early efforts to reduce unilaterally displaced hips may be indicated by some surgeons. Open reduction via an anterior approach is used; femoral shortening may assist in reducing the head and in preventing avascular necrosis from surgery. Postoperative reduction is maintained with spica casting for a short period of time and in a position of extension to assist functional standing in the future.

As mentioned above, patients with arthrogryposis can have variable deformities of the knee, including flexion deformities, hyperextension, and dislocated knees. In general, patients with extension deformities of the knees do better than fixed flexion deformities, as the extended knee allows for reasonably good standing. Physical therapy and serial casting may be of some benefit in obtaining further knee flexion in the cases of fixed extension or hyperextension of the knee. It can be a challenge to determine the proper plane of knee motion for appropriate therapy and manipulation and casting. Gentle attempts of physiotherapy and casting are encouraged to avoid risks of fracture. Once 90° of knee motion is obtained a Pavlick harness may be used to maintain reduction. An organized strategy is needed in those patients with combinations of dislocated hips and hyperextension deformities of the knees with and without clubfoot deformities. In the short term, serial long leg casting may be of some benefit in reducing the clubfoot deformity and increasing knee flexion. After patients reach 1 year of age, consider simultaneous clubfoot release and quadriceps VY plasty to obtain final clubfoot correction and further knee flexion to 100°. Short-term immobilization (5 to 6 weeks) in a long leg cast is utilized and then converted to a short leg cast so that foot correction can be maintained and knee motion can be obtained with therapy. Once knee motion is stabilized, an anterior approach and open reduction with femoral shortening will be considered in patients with a unilaterally dislocated hip.

In general, knee flexion deformities greater than 30° tend to limit ambulatory ability. Therefore, soft tissue releases, including posterior release of the hamstring muscles and joint capsule are indicated. Many of these patients will have anterior joint fibrosis and, therefore an anterior release and removal of the pulvinar from the anterior aspect of the knee is needed to obtain full knee extension. In older patients with flexion deformities, a distal femoral extension osteotomy is reasonable. Other surgical options would include anterior hemiepiphyseal stapling in actively growing individuals or consideration for external fixation and gradual joint mobilization. Progressive stretching of the knee with external fixation will improve the extension of the knee but it must be done in a gradual fashion to avoid physeal fractures; unfortunately high recurrence rates are often noted.

Patients with arthrogryposis multiplex congenita usually present with a very severe clubfoot deformity that is rigid. Treatment goals for foot deformity are to have the foot flat to allow for weight bearing and ambulation. In general, nonoperative methods for complete treatment of this deformity are met with very little success. Other foot deformities are more likely seen in patients with distal arthrogryposis (such as congenital vertical talus). The standard clubfoot release that is needed differs from than used for the idiopathic clubfoot. For example, extensive capsular releases are always needed in arthrogryposis, and it is wise to resect portions of the extrinsic tendons to prevent recurrence of deformity. After surgery and 4 months of casting, patients should be immobilized in AFOs for several years to prevent recurrence. Patients with residual deformity may be candidates for a talectomy at a later age. In rare cases, the posterior medial lateral release and second stage talectomy does not completely correct the deformities. In these cases, distal tibia extension osteotomy may be useful with residual, stiff equinus deformity.

Upper extremity function in patients with arthrogryposis is usually limited due to the shoulder contracture with internal rotation and adducted; further upper extremity limitation is due to extension contractures of the elbows. In order to improve the ability to feed oneself, it is beneficial to obtain active elbow flexion of one elbow. Extensive release of the triceps contracture and improved elbow flexion is obtainable; however ultimate active elbow flexion may not be possible due to deficient motor muscle power. Treatment may be indicated if the patient has bilateral elbow extension contractures and good triceps or

pectoralis motor function. In these patients, efforts are made to improve joint range of motion by doing posterior capsulotomy, followed by muscle transfer of the triceps or pectoralis. In general, these surgeries work better in children who are greater than 4 to 5 years of age with 4+ power and who may be compliant with the occupational therapy. As in the lower extremity, humeral osteotomies can be used at a later date in order to improve the positioning of the arm for activities of daily living.

Approximately 30% of individuals with arthrogryposis will have scoliosis. They respond poorly to brace treatment and, in general, surgery is indicated for curves that are greater than 50°.

Larsen's Syndrome

Affected individuals with Larsen's syndrome have many of the same physical exam features as patients with arthrogryposis. Larsen's syndrome may be a sporadically occurring disorder or may be autosomal dominant or autosomal recessive in inheritance. The autosomal recessive form seems to be more severe than that found in the patients with autosomal dominant inheritance. Clinical features of patients with Larsen's syndrome include multiple large joint dislocations, ligamentous laxity, and flat facies. The joints that tend to be dislocated are the knees (Figure 8-11), elbows, and hips; in addition, many patients have clubfoot deformities. Importantly, patients have very severe cervical spine kyphosis. All patients with Larsen's syndrome should have regularly scheduled cervical spine screening radiographs. A certain portion of these patients will also develop scoliosis.

Treatment of these deformities depends on the degree of dislocation of each joint. In general, upper extremity deformities and dislocation are not treated. With time and development, affected patients adapt and learn to function well with the current disability. In the lower extremity, efforts are made to improve knee range of motion in order to stand and sit. This may involve serial casting to obtain knee flexion in those patients with extension contractures. Some patients will have normal motion but will have some instability and are best treated with a knee-ankle-foot orthosis (KAFO). Surgical reconstruction for ligamentous exam may be considered. Patients with Larsen's syndrome may also have hips affected with acetabular dysplasia, subluxation, or dislocation. Efforts to reduce hips at an early age through an anterior or anterior medial approach helps patients who are highly

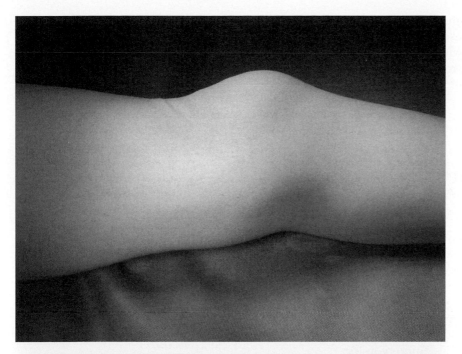

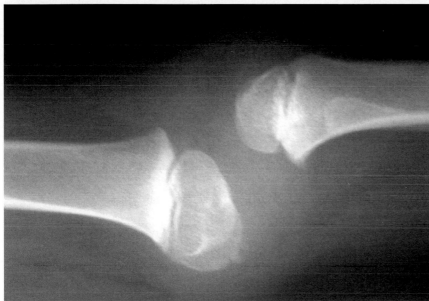

FIGURE 8-11. A 6-year-old boy with Larsen's syndrome and a dislocated knee.

functioning with a normal life span. Consideration for pelvic and femoral osteotomies may be needed in dislocated hips with severe acetabular dysplasia.

The clubfoot in Larsen's syndrome is less stiff than that in arthrogryposis multiplex congenita and is more amenable to nonoperative treatment with the Ponseti approach. Although initial improvement is probable with casting and manipulation, there may be some residual deformity, which will require later foot reconstruction or release. Alternatively, initial extensive posterior medial lateral release may be

preferred in these individuals. Try to obtain as much correction with casting before considering surgical release. Following surgery, an AFO may be beneficial for prevention of recurrent deformity.

All patients with Larsen's syndrome should have screening lateral radiographs to determine whether there is cervical kyphosis, which is apparent by radiographic midcervical kyphosis and hypoplasia of the vertebral bodies. This spinal deformity may be myelopathic and lead to complications, such as cord compromise or early death. In general, patients should be monitored for myelopathy and curve progression. In these instances, a posterior arthrodesis is indicated. With time, posterior tethering via a bone fusion will promote the cervical spine of the patient to grow into a more normal sagittal alignment.

Distal Arthrogryposis

Individuals with distal arthrogryposis have contractures of the hand and feet; the large joint dislocations and contractures seen in arthrogryposis multiplex congenita are usually not present. Patients may also have the facial flattening as seen in Larsen's syndrome. In the upper extremity, patients with distal arthrogryposis will have ulnar deviation of the fingers and flexion deformities of the IP joints. The hand has been described as a cup-like palm. Individuals with distal arthrogryposis may have severe foot deformities, including metatarsus adductus, congenital vertical talus, or clubfoot deformities. Surgery in the upper extremity is useful to improve hand function by lengthening the flexor tendons and rebalancing the extensor tendons. In general, patients with distal arthrogryposis have more severe foot deformities than hand deformities. Foot deformities in distal arthrogryposis are slightly more amenable to conservative management then in arthrogryposis multiplex congenita. Treatment of clubfeet starts with a series of clubfoot casting to try to obtain as much correction as possible. Recurrence rates seem to be less in patients with distal arthrogryposis than those in the standard arthrogryposis multiplex congenita.

Annotated Bibliography

Cerebral Palsy

Bleck EE. Cerebral Palsy. Oxford, UK: MacKeith, 1987.
A complete review of evaluation and treatment of cerebral palsy with details of the author's preferred treatment.

Bleck EE. Forefoot problems in cerebral palsy—diagnosis and management. Foot Ankle 1984;4:188.
A concise review of this often neglected topic. A good overview with concrete suggestions for management.

Boachie-Adjei O, Lonstein JE, Winter RB et al. Management of neuromuscular spinal deformities with Luque segmental instrumentation. J Bone Joint Surg 1989;71A:548.
Average 3-year follow-up of 46 patients with neuromuscular scoliosis. Twenty-two of the 46 patients with neuromuscular scoliosis. Twenty-two of the 46 patients (48%) had cerebral palsy. The authors discuss the indication for surgery, need for pelvic extension of the instrumentation and fusion, role of postoperative immobilization, role of two-stage procedures, and complications in this most difficult group of patients.

Broom MJ, Banta JV, Renshaw TS. Spinal fusion augmented by Luque-rod segmental instrumentation for neuromuscular scoliosis. J Bone Joint Surg 1989;71A:32.
Although less than half of the patients in the series had cerebral palsy, this diagnosis accounted for the largest group. With a mean follow-up of 42 months, the authors demonstrate that Luque rod segmental instrumentation with posterior spinal instrumentation is an effective treatment for patients with neuromuscular scoliosis. Failure rates were higher when 3/16-inch rods were used, and functional kyphosis occurred above the fusion when it did not extend to the upper thoracic spine.

Castle ME, Scheider C. Proximal femoral resection-interposition arthroplasty. J Bone Joint Surg 1978;60A:1051.
A simple procedure to relieve pain and maintain sitting position in severely involved patients with dislocated hips is described.

Evans EB. Knee flexion deformity in cerebral palsy. AAOS Instruct Course Lect 1971;20:42.
An extensive discussion of an approach to the evaluation and treatment of knee deformities in cerebral palsy.

Ferguson RL, Allen BL. Considerations in the treatment of cerebral palsy patients with spinal deformities. Orthop Clin North Am 1999;19:419.
Review article covering all aspects of decision making with regard to spinal deformity in patients with cerebral palsy.

Gage JR, Fabian D, Hicks R, Tashman S. Pre- and postoperative gait analysis in patients with spastic diplegia: a preliminary report. J Pediatr Orthop 1984;4:715.
A study of 20 patients with diplegia preoperatively and 6 to 18 months postoperatively. This article shows the potential benefits of gait analysis in a group of patients with complex gait abnormalities. By gait analysis criteria, 13 patients were improved, 6 were unchanged, and 1 was worsened by surgery.

Gersoff WK, Renshaw TS. The treatment of scoliosis in cerebral palsy by posterior spinal fusion with Luque-rod segmental instrumentation. J Bone Joint Surg 1988;70A:41.
Review of 33 patients with cerebral palsy who underwent posterior spinal fusion from Luque rod instrumentation at a mean follow-up of 40 months. Luque rodding accompanying posterior spinal fusion allows safe correction of the deformity, maintenance of correction, and achievement of a solid spinal fusion with minimal complications.

Hoffer MM. Management of the hip in cerebral palsy. J Bone Joint Surg 1986;68A:629.
A quick review of the range of treatments and indications for treatment of spastic hip subluxation and dislocation.

Hoffer MM, Koffman M. Cerebral palsy: the first three years. Clin Orthop 1980;151:222.
This article explicates the surgeon's role in treating the infant and young child. The comments on physical therapy are enlightening.

Hoffer MM, Stein GA, Koffman M et al. Femoral varus derotational osteotomy in spastic cerebral palsy. J Bone Joint Surg 1985;67A:1229.
The indications for and outcomes of this commonly performed procedure in 20 patients are presented. Good results, including decreased pain and maintained walking ability were found.

Kudrjavcev T, Schoenberg BS, Kurland LT, Groover RV. Cerebral palsy: survival rates, associated handicaps and distribution by clinical subtype (Rochester, MN, 1950–1976). Neurology 1985;35:900.
This review of a cohort of cerebral palsy children in Rochester, Minnesota, emphasizes the correlation between intelligence and survival and the common resolution of mild motor deficits.

Lonstein JE. Deformities of the spine in children with cerebral palsy. Orthop Rev 1981;10:33.
This article discusses incidence of scoliosis in cerebral palsy and methods of management, including seating orthoses, bracing, and surgery.

Madigan RR, Wallace SL. Scoliosis in the institutionalized cerebral palsy population. Spine 1981;6:583.
This article discusses the magnitude of the problem of scoliosis mainly in spastic quadriplegics and emphasizes the pattern of curve, the association of severe curves with severe motor involvement, and the lack of correlation of curve with hip dislocation.

Nelson KB, Ellenberg JH. Antecedents of cerebral palsy. N Engl J Med 1986;315:381.
An excellent review of factors associated with cerebral palsy derived from the study of 54,000 consecutive births at several institutions. The major predictive factors were maternal mental retardation, birth weight below 2,001 g, and fetal malformation. Breech presentation was a predictor, whereas breech delivery was not.

Neville BGR. Selective dorsal rhizotomy for spastic cerebral palsy. Dev Med Child Neurol 1988;30:391.
A quick, evenhanded review of status of this procedure at the time of its writing.

Peacock WJ, Arens LJ. Selective posterior rhizotomy for the relief of spasticity in cerebral palsy. Afr Med J 1982;62:119.
Excellent results in 15 patients with short follow-ups are presented. Indications and surgical technique are discussed.

Perry J, Hoffer MM. Pre- and postoperative dynamic electromyography as an aid in planning tendon transfers in children with cerebral palsy. J Bone Joint Surg 1977;59A:531.
A classic study demonstrating the use of dynamic EMG in improving outcomes of surgery especially about the foot and ankle for the common equinovarus deformity as well as other deformities.

Phelps WM. Long-term results of orthopaedic surgery in cerebral palsy. J Bone Joint Surg 1957;39A:53.
This is a rare long-term follow-up in cerebral palsy of 242 patients who had 500 operations. This article is part of the basis of pessimism in orthopaedic surgical treatment of this disorder. A high rate of failure of soft tissue surgery was found. Bone surgery was recommended as more predictable and lasting. The difficulty in effecting improvement in athetoids is emphasized.

Root L, Spero CR. Hip adductor transfer compared with adductor tenotomy in cerebral palsy. J Bone Joint Surgery 1981; 63A:767.
A rare study comparing two procedures at one institution is reported. Overall better results were found with adductor transfer.

Shoff H, Woodbury DF. Management of the upper extremity in cerebral palsy. J Bone Joint Surg 1985;67A:500.
A brief review of this difficult area. This article emphasizes patient selection criteria and offers specific treatment recommendations.

Sutherland DH. Gait Disorders in Childhood and Adolescence. Baltimore: Williams & Wilkins, 1984.
A classic that includes normative data as well as pathologic data on gait in cerebral palsy and other neuromuscular disorders.

Sutherland DH, Cooper L. The pathomechanics of progressive crouch gait in spastic diplegia. Orthop Clin North Am 1978; 9:143.
A superb investigation into the cause of crouch gait emphasizing the primacy of weakness of the triceps surae resulting from over lengthening of the Achilles tendon in causing this problem.

Sutherland DH, Schottstaedt ER, Larsen LJ et al. Clinical and electromyographic study of seven spastic children with internal rotation gait. J Bone Joint Surg 1969;51A:1070.
This article thoughtfully, carefully, and with explicit assumptions evaluates the clinical outcomes of treatment in this difficult patient population. Although derotational osteotomy is commonly done for internal rotation deformity, this is an excellent article exemplifying an approach to treatment and documentation of results.

Thometz JG, Simon SR. Progression of scoliosis after skeletal maturity in institutionalized adults who have cerebral palsy. J Bone Joint Surg 1988;70A:1290.
This study discusses the natural history after maturity of scolitic curves in cerebral palsy. More rapid curve progression was found in those patients with greater than 50° curves at maturity.

Winter DA. Pathologic gait diagnosis with computer-averaged electromyographic profiles. Arch Phys Med Rehab 1984;65:393.
This article has an excellent discussion of the limitations of dynamic EMGs as presently performed.

Myelomeningocele

Asher M, Olson J. Factors affecting the ambulatory status of patients with spina bifida cystica. J Bone Joint Surg 1983;65A:350.
A careful assessment of factors affecting ambulatory status in 98 patients is presented. Overall, all sacral and L5-level patients walked; thoracic through L3-level patients were general not functional ambulators.

Bazih J, Gross RH. Hip surgery in the lumbar level myelomeningocele patient. J Pediatr Orthop 1981;1:405.
This series investigated the effect of hip stability on function in 24 patients. Of those undergoing surgery to stabilize the hip, 45% failed. No functional improvement was found because of hips being located. The worst function by level were those having complications following hip surgery, mainly stiffness.

Bliss DG, Menelaus MD. The results of transfer of the tibialis anterior to the heel in patients who have a myelomeningocele. J Bone Joint Surg 1986;68A:1258.
A long-term follow-up of 46 transfers to avoid or treat the disabling calcaneus deformity resulting from triceps surae weakness. Several overcorrections requiring further surgery occurred, prompting the recommendation that spastic anterior tibialis muscles not be transferred to the calcaneus.

Bunch WH, Hakala MW. Iliopsoas transfers in children with myelomeningocele. J Bone Joint Surg 1984;66A:224.
This article describes the results of iliopsoas transfer to the greater trochanter with adductor longus weakening. Good results with few complications are presented. The authors recommended this surgical procedure to balance muscle forces about the hip and maintain hip reduction.

Dias LS, Jasty JM, Collins P. Rotational deformities of the lower limb in myelomeningocele. J Bone Joint Surg 1984;66A:215.
An excellent review of the treatment and complications of the common rotational deformities seen in ambulatory patients. Fifty children are described with 66 limbs treated. A significant number of complications occurred in tibia derotational osteotomies.

Feiwell E, Saker D, Blatt T. The effect of hip reduction on function in patients with myelomeningocele. J Bone Joint Surg 1978;60A:169.
A study of 76 patients was done with 41 patients having had no surgery on the hip and 35 having had attempts to surgically stabilize the hip. No difference in functional abilities or pain was found regardless of whether the hip was located, subluxated, or dislocated. Complications from surgery occurred in 40% of patients. A level pelvis and free hip motion were important for function.

Hall P, Lindseth R, Campbell R et al. Scoliosis and hydrocephalus in myelocele patients: the effects of ventricular shunting. J Neurosurg 1979;50:174.
Progressive scoliosis may be due to shunt malfunction. The importance of neurologic examinations at each visit is stressed.

Hoffer MM, Feiwell E, Perry R et al. Functional ambulation in patients with myelomeningocele. J Bone Joint Surg 1973;55A:137.
A review of 56 patients revealed no functional ambulators at the thoracic level and all functional ambulators at the sacral level. Lumbar level patient's walking abilities were affected by level (high, versus low), age, mental retardation, lower extremity deformities, and social situations.

Hydemann JS, Gillespie R. Management of myelomeningocele kyphosis in the older child by kyphectomy and segmental spine instrumentation. Spine 1986;12:37.

Short-term review of 12 patients treated by kyphectomy and segmental spinal instrumentation. The authors present a method of anterior fixation of the pelvis.

Lindseth RE. Treatment of the lower extremity in children paralyzed by myelomeningocele (birth to 18 months). AAOS Instruct Course Lect 1976;25:76.
A review of the early treatment of MMC with descriptive data on a large population of affected children. A simplified scheme for classifying the functional neurologic level is presented.

Lindseth RE, Stelzer L Jr. Vertebral excision for kyphosis in children with myelomeningocele. J Bone Joint Surg 1979;61A:699.
A method of kyphectomy is presented that allows continued growth of the remaining lumbar spine.

Malhotra D, Puri R, Owen R. Valgus deformity of the ankle in children with spina bifida aperta. J Bone Joint Surg 1984; 66B:381.
A review of valgus deformity of the hind foot that emphasizes that the valgus can exist in the ankle joint, subtalar joint, or both.

Mazur J, Menelaus MB, Dickens DRV et al. Efficacy of surgical management for scoliosis in myelomeningocele: correction of deformity and alteration of functional status. J Pediatr Orthop 1986;6:568.
The authors evaluated the effect of spinal fusion in 49 patients with MMC. Combined anterior interbody fusion and posterior fusion and instrumentation to the sacrum gave the best results with respect to correction of the deformity; however, the ability to ambulate was adversely affected.

McMaster MJ. Anterior and posterior instrumentation and fusion of thoracolumbar scoliosis due to myelomeningocele. J Bone Joint Surg 1987;69B:20.
The author demonstrates improved posture and function in 21 of 23 patients with MMC scoliosis treated by anterior and posterior spinal instrumentation and fusion. Indications, operative techniques, and complications are discussed.

McMaster MJ. The long-term results of kyphectomy and spinal stabilization in children with myelomeningocele. Spine 1988; 13:417.
A small series of 10 patients treated by kyphectomy and various forms of instrumentation for MMC kyphosis and followed for a mean of 7 years is presented. A long fusion from the midthoracic region to the sacrum was necessary to provide long-term stability and to prevent the development of thoracic lordosis. Operative techniques, risks, and complications are discussed.

Menelaus MB. The Orthopaedic Management of Spina Bifida Cystica. New York: Churchill Livingstone, 1980.
An excellent single source for all aspects of the aggressive treatment of this disorder derived from a large clinical experience in Melbourne, Australia.

Menelaus MB. Talectomy for equinovarus deformity in arthrogryposis and spina bifida. J Bone Joint Surg 1971;53B:468.
This study followed 41 operations in 23 children an average of 2.5 years. Principles, indications, and techniques are discussed in this short follow-up that recommends talectomy for rigid neuromuscular clubfeet.

Osebold WR, Mayfield JK, Winter RB, Moe JH. Surgical treatment of paralytic scoliosis associated with myelomeningocele. J Bone Joint Surg 1982;64A:841.
Series discussing results and evolution of treatment of scoliosis in meningomyelocele.

Samuelsson L, Eklof O. Scoliosis in myelomeningocele. Acta Orthop Scand 1988;59:122.
Review of the prevalence, type, and magnitude of scoliosis in 163 patients with MMC. Of the 163 patients 143 developed scoliosis, 21 (15%) of which were congenital in origin. Scoliosis severity increased with higher neurologic level (particularly above L3) and increasing age. Curve direction correlated with pelvic obliquity but not with hip dislocation.

Sharrard WJW. The orthopedic surgery of spina bifida. Clin Orthop 1973;92:195.
A general review of evaluation and treatment of MMC by an author with a large experience. Not all procedures described are popular now, but the approach is current.

Stillwell A, Menelaus MM. Walking ability in mature patients with spina bifida. J Pediatr Orthop 1983;3:184.
One-third of high lumbar and thoracic level patients were community ambulators in this study. This is the only report with a large number of high level patients maintaining functional walking.

Trumble T, Banta JV, Raoycroft JF et al. Talectomy for equinus deformity in myelodysplasia. J Bone Joint Surg 1985; 67A:21.
Nine patients had 17 feet corrected by talectomy. Follow-up averaged 7.4 years. Nearly all had good hind foot correction, but one-half had poor forefoot correction.

Yugue DA, Lindseth RE. Effectiveness of muscle transfers in myelomeningocele hips measured by radiographic images. J Pediatr Orthop 1982;2:121.
These authors recommend external oblique transfer to the greater trochanter and adductor transfer to the ischium to balance muscle forces about the hip. Good results are reported. The results of other procedures are desired.

Arthrogryposis Multiplex Congenita

Daher YH, Lonstein JE, Winter RB, Moe JH. Spinal deformities in patients with arthrogryposis: a review of 16 patients. Spine 1985;10:609.
Literature review and results of management of a small group of patients with arthrogryposis.

Drummond DS, Cruess RL. The management of the foot and ankle in arthrogryposis multiplex congenita. J Bone Joint Surg 1978;60B:96.
The range of treatment options is discussed. The use of primary talectomy in severe, rigid clubfoot deformities is emphasized. Follow-up to near skeletal maturity in most patients was available.

Drummond DS, MacKenzie DA. Scoliosis in arthrogryposis: multiplex congenita. J Bone Joint Surg 1978;60B:96.
In 14 patients with scoliosis, both congenital scoliosis and long C-shaped curves were observed. Progression to severe and rigid curves was typical.

Gibson DA, Urs ND. Arthrogryposis multiplex congenita. J Bone Joint Surg 1970;52B:493.
An excellent review of 114 patients treated over a 15-year period. Multiple tables help organize the complex problems and treatment of these patients.

Herron LD, Westin GW, Dawson EG. Scoliosis in arthrogryposis: multiplex congenita. J Bone Joint Surg 1978;60A:293.
Scoliosis in 18 of 88 patients with AMC was found. The curves were commonly thoracolumbar and tended to progress early despite brace or cast treatment.

Hoffer MM, Swank S, Clark D et al. Ambulation in severe arthrogryposis. J Pediatr Orthop 1983;3:293.
This article outlines criteria for identifying nonambulators, which is important in developing a treatment plan for severely involved patients.

Lloyd-Roberts GC, Lettin AWF. Arthrogryposis multiplex congenita. J Bone Joint Surg 1970;52B:494.
A review of treatment and results in 52 patients. Treatment to gain functional range in the first year is emphasized. Soft tissue rather than bone procedures are recommended in the young child.

Menelaus MB. Talectomy for equinovarus deformity in arthrogryposis and spina bifida. J Bone Joint Surg 1971;53B:468.

An in-depth discussion of the indications, technique, and complications of talectomy. The results of 41 operations are reviewed, but follow-up is short (average of 2.5 years).

Williams P. The management of arthrogryposis. Orthop Clin North Am 1978;9:67.
An aggressive, early surgical approach is presented in detail.

Wynne-Davies R, Williams PF, O'Connor JCB. The 1960's epidemic of arthrogryposis multiplex congenita. J Bone Joint Surg 1981;63B:76.
This article describes the epidemiology of this disorder. Specifically, the high number of new cases presenting in the 1960s is documented. This suggests an environmental factor as part or all of the etiology.

Muscular Dystrophies

Bieber FR, Hoffman EP, Amos JA. Dystrophin analysis in duchenne muscular dystrophy: use in fetal diagnosis and in genetic counseling. Am J Hum Genet 1989;45:362.
The use of dystrophin assay to identify an affected fetus and establish carrier status in the mother is presented. A discussion of the general use of dystrophin analysis is presented.

Brooke MH. A Clinician's View of Neuromuscular Diseases. Baltimore: Williams & Wilkins, 1986.
A superb clinician's extensive experience with the muscular dystrophies and other neuromuscular disorders is detailed in this relatively short book.

Brooke MH, Fenichel GM, Griggs RC et al. Duchenne Muscular dystrophy: patterns of clinical progression and effects of supportive therapy. Neurology 1989;39:475.
A detailed analysis of 283 boys enrolled in a prospective study. Best available data on natural history and effects of intervention except surgery of lower extremities, which was not included in the analysis.

Gutmann DH, Fischbeck KH. Molecular biology of Duchenne and Becker's muscular dystrophy: clinical applications. Ann Neurol 1989;26:189.
A review of the research that lead to the identification of the defective gene product in Duchenne and Becker muscular dystrophy. Clinical implications are discussed.

Harper PS. Congenital myotonic dystrophy in Britain. I and II. Arch Dis Child 1975;50:505.
A description of congenital myotonic dystrophy. This disorder often requires treatment of foot deformities in infancy.

Hsu JD. The natural history of spine curvature progression in the nonambulatory Duchenne muscular dystrophy patient. Spine 1983;8:771.
When the curve progresses beyond 40°, patients experience loss of sitting balance, decreased sitting tolerance, pain, decreased vital capacity, and need to use hands and arms to prop the body. Surgery is indicated to prevent these problems.

Kurz LT, Mubarak SJ, Schultz P et al. Correlation of scoliosis and pulmonary function in Duchenne muscular dystrophy. J Pediatr Orthop 1983;3:347.
Forced vital capacity peaks at the age when standing ceases. It decreased by 4% each year and with each 10-degree increase in curvature. Early spinal instrumentation is indicated to slow rate of decline of forced vital capacity.

Miller F, Moseley CF, Koreska J et al. Pulmonary function and scoliosis in Duchenne dystrophy. J Pediatr Orthop 1988;8:133.
Pulmonary function (forced vital capacity) declines most rapidly during adolescent growth spurt. Surgery does not influence the rate of pulmonary function deterioration.

Siegel IM. Diagnosis, management, and orthopaedic treatment of muscular dystrophy. AAOS Instruct Course Lect 1981;30:3.
A detailed review of the orthopaedic management of muscular dystrophy. Diagnostic information is largely outdated.

Smith AD, Koreska J, Moseley CF. Progression of scoliosis in Duchenne muscular dystrophy. J Bone Joint Surg 1989;71A:1066.
Longitudinal study of 51 boys with Duchenne muscular dystrophy followed until death without surgical treatment. All patients developed scoliosis and severe curves led to difficulty sitting, skin breakdown, and pain. When the curve exceeded 35°, the vital capacity usually was less than 40% of predicted. Spinal arthrodesis should be considered when walking becomes impossible.

Swaiman KF, Smith SA, Swaiman AF, eds. Progressive Muscular Dystrophies in Pediatric Neurology: Principles and Practice. St. Louis: CV Mosby 1989:1105.
A concise, readable review of clinical characteristics and diagnosis of these disorders.

Vignos PJ, Wagner MB, Kaplan JS et al. Predicting the success of reambulation in patients with Duchenne muscular dystrophy. J Bone Joint Surg 1983;65A:719.
A detailed approach to the selection of patients for bracing and surgery is presented.

Weimann RL, Gibson DA, Mosely CF et al. Surgical stabilization of the spine in Duchenne muscular dystrophy. Spine 1983;8:776.
Results in 24 patients with Duchenne muscular dystrophy. Discussion of natural history, curve progression and results of early surgery.

Spinal Muscular Atrophy

Aprin H, Bowen JR, MacEwen GD et al. Spine fusion in patients with spinal muscular atrophy. J Bone Joint Surg 1982;64A:1179.
A report of 22 surgical fusions. Bracing was ineffective in halting progression preoperatively. Several techniques were employed. A high rate of complications occurred.

Emery AEH. The nosology of the spinal muscular atrophies. J Med Genet 1971;8:481.
A dense review of the history and classification of these disorders and the progressive muscular dystrophies.

Evans GA, Drennan JC, Russman BS. Functional classification and orthopaedic management of spinal muscular atrophy. J Bone Joint Surg 1981;63B:516.
Fifty-four patients formed the basis of a functional grouping with differences in natural history and orthopaedic treatment among the groups. An explicit, detailed approach to the management of spine and lower extremity deformities is presented.

Schwentker EP, Gibson DA. The orthopaedic aspects of spinal muscular atrophy. J Bone Joint Surg 1976;58A:32.
Excellent review of orthopaedic problems in 50 patients with a mean age of 11.5 years. Scoliosis is the major problem with timing of surgery and complications discussed in detail. Loss of function is common after spinal stabilization. Release of lower extremity contractures is discussed.

Swaiman KF. Anterior horn cell and cranial motor neuron disease. Pediatr Neurology: Principles and Practice. St Louis: CV Mosby, 1989:1086.
A brief review of the clinical characteristics, diagnosis and pathology of these disorders.

Friedreich's Ataxia

Cady RB, Bobechko WP. Incidence, natural history and treatment of scoliosis in Friedreich's ataxia. J Pediatr Orthop 1984;4:673.
This report on 42 patients found relentless progression even after skeletal maturity, suggesting a more typical neuromuscular scoliosis that suggested in the reference by Labelle and associates in patients with this disorder.

Chamberlain S, Shaw J, Wallis J et al. Genetic homogeneity at the Friedreich ataxia locus on chromosome 9. Am J Hum Genet 1989;44:518.

Two populations with clinically different Friedreich ataxia (French Canadians and Acadians from Louisiana) were investigated by genetic linkage and found to have the same or nearly the same locus of gene abnormality on chromosome 9. This type of investigation will doubtless refine classification and improve prognostication in the future.

Labelle H, Tohme S, Duhaime JM et al. Natural history of scoliosis in Friedriech's ataxia. J Bone Joint Surg 1986;68A:564.
A follow-up of 78 patients showing similar curve pattern and progression to that found in idiopathic scoliosis. No correlation of curve progression with weakness was found. Early age of disease onset and presence of scoliosis before puberty correlated with progressive curves. Virtually all patients had curves of 10° or more.

Levitt RL, Canale ST, Cooke AJ Jr et al. The role of foot surgery in progressive neuromuscular disorders in children. J Bone Joint Surg 1973;55A:1396.
This article reemphasizes the need for triple arthrodesis to obtain and maintain a stable foot in this disorder.

Makin M. The surgical management of Friedreich's ataxia. J Bone Joint Surg 1953;35A:425.
A review of 34 patients undergoing foot surgery with an average follow-up of 7.2 years. Good results are reported using subtalar or triple arthrodesis to stabilize the foot. Tendon transfers were used as needed for foot muscle balance and toe deformities.

Hereditary Motor Sensory Neuropathies

Coleman SS. The cavo varus foot. In: Complex Foot Deformities in Children. Philadelphia: Lea & Febiger, 1983.
A thoughtful and rational approach to treatment of cavo varus. It emphasizes the different treatment options available depending on whether the hind foot is correctable or fixed in varus.

Jacobs JE, Carr CR. Progressive muscular atrophy of the peroneal type (Charcot-Marie-Tooth disease). J Bone Joint Surg 1950; 32A:27.
Forty-five patients having had foot surgery are reviewed. Sixty-six good results and 23 unsatisfactory results were obtained using a combination of soft tissue and bony procedures.

Levitt RL, Canale ST, Cooke AJ et al. The role of foot surgery in progressive neuromuscular disorders in children. J Bone Joint Surg 1973;55A:1396.
Fifteen patients with Charcot-Marie-Tooth disease or Friedriech's ataxia with foot deformity were reviewed. Soft tissue and bone procedures other than triple arthrodesis failed to maintain correction.

Smith SA. Peripheral neuropathies in children. In: Swaiman KF, ed. Pediatric Neurology: Principles and Practice. St Louis: CV Mosby, 1989:1110.
A brief review of the present classification of these disorders.

Wetmore RS, Drennan JC. Long-term results of triple arthrodesis in Charcot-Marie-Tooth disease. J Bone Joint Surg 1989;71A:417.
Thirty triple arthrodesis were followed an average of 21 years. Fourteen (47%) were considered poor results. Some bad results seem secondary to disease progression, but arthritis in adjacent joints and recurrent deformity were common. Attempts to maintain foot position without fusion seemed warranted in light of these results.

9

José A. Morcuende
Matthew B. Dobbs

Idiopathic and Heritable Disorders

A genetic and molecular revolution is happening in medicine. Lead by the Human Genome Project, genetic information and concepts are changing the way disease is defined, diagnoses are made, and treatment strategies are developed. The profound implications of actually understanding the molecular abnormalities of many clinical problems are affecting virtually all medical and surgical disciplines. Importantly, genetic technologies will increasingly drive biomedical research and the practice of medicine in the near future.

Those interested in the musculoskeletal system must be aware of the genetic cause of its inherited disorders in order to make appropriate referrals for genetic counseling and to refine the prognosis and natural history in each individual patient. Current management revolves around treatment to prevent or minimize medical complications, psychosocial support of patients and their families, and modification of the environment where appropriate. Gene discoveries will allow the development of tests to detect disease or to quantify the risk of disease. Furthermore, applying this knowledge is the best hope for developing strategies to modify the pathologic effect of the gene (drug therapy), repair the gene (gene therapy), or for approaches to restore lost or affected tissue (tissue engineering).

Instead of an empiric trial-and-error approach to therapy, it may become feasible to tailor treatment to the specific molecular malfunction.

Given the large number of inherited musculoskeletal abnormalities and the power and speed of current genetic and developmental biology information, a few selected disorders will be discussed in this chapter. The discussion will address general concepts on the genetic bases of musculoskeletal disorders, current classifications, and it will focus on the clinical characteristics of some of the most common disorders, including natural history and treatment options, and it will reflect the most recent developments in the understanding of their pathogenesis.

THE GENETIC BASES OF MUSCULOSKELETAL DISORDERS

The vertebrate skeleton is a fascinating and complex organ system, composed of 206 bones with many different shapes and sizes. Like every other organ system, the skeleton has specific developmental and functional characteristics that define its identity in biologic and pathologic terms. For normal skeletogenesis to take place, the coordination of temporal and spatial gene expression patterns is a crucial prerequisite. Any disturbances in these processes will lead to abnormalities of the skeleton.

The development of an adult organism from a single cell is an unparalleled example of integrated cell behavior. After fecundation, the single cell divides many times to produce the trillions of cells of the organism, which form structures as complex and varied as the eyes, limbs, heart, or the brain. Development is essentially the emergence of organized and specialized structures from an initially very simple group of cells. Therefore, during development, differences are generated in the embryo that leads to spatial organization, changes in form, and the generation of different cell types. Since each cell has the same genetic instructions, it must interpret this information with regard to time and space.

The vertebrate skeleton is formed by mesenchymal cells condensing into tissue elements outlining the pattern of future bones (the patterning phase). Shortly thereafter, cells within these condensations differentiate along the chondrocytic pathway. Subsequent growth generates cartilage models (anlagen)

of the future bones. The cartilage anlagen will be replaced by bone and bone marrow in a process called endochondral ossification. Finally, a process of growth and remodeling will result in a skeleton that is well adapted to its function as an organ not only for movement and internal organ protection, but also for blood cell production and regulation of calcium homeostasis.

Pattern Formation

Pattern formation is the process by which spatial and temporal arrangements of cell activities are organized within the embryo so that a well-defined structure develops. Pattern formation is critical for the proper development of every part of the organism. In the developing limb, for example, pattern formation enables the cells to know whether to make the upper arm or the fingers, and where the muscles should form.

Pattern formation in many animals is based on a mechanism where the cells first acquire a positional identity, which determines their future behavior. The ability of cells to sense their relative positions within a limited population of cells and to differentiate according to this position has been the subject of intense research. Interestingly, pattern formation in many systems has similar principles, and more striking, similar genes. It is essentially pattern formation—the size, shape, number, and arrangement of the bones—that makes human beings different from rabbits or chimpanzees.

Cell Differentiation

Cell differentiation is the process by which cells become structurally and functionally different from each other, ending up as distinct types as osteoblasts, chondrocytes, or muscle cells. Because each cell of the organism has the same genetic material, the achievement and persistence of the differentiation state depends on a series of signals that ultimately control the transcription of specific genes. In humans, the zygote gives rise to about 250 clearly distinguishable cell types.

In any organism, differentiation leads to the production of a finite number of discrete kinds of cells, each with its peculiar repertory of biochemical activities and possible morphological configurations. When cells achieve a distinctive state of differentiation, they do not transform into cells of another type. Differentiation leads to a stable, irreversible set of cellular activities.

Mutations in early patterning genes cause disorders called dysostoses: these disorders affect only specific skeletal elements, leaving the rest of the skeleton largely unaffected. In contrast, mutations in genes that are involved primarily in cell differentiation cause disorders called osteochondrodysplasias, which affect the development and growth of most skeletal elements in a generalized fashion. Many genes have important functions in both of these processes so that some inherited disorders can display features of both dysostoses and osteochondrodysplasias. Genes used during skeletal development may also be important in other organs so that when mutated, the resulting skeletal defects are part of a syndrome.

CLASSIFICATION OF MUSCULOSKELETAL DISORDERS

Broadly defined, birth defects or congenital abnormalities occur in 6% of all live births. Twenty percent of infant deaths are due to congenital anomalies. About 3% of newborns have significant structural abnormalities. At present, the cause of approximately 50 to 60% of birth defects is unknown. Chromosomal abnormalities account for 6 to 7% of the abnormalities. Specific gene mutations cause 7 to 8%. Environmental teratogens are responsible for 7 to 10% of defects. Combined genetic predisposition with environmental factors causes the remaining 20 to 25 % of congenital abnormalities.

Genetic disorders of the skeleton comprise a large group of clinically distinct and genetically heterogeneous conditions comprising more than 150 forms. Although individually rare, the different forms produce a significant number of affected individuals, with significant mortality and morbidity. Clinical manifestations range from neonatal lethality to congenital malformations, spinal and limb deformities to only mild growth retardation. Importantly, secondary complications such as early degenerative joint disease and extraskeletal organ involvement add to the burden of the disease.

Their clinical diversity makes these disorders often difficult to diagnose, and many attempts have been made to delineate single entities or groups of diseases to facilitate the diagnosis. As mentioned earlier skeletal disorders have been subdivided traditionally into dysostoses, defined as malformations of individual bones or groups of bones; and osteochondrodysplasias, defined as developmental disorders of cartilage and bone. The criteria used for their distinction has been based on a combination of clinical, radiographic, morphologic, and, in a few instances, biochemical characteristics. The modes of genetic inheritance and extraskeletal abnormalities have also been used.

Over the past 10 years, this initial broad clinical classification has progressed to the present reconsideration and regrouping of the disorders according to their molecular pathogenesis. The International Working Group on the Classification of Constitutional Disorders of Bone updated the classification in 2001. The major change was the addition of genetically determined dysostoses to the skeletal dysplasias. However, it is now becoming increasingly clear that several distinctive classifications are needed that reflect, on the one hand the molecular pathology, and on the other, the clinical signs and symptoms. Several reviews of the rapidly changing molecular basis of the skeletal dysplasias have been published, focusing either on a molecular-pathogenetic classification; on more specific aspects such as transcriptional deregulation; or on a combination of molecular-pathology and developmental biology of the musculoskeletal system. These new concepts directly link the clinical phenotype to key cellular processes of skeletal biology and should assist in providing a framework accessible to clinicians as well as basic scientists for future understanding of these disorders. It is likely that future insights will lead to reclassification.

With this regard, the "Nomenclature and Classification of the Osteochondrodysplasias," now called "Nosology," has been recently revised to reflect the molecular and pathogenetic abnormalities underlying these disorders. This classification uses similar criteria to those of the functional classification proposed in the 8th edition of *The Metabolic and Molecular Bases of Inherited Disease.*

Numerous online services allow access to public information and services relevant to the genetics of musculoskeletal disorders. One database that contains a wealth of clinical and genetic data is the Online Mendelian Inheritance in Man (OMIM). It provides free text overviews of genetic disorders and gene loci, with the correspondent mouse correlate. In general, congenital abnormalities of non-Mendelian inheritance, chromosomal abnormalities, and single case reports are not included. The total number of entries exceeds 11,000, but most importantly, it is linked to a wealth of other genetic databases allowing the users to obtain information on gene structure, map location, function, phenotype, or literature references. It is found at http://www3.ncbi.nlm.nih.gov/entrez/query.fcgi ?db/OMIM.

The logical extension of the recent success in the field of skeletal dysplasias is to establish precisely what the products of the affected genes do during skeletal development and how mutations disturb these functions to produce the characteristic phenotype. Despite the many hypotheses generated from the work in human genetics and the knowledge that has been gained from animal models, there remains a relatively poor understanding of how these genes interfere with skeletal development. Unraveling this mystery and defining it in molecular and cellular terms will be the challenge for the near future.

CLINICAL EVALUATION

With the increased availability of ultrasonographic prenatal screening, more patients with skeletal dysplasias are being diagnosed before birth. When there is suspicion of a skeletal dysplasia on ultrasound, the femoral length is the best biometric parameter. Further testing may be performed, if indicated, by chorionic villous sampling and mutation analysis.

Most skeletal dysplasias result in short stature, defined as height more than two standard deviations below the mean for the population at a given age. The resultant growth disproportion is commonly referred to as "short trunk" or "short limb." The short-limb types are further subdivided into categories based on the segment of the limb that is affected. Rhizomelic refers to shortening of the proximal part of the limb; mesomelic refers to the middle segment; and acromelic to the distal segment.

In evaluating a patient with short stature or abnormal bone development, several aspects of the medical history and the physical exam should be investigated. A history of heart disease, respiratory difficulty, immune deficiency, precocious puberty, and malabsorption should be sought because they are associated with some of these disorders. Birth length, head circumference, and weight should be recorded, and pertinent family history of short stature or dimorphism should be sought. The height and weight percentile should be determined using standard charts. The physical examination should include careful characterization of the patient facies, and presence of cleft palate, abnormal teeth, position of the ears, and extremity malformations. A thorough neurological evaluation is needed because of the frequent incidence of spinal compromise in many of these syndromes.

Following the history and physical examination, radiographs are used to identify the area of bone involvement. The so-called skeletal survey may vary from institution to institution, but it should include the following views: skull (AP and lateral); thoracolumbar spine (AP and lateral); chest; pelvis; one upper limb; one lower limb; and left hand. Flexion–extension views of the cervical spine should be ordered if instability is suspected. In some instances, imaging of other family members suspected of having the same condition may be helpful.

Laboratory tests may include calcium, phosphate, alkaline phosphatase, serum thyroxin, and protein to rule out metabolic disorders. Urine should be checked for storage products if a progressive disorder is found. Referral to a pediatric geneticist is often very helpful in reaching a diagnosis in complex cases, in providing genetic counseling to the family, and to manage the many medical problems associated with these disorders.

DEFECTS IN SKELETAL PATTERNING

Proximal Femoral Focal Deficiency

Congenital femoral deficiencies vary in severity ranging from hypoplastic femur, congenital coxa vara, congenital short femur with coxa vara, and proximal femoral focal deficiency (PFFD). This later term represents a severe disturbance in the growth of the femur with significant shortening, abnormality of the hip, and it is commonly associated to fibular deficiency. The cause is unknown, but in some cases the combination of femoral deficiency and abnormal facies is believed to be an autosomal dominant malformation.

Aitken has classified PFFD into four classes based in the radiographic evaluation of the femoral and hip involvement. In class A, a femoral head is present with an adequate acetabulum, but the femur is shortened and there is significant coxa vara. In class B, the femoral deformities are similar, but there is no connection between the femoral shaft and the femoral head. In class C, the deformities are more extensive with no femoral head with results in a poorly developed acetabulum. Finally, class D shows no development of the proximal femur or acetabulum, and the deformity is frequently bilateral.

The involved extremities in all four classes have a similar appearance and should be easily recognized. The affected site is shortened with the foot and ankle frequently at the level of the contralateral knee. The hip is flexed, abducted, and externally rotated, with flexion contracture of the knee and anterior instability secondary to absence of the cruciate ligaments (Figure 9-1). Although the hip abductors and extensors are present, they are unable to function properly because of the abnormal anatomy of the proximal femur. Frequently there is an associated fibular deficiency with or without foot deformity.

The treatment aims to compensate for the functional limitations the patient will experience, including shortening of the limb, hip function and its relationship to the alignment of the extremity, the deficiency in the muscles around the hip that will re-

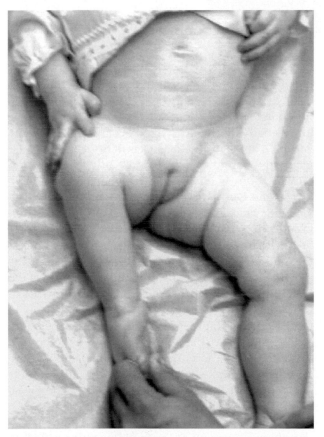

FIGURE 9-1. Proximal femoral focal deficiency. Note the affected site is shortened with the foot and ankle frequently at the level of the contralateral knee. The hip is flexed, abducted, and externally rotated with flexion contracture of the knee.

sult in a significant lurch, and the instability of the knee and foot. Therefore, there are more options and variations in the treatment of this complex deformity than in any other congenital limb deficiency.

The choice of treatment is made by the parents and the medical team after considering all surgical alternatives and functional results. If the predicted leg length discrepancy is less than 20 cm at maturity, the child may be a suitable candidate for a limb lengthening procedure. If the discrepancy is more than 20 cm, the options are prosthetic management with ankle disarticulation; ankle disarticulation and knee fusion; ankle disarticulation and femoral-pelvic fusion; rotationplasty and knee fusion; and rotationplasty and femoral–pelvis fusion.

Tibial Deficiency

Tibial deficiency is a rare type of congenital limb deficiency. It is characterized by a complete or partial absence of the tibia with bowing, limb shortening, and an intact fibula. The tibial deficiency may have a relatively normal knee and foot (intercalary deficiency), or it may be associated with absence of the medial portion of the foot (terminal deficiency). The knee may present a flexion contracture and the foot is rigidly held in varus and supination. Other findings include shortening of the femur, polydactyly and upper extremity abnormalities, and other organ systems (Figure 9-2A). The cause is unknown, but familial occurrences have been reported.

There are two classifications, both based on the radiographic findings. The simplest is that of Kalamchi and Dawe. Type I is complete absence of the tibia (Figure 9-2B). Type II is absence of the distal tibia but with a good proximal tibial portion. Type II is distal tibiofibular diastasis. An unusual type is fibular dimelia in which the tibia is absent and the fibula is duplicated.

Treatment considerations include the extent of the tibial deficiency, the magnitude of the limb shortening, the severity of the foot deformity, and importantly, the presence of active knee extension, which implies an adequate active quadriceps muscle and insertion on the tibia. Patients with a complete absence of the tibia can be treated by knee disarticulation and prosthetic fitting. Alternatively, the fibula can be fused to the femur to warrant an increase in the length of the stump and to provide a longer lever arm for the prosthesis. In patients with absence of the tibia but with a good quadriceps mechanism, the proximal fibula can be transferred to the femoral

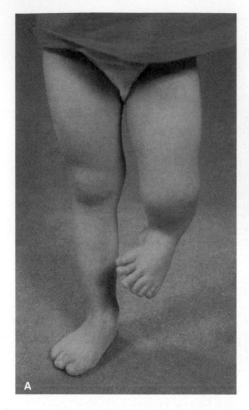

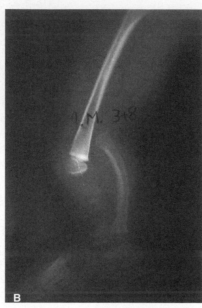

FIGURE 9-2. Tibial deficiency. **(A)** The knee may present a flexion contracture and the foot is rigidly held in varus and supination. Other findings include shortening of the femur and polydactyly. **(B)** Type I tibial deficiency with complete absence of the tibia.

notch, which will lead to a hypertrophy of the fibula. Those patients with a portion of the tibia present, a proximal tibiofibular fusion and amputation of the foot with prosthetic replacement will provide an excellent result. In cases of distal tibiofibular diastasis, a fusion of the calcaneus to the fibula is indicated.

Fibular Deficiency

The terms *fibular deficiency* or *fibular hemimelia* imply a congenital absence of all or part of the fibula, and they encompass a spectrum of abnormalities related to abnormal growth and development of the fibula. The precise cause of fibular deficiency is unknown and the deformity normally occurs sporadically. The resultant limb deficiency is usually a terminal type with associated foot abnormalities. In addition, up to 50% of the patients experience an associated femoral shortening that is variable in severity.

There have been numerous classifications mainly based on the anatomic and radiographic appearance of the deformity, but most of these classifications do not provide satisfactory guidelines for management and they do not take in account the shortening of the limb, one of the most significant factors when making management decisions. Recently, Birch and collaborators have proposed a functional classification based on the functionality of the foot and the limb length discrepancy. However, given the large variation in the different aspects of fibular deficiency, including parent's expectations, any classification only provides a general guide for management and a method for comparison of treatment results.

The clinical deformity can vary from barely detectable to severely affected. The typical characteristics include a valgus foot that often has one or several rays missing. The ankle is in valgus because of the absence of the lateral malleolus and angulation of the distal tibia. A ball-and-socket ankle has been classically described. In severe deficiencies, the foot is in rigid equinus (Figure 9-3A). There is also shortening of the femur, variable anterior bowing and shortening of the tibia, and variable valgus instability of the knee with hypoplasia of the lateral femoral condoyle and patellar abnormalities such as hypoplasia, patella alta, or subluxation (Figure 9-3B).

Treatment considerations are very complex and include management of the foot deformity as well as of the limb length discrepancy. If the foot has significant lateral deficiency and it is rigid, then amputation (Boyd or Syme type) is generally considered. Prosthetic fitting is then provided with excellent

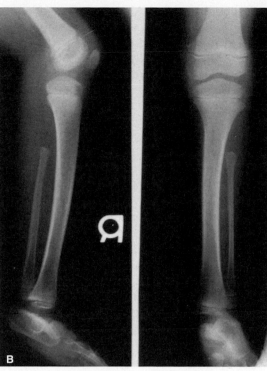

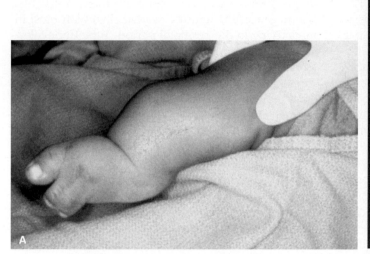

FIGURE 9-3. (A) The typical characteristics of fibular deficiency including a valgus foot with several rays missing. The ankle is in valgus and rigid equinua because of the absence of the lateral malleolus and angulation of the distal tibia. **(B)** Partial fibular deficiency.

results. In patients with a plantigrade and functional foot, the limb length discrepancy can be addressed by epiphysiodesis of the contralateral side, femoral or tibial lengthening, or a combination of techniques.

DEFECTS IN NUCLEAR PROTEINS AND TRANSCRIPTION FACTORS

Camptomelic Dysplasia

The first transcription factor discovered to cause a skeletal dysplasia was SOX9 in camptomelic dysplasia. It is a severe and rare form of dysplasia that is sometime fatal. This dominantly inherited condition is characterized by congenital bowing and angulation of long bones (camptomelia), primarily involving the tibias and femurs, and disproportionate short-limb stature. There is relative macrocephaly, distinctive face (flattened face with a high forehead), low nasal bridge, and a specific pattern of defective mineralization including areas of the spine with progressive scoliosis. There is also defective cartilage in the tracheal rings and lower respiratory tract that may cause respiratory failure. Extraskeletal features include XY sex reversal and developmental defects of the heart and kidneys.

The transcriptional targets of SOX9 include several cartilage matrix proteins such as types II and XI collagen and aggrecan. Hence, the skeletal manifestations are in part caused by decreased expression of these molecules and explain some of the phenotypic overlap with some of the severe type II collagenopathies. The bowing of the bones appears to be due to an abnormality in the formation of cartilage during fetal development (dischondrogenesis).

Treatment is symptomatic and directed to the deformities. However, there is a high degree of complications such as pseudoarthrosis and neurological complications.

Cleidocranial Dysplasia

Although the name suggests that only two bones are affected, this is a true dysplasia because there are numerous abnormalities in all parts of the skeleton, primarily those bones of membranous origin. It is transmitted as an autosomal dominant condition, and the defect is in the RUNX2 gene, which encodes for a transcription factor required for osteoblasts differentiation. Approximately two-thirds are familial and the rest are new mutations.

Typically, the disorder is identified within the first 2 years of life. Classic features include a widening of the cranium and dysplasia of the clavicles and pelvis. The patients have mildly to moderate short stature. There is bossing in the frontal parietal and occipital regions. There is maxillary micrognathism and common cleft palate and dental abnormalities. The clavicles are partially or completely absent (10% of the time). This defect causes the shoulders to look droopy, the chest to be narrow, and the neck longer. The defect may be palpable. When it is bilateral, the classic diagnostic feature is that the child can touch the shoulders together, an ability that helped one college wrestler to escape holds. Brachial plexus irritation occurs in rare occasions. The pelvis shows bilateral involvement with wide symphysis. The iliac wings appear small and coxa vara may occur, causing limitation of abduction and Trendelenburg gait. Scoliosis and syringomyelia have been described, and it is recommended to obtain a MRI in patients with progressive scoliosis.

There is no need for treatment for the clavicles. Coxa vara is treated by corrective femoral osteotomies. Scoliosis should be treated as idiopathic scoliosis. If there is brachial plexus irritation with pain and numbness, excision of the clavicular fragments can be performed to decompress it.

DEFECTS IN EXTRACELLULAR STRUCTURAL PROTEINS

Osteogenesis Imperfecta

Osteogenesis imperfecta (OI) is one of the best-known genetic skeletal disorders. At least seven discrete types have been described, ranging from mild disease with normal life expectancy to a lethal form. Approximately 80 to 90% of patients have mutations in one of the two genes encoding type I collagen (COL1A1 and COL1A2). However, in spite of the large number of mutations already identified in OI, the precise mechanisms by which different mutations cause different phenotypes are not clearly understood.

Clinical features include increased bone fragility with an increased susceptibility for fractures to occur, short stature, laxity of ligaments, hearing loss, and depending on the subtype, blue sclera, dentinogenesis imperfecta, respiratory insufficiency, excessive sweating, and early bruisability. The severity of involvement ranges from the severe cases of a crushed stillborn fetus, to an infant with multiple or unusual fractures, to an almost symptom-free adult.

The classification that is most widely accepted is the Sillence classification. Type I is a milder form of OI with onset of fractures after birth (most preschool age). Fractures heal without deformity, and their incidence decreases after puberty. Type I patients are further divided into two subgroups based on the presence of dentinogenesis imperfecta. Type II demonstrates more severe involvement (dark blue sclera, concertina femurs, beaded ribs) with most infants dying in the perinatal period. Type III develops severe progressive deformities in the extremities and spine, and these patients usually have in utero fractures and many die in infancy and early childhood from respiratory insufficiency. These patients have normal sclerae and hearing. Type IV demonstrates severe osteoporosis, bowing of the bones, and increased susceptibility to fractures, but they lack blue sclera. Many of these patients have short stature. The most severely affected surviving patients often have this type of disease. Type IV patients are also subdivided based on the presence or lack of dentinogenesis imperfecta. Type V patients have bone fragility, but not blue sclera or dentinogenesis imperfecta. These patients are characterized by three distinctive features: the presence of hypertrophic callus formation at fracture sites, calcification of the interosseous membranes between the bones of the forearm, and the presence of a radio-opaque metaphyseal band immediately adjacent to the growth plates on radiograph. Type VI patients have moderate deformity, not blue sclera or dentinogenesis imperfecta. The distinctive features of this OI type VI are the fish scale-like appearance of the bone lamellae and the presence of excessive osteoid upon histological examination.

Radiographically, patients with OI demonstrate osteopenia though it varies in its severity according to the severity of involvement. Type I patients have minimal alterations with thinning of the cortices and decreased trabecular bone. In type II patients there is bone shortening and widening, and they have "crumpled concertina" appearance. Type III patients have narrow diaphyses with increased flaring and enlargement of the metaphyses and epiphyses. Typically the long bones are deformed due to multiple fractures. Pelvic radiographs demonstrate protrusio acetabuli. Spine radiographs demonstrate platyspondyly, biconcave vertebrae, and varying degrees of scoliosis, kyphosis, or spondylolisthesis. Some patients will have cranial osteoporosis with wormian bones and flattening of the occiput (tam-o'-shanter skull).

There is no specific treatment to correct the basic mutant gene defect in OI. The treatment of OI has been focused on maximizing patient's function, preventing deformity and disability as a result of recurrent fractures, correcting deformities that have developed, and monitoring potential complicating conditions associated with OI.

The treatment of fractures in patients with OI is sometimes difficult. Fractures heal readily, often with exuberant callus, but this is plastic and easily deformed. As a result, bone deformities and shortening occur. Closed treatment is often used with lightweight splints or braces. Devices such as the parapodium may help a child to acquire an upright position. When conservative treatment fails, intramedullary rodding is indicated. In addition, multiple corrective osteotomies with intramedullary fixation have been accepted for managing recurrent fractures (Figure 9-4). Scoliosis treatment in patients with OI still remains a challenge.

Based on recent advances in the understanding of the underlying biology of this disorder, the medical treatment of OI is undergoing major improvements. Two new approaches have been studied; one using bisphosphonates and the other using bone marrow transplantation.

Bisphosphonates are synthetic analogs of pyrophosphate that inhibit bone resorption, therefore increasing bone mass overtime. They have been extensively used in adults with osteoporosis, but they have recently explored in children. Several cohort studies of patients with OI have demonstrated improved bone mass after the administration of intravenous pamindronate. This increase in bone mass is mainly due to an increase in the thickness of the cortex, which resulted in a significant reduction of fracture rates. Fracture healing was not affected; neither was longitudinal bone growth. Patients undergoing treatment also described less fatigue and less chronic pain, and they had minimal side effects. Although very encouraging, many questions still need to be resolve regarding when to start treatment, duration, long-term efficacy, and the safety of the treatment.

The second approach has been the use of bone marrow transplantation. Bone marrow contains nonhematopoietic mesenchymal stem cells (MSC) that can differentiate, among other cell types, into osteoblasts. The results are very encouraging and demonstrated good engraftment of the cells in vivo with improvement of the osteopenic phenotype.

Marfan Syndrome

Marfan syndrome is an autosomal dominant disorder that has an estimated incidence of approximately

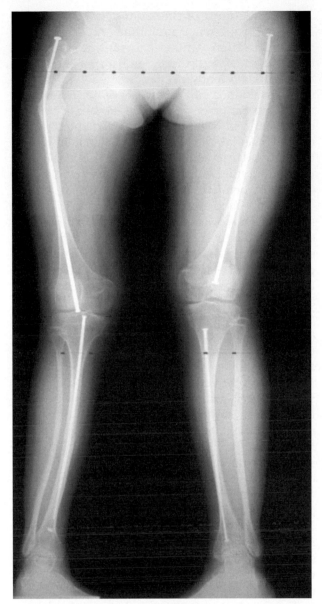

FIGURE 9-4. Osteogenesis imperfecta, type I. Treatment by intramedullary rodding.

1 in 10,000. Approximately 25% of cases occur in the absence of a family history representing new mutations. The syndrome involves many systems (skeletal, ocular, cardiovascular, pulmonary, skin and integument, and dura), but its more prominent manifestations are skeletal, ocular, and cardiovascular. Mutations in the gene encoding type 1 fibrillin (FBN1) have been reported in Marfan syndrome patients. Fibrillin-1 represents the major component of microfibrils, which are found in many types of connective tissue, including bone. To date over 500 mutations have been identified in the FBN1 gene.

Three categories of mutations have been described: (1) missense mutations, (2) small insertion or deletions, mutations causing premature termination of translation, and (3) exon-skipping mutations. Presently no definite genotype/phenotype correlations have been identified. To facilitate the identification of different mutations, a "Marfan database" has been developed that includes not only molecular but also clinical data. It is only through a large collaborative international effort that genotype and phenotype correlations will eventually be identified.

Although no specific therapy exists for Marfan syndrome, it is of great importance to confirm or exclude the diagnosis in family members at risk as early as possible because of the potential fatal complications of the disease (aortic dissection and rupture). At present, diagnosis for most cases is still based on thorough clinical examination, including measurements of body proportions, echocardiography of the aorta, slit-lamp ophthalmologic evaluation, and radiographs. In the absence of a family history, patients are diagnosed based on involvement of the skeletal system and two other systems with at least two major manifestations (ectopia lentis, aortic dilation/dissection, dural ectasia, or molecular data). In the presence of a positive family history, an affected person should display one major criterion in an organ system and involvement of a second system. Within a given family, however, considerable heterogeneity may be present. It is not uncommon for milder involved patients to have the diagnosis go unrecognized until another family member is diagnosed. The phenotype of the Marfan syndrome remains incompletely defined. Most manifestations are age dependent and are difficult to quantify. Molecular data are becoming increasingly important to better characterize Marfan syndrome and to study its natural history.

A variety of skeletal manifestations may be present in patients with Marfan syndrome. Most characteristic is tall stature and disproportionately long, thin limbs (dolichostenomelia). This can be confirmed by demonstrating a smaller than normal upper segment (head to pubic symphysis) to lower segment (pubic symphysis to plantar surface) ratio or an arm span that exceeds the patient's total height by at least 7.5 cm. Patients frequently have arachnodactyly (abnormally long and slender digits) and ligamentous laxity. This combination of joint laxity and long digits results in several clinical signs that are indicative of, but not pathognomonic , for Marfan syndrome. One such sign is the thumb sign described by Steinberg. This is positive if the opposed thumb projects past the ulnar border of the clenched fist. The wrist sign is the ability of the patient to encircle the opposite wrist with the thumb and small finger, with the thumb overlapping the distal phalanx of the small finger. The crossover leg sign is the ability of the patient to touch the floor with the foot of the crossing-over leg. Joint laxity is another hallmark of the disease, and many patients have recurrent instability of the patella, shoulder, hip, and thumb. Marked flatfeet (pes planovalgus), genu valgum, and genu recurvatum are typical.

Approximately 66% of patients have pectus excavatum (chest depression) or pectus carinatum (pigeon chest). The chest wall deformities in Marfan patients are due to longitudinal overgrowth of the ribs. A severe pectus deformity can become clinically significant by reducing total lung capacity, forced vital capacity, and forced expiratory volume. Additionally, the occurrence of a severe pectus deformity in association with scoliosis may further compromise the lung capacity of patients with Marfan syndrome. It is recommended that patients with Marfan syndrome have repair of the pectus deformity done after skeletal maturity to minimize the chance of recurrence with longitudinal growth of the ribs.

Spinal deformities are a frequent finding in patients with Marfan syndrome. Abnormalities include thoracic lordosis, thoracolumbar kyphosis, flat-back deformity, and spondylolisthesis. Scoliosis is one of the most common and important manifestations of Marfan syndrome from an orthopaedic perspective with an incidence of 62%. The curve pattern frequently is either a single right thoracic curve or a double major curve pattern. The thoracic curve is most commonly lordoscoliotic. The thoracolumbar junction is prone to kyphosis, probably related to the underlying ligamentous laxity. The treatment regimen for scoliosis in Marfan syndrome and adolescent idiopathic scoliosis is similar but the results of treatment are often different. Specifically, scoliosis in Marfan syndrome has a higher tendency toward progression and responds less well to bracing than adolescent idiopathic scoliosis. Both family and physician should be aware of these facts. In addition, back pain is frequently associated with scoliosis in Marfan syndrome.

Bracing is recommended for curves between 15° and 25°. Spinal fusion with autogenous bone graft and rigid internal fixation should be considered in patients with curves that have progressed beyond 40° (Figure 9-5A,B). The surgeon should

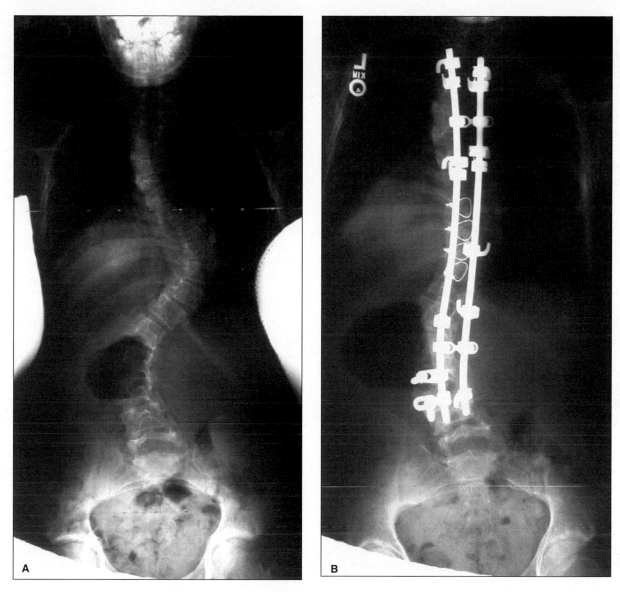

FIGURE 9-5. (A) and **(B)**. Scoliosis in a patient with Marfan syndrome. The deformity was treated by posterior spine fusion and instrumentation.

be aware that there is significantly smaller pedicle widths and laminar thickness in patients with Marfan syndrome as well as widened interpedicular distances in the lumbar spine. These osseous vertebral anomalies may be responsible for some reported postoperative complications including fracture dislocation and pseudarthrosis. Preoperative cardiac evaluation is critical and frequently determines whether a patient is a suitable candidate for extensive spine surgery.

Planovalgus foot deformity is common in Marfan syndrome and is postulated to be due to increased ligamentous laxity resulting from underlying connective tissue pathology. Acetabular protrusio can be seen radiographically in as many as half of patients with Marfan syndrome. Patients can be asymptomatic or have symptoms of hip pain and stiffness. Because of the lack of a direct relation between protrusio and hip symptomatology treatment recommendations are difficult to make.

Dural ectasia, a widening of the dural sac, has a reported incidence of 63% in Marfan syndrome and can result in back pain and headaches. It usually occurs in the most caudal portion of the spinal column causing bone erosion and anterior meningoceles. Dural ectasia is thought to result from fibrillin deficiency resulting in weakness of the dural sac. There has been a reported direct correlation between the size of the dural ectasia and the presence of pain. Posterior laminectomy has been used as a means of relieving back pain thought to be secondary to dural ectasia.

The hallmark of ocular involvement is ectopia lentis (dislocated lens) due to lax suspensory ligaments. The dislocation is superior and lateral and may not be recognized unless a slit-lamp examination is performed. Ectopia lentis occurs in more than half of involved patients. Other ocular manifestations include myopia, retina detachments, strabismus, cataract, and glaucoma.

Multiple cardiovascular abnormalities exist in patients with Marfan syndrome and are the most common cause of death in this patient group. For this reason a complete cardiology workup should be done on all Marfan syndrome patients that includes an electrocardiogram and echocardiogram. The most serious complication is dilation of the ascending aorta and associated aortic regurgitation. This often leads to a dissecting aortic aneurysm. Mitral valve prolapse and mitral valve regurgitation are the most common significant cardiac problems in children. Many patients are being treated with medications in an attempt to delay the onset of serious cardiovascular abnormalities.

Multiple Epiphyseal Dysplasia

Multiple epiphyseal dysplasia (MED) is one of the most widely known and commonly occurring skeletal dysplasia. It is most commonly inherited in an autosomal dominant fashion though autosomal recessive forms have been described as well. Its prevalence is estimated at 1 in 10,000 individuals. The predominant feature of multiple epiphyseal dysplasia is the delayed and irregular ossification of numerous epiphyses. In most cases there is pain and stiffness in the joints, with hips and knees being most commonly affected. In general, affected patients have mild short stature and early onset osteoarthritis.

Historically, it was described as occurring in two separate forms: Ribbing's dysplasia, having mild involvement, and Fairbanks dysplasia, a more severe type. However, with the current genetic understanding, multiple epiphyseal dysplasia is now considered to represent a continuous spectrum from mild to severe and these eponyms have been abandoned.

Multiple epiphyseal dysplasia shows considerable genetic heterogeneity. To date, mutations have been reported in 40 patients or families with multiple epiphyseal dysplasia, and 15 of these are allelic with pseudoachondroplasia and result from mutations in the gene encoding cartilage oligomeric matrix protein (COMP). MED can also result from mutations in the genes encoding the α1, α2, and α3 chains of type IX collagen, COL9A1, COL9A2, COL9A3, respectively. Furthermore, mutations in the gene encoding matrilin-3, a member of the matrilin family of extracellular oligomeric proteins, can cause a distinctive mild form of MED. Finally, it has been demonstrated that a form of recessively inherited MED, with a distinctive clinical presentation including clubfoot and bilateral double-layered patellae, can result from mutations in the solute carrier family 26, member 2 gene (SLC26A2). Therefore, MED is one of the more genetically heterogeneous of the bone dysplasias.

Patients typically present in early adolescence because of joint stiffness and contractures, lower extremity pain, angular deformities of the knees, gait disturbance, or short stature. Depending on the severity of the epiphyseal dysplasia, symptoms may develop as early as 4 or 5 years. It is not uncommon, however, for patients with milder forms to go unrecognized until young adult life. Most patients have minimal short stature and are above the third percentile for standing height; so true dwarfism is not present. The face and spine are normal. There are no associated neurologic findings. Intelligence is not affected. The epiphyses of the upper extremities can be involved but patients rarely complain of any significant symptoms in this area. Mild limitation of motion in the elbow, wrist, and shoulder is occasionally found.

The principal finding on radiographs is a delay in the appearance of the ossification centers. When the epiphyses do appear, they are fragmented, mottled, and flattened. The more fragmentation there is in the capital femoral epiphysis, the earlier onset of osteoarthritis (Figure 9-6).

The proximal femur is most often affected and its appearance may be easily confused with those of bilateral Legg-Calvé-Perthes disease. Several radiographic clues may be helpful in differentiating the two. In Legg-Calvé-Perthes disease, usually one hip is involved before the other, so that each hip is in a different stage of the disease. This is not the case in MED. In addition, acetabular changes are primary in MED and are more pronounced. Metaphyseal cysts are seen in Legg-Calvé-Perthes disease, but not in MED. Radiographs of the knees, ankles,

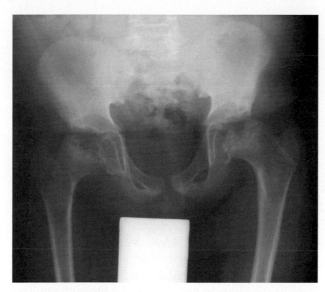

FIGURE 9-6. Multiple epiphyseal dysplasia. Radiograph of the pelvis demonstrating a fragmented, mottled, and flattened femoral head, and corresponding changes in the acetabulum.

shoulders, and wrists should be obtained in any child when the diagnosis of Legg-Calvé-Perthes disease is being entertained to rule out MED.

Coxa vara occurs in some patients. Radiographs of the knees often demonstrate flattening of the femoral condyles as well as a genu valgum deformity. Osteochondritis dessecans may be superimposed. Lateral radiographs of the knees demonstrate a double-layered patella in some patients. When this is present, it is characteristic for MED. The ankles in MED are also in valgus due to deformity in the talus predominantly. Upper extremity involvement is less severe. The metacarpals and phalanges usually are short with irregular epiphyses. MED is distinguished from spondyloepiphyseal dysplasia by the absence of severe vertebral changes. Mild endplate irregularities may be present.

Hip pain or subluxation is a common reason patients with MED seek orthopaedic care in adolescence. Containment surgery can be considered for those hips that show progressive subluxation. Although the principle of coverage is the same as that used in Perthes disease, there is often preexisting coxa vara in hips with MED, which contraindicates use of a proximal femoral varus osteotomy. In those cases, a shelf acetabular augmentation can improve coverage of the misshapen femoral head. If hinge abduction is present on arthrography, a valgus proximal femoral osteotomy may improve congruency and therefore

relieve pain. Osteotomies may be helpful in realigning angular deformities at the knees. For optimal surgical correction, the site of the deformity must be ascertained preoperatively as either the distal femur, proximal tibia, or both. Degenerative joint disease is the biggest problem, and it usually occurs in the second or third decade. If the femoral head is well formed at maturity, the onset of arthritis is delayed. The hip is the most common location of arthritis in this patient group and often leads to total joint arthroplasty.

Pseudoachondroplasia

Pseudoachondroplasia is a form of short-limbed dwarfism that has a prevalence of approximately four per million, making it one of the more common skeletal dysplasias. It is characterized by involvement of both the epiphyses and metaphyses with affected individuals having significantly short stature and a predisposition to premature osteoarthritis. The spine is also involved with this disorder.

Pseudoachondroplasia is usually transmitted as an autosomal dominant trait. The molecular genetics of pseudoachondroplasia have been extensively studied and it now appears that this disease results almost exclusively from mutations in the gene encoding cartilage oligomeric matrix protein (COMP). The COMP gene consists of 19 exons, and the majority of mutations to date (95%) are clustered within exons 8 to 14, which encode the type III repeats. The fact that most of these mutations are in the conformationally sensitive type III repeats indicates that this region is critical for protein function. The remaining 5% of mutations are in exons 16 and 18, which encode specific segments of the C-terminal globule.

The cell-matrix pathology of pseudoachondroplasia resulting from COMP mutations has been well documented. Abnormal COMP is retained within the rough endoplasmic reticulum of cartilage, tendon, and ligament cells. This results in the secondary retention of type IX collagen, chondroitin sulfate proteoglycan 1 (aggrecan), and link protein. This retention of proteins leads to a reduction in the amount of these molecules available for interactions within the extracellular matrix of cartilage resulting in cell death and the phenotypic picture of pseudoachondroplasia. Additional studies are needed to delineate the mechanism leading to excessive retention of proteins in order to develop treatment modalities.

Pseudoachondroplasia is a relatively straightforward disease to provide molecular diagnosis for because it results almost exclusively from mutations along a very compact region in the COMP gene. Molecular diagnosis for pseudoachondroplasia is currently provided on a commercial basis (www.genetests.com) and also as part of the service provision of the European Skeletal Dysplasia Network (ESDN) for research and diagnosis (www.esdn.org).

Children with pseudoachondroplasia are normal at birth and are usually diagnosed at 2 years of age after the onset of a waddling gait and at the time rhizomelic shortening becomes noticeable. Adult height ranges from 106 to 130 cm. Growth curve charts specific to pseudoachondroplasia are available. The clinical features are limited to the skeleton. The skull and facies in pseudoachondroplasia are normal, and this is helpful in differentiating it from achondroplasia, in which frontal bossing and midface hypoplasia are present. Abnormalities of the lower extremities are common and include genu valgum and varum deformities. Some patients develop windswept deformity of the knees, in which genu valgum is present on one side and genu varum on the other. The joints are extremely lax, especially in childhood and adolescence, and there is a predisposition to early osteoarthropathy. The large weight-bearing joints (hips and knees) are the ones most often affected, and approximately one-third of patients need total hip replacement by their mid-30s. Scoliosis may occur in adolescence but is generally not severe. Cervical spine instability is seen in 10 to 20% of individuals (Figure 9-7). Development milestones and

intelligence are normal and premature mortality is not a reported problem.

Typical radiographic changes include small, irregular epiphyses and metaphyseal changes. Hand radiographs reveal delayed epiphyseal ossification resulting in delayed bone age. In the long bones, these changes are seen as epiphyseal ossification delay. When the epiphyses do ossify, they appear irregular and fragmented. The hip and knee are most severely affected (Figure 9-8). In the pelvis, there is delay in ossification of the capital femoral epiphysis, and when ossified they are small and flattened. The femoral heads may resemble what is seen in other spondyloepiphyseal dysplasias or bilateral Legg-Calve-Perthes disease. Sclerosis and irregularity of the acetabular roof are commonly observed. Subluxation of the hips often occurs and degenerative arthritis develops in response to the incongruity. The vertebral changes in pseudoachondroplasia are characteristic and consist of anterior beaking in childhood that resolves in adolescence. The interpedicular distance in the lumbar spine is normal in pseudoachondroplasia, unlike achondroplasia. Odontoid hypoplasia may be present resulting in atlantoaxial instability.

Patients with pseudoachondroplasia often have significant angular deformities of the lower extremities that require corrective osteotomies. Careful preoperative assessment is necessary to properly realign the mechanical axis through the hip, knee, and ankle. For instance, in genu varum associated with

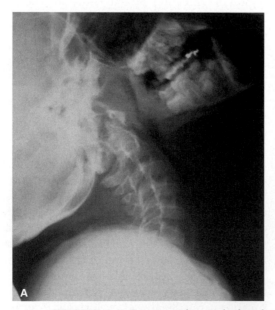 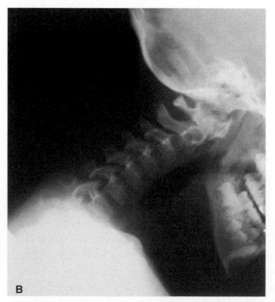

FIGURE 9-7. Patient with pseudochondroplasia and cervical spine instability.

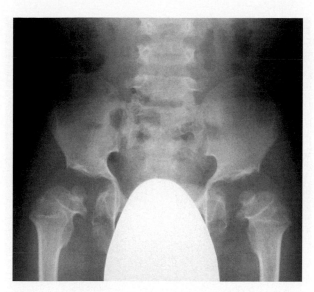

FIGURE 9-8. Patient with pseudoachondroplasia at age 8. Radiograph of the pelvis with severe proximal femoral and acetabular deformities.

DEFECTS IN SIGNAL TRANSDUCTION MECHANISMS

Achondroplasia Group

Achondroplasia is by far the most common chondrodysplasia in humans, occurring in about 1 in 30,000 live births. A single gene defect (a mutation in the FGFR3 gene) has been established for this disorder. Initial reports, confirmed subsequently in many other laboratories, demonstrated that more than 97% of patients with achondroplasia carried the same mutation, a G to A change at nucleotide 1138, and that the remaining patients had a G to C change at the same nucleotide. Very recently it has been demonstrated that, as previously expected, FGFR3 mutations in sporadic cases of achondroplasia occur exclusively on the parentally derived allele.

Since the FGFR3 mutation in achondroplasia was recognized, similar observations regarding the conserved nature of FGFR3 mutations and resulting phenotype have been made regarding hypochondroplasia, the lethal thanatophoric dysplasia, SADDAN (severe achondroplasia with developmental delay and acanthosis nigricans), and recently two craniosynostosis disorders: Muenke coronal craniosynostosis and Crouzon syndrome with acanthosis nigricans. More importantly, the relationship between mutations in the FGFR3 gene and other FGFR genes, and the phenotypes that result from these mutations have improved our understanding of these disorders, and it has been observed that there is a highly conserved relationship between mutations at a particular amino acid and the resulting phenotype. The skeletal manifestations of achondroplasia are related to a defect in endochondral bone formation. The resulting growth disturbances are variable, affecting proximal segments to a greater extent than the distal segments of the limbs (rhizomelia), and with relatively minor involvement of the growth of the spine.

Achondroplasia is recognized at birth, and the appearance of a person with achondroplasia has numerous features that are uniform and predictable. Intelligence is normal, and life expectancy is not significantly diminished. The predicted adult height is 132 cm for men and 122 cm for women. Obesity is more common than in the general population. Developmental milestones are met later in children with achondroplasia than the average-stature children.

achondroplasia, the deformity is present solely in the tibia; however, in pseudoachondroplasia the deformity is often present in both the femur and the tibia, requiring osteotomies in both the distal femur and the proximal tibia. Care must also be taken in assessing the contribution of ligamentous laxity to the bowing deformity. After corrective osteotomy, recurrence of the deformity with growth is not uncommon.

Premature osteoarthritis of the hip in early adulthood is a frequent problem in pseudoachondroplasia. Patients with symptomatic subluxation or incongruity may benefit from a realignment osteotomy of the proximal femur. Varus osteotomy of the proximal femur usually creates more incongruity. If hinge abduction is present, demonstrated by the femoral head levering out of the joint with abduction of the hip, a proximal femoral valgus osteotomy may improve joint congruity and improve abductor function. Before performing a proximal femoral valgus osteotomy, preoperative arthrography should be performed to demonstrate improved congruity with 15° to 20° of flexion and adduction of the femur. Abduction of the hip should demonstrate hinge abduction of the femoral head. Reconstructive pelvic osteotomies, such as the Salter osteotomy or the triple innominate osteotomy of Steel, are contraindicated in pseudoachondroplasia because a concentric reduction is not present preoperatively, which is a prerequisite for these osteotomies. Salvage procedures such as the shelf augmentation or the Chiari osteotomy can be done in select cases. As many as 50% of adult patients have undergone total hip arthroplasty.

There is enlargement of the cranium with frontal bossing, midface hypoplasia, flattening of the nasal bridge, and prominent mandible. The foramen magnum is frequently narrowed and it is associated with neurological complications from compression of the brain stem (quadriparesis, spasticity, sleep apnea and respiratory insufficiency, and sudden death). The spine length is in the lower range of normal whereas the extremities are much shorter than normal, with the proximal segments—the humeri and femora—the most foreshortened (rhizomelic). There is kyphosis of the thoracolumbar junction during infancy, and it usually improves with increasing age. Scoliosis is rare. Hyperlordosis of the lumbar spine increases with age, and there is a high incidence of symptomatic spinal stenosis (narrowing of the interpedicular distances with shortening of the pedicles). Clinically, patients will present with low back and leg pain, paresthesias, dysesthesias, weakness, or bowel and bladder incontinence.

There is limitation of extension of the elbows and some patients may have asymptomatic radial head dislocations. Patients have a classic "trident hand" characterized by a persistent space between the long and ring fingers. The main functional limitations of the upper extremities are related to shortening of the humeri, which lead to difficulties in personal hygiene and dressing. Radiographically, the pelvis is broad with a diminished vertical height. The iliac crest has a square appearance and the superior acetabular roof is horizontal. There is flaring of the distal femoral metaphysis. Genu varum is very common, with ligamentous laxity and the fibula overgrow the tibia. Internal tibial torsion is common with varus of the ankle (Figure 9-9).

Children with achondroplasia should be closely monitored in the first 2 years of life for signs of foramen magnum stenosis. If the diagnosis is made and symptoms are persistent, decompression of the brain stem is indicated. In some patients associated hydrocephalus will require shunting. Problems of the ear, nose, and throat are frequent secondary to the facial abnormalities. Recurrent otitis media may result in hearing loss, thus early hearing screening should be performed. Maxillary hypoplasia leads to dental crowding and malocclusion, which may require orthodontic treatment. Sleep apnea treatment, if necessary, begins with adenotonsillectomy and may progress to include more complex procedures.

The main orthopaedic problems include thoracolumbar kyphosis, spinal stenosis, shortening of the extremities and angular deformities of the knees.

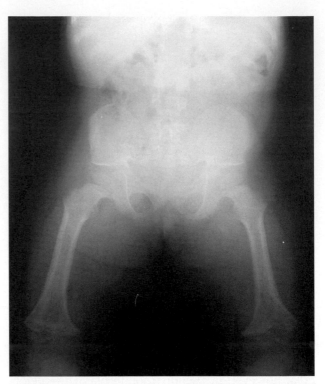

FIGURE 9-9. Characteristic radiographic appearance of achondroplasia.

Kyphosis is noncongenital and it is centered in the thoracolumbar junction. Treatment may be indicated to prevent further development of the deformity and to assist in those that do not correct with time (bracing); and in adulthood, to correct surgically those cases in which kyphosis contribute to symptomatic spinal stenosis. Spinal stenosis is the most serious problem and usually develops in the third decade of life. Spinal decompression is indicated as soon as the diagnosis is made. Limb lengthening remains controversial but is gradually gaining greater acceptance. If the lower extremities are lengthened, the humeri should be lengthened also to facilitate personal care. Treatment of the genu varum usually requires surgery because bracing is not effective. Fibular head epiphysiodesis, fibular shortening, and tibial osteotomies can be performed to correct the deformity usually not until age 4 at the earliest. Interestingly, severe degenerative arthritis is not common in adults with achondroplasia.

Vitamin D-Resistant Rickets

Vitamin D-resistant rickets, also know as familial hypophosphatemic rickets, encompasses a group of disorders in which dietary intake of vitamin D is insufficient to achieve normal mineralization of the growing bone. There are four types of vitamin D–resistant rickets: phosphate diabetes (i.e., failure of the reabsorptive mechanism for phosphate); failure of production of 1, 25-vitamin D (i.e., vitamin dependent rickets); end-organ insensitivity to 1, 25 vitamin D, and renal tubular acidosis.

Historically, patients with these disorders were first differentiated on the basis of their resistance to the ordinary treatment doses of vitamin D and were found to have normal or near normal levels of calcium, PTH, and vitamin D, but significantly decreased serum phosphate and abnormal urinary excretion for phosphate, water, amino acids, glucose, bicarbonate, ketone bodies, and glycine.

The condition usually becomes symptomatic between 1 and 2 years of age, and the disease is suspected because of the family history, laboratory determination of phosphorus concentrations can lead to the diagnosis in infants as young as 3 months. The usual presenting complaints are delayed walking, short stature, and angular deformities of the lower extremities (genu varum, although genu valgum may happen in some cases). Systemic manifestation such as irritability and apathy are minimal. The "rachitic rosary" may also occur. Spinal stenosis and kyphosis has been described. Radiographically there is marked increase in axial height and widening of the growth plates, cupping, and thin and indistinct cortices and fuzzy, poorly defined trabecular bone (osteopenia).

Coxa vara may be present as well as lateral bowing of the femur and tibia. Looser lines can be seen in the rib cage of a child with florid rickets, resulting from accumulation of osteoid in the bone matrix.

Medical treatment is best managed by a pediatric nephrologist with expertise in metabolic bone disease. The usual treatment consists of oral neutral phosphate replacement and the administration of vitamin D, and the correction of the metabolic abnormality present. The orthotic management to correct the lower extremity deformities has proven ineffective. If patients experience pain and increased deformities, surgical correction of the angular deformities should be performed. Multilevel osteotomy is usually required with intramedullary fixation or external fixation. Because of a high risk of recurrences in the younger patient, surgery should not be performed in early childhood.

DEFECTS IN METABOLIC MACROMOLECULAR DEGRADATION

Mucopolysaccharidoses

Mucopolysaccharide excretion in the urine characterizes this group of genetic disorders, and these disorders are among the first skeletal dysplasias to be described and also among the first to be understood at the biochemical level. There are at least 13 types (Table 9-1), and each type produces a particular

TABLE 9-1.
Mucopolysaccharidoses

Designation	Name	Enzyme Defect	Stored Substance
MPS I	Hurler/Scheie	α-L-iduronase	HS+DS
MPS II	Hunter	iduronase-2-sulfate	HS+DS
MPS IIIA	Sanfilippo A	heparin-sulfatase	HS
MPS IIIB	Sanfilippo B	α-N-acetylglucosamine	HS
MPS IIIC	Sanfilippo C	acetyl-CoA:α-glucosamine-N-acetyl transferase	HS
MPS IIID	Sanfilippo D	glucosamine-6-sulfatase	HS
MPS IVA	Morquio A	N-acetyl-galactosamine-6-sulfate sulfatase	KS, CS
MPS IVB	Morquio B	β-D-galactosidase	KS
MPS IV C	Morquio C	unknown	KS
MPS V	Formerly Scheie, no longer in use		
MPS VI	Maroteux-Lamy	arylsulfatase B	DS, CS
MPS VII	Sly	β-D-glucuronidase	CS, HS, DS
MPS VIII		glucuronate-2-sulpitase	CS, HS

sugar in the urine because of a specific enzyme defect. The incidence is about 1 in 20,000 live births.

The intracellular degradation of sulfated glycosaminoglycans (heparin sulfate, dermatan sulfate, keratan sulfate, and chondroitin sulfate) by lysosomal enzymes is abnormal leading to intracellular accumulation of these incompletely degraded compounds in the lysosomes themselves. They are classified based on their enzyme deficiency and the type of substance that accumulates. The most common types are Morquio's and Hurler's syndromes.

The incomplete product progressively accumulates in the tissues such as the brain, the viscera, and the joints. This unremitting process leads to the clinical progression of the disorders. The child is normal at birth, being biochemically detectable by 6 to 12 months of age, and clinically symptomatic by 2 years of age. All these disorders lead to abnormally short stature. And in some cases, there is severe mental retardation (Hurler's, Hunter's, and Sanfilippo's). There are also abnormalities of the skull (enlarged, with thick calvarium) and facies (coarse, gargoyle), and deafness. In some cases there is hepatosplenomegaly and cardiovascular abnormalities. Radiographically, the clavicles are broad and the scapulae are short and stubby. The vertebral bodies are ovoid and scoliosis and kyphosis are frequent (Figure 9-10). There is acetabular dysplasia, coxa valga, and the iliac wings are flared.

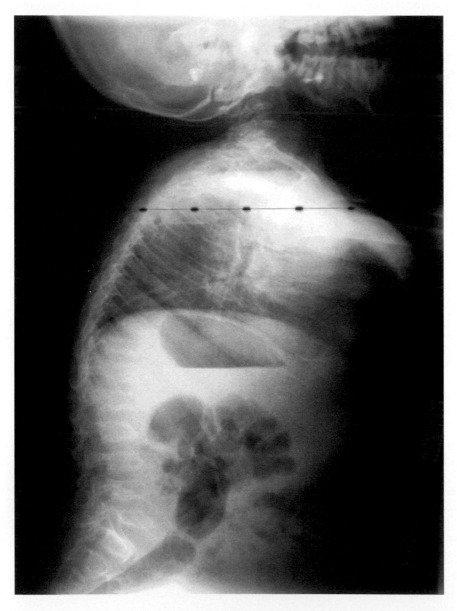

FIGURE 9-10. Spine of a patient with Morquio's. Platyspondyly with anterior beaking and mild kyphosis of the thoracolumbar junction.

The clinical course is variable, but most patients die in the first two decades of life if untreated. Treatment is evolving and some of these disorders have been treated successfully with bone marrow transplantation. The preferred donor is an HLA-identical sibling. Following successful transplantation, accumulation of the mucopolysaccharide stops, and there is improvement in the coarse facies, hepatosplenomegaly, and partially in the hearing. Research is currently under way in the field of gene therapy for some of these syndromes.

Orthopaedic treatment is directed to correct the functionally impairing musculoskeletal deformities. Hip flexion contractures and dysplasia often require surgical reconstruction, including reduction, femoral and pelvis osteotomies. Cervical instability may be present and C1–C2 fusion and halo immobilization may be necessary. Kyphosis requires orthotic treatment or even surgical spine fusion. Genu valgus may be treated with corrective osteotomies.

DEFECTS IN TUMOR SUPPRESSOR GENES

Hereditary Multiple Exostoses

Hereditary multiple exostoses (HME), or diaphyseal aclasia, is a highly penetrant, autosomal dominant trait characterized by slightly stunted growth of long bones and multiple osteochondromas. Osteochondromas are cartilage-capped excrescences of bone that develop at the growth plate level during growth. These osteochondromas are indistinguishable morphologically from the solitary cases. HME has an incidence of about 1 in 50,000 live births. The median age at the time of diagnosis in affected individuals is approximately 3 years. By the second decade of life, nearly all affected individuals will have exostoses as the penetrance of the disorder has been found to be 96 to 100%. Many patients with HME require resection of the lesions due to a mass effect or neurovascular impingement symptoms. Importantly, up to 3% of patients with HME will eventually develop a malignant chondrosarcoma.

Over the last decade, advances in molecular biology and genetics have permitted a better understanding into the molecular players underlying these lesions. Linkage analysis has located three etiological genes for HME, EXT1, EXT2, and EXT3. Interestingly, mutations in any of these genes demonstrate very similar clinical manifestations. These EXT loci have defined a new class of putative tumor suppressor genes, to which have been recently added three related genes, EXTL1, EXTL2, and EXTL3.

Because both HME and sporadic osteochondromas have been associated with loss of heterozygosity at one or more of the EXT loci, a neoplastic model of pathogenesis has been suggested. The Knudson "two-hit" theory of carcinogenesis derived from familial retinoblastoma has been applied to HME. Both copies of the EXT1 gene have been observed to be deleted and gene losses and mutations have been observed in chondrosarcomas arising from osteochondromas. However, it is still unclear how EXT1 and EXT2 can function as tumor suppressors.

Patients present with several hard, knobby lumps near the joints. Numerous sites can be involved, typically five or six exostoses can be found in the upper and lower extremities. The most common locations are distal femur (70%), proximal tibia (70%), humerus (50%), and proximal fibula (30%). Over time, the extremities will shorten in relation to the trunk, and legs will grow unequally. As the lesions enlarge, they may cause discomfort secondary to mechanical pressure to adjacent soft tissues and muscles. They rarely cause neurological dysfunction. Often, patients complain of an undesirable cosmetic appearance. Valgus deformity of the knee and ankle are not uncommon, and osteochondromas of the proximal femur may lead to dysplasia of the hip, which may require corrective osteotomies. In adults, sarcomatous transformation will present as a painful and enlarging mass in an area of previous deformity.

Treatment for multiple hereditary exostoses is surgical excision. However, not all the exostoses should be removed. Established indications for surgery include growth disturbances leading to angular deformities or hip dysplasia; functional limitation of joint range of motion; spinal cord compression with neurological compromise; painful mass and obvious cosmetic deformity, and rapid increase in the size of the lesion. Deformities in the forearm should be treated early to prevent further progression and to reduce disability. Knee osteotomies are associated with a high incidence of peroneal nerve palsy.

Annotated Bibliography

Classification

Carey JC, Viskochil DH. Status of the human malformations map: 2002. Am J Med Genet 2002;115:205.
  Summary update of the mapped and cloned genes that are important in the cause of human malformations and syndromes.

Hall CM. International nosology and classification of constitutional disorders of bone (2001). AM J Med Genet 2002;113:65.

An update in the international classification of bone disorders with inclusion of the osteochondrodysplasias and dysostoses.

Hermanns P, Lee B. Transcriptional dysregulation in skeletal malformation syndromes. Am J Med Genet 2001;106:258.
Mutations in transcription factors result in an array of defects affecting craniofacial, appendicular, and axial skeletal development.

Kornak U, Mundlos S. Genetic disorders of the skeleton: a developmental approach. Am J Hum Genet 2003;73:447.
The authors present a classification based on a combination of molecular pathology and embryology, taking into account the importance of development for the understanding of bone disease.

Superti-Furga A, Bonafe L, Rimoin DL. Molecular-pathogenetic classification of genetic disorders of the skeleton. J Am Med Genet 2001;106:282.
The authors present a classification based on the molecular and pathogenetic aspects of the disorders of the skeleton, with an attempt to identify the metabolic pathways, signaling cascades, and regulatory networks underlying these disorders.

Proximal Femoral Focal Deficiency

Aitken GT. Proximal femoral focal deficiency: definition, classification, and management. In: Proximal Femoral Focal Deficiency: A Congenital Abnormality. Washington, DC: National Academy of Sciences, 1969:1.
Classic article on the clinical and radiographic characteristics of PFF, with a discussion on its classification and treatment guidelines.

Epps CH. Current concepts review: proximal femoral focal deficiency. J Bone Joint Surg 1983;65A:867.
Excellent review on the etiology, classification, and management of PFFD.

Kalamchi A, Cowell HR, Kim KI. Congenital deficiency of the femur. J Pediatr Ortho 1985;5:129.
The authors present a classification of PFFD based on 60 patients. Recommendations for treatment are discussed.

Koman LA, Meyer LC, Warren FH. Proximal femoral focal deficiency: natural history and treatment. Clin Ortho Rel Res 1982;162:135.
The authors discussed the natural history of the deformity and options of treatment.

Sener G, Yigiter K, Bayar K, Erbahceci F. Effectiveness of prosthetic rehabilitation of children with limb deficiencies present at birth. Prosthet Orthot Int 1999; 23:130.
Discussion of the most important aspect of prosthetic rehabilitation in children with limb deficiencies.

Tibial Deficiency

Brown FW. Construction of a knee joint in congenital total absence of the tibia (paraxial hemimelia tibia). J Bone Joint Surg 1965;47A:695.
Classic description of the fibular transfer for complete tibial deficiency.

Jones D, Barnes J, Lloyd-Roberts GC. Congenital aplasia and dysplasia of the tibia with intact fibula: classification and management. J Bone Joint Surg 1978;60B:31.
The authors propose a classification with recommendations for treatment based in a review of 20 patients.

Kalamchi A, Dawe RV. Congenital deficiency of the tibia. J Bone Joint Surg 1985;67B:581.
Revised classification of tibial deficiency based on its radiographic appearance. Results of treatment of 21 patients are presented.

Loder RT, Herring JA. Fibular transfer for congenital absence of the tibia: a reassessment. J Pediatr Orthop 1987;7:8.
The authors examine 87 cases from the literature using the minimal requirements for a good result. They found that 53 of the 55 cases of Jones type I had a poor result. It emphasizes the need for strong, active knee extension.

Shoenecker PL, Capelli AM, Millar EA et al. Congenital longitudinal deficiency of the tibia. J Bone Joint Surg 1989;71A:278.
The authors reviewed the treatment results of 57 patients (71 limbs) with tibial deficiency. An ablative procedure was performed on 61 of the limbs. Brown's procedure yielded less than satisfactory results.

Fibular Deficiency

Achterman C, Kalamchi A. Congenital deficiency of the fibula. J Bone Joint Surg 1979;61B:133.
The authors present a classification for fibular deficiency with recommendations for treatment.

Birch JG, Lincoln TI, Mack PW. Functional classification of fibular deficiency. In: Herring JA, Birch JG eds. The Child with a Limb Deficiency. Rosemont, IL: American Academy of Orthopaedic Surgeons, 1998;161.
The authors present a functional classification of fibular deficiency and recommend treatment option for each type.

McCarthy JJ, Glancy GL, Chang FM et al. Fibular hemimelia: comparison of outcome measurements after amputation and lengthening. J Bone Joint Surg 2000;82:1732.
The purpose of our study was to compare the outcome after amputation with that after tibial lengthening, specifically with regard to activity restrictions, pain, satisfaction, complications, number of procedures, and cost, in children with fibular hemimelia. The study demonstrated that children who undergo early amputation are more active, have less pain, are more satisfied, have fewer complications, undergo fewer procedures, and incur less cost than those who undergo lengthening.

Epps CH Jr. Schneider PL. Treatment of hemimelias of the lower extremity. Long-term results. J Bone Joint Surge 1989;71A:273.
Review of 33 patients treated with contemporary methods. The authors concluded that surgical treatment and prosthetic rehabilitation yield excellent results, both short and long term.

Herring JA. Syme's amputation for fibular hemimelia: a second look in the Ilizarov era. Instructional Course Lectures 1992;41:435.
Discussion of the results of Syme's amputation in fibular deficiency.

Hootnick D, Boyd NA, Fixsen JA et al. The natural history and management of congenital short tibia with dysplasia or absence of the fibula. J Bone Joint Surg 1977;59B:267.
The authors note that the leg length discrepancy remains constant throughout childhood.

Stanitski DF, Stanitski CL. Fibular hemimelia: a new classification system. J Pediat Orthop 2003;23:30.
A new classification system for fibular hemimelia is proposed based on the authors' experience with 32 patients (33 involved limbs) representing a spectrum of involvement. The data demonstrate the broad and unpredictable relationships among the fibula, ankle, and foot in this disorder. Because of this variability and unpredictability of the multiple relationships, limb salvage criteria should also include the nature of the foot and ankle and not merely depend on the length discrepancy or the presence or absence of the fibula.

Westin GW, Sakai DN, Wood WL. Congenital longitudinal deficiency of the fibula. J Bone Joint Surg 1976;58A:492.
Follow-up study of Syme's type amputation for fibular deficiency with severe shortening of the limb and equinovalgus deformity of the foot and ankle.

Camptomelic Dysplasia

Cheema JI, Grissom LE, Harcke HT. Radiographic characteristics of lower-extremity bowing in children. Radiographics 2003;19:204.
This article reviews lower-extremity bowing conditions in infants and children. Recognition of these pathologic conditions is important for differentiating those that will resolve spontaneously from those that require surgery or other treatment.

Coscia MF, Bassett GS, Bowen JR et al. Spinal abnormalities in camptomelic dysplasia. J Pediatr Orthop 1989;9:6.
Significant spinal abnormalities were found in eight patients (average age of 6 years, 5 months) with camptomelic dysplasia. This study clarifies that patients with camptomelic dysplasia are surviving longer than previously expected and therefore should have their spinal deformities treated aggressively.

Cleidocranial Dysplasia

Golan I, Baumert U, Hrala BP, Mussig D. Dentomaxillofacial variability of cleidocranial dysplasia: clinicaoradiological presentation and systematic review. Dentomaxillofac Radiol 2003;32:347.
Review of authors' series (24 patients) and from the literature (259 cases) with documentation of the most common caraniofacial abnormalities observed in these patients.

Tessa A, Salvi S, Casali C et al. Six novel mutations of the RUNX2 gene in Italian patients with cleidocranial dysplasia. Hum Mutat 2003;22:104.
Report of clinical and molecular findings in 14 patients with this condition.

Otto F, Kanegame H, Mundlos S. Mutations in the RUNX2 gene in patients with cleidocranial dysplasia. Hum Mutat 2002; 19:209.
Review of the genetics abnormalities leading to this condition.

Cooper SC, Flaitz CM, Johnston DA et al. A natural history of cleidocranial dysplasia. Am J Med Genet 2001;104:1.
Review of clinical characteristics and a more complete delineation of clinical complications associated with this condition. Management recommendations based on the results of this study are included.

Mundlos S. Cleidocranial dysplasia: clinical and molecular genetics. J Med Genet 1999;36:177.
Review of the clinical and molecular aspects of this condition.

Osteogenesis Imperfecta

Benson DR, Donaldson DH, Millar EA. The spine in osteogenesis imperfecta. J Bone Joint Surg 1978;60A:925.
The incidence and severity of spinal deformities in patients with this condition varies with age (26% < 5 years and 80% for those older than 12).

Chamberlain JR, Schwarze U, Wang PR et al. Gene targeting in stem cells form individuals with osteogenesis imperfecta. Science 2004;303:1198.
The authors have used adeno-associated virus vectors to disrupt dominant-negative mutant COL1A1 genes in MCS from individuals with this condition, demonstrating successful gene targeting.

Gamble JG, Studwick WJ, Rinsky LA et al. Complications of intramedullary rods in osteogenesis imperfecta: Bailey-Dubow rods versus nonelongating rods. J Pediatr Orthop 1988;8:645.
Evaluation of these two techniques with a complication rate of 69% for the Bailey-Dubow and 55% for the rigid rods.

Niyibizi C, Wang S, Mi Z, Robbins PD. Gene therapy approaches for osteogenesis imperfecta. Gene Ther 2004;11:408.
Review of the molecular changes seen in osteogenesis imperfecta, the current treatment options and the gene therapy approaches being investigated as potential future treatments for this condition.

Rauch F, Glorieux FH. Osteogenesis imperfecta. Lancet 2004; 363:1377.
Most current review of this condition and new methods of management.

Sillence DO. Osteogenesis imperfecta: an expanding panorama of variants. Clin Orthop 1981;159:11.
Description of clinical features of this condition emphasizing its heterogeneity and proposal of a classification.

Wynne-Davies R, Gormley J. Clinical and genetic patterns in osteogenesis imperfecta. Clin Orthop 1981;159:26.
Description of clinical features and genetic patterns in this condition that can help in its classification.

Marfan Syndrome

Ahn NU, Sponseller PD, Ahn UM et al. Dural ectasia is associated with back pain in Marfan syndrome. Spine 2000; 25:1562.
A cross-sectional study comparing the prevalence and size of dural ectasia in patients with Marfan syndrome with or without pain.

De Paepe A, Devereux RB, Dietz HC et al. Revised diagnostic criteria for the Marfan syndrome. Am J Med Genet 1996;62:417.
In this paper the authors proposed a revision of diagnostic criteria for Marfan syndrome and related conditions.

Morse RP, Rockenmacher S, Pyeritz RE et al. Diagnosis and management of infantile Marfan syndrome. Pediatrics 1990;86:888.
The experience of the authors with 22 severely affected infants diagnosed with Marfan syndrome. Morbidity and mortality may be high during infancy and prompt recognition can facilitate management and counseling.

Pereira L, Levran O, Ramirez F et al. A molecular approach to the stratification of cardiovascular risk in families with Marfan's syndrome. N Engl J Med 1994;331:148.
The goal of this study was to develop a widely applicable method of molecular diagnosis. The results demonstrated that the various clinical phenotypes may be due not to the single fibrillin mutations, but rather to different genetic alterations.

Phornphutkul C, Rosenthal A, and Nadas AS. Cardiac manifestations of Marfan syndrome in infancy and childhood. Circulation 1973;47:587.
Description of the clinical features associated with the cardiac abnormalities in this condition.

Sponseller PD, Hobbs W, Riley LH III et al. The thoracolumbar spine in Marfan syndrome. J Bone Joint Surg 1995;77A:867.
This study analyzed the prevalence, inheritance, progression, and functional implications of spinal deformity in Marfan syndrome.

Wenger DR, Ditkoff T J, Herring JA et al. Protrusio acetabuli in Marfan's syndrome. Clin Orthop 1980;147:134.
This study evaluates the prevalence of protrusio acetabuli in this condition.

Multiple Epiphyseal Dysplasia and Pseudoachondroplasia

Briggs MD, Chapman KL. Pseudoachondroplasia and multiple epiphyseal dysplasia: mutation review, molecular interactions, and genotype to phenotype correlations. Hum Mutat 2002;19:465.
Excellent review of the molecular abnormalities of these conditions, and discussion of the correlation between genotype and phenotype.

Cooper RR, Ponseti IV, Maynard JA. Pseudoachondroplastic dwarfism: a rough-surfaced endoplasmic reticulum storage disorder. J Bone Joint Surg 1973;55A:475.
Description of the ultrastructural abnormalities that differentiates this disorder from other skeletal dysplasias.

Crossan JF, Wynne-Davies R, Fulford GE. Bilateral failure of the capital femoral epiphysis: bilateral Perthes disease, multiple epiphyseal dysplasia, pseudoachondroplasia, and spondyloepiphyseal dysplasia congenita and tarda. J Pediatr Orthop 1983;3:297.
The authors conclude that Perthes disease can be differentiated radiographically from other skeletal dysplasias.

Fairbank T. Dysplasia epiphysialis multiplex. Br J Surg 1947;34:225.
Classic article describing the clinical and radiographic characteristics of this condition.

McKeand J, Rotta J, Hecht JT. Natural history study of pseudoa-chondroplasia. Am J Med Genet 1996;63:406.
This study delineates the natural history of this condition based on the follow up of 79 patients. Premature osteoarthritis was the major health problem for these individuals.

Treble NJ, Jensen FO, Bankier A et al. Development of the hip in multiple epiphyseal dysplasia. Natural history and susceptibility to premature osteoarthritis. J Bone Joint Surg 1990;72B:1061.
Premature osteoarthritis was a frequent outcome and was almost inevitable before the age of 30 years in those with incongruent hips.

Achondroplasia

Hall JG. The natural history of achondroplasia. Basic Life Sci 1988;48:3.
A review of the long term problems in this condition.

Lutter LD, Lonstein JE, Winter RB, Langer LO. Anatomy of the achondroplastic lumbar canal. Clin Orthop 1977;126:139.
A description of the anatomic variations of the lumbar spine in patients with this condition.

Maynard JA, Ippolito EG, Ponseti IV, Mickelson MR. Histochemistry and ultrastructure of the growth plate in achondroplasia. J Bone Joint Surg 1981;63A:969.
Detailed analysis of the histological and ultrastructural abnormalities of the growth plate in this condition.

Ponseti IV. Skeletal growth in achondroplasia. J Bone Joint Surg 1970;52A:701.
Classic paper on the growth disturbances in this condition based on histological and radiographic observations.

Shiang R, Thompson LM, Zhu YZ et al. Mutations in the transmembrane domain of FGFR3 cause the most common genetic form of dwarfism, achondroplasia. Cell 1994;78:335.
Description of the genetic abnormality underlying this condition.

Vitamin D–Resistant Rickets

Choi IH, Kim JK, Chung CY et al. Deformity correction of knee and leg lengthening by Ilizarov method in hypophosphatemic rickets: outcomes and significance of serum phosphate level. J Pediatr Orthop 2002;22:626.
The authors evaluated 14 patients with this condition and found that the healing index correlated with the biochemical parameters. They suggested a serum phosphate of 2.5 mg/dL as the cutoff point for surgical indications.

Habener JF, Mahaffey JE. Osteomalacia and disorders of vitamin D metabolism. Ann Rev Med 1978;29:327.
Review of the pathogenic mechanism, clinical and laboratory features of these conditions, and discussion on the differential diagnosis.

Kato S, Yoshizazawa T, Kitanaka S et al. Molecular genetics of vitamin D-dependent hereditary rickets. Horm Res 2002;57:73.
Review of the most current understanding of the molecular abnormalities in these conditions.

Mankin HJ. Metabolic bone disease. J Bone Joint Surg 1994;76A:760.
Review article on the different metabolic bone conditions and their orthopaedic implications.

Parfitt AM. Hypophosphatemic vitamin D refractory rickets and osteomalacia. Orthop Clin North Am 1972;3:653.
Review of the clinical and laboratory features of this condition.

Mucopolysaccharidoses

Muenzer J. The mucopolysaccharidoses: a heterogeneous group of disorders with variable pediatric presentations. J Pediatr 2004;144:S27.
Review of the most current understanding in these conditions with discussion of the clinical features and management strategies.

Sauer M, Grewal S, Peters C. Hematopoietic stem cell transplantation for mucopolysaccharidoses and leukodystrophies. Clin Pediatr 2004;216:163.
Recent update on the use of stem cell transplantation for these disorders.

Wraith JE, Clarke LA, Beck M et al. Enzyme replacement therapy for mucopolysaccharidosis I: a randomized, double-blind, placebo-controlled, multinational study of recombinant human alpha-L-iduronidase (laronidase). J Pediatr 2004;144:581.
This study confirms that laronidase significantly improves respiratory function and physical capacity, reduces glycosaminoglycans storage, and has a favorable safety profile.

Hereditary Multiple Exostoses

Ballantyne JA, Simpson Ah, Porter DE et al. Wrist and forearm dysfunction in hereditary multiple exostosis. J Hand Surg 2003;28 (Suppl 1):26.
Description and management strategies of wrist and forearm dysfunction in patients with this condition.

Hall CR, Cole WG, Haynes R et al. Reevaluation of a genetic model for the development of exostosis in hereditary multiple exostosis. Am J Med Genet 2002;112:1.
Review of the current understanding of the molecular abnormalities and their pathogenic implications for this condition.

Noonan KJ, Feinberg JR, Levenda A et al. Natural history of multiple osteochondromatosis of the lower extremity and ankle. J Pediatr Orthop 2002;22:120.
The authors evaluated 38 patients with an average age of 42 years at follow up. They found measurable decreases in ankle function and suggest that correction or prevention of excessive tibiotalar tilt may be warranted to improve outcome.

Porter DE, Benson MK, Hosney GA. The hip in hereditary multiple exostoses. J Bone Joint Surg 2001;83B:988.
The authors define the characteristics of dysplasia and coxa valga in this condition by radiological analysis of 24 hips.

Zak BM, Crawford BE, Esko JD. Hereditary multiple exostoses and heparan sulfate polymerization. Biochem Biophys Acta 2002;1573:346.
An overview of HME, the EXT family of proteins, and possible models for the relationship of altered HS synthesis to the ectopic bone growth characteristic of the disease.

10

Kristy L. Weber
Joseph A. Buckwalter

Musculoskeletal Neoplasms and Disorders That Resemble Neoplasms

EVALUATION OF A PATIENT
  WITH A BONE OR SOFT
  TISSUE LESION
  Clinical
  Laboratory Studies
    and Radiographic Evaluation
  Biopsy Considerations

DISORDERS THAT RESEMBLE
  NEOPLASMS
  Bone Disorders
  Soft Tissue Disorders
BENIGN NEOPLASMS
  Benign Bone Neoplasms
  Benign Soft Tissue Neoplasms

MALIGNANT NEOPLASMS
  Malignant Bone Neoplasms
  Malignant Soft Tissue Neoplasms
METASTATIC NEOPLASMS
SUMMARY

Neoplasms and lesions that resemble neoplasms often present difficult diagnostic and treatment dilemmas. The anatomic location, tissue of origin, clinical presentation, and behavior of these lesions varies greatly. They may appear in any region of the musculoskeletal system; consist of or involve almost any tissue including bone, cartilage, fibrous tissue, bone marrow, lymphoid tissue, nerve, and blood vessel; and arise in patients of any age. They may destroy normal tissue and cause dramatic signs and symptoms including intolerable pain, massive swelling, severe disability, and pathologic fracture, or they may have little effect on normal tissues and remain asymptomatic. They vary in natural history from lesions that spontaneously regress to those that rapidly spread and lead to death despite early diagnosis and aggressive treatment. Despite their diversity, benign and malignant neoplasms and lesions that resemble neoplasms can have similar clinical and radiographic presentations.

Many of the lesions that resemble neoplasms occur frequently, cause minimal discomfort or disability, and can be treated without surgery. Musculoskeletal neoplasms present more complex problems. Because of their rarity and variability in presentation and behavior, few physicians have extensive experience with these problems. A standardized approach cannot always be applied to each patient

267

with symptoms, signs, or imaging studies that suggest the presence of a musculoskeletal neoplasm. In many instances, optimal care requires a multidisciplinary team of physicians, including orthopaedic surgeons, radiologists, pathologists, medical oncologists, and radiation oncologists. For these reasons, orthopaedic surgeons and other specialists with additional training in the treatment of malignant and aggressive benign neoplasms of the musculoskeletal system should provide the definitive care for most patients with these rare, complex problems.

Patients with musculoskeletal neoplasms are not always easily distinguished from patients with disorders that resemble neoplasms when they first seek medical attention. These lesions often come to the patient's or physician's attention because of nondiagnostic symptoms, signs, and abnormalities on imaging studies; as a result most patients with musculoskeletal neoplasms first present to generalists rather than orthopaedic surgeons with special experience in the treatment of these problems. It is important for the initial treating physician to determine whether a lesion is present and whether to refer the patient to an orthopaedic surgeon. The orthopaedist then must decide whether to recommend observation and symptomatic treatment, further laboratory and imaging studies, biopsy, or definitive treatment.

To provide an overview of the information necessary to identify musculoskeletal neoplasms and disorders resembling neoplasms and make initial decisions concerning diagnosis and treatment, this chapter first reviews the clinical presentation of these disorders. Subsequent sections summarize the more common disorders that resemble neoplasms, as well as benign, malignant, and metastatic neoplasms of the musculoskeletal system (Table 10-1 and 10-2).*

EVALUATION OF A PATIENT WITH A BONE OR SOFT TISSUE LESION

Bone and soft tissue neoplasms or musculoskeletal lesions that resemble neoplasms usually come to the attention of the patient or physician because of pain, swelling, or loss of musculoskeletal function. For benign, indolent lesions, a physical examination or imaging study performed for other reasons may identify the presence of a neoplasm.

Clinical

History

It is important to elicit a complete verbal history and ask specific questions to clarify the patient's symptoms and presentation. For bone lesions, pain is usually the primary symptom, but the type and

---

*The references included in the bibliography provide more detailed information concerning the diagnosis and treatment of these lesions.

TABLE 10-1.
Common Musculoskeletal Disorders That Resemble Neoplasms and Benign Neoplasms

Disorders That Resemble Neoplasms		Benign Neoplasms	
Bone	*Soft Tissue*	*Bone*	*Soft Tissue*
Diffuse osteopenia caused by metabolic bone disease	Muscle contusion/ tear/hematoma	Osteoma	Lipoma
Stress fracture	Myositis ossificans	Osteoid osteoma	Hemangioma
Brown tumor of hyperparathyroidism	Nodular fasciitis	Osteoblastoma	Glomus tumor
	Traumatic fat necrosis	Osteochondroma	Lymphangioma
Osteomyelitis	Traumatic neuroma	Enchondroma	Neurolemmoma
Infantile cortical hyperostosis	Soft tissue abcess	Periosteal chondroma	Solitary neurofibroma
Paget's disease	Ganglion cyst	Chondroblastoma	Neurofibromatosis
Bone infarct	Intramuscular myxoma	Chondromyxoid fibroma	Desmoid tumor
Bone island		Giant cell tumor of bone	Elastofibroma
Simple bone cyst		Desmoplastic fibroma	Giant cell tumor of tendon sheath
Aneurysmal bone cyst		Hemangioma	Pigmented villonodular synovitis
Fibrous cortical defect/ nonossifying fibroma		Langerhans cell histiocytosis	Synovial chondromatosis
Fibrous dysplasia			

TABLE 10-2.
Common Malignant Musculoskeletal Neoplasms and Metastatic Neoplasms

Malignant Neoplasms		Metastatic Neoplasms
Bone	*Soft Tissue*	
Multiple myeloma	Liposarcoma	Breast
Lymphoma	Malignant fibrous histiocytoma	Prostate
Ewing's sarcoma	Fibrosarcoma	Lung
Osteosarcoma	Synovial sarcoma	Kidney
Chondrosarcoma	Neurofibrosarcoma	Thyroid
Fibrosarcoma	Rhabdomyosarcoma	Gastrointestinal tract
Malignant fibrous histiocytoma	Malignant vascular tumors	
Malignant vascular tumors	Epithelioid sarcoma	
Adamantinoma	Clear cell sarcoma	
Chordoma		

pattern of pain varies. Musculoskeletal lesions can cause symptoms that range from excruciating, sharply localized pain to vague discomfort or a sense of fullness, weakness, abnormal sensation, or stiffness. When aggressive benign or malignant musculoskeletal neoplasms cause pain, patients commonly describe the pain as a progressive, deep aching that interferes with normal activities, awakens them at night, or disrupts sleep. Activity-related pain alone is more consistent with inflammation or injury. Often, rest does not relieve tumor-related pain, and occasionally the pain may be referred to a more distal location. For example, a tumor involving the hip may either cause radiating pain from the thigh to the knee or pain limited to the ipsilateral knee. A tumor of the cervical spine may cause radiating pain down the arm, and neoplasms of the lumbar spine or pelvis may cause discomfort in the buttock, thigh, or leg. The physician should not be fooled by referred pain when performing a clinical or radiographic evaluation. For example, it is not unusual for a patient with a proximal femoral lesion to complain of knee pain, and subsequently have extensive studies of the knee before radiographs of the proximal femur reveal the presence of the lesion responsible for their symptoms.

Benign and malignant soft tissue neoplasms are not generally painful, and this often leads to denial by the patient and a delay in diagnosis. A thorough clinical history can often provide clues to whether a lesion is benign or malignant, especially in the soft tissues. It is important to ask how long the pain or a mass has been noted. A long-standing mass is less likely to be malignant, but rare malignant lesions,

such as a synovial sarcoma, grow slowly over months or years. An enlarging mass is more worrisome than a small, stable mass, but some soft tissue sarcomas such as an epithelioid sarcoma or clear cell sarcoma can present as small nodules along the tendon sheaths of the hands and feet. A history of trauma might signify the presence of myositis ossificans. It is important to ask about a personal history of cancer, as carcinomas can metastasize to the bone or soft tissues. A family history of masses might suggest an inherited disorder such as neurofibromatosis.

Physical Examination

Many soft tissue and some bone neoplasms cause diffuse swelling or a firm, well-defined mass. Others produce only a slight increase in limb circumference. Infrequently, the reaction of normal tissues to a tumor near a synovial joint causes an effusion, and bleeding into a tumor produces a hematoma, but physicians should be alert to the underlying problem. Tumors confined within bone cannot be palpated, and deep soft tissue tumors may produce little or no increase in limb circumference. This is a particular problem with deep soft tissue tumors of the pelvis, thigh, hip, and shoulder. These lesions can reach substantial size without producing an easily palpated mass, particularly in obese or muscular patients. For these reasons, lack of a palpable mass or measurable swelling does not eliminate the possibility of a musculoskeletal neoplasm. Masses worrisome for malignancy are large (>5 cm), firm, deep, fixed, and proximal in the extremities. A rock-hard mass is typical of a benign, but aggressive, desmoid tumor. Small superficial nodules in the hand include the possibility of an epithelioid sarcoma, and nodules along the tendon sheath may be a clear cell sarcoma. It is important to examine the entire extremity for additional masses, as malignant soft tissue tumors can have satellite lesions or regional nodal metastasis.

Occasionally, patients with musculoskeletal tumors present with a primary complaint of loss of musculoskeletal function. The loss of function associated with tumors may result from pain, neurologic deficit, pathologic fracture or restriction of joint motion. Neurologic deficits may progress slowly as in a patient with a large soft tissue sarcoma of the posterior thigh gradually compressing the sciatic nerve. More commonly, the neurologic deficits may occur acutely as in the sudden compression of the spinal cord or nerve roots resulting from rapid enlargement of a primary or metastatic vertebral tumor.

Physicians should suspect the presence of a neoplasm in any patient that develops a fracture following minor trauma. If the mechanism of injury does not correlate with the fracture, there should be a high suspicion of an underlying pathologic process. Some patients report pain at the site of the fracture before the injury. Plain radiographs often show a bony irregularity or lytic lesion, but these irregularities may be difficult to identify. The neoplasm may cause a diffuse decrease in bone mass and density instead of a localized abnormality. Thus, even when the radiographs do not show an obvious lesion, patients who sustain a fracture following minimal trauma should be carefully evaluated for the presence of a neoplasm. If a pathologic fracture secondary to an underlying malignant bone tumor is not recognized, the surgical treatment could compromise the limb or life of the patient.

Laboratory Studies and Radiographic Evaluation

The majority of neoplasms and lesions resembling neoplasms cannot be identified with routine laboratory studies. There are few serum markers available of diagnostic or prognostic significance for patients with musculoskeletal tumors. Elevated white blood cell counts and erythrocyte sedimentation rates (ESR) are usually indicative of infection, but these values can be elevated in tumors such as Ewing's sarcoma. Often alkaline phosphatase is elevated in metastatic bone disease or Paget's disease. Patients with multiple myeloma often have a marked anemia and an abnormal serum and urine protein electrophoresis.

Plain radiographs are often the only study necessary to diagnose benign bone lesions. Many have a classically described appearance, and more elaborate imaging is not helpful. Occasionally, radiographs performed for a different reason reveal an unsuspected bone lesion. The majority of these incidentally noted findings are benign. For patients with a soft tissue mass, the plain radiographs may reveal helpful soft tissue shadows or calcifications within the lesion, such as are occasionally found in hemangiomas and synovial sarcomas. For patients with bone lesions, it is important to evaluate radiographs in two planes, and for those with metastatic disease, the entire bone should be imaged to rule out the possibility of additional lesions.

A technetium bone scan is used to identify additional skeletal lesions without performing multiple radiographs. In rapidly growing lesions with minimal osteoblastic response such as multiple myeloma and some metastatic bone tumors, the bone scan is not reliable and a skeletal survey should be performed instead. For patients with multiple osteochondromas or Langerhans cell histiocytosis, skeletal surveys are also preferred over bone scans in order to better define the characteristics of specific lesions. In recent years, FDG-PET scans are gaining in importance for staging patients with metastatic disease and following the effects of systemic treatment.

Three dimensional studies such as computed tomography (CT) and magnetic resonance imaging (MRI) are frequently used to evaluate musculoskeletal neoplasms. The CT scan is useful in defining the bony anatomy, the integrity of the cortex surrounding a lesion, and calcification within a lesion. The MRI scan is useful when evaluating patients with malignant bone or soft tissue tumors. The multiple magnetic sequences now available can accurately delineate the extent of marrow involvement of bone tumors and the effect of soft tissue masses on surrounding visceral or neurovascular structures.

Biopsy Considerations

After the clinical and radiographic evaluation of a patient with a suspected bone or soft tissue lesion is complete, the physician should have a general idea of whether the lesion is benign or malignant.

Unless the radiographic appearance is classic for a benign lesion, a biopsy is needed to make a definitive diagnosis. Only a radiologist or orthopaedic surgeon with training and expertise in performing biopsies should do this procedure. Options include a fine needle aspiration, core biopsy, or an open incisional biopsy. The diagnosis of these rare musculoskeletal lesions should be made at institutions with trained musculoskeletal pathologists, especially in situations where needle biopsies are utilized. All biopsies should be performed with oncologic principles in mind to minimize contamination of surrounding tissues and allow the best chance of limb-sparing surgery if the lesion is malignant.

DISORDERS THAT RESEMBLE NEOPLASMS

Musculoskeletal disorders that resemble neoplasms, or tumor simulators, occur more frequently than neoplasms. The symptoms, signs, and imaging studies of metabolic bone diseases, musculoskeletal injuries, infections, developmental disorders and diseases of unknown etiology may closely resemble neoplasms. For example, a stress fracture can mimic a bone-forming neoplasm, and myositis ossificans can resemble a sarcoma. Osteomyelitis and Ewing's sarcoma are often difficult to distinguish based on the history, physical findings, and plain radiographs.

Bone Disorders

Diffuse Osteopenia Caused by Metabolic Bone Disease

Metabolic bone diseases, most commonly osteoporosis, osteomalacia, and various forms of hyperparathyroidism, decrease bone density and strength and thereby increase the probability of fracture. Some pathologic fractures associated with nonneoplastic causes of osteopenia may be difficult to distinguish from pathologic fractures due to diffuse lysis from multiple myeloma or metastatic carcinoma.

Vertebral compression fractures, collapse, or wedging of vertebral bodies in patients with osteopenia occur frequently and can present difficult diagnostic problems. Common nonneoplastic conditions that cause osteopenia and predispose older patients to vertebral compression fractures include osteoporosis and osteomalacia; neoplasms, especially multiple myeloma and metastatic carcinoma, may produce similar clinical, physical, and radiographic findings. Many vertebral compression fractures associated with nonneoplastic causes of osteopenia require only symptomatic treatment, but untreated vertebral fractures due to neoplastic disease can lead to progressive pain and neurologic compromise.

The presence of osteopenia due to metabolic bone disease may present as a pathologic fracture or after radiographs are taken for evaluation of another problem and show decreased bone density. Clinical evaluation and standard laboratory tests can help identify the probable cause of diffuse osteopenia. Well-nourished elderly patients with diffuse osteopenia but a normal blood count, erythrocyte sedimentation rate (ESR), serum calcium, and serum phosphorus usually have osteoporosis, but a bone biopsy may be necessary to rule out osteomalacia and make a definitive diagnosis. Elevated serum calcium and depressed serum phosphorus suggest the possibility of hyperparathyroidism, and an elevated ESR with anemia suggests the possibly of neoplastic disease such as multiple myeloma.

Stress Fracture

A stress or fatigue fracture is a localized osteoblastic reaction of bone without apparent disruption of the cortex. It usually causes pain and may cause radiographic changes that imitate bone-forming tumors. They occur in children, adults, and the elderly. In children, stress fractures may resemble osteosarcomas; in older people stress fractures may resemble metastatic tumors. Biopsy of a stress fracture reveals cellular tissue with extensive new bone formation that may be difficult to distinguish from tissue found in a malignant bone-forming neoplasm.

Stress fractures presumably result from fatigue failure of bone or a localized reaction of bone to repetitive loading. Common sites include the metatarsals, tibia, fibula, femur, pelvis, and lamina of the lumbar vertebrae. Stress fractures often occur in young active individuals with normal bone, but they also present in patients with osteopenia from osteoporosis or osteomalacia and in those with neoplasms. The pain associated with a stress fracture usually increases with activity and decreases with rest. In the early phases of a stress fracture or stress reaction of bone, plain radiographic studies may not show obvious abnormalities, but a bone scan will demonstrate increased uptake at the site of new bone formation. At later stages plain radiographs may or may not reveal a fracture line, but they usually show periosteal new bone formation that extends as a dense line into the medullary cavity of the bone. Stress fractures usually heal with restriction of activity or immobilization.

Brown Tumor of Hyperparathyroidism

Patients with hyperparathyroidism can develop localized, expansile, destructive bone lesions called brown tumors. They mimic neoplasms because of diffuse bone resorption similar to neoplastic and non-neoplastic osteopenia. The focal, destructive lesions occur within the diaphysis or metaphysis of long bones where they resorb the medullary cancellous bone and expand the bone cortex. They may reach a large size and lead to pathologic fractures. Because of their radiographic appearance and histologic picture of multiple giant cells, hemorrhage, and fibrous tissue, brown tumors can be mistaken for giant cell tumors (GCTs) of bone. Unlike patients with GCTs, those with hyperparathyroidism often have a history consistent with hyperparathyroidism—an elevated serum calcium, depressed serum phosphorous, elevated parathyroid hormone, and radiographic changes of diffuse bone resorption. The bone disease associated with hyperparathyroidism usually resolves following successful treatment of the underlying disorder.

Osteomyelitis

Osteomyelitis is an infection of bone usually due to bacteria and can cause pain, systemic symptoms, physical findings and radiographic changes (bone destruction combined with new bone formation and prominent periosteal reaction) that closely resemble tumors including osteoid osteoma, eosinophilic granuloma, Ewing's sarcoma, lymphoma, and osteosarcoma (Figure 10-1, Figure 10-2). Histologic examination of infected bone reveals inflammatory cells, necrotic bone, and new bone formation (Figure 10-3). Some patients with osteomyelitis have systemic symptoms including fever, weight loss, and fatigue, while others are nearly asymptomatic.

Typically, hematogenous osteomyelitis involves the metaphysis of long bones, but it can occur in any location. A definitive diagnosis of osteomyelitis depends on a positive culture of the infecting organism. Biopsies of presumably infected bone show nonspecific inflammation with regions of new bone

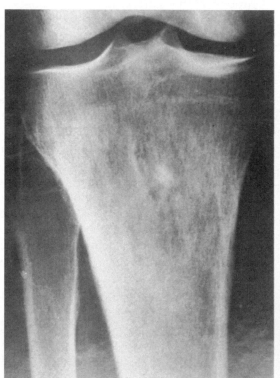
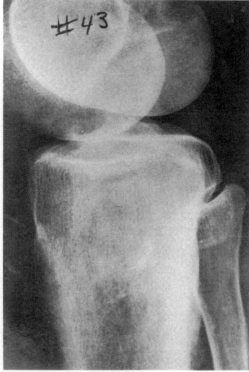

FIGURE 10-1. Radiographs showing osteomyelitis of the proximal tibia with irregular bone destruction and formation.

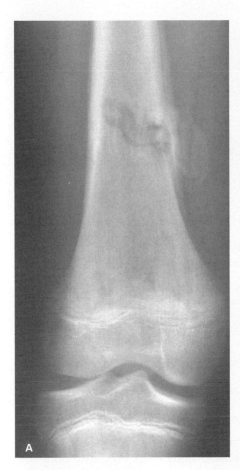
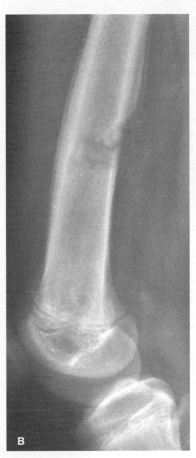
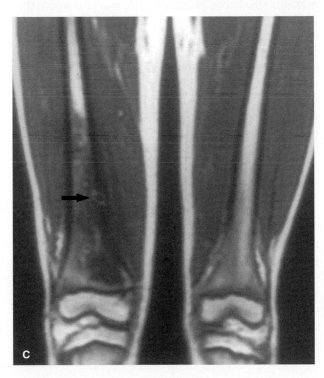

FIGURE 10-2. (A) and **(B)** Radiographs showing osteomyelitis of the distal femur. Periosteal new bone increases the diameter and density of the bone. **(C)** An MRI reveals the extensive marrow signal change (*arrow*).

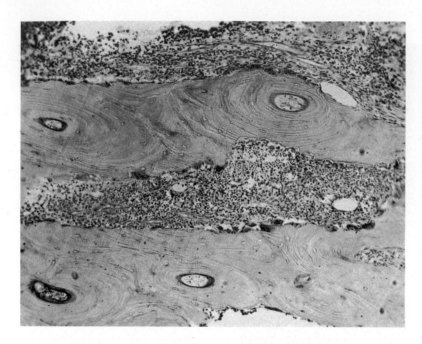

FIGURE 10-3. Low power histologic section of infected bone. Inflammatory cells fill the marrow space, and osteoclasts resorb adjacent bone. The areas with no osteoclasts indicate necrotic bone.

formation that could result from infection by a variety of organisms, but these same processes can be found near bone tumors. In addition to antibiotic therapy, treatment of osteomyelitis usually requires surgical debridement.

If treatment does not eradicate the infection, a chronic draining sinus may develop from the underlying site. Some patients, after years of sinus drainage, develop squamous cell carcinoma in the sinus tract. These malignancies can be detected by a change in the amount or odor of the drainage, a friable, vascular, enlarging mass, and subsequent bone destruction. Treatment of these secondary carcinomas requires wide resection or amputation.

Infantile Cortical Hyperostosis (Caffey's Disease)

Infantile cortical hyperostosis, a rare idiopathic disorder that causes rapid periosteal new bone formation, occurs most frequently in children under 6 months of age. Common sites include the diaphysis of long bones, ribs, mandible, and scapula. Fever, leukocytosis, and an increased ESR often accompany the periosteal new bone formation. Tenderness of the involved bones and palpable swelling of the periosteum precede radiographic changes. Once new bone formation begins, radiographs show multiple layers of periosteal new bone (Figure 10-4). The clinical presentation and radiographic changes resemble osteomyelitis, syphilis, Vitamin A toxicity, Vitamin C deficiency, trauma, and Ewing's sarcoma.

The patient may have multiple remissions and exacerbations, but the disorder eventually resolves and the bones remodel to a normal configuration.

Paget's Disease (Osteitis Deformans)

Paget's disease, an idiopathic disorder characterized by increased bone resorption and bone formation, produces characteristic bone lesions that cause pain, deformity, and fracture. It either occurs in one bone (monostotic Paget's disease) or multiple bones (polyostotic Paget's disease). It varies in severity from an isolated, asymptomatic bone lesion to crippling deformities of multiple bones. The clinical and radiographic presentation of Paget's disease may resemble neoplasms such as metastatic carcinoma. Paget's disease rarely occurs before age 20, and most patients are over age 50. It can affect any part of the skeleton, although it frequently appears in the pelvis, femur, skull, tibia, and spine. It is one of the few disorders that causes bone enlargement.

Radiographically, Paget's disease proceeds through three phases: a purely lytic phase, a mixed lytic and blastic phase, and a blastic phase (Figure 10-5). The early bone lysis results from extensive osteoclastic bone resorption. The blastic changes correspond to a decrease in bone resorption and increase in formation of new dense bone with an irregular mosaic pattern. The earliest phase of Paget's disease appears radiographically as a wedge, flame,

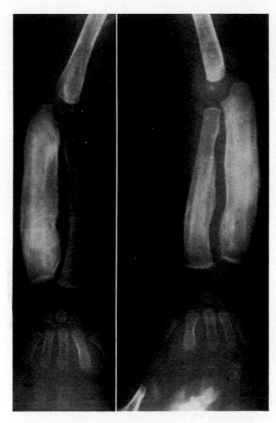

FIGURE 10-4. Radiographs showing characteristic laminations of subperiosteal new bone about the radius and ulna in a patient with infantile cortical hyperostosis.

or V-shaped region of bone lysis at the end of a long bone. Later the cortical bone and medullary trabeculae become more dense, enlarged, and irregular. Some regions of the bone become extremely dense, obliterating the areas of lysis. Histologic examination of pagetoid bone reveals an irregular or "mosaic" pattern of bone formation and fibrovascular tissue filling the marrow spaces (Color Figure 10-1).

Pagetoid bone lacks the strength of normal bone. As a result it deforms and fractures more easily. Patients with Paget's disease may develop primary malignancies such as osteosarcoma in the abnormal bone that spread rapidly and portend an extremely poor prognosis. Increasing localized pain, a soft tissue mass, radiographic evidence of bone destruction (Figure 10-6), or a pathologic fracture suggest the possibility of malignant degeneration.

Bone Infarct/Avascular Necrosis

Bone infarcts are areas of avascular bone within the medullary canal, and their actual incidence is unknown. They occasionally cause pain. Avascular necrosis may occur following traumatic or surgical

interruption of the blood supply to a portion of the bone or in association with corticosteroid use, radiation therapy or sickle cell anemia. Idiopathic bone infarcts occur in the absence of any underlying medical condition or known cause. Common sites for bone infarcts include the femoral head, femoral condyle, talus, carpal navicular, and metaphyses of the long bones, but the process can occur in any region of the skeleton.

The radiographic appearance is of an area of irregular increased density within the medullary canal that resembles an enchondroma or low grade chondrosarcoma. They have a classic, serpiginous appearance on MRI scan. Necrosis of small regions of bone marrow may be painful but does not significantly weaken the bone. However, necrosis of load-bearing subchondral regions with subsequent vascular invasion and resorption of necrotic bone can lead to structural collapse, particularly in the femoral head, humeral head, and talus. Degenerative joint disease develops following collapse of the articular surface. Rarely, a malignant fibrous histiocytoma can develop in or near bone infarcts, especially the idiopathic, metaphyseal infarcts of long bones.

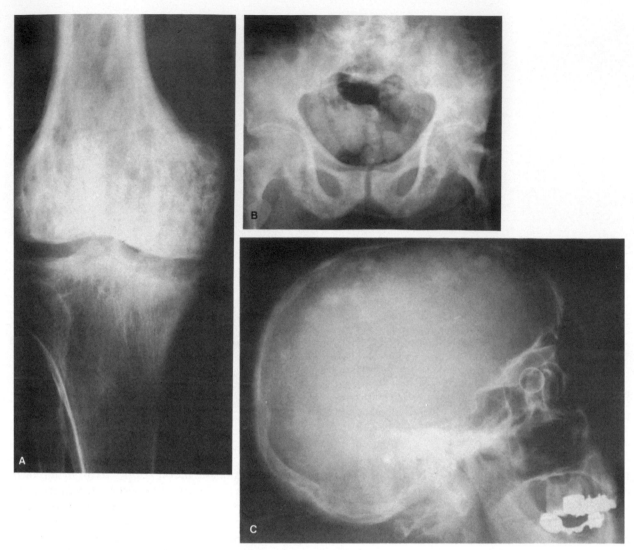

FIGURE 10-5. Radiographs showing the lytic and blastic changes of Paget's disease in the **(A)** distal femur, **(B)** pelvis, and **(C)** skull.

Metaphyseal bone infarcts usually require only symptomatic treatment, but subchondral infarcts that cause articular surface collapse often require surgical intervention. The indications and long-term results of surgical procedures intended to revascularize or decompress large areas of subchondral bone necrosis are controversial.

Bone Island

Bone islands consist of discrete areas of mature lamellar bone within the medullary cavity. On radiographic studies they are rounded lesions less than two centimeters in size located within cancellous bone (Figure 10-7). Occasionally they resemble osteoblastic metastasis. Because they are asymptomatic, bone islands are usually identified as incidental findings on plain radiographs or other imaging studies. They do not require treatment.

Simple Bone Cyst

Simple, or unicameral, bone cysts consist of fluid-filled cavities within bone lined by a thin layer of fibrous tissue. They occur most commonly in children less than 15 years of age. Approximately 50% occur in the proximal humeral metaphysis. Other common sites include the proximal femur

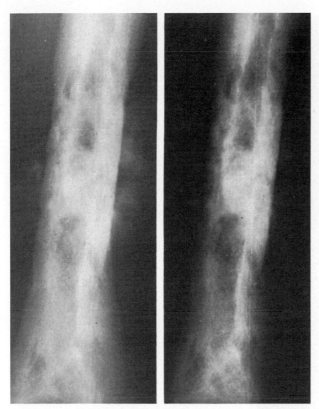

FIGURE 10-6. Radiographs showing a femoral osteosarcoma arising in pagetoid bone. The tumor has formed new bone and extended through the cortex.

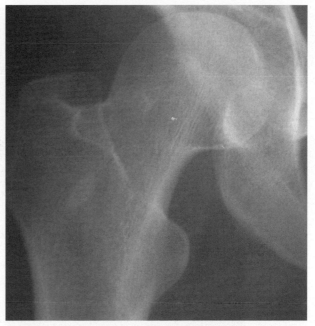

FIGURE 10-7. Radiograph showing a small bone island in the proximal femur. It is sclerotic and incites no surrounding reaction.

and iliac wing. They may cause slight expansion of bone and thinning of the cortex. As a result patients often present with a pathologic fracture through the cyst. Some cysts may be discovered incidentally when radiographs are taken for other reasons.

Radiographically, simple bone cysts are centrally located, lucent lesions of the metaphysis (Figure 10-8). As new bone in skeletally immature patients grows away from the cyst, the lesion may eventually reside in the diaphysis. Unicameral cysts that present as central, lytic lesions of the proximal humerus or proximal femur in young children have a classic appearance that does not require further imaging or biopsy. However, cysts in other locations or those that lack characteristic radiographic features may mimic other musculoskeletal lesions including aneurysmal bone cysts, fibrous dysplasia, and osteosarcoma. More aggressive lesions can be eliminated based on the histologic appearance of a large cystic lesion with innocuous cells in the lining tissue. Simple cysts resolve as patients reach skeletal maturity, but they can cause multiple pathologic fractures during growth, especially when they are noted at a very young age. The

fractures cause skeletal deformity, especially when they occur in the proximal femur. Most fractures through simple cysts heal rapidly with closed treatment (Figure 10-9). The current recommended treatment of simple cysts includes observation with restriction of activity and steroid injections. Intralesional curettage and bone grafting is generally reserved for large cysts at high risk for fracture in the proximal femur.

Aneurysmal Bone Cyst

Aneurysmal bone cysts (ABCs) consist of blood-filled cavities lined by fibrous septae that include giant cells and areas of osteoid but no true endothelial cells (Color Figure 10-2). Approximately 85% of patients with ABCs present before age 20. The most common symptoms are pain, swelling, and tenderness on palpation of the involved bone. ABCs commonly involve the metaphysis of long bones, posterior elements of the vertebrae, pelvis, or scapula, but they can occur throughout the skeleton (Figure 10-10). ABCs can grow rapidly and frequently cause pathologic fractures. When located in the spine, they can cause neurologic compromise.

Plain radiographs show a lytic lesion causing marked expansion of the involved bone and occa-

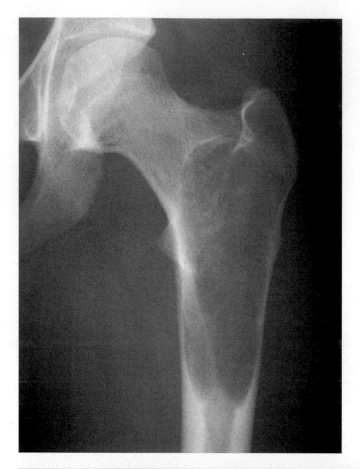

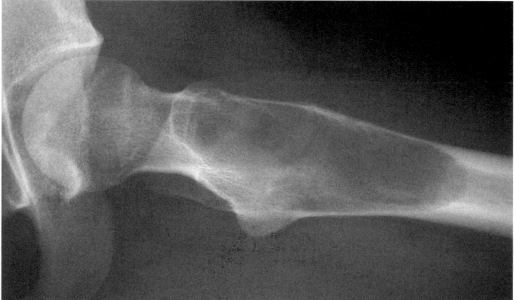

FIGURE 10-8. Radiographs showing a unicameral (simple) bone cyst of the proximal femur at risk for pathologic fracture. Notice the symmetrical metadiaphyseal location of the cyst.

expanding and begin to ossify after reaching a certain size or they may regress spontaneously. Standard treatment is a confirmatory biopsy followed by intralesional curettage and bone grafting.

Fibrous Cortical Defect and Nonossifying Fibroma

Fibrous cortical defects (metaphyseal fibrous defects) and nonossifying fibromas are lytic bone lesions that consist of fibroblasts arranged in whirled bundles with scattered giant cells and regions of histiocytes. They are commonly discovered incidentally on plain radiographs. They rarely appear in children younger than 2 years of age or in adults over 20 years of age. They develop in the metaphysis and, as the bone grows, they gradually seem to move toward the diaphysis. When patients near skeletal maturity, the lesions ossify or completely disappear. Most authors refer to large fibrous cortical defects that extend into the intramedullary region of the bone as nonossifying fibromas.

Radiographically, these are sharply circumscribed, radiolucent, eccentric, or intracortical lesions of long bones (Figure 10-12). Except for rare pathologic fractures, they do not cause pain. The diagnosis can usually be made based on their distinctive radiographic appearance. These lesions heal spontaneously, so they do not require treatment unless a pathologic fracture has or is likely to occur. In these situations, intralesional curettage and bone grafting allows definitive healing of the lesion.

Fibrous Dysplasia

Fibrous dysplasia is metaplastic bone formation consisting of irregularly arranged bone trabeculae in bland fibrous tissue (Figure 10-13) and is among the most common lesions of bone. It can weaken bone and lead to a pathologic fracture, and it may have a radiographic appearance that resembles a more aggressive tumor. In some patients it involves a single bone (monostotic fibrous dysplasia), but in others it involves multiple bones (polyostotic fibrous dysplasia). The severity of the disorder ranges from isolated small lesions that remain asymptomatic to lesions that cause repeated pathologic fractures and deformity of multiple bones. Although most authors consider fibrous dysplasia a developmental disorder rather than a neoplasm, it can destroy or expand normal bone and frequently recurs following curettage and bone grafting.

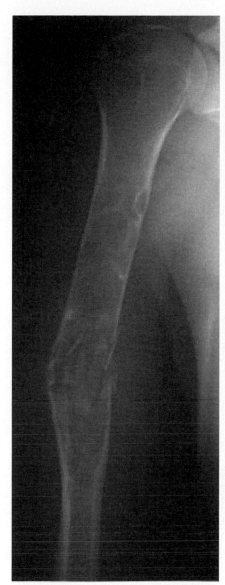

FIGURE 10-9. Radiograph showing an extensive simple bone cyst of the humerus with a pathologic fracture and mild displacement.

sional periosteal new bone formation (Figure 10-11). An MRI scan often reveals fluid-fluid levels. Aggressive benign neoplasms such as giant cell tumors and primary malignant neoplasms such as telangiectatic osteosarcoma can have a similar radiographic appearance.

ABCs frequently occur in association with primary bone lesions including fibrous dysplasia, giant cell tumor, simple bone cyst, eosinophilic granuloma, nonossifying fibroma, chondroblastoma, osteoblastoma, and occasionally osteosarcoma. They may stop

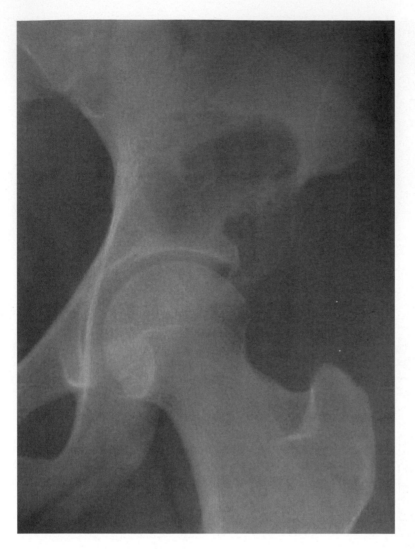

FIGURE 10-10. Radiograph of the hip showing an expansile, lytic lesion in the acetabulum consistent with an aneurysmal bone cyst.

Fibrous dysplasia occurs in children and is often discovered because of pain, pathologic fracture, or skeletal deformity. Plain radiographs show circumscribed areas of decreased bone density having a ground glass or "shower door glass" appearance. Because fibrous dysplasia can thin and expand the cortex concentrically or eccentrically, the lesions may resemble unicameral or multilocular cysts (Figure 10-14).

Fibrous dysplasia commonly affects the ribs, vertebrae, femur, tibia, humerus, and maxilla (Figure 10-15). When fibrous dysplasia involves the proximal femur, the resulting weakening of the bone may lead to progressive microfractures and is referred to as a "Shepherd's crook deformity" (Figure 10-16).

Fibrous dysplasia begins during childhood and may progressively enlarge. The lesions often become less active or inactive at skeletal maturity, but they can grow in adults. In some patients, polyostotic fibrous dysplasia occurs in association with precocious puberty and darkly pigmented skin lesions in a disorder called McCune-Albright syndrome. Several case reports have described the appearance of malignant tumors in regions of fibrous dysplasia, although malignant transformation is extremely rare. Most patients with small lesions of fibrous dysplasia do not require treatment. Patients with pathologic fractures or progressive skeletal deformity require curettage, bone grafting, and skeletal stabilization. Recently, bisphosphonates have been used with documented pain relief in a subset of patients.

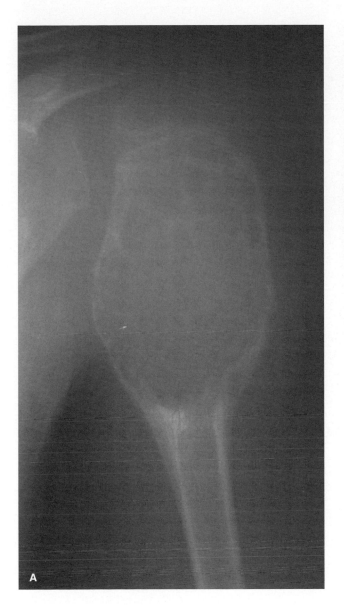

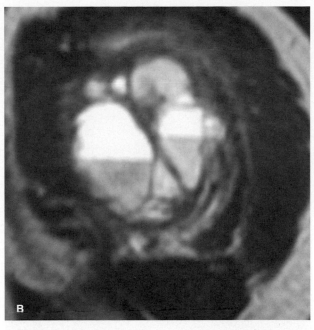

FIGURE 10-11. A large aneurysmal bone cyst in the proximal humerus is shown by **(A)** radiograph and **(B)** MRI scan. Note the expansile nature of the lesion as well as the fluid-fluid levels.

Soft Tissue Disorders

Muscle Contusions, Tears, and Intramuscular Hematomas

Muscle contusions and tears may result in soft tissue masses that resemble neoplasms. The hemorrhage that results from these injuries causes swelling, and the muscle that retracts from the site of a tear may form a discrete mass. Initially the muscle damage, inflammation, and hemorrhage causes pain and weakness. As the tissue heals the pain resolves, but a mass can remain for several months.

Muscle contusions result from direct trauma that ruptures blood vessels and damages muscle cells. Common sites of muscle contusion include the deltoid, brachialis, biceps, and quadriceps muscle bellies. Muscle tears usually result from contraction of the muscle against resistance. They often occur at the musculotendinous junction, and common sites include the hamstrings, quadriceps, and biceps muscles.

Most intramuscular hematomas gradually resolve, but some become organized and remain as firm, intramuscular masses. These organized hematomas may mimic intramuscular neoplasms on

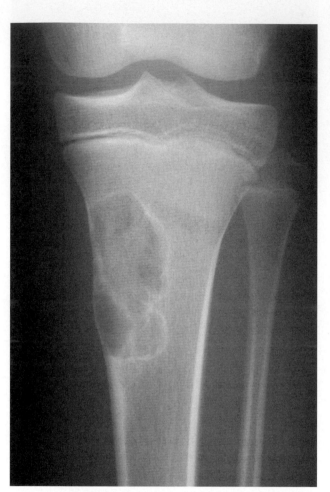

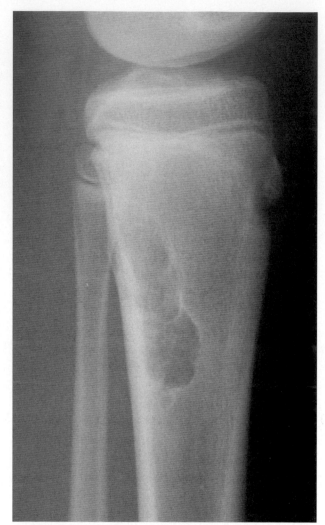

FIGURE 10-12. Radiographs showing a nonossifying fibroma in the proximal tibia. Note the sclerotic rim and eccentric location of the lesion.

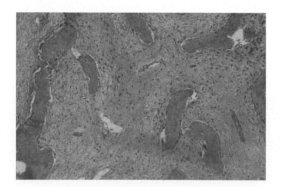

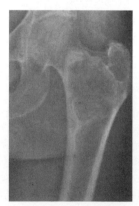

FIGURE 10-13. A histologic section of fibrous dysplasia reveals woven bone trabeculae surrounded by a fibrous tissue stroma. Unlike other bone-forming lesions, fibrous dysplasia forms metaplastic bone directly from the stroma.

FIGURE 10-14. A radiograph reveals fibrous dysplasia of the proximal femur. Note the mottled density of the neoplastic bone. It has a well-circumscribed benign appearance.

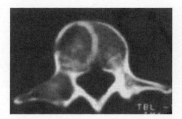

FIGURE 10-15. A CT scan of the spine reveals an area of fibrous dysplasia in the vertebral body. The lesion is well-circumscribed with no soft tissue mass.

physical examination and MRI scans. Most patients identify a specific traumatic episode followed by pain, swelling, weakness, and ecchymosis, but not all patients have a definite history of trauma. In individuals with muscle tears, the physical examination often reveals a muscle defect or retraction. Muscle tears and intramuscular hematomas can be treated by gentle stretching and restriction of heavy activity. In the absence of trauma, deep intramuscular hematomas are unlikely and may be difficult to distinguish from neoplasms without performing a biopsy. Further workup is necessary if the MRI appearance is indeterminate or the mass is enlarging.

Myositis Ossificans

Occasionally single or repetitive blunt muscle trauma causes myositis ossificans, formation of benign bone, cartilage, and fibrous tissue within contused muscle. This poorly understood condition begins following muscle damage with hemorrhage and inflammation. During the initial stages it causes pain or tenderness along with diffuse swelling and may be confused with a malignant soft tissue tumor, parosteal osteosarcoma, or benign lesions such as nodular fasciitis. As the inflammation subsides, pain and tenderness decrease, but a firm mass containing bone usually remains.

Myositis ossificans most frequently occurs in adolescents and young adults. Common sites include the quadriceps, adductors, deltoid, and brachialis muscles. Mineralization begins within the lesion approximately 4 to 6 weeks after injury and proceeds from the periphery toward the center.

Radiographically the lesions initially consist of an area of soft tissue swelling that becomes progressively mineralized to contain bone (Figure 10-17). Microscopic examination reveals a distinct zonal pattern reflecting the gradations of cellular maturation (Figure 10-18). The inner region of the lesion

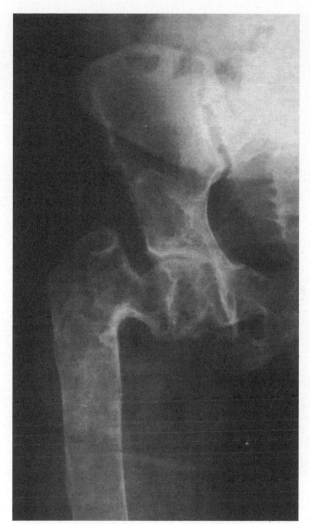

FIGURE 10-16. Extensive fibrous dysplasia of the proximal femur produces a characteristic Shepherd's crook deformity from multiple microfractures over time.

contains immature, rapidly proliferating fibroblasts along with inflammatory cells and occasional giant cells. A zone of poorly defined osteoid trabeculae with fibroblasts and osteoblasts surrounds this region and, in the peripheral areas, the osteoid mineralizes into mature lamellar bone. Current initial treatment of myositis ossificans includes restriction of activity and gentle stretching to prevent contractures. The mass is only removed in symptomatic cases after the appearance is completely mature.

Nodular Fasciitis

Nodular fasciitis or pseudosarcomatous fasciitis consists of a proliferation of fibroblasts, capillar-

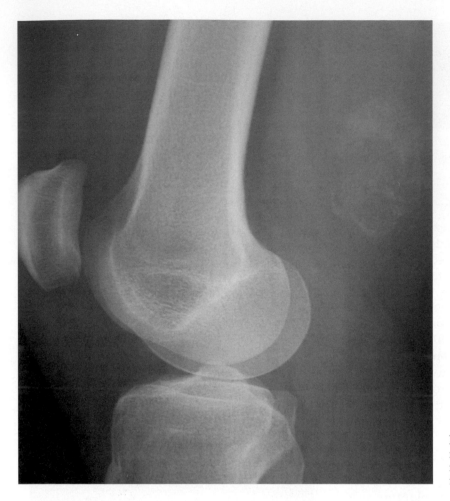

FIGURE 10-17. A lateral radiograph reveals myositis ossificans in the posterior thigh musculature. It gradually ossifies as it matures.

ies, and inflammatory cells that produce a tender soft tissue mass most often in the subcutaneous tissues and infrequently within muscle. It develops most commonly in adolescents and young adults and occasionally enlarges rapidly. The cause of this rare disorder remains unknown, but it appears to be an inflammatory process instead of a neoplasm. Simple excision of the mass is usually sufficient to provide a definitive diagnosis and local control.

Traumatic Fat Necrosis

Blunt trauma to subcutaneous fat can result in cell death, hemorrhage, and inflammation. As the inflammation subsides it can leave a firm plaque-like mass consisting of scar tissue and fat that persists long after the injury. A history of injury and a subcutaneous location of the mass usually suggests the diagnosis of traumatic fat necrosis.

Traumatic Neuroma

Partial or complete transection of a peripheral nerve causes proliferation of nerve tissue that can form firm, usually mobile, nodules. These traumatic neuromas may grow to moderate size and cause intense discomfort. A history of trauma or previous surgery combined with paresthesias or a Tinel's sign in the region of the mass helps establish the clinical diagnosis of posttraumatic neuroma. Neuromas that develop in the surgical site after resection of a soft tissue neoplasm may be difficult to distinguish from recurrent tumor without a biopsy.

Soft Tissue Abscess

A soft tissue abscess may resemble a neoplasm. These uncommon lesions develop from open wounds or by direct extension of infection from

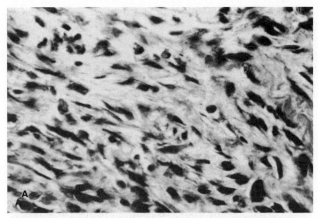

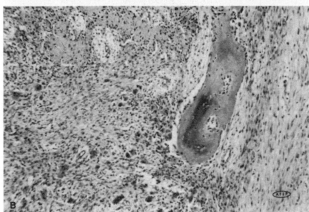

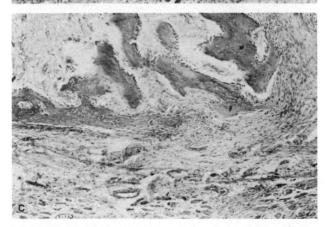

FIGURE 10-18. Light micrographs of myositis ossificans. **(A)** The cellular inner zone illustrates numerous cells with occasional atypical mitotic figures and variations in size and shape of the cells. The histologic appearance is sarcomatous. **(B)** The middle zone shows osteoid formation with a fibrovascular background. The cellular pattern is uniform. **(C)** The outer zone illustrates mature, well-oriented peripheral bone. The fibrous stroma appears more mature than at the center of the lesion. (Courtesy of Dr. William Bacon)

adjacent structures including bones and joints. They can result from hematogenous spread of organisms, especially in immunocompromised patients or those with diabetes mellitus. Most bacterial soft tissue abscesses cause exquisite tenderness, erythema, and fever, but most tuberculous abscesses (cold abscesses) cause minimal tenderness and may not produce systemic symptoms. Indolent abscesses may be difficult to distinguish from a neoplasm without a biopsy. The treatment of a musculoskeletal soft tissue abscess includes tissue cultures, surgical drainage, and antibiotics.

Ganglion Cyst

Ganglion cysts are unilocular or multilocular collections of translucent fluid or gelatinous myxoid tissue surrounded by fibrous tissue. They can occur in patients of any age and are located in a superficial location adjacent to synovial joints or tendon sheaths. They are commonly found near the wrist, hand, and knee. Occasionally those that develop near the knee grow to a large size and dissect through the surrounding soft tissues. Enlargement of the limb or swelling caused by these unusual ganglia may suggest the presence of a neoplasm. Although aspiration can remove the fluid from a ganglion cyst, surgical resection is currently the most predictable method of eradicating symptomatic lesions.

Intramuscular Myxoma

Intramuscular myxomas are solid soft tissue masses consisting of an abundant, gelatinous, myxoid matrix containing few cells and occasional cystic areas that resemble ganglia. Clinically, they are painless, fluctuant, mobile intramuscular masses that occur in patients between the ages of 40 and 70 years. When multiple myxomas are associated with monostotic or polyostotic fibrous dysplasia, it is referred to as Mazabraud's syndrome.

Myxomas may enlarge slowly or remain unchanged for many years. Because of their deep, intramuscular location in the thigh, shoulder, buttock, or arm, they cannot be easily distinguished from soft tissue sarcomas by clinical evaluation. They are well defined and have low signal relative to muscle on T1-weighted MR images. Treatment of symptomatic or enlarging lesions is by simple excision.

BENIGN NEOPLASMS

Benign neoplasms of bone and soft tissue occur much more commonly than malignant neoplasms. Benign lesions result from cell proliferation and matrix synthesis that produces new tissue, but their behavior varies considerably. Many enlarge to a certain size during skeletal growth and then remain unchanged indefinitely; thus, they might be considered developmental disorders rather than neoplasms. Lesions that follow this pattern include osteochondromas, enchondromas, lymphangiomas, and hemangiomas. Benign lesions including GCTs of tendon sheath, elastofibromas, and pigmented villonodular synovitis may represent inflammatory or reactive disorders, but lesions such as GCTs of bone and osteoblastomas are more aggressive neoplasms.

Because of their differences in behavior, benign proliferative lesions require varied treatments. Most osteochondromas and enchondromas do not require surgical treatment, but GCTs and osteoblastomas require intralesional curettage or resection. The more aggressive benign tumors invade and destroy normal tissue and may be difficult to distinguish from low-grade malignant neoplasms. Some of these benign lesions such as GCT and chondroblastoma can metastasize to the lungs despite their histologic appearance.

Benign Bone Neoplasms

Osteoma

Osteomas, similar to bone islands, consist of mature bone. They form on endosteal and periosteal bone surfaces and occur most commonly in the mandible, flat bones of the skull, and tibia in adolescents and young adults. On plain radiographs they appear as dense nodules of bone. Patients may notice a firm bony mass or the lesion may be detected as an incidental finding on plain radiographic studies. Osteomas do not require treatment.

Osteoid Osteoma

Osteoid osteomas are small, bone-forming lesions consisting of a central nidus less than 2 cm in diameter containing capillaries, osteoclasts, and osteoblasts forming large volumes of disorganized osteoid (Color Figure 10-3). A larger region of reactive new bone formation matures to become dense, lamellar bone around the central region. A thin rim of granulation tissue may separate the central osteoid-forming region from the dense, reactive bone.

Most osteoid osteomas occur in children, adolescents, or adults less than 30 years old. They cause considerable pain, classically worse at night. Typically aspirin provides better pain relief than other medications. Osteoid osteomas occur most frequently in the diaphysis and metaphysis of long bones, but they can develop in any bone. When they occur near synovial joints, effusions, muscle spasms, and contractures may be apparent. The pain will eventually resolve if aspirin or anti-inflammatory medications are taken for a prolonged period of time, but most lesions are now treated with radiofrequency ablation (RFA). In some vertebral lesions where RFA is unsafe near the spinal cord, resection or surgical burring of the area may be indicated.

Radiographs reveal osteoid osteomas to be small, dense regions rimmed by a thin lucent ring within a region of mature bone (Figure 10-19). Occasionally, they appear only as small, lucent areas surrounded by dense bone as the increased density of the reactive bone hides the central lesion on plain radiographs. In these instances, CT scans are the procedure of choice to identify the nidus (Figure 10-20).

Osteoblastoma

Like the central region of an osteoid osteoma, osteoblastomas consist of osteoblasts, osteoid, and blood vessels (Figure 10-21). They are benign, bone-forming neoplasms larger than osteoid osteomas that can expand and destroy bone. Most osteoblastomas are painful and occur in patients less than 30 years of age. The pain is usually less severe than that associated with an osteoid osteoma. They occur in the metaphysis or diaphysis of long bones or the posterior elements of the vertebrae (Figure 10-22, Figure 10-23).

Radiographically they are lucent lesions surrounded by a thin rim of reactive bone. The central lucent area often contains areas of mineralization. The differential diagnosis of an osteoblastoma includes osteosarcoma, giant cell tumor, and osteoid osteoma.

The behavior of osteoblastomas varies from slow enlargement to rapid aggressive growth that resembles the behavior of an osteosarcoma. Occasionally they cause pathologic fractures. Surgical resection or meticulous intralesional curettage provides local control.

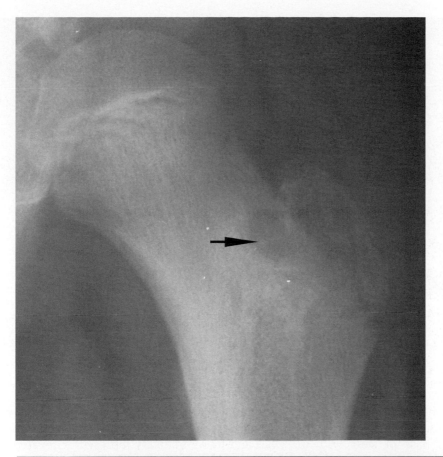

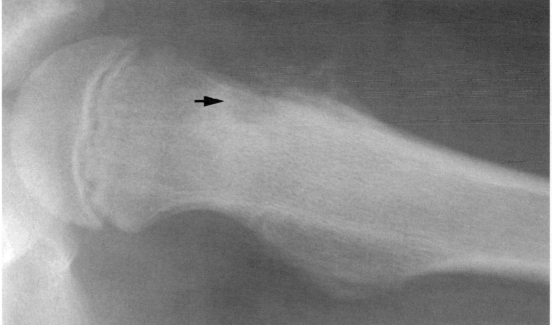

FIGURE 10-19. Radiographs of the proximal femur reveal a small lucency in the lateral femoral neck (*arrow*) consistent with an osteoid osteoma. There is mild surrounding sclerosis.

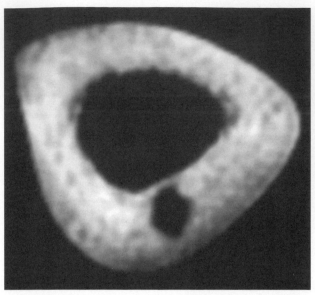

FIGURE 10-20. The nidus of an osteoid osteoma is best visualized on a thin-cut CT scan.

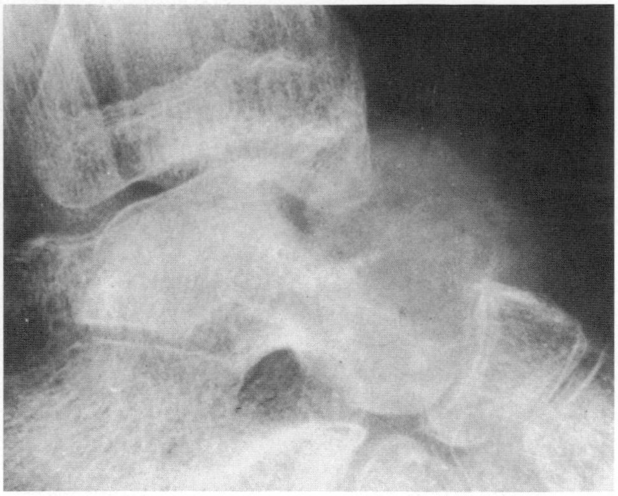

FIGURE 10-22. A radiograph of an osteoblastoma reveals an osteolytic, expanding tumor that has eroded the cortex of the talus and expanded into the surrounding soft tissues. It is surrounded by a thin shell of bone. Scattered, minute opacities throughout the tumor represent new bone. (Pochaczevsky R, Ven YM, Sherman RS. The roentgen appearance of benign osteoblastoma. Radiology 1960;75:429)

Osteochondroma

An osteochondroma, or osteocartilagenous exostosis, is one of the most common benign bone tumors. It consists of a bony base or stalk with a cartilage cap that projects from the normal bone away from a nearby joint (Figure 10-24). A fibrous tissue capsule or bursa typically covers the cartilage surface. Osteochondromas may develop from proliferation of cartilage-forming periosteal cells or from a defect in the fibrous tissue surrounding a physis and therefore likely represent a developmental disorder instead of a neoplasm. Common locations include the metaphysis of the proximal tibia, distal femur, distal tibia, distal fibula, proximal femur, and proximal humerus. They also can develop from flat bones of the pelvis and scapula.

Osteochondromas commonly present as solitary or multiple firm, fixed, asymptomatic bony masses. Most affected patients have a solitary osteochondroma, but some individuals have a hereditary disorder that causes multiple osteochondromas. This disorder, multiple hereditary exostoses (MHE), is transmitted as an autosomal dominant trait with a high degree of penetrance and can cause marked skeletal deformity and disability. Most patients recognize the presence of multiple lesions before 20 years of age. Severely affected people develop considerable skeletal deformity.

The appearance on a plain radiograph establishes the diagnosis of an osteochondroma. The bony base of the lesion extends directly from the medullary canal of normal bone (Figure 10-24). During skeletal growth the lesions enlarge with the surrounding bone, and they stabilize with skeletal maturity. As the bone component of an osteochondroma forms by enchondral ossification, growing osteochondromas typically have a

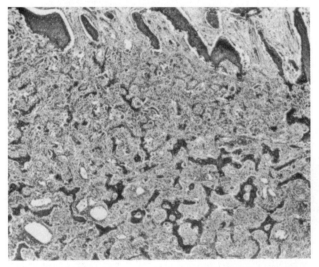

FIGURE 10-21. Low power histologic section of an osteoblastoma shows new bone trabeculae lined by neoplastic cells.

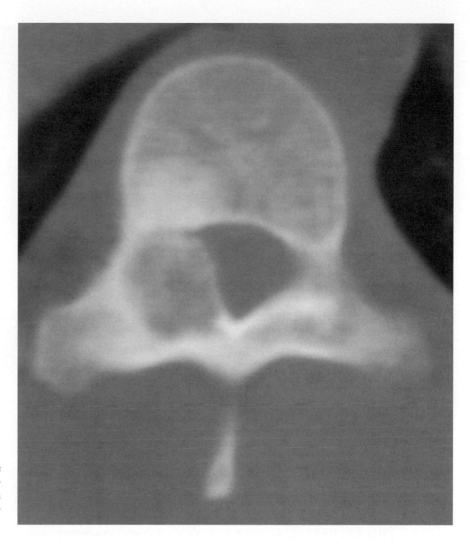

FIGURE 10-23. A CT scan of the spine reveals an osteoblastoma appearing in the posterior elements, a common location for this aggressive lesion.

large cartilaginous component. As the lesions mature, the cartilage component decreases until the osteochondroma consists primarily of bone.

Occasionally an osteochondroma fractures through its bony stalk or develops an overlying soft tissue bursa. In these instances it may cause pain. Enlargement of an osteochondroma may cause adjacent nerve compression or skeletal deformity. Rarely, a chondrosarcoma develops from an osteochondroma. This is more common in patients with multiple lesions. Malignant transformation occurs more frequently in osteochondromas of flat bones, particularly the pelvis and scapula. This phenomenon should be suspected when an osteochondroma causes pain or enlarges in an adult. The main treatment for an osteochondroma is observation until the patient reaches skeletal maturity. Patients with MHE are followed yearly with skeletal surveys. Surgical resection is only indicated when there is

neurologic compromise, abnormal growth, skeletal deformity, or decreased motion of the adjacent joint.

Enchondroma

An enchondroma is a benign hyaline cartilage lesion located in the medullary cavity of otherwise normal bones. It frequently occurs in the bones of the hands and feet but may appear in any bone including the femur, tibia, and humerus (Figure 10-25). It is generally considered an asymptomatic, indolent lesion. It is most frequently noted when obtaining radiographs to evaluate impingement of the shoulder or degenerative arthritis of the knee.

Plain radiographs reveal a central, well-circumscribed lucent region that may be mineralized. Enchondromas resemble bone infarcts. Further imaging studies are not necessary, but enchondromas normally show increased activity on a bone

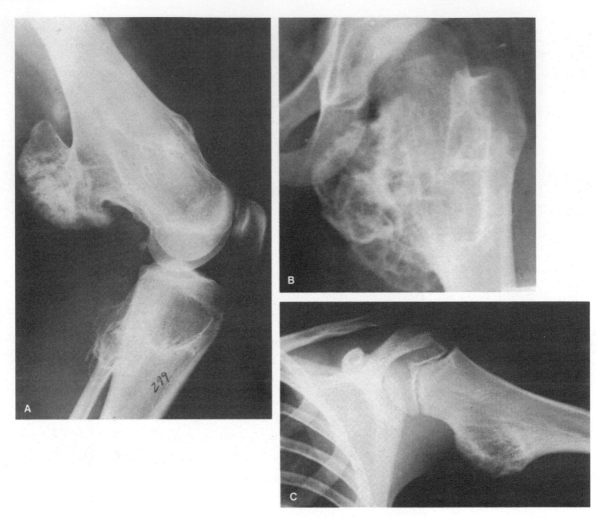

FIGURE 10-24. Plain radiographs showing typical osteochondromas of long bone metaphyses. Notice that the bony bases of the lesions extend directly from normal bone and that the medullary cavity of the normal bone extends into the lesion. Plain radiographs do not show the cartilage portion of an osteochondroma, so the lesions may be larger than visualized on the plain radiographic images. Osteochondromas are shown of the **(A)** distal femoral and proximal tibial metaphyses in a patient with multiple hereditary exostoses, **(B)** the proximal femoral metaphysis, and **(C)** the proximal humeral metaphysis.

scan. During skeletal growth the lesions may slowly enlarge. Following completion of normal growth, they cease to enlarge and the cartilage component calcifies to give a stippled radiographic appearance (Figure 10-26). In extremely rare cases, a chondrosarcoma can develop from an enchondroma. Because enchondromas are usually asymptomatic and do not enlarge after skeletal maturity, a lesion that causes pain or enlarges in an adult strongly suggests the possibility of malignant transformation. It is important to eliminate other causes for pain before attributing symptoms to an enchondroma.

Some patients have Ollier's disease, or multiple enchondromas, which causes severe deformity and stunting of growth. These patients have an increased probability of malignant transformation of an enchondroma. Maffucci's syndrome is a condition where multiple enchondromas occur in association with multiple hemangiomas. These patients have an increased probability of developing a chondrosarcoma or other visceral malignancies. Enchondromas generally do not require surgical treatment.

Periosteal Chondroma

A periosteal chondroma is a rare, subperiosteal lesion consisting of hyaline cartilage. It forms between the cortical bone and overlying periosteum,

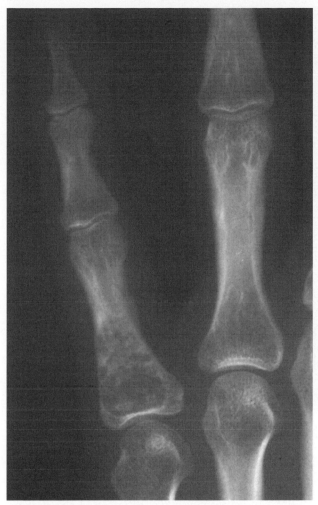

FIGURE 10-25. A radiograph reveals an enchondroma of the proximal phalanx with a stippled appearance. These lesions are the most common bone tumors found in the hand. They can be expansile and often fracture.

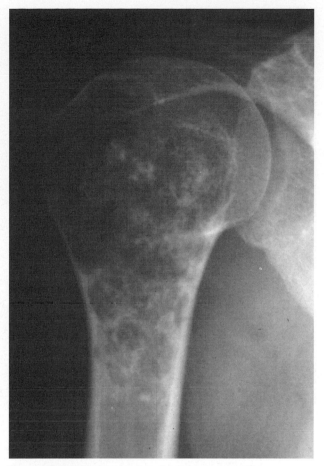

FIGURE 10-26. A radiograph of the proximal humerus reveals a calcified enchondroma. There is no expansion of the bone or soft tissue mass.

often creating an indentation in the bone surface and a smooth bulge of periosteum-covered cartilage that projects into the soft tissues. Most patients are young or middle-aged adults. Presumably periosteal chondromas develop from proliferation of cartilage-forming periosteal cells. They occur most frequently in the proximal humeral metaphysis, phalanges, metacarpals, and metatarsals.

They usually present as a solitary, painful mass or as an incidental radiographic finding. Radiographs show a scalloped depression in the bone cortex and may show the faint image of a soft tissue mass containing speckled regions of calcification. Periosteal chondromas can slowly enlarge, but they have not been shown to be aggressive. For symptomatic or enlarging lesions, surgical resection provides definitive local control.

Chondroblastoma

A chondroblastoma is a benign cartilage tumor consisting of regions or "islands" of densely packed polyhedral cells called chondroblasts admixed with fibrous tissue and chondrocytes forming a cartilage matrix (Color Figure 10-4). In some areas the cartilage matrix mineralizes creating a distinctive "chicken wire" pattern, while other regions contain large numbers of giant cells. Chondroblastomas involve the epiphysis of long bones in patients with open physes. They occur most commonly in the proximal humerus, distal femur, proximal tibia, and proximal femur. Most patients present with pain and local tenderness. Occasionally they have swelling, limitation of joint motion, and an effusion.

Radiographs typically show an eccentric, epiphyseal lucency with punctate calcifications. A sclerotic rim surrounds the lucent area (Figure 10-27). The lesions rarely involve more than half of the epiphysis and only occasionally extend into the

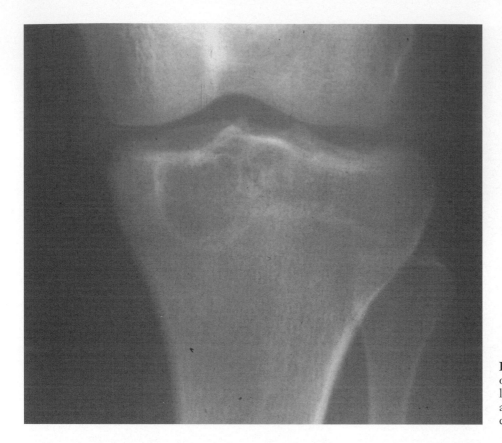

FIGURE 10-27. A radiograph of the proximal tibia reveals a lytic lesion in the epiphysis with a sclerotic rim consistent with a chondroblastoma.

metaphysis. Intralesional curettage and bone grafting is indicated for a chondroblastoma, but occasionally these lesions recur in the bone or surrounding soft tissues. Rarely chondroblastomas metastasize to the lungs.

Chondromyxoid Fibroma

A chondromyxoid fibroma (CMF) is a rare, benign, cartilage tumor consisting of fibrous, cartilaginous and myxoid tissues in variable proportions (Figure 10-28). Most present in older adolescents and young adults. It occurs most commonly in the metaphysis of the tibia as well as the pelvis and scapula (Figure 10-29). CMFs may be discovered as an incidental finding on a plain radiograph or because of mild to moderate pain. In some locations they form a palpable mass, but they rarely cause pathologic fractures. Plain radiographs demonstrate an eccentrically located lytic lesion with smooth sclerotic margins. Treatment by intralesional curettage or resection provides local control.

Giant Cell Tumor

Giant cell tumor (GCT) is a benign but aggressive lesion consisting of osteoclast-like giant cells,

fibroblast-like stromal cells, and blood vessels (Figure 10-30). Patients with GCTs are usually between 30 and 45 years of age with a female predominance. Unlike chondroblastomas, most GCTs occur after physeal closure in the involved bone. They can cause pain, swelling, and pathologic fracture, and aggressive lesions cause extensive destruction of normal tissue. They occur in the epiphysis of long

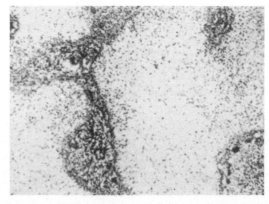

FIGURE 10-28. Light micrograph showing a chondromyxoid fibroma. The lesion consists of lobules of myxoid cartilage matrix surrounded by vascular fibrous tissue. The cell density of the lobules increases towards the periphery.

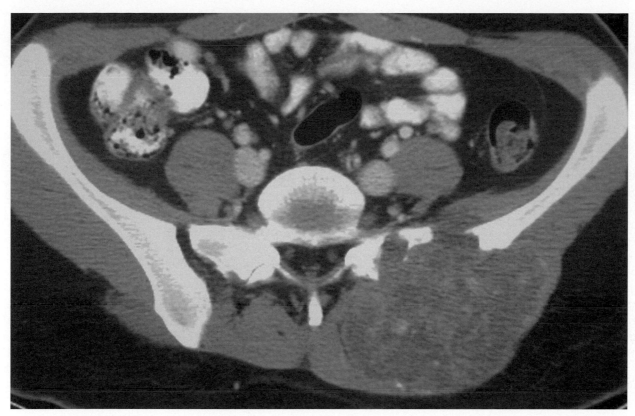

FIGURE 10-29. A CT scan of the pelvis reveals an aggressive lesion in the posterior ilium and lateral sacrum. There are visible calcifications within the lesion. This is a common location for a chondromyxoid fibroma.

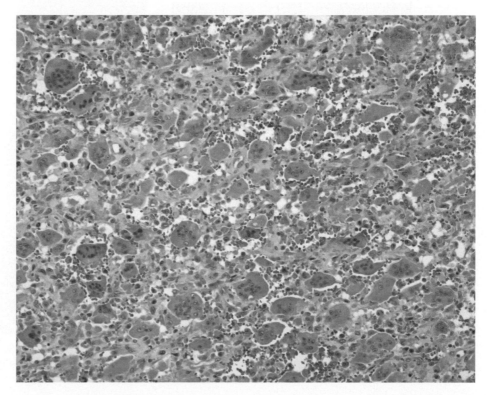

FIGURE 10-30. Histologic section of a giant cell tumor reveals multinucleated giant cells, fibroblast-like stromal cells, and blood vessels.

bones and extend into the metaphysis. GCTs abut the subchondral surface of the adjacent joint. Common sites include the tibial plateau, femoral condyle, distal radius, and humeral head (Figure 10-31).

Plain radiographs demonstrate lucent, eccentric, expansile lesions that thin or fracture the overlying cortex (Figure 10-32). The differential diagnosis of GCT includes ABC, chondroblastoma, Brown tumor of hyperparathyroidism, and nonossifying fibroma. The radiographic appearance of aggressive GCTs can resemble a sarcoma. Rarely, giant cell tumors appear in multiple sites or produce benign lung metastases.

When possible, GCTs are treated with thorough intralesional curettage using a high-speed burr followed by cementation or bone grafting. Frequently, adjuvants such as phenol, cryotherapy, or argon beam coagulation are used to extend the zone of treatment. There is a 10 to 20% risk of local recurrence. In aggressive lesions with extensive bone destruction, resection of the joint is necessary followed by reconstruction using either an allograft or metal prosthesis.

Desmoplastic Fibroma

A desmoplastic fibroma is a bone lesion consisting of dense benign fibrous tissue. These rare lesions behave as low-grade malignant neoplasms and may be mistaken for a fibrosarcoma of bone. They can aggressively destroy bone and invade surrounding soft tissues. Desmoplastic fibromas usually appear in patients younger than 30 years of age. They may cause aching pain, swelling, and rarely, pathologic fractures.

Radiographically they are lytic lesions that occasionally produce bone expansion. Although they do not metastasize and their clinical behavior varies, they frequently recur unless excised with a margin of normal tissue.

Hemangioma of Bone

Hemangiomas are collections of blood vessels within bone (Figure 10-33) and often occur in vertebral bodies. They may represent a developmental disorder or a neoplasm. Generally, they remain within the medullary cavity. Plain radiographs reveal regions of generalized decreased bone density with abnormally prominent bone trabeculae. Most of these

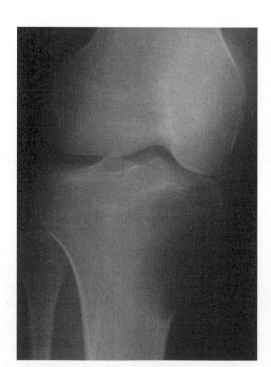 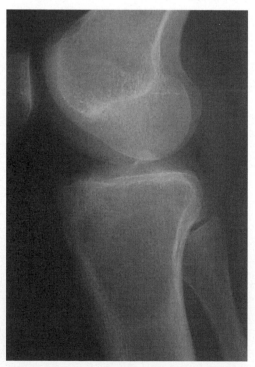

FIGURE 10-31. Radiographs of the proximal tibia reveal an eccentric, lytic lesion with no sclerotic border located in the epiphysis or metaphysis. It is consistent with a giant cell tumor.

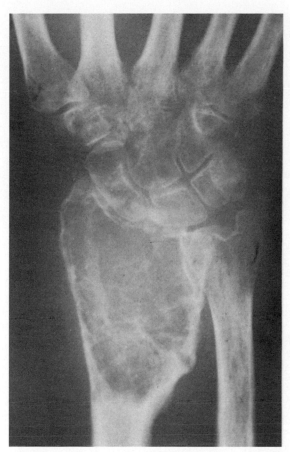

FIGURE 10-32. A giant cell tumor of the distal radius has expanded the cortex.

lesions are asymptomatic and detected as an incidental finding, thereby requiring no surgical treatment. However, occasionally vertebral hemangiomas are associated with pain and neurologic deficits.

Langerhans Cell Histiocytosis

The bony lesions of Langerhans cell histiocytosis (LCH) consist of histiocytes admixed with eosinophils, lymphocytes, and neutrophils (Figure 10-34). They cause bone destruction and a surrounding reaction that mimics benign and malignant neoplasms as well as osteomyelitis. They can lead to pathologic fractures and, in children, collapse of a vertebral body, called vertebra plana (Figure 10-35). Plain radiographs of the lesions vary from sharply circumscribed, round or oval lucent regions to extensive, permeative bone destruction (Figure 10-36).

The age at diagnosis and severity of the disease previously separated LCH into three overlapping disorders. Two disorders, Letterer-Siwe and Hand-Schüller-Christian, involved multiple tissues and affected young children. A solitary bony lesion (eosinophilic granuloma) was more common in older children and young adults. More recently, LCH has been referred to as a spectrum of disease with varying degrees of severity and bone

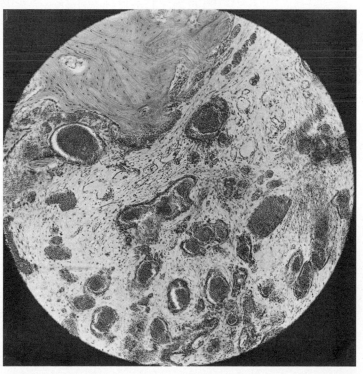

FIGURE 10-33. A histologic section of an intraosseous hemangioma reveals blood vessels admixed with fibrous tissue within the bone.

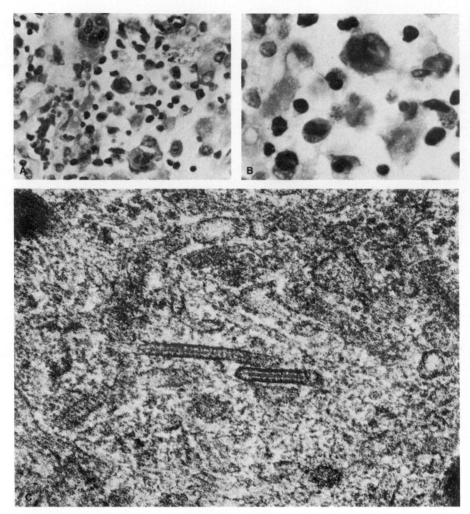

FIGURE 10-34. Cytologic features of Langerhans cell histiocytosis. **(A)** Smear of aspiration specimen shows an admixture of abundant histiocytes, containing either single or multiple nuclei. These nuclei often contain lipid-filled vacuoles and hemosiderin-like pigment. Also shown are eosinophils, lymphocytes, and neutrophils (×460). **(B)** Higher magnification. The histiocytes are irregularly shaped with ill-defined outlines, and they contain an eccentric, large, indented, finely creased nucleus with delicate chromatin, surrounded by abundant, delicate, pink-staining cytoplasm that contains granular material. The histiocytes sometimes have a loose syncytial appearance, often possess long cytoplasmic processess, and appear to fuse to form giant cells (×1150). **(C)** Ultramicroscopic features of Langerhans cell histiocytosis shows characteristic Langerhans granules. The electron micrograph shows the tubular inclusions within the cytoplasm of a typical histiocyte of eosinophilic granuloma. These are invariable features of this disease. They may be found in any condition in which the pathologic process is associated with a reactive histiocytosis (×140,000). (Katz R, Silva EG, de Santos LA et al. Diagnosis of eosinophilic granuloma of bone by cytology, histology, and electron microscopy of transcutaneous bone-aspiration biopsy. J Bone Joint Surg 1980;62A:1284)

or soft tissue involvement. The more severe forms of LCH cause systemic illness in young children, and these patients rarely present with skeletal involvement alone. In contrast, patients with a solitary eosinophilic granuloma seek medical attention because of bone pain, a pathologic fracture, or because the lesion was discovered incidentally.

Most patients with the most severe form of LCH present at less than 2 years of age with an acute onset

of the disease that may include hepatosplenomegaly, lymphadenopathy, rash, bleeding diathesis, anemia, and occasionally exophthalmos and diabetes insipidus. Patients with a more chronic from of disseminated histiocytosis usually present before age 5 and may develop otitis media, diabetes insipidus, exophthalmos, fever, hepatosplenomegaly, lymphadenopathy, anemia, and disturbances of liver function. These disseminated forms of the disease

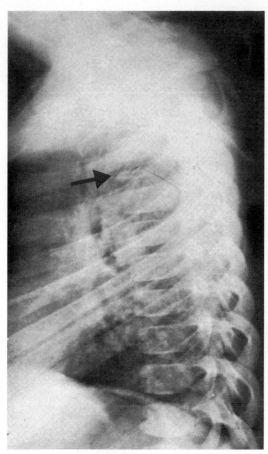

FIGURE 10-35. Radiograph showing an eosinophilic granuloma that has caused collapse of the T5 vertebral body (vertebra plana). These lesions usually resolve spontaneously and, if a sufficient period of growth remains, the vertebral body regains normal size.

have historically had a high mortality rate despite treatment. However, new chemotherapy regimens have been successful in improving the overall survival of these patients in recent years.

A solitary eosinophilic granuloma can occur in children, adolescents, and young adults, although most patients present before age 10. The primary symptom is localized pain. It occurs in the diaphysis or metaphysis of long bones and can stimulate a periosteal reaction that resembles osteomyelitis or Ewing's sarcoma. Patients may have a solitary lesion, multiple lesions simultaneously, or a succession of lesions over years. Some patients that present with an isolated bone lesion later develop multiple lesions or more diffuse systemic involvement. Eosinophilic granulomas involving bone heal spontaneously, but establishing the diagnosis, relieving pain, or preventing pathologic fracture may require intervention before this occurs. Steroid injection is

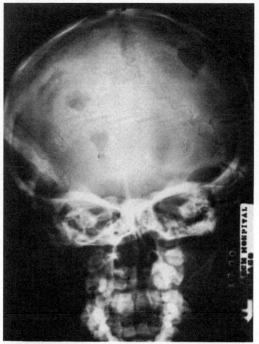

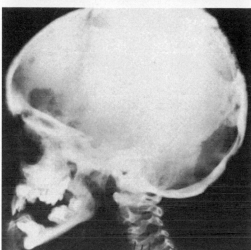

FIGURE 10-36. Radiographs showing disseminated Langerhans cell histiocytosis involving the skull. The lesions are seen as well-circumscribed lytic bone defects.

the treatment of choice with intralesional curettage reserved for persistent lesions.

Benign Soft Tissue Neoplasms

Lipoma

A lipoma is a common, benign neoplasm consisting of mature fat. It rarely develops in individuals less than 20 years of age, and it becomes more common in the fifth and sixth decades. Lipomas occur in both the superficial subcutaneous and deep soft tissues. Superficial lipomas occur frequently on the back, shoulder, neck, and proximal regions of the arms and legs. Lipomas that develop deep in the muscle fascia (usually within muscle) can occur in almost any muscle but appear most frequently in the large muscles of the limbs, back, and pelvis. Lipomas present as asymptomatic, slowly growing, mobile soft tissue masses. Occasionally large lipomas compress peripheral nerves and cause pain.

Plain radiographs show lipomas as distinct radiolucent masses, but an MRI shows a classic appearance of a lesion bright on T1-weighted images that also suppresses with fat suppression sequences (Figure 10-37). Left untreated, some tumors become large enough that patients have difficulty finding suitable clothing. Simple excision successfully removes the lipoma with a low risk of recurrence.

Soft Tissue Hemangioma

Hemangiomas consist of abnormal collections of blood vessels. It is not clear if they result from a disturbance in tissue development or actual neoplasia. More than 80% of these lesions first appear in people younger than 30. They present as slowly enlarging soft tissue masses, and many patients have pain or vague discomfort in the region of the hemangioma for years before diagnosis. Hemangiomas occur most frequently in the skin and subcutaneous tissues where they form soft masses with a blue appearance. These superficial lesions may be present at birth or develop during childhood and adolescence. The clinical appearance of these lesions is diagnostic.

Deep soft tissue or intramuscular hemangiomas are more difficult to diagnose and may resemble

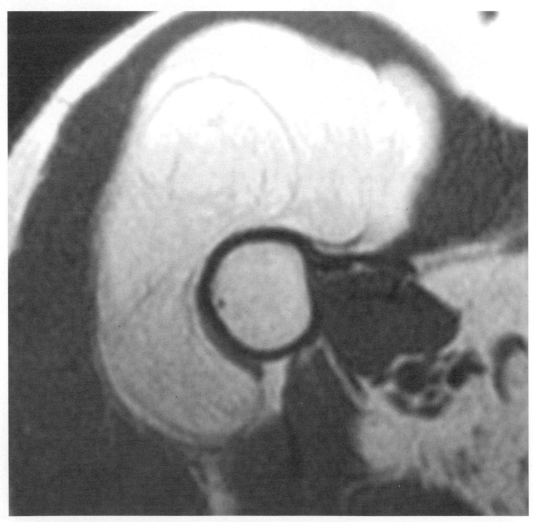

FIGURE 10-37. An axial MRI of the proximal arm reveals a lipoma deep to the deltoid muscle. It has a signal similar to the superficial adipose tissue.

malignant neoplasms. They consist of blood vessels, fibrous tissue, and adipose tissue. They may appear in any muscle but most commonly involve the lower extremity, particularly the thigh muscles. They do not cause skin discoloration unless they extend into the subcutaneous tissues. Small deep lesions may be difficult to identify without performing an MRI of the involved muscle (Figure 10-38). Although many hemangiomas remain confined to muscle, these lesions can erode adjacent bone or surround nerves and blood vessels.

In most instances, surgery is not appropriate because these lesions do not metastasize. They have not been shown to become malignant even in patients with large lesions, and they generally do not enlarge after skeletal maturity. Recurrence of

the hemangioma often follows surgical treatment. In some cases, successful surgical excision of small, superficial hemangiomas can be performed, but a more recent option is embolization or sclerotherapy of symptomatic lesions. This treatment is usually performed by an interventional radiologist. Other options for treatment of symptomatic, inoperable hemangiomas include anti-inflammatory use and compression stockings.

Rarely, a patient is born with a hemangioma that extends throughout the soft tissues of an extremity. This disorder, congenital hemangiomatosis, increases the circumference and length of the involved extremity and may cause significant deformity. During childhood the discrepancy in size between the normal and involved extremities may

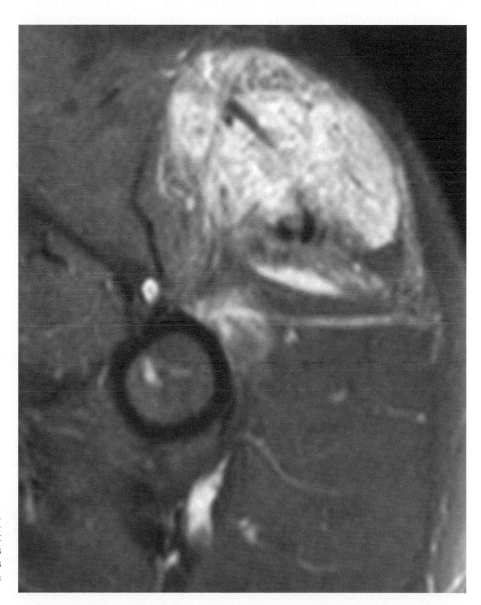

FIGURE 10-38. An axial MRI of the proximal arm reveals a soft tissue hemangioma. It contains both fluid and adipose elements and is diffusely present within the muscle.

increase and, in some patients, amputation may be appropriate.

Glomus Tumor

A glomus tumor consists of capillary-sized blood vessels surrounded by layers of polygonal cells called pericytes. Fine unmyelinated nerve fibers run between the blood vessels. These tumors occur in young adults and usually form soft, vascular masses no more than a few millimeters in diameter. Patients with glomus tumors characteristically report episodes of intense pain in the region of the tumor. Many of these episodes follow minor trauma. The tumor can be found in multiple locations, but it typically develops in the nail bed of a finger or toe where it may be seen through the nail as a small, blue nodule. Surgical excision eradicates most glomus tumors.

Lymphangioma

A lymphangioma is a mass formed primarily from lymphatic vessels and lymphoid aggregates that rarely affects the musculoskeletal system. These lesions are discovered in newborns or infants. More than 50% present at birth, and over 90% present by the age of 2 years. Parents or physicians can recognize the presence of a lymphangioma because of a fluctuant soft tissue mass that may fluctuate in size. The lesions rarely cause pain at rest but may be associated with discomfort following trauma or exercise. Large lymphangiomas may cause disfigurement or interfere with musculoskeletal function. Most lymphangiomas involving the trunk or limbs occur in the superficial tissues of the axilla or upper extremity. It is not certain if these lesions form by neoplastic proliferation of lymph vessels or represent hamartomas or lymphangiectasis. They are benign but may enlarge by accumulation of fluid.

Surgical excision can be curative for small lesions; but attempts to excise large lesions frequently lead to complications including infection and wound healing problems.

Neurolemmoma (Benign Schwannoma)

A neurolemmoma is a benign encapsulated proliferation of nerve sheath cells. It can occur at all ages but reaches a peak incidence in patients between the ages of 20 and 50 years. It most commonly develops in the larger nerves of the head, neck, and flexor surfaces of the upper and lower extremities. It grows slowly and rarely causes pain or neurologic deficits unless it becomes quite large. Palpation or compression of a neurolemmoma usually causes paresthesias. Malignant transformation of a neurolemmoma is rare. Neurolemmomas tend to expand within a nerve sheath without infiltrating between nerve fibers, so they can often be safely removed without sacrificing nerve function.

Solitary Neurofibroma

Solitary neurofibromas and neurolemmomas share many clinical and histologic features. Presumably, they both originate from the Schwann cell but, theoretically, neurolemmomas consist of a more homogeneous population of cells and have distinct capsules. They can both develop from major nerves and have similar clinical presentations but, unlike neurolemmomas, neurofibromas also develop from small, unmyelinated nerves. In some instances it is difficult to identify a clear relationship between a neurofibroma and a nerve. Neurofibromas also tend to grow in and around individual nerve fibers rather than compressing or displacing them as is the case with neurolemmomas. This entwining growth often makes it difficult to resect a neurofibroma without causing neurologic damage.

Isolated neurofibromas occur most frequently in individuals between the ages of 20 and 30 and appear as superficial lesions in the dermis or as deep soft tissue masses. They usually remain asymptomatic. However, some may grow slowly and cause a neurologic deficit. Occasionally, a solitary neurofibroma becomes malignant. Surgical excision of a neurofibroma is curative.

Neurofibromatosis (von Recklinghausen's Disease)

Neurofibromatosis, a genetically determined disorder, causes neurofibromas (Figure 10-39), acoustic neuromas, café-au-lait spots and skeletal deformities including scoliosis, kyphosis, pseudarthrosis and asymmetrical enlargement of limbs. Neurofibromatous tissue may form discrete masses like those seen in patients with solitary neurofibromas or plexiform neurofibromas, which are diffuse lesions that extend throughout normal tissues without a definite margin (Figure 10-40).

Neurofibromatosis develops as an autosomal dominant inheritance pattern with a high degree of penetrance, but approximately 50% of patients present as new mutations. The severity of neurofibromatosis varies among patients: some have café-au-lait spots with or without neurofibromas, and others have extensive, disfiguring neurofibromas and severe

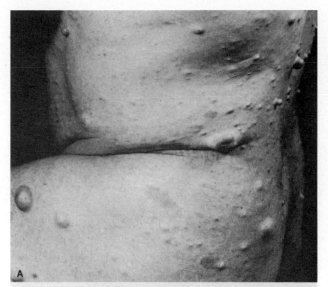

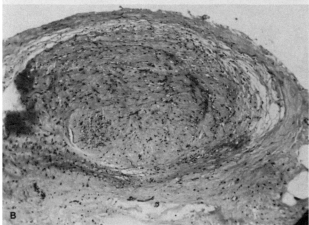

FIGURE 10-39. Neurofibromatosis. **(A)** Typical multiple subcutaneous tumor nodules. These nodules are composed of nerve tissue covered by areolar tissue and skin. **(B)** Low power magnification of enlarged nerve fiber removed from a plexiform neurofibromatous mass. (McCarroll HR. Clinical manifestations of congenital neurofibromatosis. J Bone Joint Surg 1950;82A:601)

skeletal deformity (Figure 10-41, Figure 10-42). In severely affected patients or those with a family history of neurofibromatosis, the diagnosis is often apparent at birth. In others, multiple neurofibromas appear during childhood or adolescence and progressively enlarge.

In addition to the problems caused by skeletal deformities, patients with neurofibromatosis have a higher risk of secondary malignant transformation of a lesion. Patients who have had the disease for over 10 years are at the greatest risk. Rapid enlargement of a neurofibroma or increasing pain in a neurofibroma suggest the possibility of malignant change. Despite radical surgical excision and aggressive adjunctive treatment, the prognosis for patients with malignant nerve sheath tumors in the setting of neurofibromatosis remains poor.

Desmoid Tumor

Similar to a desmoplastic fibroma found in bone, desmoid tumors in the soft tissues consist of dense, proliferating fibrous tissue. They rarely affect infants or the elderly and occur most commonly in people between 25 and 35 years of age. They present as rock-hard, painless masses. With time they may cause discomfort, nerve compression, and muscle weakness. Large lesions can restrict joint motion. The tumors are usually located deep in the musculature of the shoulder, chest wall, back, or thigh. They often lie within muscle, but they can extend along fascial planes and appear in multiple sites within a single limb. These lesions do not metastasize, but they can aggressively invade normal tissue including bone, and they occasionally develop in old scars.

Desmoid tumors do not follow a predictable pattern of behavior. Their aggressiveness has led some authors to call them well-differentiated fibrosarcomas,

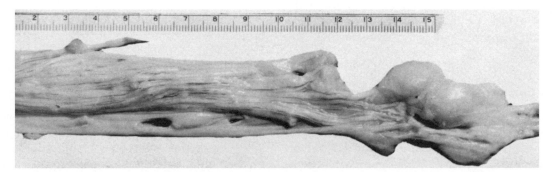

FIGURE 10-40. Neurofibromatosis. Multiple nerve root involvement at cauda equine. The patient died at 42 years of age of sarcomatous degeneration of a neurofibroma of the brain. (Courtesy of Pathology Department, Mount Sinai Hospital, Chicago)

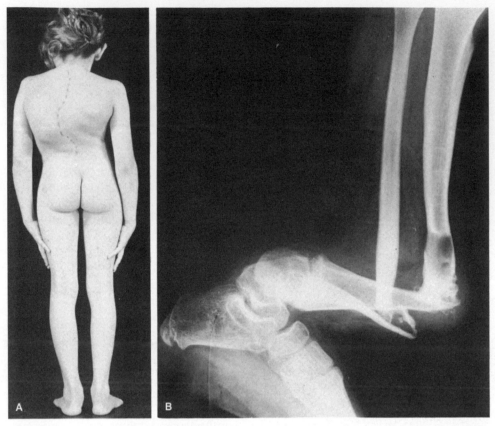

FIGURE 10-41. Neurofibromatosis. **(A)** Congenital thoracic scoliosis in a child. The angulation is acute and usually rapidly progressive and disabling. Fusion should be done promptly. **(B)** Pseudoarthrosis of tibia at site of a cystic lesion. (McCarroll HR. Clinical manifestations of congenital neurofibromatosis. J Bone Joint Surg 1950;82A:601)

but an occasional desmoid tumor ceases growing or even spontaneously regresses. If possible these tumors should be treated by wide surgical excision, which is often difficult. With less than a wide excision, the lesions frequently recur. Radiation therapy has been used in cases with an inadequate surgical margin or at the time of local recurrence. More recently there are low-dose chemotherapy regimens available that may provide benefit and allow surgery to be avoided in anatomically difficult areas. Amputation is to be avoided if possible as this is a benign tumor.

Elastofibroma

An elastofibroma is an ill-defined, firm mass of fibrous tissue containing elastic fibers that occurs in the soft tissues between the scapula and chest wall of elderly people. It may result from repetitive mechanical trauma rather than a neoplastic process, but this hypothesis has not been proven. This lesion causes mild tenderness, pain, and occasional restriction of scapulothoracic motion. It does not adhere to the skin and can often be palpated in the lower subscapular area deep to the rhomboid and latissimus dorsi muscles where it is firmly fixed to the chest wall. An elastofibroma grows slowly and can be treated by surgical excision.

Giant Cell Tumor of Tendon Sheath

A giant cell tumor of tendon sheath consists of multinucleated giant cells, inflammatory cells, histiocytes, and fibroblasts. It develops in or near synovial joints, bursae, and tendon sheaths and may represent a reactive inflammatory process or a benign neoplasm. It most frequently develops in people between 30 and 50 years of age. It commonly appears in the hand and less commonly in the foot, ankle, and knee. Physical examination reveals a firm, small, lobulated mass fixed to the underlying tissues or tendon sheaths. Occasionally it can erode bone. This tumor may grow slowly and recur following surgical excision.

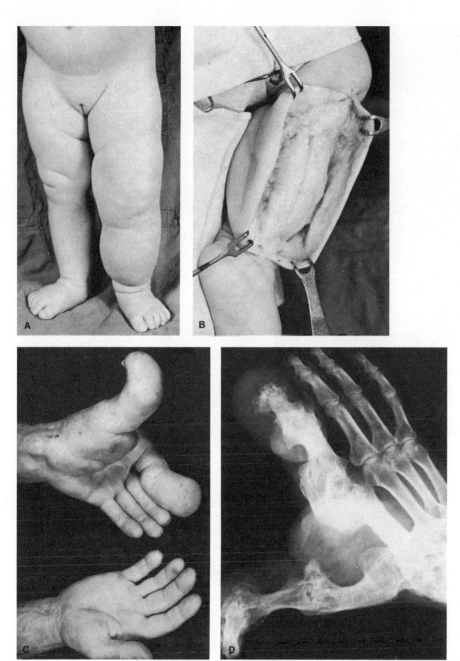

FIGURE 10-42. Neurofibromatosis. **(A)** Diffuse soft tissue hypertrophy and increased length of the lower extremity. **(B)** A typical tumor mass of hypertrophied soft tissue is exposed at operation. It is not encapsulated and is superficial to the deep fascia. **(C)** and **(D)** Hypertrophy of the left thumb and index finger and corresponding portion of the hand. (McCarroll HR. Clinical manifestations of congenital neurofibromatosis. J Bone Joint Surg 1950;82A:601)

Pigmented Villonodular Synovitis

Pigmented villonodular synovitis (PVNS) consists of proliferating synovial tissue containing histiocytes, fibroblasts, multinucleated giant cells, and capillaries that can destroy dense fibrous tissue, form soft tissue masses, and invade bone. Like GCT of tendon sheath, PVNS may represent a reactive inflammatory process or a benign neoplasm. It occurs most commonly in adolescents and young adults in large synovial joints including the knee, hip, and ankle, although it also occurs in smaller synovial joints,

tendon sheaths, and bursae. It can occur in a focal or diffuse form. Most patients present with a swollen joint and give a history of recurrent effusions. Plain radiographs initially show erosions on both sides of a joint (Figure 10-43). There is periarticular bone destruction and degenerative joint disease in the later stages. The MRI appearance of PVNS is a low signal on both T1- and T2-weighted images. Occasionally it presents as solitary or multiple soft tissue nodules near a joint and can resemble GCT of tendon sheath.

PVNS requires simple excision of the focal type or complete open or arthroscopic synovectomy for

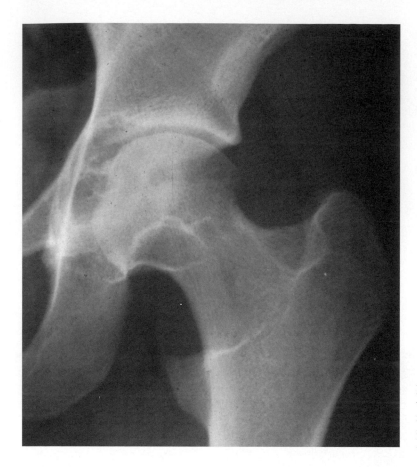

FIGURE 10-43. A radiograph of the hip reveals lytic lesions on both sides of the joint and mild degenerative changes consistent with an active synovial process such as pigmented villonodular synovitis (PVNS).

the diffuse type. Local recurrence is common. Adjuvant chemotherapy and radiation have been tried with variable success.

Synovial Chondromatosis

Synovial chondromatosis is a collection of hyaline cartilage nodules within the synovium of large joints. It occurs most frequently in young adults. Patients present with pain, mechanical symptoms, and an enlarging mass. Most patients develop loose fragments of cartilage within the joint, but some patients form an enlarging mass of proliferating chondrocytes in the periarticular tissues. Radiographs reveal speckled calcifications within the joint or in the soft tissues around a joint. The current treatment of synovial chondromatosis includes complete synovectomy and removal of any cartilaginous loose bodies.

MALIGNANT NEOPLASMS

Primary malignant musculoskeletal neoplasms occur much less frequently than benign lesions. Unlike their benign counterparts, malignant tumors have the capacity to cause disseminated disease and death. Some malignant neoplasms develop in or near previously existing benign lesions such as osteochondromas (multiple hereditary exostoses), enchondromas (Ollier's disease and Maffucci's syndrome), chronic draining osteomyelitis, bone infarcts, Paget's disease, and neurofibromas (neurofibromatosis). The development of a malignant neoplasm presumably results from overexpression of preexisting malignant potential (Ollier's disease). In spontaneous cases of malignancy, the development presumably results from an alteration in the normal cells near the lesion (bone infarcts).

Primary malignant bone tumors vary in their clinical presentation. For example, multiple myeloma frequently causes generalized weakness and bone pain without a mass in elderly, debilitated people, whereas osteosarcoma commonly causes sharply localized bone pain with a soft tissue mass in children and adolescents without systemic symptoms. Current treatment of these neoplasms also varies from systemic chemotherapy and radiation used for multiple myeloma to preoperative chemotherapy and surgery used for osteosarcoma.

In contrast with malignant bone tumors, most soft tissue sarcomas vary less in clinical presentation and current treatment. Most present as a painless mass. Wide surgical excision of primary bone and soft tissue tumors is the recommended treatment with or without adjuvant chemotherapy and radiation.

Malignant Bone Neoplasms

Multiple Myeloma

Multiple myeloma, the most common primary bone tumor, consists of malignant plasma cells (Color Figure 10-5). The disease rarely occurs before the fifth decade of life. In many patients the malignant cells extend throughout the bone marrow (BM), so a BM aspiration provides diagnostic tissue. Most patients have moderate to severe anemia, an elevated ESR, and an abnormal serum protein electrophoresis and immunoelectrophoresis. Occasionally, patients present with a solitary focus of plasma cells referred to as a plasmacytoma. These individuals usually develop diffuse disease after a latent period of up to 5 to 10 years.

Most patients with multiple myeloma have bone pain that is diffuse or localized to regions of bone destruction. Because the disease often involves the vertebral bodies, patients can develop back pain and vertebral compression fractures. In addition, many affected individuals have systemic symptoms including weakness, fatigability, and weight loss. The radiographic features of multiple myeloma vary from multiple "punched out" areas of bone destruction often in the skull and pelvis (Figure 10-44), to diffuse osteopenia difficult to distinguish from that secondary to metabolic bone disease. In the early stages of multiple myeloma, radiographs may not show any changes. An osteoblastic reaction to multiple myeloma is rare, so bone scans may be falsely negative. Pathologic fractures due to multiple myeloma commonly occur in the vertebral bodies but may occur throughout the skeleton. Radiation alone can effectively treat a plasmacytoma, and chemotherapy with radiation is the treatment of choice for disseminated disease. Recently, stem cell transplant has been used with success in many patients.

Lymphoma

Lymphoma of bone is comprised of malignant histiocytes and occurs in middle-aged patients. The appearance of a lymphoma, also called a reticulum cell sarcoma, frequently resembles a Ewing's sarcoma. However, a lymphoma contains a network or reticulum of fine matrix fibers that appear as thin dark threads when stained with a silver or reticulum stain (Figure 10-45).

A lymphoma involving bone can cause pain or a pathologic fracture. Plain radiographs show extensive, permeative lesions that often extend throughout the bone. The regions of bone destruction have an irregular appearance that blends with normal bone. Occasionally plain radiographs appear normal, but a bone scan is positive and an

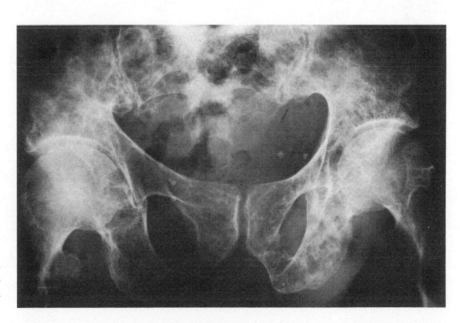

FIGURE 10-44. Radiograph showing the multiple punctate lucent defects in the pelvis of a patient with multiple myeloma.

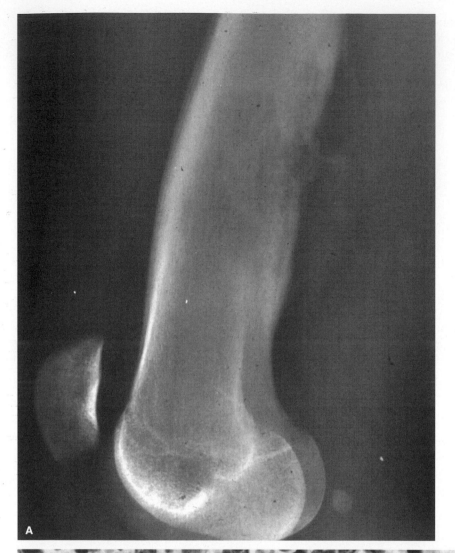

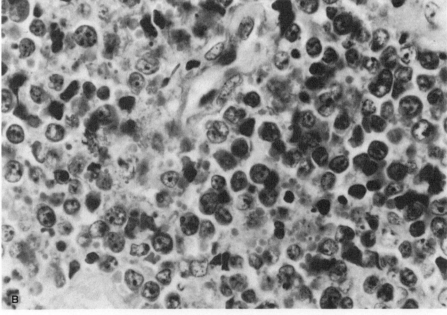

FIGURE 10-45. (A) A lateral radiograph of the distal femur in a patient with lymphoma reveals subtle permeative destruction. **(B)** A histologic section shows the population of round cells that form the neoplasm. (Histology courtesy of Dr. A.G. Huvos)

MRI scan shows a large soft tissue mass. The majority of lymphomas involve bone as part of a systemic presentation. These patients are treated with chemotherapy as well as radiation to the bony site. Isolated lymphoma of bone is rare but can be treated with radiation with or without surgery.

Ewing's Sarcoma

Ewing's sarcoma, a highly malignant tumor of bone, consists of densely packed, distinctive, small round cells of uncertain origin. The light microscopic appearance is similar to other small round cell tumors; however, recent molecular tests have a high sensitivity for an accurate diagnosis. Ewing's sarcoma occurs more frequently in males and in patients younger than 20 years of age. The tumor may appear in any bone or occasionally in the soft tissues, but most present in the pelvis and lower extremities. The tumor usually causes pain and may enlarge rapidly to produce significant soft tissue swelling and occasional pathologic fractures. Some patients with Ewing's sarcoma have systemic symptoms such as fever, generalized weakness, and laboratory abnormalities including anemia and an elevated ESR. It is important to differentiate the clinical presentation from osteomyelitis.

Plain radiographs show a diffuse, permeative lesion that stimulates a layered periosteal reaction (Figure 10-46). In long bones Ewing's sarcoma usually involves the diaphysis, but it may extend into the metaphysis. In flat bones such as the pelvis or scapula, it can involve the entire bone. The radiographic appearance of Ewing's sarcoma may resemble osteomyelitis, lymphoma, osteosarcoma, eosinophilic granuloma, and metastatic carcinoma. The tumors often break through the cortex and periosteum with invasion of the soft tissues at the time of diagnosis (Figure 10-46).

The current standard treatment for Ewing's sarcoma is systemic chemotherapy. Local control is usually obtained with wide surgical resection. Radiation is also effective and is indicated for unresectable lesions.

Osteosarcoma

The presence of malignant cells producing osteoid identifies a tumor as an osteosarcoma (Color Figure 10-6). The matrix of a typical osteosarcoma consists of osteoid that may or may not mineralize. Other osteosarcomas synthesize a cartilaginous or fibrous matrix, and a rare subtype forms large vascular channels. These neoplasms occur most frequently

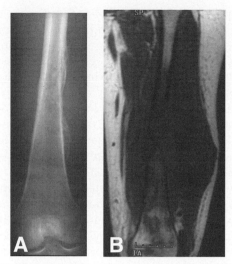

FIGURE 10-46. (A) A radiograph and **(B)** an MRI scan of a patient with Ewing's sarcoma of the femur. Note the subtle destruction and periosteal reaction on the radiograph as well as the large soft tissue mass on the MRI scan.

in the second decade of life with an additional peak in patients 70 to 80 years of age. Osteosarcomas cause progressively increasing pain. At the time of diagnosis many extend through the bone cortex and produce a firm soft tissue mass (Figure 10-47). They can

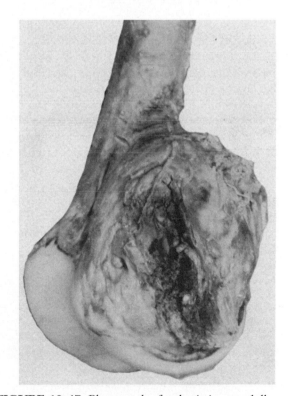

FIGURE 10-47. Photograph of a classic intramedullary osteosarcoma of the distal femur. Notice how the neoplasm has broken through the bone and formed a large soft tissue mass.

develop in association with Paget's disease or following radiation therapy and, in these situations, have an extremely poor prognosis. Osteosarcomas develop in the metaphysis of long bones, especially the distal femur, proximal tibia, and proximal humerus, although they can be found in any bone (Figure 10-48). Less commonly osteosarcomas can develop on the surface of the bone (periosteal and parosteal osteosarcomas). A rare type of osteosarcoma develops in the soft tissues (extraosseous osteosarcoma).

On plain radiographs, osteosarcomas appear as regions of permeative bone destruction and irregular new bone formation (Figure 10-48); although, tumor osteoid does not always mineralize, so occasionally there is no evidence of new bone formation. The radiographic appearance of a telangiectatic osteosarcoma containing large vascular channels may resemble the bone changes seen in an ABC. Parosteal osteosarcomas mineralize so densely that they appear as sclerotic masses on the surface of the bone.

Classic osteosarcomas that originate within bone behave aggressively. They rapidly destroy normal bone, invade soft tissue, and frequently metastasize to the lungs. The current treatment for these tumors is systemic multiagent chemotherapy followed by surgical resection with a wide margin.

Periosteal osteosarcomas occur on the cortical surface of long bones most often in young adults. They erode the cortex producing a shallow cavity and reactive periosteal new bone formation. Some produce radiographic changes that resemble a periosteal chondroma, but the osteosarcoma creates a more irregular bony margin that suggests the presence of a malignant tumor. As a periosteal osteosarcoma grows, it extends into the soft tissues, and ossification may appear within the enlarging mass. Eventually the lesions grow into the medullary cavity. Patients with a periosteal osteosarcoma often present after they notice a firm, fixed, slowly enlarging mass. This type of osteosarcoma is an intermediate grade malignancy. Surgical resection with or without chemotherapy is the standard treatment.

Parosteal osteosarcoma has a better prognosis than classic intramedullary or periosteal osteosarcoma. Most parosteal osteosarcomas involve the

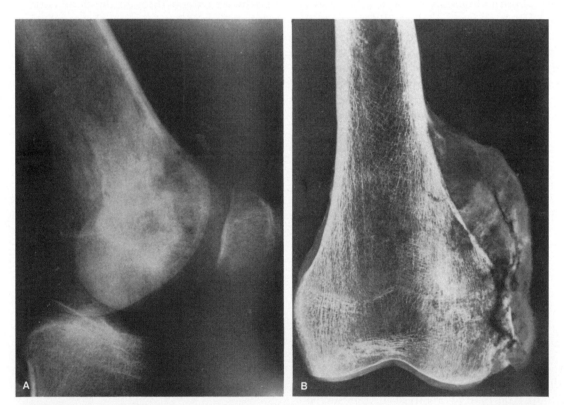

FIGURE 10-48. Radiographs of a distal femoral osteosarcoma. **(A)** Lateral view of the distal femur showing the irregular bone destruction and bone formation that gives the bone a mottled appearance. **(B)** A radiograph of the resected specimen after removal of the soft tissues. This view reveals destruction of the cortex and development of a soft tissue mass. Notice the new bone formation in the soft tissue mass.

femur, humerus, or tibia with the vast majority occurring on the posterior aspect of the distal femur (Figure 10-49). These tumors grow slowly over years, and the patient may notice swelling but little discomfort. Plain radiographs reveal dense mineral deposits within the tumor. It lies directly on the cortical surface and occasionally extends into the medullary canal. The radiographic differential diagnosis includes myositis ossificans, periosteal osteosarcoma, and osteochondroma. Wide surgical excision without chemotherapy is necessary for local control.

An extraosseous osteosarcoma is a soft tissue tumor that contain regions of ossification. It occurs in young adults near the shoulder and pelvis. These rare lesions are treated by surgical resection with or without adjuvant chemotherapy and radiation similar to the treatment of a soft tissue sarcoma.

Chondrosarcoma

A chondrosarcoma is a malignant tumor consisting of chondrocytes in a cartilaginous matrix (Color Figure 10-7). It may develop from an enchondroma or osteochondroma but occurs more commonly in bones with no known preceding cartilage lesion. Chondrosarcomas occur in adults and the elderly most commonly in the pelvis, scapula, humerus, femur, and tibia. Patients with multiple

hereditary exostoses, Ollier's disease and Maffucci's syndrome have a higher risk for malignant transformation of a cartilaginous lesion.

Chondrosarcomas vary considerably in their behavior: some enlarge rapidly, aggressively invade normal tissue, metastasize, and cause death, but most are low grade tumors that enlarge slowly, cause little damage to adjacent tissues, and metastasize only after many years. They vary in their histologic appearance from lesions that resemble normal hyaline cartilage to lesions consisting of poorly differentiated cells that fail to produce a typical hyaline cartilage matrix. These differences in the histologic appearance of chondrosarcoma led to a three-tiered classification of chondrosarcoma based on its resemblance to normal hyaline cartilage (Figure 10-50). The grade of the tumor is a strong predictor of its behavior. Rare subtypes include mesenchymal, dedifferentiated, and clear cell chondrosarcoma.

Chondrosarcomas may arise within the bone (central chondrosarcoma) or from the surface of the bone (peripheral chondrosarcoma). Plain radiographs reveal bone destruction as well as mineralization within the tumor (Figure 10-51). Peripheral chondrosarcomas may resemble osteochondromas on plain radiographs, although they commonly show bone destruction and irregular calcification of the cartilage cap. MRI and CT scans of these lesions

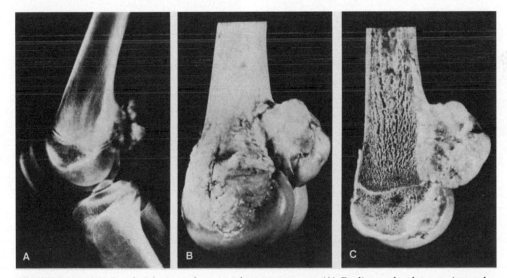

FIGURE 10-49. Grade I lesion of parosteal osteosarcoma. **(A)** Radiographs show an irregular ossified mass with prominent lucency indicating a large amount of fibrous and cartilaginous tissue. The subjacent cortex is sclerotic. **(B)** Typical external appearance. This is the most common location of the tumor on the posterior aspect of the distal end of the femur at the popliteal area. **(C)** Sagittal section shows that this tumor merges imperceptibly with the cortex along its entire base. The underlying cortical bone is thickened. (Ahuja SC, Villacin AB, Smith J et al. Juxtacortical (parosteal) osteogenic sarcoma. J Bone Joint Surg 1977;59A:632)

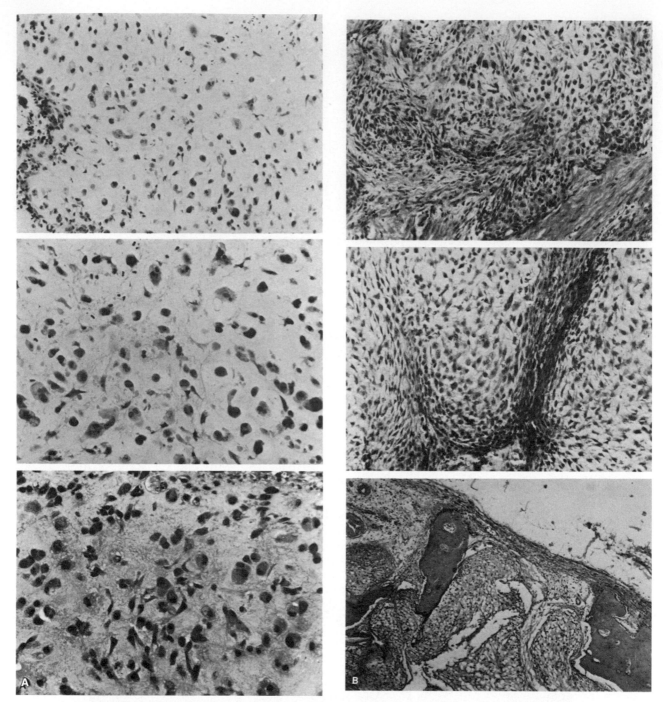

FIGURE 10-50. Light micrographs showing the variability in the histologic appearance of chondrosarcomas. **(A)** The histologic appearance of grade I and grade II chondrosarcomas. (*Top and middle*) Grade I changes include increased cell density and increased variability cell size, shape and staining. (*Bottom*) Grade II changes include more advanced cellular pleomorphism. **(B)** The histologic appearance of grade III chondrosarcomas. (*Top and center*) Dedifferentiation toward fibrosarcoma at the periphery of chondrosarcomatous lobules. (*Bottom*) Lobules of malignant cartilage penetrate bone, demonstrating the ability of these lesions to destroy normal bone. (Dahlin DC, Salvador AH. Chondrosarcomas of bones of the hands and feet: a study of 30 cases. Cancer 1974:34:755)

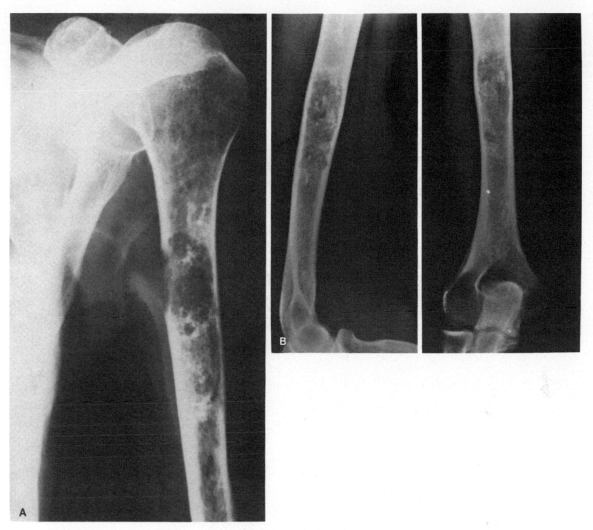

FIGURE 10-51. Plain radiographs showing central chondrosarcomas. These lesions cause bone destruction and produce regions of mineralization. **(A)** A central chondrosarcoma of the humerus showing an irregular area of central bone destruction with mineralization and erosion of the medial cortex. **(B)** Radiographic features include osteolysis, scalloping endosteal erosion of inner cortex, central areas of calcification, and no reactive bone formation about the periphery.

may show increased thickness of the cartilage cap suggesting the presence of malignancy. Because plain radiographs do not accurately show the cartilage component of these tumors, they may be considerably larger than they appear. Central chondrosarcomas appear as regions of bone destruction with areas of calcification. Frequently they extend further in the medullary cavity than the plain radiographs suggest. They can break through the cortex and form large soft tissue masses. There is usually no reactive bone formation.

Most chondrosarcomas eventually cause pain, but some cause little or no discomfort despite reaching large size, especially within the pelvis (Figure 10-52). Peripheral and central chondrosarcomas that extend into the soft tissues form firm, fixed masses. In some patients, a mass may have been present for years. Wide surgical excision is necessary and offers the best possibility of cure, as radiation and chemotherapy have not proven to be effective methods of treatment for chondrosarcoma. Locally recurrent disease is common and may be difficult to treat.

Fibrosarcoma

A fibrosarcoma is one of the most uncommon malignant bone tumors. Like a fibrosarcoma of soft tissue, it consists of fibroblasts and a collagenous matrix. These tumors occur over a wide age range

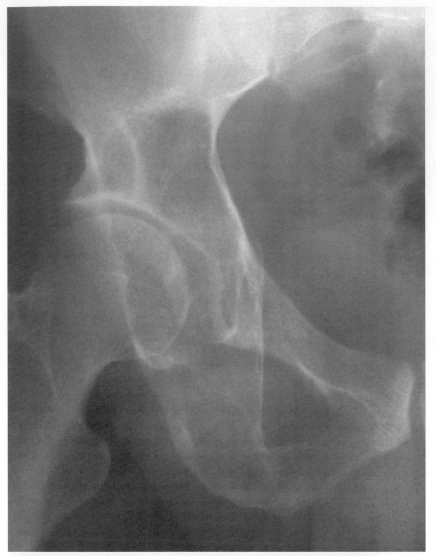

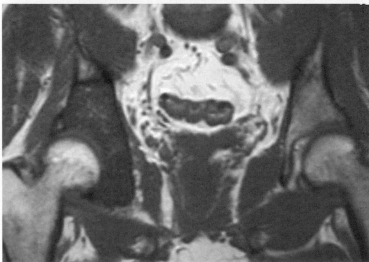

FIGURE 10-52. (A) A plain radiograph and **(B)** MRI of the pelvis reveal a lesion in the right periacetabular region consistent with a chondrosarcoma. These tumors frequently occur in the pelvis as lytic lesions and can become destructive with large soft tissue masses that may go unrecognized given their deep location.

and may appear in any part of the skeleton. Most of them cause pain and swelling. They may occur in association with Paget's disease, fibrous dysplasia, bone infarcts, or following radiation therapy. Plain radiographs show irregular, mottled bone destruction with occasional regions of reactive new bone formation around the periphery. Wide surgical excision is the currently accepted treatment, and neoadjuvant chemotherapy has been used for some patients.

Malignant Fibrous Histiocytoma

A malignant fibrous histiocytoma (MFH) is a highly malignant tumor consisting of the same cell types found in MFH of soft tissues such as giant cells, fibroblasts and histiocytes. It is much more commonly found in the soft tissues but can occur in bone. These tumors occur in patients of any age and have also been reported in association with Paget's disease, bone infarcts, and radiation therapy. Patients have pain, and plain radiographs show irregular bone destruction. They are treated with the same chemotherapy regimen as is used for osteosarcoma. Wide surgical resection is indicated following neoadjuvant chemotherapy.

Malignant Vascular Tumors

All malignant vascular tumors in bone contain capillaries formed by malignant cells, but they vary in their predominant cell type. In hemangioendotheliomas, capillary endothelial cells are the predominant cell type, whereas in hemangiopericytomas, pericytes are the predominant cell type. Hemangioendotheliomas occur more frequently in bone, and hemangiopericytomas occur more frequently in the soft tissues. An angiosarcoma refers to the most malignant form of hemangioendothelioma or hemangiopericytoma.

Malignant vascular tumors can appear in most regions of the skeleton, and occasionally occur in multiple sites within the same limb. They usually produce pain, and radiographs show evidence of bone destruction. Surgical resection and chemotherapy are indicated for high grade solitary lesions. Radiation therapy is frequently the sole treatment for hemangioendothelioma involving multiple areas within the same bone.

Adamantinoma

An adamantinoma is a rare neoplasm consisting of islands or strands of epithelial-like cells surrounded by fibrous tissue (Color Figure 10-8).

It is almost exclusively found in the tibial diaphysis. It tends to follow a prolonged course and occurs in individuals between late adolescence and middle age. Most adamantinomas cause mild to moderate discomfort and a palpable mass over the anterior tibial border. Radiographically, they cause irregular, bubbly bone destruction of the anterior cortex (Figure 10-53). The lesion may be confined to the cortex of the bone.

Wide resection of the tumor is the recommended treatment. The diaphysis is most commonly affected, so an intercalary allograft is often the reconstruction of choice. Chemotherapy and radiation have no role in treatment. Patients can develop late pulmonary metastasis.

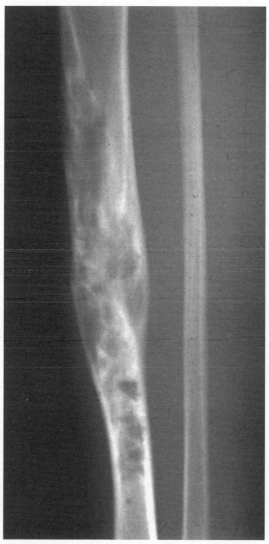

FIGURE 10-53. A radiograph of the tibia reveals a lytic, bubbly lesion involving the cortex consistent with an adamantinoma.

Chordoma

A chordoma consists of malignant cells derived from notochordal rests (Color Figure 10-9). It may occur throughout the spine but is most frequently noted in the sacrococcygeal region or at the base of the skull. These tumors rarely occur in individuals less than 30 years of age. Most chordomas grow slowly, and patients present with pain, bowel dysfunction, or neurologic symptoms. Plain radiographs of chordomas typically show irregular midline bone destruction. Small lesions are often difficult to recognize on plain radiographs due to overlying shadows. A CT or MRI scan is preferred to better define the anatomical extent of the tumor (Figure 10-54). Chordomas often have a large presacral mass that can be identified on a rectal examination. A wide surgical margin is necessary to achieve local control, but this is difficult given the anatomic location. Nerve roots or visceral structures involved by the chordoma should be sacrificed to obtain an adequate resection. Radiation can be helpful for areas where margins are positive or for locally recurrent disease. Chemotherapy has not been effective in the treatment of this tumor.

Malignant Soft Tissue Neoplasms

Malignant soft tissue neoplasms, such as fibrosarcoma and neurofibrosarcoma, are named for their presumed cell of origin. However, for many lesions such as synovial sarcoma and epithelioid sarcoma, the cell of origin is unknown. Other soft tissue sarcomas consist of undifferentiated cells that cannot be identified with a specific tissue. Although soft tissue sarcomas differ in basic cell type, they have similar clinical presentations, radiographic appearances, and treatment. They usually present as firm, painless masses. MRI scans are extremely accurate in elucidating the size and anatomic location of a soft tissue tumor, but they cannot reliably distinguish between histologic subtypes or between benign and malignant neoplasms. Soft tissue sarcomas appear as heterogeneous masses that are often large and deep to fascial planes (Figure 10-55). The current treatment of soft tissue sarcomas consists of wide surgical resection and preoperative or postoperative radiation. The use of chemotherapy is the standard of care for patients with rhabdomyosarcoma but is controversial for adults with soft tissue sarcomas. There is a high risk of pulmonary metastasis for large, deep, high grade tumors.

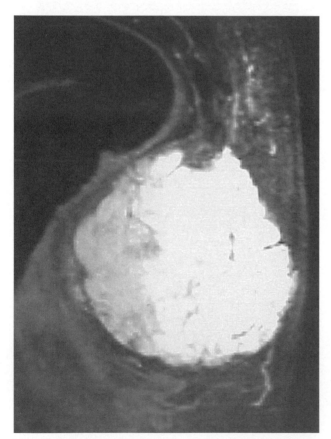

FIGURE 10-54. A sagittal MRI reveals a large lesion emanating from the lower sacrum with a large presacral mass consistent with a chordoma.

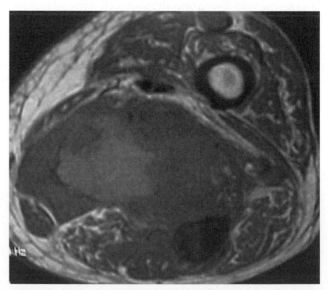

FIGURE 10-55. An MRI of the thigh reveals a large, inhomogeneous soft tissue mass consistent with the appearance of multiple different histologic subtypes of soft tissue sarcoma.

Malignant Fibrous Histiocytoma

Malignant fibrous histiocytoma is the most common soft tissue sarcoma and, similar to its rare bony counterpart, consists of malignant fibroblasts and histiocytes as well as giant cells and occasionally inflammatory cells. The majority of soft tissue MFHs present as painless, enlarging masses in people between 50 and 70 years of age. They occur most frequently in the deep soft tissues of the lower extremity.

Liposarcoma

Liposarcomas are malignant tumors of fat cells with a variable histologic appearance. They are the second most common soft tissue sarcoma. They frequently reach a large size and have a peak incidence in people between 40 and 60 years of age. Most liposarcomas of the extremities lie deep within the soft tissues, especially in the quadriceps muscle and popliteal fossa. Other common locations include the shoulder and calf. Patients usually detect liposarcomas because of a mass or increase in size of the limb. The clinical behavior of these tumors varies based on their grade.

Fibrosarcoma

Soft tissue fibrosarcomas consist of malignant fibroblasts. They occur in patients of any age but appear most frequently in those between 30 and 55 years of age. They can occur throughout the soft tissues, most frequently in the thigh. Usually they present deep within the soft tissues and as an enlarging mass. Only rarely do they cause significant discomfort before reaching a large size. Occasionally fibrosarcomas arise in tissues previously treated with radiation or in burn scars.

Synovial Sarcoma

Despite the name, cells forming synovial sarcomas do not originate from the synovium. These tumors consist of two morphologically distinct cell types: epithelial-like cells that assume a cuboidal or columnar form and fibroblast-like spindle cells. The combination of these two cell types creates a distinctive biphasic pattern: the spindle cells surround islands and strands of epithelial cells (Color Figure 10-10). Some synovial sarcomas only contain the spindle cells and are referred to as monophasic synovial sarcomas.

Synovial sarcomas occur most frequently in young adults between 15 and 35 years of age and rarely appear in individuals over 50 years of age. They present as discrete masses or diffuse swelling, and they often cause discomfort. These tumors grow quite slowly, and many patients have symptoms for years before biopsy or excision demonstrates the presence of the tumor. Synovial sarcomas appear most frequently in the extremities, usually in periarticular regions or near tendon sheaths, bursae and joint capsules. It is extremely uncommon to find synovial sarcomas within a joint.

Plain radiographs may show scattered areas of calcification within a synovial sarcoma. These tumors can metastasize to regional lymph nodes. In some series, chemotherapy adds to the effectiveness of surgery and radiation.

Neurofibrosarcoma

Neurofibrosarcomas (also referred to as malignant peripheral nerve sheath tumors) arise from peripheral nerve sheath cells or from neurofibromas. Most occur in patients between 20 and 50 years old. They present as enlarging masses that may or may not cause pain. Patients with neurofibromatosis (von Recklinghausen's disease) have a significantly increased risk of developing a neurofibrosarcoma, and this underlying disease may predispose them to a worse prognosis than those who develop this tumor spontaneously. Like other soft tissue sarcomas, surgical excision is the best treatment for this disorder. Unfortunately, some of the tumors assume a diffuse form that makes wide resection almost impossible. In addition, when major neurologic structures such as the brachial plexus are involved, amputation may be the best surgical option.

Rhabdomyosarcoma

Rhabdomyosarcomas arise in or near skeletal muscle and consist of cells that form myofibers. There are different histologic subtypes with different prognoses. They are the most common soft tissue sarcomas in children and adolescents. Most of these tumors present as enlarging, deep masses closely associated with muscle and can metastasize to regional lymph nodes. They rarely cause pain or tenderness. A combination of surgical excision, radiation therapy, and chemotherapy are used to treat patients with this tumor.

Malignant Vascular Tumors

Malignant vascular neoplasms account for only a small percentage of soft tissue sarcomas. Like their bony counterparts, malignant vascular tumors of soft tissue form capillaries and vary in their predominant cell type. Hemangiopericytomas occur more frequently in the soft tissues than in bone. Some malignant vascular neoplasms arise in the superficial tissues and skin, but others develop in the deep soft tissues and closely resemble other soft tissue sarcomas. In some vascular sarcomas, a wide surgical margin is difficult to achieve given their diffuse nature.

Epithelioid Sarcoma

Epithelioid sarcomas consist of malignant round cells of mesenchymal origin, inflammatory cells, and capillaries. These neoplasms occur most commonly in young adults and often develop in the hand or foot. They are the most common soft tissue sarcomas of the hand. Epithelioid sarcomas present as small, tender masses fixed to tendon sheaths, periarticular tissues, and fascia. Because their clinical presentation differs from other soft tissue tumors and because there are inflammatory cells in the lesion, these tumors are frequently mistaken for nonspecific inflammatory processes even after a biopsy. The current treatment of these tumors is wide surgical excision. Regional lymph node metastases are common, and patients are at high risk for eventual lung metastasis.

Clear Cell Sarcoma

A clear cell sarcoma consists of large malignant cells with clear cytoplasm resembling swollen chondrocytes. It occurs in older adolescents and young adults and presents as a slowly growing, fixed mass. It is the most common malignant soft tissue tumor of the foot. Like epithelioid sarcomas, clear cell sarcomas may involve periarticular tissues and tendon sheaths and spread to regional lymph nodes. The current treatment is wide excision, and there are no effective options for chemotherapy. Patients with this disease have a poor prognosis unless the tumor is discovered before it metastasizes.

METASTATIC NEOPLASMS

Skeletal metastases from carcinomas occur far more frequently than primary bone tumors. Malignant cells grow within the bone, replace normal bone marrow, and usually cause bone destruction. Prostate and some breast cancer metastases stimulate neoplastic bone formation. Nearly all malignant tumors have

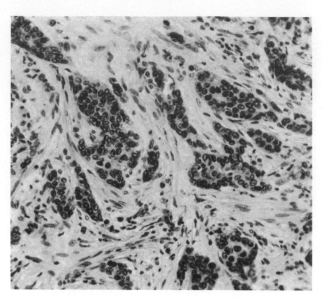

FIGURE 10-56. A histologic section showing a metastatic carcinoma of the breast. The lesion consists of islands of neoplastic epithelial cells surrounded by reactive fibrous tissue.

the ability to metastasize to bone, but carcinomas of the breast, lung, prostate, kidney, and thyroid are the most common. Approximately 50% of patients with breast, lung, or prostate cancer eventually develop bone metastasis. Examination of the skeletal metastases reveals cells similar to those in the primary neoplasm (Figure 10-56, Figure 10-57, Figure 10-58). Soft tissue sarcomas and primary bone tumors can metastasize to bone, but this is extremely rare.

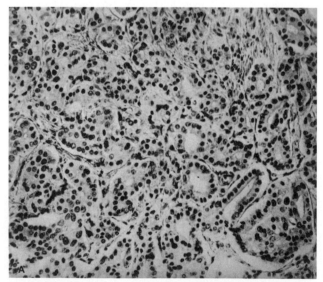

FIGURE 10-57. A histologic section showing metastatic prostate carcinoma. The lesion consists of gland-forming epithelial cells.

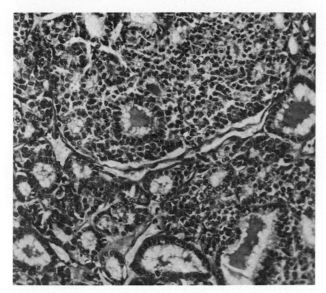

FIGURE 10-58. A histologic section of metastatic carcinoma of the thyroid gland. Note the filled spaces with a similar appearance to native thyroid tissue.

Metastatic bone lesions are painful and frequently cause pathologic fractures (Figure 10-59). They occur most commonly in the vertebrae, pelvis, ribs, and proximal appendicular skeleton (Figure 10-60, Figure 10-61). Although bone metastases occur primarily in adults over 45 years of age, neuroblastomas can metastasize to bone in children. Most patients with

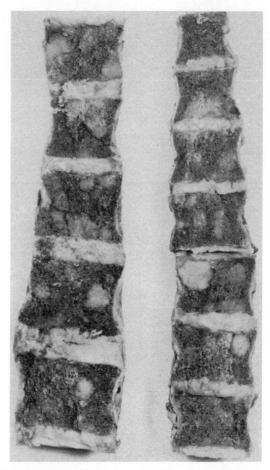

FIGURE 10-60. Thoracic and lumbar vertebra with multiple metastasis from breast carcinoma. The roughly spherical metastatic lesions have replaced bone marrow in part of every vertebral body.

bone pain or a pathologic fracture from skeletal metastases have a known primary malignant tumor, but occasionally the skeletal metastasis is the first indication of a primary malignancy. For this reason, the possibility of metastatic carcinoma should be investigated in middle-aged and older patients with a destructive bone lesion.

In patients with metastatic bone disease, the tumor must destroy 30 to 50% of the bone before a plain radiograph reveals the lesion. A technetium bone scan offers a more sensitive method of detecting metastatic disease, although it may not be reliable for rapidly destructive lesions such as multiple myeloma or renal cell carcinoma. Most metastases destroy bone, but those from prostate and breast cancers can stimulate bone formation and appear as regions of increased bone density on plain radiographs. If plain radiographs or bone scans fail to demonstrate suspected bone metastasis, an MRI

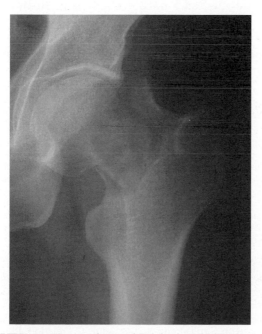

FIGURE 10-59. A radiograph of the hip showing a pathologic fracture from metastatic renal cell carcinoma.

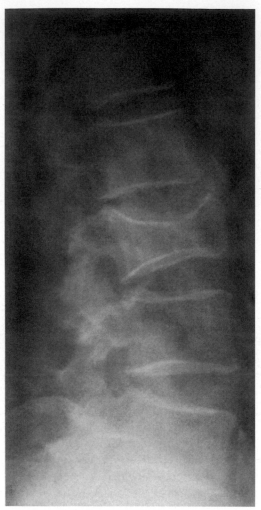

FIGURE 10-61. Radiograph showing a pathologic compression fracture of a vertebral body caused by metastatic breast carcinoma.

in patients with lytic bone metastasis and inhibit osteoclast-mediated bone destruction.

SUMMARY

Lesions that resemble neoplasms, benign neoplasms, primary malignant neoplasms, and metastatic neoplasms (Tables 10-1 and 10-2) can involve all areas of the musculoskeletal system. They vary in clinical behavior from developmental disturbances that resolve spontaneously to benign neoplasms that can grow and destroy bone to highly malignant tumors that cause death, despite aggressive treatment.

Because these tumors are rare, many physicians may not suspect neoplastic disease in a patient with vague discomfort, swelling, loss of musculoskeletal function, or incidental radiographic abnormalities. In addition, common benign lesions of the musculoskeletal system may initially resemble malignant lesions.

Patients with signs, symptoms, or abnormalities on imaging studies that suggest the presence of a musculoskeletal tumor should have a careful evaluation. Based on this evaluation the physician must decide if the patient can be observed and treated symptomatically or if the patient should have further testing, referral, or treatment. Conditions requiring immediate treatment include pathologic fractures, impending pathologic fractures, neurologic deficits, and uncontrolled pain. In most instances, the definitive evaluation and biopsy of a lesion that may be malignant should be performed by an orthopaedic surgeon with experience in the management of these problems.

scan may provide more detailed information. In a small subset of these patients, biopsy of the bone lesion shows a poorly differentiated metastatic carcinoma, and physical examination, imaging studies and laboratory studies will not identify the primary lesion.

Operative treatment of metastatic bone disease can preserve musculoskeletal function and relieve pain. Options include prophylactic internal fixation or prosthetic reconstruction of involved bones to prevent pathologic fractures. New implants and techniques are available to provide durable reconstructions. Methyl methacrylate is often used as a local adjuvant to add strength to the metal construct. Postoperatively, radiation is often effective in maintaining local control. Bisphosphonates are now used routinely

Annotated Bibliography

Enneking WF. Musculoskeletal Tumor Surgery. New York: Churchill Livingstone, 1983.
The author reviews the clinical presentation and surgical treatment of bone and soft tissue neoplasms. The first section of the book discusses the presentation, natural history, and staging of musculoskeletal neoplasms. The second section explains how different anatomic locations affect the presentation, progression. and treatment of these neoplasms, and the last section covers specific types of neoplasms.

Enzinger FM, Weiss SW. Soft Tissue Tumors. 3rd Ed. St Louis: Mosby, 1995.
The authors provide in-depth discussions of benign and malignant neoplasms of the musculoskeletal soft tissues and lesions of the soft tissues that resemble neoplasms.

Frassica FJ, McCarthy EF. Pathology of Bone and Joint Disorders with Clinical and Radiographic Correlation. Philadelphia: W. B. Saunders, 1998.
An orthopaedic oncologist and musculoskeletal pathologist have combined talents to provide an excellent teaching guide for diagnosis

of musculoskeletal conditions. *This book is limited to disorders of bone including neoplasms, infection, fractures, and metabolic bone disease. It is well illustrated with radiographs and classic histology for all conditions discussed.*

Mirra JM. Bone Tumors: Clinical, Radiologic, and Pathologic Correlations. Philadelphia: Lea & Febiger, 1989.
This detailed text presents the clinical, radiologic, and pathologic characteristics of bone tumors. The author also summarizes the course and treatment of each neoplasm.

Sim FH, ed. Diagnosis and Management of Metastatic Bone Disease: A Multidisciplinary Approach. New York: Raven, 1988.
The authors of this book provide an excellent review of the diagnosis and treatment of metastatic bone disease. They include discussions of clinical findings, laboratory tests, imaging studies, and biopsy in the sections on diagnosis. The chapters devoted to treatment include the general principles of surgical and nonsurgical management and the specific approaches to metastases in different parts of the skeleton and to particular types of metastatic neoplasms.

Springfield D, Simon MA, eds. Surgery for Bone and Soft Tissue Tumors. Philadelphia: Lippincott-Raven, 1998.
The editors compiled a group of experts in the field to provide the most recent comprehensive overview of the diagnosis and treatment of benign and malignant bone and soft tissue tumors. Surgical approaches are outlined for each area of the musculoskeletal system. There is a separate section on metastatic bone disease.

Wold LE, Adler C-P, Sim FH et al. Atlas of Orthopaedic Pathology. 2nd Ed. Philadelphia: W. B. Saunders, 2003.
This updated well-illustrated atlas summarizes the symptoms, signs, radiographic features, pathologic features, differential diagnosis, and treatment of orthopaedic tumors and lesions that resemble tumors.

III

Regional Disorders of the Musculoskeletal System

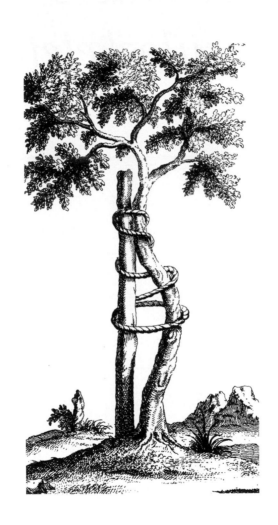

11

Eric T. Jones
John C. France

The Neck

TORTICOLLIS

Torticollis, or wry neck, a common clinical symptom and sign found in a variety of situations, is a rotational deformity of the upper cervical spine that causes a turning and tilting of the head (Figure 11-1). The head is tilted to the involved side and the chin rotated to the opposite side. This is most often seen in the newborn period. It is often associated with deformity of the head (plagiocephaly). If torticollis is present in the newborn period, the usual cause is congenital muscular torticollis. Roentgenograms of the cervical spine, however, should be obtained to exclude other less common congenital conditions, such as fixed or bony torticollis resulting from Klippel-Feil syndrome, or other anomalies of the atlantoaxial portion of the cervical spine.

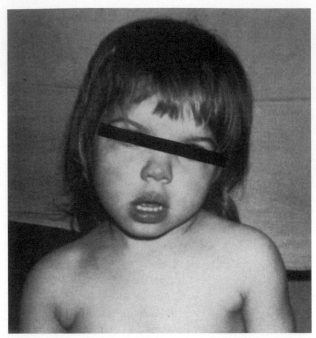

FIGURE 11-1. Torticollis is head tilt with rotation. Congenital muscular torticollis and rotatory subluxation of the atlas on the axis are the two most common causes in children. Facial asymmetry is present.

Torticollis may also be seen following a childhood upper respiratory tract illnesses. When torticollis is present after the newborn period one should be highly suspicious of a problem in the upper cervical spine as 50% of the rotation of the cervical spine occurs at C1-C2. Therefore, conditions that would cause a rotational deformity are likely present at the atlantoaxial level.

Congenital Muscular Torticollis (Congenital Wry Neck)

Congenital muscular torticollis is usually discovered in the first month of life. It presents as unilateral

tightness of the sternocleidomastoid muscle. Seventy-five percent of the involved muscles are on the right side. There may be a palpable mass "tumor" that is generally nontender, firm to soft and mobile beneath the skin, and attached to or located within the body of the sternocleidomastoid muscle. This mass often enlarges during the first 4 to 6 weeks of life and then gradually decreases in size. By 4 to 6 months of age, the mass is usually absent, and the only clinical findings that may remain are the contracture of the sternocleidomastoid muscle and the torticollic posture with the head tilted toward the involved side and the chin rotated toward the opposite shoulder.

Differential Diagnosis

The causes of torticollis is diverse, and identifying the cause can pose a difficult diagnostic problem. Radiographs are often difficult to obtain because the mastoid overlies the upper cervical spine. A radiograph of the cervical spine taken as a lateral to the skull can image the atlantoaxial region where the problem usually exists.

If congenital muscular torticollis is not present, there may be an odontoid anomaly, C1-C2 instability, Klippel-Feil syndrome, and so forth (Table 11-1). All children with torticollis should be evaluated with roentgenograms to exclude bony abnormality or fracture. Roentgenographic evaluation may be difficult in any child with a rotational deformity, but this is particularly true in the neonate.

Clinical and Radiographic Features

If torticollis is noted in the weeks following delivery, the usual cause is congenital muscular torticollis. If the child is less than 2 months of age, the palpable lump usually is diagnostic. Congenital

TABLE 11-1.
Differential Diagnosis of Torticollis

Congenital	Neurologic	Inflammatory	Traumatic
Congenital muscular torticollis	Ocular dysfunction	Lymphadenitis of the neck	Fractures, subluxations, dislocations of the cervical spine, particularly C1-C2
Klippel-Feil syndrome	Syringomyelia	Spontaneous hyperemic atlantoaxial rotatory subluxation	
Basilar impressions	Spinal cord or cerebellar tumors (posterior fossa)		
Atlantooccipital fusion	Bulbar palsies	Upper respiratory tract infection	
Pterygium colli (skin webs)		Post-tonsillectomy	
Odontoid anomalies			

muscular torticollis is painless, is associated with a contracted sternocleidomastoid muscle, and is unaccompanied by any bony abnormalities or neurologic deficit. Any findings of pain or neurologic deficit should lead one to seek out other causes. Soft tissue problems are less common and include abnormal skin webs or folds (pterygium colli). Tumors in the region of the sternocleidomastoid include brachial cleft cyst and teratomas, which are rare but should be considered.

In later childhood, bacterial or viral pharyngitis and involvement of the cervical nodes is the primary cause of torticollis. Spontaneous atlantoaxial rotatory subluxation may follow an acute pharyngitis. Radiographic confirmation is difficult, and computed tomographic (CT) scans and magnetic resonance images (MRIs) may be necessary for diagnosis. If torticollis goes untreated for more than several weeks, there may be secondary soft tissue deformities that result in fixed rotatory subluxation.

Traumatic causes should be considered and excluded as part of the evaluation. Torticollis most commonly follows injury to the C1-C2 level. Fractures of the odontoid may not be apparent in the initial radiographic views; if a high index of suspicion is present, special radiographic studies should be undertaken. Children with bone dysplasias, such as Morquio's disease, spondyloepiphyseal dysplasia, and Down syndrome, have a high incidence of C1-C2 problems and should be evaluated if torticollis is present.

Neurologic problems, particularly space-occupying lesions of the central nervous system, such as tumors of the posterior fossa or spinal column and syringomyelia, may be accompanied by torticollis. Generally, there are additional neurologic findings such as long tract signs, weakness in the upper extremities, and hearing or visual problems that may also cause head tilt.

Pathoanatomy

Congenital muscular torticollis is believed to be caused by local trauma to the soft tissues of the neck just before or during delivery. Two-thirds of children are associated with difficult labor and delivery, and these children often have had breech or difficult forceps deliveries. Torticollis can occur after otherwise normal delivery, however, and has been reported following cesarean section. The fibrosis in the muscle may be due to venous occlusion and pressure on the neck in the birth canal because of cervical and skull position. The persistent clinical deformity is probably related to the ratio of fibrosis in the muscle to the remaining functional muscle. If sufficient normal muscle is present, it usually stretches with growth, and the child does not develop torticollis. In three of four children, the lesion is on the right side. Up to 20% of these children have congenital dysplasia of the hip associated with torticollis.

Natural History

If the condition is not treated, considerable cosmetic deformities of the face and skull can result, including asymmetry of the eyes and ears. Flattening of the face on the side of the contracted sternocleidomastoid may be impressive and is due to the position of the head when the child sleeps. If the child sleeps prone, it is more comfortable to have the affected side down. The face on the affected side remodels to conform to the surface. In children who sleep supine, the modeling of the contralateral aspect of the skull is evident.

Treatment

Excellent results can be obtained in most patients with stretching exercises. The exercises include positioning the ear opposite the contracted muscle to the shoulder and also stretching the chin to the shoulder on the opposite side. When adequate stretching has been obtained in the neutral position, these maneuvers should be repeated with the neck extended. Other measures include positioning of crib toys so the sternocleidomastoid are stretched when trying to reach and grasp. If exercises are unsuccessful, surgical resection may be required to release a portion of the tendon at the clavicular attachment. Surgery is usually performed before school age. Asymmetry of the skull and face corrects as long as adequate growth potential remains after the deforming force of the sternocleidomastoid is removed. The results of surgery are usually good with a low incidence of complications and recurrence, although some children require a repeat procedure during adolescence. More severe deformities may require both proximal and distal sternocleidomastoid release.

Rotatory Subluxation of Childhood

A common condition present in children is Cl-C2 rotatory subluxation or Cl-C2 rotatory displacement (rotatory subluxation of childhood; Figure 11-2).

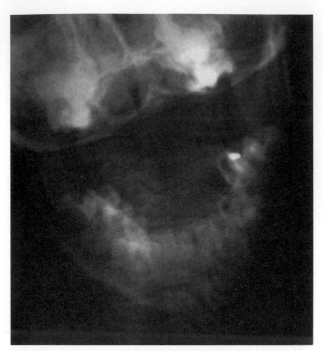

FIGURE 11-2. Rotatory subluxation, C1 on C2. This open mouth view is consistent with atlantoaxial rotatory subluxation. There is tilt of the skull as well as a shift of the lateral masses of C1 on C2, with overlap of the lateral mass of C1 on C2 on the left side. Cineradiography or dynamic CT scan is the best method to confirm fixed rotatory subluxation of C1 on C2.

This condition may occur following trivial trauma or a viral upper respiratory tract inflammatory condition but also can occur following tonsillectomy or other oral pharyngeal surgery. Grisel's syndrome is not a cervical infection but a rotatory displacement of C1-C2 secondary to local inflammation, which can allow capsular or synovial interposition of tissue at the atlantoaxial level.

Clinical Features

Symptoms and signs of rotatory subluxation include local muscle spasm, torticollis, and pain on cervical motion. Usually the range of motion is not significantly altered, but motion is uncomfortable if moved from the torticollic position. This condition occurs most commonly in children 3 to 12 years of age. There is no spasm or contracture of the sternocleidomastoid muscle. The sudden onset of torticollis in this age group or in adults should lead to radiographs of the upper cervical spine. If these are not rewarding, further radiographic studies should be done in this area to look for the cause of torticollis.

If the torticollis develops rather slowly, consider either some type of central nervous system tumor or a visual abnormality. As children compensate for various abnormal vision-related problems, they may tilt their head to be more comfortable with the image.

Treatment

In most cases, the torticollis resolves in a few days with or without treatment. Occasionally, it becomes fixed and requires treatment. Most patients are in between these extremes and may require anti-inflammatory medication, soft collar, or head halter traction to resolve the torticollis. Treatment should be persistent and early to avoid the fixed rotatory problem. If the torticollis becomes fixed, in situ fusion may be indicated.

Spasmodic Torticollis

This is an uncommon condition that may be present in adults with painful spasms producing a wry neck deformity. Radiographic studies are normal. The cause is idiopathic; however, electromyelographic studies show involvement of many muscles in the area, including the sternocleidomastoid, trapezius, and splenius. This condition is resistant to the usual forms of treatment, including surgery. Often these patients have concomitant or develop severe psychiatric disturbances.

Treatment consists of intradural section of the spinal accessory nerves and the first three anterior cervical nerve roots. Minimal involvement on one side and severe involvement on the other may require nerve root section on one side only. When the pain is intense and bilateral and many muscles are at fault, section of the fourth anterior cervical nerve root may be added without fear of compromising diaphragmatic function. Postoperatively, neck function is weak but the patient's painful spasms have improved.

Neuritis of the spinal accessory nerve can present much like spasmodic torticollis (Figure 11-3). This condition is, however, temporary and usually resolves in a few weeks with application of heat, rest, and, occasionally, local injection of the spinal accessory nerve.

STIFF NECK

A stiff neck may be caused by trauma or can follow exposure to direct cool air on the neck. There are multiple causes for neck stiffness, and many of these

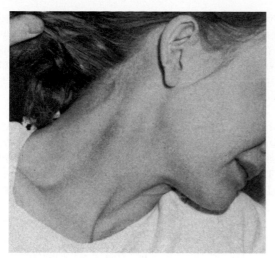

FIGURE 11-3. Acute torticollis due to neuritis of the spinal accessory nerve. The severely painful spasms were unilateral, temporary, and relieved by infiltration of the nerve with a local anesthetic. In contrast, spasmodic torticollis is bilateral, persistent or intermittent, and unaffected by injection of the nerve.

problems may come from the degenerative processes discussed later. Patients may present with torticollis that lasts for several days or more. A significant amount of discomfort is commonly associated with any motion of the cervical musculature leading one to rotate the thorax with the head. This condition is more commonly seen in adolescents and young adults than in older patients. The exact cause is variable and often not identified. Causes can include muscle spasm, early disc herniation, multiple sclerosis, rheumatoid arthritis, primary or metastatic neoplasm, and vertebral osteomyelitis.

Clinical Features

Symptoms may last for only a few days to a few weeks. The area of discomfort may be the entire neck but is usually located in the paraspinous muscles posteriorly and in the occipital area. Often patients are tender to palpation and with any passive or active motion is painful. Lying down, using traction or cervical collars, or employing other measures to relax the cervical muscles are the only methods that tend to give any relief from the complaint. Associated symptoms such as nausea, dizziness, or headache may accompany the neck discomfort. Patients with this problem are usually obvious because when they turn their head, they turn their entire body, or they may use their hands for support of

their head with any active movement. Pain may be referred to the scapula, occipital area, or the shoulders, and there may be diffuse tenderness in the area of the trapezius.

Radiographic Studies

Following a history and physical examination, radiographic evaluation should include anteroposterior (AP) and lateral flexion-extension radiography to evaluate the bony portions of the cervical spine. Early with muscle spasm, there is loss of cervical lordosis as seen in the lateral cervical spine radiograph. There is little movement of the cervical spine on motion studies, which are often not helpful in evaluating for stability or injury because patients guard the spine against attempts at motion. Depending on history and physical examination, other studies (e.g., myelogram or MRI) may be important to arrive at the exact diagnosis for a stiff neck.

Natural History

Depending on the cause of the problem the condition usually is self-limiting and responds to rest and anti-inflammatory agents. The problem may clear without treatment. If one of the more significant degenerative, infectious, or neoplastic processes are found, treatment should be appropriate to that condition.

In general, if all early studies and physical examination are within normal limits, treatment usually consists of application of heat, nonsteroidal anti-inflammatory medication, and a soft collar or supine cervical traction to relax cervical musculature.

DEGENERATIVE AND HERNIATED INTERVERTEBRAL DISC DISEASE

Degenerative problems of the cervical spine generally occur in the middle or later years of life. Cervical disc degeneration can be manifested as axial pain, radiculopathy, or myelopathy. The process can be acute as seen with disc herniations and cause symptoms resembling those of an acute lumbar disc herniation (i.e., clear radicular pattern of pain, motor, and sensory deficits); the clinical picture may also be more indolent from chronic cervical disc degeneration and may be confusing. Several terms are commonly used to describe the degenerative cervical spine. The most frequent term is *cervical spondylosis;* other synonyms are *osteoarthritis, osteoarthrosis, chronic herniated disc, chondroma,* and *spur formation.*

Incidence

Kelgren found that 82% of people age 55 and older have radiographic evidence of cervical degeneration. Degeneration of cervical discs is a natural process associated with aging, which is difficult to distinguish from the disc disease that is a deteriorative process and may produce pain. DePalma reported that in people older than 70 years, 72% had severe radiographic abnormalities. Rothman found myelographic abnormalities were common in asymptomatic patients. Abnormalities were seen in 21% of cervical myelograms, 24% of lumbar myelograms, and 8% of lumbar and cervical myelograms. Thus, no clear correlation exists between radiographic changes and symptoms. Radiographically, the most frequently involved level is C5-C6 followed by C6-C7, and C4-C5. Upper-level (occiput-C3) involvement is less common.

Clinical Features

Patients usually present with either pain or neurologic dysfunction (i.e., radiculopathy or myelopathy). Radiculopathy—root compression—is a lower motor neuron problem and is manifested by pain in the distribution of a nerve root. It can be associated with neck pain, sensory deficit, and motor deficiency. Ideally, these findings would all correlate with a specific root but at times can be more vague with some overlap of adjacent roots as demonstrated by Marzo et al. The associated reflex may be diminished. Myelopathy involves compression of the spinal cord, and thus, it can effect the upper and lower extremities with a mixture of upper and lower motor neuron lesions. Patients with myelopathy do not necessarily complain of pain. The hallmark is extremity dysfunction such as hand clumsiness with fine motor tasks and gait instability.

Pain production is multifactorial. Nerve roots may be directly compressed. Osteophytes, which develop as a reaction to the process of degenerative disc disease extending across the posterior and posterolateral aspect of the vertebral bodies, may cause

direct compression. An inflammatory component of the neuroelements may be a more significant cause of pain than actual mechanical changes. Studies have shown that compression of a normal nerve root results in paresthesia while compression of an inflamed root results in pain.

The spondylotic spine may be hypermobile, resulting in instability. This can usually be identified on lateral flexion and extension radiographs. Anterior-posterior movement of one vertebral body on another of 3.5 mm or greater in the adult is considered abnormal. Traction (horizontal) osteophytes may be an indicator of hypermobility.

Spinal cord compression occurs when the dimensions of the spinal canal itself becomes compromised by bone or soft tissue hypertrophy. In addition, the canal may be congenitally narrow. Hyperextension in the spondylotic cervical spine may cause further compromise with inward bulging of the posterior ligamentum flavum and by disc protrusion. Ischemic changes of the spinal cord may result from compression of its blood supply as the vessels pass through the pia mata. The vertebral artery, which ascends through an osseous canal formed by the foramen transversarium in the transverse processes of the sixth to the second cervical vertebrae, may be compressed creating a constellation of symptoms from the cerebellum, posterior fossa or brainstem.

Arthrosis of the facet joints in the spondylotic cervical spine may be a source of a dull, aching axial pain or radiating pain secondary to direct nerve root compression. Likewise, the pathophysiological changes that occur within the aging disc may be a direct source of axial pain. Additional mechanical sources of pain are microfractures in the vertebral bodies and pseudarthrosis of the cervical spine.

The differential diagnosis (Table 11-2) of neck pain must include tumors, either primary such as osteoid osteomas or metastatic. A pancoast (superior sulcus) tumor in the apex of the lungs can mimic neck pain or create neurological deficits within the lower brachial plexus that can be confused with cervical disease. Additional causes of neck pain are compressive lesions of the brachial plexus and shoulder pathology.

Vertebral artery compression must be considered in the differential diagnosis and may result in vertebral artery syndrome. The symptoms are intermittent in nature and include headaches, vertigo, tinnitus, and momentary loss of consciousness particularly when associated with extension or rotation

TABLE 11-2.
Cervical Radiculopathy: Differential Diagnosis

Carpal tunnel syndrome
Ulnar nerve compression palsy
Tardy ulnar palsy
Thoracic outlet
Cervical pain syndrome
Brachial plexopathy
Shoulder soft tissue and articular pain syndromes
Shoulder hand syndrome
Infection and inflammation
Developmental abnormalities
Vascular malformations
Neoplasms

maneuvers of the head and neck. The patient may experience dizziness, ataxia, headaches, nystagmus, and visual aberrations. Vertebral artery compression syndrome resulting by ingrowth of osteophytes from the lateral aspect of the vertebral bodies are more common than realized.

Thoracic outlet syndrome may cause neck pain. The patient may experience supraclavicular pain with radiation to the arm increased by use of the arm. There may be a history of paresthesia, particularly in the ulnar distribution, and blanching or coldness of the fingers. Physical examination may reveal tenderness about the brachial plexus and a positive Adson test in which patients place their hands on the thighs in a sitting position, turn the head to the side, and inhale deeply, resulting in a reproduction of the symptoms. Other peripheral compressive neuropathies, such as cubital tunnel syndrome and carpal tunnel syndrome, can be confused with cervical radiculopathies.

Posterior head and neck pain may result from greater occipital nerve neuralgia in which the posterior primary ramus of the C2 nerve becomes irritated or inflamed. Physical examination may reveal subjective paresthesia to percussion. The patient may experience limited neck motion, and symptoms may be reproduced by vertical loading or by maintaining the neck in extension.

Cervical Radiculopathy

Cervical radiculopathy is most common between ages 40 and 70. The onset of pain is insidious or sudden, and there may or may not be a history of trauma. The location of pain varies with the nerve root involved. Referred pain and soreness in the

intrascapular region via the dorsal ramus of C6, or suboccipital headache secondary to greater occipital nerve involvement may occur (Table 11-3). The pain of cervical radiculopathy may be described as dull, aching, boring, and related to neck motion. It may or may not be related to sneezing or coughing. Extension with ipsilateral tilt of the neck, Spurling's sign, may exacerbate the arm symptoms. Patients sometimes get relief by placing their arm on top of their head, relaxing any root tension.

Myelopathy

Cervical myelopathy secondary to chronic disc degeneration with posterior osteophyte formation is the most common cause of spinal cord dysfunction in patients older than 55 years. The patient may present with a stooped wide based or spastic gait and complain of weakness and clumsiness in the hands. Pain may not even be present, although many of these patients include axial or radicular pain. The symptoms may be dynamic with paresthesias into the upper extremities on flexion and extension, L'hermittes's sign.

The clinical examination often reveals signs of upper motor neuron involvement in the lower extremities, and a combination of upper and lower motor neuron involvement in the upper extremities. In other words, the lower extremities are spastic with increased deep tendon reflexes and a positive or upgoing Babinski test. They often have several beats even sustained clonus. The upper extremities show weakness and atrophy. A Hoffmann's reflex is frequently positive. Several proposed mechanisms describe the pathophysiology of cervical myelopathy. Anterior compression of the spinal cord results from posterior osteophytes. Posterior compression may result by infolding of the ligamentum flavum particularly in extension. Nutritional and vascular involvement with decreased blood supply through the spinal arteries resulting in ischemic changes to the spinal cord has been identified.

Roentgenographic Features

Plain radiographs of the spine provide a clue to the level or levels of spine disease that may be responsible for the radicular syndrome in cervical spondylosis. Studies can include AP, bilateral obliques, lateral, odontoid open mouth, and lateral flexion and extension views (Figure 11-4). Look for

TABLE 11-3.
Cervical Radiculopathy

Nerve Root	Disk Level	Sensory and Pain Symptoms	Motor and Reflex
C3	C2–C3	Pain and numbness in back of neck, especially around ear	No changes; electromyelographic findings only
C4	C3–C4	Pain and numbness in back of neck; radiation to intrascapular area and down anterior chest	No changes; electromyelographic findings only
C5	C4–C5	Pain radiating from side of neck to supraspinous shoulder; numbness chevron or middeltoid (axillary nerve) area	Deltoid weakness; shoulder abduction; biceps reflex
C6	C5–C6	Pain lateral arm and forearm, into thumb and index; numbness tip of thumb and first dorsal interosseous muscle	Weak biceps, elbow flexion and supination; wrist extension; brachioradialis reflexes
C7	C6–C7	Pain middle of forearm to long finger; index and ring may be involved	Triceps elbow extension; finger extension, wrist flexion; triceps reflex
C8	C7–T1	Pain medial forearm to ring and little fingers; numbness ulnar side of ring finger and little finger	Triceps elbow extension, finger flexion at metacarpophalangeal joints and distal joints; reflex—none
T1	T1–T2	Medial arm	Finger intrinsics, dorsal interrossei, abduction, and palmar interrossei adduction; reflex—none

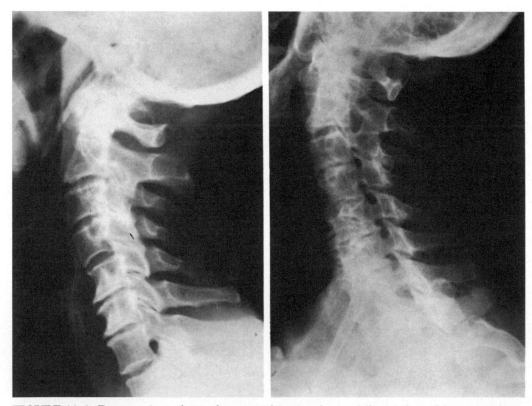

FIGURE 11-4. Degenerative arthritic changes in the cervical spine following loss of disc material particularly between C5 and C6. However, the oblique view shows spur formation encroaching on the intervertebral foramina from C3 to C7, which can cause nerve root symptoms.

evidence of foraminal encroachment, vertebral malalignment, sclerosis, facet joint subluxation, osteophyte protrusions, destructive changes within the disc or vertebral body, and ossification of the posterior longitudinal ligament. Canal dimensions can be inferred by measuring the Torg ratio of canal width (posterior vertebral body to posterior laminar line) to vertebral body, with anything less than 0.8 is considered stenosis. Further evaluation may include MRI, myelography using water-soluble contrast followed by contrast-enhanced CT scanning. An extension lateral view taken during the myelogram may illustrate infolding of the ligamentum flavum and dynamic encroachment in the spinal canal.

Computed Tomographic Scans

High-quality CT scans are extremely useful in assessing the size of the neuroforamina, which are normally 5 to 8 mm in vertical diameter. Scans must be performed using thin overlapping slices, appropriate bone windows, and reconstructions in the parasagittal plain to show the neuroforamina in profile. A noncontrasted CT scan is also very useful in delineating bone from soft tissue in planning a decompressive procedure.

Myelography

For many investigators, water-soluble contrast myelography in combination with CT scanning remains the securest way of defining root sleeve pathology (Figure 11-5). It must be remembered that myelography does not define the most lateral component of the neuroforaminal encroachment because the subarachnoid space does not extend out to the full extent of the neuroforamen along with the nerve roots. Myelography with flexion and extension views can demonstrate dynamic cord compression related to bulging of the posterior longitudinal ligament and ligamentum flavum, or to spinal instability.

MRI

MRI scanning has become the gold standard in evaluating the cervical spine. Although CT scanning is still better at delineating bone from soft tissue, the MRI is far superior in defining soft tissue anatomy (Figure 11-6). The disc material and nerve anatomy can be seen as well as demonstrating pathophysiological effects such as "gliosis" associated with chronic

spinal cord compression. Be careful in assessing the amount of canal compromise on T2-weighted image because the degree of stenosis can be overestimated. Under those circumstances a CT or myelogram can be a complimentary study. Infections, hematomas, and tumors are also much better visualized by MRI.

Diskography

The internal structure of the disk can be outlined by injecting it with a radiopaque substance, thus obtaining a cervical diskogram (Figure 11-7). Distinctive diskogram determinations are dynamic tension on injection, the actual diskogram appearance on radiograph, and the reproduction of pain response. In the cervical spine, reproduction of clinical symptoms with injection is more important than the actual descriptive interpretation of the diskogram. Diskography is not a routine diagnostic procedure. It is important, however, to recognize that abnormal diskograms and pain produced locally and at a distance by injecting can be demonstrated in some

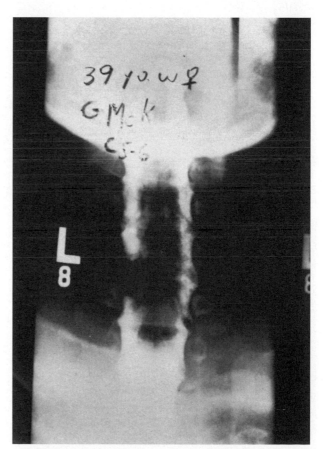

FIGURE 11-5. Cervical myelogram demonstrating herniated disc with left C5-C6 nerve root compression.

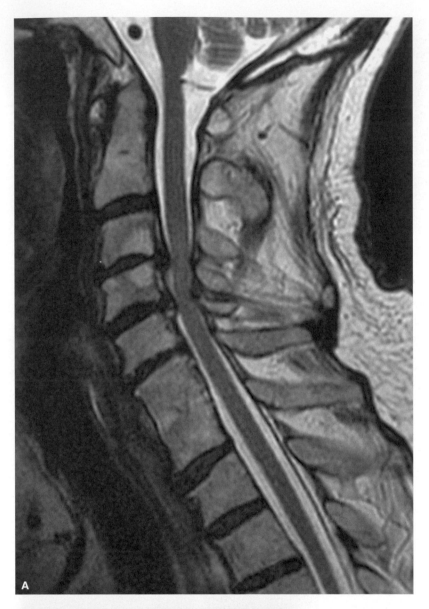

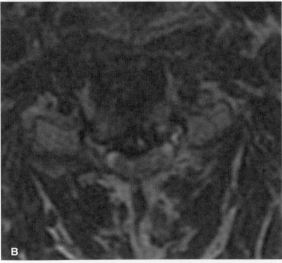

FIGURE 11-6. (A) A sagittal T2-weighted MRI scan of the cervical spine demonstrates chronic disc protrusions at C3-C4 and C4-C5 along with infolding of the ligamentum flavum at those same levels. This is typical of cervical spondylosis and the resultant cord compression has created "gliosis" changes within the cord as illustrated by the increased signal intensity within the cord at the C3-C4 disc level. **(B)** The corresponding T2 axial images at C3-C4 in the same patient further defines the degree of cord deformity from the compression.

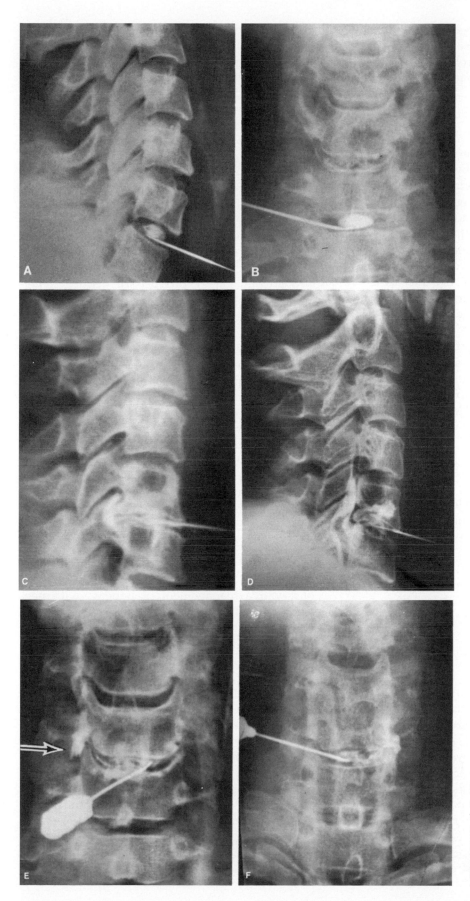

FIGURE 11-7. Normal cervical diskograms: **(A)** lateral view; **(B)** AP view. **(C)** "Mushroom" diskogram. (Dye around the posterior osteophyte beneath the posterior longitudinal ligament.) **(D)** Massive posterior disc rupture. **(E)** and **(F)** Examples of unilateral disc rupture.

asymptomatic people. The percentage of false-positive examinations increases with advanced age. The procedure itself, therefore, is not infallible proof of an abnormal symptom.

Other Diagnostic Studies

Electrodiagnostic studies may be useful in establishing the diagnosis particularly by documenting the distribution of involvement, and distinguishing peripheral entrapment syndromes and generalized peripheral neuropathy, from radiculopathy. Nerve conduction studies can indicate that the nerve lesions are axonal rather than demyelinated. Conduction velocities within the involved nerve are normal or reduced in proportion to the degree of axonal loss.

Electromyography is a motor study not a sensory study. It takes 4 to 28 days for electromyelographic (EMG) changes to develop in acute radiculopathy. One-third of patients have abnormalities in only the arm muscles, one-third are abnormal in only the paraspinal muscles, and one-third have electrical abnormalities in both paraspinal and arm muscles. The EMG is an electronic extension of the physical examination.

Local Injection

In older patients with multiple levels of abnormality shown on radiologic and other imaging studies in whom cervical radiculopathy cannot be localized, injection of local anesthetic into the interspace under fluoroscopic control and injections of local anesthetic into the facet joints may be useful in localizing the pain syndrome.

Pathoanatomy

Several factors should be considered in cervical disc degeneration, including physical stress, biochemical abnormalities, genetic defects, psychophysiologic effects, and autoimmune processes.

Biochemical changes precede structural changes. With aging, there is decreased water content of the disc and diminished water-binding capacity. Collagen, the main structural component of the disc, increases, and its orientation and pattern change with age. These and other biochemical changes lead to a loss of the gel behavior of the nucleus and a loss of the desired biomechanical properties of the annulus, which becomes weakened and inelastic. The

mechanical properties change from liquid to solid. Radiographically, this is manifested by gradual narrowing of the cervical disc space, sclerosis of the vertebral bodies, and the presence of osteophytes.

Deterioration of a cervical disc may result in acute nuclear herniation, annular protrusion or bulging, and diffuse degenerative changes. Degenerative changes commonly seen include osteophytes, both anterior and posterior, fissures in the discs, nuclear extrusion, abnormality and sclerosis at the joints of Luschka, foraminal narrowing, rounding of the anterosuperior vertebral bodies, and disc space narrowing.

The neuroforamen may be compromised as the disc space narrows. Encroachment into the neuroforamina may be caused by the joints of Luschka (uncovertebral joints), products of disc, or hypertrophic or subluxed facet joints. Osteophytes may develop posteriorly and extend across the entire width of the vertebral body as a protuberant ridge. Additionally, the posterior longitudinal ligament may become hardened or calcified. Hypertrophy of the ligamentum flavum may also occur, which, on hyperextension, results in a rigid encroachment or bulging into the spinal canal with resultant compression on the posterior aspect of the thecal sac. The average spinal canal diameter between C3 and C6 is 17 mm. Degenerative changes in the cervical spine may result in a decreased canal diameter, thus reducing the space available for the cord (SAC). A SAC of 11 mm or less implies spinal cord compression.

Treatment

Conservative management of patients with neck pain involves the use of rest and splinting. Often a soft cervical collar is adequate to provide gentle support. Philadelphia collars and other rigid cervical collars are frequently not well tolerated. Gentle traction using 5 to 10 lb with a head halter and a neutral position of flexion-extension to open up the neuroforamina may be of value. Traction applied in either flexion or extension may aggravate the patient's pain problem. Salicylates and the application of hot moist packs may be effective.

Cervical epidural steroid injections can prove useful in treatment of radiculopathy. Approximately 80% of radiculopathy patients can be successfully treated nonoperatively.

Surgical treatment for radiculopathy is usually indicated if there has been a documented failure of appropriate nonoperative treatment or if there is progressive neurologic deficit with a radiculopathy. Options are anterior or posterior decompression with or without fusion (Figure 11-8), depending on location and type of compressive pathology. Cervical myelopathy resulting from degenerative spondylosis or disc herniation is typically treated surgically. Patients presenting with cervical myelopathy seldom improve with nonoperative management and roughly one-third will continue to deteriorate, sometimes suddenly with hyperextension. The intent of surgical decompression in myelopathy patients is to prevent progression with neurological improvement being secondary and unpredictable. Because one cannot foresee those patients that will deteriorate while being treated nonoperatively, surgical management is favored. Options are anterior decompression via corpectomy, diskectomy, and fusion versus posterior complete laminectomy and decompression. In the case of multilevel disease (3 or more levels), open door hinged laminoplasty, in which the lamina is cut

on one side and hinged on the other side to create a flap-type opening and thus expand the spinal canal, has been gaining favor (Figure 11-9). Open-door laminoplasty for multiple-level decompression seems to prevent postoperative swan-neck-type deformities, which sometimes occur after extensive multilevel posterior laminectomies.

KLIPPEL-FEIL SYNDROME

Klippel-Feil syndrome includes all individuals with congenital fusion of the cervical vertebrae whether it be two segments or the entire cervical spine. The incidence is less than 1% of the population.

The cause is unknown; however, embryologically congenital cervical fusion represents a failure of the normal segmentation of the cervical somites during the third to 8th week of life. There can be congenital blocked vertebrae with complete fusion of two or more adjacent vertebral bodies or a congenital bar with partial fusion of two or more vertebrae. This syndrome is usually most apparent in children in the posterior elements and radiographically may appear as a bar between the bones (Figure 11-10). The embryologic abnormality is not limited to the cervical spine.

Children with Klippel-Feil syndrome, even those with minor cervical fusions, may be at risk for other less apparent but serious defects in the genitourinary, nervous, and cardiopulmonary systems. Many have hearing impairment. These hidden abnormalities may be far more detrimental to the child's general well-being than the deformity of the neck.

Clinical Findings

Most patients appear normal without any abnormal clinical appearance. There is, however, a classic syndrome triad that includes a low posterior hairline, a short neck, and limitation of head and neck motion. The limitation of motion is predominantly in lateral side bending. Despite severe congenital fusion, many with this syndrome are able to maintain a deceptively good range of motion. Associated conditions, which are commonly seen when congenital cervical fusion is present, include Sprengel's deformity, scoliosis, deafness, synkinesis, and hand, renal, and cardiac deformities. Individuals with this syndrome may present because of an incidental radiologic finding or in association with the workup of other conditions or because of cosmetic concerns about their neck web or low hairline.

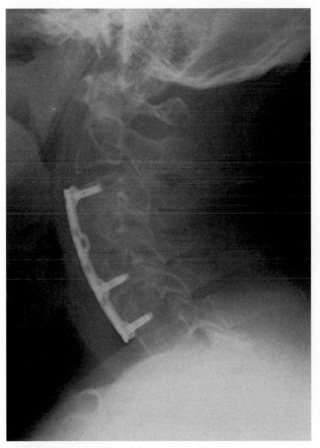

FIGURE 11-8. A lateral radiograph demonstrating an anterior cervical fusion with plating done in conjunction with a corpectomy and C5-C6 diskectomy used to decompress the spinal cord in a patient with cervical myelopathy.

Radiographic Findings

The fixed bony deformities often prevent classic positioning for AP, lateral, and oblique views of the cervical spine. Often there are overlapping shadows from the mandible, occiput, and mastoid areas. Lateral flexion-extension views, CT scans, and other studies may be necessary to fully evaluate the cervical spine deformity. If pain is present (as may be evident in older patients with this problem), serial lateral flexion-extension views may be necessary to evaluate for segmental instability with blocked motion at other levels. Other special studies, such as cineradiography, CT scans, and MRIs, may be necessary in certain situations.

If fusion is suspected in a child, it may be evident on flexion-extension views; however, there may be persistent cartilaginous endplates, which look as if they are normal disc spaces. As the vertebral body completes its ossification, the fusion often becomes obvious.

Usually, no neurologic problems are associated with Klippel-Feil syndrome; however, there can be radiculopathy, myelopathy, quadriplegia, and sudden death from abnormal motion in the neck.

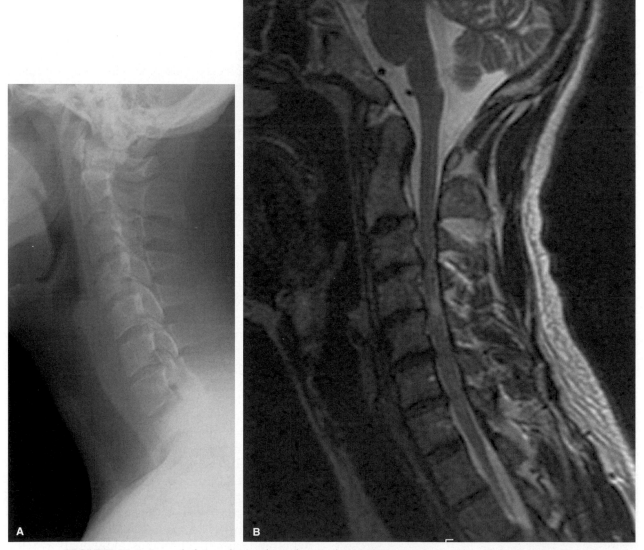

FIGURE 11-9. Lateral plain radiographs and sagittal T2 MRI in a patient with multilevel congenital cervical stenosis with associated spondylosis causing severe cord compression, including signal change within the cord, in a patient with spastic gait and clumsy hand consistent with cervical myelopathy **(A, B)**. Because of the multilevel nature of the problems the treatment selected was a posterior laminoplasty with excellent recovery of neurological complaints **(C, D)**.

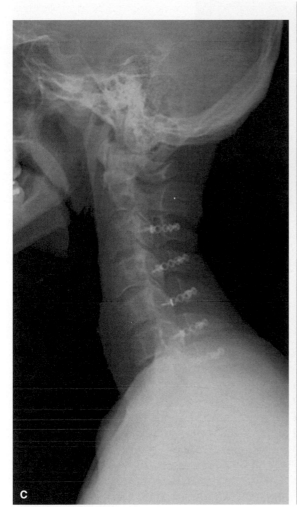
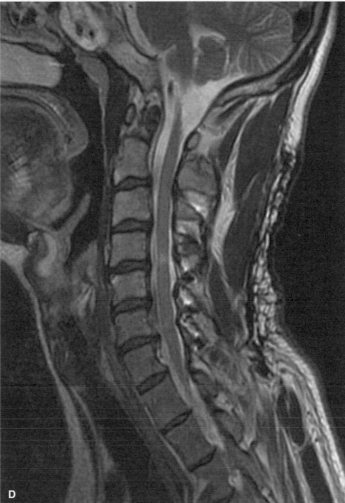

FIGURE 11-9. *(Continued)*

Associated Conditions

Scoliosis or kyphosis is commonly associated with this syndrome. Spinal deformity may be present in up to 60% of patients with Klippel-Feil syndrome. There is a 20% incidence of renal abnormalities reported in patients with congenital scoliosis. Usual evaluation of Klippel-Feil syndrome includes an ultrasound of the kidneys and, if there is any doubt about a diagnosis, an intravenous pyelogram.

Treatment

Treatment, in general, is directed at the symptoms that may be associated with Klippel-Feil syndrome. Few children are symptomatic, and most patients who develop symptoms are in at least the second or third decade of life. Usually patients with Klippel-Feil syndrome can be expected to lead a normal, active life with only minor restrictions. Many of the severely involved patients may require fusion of abnormally mobile levels.

JUVENILE RHEUMATOID ARTHRITIS

Cervical spine involvement in juvenile rheumatoid arthritis (JRA) is usually limited to polyarticular and systemic JRA. The major problem associated with the cervical spine in JRA is slow, progressive, clinical stiffness and anatomic fusion of segments of the cervical spine. The usual reason to evaluate this problem early is to provide cervical protection during the active stage of the disease to direct the iatrogenic fusion of segments to a position of function.

Involvement of the cervical spine in JRA is common, with an occurrence of 60 to 70% in patients

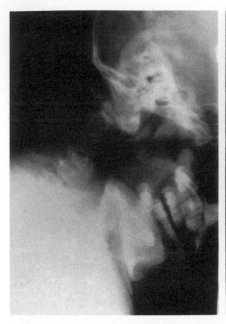 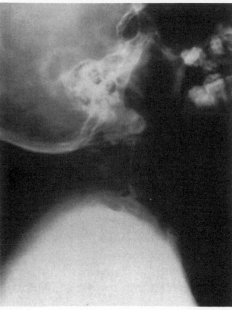

FIGURE 11-10. Lateral flexion-extension radiographs of a 10-year-old child with occipital and shoulder pain. There is fusion of C2-C4 (Klippel-Feil syndrome), the odontoid is absent, and motion of C1 on C2 is abnormal.

with the disease. Radiographic evidence of cervical spine abnormalities have been found in 27 to 80% of children with JRA.

Clinical Features

Neck pain is a frequent complaint in children with JRA. The pain is characteristically in the posterior area of the neck, radiating up into the occipital area and down into the shoulders and is worse with any motion of the head and neck. Usually the pain and loss of motion occur before the radiographic abnormalities, although severe neck pain is not common in the juvenile form of this disease.

Signs of neurologic change, either radicular, compressive, or myelopathic, are rare. They may occur in those few children with C1-C2 instability or with one motion segment following spontaneous fusion above and below.

Origins

As in joint destruction in other anatomic areas, there is inflammation of synovial tissues that spread to involvement of the supporting ligamentous structures around the cervical spine. Synovial joints in the cervical spine include the posterior apophyseal joints, which rapidly become ankylosed with developing arthrosis, and the area around the odontoid both in the anterior articulation with the ring of C1 as well as with the transverse ligament. This results in the radiographic apple core odontoid.

The upper cervical spine may be involved in JRA just as in adult rheumatoid arthritis. Early changes consist of erosion of the odontoid or the so-called apple core odontoid. There may be apparent C1-C2 instability because of narrowing of the odontoid from this process. There is erosion of the odontoid at the level of the synovial membrane with the transverse ligament.

With long-standing rheumatoid disease, C1-C2 instability may be evident because of attrition or fracture of the odontoid. There may also be collapse of the C1-C2 facet area laterally, resulting in torticollis or abnormal positioning.

The most common problem in juvenile arthritis is apophyseal joint ankylosis resulting from inflammatory disease of the facet joints (Figure 11-11). There may be decreased height secondary to this fusion if it occurs when the growth plates are still open. Spontaneous fusion usually has no associated neurologic problems. There may be decreased size of the vertebral body, but the spinal canal is not compromised. Subluxation and instability may be a problem because of segmental fusion and abnormal motion occurring at fewer mobile levels.

Natural History

The ankylosis of the apophyseal joints in the cervical spine, particularly the joints between the second and third cervical vertebrae, is considered characteristic of JRA. As these areas fuse, the mechanical cervical pain improves but results in an inability to move the

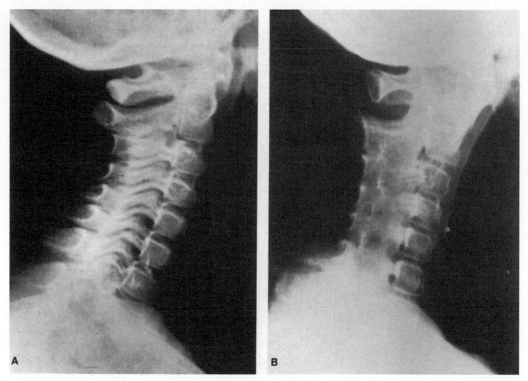

FIGURE 11-11. (A) Radiograph of a 9-year-old child with neck pain and polyarticular juvenile rheumatoid arthritis, illustrating early sclerotic change in posterior cervical joints. **(B)** Radiograph of the same patient 13 months later shows complete ankylosis of the apophyseal joints of the cervical spine typical of juvenile arthritis.

neck. This may result in instability if there are levels between fused segments that become hypermobile. The usual course of the cervical spine disease parallels the systemic course of the disease and also usually correlates with the severity of involvement of the individual patient. The stiffness of the cervical spine usually results in stiffness in extension and is a common early finding in polyarticular or systemic onset juvenile arthritis. Severe neck pain or torticollis is not common. When a severe amount of pain or torticollis is present, look for either a fracture or infection as the cause of that complaint.

Treatment

The treatment for cervical spine involvement in JRA consists of splinting the neck in a functional position. The patient should be encouraged to sleep without a pillow or in a position with a small amount of flexion. A cervical collar, either hard or more commonly soft, is the usual treatment method. Occasionally, surgical treatment for instability is required to further fuse areas of the cervical spine. Rarely, atlantoaxial subluxation requiring surgery may be present.

RHEUMATOID ARTHRITIS

Involvement of the cervical spine in adults with rheumatoid arthritis varies significantly from the juvenile counterpart. Stiffness is the rule in JRA, whereas looseness and instability is frequently a problem in adults who have cervical spine involvement. Only rarely is there autofusion of the subaxial spine as in JRA. Adults tend to develop instability patterns that generally fall into one of three types; occipital cervical settling (basilar invagination), atlantoaxial (C1-C2) instability, or subaxial subluxation. Atlantoaxial subluxation is probably the most common and significant manifestation of involvement of the cervical spine. Its incidence has been estimated to be somewhere between 25 to 60% of patients with rheumatoid arthritis. About 33% of patients with rheumatoid arthritic involvement demonstrate C1-C2 subluxation on flexion-extension radiographs. These patterns can occur in combination or as isolated areas of disease. The patients with severe erosive extremity disease and nodules are at greatest risk for cervical involvement.

Clinical Features

Neck pain is a frequent complaint in rheumatoid arthritic patients regardless of the radiographic findings. This pain can be suboccipital indicating upper cervical disease or more generalized. The most significant concern is that of myelopathy, which is manifested by upper extremity dysfunction, paresthesias, and gait instability. If these symptoms are secondary to cord compression, they may not be associated with pain. Some patients will also have radiculopathy from root compression and can complain of upper extremity radiating pain in that root distribution.

Because many of these patients have advanced disease in their extremities, such as contractures and joint instability, their hand function and gait can be difficult to accurately assess. Often the patient can distinguish progressive dysfunction secondary to neurologic impairment as opposed to peripheral extremity disease progression. Particular attention should be paid to identifying signs of spasticity such as hyperreflexia, Hoffmann's sign, clonus, and Babinski sign. If the cord compression is due to basilar invagination, there may be brain stem manifestations such as dysphagia, nystagmus, or other cranial nerve findings. Consider the possibility of peripheral neuropathies, which are also common in rheumatoid patients. Another less common manifestation of instability is vertebral artery insufficiency resulting from intermittent mechanical blockage.

Diagnostic Studies

Atlantoaxial subluxation is usually best seen on the lateral flexion view (Figure 11-12). The atlantodental interval (ADI) is measured from the anterior surface of the odontoid to the posterior surface of the anterior ring of C1. Flexion-extension views can identify how much motion is present at that level. The ADI is thought to be abnormal when greater than 3 mm in an adult and greater than 5 mm in a child. Perhaps a better indication of the potential for neurological involvement is the space available for the cord (SAC), measured from the posterior cortex of the odontoid to the anterior cortex of the posterior C1 ring. This can also be called the posterior atlanto-dens interval (PADI). Measurement of 14 mm or less indicate significant risk for neurologic

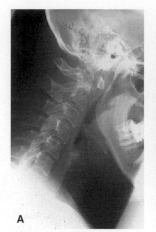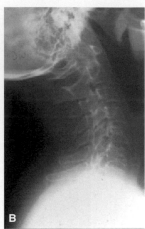

FIGURE 11-12. Lateral flexion **(A)** extension **(B)** cervical radiographs demonstrating instability at the C1-C2 junction.

involvement. MRI flexion-extension views may also be helpful in cord compression because these views allow better visualization of the soft tissues such as the cord itself and pannus formation anterior to the cord at C1 odontoid joint. If the pannus is large enough, it alone can create cord compression.

Basilar invagination may be difficult to accurately assess with plain radiographs and may be better seen on an MRI or CT scan. Similar measurements can be made for translocation of the odontoid into the foramen magnum. This is usually done by measuring the McGregor line as well as the Chamberlain line to determine the degree of odontoid projection (Figure 11-13). The line drawn across the foramen magnum described by McRae should be well above the tip of the odontoid process. It is often difficult to visualize the pertinent structures at the base of the skull. Under those circumstances Ranawat's line can be useful. Cervicomedullary angle measured via a sagittal MRI scan can also be used and anything less than 135° signifies neurological risk to the patient (Figure 11-14). This measures with a line parallel to the brainstem and intersecting a second line parallel to the cervical cord. This disease is a systemic disease, so nearly all elements of the cervical spine are involved, including the bone ligaments, capsules, and so forth. Further changes can occur if the patient has been using steroids. The severity of cervical spine involvement usually parallels the severity of the disease.

Natural History

The natural history of involvement of the upper cervical spine is somewhat controversial. The greatest concern with regard to natural history of the cervical

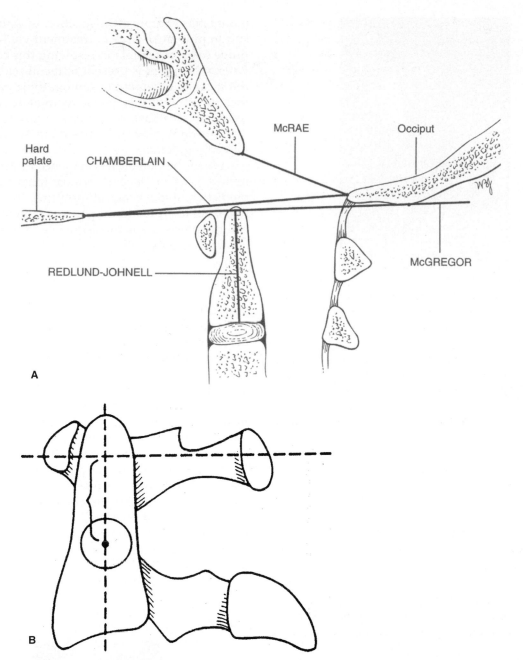

FIGURE 11-13. (A) Drawing of lines for measurements of basilar invagination. Chamberlain's line: odontoid tip > 6 mm above the line. McRae's line: odontoid tip above this line. McGregor's line: males, odontoid tip > 8 mm above the line; females, odontoid tip > 9.7 mm above the line. Redlund-Johnell distance: males < 34 mm; females, < 29 mm. **(B)** The distance described by Ranawat and associates is between the sclerotic ring, which represents the pedicle of the axis, and the transverse axis of the atlas, as measured along the longitudinal axis of the odontoid process. As this distance becomes shorter, the severity of cranial settling increases. Normal values are 17 mm + 2 in females. (Reprinted with permission from Clark CR, Goetz DD, Menezes AH. Arthrodesis of the cervical spine in rheumatoid arthritis. J Bone Joint Surg 1989;71A:381–392)

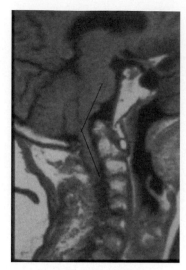

FIGURE 11-14. A midline sagittal MRI reveals basilar invagination with the odontoid extending into the foramen magnum and a decrease in the cervicomedullary angle to 135°.

disease is to predict those patients that are at risk to develop progressive myelopathy. Once a patient is identified with extremity dysfunction from myelopathy, any improvement in function as a result of surgical treatment is unpredictable, thus it is ideal to identify these patients at risk prior to or early in their course of myelopathy. Boden et al analyzed patients based on the PADI and found that a measurement of 14 mm or less was predictive of paralysis and surgical treatment was warranted even in patients thus far asymptomatic.

In addition to myelopathic syndromes, these patients are at risk for sudden death due to upper cervical cord compression above the root supply to the diaphragm (C3, C4, C5). Once a patient develops myelopathy from upper cervical disease, the risk of sudden death is significant as demonstrated on autopsy studies by Delamarter, Dodge, and Bohlman.

Treatment

A protective soft collar or firm collar may help provide some degree of comfort. A firm Philadelphia collar may give some support. However, there may be skin sensitivity and difficulty in using the collar and it does not protect from progressive neurological deterioration nor death. Thus, it is a symptomatic treatment for pain component only.

The indications for surgical intervention are (1) pain, (2) neurologic dysfunction, and (3) radiographic

parameters. Because the location of pain is difficult to pinpoint, surgical treatment via fusion can prove to be unreliable in resolving this complaint. Thus, when pain is present in the absence of neurological involvement or radiographic parameters then every effort is made to treat it nonoperatively. If recalcitrant to nonoperative treatment then fusion is generally carried out at the most involved segments.

When the patient has evidence of neurological involvement or specific radiographic parameters predictive of neurological problems, then the only treatment likely to aid the patient is surgical. In general the procedure is to adequately decompress the neural elements, either by directly removing the compressive structure or indirectly by realigning the spinal canal. In order to maintain the decompression and prevent recurrence a fusion is warranted in essentially all of these patients.

Atlantoaxial instability can be treated with a posterior C1-C2 arthrodesis using one of many techniques (Figure 11-15). Techniques that provide the best immediate stability are favored in order to avoid the need for postoperative halo immobilization. Basilar invagination can be more difficult to treat. If the occipital migration can be reduced via traction then a simple occipital cervical posterior fusion may be adequate, occasionally including posterior C1 laminectomy. If this cannot be accomplished then a similar posterior fusion can be utilized followed by direct decompression of the anterior cord with an odontoid resection. For subaxial subluxations the surgical technique is generally a posterior fusion. A laminectomy decompression is included if the anatomic alignment of the segment cannot be restored with the fusion.

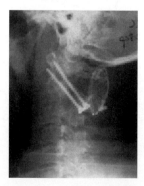

FIGURE 11-15. One technique of posterior atlantoaxial (C1-C2) fusion using transarticular screws in combination with a Brooks wiring. This allows for enough immediate stability to avoid the need for postoperative halo immobilization.

Complications of Treatment

These patients often have numerous comorbidities making their medical complications rates high. In addition they tend to be osteopenic with poor tissue quality giving risk to frequent instrumentation related complications. The mortality rates within a year of surgery on the cervical spine, particularly the upper cervical spine in patients with rheumatoid arthritis, range as high as 50%. These patients have a high incidence of failure of fusion and a tendency to resorb bone graft particularly in upper cervical fusion. Infection rates, wound healing problems, and difficulty with postoperative immobilization are other significant problems in the treatment of this condition. Adjacent segment instability can be a late problem particularly given the predisposition to instability in these patients.

Annotated Bibliography

Torticollis

Cheng JCY, Au AWY. Infantile torticollis: a review of 624 cases. J Pediatr Orthop 1994;14:802–808.
An article that reviews 624 cases of infantile torticollis treated over a period of 7 years. Ninety-seven percent of all cases resolved with a passive stretching exercise program.

Coventry MB, Harris LE. Congenital muscular torticollis in infancy: some observations regarding treatment. J Bone Joint Surg 1959;41A:815.
This is an excellent classic review of 35 patients with congenital muscular torticollis. The physical and pathologic findings and treatment with follow-up are well recorded.

MacDonald D. Sternomastoid tumor and muscular torticollis. J Bone Joint Surg 1969;51B:432.
This article evaluates the relation between the sternomastoid tumor and congenital muscular torticollis. It reviews the etiology and pathogenesis of the condition and presents the cases of 152 children with torticollis.

Tien C, SU J, Lin G, Lin S. Ultrasonographic study of the coexistence of muscular torticollis and dysplasia of the hip. J Pediatr Orthop 2001;21:343.
This article demonstrates that DDH coexists with torticollis about 17% of the time and that in cases that they found of treated DDH they found torticollis in about 85% of the time.

Wycis HT, Moore JR. The surgical treatment of spasmodic torticollis. J Bone Joint Surg 1954;36A:119.
This article describes the surgical treatment for spasmodic torticollis and discusses the differential diagnosis and how to arrive at the diagnosis of true spasmodic torticollis.

Rotatory Subluxation

Phillips WA, Hensinger RN. The management of atlantoaxial subluxation in children. J Bone Joint Surg 1989;71A:664.
This is a retrospective review of 23 children treated for atlantoaxial rotatory subluxation. In children seen less than 1 month after the onset of symptoms the subluxation was able to be reduced either spontaneously or with traction. Of the other seven children seen more than a month after the onset of symptoms, three eventually needed C1-C2 fusion. Dynamic CT scans made in maximum rotation to each side proved to be an excellent method of documenting the presence of rotatory subluxation.

Cervical Herniated Discs and Degenerative Disease

An HS. Section 1. Degenerative cervical disorders. Instr Course Lectures, Spine 2003; 5–58. Rosemont, IL: American Academy of Orthopaedic Surgeons.
This book offers an excellent up-to-date review of cervical degeneration pathology, clinical findings, a variety of treatment techniques, and complications. Each chapter is written by experts and addresses an aspect of cervical degenerative disease in detail.

DePalma AF, Rothman RH, Levitt RL, et al. The natural history of severe cervical disc degeneration. Acta Orthop Scand 1972; 43:392–96.
Natural history of symptomatic and assymptomatic radiographic degenerative disc disease.

Geck MJ, Eismont FJ. Surgical options for the treatment of cervical spondylotic myelopathy. Orthop Clin North Am 2002; 33(2):329–48.
A review of the various surgical treatment options for myelopathy resulting from cervical spondylosis and offers a guide as to the procedure that would best address the patients' pathology.

Malloy KM, Hilibrand AS. Autograft versus allograft in degenerative cervical disease. Clin Orthop 2002;394:27–38.
A review of the literature and techniques of cervical fusion comparing allograft versus autograft. Iliac crest and fibula graft are discussed for reconstruction of the anterior column supports of the cervical spine.

Marzo JM, Simmons EH, Kallen F. Intradural connections between adjacent cervical spinal roots. Spine 1987;12(10):964–968.
A cadaveric study that demonstrates the extent of intradural connections between adjacent nerve roots that offers anatomic evidence supporting the common clinical finding of motor, sensory, or reflex changes that are frequently noted at levels cephalad or caudal to the radiographically identified root of compression.

Rechtine GR. Nonsurgical treatment of cervical degenerative disease. Instr Course Lect 1999:48:433–435.
A comprehensive review of nonoperative treatment strategies for cervical degenerative disease.

Rothman RH, Rashbaum RF. Pathogenesis of signs and symptoms of cervical disc degeneration. AANS Instructional Course Lectures 1978:27:203–15.
Instructional course on signs, symptoms, and diagnoses of cervical disc disease. Many patients have abnormal radiographic findings that are not associated with symptoms.

Shafaie FF, Wippold FJ II, Goado M et al. Comparison of computed tomography, myelography and magnetic resonance imaging in the evaluation of cervical spondylotic myelopathy and radiculopathy. Spine 1999;24(17):1781–1785.
This is a retrospective radiographic study done blindly and in a random fashion to assess the concordance rates between the interpretations of the two radiographic studies in 20 patients.

Zeidman SM, Ducker TB, Raycroft J. Trends and complications in cervical spine surgery: 1989–1993. J Spinal Disord 1997;10(6): 523–526.
Data collection on 4,589 patients operated on by 35 surgeons is reviewed to assess diagnosis, procedure, and complications.

Klippel-Feil Syndrome

Hensinger RN, Lang JE, MacEwen GD. Klippel-Feil syndrome: a constellation of associated anomalies. J Bone Joint Surg 1974;56A:1246.
This is an evaluation of 50 patients with Klippel-Feil syndrome to evaluate associated anomalies. Less than half had the classic triad,

more than half had scoliosis, and a third had renal anomalies. All patients with Klippel-Feil syndrome were found to be at risk for having other serious but less apparent anomalies including the Sprengel deformity, impairment of hearing, and congenital heart disease.

Pizzutillo PD. Klippel-Feil syndrome. The cervical spine. Philadelphia: JB Lippincott, 1998.
This chapter is the best single reference for reviewing Klippel-Feil syndrome. The triad of short-neck, low posterior hairline, and limited range of motion, as well as other clinical findings in Klippel-Feil syndrome are discussed thoroughly. The history, embryology, associated problems, natural history, and treatment are also discussed.

Suh SW, Sarwark JF, Vora A et al. Evaluating congenital spine deformities for intraspinal anomalies with magnetic resonance imaging. J Pediatr Orthop 2001;21:525.
This study looking at multiple and congenital spine deformities found that 32% of their patients had no symptoms although there was intraspinal pathology found on MRI. It is their recommendation that all patients with congenital deformity as torticollis have an MRI.

Juvenile Rheumatoid Arthritis

Espada G, Babini JC, Maldonado-Cocco JA et al. Radiologic review: the cervical spine in juvenile rheumatoid arthritis. Semin Arthritis Rheum 1988;17:185.
This is a good radiographic review of involvement of the cervical spine in juvenile rheumatoid arthritis. The most common radiographic abnormality found was apophyseal joint fusion, with paraspinal calcifications and growth disturbance being next in frequency. About 20% of patients in this study of 120 had atlantoaxial subluxation or odontoid erosion.

Hensinger RN, DeVito PD, Ragsdale CG. Changes in the cervical spine in juvenile rheumatoid arthritis. J Bone Joint Surg 1986;68A:189.
This article sought evidence of disease in the cervical spine in 121 patients with juvenile rheumatoid arthritis. The authors reported that clinical stiffness and radiographic changes occurred most commonly in patients with polyarticular-onset disease and system-onset disease. Despite extensive roentgenographic involvement of the cervical spine, neck pain was not a common complaint.

Rheumatoid Arthritis

Boden SD, Dodge LD, Buhlman HH et al. Rheumatoid arthritis of the cervical spine: a long-term analysis with predictors of paralysis and recovery. J Bone Joint Surg 1993;75A:1282–1297.
This is an analysis of radiographic parameters that may be predicative of neurologic deterioration in patients with cervical disease due to rheumatoid arthritis. It reinforces the use of the posterior atlanto dems interval (PADI less than 14 mm) as an indication for surgical intervention.

Casey AT, Crockard HA, Pringle J et al. Rheumatoid arthritis of the cervical spine: current techniques for management. Orthop Clin North Am 2002;33(2):291–309.
This is a review article offering an algorithm for treatment decision in the cervical patient affected by rheumatoid arthritis.

Delmarter RB, Dodge L, Bohlman HH et al. Postmortem neuropathelogic analysis of eleven patients with paralysis secondary to rheumatoid arthritis of the cervical spine. Orthop Trans 1988;12:54.
In this study 10 of 11 patients with cervical myelopathy due to rheumatoid disease were identified as having cervical cord compression as their main cause of death on postmortem study.

Halla JT, Hardin JG, Vitek J et al. Involvement of the cervical spine in rheumatoid arthritis. Arthritis Rheum 1989;32:652.
This article summarizes the radiographic involvement of the cervical spine in rheumatoid arthritis and focuses on the use of special studies such as CT and MRI in evaluating these patients both for patterns of involvement as well as in treatment.

Monsey RD. Rheumatoid arthritis of the cervical spine. J Am Acad Orthop Surg 1997;5(5):240–248.
An excellent review article covering the various common definitions, clinical manifestations, natural history, and treatment options.

Riew KD, Hilibrand AS, Palumbo MA et al. Diagnosing basilar invagination in the rheumatoid patient: the reliability of radiographic criteria. J Bone Joint Surg 2001;83A(2):194–200.
This article analyzed cervical radiographs of 131 rheumatoid patients to assess them for basilar invagination using a variety of radiographic measurement. It offers insight into which ones appear to be the most reliable and directive in further radiographic assessment.

12

Edward W. Lee
Evan L. Flatow

The Shoulder and Arm

BIRTH PALSY

Birth palsy is a traumatic injury to the brachial plexus resulting in partial or complete paralysis of the upper extremity, usually occurring secondary to perinatal complications. These injuries occur in 0.1 to 0.4% of live births. Development of a plexus injury may be related to a number of factors such as intrauterine positioning, mismatch between infant size and the vaginal outlet, and the child's ability to self-protect during a difficult delivery. These scenarios may include multiparous pregnancy, prolonged labor, large size for gestational age, fetal hypotonia secondary to fetal distress or maternal sedation, shoulder dystocia in vertex deliveries, and arm and head extractions during breech presentations.

In predicting outcome, it is important to localize the lesion. Partial injury to the plexus is most common and occurs at the upper roots (C5-C6) resulting in Erb's palsy. Weakness in shoulder abduction, external rotation, elbow flexion, and forearm supination result in the characteristic "waiter's tip" posture of the upper extremity.

Complete brachial plexus involvement is typically the result of root avulsions from the spinal cord and consequently have a poorer prognosis. In addition to the extremity paralysis, these preganglionic lesions manifest unilateral Horner's syndrome (anhydrosis, miosis, ptosis) from injury to the cervical sympathetic chain, paralysis of the hemidiaphragm from phrenic nerve injury, and asymmetric tonic neck and Moro reflexes.

The least common form of plexus birth injury is Klumpke's paralysis involving the lower spinal roots (C7-T1). Findings include absence of the palmar grasp reflex and weakness of hand and wrist flexors as well as hand intrinsics resulting in a claw-hand deformity.

Clinical and Radiographic Features

Directed physical examination is the most reliable method of determining the nature of the injury. Gross inspection of the infant may demonstrate partial or complete paralysis of the affected limb. Provocative testing by eliciting neonatal reflexes to induce elbow, wrist, and digital extension may be used. The Moro reflex is demonstrated by placing the infant face up on a soft, padded surface. The head is gently lifted to remove the body weight from the pad. The head is then released suddenly but quickly supported. The infant may have a "startled" look as the arms fling out sideways with the palms up and the thumbs flexed. As the reflex ends, the infant draws the arms back to the body, elbows flexed, and then relaxes. Unilateral absence of the Moro reflex may indicate neural or bony injury. Similarly, the asymmetric tonic neck reflex, activated by turning the head to one side, may be used to elicit upper extremity movement. As the head turns, the arm and leg on the same side extends while the opposite limbs bend.

Osseous injuries to the shoulder girdle should be sought as the cause of the paralysis or as a coexisting injury. Soft tissue swelling may indicate a fracture of the clavicle or the proximal humeral physis. Fractures of the clavicle are often initially unappreciated, being discovered as a lump over the site of injury at about 10 days after birth. Findings in proximal humeral physeal fractures can be subtle, such as irritability with attempted arm movement or pseudoparalysis. Plain films of the shoulder should be obtained with comparison views of the opposite side. Because the proximal humeral ossification centers do not coalesce until about 5 to 7 years of age, other studies may be necessary to confirm the diagnosis; arthrography, ultrasound, and magnetic resonance imaging (MRI) have been used to help delineate the position of the largely cartilaginous proximal humeral fragment.

The use of invasive and noninvasive diagnostic tools has attempted to differentiate between root avulsions and extraforaminal ruptures. One study examined the results of myelography, myelography combined with computed tomography (CT), and MRI and comparing them with operative findings in infants. CT myelography demonstrated a true-positive rate of 94%; similar results were obtained with MRI with the additional advantage of permitting more distal visualization of the plexus.

Electromyography (EMG) and nerve conduction velocities (NCV) have also been used to further define the extent of the neurological deficit. In the early postinjury period, documentation of nerve recovery can be performed; however, the presence of motor activity in a given muscle unit may not accurately reflect the extent of useful motor function. Multiple investigators in helping to predict functional outcome have emphasized the importance of serial clinical examinations. Gilbert and Tassin first described the importance of monitoring the return of biceps function as an indicator of overall neurologic recovery. They noted that if normal biceps function did not return by 3 months of age, the outcome at 2 years of age was abnormal. Michelow et al. found increased accuracy in predicting outcome by combining elbow flexion with return of wrist, finger, and thumb extension and shoulder abduction. A general consensus exists that total plexus or C5-C7 involvement, or the presence of Horner's syndrome, predict a poorer prognosis for spontaneous recovery.

Treatment

In the early postinjury period while awaiting neurologic recovery, nonsurgical treatment is directed at preserving joint motion. Daily passive motion of all affected joints should be performed with adjunctive splinting as necessary to prevent contracture. Conservative measures should be continued until sufficient motor recovery has occurred or the child is able to cooperate with a postoperative regimen following a reconstructive procedure.

Controversy remains in regard to the indications for and timing of operative intervention for brachial plexus injuries. The timing of plexus exploration with microsurgical nerve graft reconstruction or nerve transfers for upper root avulsions is based on the overall extent of injury and return of biceps function. Infants with total plexus involvement with Horner's syndrome and no return of biceps function at 3 months or partial plexopathy with no return of biceps function between 3 and 6 months may be considered for surgical intervention.

Chronic untreated or incompletely recovered plexopathies may develop significant contractures impairing activities of daily living. Upper-trunk lesions result in weak external rotators against intact internal rotators and adductors; this imbalance may lead to posterior glenohumeral subluxation or dislocation with secondary glenohumeral changes. In an attempt to avert this complication, a subscapularis muscle slide has been described to increase passive external rotation at 1 year of age for those unresponsive to physical therapy.

In the slightly older child with an internal rotation contracture, external rotator and abductor weakness, and posterior glenohumeral subluxation without significant glenoid deformity, the Sever-L'Episcopo procedure has been successfully performed to address the anterior contracture in addition to providing active external rotation. First, open release of the anterior capsule with division of the subscapularis and pectoralis major increase passive external rotation. Second, transfer of the teres major and latissimus dorsi tendons to the rotator cuff permits active external rotation.

If osseous deformity with flattening of the humeral head and posterior glenoid is present from chronic subluxation or dislocation, a derotational osteotomy of the proximal humerus becomes a reasonable option. A transverse osteotomy is performed followed by external rotation of the distal segment to improve the utility and function of the existing arc of motion by rotating it into a more central position.

Multiple studies have demonstrated glenohumeral arthrodesis improves stability and function of the upper extremity after brachial plexus injuries with a resultant flail shoulder. Despite the loss of glenohumeral motion, residual scapulothoracic and elbow motion reliably permit activities at waist and midelevation levels.

Symptomatic glenohumeral arthrosis following a chronic plexus injury may require prosthetic replacement. Patients suffering from debilitating pain unresponsive to conservative measures including anti-inflammatory medications and activity modification may benefit from a joint replacing procedure. However, given that resultant motion and glenohumeral stability is highly dependent on the integrity and function of the surrounding rotator cuff and deltoid musculature, pain relief is a more reliable surgical goal.

DEGENERATIVE AND PAINFUL CONDITIONS OF THE ACROMIOCLAVICULAR JOINT

The acromioclavicular (AC) joint is a freely movable, or diarthrodial, joint that connects the distal clavicle medially to the acromial facet laterally. Between the articular cartilaginous surfaces is a fibrocartilaginous meniscal disc of variable size and shape and whose biomechanical role is poorly understood.

The synovial-lined joint capsule is reinforced by a number of surrounding ligaments. In their biomechanical study of the capsular and ligamentous structures of the AC joint, Fukuda et al. induced fixed displacements and rotations, and recorded the forces and torques required to produce them. The thicker superior and thinner inferior acromioclavicular ligaments, in conjunction with the capsule, are predominantly responsible for AC joint stability in the anteroposterior as well as in the superior-inferior plane with small displacements. The coracoclavicular ligaments, consisting of the conoid and trapezoid ligaments, provide further stability to the AC joint with larger displacements. The conoid provides the greatest contribution to superior translation (62%) and the trapezoid resists most (75%) of the axial compressive loads (as in weight lifting). In all degrees of displacement, the primary restraint to posterior clavicular translation is the AC capsule and ligaments.

Motion about the AC joint has historically provided some confusion with the seemingly contradictory observations of clavicular rotation with arm elevation and the little observed motion between the acromion and clavicle. The clavicle does, indeed, rotate 40 to 50° during full overhead elevation; however, the scapula simultaneously rotates during this "synchronous scapuloclavicular" motion resulting in very little relative rotation (5 to 8°) at the AC joint.

Origins

As with other joints in the body, the AC joint is subject to inflammatory and degenerative processes. Primary osteoarthritis of the AC joint appears to be related to the normal aging process. The relatively small surface area of this joint is subject to high loads and shear stresses with disc degeneration occurring as early as the second decade and degenerative changes by the fourth decade in the majority of specimens obtained from 151 patients.

In spite of these findings, symptomatic primary osteoarthritis of the AC joint is relatively uncommon. In the evaluation of pain around the shoulder, consider other possible coexisting conditions. AC arthrosis may be only one of a number of pathologic disorders such as rotator cuff impingement or glenohumeral arthritis resulting in the symptom complex. Similarly in rheumatoid arthritis, a recent prospective study of 74 patients demonstrated that although the AC joint was affected more often than the glenohumeral articulation, both joints were affected in almost half (42%) of the cohort.

Acute or repetitive injury can result in post-traumatic arthritis. Acromioclavicular sprains and separations and fractures of the clavicle, particularly those with intra-articular extension, can produce a painful joint. Osteolysis following repetitive microtrauma has gained increased recognition as a potential source of AC joint symptoms. Most commonly associated with weight-lifting activities, the so-called "weightlifter's clavicle" may result from repeated injury to the subchondral bone resulting in microfractures. The resorptive response following this trauma produces the characteristic osteolysis.

Clinical and Radiographic Features

The patient with isolated AC joint symptoms typically report discomfort and aching along the anterior and superior aspect of the shoulder. Occasionally, the pain may radiate into the trapezius, deltoid, and down the arm; irritation of the AC joint has been shown to mimic symptoms similar to cervical radicular pain.

Common daily activities elicit and exacerbate the pain. Reaching overhead to high shelves, behind the back to a back pocket or to unhook a bra, or to the opposite shoulder or axilla for daily hygiene increase contact between the acromial and clavicular facets. Pain at night may also occur, disrupting sleep when the patient rolls onto the affected shoulder.

A patient may also have a history of more physically demanding heavy-load or repetitive overhead activities resulting in or exacerbating the pain. These patients may include laborers, throwers, golfers, swimmers, and racquet-sport athletes. Weight-training individuals often report onset of symptoms after bench pressing, dips on the parallel bars, and push-ups.

Physical examination may initially reveal joint prominence and asymmetry secondary to osteophyte formation or synovitis. Localized tenderness over the AC joint is present, and pain may be reproduced with certain provocative maneuvers such as adducting the arm across the body to the opposite shoulder (the cross-body adduction test) or placing the shoulder into internal rotation with the hand behind the back (Figure 12-1).

Glenohumeral and scapulothoracic motion are usually largely unaffected. With the exception of chronic cases that may develop some loss of terminal internal rotation and cross-body adduction, passive motion is rarely limited other than by discomfort. Greater restrictions in motion may indicate underlying capsular tightness or glenohumeral arthrosis.

A complex or unclear clinical picture can be clarified with direct local anesthetic injection into the AC joint. Elimination of symptoms several minutes following an injection may serve as a very useful diagnostic tool as well as a reliable indicator of probable success or failure with a distal clavicle excision procedure.

Anteroposterior (AP) and axillary views of the AC joint are usually sufficient for initial radiographic evaluation. The Zanca view provides an unobstructed AP view of the AC joint by angling the x-ray beam 10 to 15° cephalad. Stress views obtained with traction or weights on the affected extremity are not routinely indicated in evaluation of degenerative AC joint disorders but may be useful in diagnosis of AC joint instability following trauma.

The radiographic findings will depend on the underlying pathological process. Degenerative disease manifests itself similarly to other joints with narrowing of the joint space, subchondral cysts and sclerosis, and osteophyte formation (Figure 12-2). In contrast, osteolysis of the distal clavicle may demonstrate relative osteopenia, widening or tapering of the distal clavicle, and expansion of the joint space (Figure 12-3).

Three phase technetium-99m bone scans may be useful in cases where plain radiographic findings do not correlate with the clinical examination. In the active patient whose history and physical exam are inconsistent with radiographic findings,

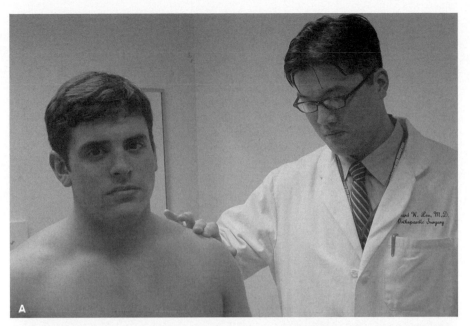

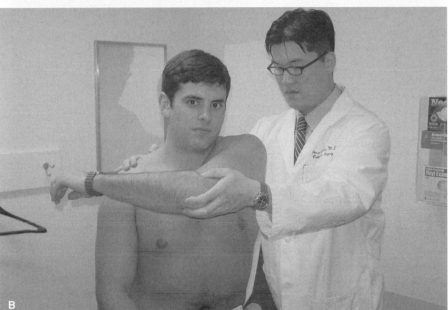

FIGURE 12-1. (A) Palpation of the acromioclavicular (AC) joint; **(B)** cross-body adduction test elicits pain with AC arthritis and osteolysis.

bone scintigraphy may detect subtle osteolysis as well as infectious or neoplastic conditions.

Treatment

The initial approach to a symptomatic degenerative or osteolytic AC joint is nonoperative treatment. Activity modification, heat, and nonsteroidal anti-inflammatory medications along with judicious use of intra-articular steroid injections may adequately alleviate symptoms. Physical therapy, while not directly addressing the AC joint pathology, may be useful as an adjunct to decrease or prevent restricted motion as well as address any associated rotator cuff disease. Although some authors recommend 6 months prior to initiating operative treatment, this must be adjusted to the patients' activity level, symptoms, and degree of disability.

If a course of nonoperative treatment has failed, surgical intervention may be considered. Open distal clavicle excision was first described independently by Mumford and Gurd in 1941 and remains a reliable procedure allowing direct

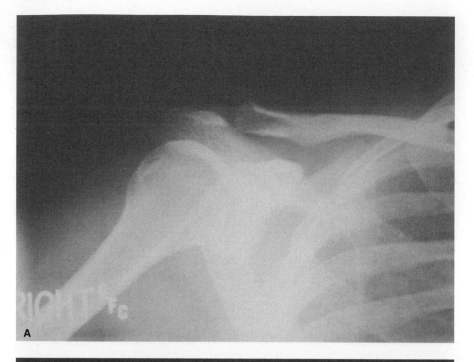

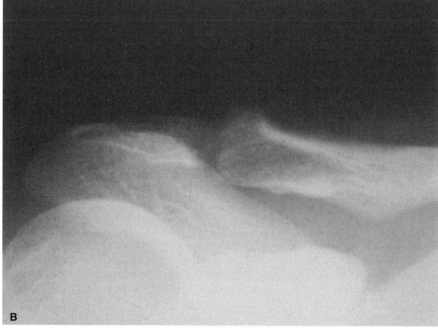

FIGURE 12-2. (A) and **(B)** Anteroposterior view of an arthritic AC joint with joint space narrowing and superior osteophyte formation.

visualization of the AC joint ensuring adequate bone removal.

As the technology has evolved and more procedures are performed arthroscopically, the technique of arthroscopic distal clavicle resection has become more common. Esch et al. described a subacromial approach to excision of the distal clavicle in patients undergoing a subacromial decompression procedure. A superior direct approach to the AC joint was subsequently developed with the theoretical advantage of preserving subacromial and capsular anatomy (Figure 12-4). The advantages of either arthroscopic approach over open resection are reduced morbidity with smaller incisions and avoidance of detaching the deltoid and trapezius. However, more technical skill is required in addition to the potentially higher risk of inadequate resection (Figure 12-5).

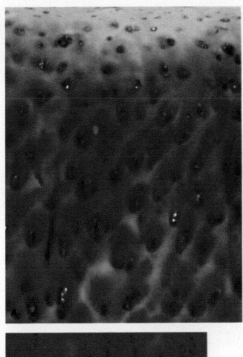

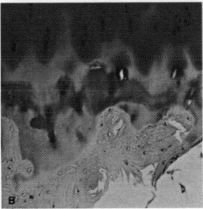

COLOR FIGURE 1-1. Normal adult (70-year-old patient) human cartilage stained with safranin-O to specifically demonstrate, by the intensity of the stain, the concentration of glycosaminoglycans; counterstained with hematoxylin. (*Top*) Superficial zone: elongated cells are arranged with the long axis parallel to articular surface. The acellular bright line at the articular surface is the lamina splendens. The matrix does not stain with safranin-O. Transitional zone: rounded cells are in random arrangement; some cells are in pairs. This zone stains with safranin-O. Radial zone: rounded cells are in short columns arranged perpendicular to the articular surface. The zone stains with safranin-O. (*Bottom*) Basilar portion. The cell columns of the radial zone are surrounded by an intensely stained matrix indicating an increased concentration of glycosaminoglycans at this level. The "tidemark" separates the radial from the calcified zone. Calcified zone: rests on the subchondral bony endplate. (× 100) (Courtesy of Dr. Charles Weiss)

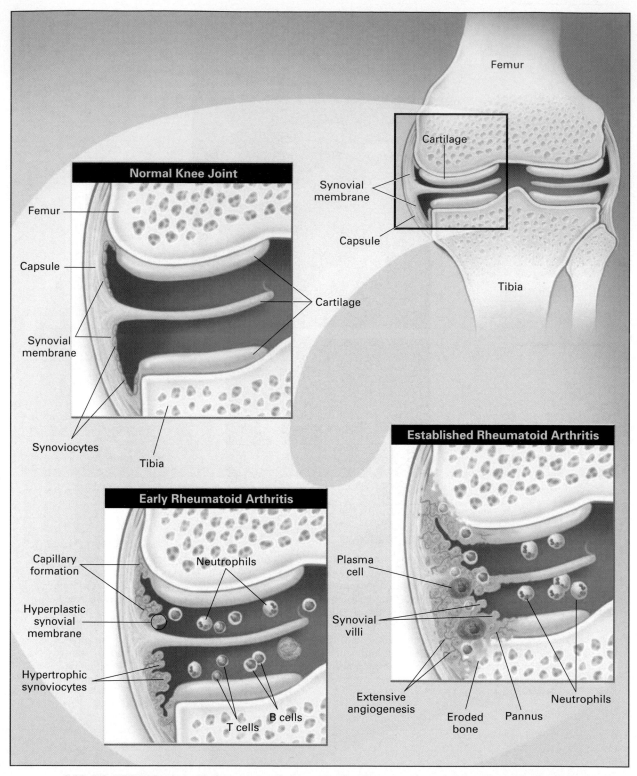

COLOR FIGURE 6-1. Pathogenesis of rheumatoid arthritis. (Adapted from the New England Journal of Medicine, Vol. 344, No. 12. Copyright © 2001 Massachusetts Medical Society. All rights reserved.)

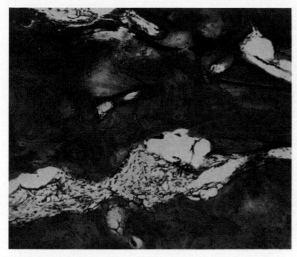

COLOR FIGURE 10-1. Histologic section showing pagetoid bone. The thick trabeculae have an irregular or "mosaic" structure instead of the normal lamellar structure. Fibrovascular tissue replaces the marrow.

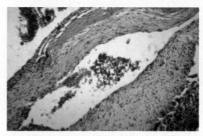

COLOR FIGURE 10-2. Histologic section of an aneurysmal bone cyst. The cyst lining is comprised of fibrous tissue containing benign giant cells. It surrounds blood-filled cavities.

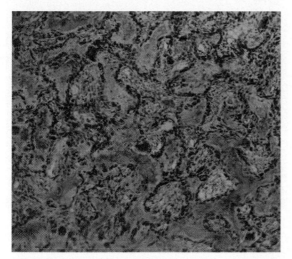

COLOR FIGURE 10-3. Histologic section of an osteoid osteoma. The lesion consists of abundant osteoid, osteoblasts, fibroblasts, and blood vessels.

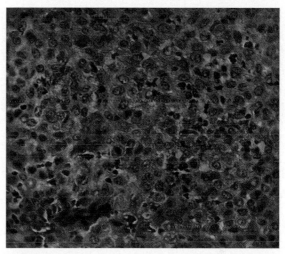

COLOR FIGURE 10-4. High power histologic section of a chondroblastoma. The lesion consists of densely packed round and polyhedral cells with large vesicular nuclei and giant cells.

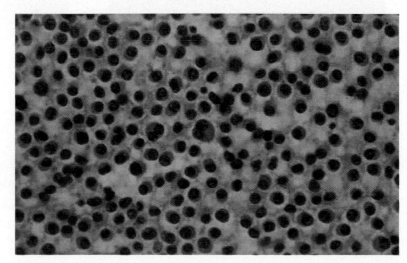

COLOR FIGURE 10-5. High power histologic section of multiple myeloma. The lesion consists of plasma cells with round eccentrically placed nuclei. Within the nuclei the chromatin forms dark clumps usually arranged around the periphery of the nuclear membrane like the hour markers on a clock face.

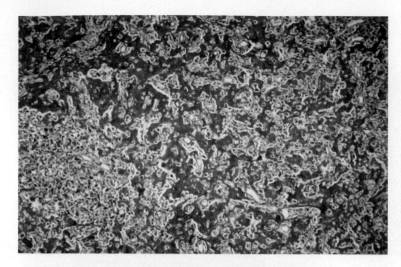

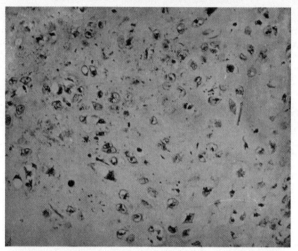

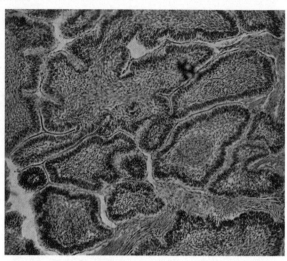

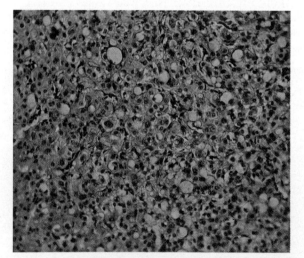

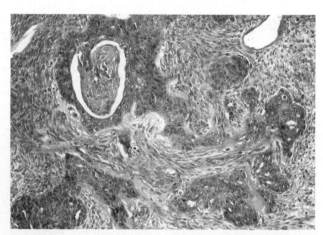

COLOR FIGURE 10-6. Histologic section of an osteosarcoma. The lesion consists of pleomorphic, malignant osteoblasts forming poorly organized immature bone.

COLOR FIGURE 10-7. Histologic section of a chondrosarcoma showing the malignant chondrocytes and the matrix they have synthesized. The cellular features of chondrosarcoma include pleomorphism, increased cell density, and binucleate cells.

COLOR FIGURE 10-8. Histologic section of an adamantinoma. The neoplasm consists of islands of epithelial-like cells surrounded by fibrous tissue.

COLOR FIGURE 10-9. Histologic section of a chordoma. The neoplasm consists of large polyhedral (physaliferous) cells formed into epithelial-like cords, clusters, and sheets. The cells have abundant cytoplasm and well-defined nuclei.

COLOR FIGURE 10-10. Histologic section of a biphasic synovial sarcoma. Note the glandular pattern intermixed with the fibrous stroma.

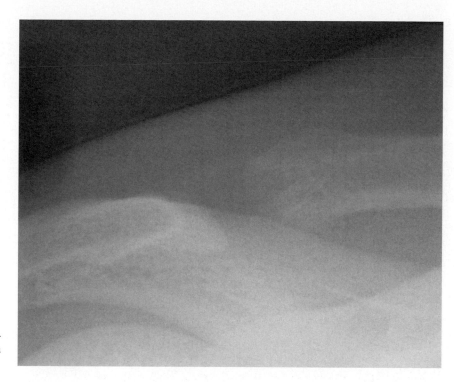

FIGURE 12-3. Osteolysis of the distal clavicle demonstrating osteopenia and widening of the joint space.

Complications

The complications of treatment are similar for both open and arthroscopic distal clavicle resection. Persistent pain or weakness can occur and may be attributable to diagnostic error, inadequate bone resection, or joint instability.

DEGENERATIVE OSTEOARTHRITIS OF THE GLENOHUMERAL JOINT

Causes and presentation of glenohumeral osteoarthritis share the same characteristics as that of degenerative arthroses elsewhere in the body. In all diarthrodial joints, hyaline cartilage provides a congruent, smooth bearing surface with a coefficient of friction 10 to 100 times less than that of ice on ice. In the osteoarthritic shoulder, however, distortion of the articular surfaces and joint orientation in addition to soft tissue contractures can lead to pain and loss of function.

Epidemiology, Origins, Pathoanatomy

About 5 to 10% of patients with shoulder pain manifest glenohumeral degenerative joint disease. In primary osteoarthritis, a source cannot be identified but may result from a combination of genetic and environmental factors resulting in articular cartilage injury. Several secondary forms of arthritis have been described in the shoulder including posttraumatic, rheumatoid, inflammatory, post-instability repair, and rotator cuff arthropathy. The incidence of shoulder osteoarthritis is higher in women and appears to increase with age for the typical patient in the sixth or seventh decade of life.

The anatomic findings of glenohumeral osteoarthritis were well characterized by Neer with the gross pathologic findings similar across most of the patient population. Articular cartilage loss with eburnation and sclerosis of the bone is most pronounced in the area of the humeral head that contacts the glenoid between 60 and 100° of abduction. Subarticular cysts may be present. Large peripheral osteophytes occur most commonly at the inferior margin of the joint, blocking rotation and enlarging the diameter of the head (Figure 12-6).

The glenoid is typically smooth but eburnated with marginal osteophytes. These excrescences are easily palpated but usually obscured from direct view by the overlying capsular and ligamentous structures. Posterior glenoid wear is a common finding in conjunction with an internal rotation contracture and posterior subluxation of the humeral head.

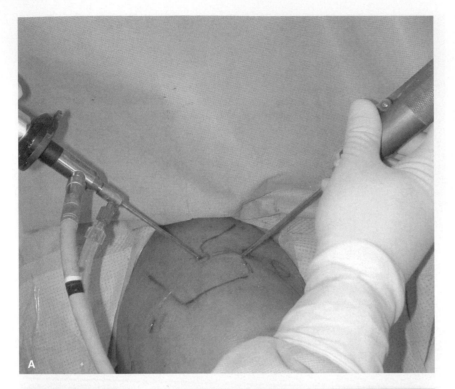

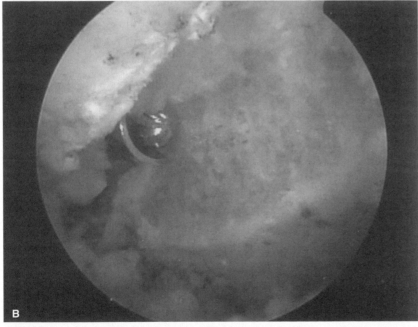

FIGURE 12-4. (A) Arthroscopic distal clavicle resection from a superior (direct) approach; **(B)** Resection of the distal clavicle viewed from the subacromial space.

Clinical Features

Patients frequently present with an insidious onset of pain over the course of several months to years. Pain localized to "deep" in the joint or along the anterior and lateral deltoid is common, although patterns vary. Symptoms may initially be merely a nuisance but ultimately can become debilitating. Maneuvering the affected extremity in space to perform basic activities such as daily hygiene may become difficult, secondary to pain and loss of motion. Interference with sleep may also occur with pain at rest and at night, often with the patient rolling onto the affected side.

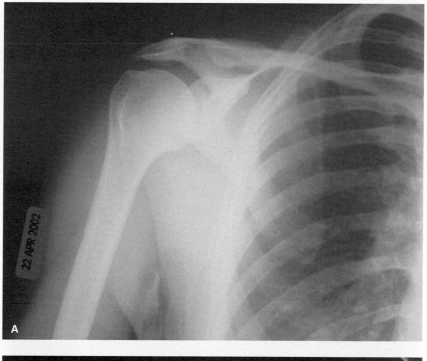

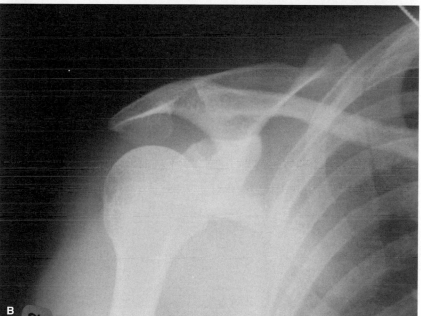

FIGURE 12-5. (A) and **(B)** Postoperative anteroposterior views after distal clavicle resection.

On examination, active and passive motion are often restricted with a relative compensatory increase in scapulothoracic motion. Contracture of the surrounding soft tissues, distortion of the bony anatomy, osteochondral loose bodies, and pain may all contribute to the loss of motion. Movement may elicit palpable and audible crepitation or grating as the articular surfaces devoid of cartilage rub against one another. Joint line tenderness with palpation is common with the posterior margin usually more pronounced due to less overlying soft tissue. Aside from weakness due to pain inhibition and disuse, strength is usually well-preserved with a low incidence of tears of the rotator cuff in association with osteoarthritis.

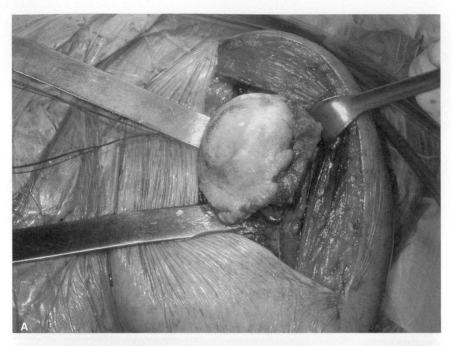

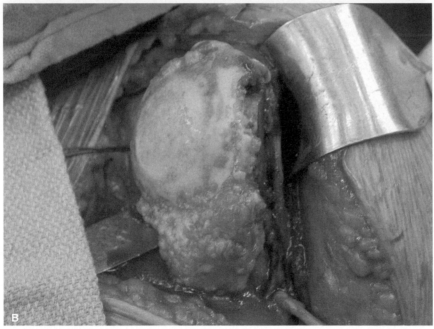

FIGURE 12-6. (A) and **(B)** Intraoperative photographs of glenohumeral arthritis with flattening of the head, loss of articular cartilage, eburnation of the subchondral bone, and large peripheral osteophytes.

Radiographic Features

Patients with degenerative glenohumeral osteoarthritis share similar roentgenographic features. Plain radiographs in the AP and axillary planes are usually sufficient to evaluate the extent of disease. The absence of articular cartilage manifests as a loss of the joint space along with sclerosis of the subchondral bone and subarticular cysts in both the humerus and glenoid. Flattening of the humeral head and large peripheral osteophyte formation, particularly along the anterior and inferior margins, results in an apparent increase in the head diameter. Although rotator cuff tears are uncommon in primary osteoarthritis, as previously mentioned, maintenance of the subacromial space provides a simple initial indicator of rotator cuff integrity (Figure 12-7).

Assessment of glenoid bone stock is crucial in preoperative planning. The AP view is useful in determining the amount of medial glenoid bone loss. Posterior glenoid bone erosion is common and is best visualized on the axillary view. The

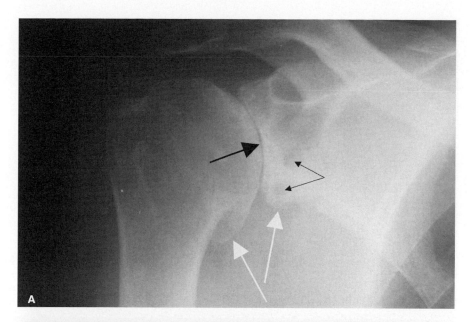

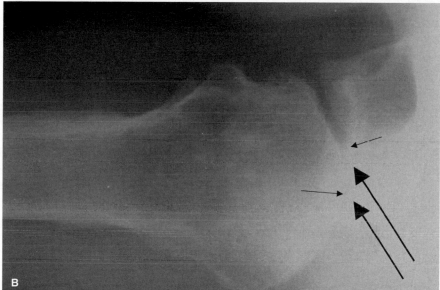

FIGURE 12-7. Glenohumeral osteoarthritis. **(A)** Anteroposterior radiograph demonstrating joint space narrowing (*large black arrow*), osteophyte formation (*large white arrows*), and subchondral cysts (*small black arrows*). **(B)** Axillary view showing typical posterior glenoid wear (*large black arrows*) and posterior subluxation of the humeral head. The small black arrows indicate normal points of contact between the head and the glenoid.

combination provides crucial information in predicting the ability to resurface the glenoid. Although not routine in the initial workup of primary osteoarthritis, an MRI, usually obtained to determine the status of the rotator cuff, or CT, may also yield additional information about glenoid alignment and bone quantity (Figure 12-8).

Treatment

Symptomatic osteoarthritis may adequately respond to an initial trial of conservative treatment. Judicious use of oral anti-inflammatory medications, taken with the caveat of possible gastrointestinal and renal side effects, may make symptoms tolerable. Activity modification may diminish exacerbating events but can be difficult or impossible to institute when symptoms are elicited with activities of daily living. Intraarticular steroid injections may provide longer lasting relief but remain unpredictable in duration and carry the catastrophic risk of infection. Aside from maintaining generalized strength and conditioning of the muscles, physical therapy has no formal role in treatment and may in fact worsen symptoms.

Surgical treatment is reasonable after failure of nonoperative therapy. Several options have been described ranging from arthroscopic debridement to prosthetic arthroplasty with distinct indications for each intervention.

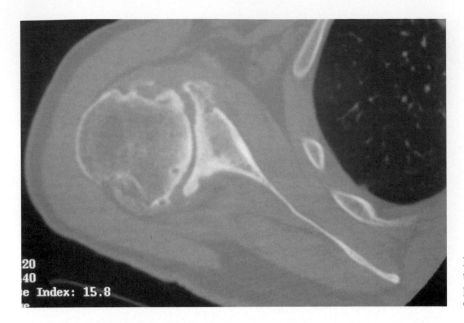

FIGURE 12-8. Axial CT image of the glenohumeral joint demonstrating posterior glenoid wear and subchondral sclerosis and cyst formation.

Arthroscopic debridement has had mixed results with the extent of disease as a primary influence on outcome. Success with this technique has been demonstrated in patients with evidence of early osteoarthritis. One study found arthroscopy as a reasonable option when the humeral head remains concentric within the glenoid and where some joint space remains on the axillary radiograph. Another group found that patients with Outerbridge IV changes could gain significant improvement in pain relief and function with results deteriorating with lesions greater than 2 cm in diameter.

Arthrodesis is seldom, if ever, an accepted treatment for glenohumeral osteoarthritis. Appropriate situations may include painful arthritis with permanent loss of motor function (i.e., brachial plexus injuries or insufficiency of the deltoid and rotator cuff), chronic infection, failed revision arthroplasty, severe refractory instability, or bone loss following tumor resection. In the young patient who is likely to place excessive demands on a prosthesis with heavy manual labor, consider an arthrodesis. Although it remains a viable salvage procedure to achieve pain relief, fusion results in significant functional limitations such as loss of internal and external rotation and use of the extremity above shoulder level.

Resection arthroplasty also has limited utility in treatment of glenohumeral osteoarthritis. This treatment modality, now essentially reserved for failed arthroplasty with extensive bone loss and salvage after severe infection, results in limited motion and variable pain relief.

Prosthetic arthroplasty, either replacement of only the humeral head (hemiarthroplasty) or the head and the glenoid (total shoulder replacement), remains the treatment of choice for most cases of degenerative osteoarthritis of the glenohumeral joint. In the early 1950s, Neer introduced his technique and design for humeral head replacement for complex shoulder fracture-dislocations. Current technology includes a polyethylene glenoid component and adaptation of the humeral prosthesis with most modern systems providing an array of modular stem and head sizes (Figure 12-9).

Unconstrained prosthetic arthroplasty provides predictable pain relief as well as functional improvement with an intact functional rotator cuff and appropriate physical therapy. Both total shoulder replacement and hemiarthroplasty can reliably provide improvement in pain in more than 90% of patients; however, humeral head replacement alone may result in less pain relief, relief that deteriorates with time, and inferior functional outcomes (Figure 12-10).

Complications

Although the results of shoulder arthroplasty are good to excellent in the vast majority of cases, potential complications are a concern with any prosthetic reconstruction. With an overall incidence reported to

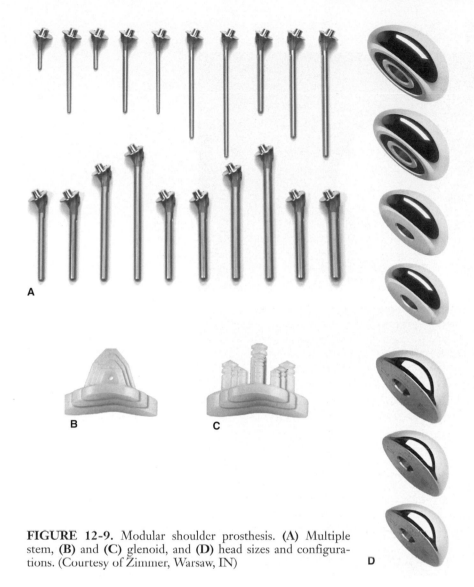

FIGURE 12-9. Modular shoulder prosthesis. **(A)** Multiple stem, **(B)** and **(C)** glenoid, and **(D)** head sizes and configurations. (Courtesy of Zimmer, Warsaw, IN)

be approximately 14%, problems may occur, including instability, rotator cuff tear, glenoid and humeral component loosening, intraoperative fracture, nerve injury, and infection. Revision surgery can successfully manage many of these causes of failed shoulder arthroplasty, but overall results are inferior compared to primary procedures.

OSTEONECROSIS OF THE HUMERAL HEAD

Osteonecrosis, also referred to as aseptic or avascular necrosis, is a condition caused by a vascular insult leading to death and collapse of the bone. Although more commonly affecting the femoral head and similar in many respects, osteonecrosis of the proximal humerus is a distinct entity with different clinical manifestations.

Origins

Any injury or disease process that results in interruption of the blood supply to the humeral head can lead to osteonecrosis. Reported causes include trauma, corticosteroid use, alcohol abuse, radiation, dysbarism, cigarette smoking, and systemic diseases such as Gaucher's disease, rheumatoid arthritis, systemic lupus erythematosus, and infection with human immunodeficiency virus. Sickle cell hemoglobinopathy is the most common cause

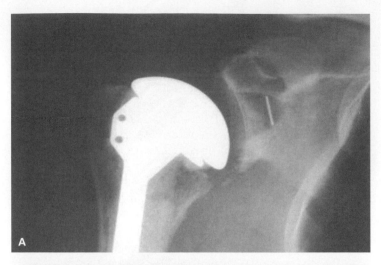

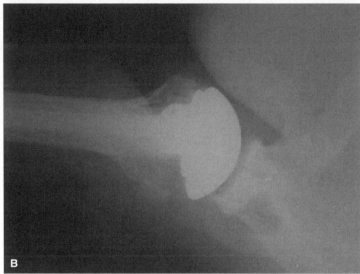

FIGURE 12-10. Total shoulder arthroplasty. **(A)** Anteroposterior and **(B)** axillary radiographs of a total shoulder prosthesis.

of osteonecrosis worldwide. Occasionally, no cause can be identified.

Clinical Features

A patient's symptoms and physical findings may reflect the extent of disease. Patients will typically present with pain that is not well localized and worse with activity. Night pain and pain at rest may occur but not as commonly as with other disorders of the shoulder, such as osteoarthritis or rotator cuff disease. Active motion may be affected early in the disease process by pain inhibition, but passive motion is

often preserved unless capsular contracture and secondary osteoarthritis are present. Strength is usually preserved except in those cases with underlying cuff pathology or systemic disease affecting the muscles.

Radiographic Features

Radiographic workup should initially consist of plain radiographs in orthogonal planes. Cruess's modification of the Ficat-Arlet classification of osteonecrosis of the femoral head is the most widely used system for evaluation and treatment planning. The continuum ranges from stage I where changes are not visible on plain radiographs; stage II characterized by focal sclerosis; stage III with subchondral collapse and loss of the head's spherical contour (the crescent sign); stage IV with an area of collapsed articular surface; and stage V with signs of secondary arthritis on both the humeral and glenoid surfaces (Figure 12-11). Signal intensity on MRI depends on water and fat variations and therefore can reveal osteonecrosis prior to radiograph changes (Figure 12-12). Bone scanning has been used for early detection of the disease, but recent work has called its utility into question with failure to detect more than half of the lesions identified by MRI and histology.

Natural History

Disease progression and symptom development is varied with relationship to etiologic factors and extent of involvement. In general, clinical progression is slow with most patients presenting with advanced radiographic changes. Patient with sickle cell disease tend to have the most benign course. Corticosteroid-induced osteonecrosis appears to fare better than posttraumatic causes with Hattrup and Cofield finding almost twice as many trauma-related cases requiring arthroplasty at 3 years after diagnosis.

Treatment

A course of nonoperative treatment should initially be instituted with oral anti-inflammatory medication and physical therapy for range of motion and strengthening exercises. These interventions are often more successful in the shoulder than in the hip for several reasons. The glenohumeral joint is not subjected to the same weight-bearing forces, the articulation is less conforming than the acetabulum and can tolerate greater deformity, and scapulothoracic motion can partially compensate for lost glenohumeral motion.

If nonsurgical options have failed, several forms of operative management may provide relief of symptoms. Core decompression has been described with some good results in earlier stages of disease. LaPorte et al. reported their experience with 63 shoulders followed for an average of 10 years. Results demonstrated success rates as high as 94% for stage I disease and falling precipitously to 14% for stage IV osteonecrosis.

Prosthetic replacement, either hemiarthroplasty or total shoulder arthroplasty, may be appropriate in stage IV and V disease and select patients with stage III involvement (Figure 12-13). Glenoid resurfacing is used when the glenoid is involved with substantial secondary arthritis. In a recent study, 88

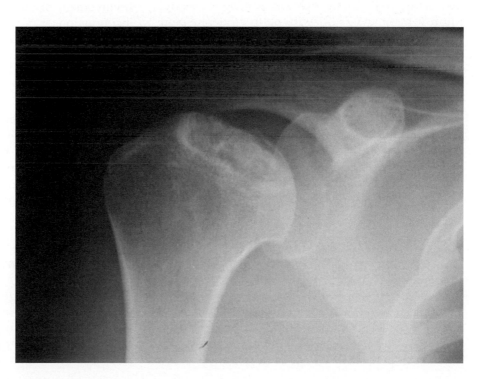

FIGURE 12-11. Avascular necrosis of the humeral head with collapse of the subchondral bone.

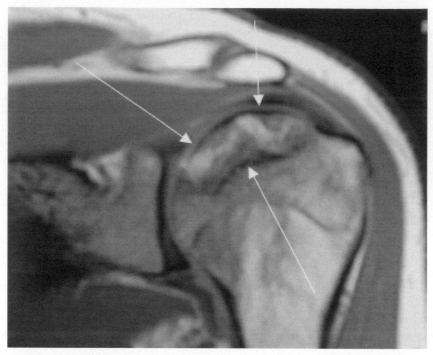

FIGURE 12-12. Coronal MRI image of avascular necrosis of the humeral head (*depicted by white arrows*).

shoulders followed for an average of 8.9 years were treated with either hemiarthroplasty or total shoulder arthroplasty with 79.5% reporting subjective improvement and 77.3% with no to moderate pain. Inferior clinical results were noted in posttraumatic osteonecrosis and superior results in corticosteroid-induced disease.

Careful evaluation should be performed prior to initiating operative treatment and should be based on patient function, symptomatology, and radiographic findings. Rutherford and Cofield reviewed the data on 33 shoulders and concluded that even with extensive radiographic changes (stage IV and V), mild symptoms will not necessarily progress and can be treated nonoperatively.

RHEUMATOID ARTHRITIS

Rheumatoid arthritis (RA) is a chronic, systemic inflammatory disease with formation of destructive, hyperplastic synovium or pannus. The inflammation results in erosive, symmetrical polyarthritis with approximately 91% of patients with long-standing disease developing shoulder symptoms.

Clinical Features

Involvement of the shoulder may present with an insidious onset of pain, swelling, and loss of motion. All synovial-lined joints may be affected including the acromioclavicular, sternoclavicular, and glenohumeral joints, although the latter can be the only symptomatic location in up to two-thirds of patients.

Initially, pain may restrict active motion while preserving passive motion. Development of soft tissue contracture and bony destruction may eventually affect passive motion as well. Strength may deteriorate with muscle atrophy and rotator cuff disease, which is found in as high as 75% of patients with RA.

Radiographic Features

Radiographic changes are variable with early involvement exhibiting only minimal findings with more extensive changes late in the course of disease. Plain radiographs may reveal only osteopenia of the humeral head and glenoid. Symmetrical

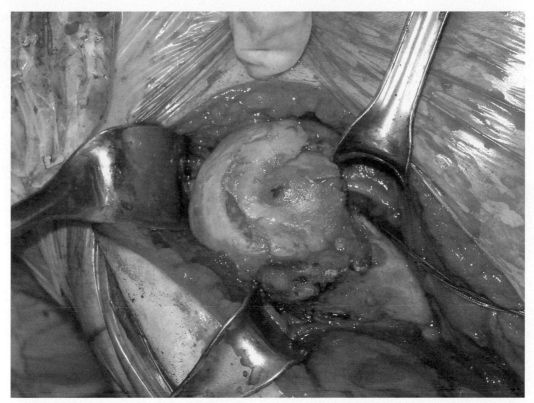

FIGURE 12-13. Intraoperative photograph of avascular necrosis of the humeral head. Note the collapse of the articular surface.

marginal erosions along the inferior humeral head and subchondral cysts develop and may eventually involve large portions of the head. Glenoid destruction occurs with disease progression demonstrating central or peripheral erosions (Figure 12-14). Osteosclerosis and osteophytosis is uncommon in RA and typically reflects quiescence of the inflammation and development of secondary osteoarthritis.

Superior migration of the humeral head may result from incompetence of the rotator cuff. Continued contact between the head and the undersurface of the acromion can produce erosion and thinning of the acromion process and possible fracture (Figure 12-15).

MRI is useful in delineating the soft tissue component of the disease. The extent of synovial proliferation and joint effusion can be visualized. More importantly, the integrity of the rotator cuff can be determined with pathology ranging from mild inflammation to full-thickness tears.

Bone destruction and alteration in the normal osseous architecture is best evaluated with CT scan. In the preoperative planning process, quantification of bone loss, particularly when considering implantation of a glenoid component, may be necessary; CT scan has been shown to provide superior characterization of bony defects compared to conventional radiography.

Treatment

Initial nonsurgical management of rheumatoid arthritis affecting the shoulder is appropriate in the early phases of disease with minimal bony destruction. Physical therapy may be helpful in maintaining active and passive motion during acute exacerbations and gradually adding resistive exercises to preserve strength.

Optimization of medical therapy is the primary means of controlling the disease process prior to development of extensive radiographic changes and severe symptoms unresponsive to conservative measures. Limited trials of corticosteroid injections may be useful in reducing the symptoms of acute inflammation unresponsive to oral medications aimed at the underlying disease process. Communication with the patient's rheumatologist is essential prior to embarking on surgical treatment. When the rheumatologist's medical armamentarium of nonsteroidal anti-inflammatory medications, antimetabolic drugs, steroids, and disease-modifying drugs has been exhausted, surgical intervention should be considered. However, once joint destruction is demonstrated, early replacement before loss of the rotator cuff and glenoid vault preclude glenoid resurfacing should be considered.

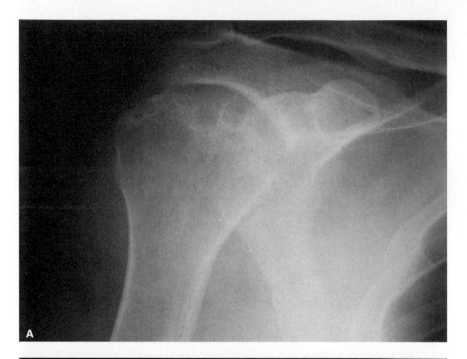

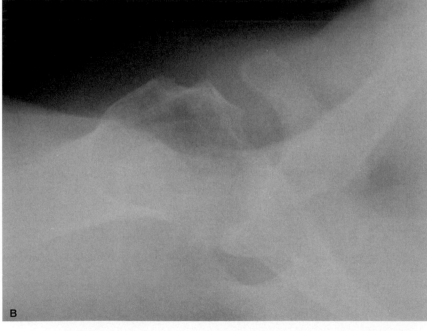

FIGURE 12-14. (A) Anteroposterior and **(B)** axillary views demonstrating rheumatoid arthritis of the glenohumeral joint. Narrowing of the joint space, large subchondral cysts, and medialization of the glenoid are typical. Note the absence of large peripheral osteophytes commonly seen with osteoarthritis.

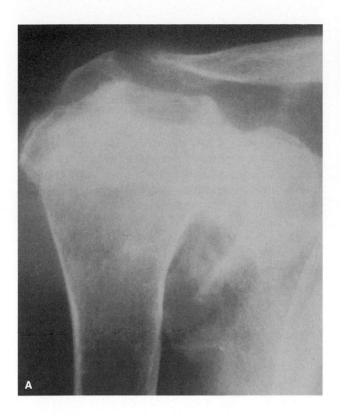

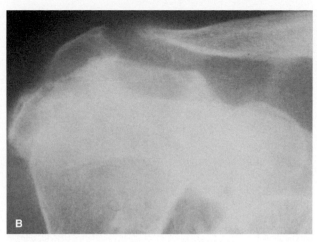

FIGURE 12-15. **(A)** and **(B)** Destructive rheumatoid arthritis with superior migration of the humeral head and erosion of the acromion and distal clavicle.

In patients with joint swelling and pain but relative preservation of the glenohumeral articular surfaces, bursectomy and synovectomy may be useful. Synovectomy may also help slow disease progression in aggressive cases of synovitis.

Hemiarthroplasty or total shoulder arthroplasty should be considered for patients with severe pain and functional limitation unresponsive to more conservative modalities. The indications for humeral head replacement are an irreparable rotator cuff tear or inadequate glenoid bone stock precluding adequate fixation of the polyethylene component (Figure 12-16). Most patients who undergo prosthetic arthroplasty for RA can expect some pain relief and improvement in shoulder function, but results are less reliable than in the treatment of osteoarthritis.

POSTTRAUMATIC GLENOHUMERAL ARTHRITIS

Glenohumeral arthritis as a sequelae of traumatic injury can develop from a number of differing mechanisms. Commonly, arthritis can develop as a result of a proximal humerus fracture treated opera-tively or nonoperatively. Glenohumeral instability also may result in degenerative changes either as a result of the trauma itself or, more frequently, from the surgical treatment.

Clinical Features

The presenting symptoms of posttraumatic arthritis are similar to other forms of degenerative arthritis of the shoulder. Pain level is variable but is usually the primary complaint. Motion may be restricted by pain, bone deformity, and contractures of the surrounding capsule and rotator cuff. Strength may be compromised as well from injury to the rotator cuff and deltoid or from alterations in rotator cuff attachments seen in proximal humerus malunions and nonunions. Neurologic injury should always be considered and appropriate evaluation with an EMG should be performed if there is clinical suspicion.

Radiographic Features

The radiographic findings are varied and depend on the underlying inciting injury. Fractures of the

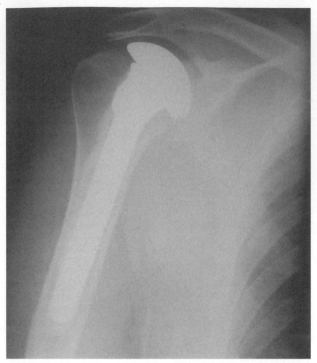

FIGURE 12-16. Postoperative anteroposterior radiograph of Figure 12-14 after hemiarthroplasty.

proximal humerus may demonstrate malunion or nonunion of the tuberosities, head segment, or surgical neck or articular surface collapse from posttraumatic osteonecrosis. Arthritis resulting from anterior instability may show a Hill-Sachs lesion on the posterolateral humeral head, a so-called Reverse Hill-Sachs lesion on the anteromedial head in posterior dislocations, persistent anterior or posterior subluxation with corresponding glenoid bone loss, or a chronic dislocation with bony injury to the humerus and glenoid. The presence of metallic implants used for fracture fixation or instability repair have the potential to encroach on the glenohumeral joint and may be evident on radiographic examination.

Further testing with CT or MRI may be useful in preoperative planning in more complex cases where the normal anatomical relationships have been distorted by the injury.

Treatment

A course of nonoperative therapy should be attempted as an initial form of treatment. Activity modification, gentle exercises, and anti-inflammatory medications may provide enough symptomatic relief to avoid surgical intervention.

Operative intervention is warranted if nonoperative therapy has failed. When arthritis has developed secondary to fracture nonunion or malunion, osteotomies or soft tissue procedures alone will not address the articular incongruity. Humeral head and glenoid articular destruction would likely most benefit from prosthetic replacement. In cases of arthritis following instability repair, mild arthritic change and significant loss of external rotation due to tightening of the anterior soft tissue structures may benefit from anterior releases. Studies examining arthroplasty for arthritis following instability repairs have shown reduction in pain and improved function but high rates of revision surgery secondary to instability, component failure, and pain due to an unresurfaced glenoid at long-term follow-up. The difficulties following previous injury or surgery including extensive scarring and distortion of the normal bony and soft tissue anatomical relationships make these cases challenging for even the most experienced of surgeons.

ROTATOR CUFF TEAR ARTHROPATHY

A massive chronic full-thickness rotator cuff tear and collapse of the subchondral bone of the humeral head are the hallmarks of a clinical entity termed *cuff-tear arthropathy* by Neer. A diagnosis of rotator cuff-tear arthropathy (RCTA) requires the aforementioned findings in addition to progressive bone loss of the glenohumeral joint, coracoacromial arch, and the distal clavicle.

Origins

The findings of Neer et al. suggested that the precipitating event in RCTA was, as its name suggests, the massive, untreated rotator cuff tear. They noted, however, that only 4% of shoulders with full-thickness cuff tears progressed to RCTA. Thus, aside from pure mechanical dysfunction, other possible contributing factors must be involved to account for the pathologic findings (Figure 12-17).

Normally, the rotator cuff stabilizes the head against the glenoid and provides the mechanism for rotation of the glenohumeral joint. Full-thickness tears of the cuff may disrupt these functions as well

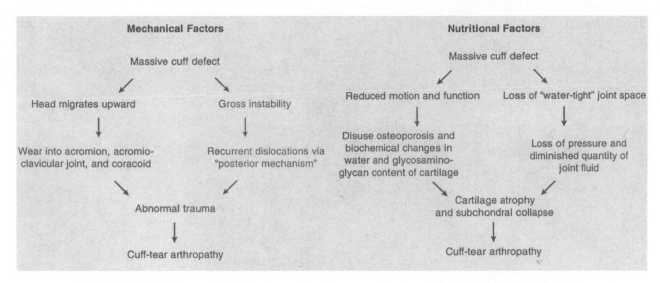

FIGURE 12-17. Proposed mechanisms of development of rotator cuff-tear arthropathy. (From Neer CS II, Craig EV, Fukuda HA. Cuff-tear arthropathy. J Bone Joint Surg 1983;65r:1232–1244.)

as provide a conduit for escape of synovial fluid essential for cartilage nutrition.

Studies in the rheumatology literature have emphasized the role of crystal deposition and the subsequent inflammatory cascade and injury in the pathogenesis of a clinically similar disease. McCarty et al. hypothesized that diseased synovium and cartilage release basic calcium phosphate crystals in shoulders clinically similar to RCTA but what they termed Milwaukee shoulder syndrome. The ensuing inflammatory response results in injury to the rotator cuff and articular cartilage.

Although the precise cause still remains unclear, these differing theories may in fact represent a single disease entity.

Clinical Features

Patients with cuff-tear arthropathy will often present with predictable symptoms related to arthritis and cuff deficiency. A long history of progressively worsening pain and stiffness is typical. Both active and passive motion may be affected secondary to joint incongruity, pain, and lack of a competent rotator cuff. Dislocation or rupture of the tendon of the long head of the biceps occurs in most patients and may be detected on exam. Many patients also exhibit significant shoulder swelling resulting from synovial fluid communication between the gleno-

humeral joint and subacromial bursa (*fluid sign*). Aspiration of this fluid may reveal a bloody or blood-streaked effusion. Large ecchymoses down the arm are not unusual, and often spur fruitless workups for clotting abnormalities. Shoulder girdle muscular atrophy, weakness, and loss of active and passive motion will be evident resulting from disuse, pain, joint incongruity, and the large rotator cuff tear.

Radiographic Features

Destructive, arthritic changes of the osseous structures of the shoulder are characteristic of RCTA. Early in the disease process, radiographic changes may only reflect a large rotator cuff tear with proximal humeral migration and abutment against the undersurface of the acromion. Progression will involve extensive erosion of the proximal humerus and narrowing of the glenohumeral joint (Figure 12-18). A standard axillary radiograph may reveal subluxation or dislocation of the proximal humerus.

Additional imaging will most often not be necessary. MRI is typically not indicated in the evaluation of RCTA, given the drastic changes seen on plain radiography suggestive of a massive, chronic rotator cuff tear. Similarly, CT scan does not have specific utility in preoperative planning aside from assessment of bone loss.

Treatment

As in most conditions affecting the shoulder, a trial of nonoperative management is reasonable. Oral nonsteroidal anti-inflammatories, limited trials of intra-articular cortisone, activity modification, and gentle exercises may provide some symptomatic relief.

Several surgical options have been described for treatment of the cuff-deficient arthritic shoulder.

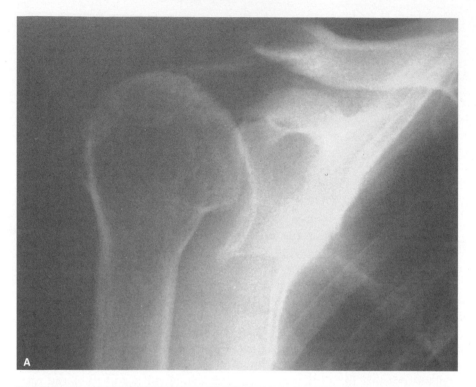

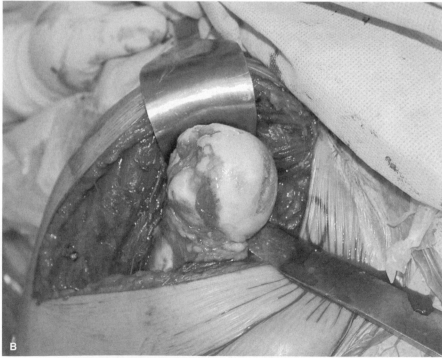

FIGURE 12-18. (A) Anteroposterior radiograph of cuff-tear arthropathy with superior migration of the head and arthritic changes of the glenohumeral joint. **(B)** Intraoperative photograph with erosion of the articular surface and absence of the rotator cuff.

Arthrodesis, now considered a salvage procedure by most surgeons, may rarely be indicated in the setting of the arthritic shoulder with an irreparable cuff tear and an incompetent deltoid. Constrained shoulder arthroplasty, involving a coupled humeral and glenoid articulation, theoretically provided a stable fulcrum around which the remaining deltoid could rotate the humerus. However, the tremendous stresses generated from this construct have been shown to lead to rapid component loosening, catastrophic implant failure, and fracture.

Nonconstrained prosthetic shoulder arthroplasty is currently the surgical treatment of choice for this patient population with pain relief as the primary goal. Despite providing a painless articulation with prosthetic replacement, the remaining cuff defect will result in a persistently weak shoulder. Multiple studies examining the results of total shoulder arthroplasty have emphasized the importance of the rotator cuff in centering the humeral head on the glenoid during active motion. Loss of this stabilization effect from an unrepaired or irreparable cuff tear has been shown to result in eccentric loading and early failure of the glenoid component. Although every attempt should be made at reconstructing the rotator cuff, it is now recommended that large defects with proximal humeral migration should be treated with hemiarthroplasty alone with preservation of the coracoacromial arch to prevent anterosuperior migration of the component (Figure 12-19).

In the early 1990s, Grammont introduced a reverse shoulder prosthesis with a concave humeral articulation and a spherical glenoid. Early results in Europe have been promising with respect to stability and function, however, glenoid survival remains a concern. Long-term experience with this prosthesis is lacking, and it has only recently been approved for use in the United States.

ROTATOR CUFF DISEASE

Diseases of the rotator cuff involve a continuum of disorders ranging from subacromial bursitis and tendinosis to full-thickness tears. Proper diagnosis and treatment of these disorders is based on an understanding of the basic anatomy and function of the rotator cuff as well as the intrinsic and extrinsic factors associated with cuff tendon degeneration.

Anatomy and Function

The glenohumeral joint is a diarthrodial ball-and-socket-type articulation with tremendous capacity for motion in multiple planes. This motion is

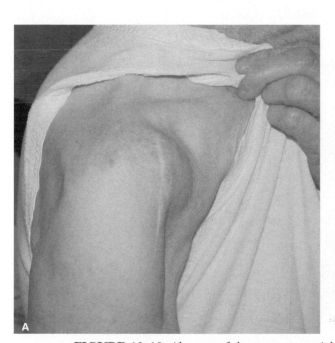 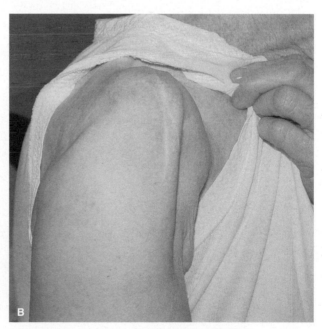

FIGURE 12-19. Absence of the coracoacromial arch and injury to the deltoid leads to anterior-superior ascent of the shoulder prosthesis. **(A)** At rest and **(B)** with attempted glenohumeral motion.

obtained through the sacrifice of joint stability. Often likened to a "golf ball on a tee," the humeral head articulates with the small, shallow glenoid surface. The labral, capsuloligamentous, and musculotendinous structures surrounding the joint provide compensation for the lack of inherent bony restraint.

The rotator cuff is composed of four musculotendinous units that provide multiple functions including motion about the axis of the joint. The subscapularis, which originates on the anterior surface of the scapula and inserts onto the lesser tuberosity of the humerus, provides internal rotation, particularly at the end range of motion. The supraspinatus originates from the supraspinatus fossa of the scapula, and inserts on the greater tuberosity of the humerus and contributes to shoulder abduction. External rotation power is produced solely by the infraspinatus and teres minor, both of which originate from the scapula and insert onto the greater tuberosity.

Despite its ascribed name, current understanding of rotator cuff function has emphasized its role as a prime stabilizer of the humeral head rather than its motor function. The cuff compresses the joint and provides resistance to sliding and translation during dynamic activity. In midrange positions of the shoulder when passive soft tissue restraints are lax, almost all stability is imparted by cuff function (Figure 12-20).

Pathogenesis

Extrinsic mechanical and intrinsic factors have both been proposed as the origin of rotator cuff disease. No one unifying theory exists addressing their relative contributions to these conditions.

The mechanism of external impingement is based on compression of the rotator cuff between the unyielding surfaces of the humerus and coracoacromial arch, which is composed of the coracoid, coracoacromial ligament, and the anterior acromion (Figure 12-21). Inherent morphologic variations of the acromion (flat, curved, or hooked) (Figure 12-22) or age-related acromial spur formation may contribute to the role of mechanical-based pathology of the rotator cuff. Biomechanical

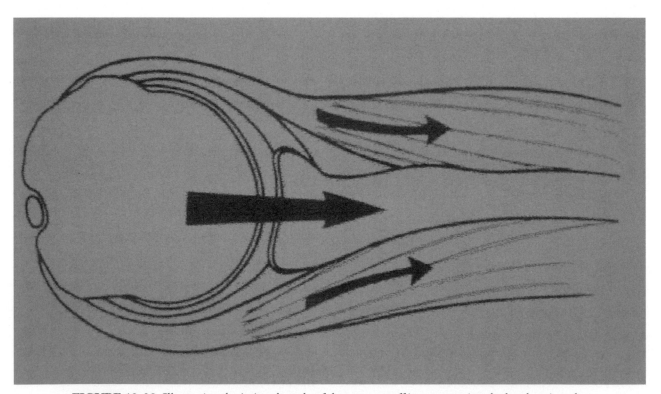

FIGURE 12-20. Illustration depicting the role of the rotator cuff in compressing the head against the glenoid.

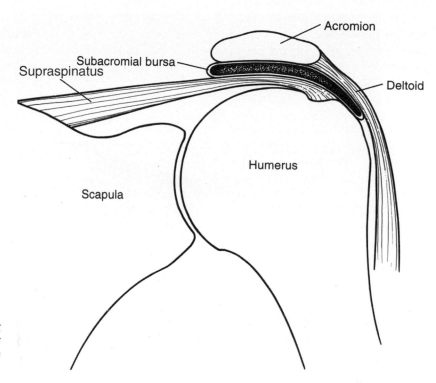

FIGURE 12-21. Illustration depicting the normal relationship of the rotator cuff between the humeral head and the acromion.

analysis has demonstrated a correlation between a hooked acromion and increased contact with the underlying cuff. Furthermore, contact of the acromial undersurface has also been shown to occur predominantly with the supraspinatus, consistent with the majority of pathology originating in this location. More recent studies have described the entity of internal impingement where the articular-sided surface of the cuff repetitively contacts the glenoid rim. Tensile overload and subtle glenohumeral instability can result in repeated microtrauma in the overhead throwing athlete in the absence of external, or subacromial, impingement.

Intrinsic properties of the rotator cuff have been the focus of other studies examining the causes of rotator cuff disease. Higher incidence of articular-sided partial-thickness rotator cuff tears may be partially explained by histologic studies demonstrating variations in collagen with thinner, less uniform bundles near the articular surface. Thicker, longitudinally oriented fibers found near the bursal surface were found to have an ultimate failure stress twice as high as those found near the articular side. Tenuous vascularity along the articular surface of the cuff shown in injection studies has also been suggested as a factor in the pathogenesis of undersurface partial tears.

Clinical Features

The symptom characteristics of rotator cuff disease may be somewhat variable depending on the duration and extent of tendon involvement. The patient will typically have a history of slowly escalating pain or pain arising acutely from a single traumatic event. A dull ache in the anterior and lateral deltoid is typical, often with radiation down the arm to the elbow. Occasionally, the pain may radiate into the trapezius and parascapular musculature, but these findings should alert the examiner to possible cervical spine pathology; an examination of the neck is essential to rule out other causative or potentiating sources of shoulder complaints. Symptoms may initially occur only with vigorous activities such as lifting or sports requiring motion above shoulder level. A painful arc of motion between 60 and 120° of elevation is present in most patients. Early in the course, rest and occasional use of anti-inflammatory medication may provide significant relief. Secondary stiffness can develop from inflammation and immobility of the shoulder due to pain inhibition, although stiffness is surprisingly uncommon with full-thickness tears. Eventually, pain may progress to symptoms at rest or with use of the extremity for daily activities such as brushing the

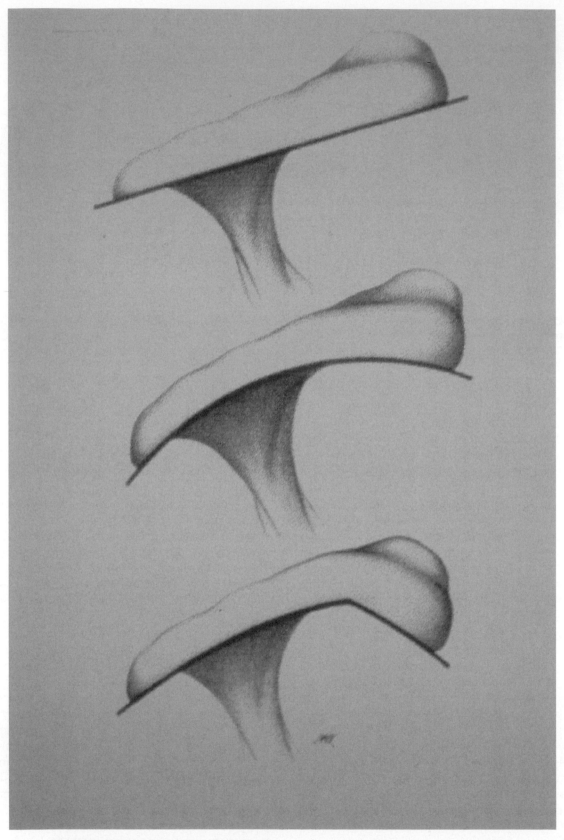

FIGURE 12-22. Illustration depicting flat, curved, and hooked acromial morphologies.

teeth, combing the hair, reaching the perineum, unhooking a bra, or even donning a coat. Pain preventing or interrupting sleep is common, particularly when rolling onto the affected side.

Physical exam findings are essential to accurately assess the status of the rotator cuff. The presence and severity of certain provocative maneuvers and signs will often aid in determining the degree of rotator cuff injury.

Abnormalities in the normal contour of the shoulder girdle may be found on visual inspection. Atrophy in the supraspinatus or infraspinatus fossae may indicate chronic massive tearing of the associated tendons or compression of the suprascapular nerve. Loss of the rotator cuff's compressive function may result in anterosuperior prominence of the humeral head. Associated proximal rupture of the long head of the biceps is identified as a painless soft tissue bulge along the upper arm (Popeye muscle). A discrete fluid-filled mass or swelling around the shoulder may also become evident with full-thickness tears as synovial fluid escapes into the subacromial space (fluid sign).

The diagnostic challenge is often in distinguishing pain from mechanical impingement from other sources of shoulder pain. The Neer impingement sign (Figure 12-23) (pain with forced passive forward elevation) and Hawkins sign (Figure 12-24) (pain with internal rotation and 90 degrees of forward elevation) may reproduce symptoms. Diminution of pain on repeat testing after injection of 10 mL of 1% lidocaine into the subacromial space (the impingement test) is useful not only in verifying the diagnosis as well as discerning it from other causes of shoulder pain but also in obtaining a more accurate measure of strength inhibited by pain.

Strength is highly dependent on the specific tendons involved and their degree of integrity (Figure 12-25). Strength is generally preserved with partial tears but can be falsely diminished by pain. External rotation lag signs may help differentiate partial from full-thickness tears; the inability to hold the affected extremity in external rotation in abduction or at the side is highly suggestive of a complete tear (Figure 12-26). The hornblower's sign, an inability to externally rotate the elevated arm, is another indication of significant pathology of the posterior cuff (Figure 12-27). Patients with large cuff tears may also shrug the affected shoulder in an attempt to elevate the arm (Figure 12-28). Tears of the subscapularis are often missed but can be detected by noting a loss of terminal internal

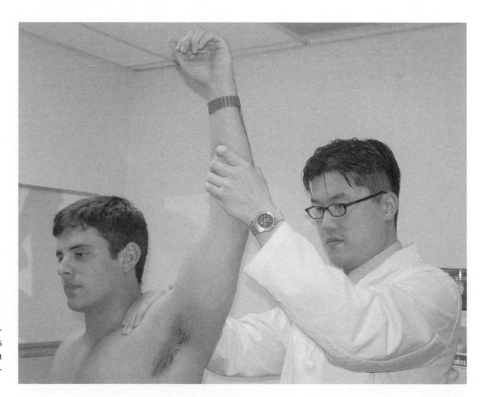

FIGURE 12-23. Neer impingement sign. As one hand stabilizes the scapula, pain is elicited with forced passive elevation of the affected extremity.

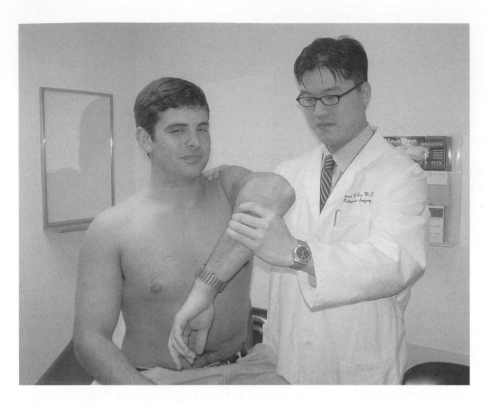

FIGURE 12-24. Hawkins sign. Forward flexion and internal rotation elicits shoulder pain.

rotation strength, increased passive external rotation as compared to a normal contralateral side, and inability to perform the belly-press and Gerber liftoff tests (Figure 12-29).

Radiographic Features

Plain radiographic studies should include AP views in the plane of the scapula and glenohumeral joint as well as an axillary lateral. Subtle findings suggestive of rotator cuff pathology such as an acromial or AC joint spur, cystic changes in the greater tuberosity, or a sourcil (or eyebrow) sign with sclerosis on the undersurface of the acromion to unequivocal signs, such as proximal humeral migration, may be evident on radiographs. Certain specialized views, including the supraspinatus outlet (Figure 12-30) (10 to 15° caudal tilt lateral scapular view) and Zanca (10 to 15° cephalic tilt AP coronal view), may also be obtained to look specifically for outlet narrowing and AC joint degeneration.

Because information about the integrity of the rotator cuff can only be inferred from plain films, additional imaging modalities are crucial in the evaluation of rotator cuff disease. Arthrography has been considered the gold standard for diagnosis of rotator cuff tears. Though highly accurate, it remains an uncomfortable, invasive test with less

utility in determining the size of full-thickness tears or the presence of partial tears. For these reasons, it has been largely supplanted by other techniques.

Ultrasonography has been gaining more interest in the diagnosis of rotator cuff disorders. This noninvasive and relatively inexpensive technology has been shown to be accurate in detecting and determining the size of larger full-thickness tears. The problems have included a high dependence on operator experience and detection of smaller tears. However, modern equipment and addition of dynamic images have increased the accuracy.

Magnetic resonance imaging (MRI) is the mainstay of radiographic diagnosis of rotator cuff pathology. The advantages of MRI are numerous and include noninvasiveness; capacity to detect full-thickness, partial-thickness, and intrasubstance tears; and ability to measure tear size and extent of retraction (Figure 12-31). In addition, MRI can evaluate other associated abnormal conditions such as degenerative acromioclavicular or glenohumeral changes, muscle atrophy and fatty degeneration, capsular and labral pathology, biceps rupture or dislocation, and ganglion cysts (Figure 12-32). Through compression of the suprascapular nerve, these ganglion cysts may produce signs and symptoms mimicking those of a rotator cuff tear. Experience of the reader and the quality of the equipment limit the study's accuracy. Furthermore, long study

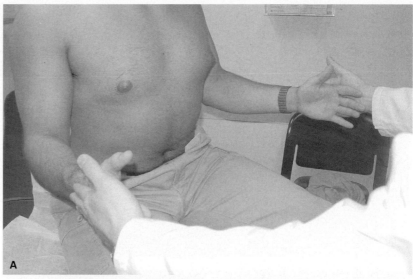

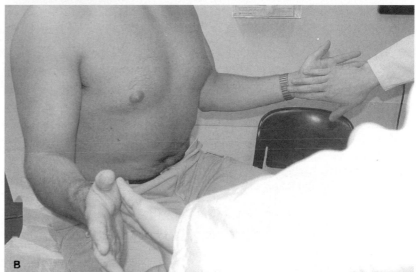

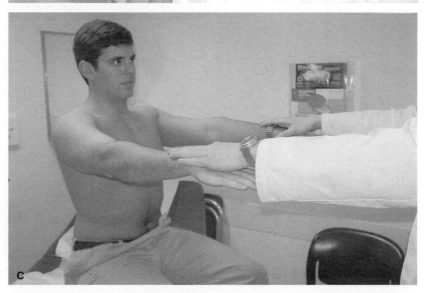

FIGURE 12-25. Manual strength testing in **(A)** external rotation, **(B)** internal rotation, and **(C)** forward elevation.

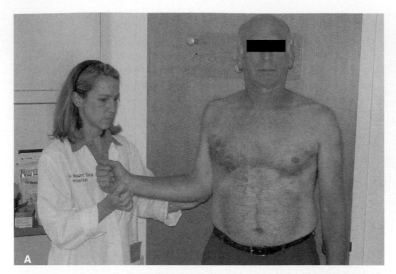

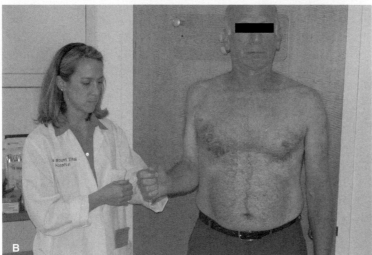

FIGURE 12-26. External rotation lag sign. **(A)** The affected extremity is held in external rotation; **(B)** the patient is unable to actively hold this position due to a full-thickness rotator cuff tear.

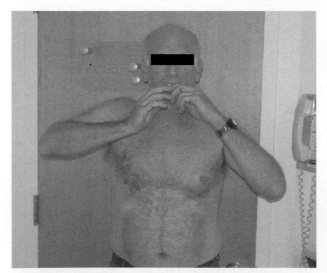

FIGURE 12-27. Hornblower's sign. The patient is unable to externally rotate the elevated arm due to a full-thickness rotator cuff tear involving the teres minor.

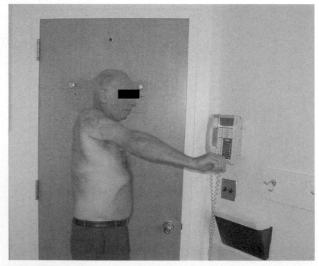

FIGURE 12-28. Attempted forward elevation with a large rotator cuff tear. The patient will commonly shrug the shoulder in an effort to compensate for the loss of active elevation.

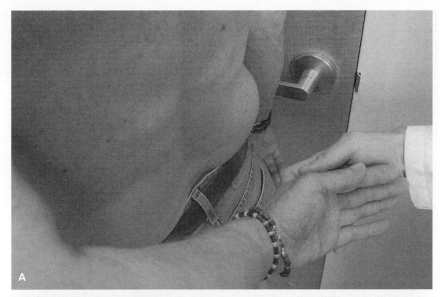

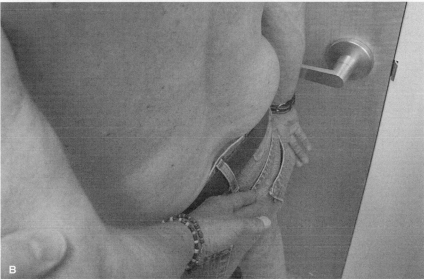

FIGURE 12-29. Rupture of the sub-scapularis (*left side*) with loss of terminal internal rotation. **(A)** and **(B)** Gerber lift-off test: a positive test is an inability to hold the affected extremity off the back; **(C)** the belly-press test: a positive test is an inability to press the hand in toward the abdomen and keeping the wrist straight. Normally, one performs this maneuver using the subscapularis to internally rotate the arm. With a subscapularis-deficient shoulder, the wrist is flexed to orient the arm and set the posterior deltoid to perform this function.

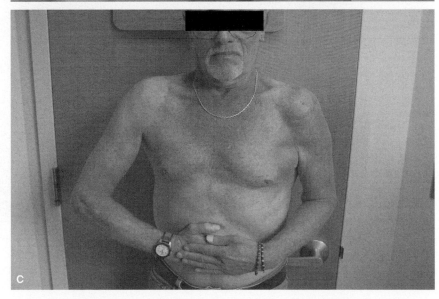

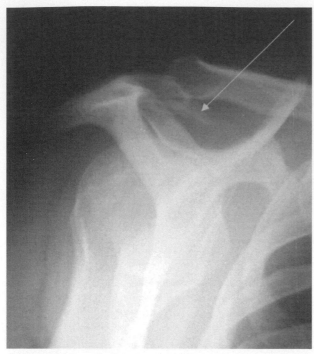

FIGURE 12-30. Large outlet spur impinging on the subacromial space (*white arrow*).

times and the confined space in the machine may be intolerable to some patients.

Natural History

Cadaveric studies have estimated a prevalence of full-thickness rotator cuff tears ranging from 7 to 40%. Radiographic imaging studies of asymptomatic patients have shown that rotator cuff tears are an age-related phenomenon with a significantly higher prevalence in individuals older than 60 years of age. Of course, the tears of clinical significance are those that become symptomatic.

Although the reasons why some asymptomatic tears develop symptoms remain unclear, recent study has suggested that many asymptomatic tears will become symptomatic as well as demonstrate progression of tear size (Figure 12-33). Furthermore, studies have shown that rotator cuff tears do not heal spontaneously. Over time, irreversible tendon and muscle degeneration can occur with profound effects on the likelihood of success with treatment.

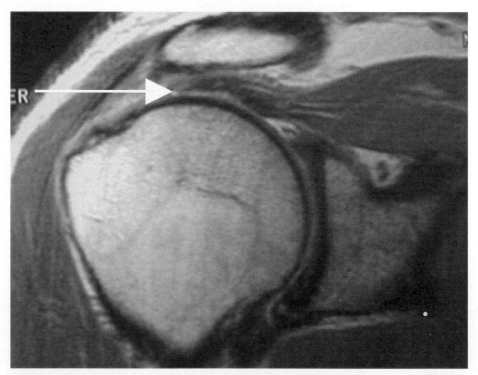

FIGURE 12-31. Coronal MRI image of a full-thickness rotator cuff tear with retraction half way to the glenoid rim. The white arrow is pointing to the tendon edge.

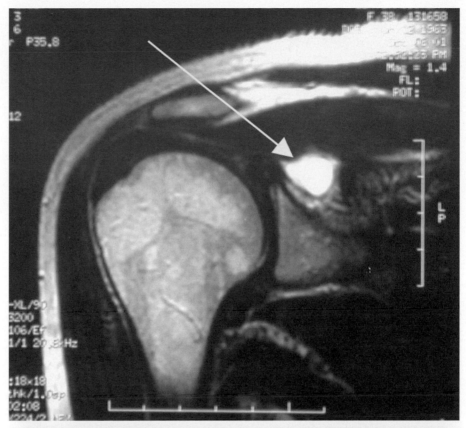

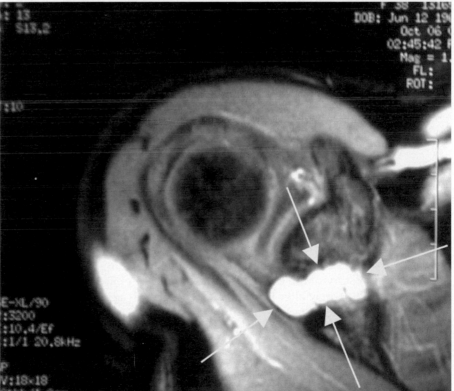

FIGURE 12-32. Coronal **(A)** and axial **(B)** MRI images of a ganglion cyst (*white arrows*) compressing the suprascapular nerve.

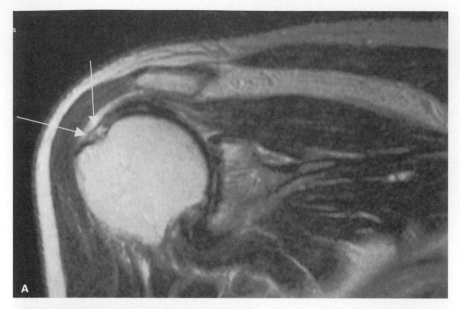

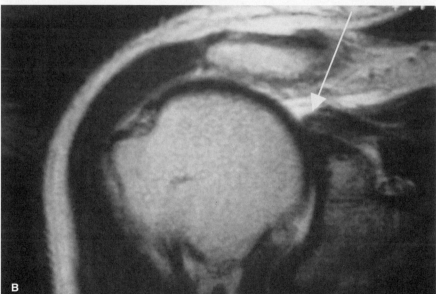

FIGURE 12-33. **(A)** Coronal MRI image of a partial-thickness rotator cuff tear (*white arrows*). **(B)** Three years later, MRI of the same patient demonstrating a full-thickness tear of the rotator cuff with retraction of the supraspinatus tendon (*white arrow*) to the glenoid rim.

Treatment

Therapeutic decision making in the treatment of rotator cuff disorders should be based on knowledge of the natural history of the disease and how a particular intervention may alter its course.

Patients presenting early with outlet impingement and intact cuffs with tendinosis or partial-thickness tears are almost universally treated with an initial course of nonoperative therapy. Inflammation is controlled with activity modification, oral anti-inflammatory medication, judicious use of subacromial corticosteroid injections, and physical therapy aimed at regaining motion and strengthening of the rotator cuff and periscapular musculature. Although studies have suggested that most partial-thickness tears will continue to enlarge with time, the role of operative treatment in modifying disease in this stage is unclear. There is no universal agreement that surgical debridement of a partially torn cuff relieves pain or stimulates a sufficient healing response. Furthermore, the permanent changes in tendon and muscle quality associated with larger, more chronic tears are not present. Thus, although nonoperative care runs a risk of prolonged pain and progression to larger tears, irreversible injury due to delayed surgical intervention is unlikely.

Surgical care should be considered with failure of nonoperative treatment in these early stages after a course of approximately 6 to 12 months. Treatment includes anterior acromioplasty for impingement lesions and debridement or tear completion and repair of partial tears. The rationale for removal of the anterior acromial spur is to eliminate the pathologic compression of the cuff. As previously mentioned, tear debridement has been met with mixed results. Tear completion and subsequent repair has been advocated in more extensive partial tears (more than 50% of the cuff thickness) with significantly better results reported as compared to debridement alone.

Treatment of symptomatic full-thickness tears is based on several factors including severity and duration of symptoms, patient activity level and goals, and tear size, chronicity, and location. Although a trial of nonoperative treatment is not unreasonable with smaller, minimally symptomatic tears or massive, chronic tears with irreversible tendon and muscle degeneration, anterior acromioplasty and rotator cuff repair remain the mainstays of treatment for most symptomatic full-thickness lesions (Figure 12-34). Results have been shown to be good or excellent in as many as 95% of patients with preoperative tear size as the primary predictor of outcome. Pain relief is a reliable goal with less consistent return of function with larger tear sizes. Some authors have recommended the use of tendon transfers in the presence of larger, chronic, retracted tears with associated fatty degeneration and muscle atrophy. Transfers of the latissimus dorsi or teres major for infraspinatus and supraspinatus loss and pectoralis major transfer for irreparable subscapularis ruptures have been described for massive tears and in those who have undergone a failed primary repair with local tissue.

Although conventional open treatment for rotator cuff repair and acromioplasty remains the standard, less invasive techniques are becoming more widely used. Arthroscopic subacromial decompression in conjunction with arthroscopically assisted or mini-open repair or all-arthroscopic rotator cuff repair offer distinct advantages over traditional methods with indications identical to those for open techniques. These advantages include smaller incisions, avoidance of deltoid detachment, shorter hospital stays, and ability to inspect the glenohumeral joint and treat pathologic entities such as articular-surface partial cuff tears, labral tears, biceps lesions, and arthritic lesions of the glenoid and humeral head. These methods are technically demanding but early results are promising with patient satisfaction approaching that or equal to formal open procedures (Figure 12-35).

Postoperative rehabilitation is extremely important to the success of all of the surgical treatment options. Early passive motion is instituted and continued for approximately 6 weeks at which time patients begin active range-of-motion exercises. Strengthening exercises are added at about 3 months from surgery and continue until 1 year when the patient can expect maximal improvement.

LESIONS OF THE BICEPS TENDON/BICEPS ORIGIN

The biceps, as its name implies, is composed of two heads: the short head originating from the coracoid process and the long head from within the glenohumeral joint, both which combine at the level of the deltoid insertion to form the muscle proper. As the long head exits the glenohumeral joint, it traverses through the rotator interval, a triangular portion of the shoulder capsule between the supraspinatus and subscapularis tendons, and enters the bicipital groove of the humerus.

The function of the biceps tendon as it relates to the kinematics of the glenohumeral joint has been extensively studied but not entirely understood. Some authors have proposed that it acts as a depressor of the humeral head and anterior stabilizer of the glenohumeral joint. More recent attention has been given to lesions of the superior labrum at the biceps origin as a source of subtle glenohumeral joint instability and pain.

Pathogenesis

Because of the proximity of the biceps tendon to the rotator cuff, degeneration of the biceps tendon is thought to occur much in the same way as mechanical

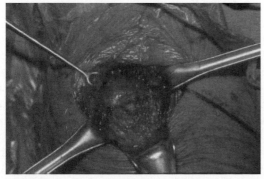

FIGURE 12-34. Intraoperative photograph of an open rotator cuff repair with suture fixation of the tendon to bone.

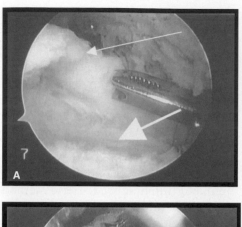
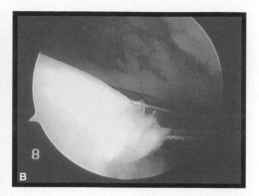
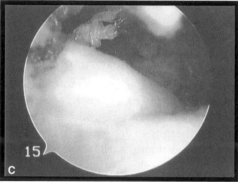

FIGURE 12-35. Arthroscopic rotator cuff repair. **(A)** Retracted tendon edge (*small arrow*) and greater tuberosity (*large arrow*); **(B)** grasper pulling the tendon laterally to the prepared bone bed on the greater tuberosity; **(C)** completed repair held with sutures.

impingement of the cuff beneath the coracoacromial arch. The role of other factors such as failure from tensile overload or vascular insufficiency is unclear although pathologic findings of the distal tendon have been found with normal segments proximally where mechanical degeneration would be expected (Figure 12-36).

Disorders of the biceps origin have gained more attention with increasing recognition of this entity using arthroscopy. The term *SLAP lesion* (superior labrum anterior and posterior lesions) was introduced by Snyder et al. to characterize injuries of the superior labrum and biceps anchor (Figure 12-37). These lesions have been postulated to occur in various ways including sudden deceleration of the flexed elbow in the follow-through stages of throwing and shearing of the glenoid rim from a fall on the outstretched hand. Disruption of this complex has been shown to increase humeral head translation and secondarily compromise important static restraints to shoulder stability.

Clinical Findings

Pain is typically the presenting complaint of biceps tendinopathy. Anterior shoulder pain at the bicipital groove may be found while associated cuff disease or glenohumeral instability may produce a vaguer, diffuse pain. Painful clicks with shoulder motion may indicate disorders of the labrum and biceps origin.

Provocative testing may help isolate symptoms to the biceps tendon. Speed's test is performed by elevation of the extended, supinated arm against resistance. Yergason's test may elicit symptoms by having the patient supinate the forearm against

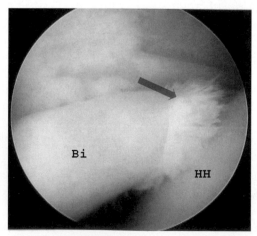

FIGURE 12-36. Arthroscopic image of humeral head (HH) and fraying (*black arrow*) of the biceps tendon (Bi).

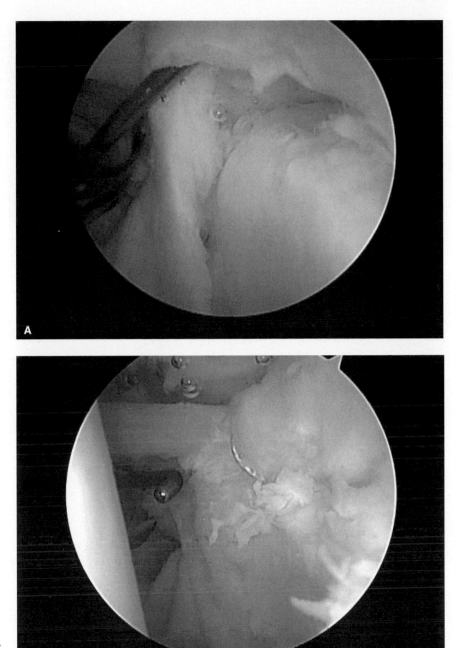

FIGURE 12-37. (A) Arthroscopic image of a SLAP lesion. **(B)** Arthroscopic repair of a SLAP lesion.

resistance with the elbow flexed to 90°. O'Brien's test (active compression test) is utilized to isolate SLAP lesion-related pain from other sources. The shoulder is internally rotated, flexed to 90° and adducted 10 to 15°. Pain that occurs with resisted elevation in this position and diminishes with testing in external rotation signifies a positive test.

As degeneration of the tendon progresses, rupture of the long head of the biceps may occur with retraction of the distal segment through the bicipital groove. The loss amounts to little more than a cosmetic deformity in the arm (Popeye muscle) and a minimal loss in supination and elbow flexion strength (Figure 12-38). In fact, removal of the diseased intra-articular portion of the tendon, either through spontaneous rupture or surgical resection, generally results in improvement of pain.

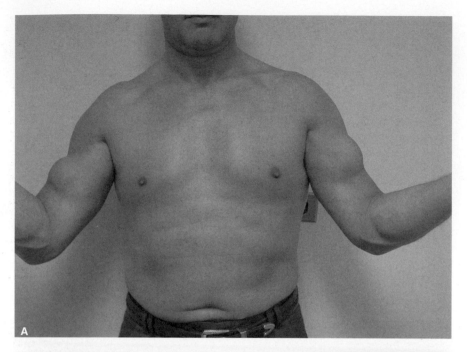

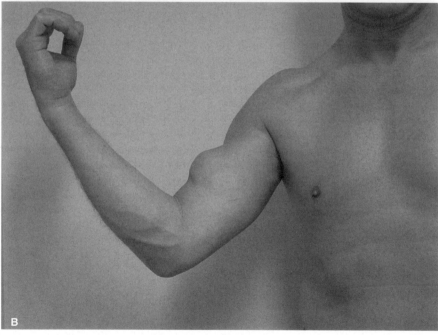

FIGURE 12-38. Popeye muscle. **(A)** and **(B)** Rupture of the long-head of the biceps (*right side*) with distal retraction of the muscle belly into the arm.

Treatment

Biceps pathology rarely occurs in isolation, and as previously mentioned, may be associated with rotator cuff disease or glenohumeral instability. Initial conservative treatment should address these underlying disorders in conjunction with alleviating the acute symptoms. Oral nonsteroidal anti-inflammatory medication and avoidance of exacerbating activities

followed by a physical therapy regimen emphasizing shoulder and periscapular strengthening may provide relief.

If symptoms persist, surgical options may be considered. Options for operative care entail debridement, tenotomy, or tenodesis of the biceps tendon. Tenotomy simply involves transection of the intra-articular portion of the tendon, either arthroscopically or during an open procedure for concomitant pathology. This approach is particularly attractive for older, lower demand patients who are willing to accept the resultant deformity and prefer a faster return to activity, although tenodesis may be preferable in the younger, more active individual.

Several methods of tenodesis have been described from suturing the tendon back on itself or to adjacent soft tissue structures to locking the distal segment into the humeral head using a bone tunnel and interference screw fixation. The effect of tenotomy on the purported stabilizing function of the biceps is unknown. Isolated biceps tendinopathy with no evidence of coexisting shoulder pathology, such as impingement of glenohumeral instability, is rare. Results of isolated biceps release (tenotomy) or tenodesis have been mixed implying that there are various mechanisms of biceps-related pathology.

Disorders of the biceps origin and labrum are treated arthroscopically. Simple fraying of the labrum with a stable biceps anchor is typically treated with debridement. Detachment of the superior labrum and biceps origin is best treated with reattachment to the glenoid rim with bioabsorbable tacks or suture anchors to restore the stabilizing effect on the glenohumeral joint. Tears of the biceps tendon extending from the labrum are debrided, but may require repair or tenodesis if a significant portion of the tendon is torn or degenerated.

FROZEN SHOULDER

The term *frozen shoulder*, as it will be used here, has been broadly applied to a wide range of disorders that result in a stiff and painful shoulder. Although attempts in the literature have been made to differentiate these entities, confusion still exists as to the proper terminology. In terms of treatment, it may be useful to categorize the stiff and painful shoulder into conditions that primarily result from pericapsular scarring and adhesions in contrast to contraction of the glenohumeral capsule, with extracapsular structures secondarily involved.

Origins

The idiopathic form of shoulder motion loss due to capsular contractures and adhesions was termed *adhesive capsulitis* by Neviaser based on the observed pathoanatomy. The pathogenesis of this disease remains unclear with several systemic disorders, such as diabetes mellitus, cardiovascular disease, mastectomy, or other operations about the chest and shoulder, found in association with this form of stiffness. Patients with diabetes mellitus, in particular, are more prone to bilateral involvement that is extremely resistant to all forms of treatment.

Capsular contracture may also result secondary to an underlying disorder such as voluntary immobilization from rotator cuff tendonitis or tear or bicipital tenosynovitis. These forms of secondary stiffness and pain are often difficult, if not impossible, to clinically discern from the primary or idiopathic type.

In contrast, shoulder stiffness and pain due to trauma or surgery will typically result in scarring of the extra-articular tissues and tissue planes. Fractures of the proximal humerus, treated operatively or nonoperatively, or surgery for instability, for example, may cause shortening or contracture of the pericapsular tissues and present with a clinical picture very similar to other etiologies.

Clinical Features

Demographically, patients with idiopathic stiffness are usually females between the ages of 40 and 60 years with the nondominant arm more commonly involved. As mentioned previously, patients with diabetes mellitus tend toward bilateral involvement. Motion loss must be carefully documented to assess severity and track progress with both active and passive motion deficits found on examination. Patients may exhibit compensatory increases in scapulothoracic motion or trunk lean and should be carefully identified to accurately measure pure glenohumeral motion loss (Figure 12-39).

Detailed history is essential and may reveal concomitant disorders or potential etiologic sources. History of systemic disease, trauma or previous surgery, or a long-standing rotator cuff tear with pain and normal motion at a prior office visit may provide a likely cause for the current stiffness. Similarly, in patients with a noncontributory history, symptom patterns may suggest or mimic other underlying disorders such as rotator cuff disease, although the stiffness and associated pain often may mask other clinical findings.

Patterns of motion loss may vary with different causes of stiffness. Adhesive capsulitis or capsular stiffness secondary to other processes typically result in global loss of motion. Postsurgical or posttraumatic stiffness may present with motion loss in all planes or with stiffness in some planes although sparing other ones. Discriminating between these types will help guide specific treatment.

Radiographic Features

Plain radiographs of the shoulder are typically not helpful in diagnosis or determination of cause in frozen shoulder but may identify other associated abnormalities such as fracture, arthritis, metal implants, or neglected dislocations, which may contribute to the clinical findings.

Historically, arthrography has been used to confirm a diagnosis of adhesive capsulitis with obliteration of the axillary fold seen with contrast infusion. However, little correlation has been demonstrated between arthrographic findings and motion loss. In addition, the invasive nature of the test has decreased its utility.

MRI may be used in cases when other associated disorders are suspected. Rotator cuff or labral tears can be readily detected. Use of MR imaging to define specific pathologic findings consistent with capsular contracture such as capsular or synovial thickening and decrease in capsular volume, however, has been inconclusive.

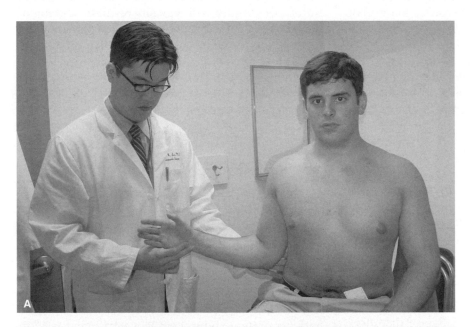

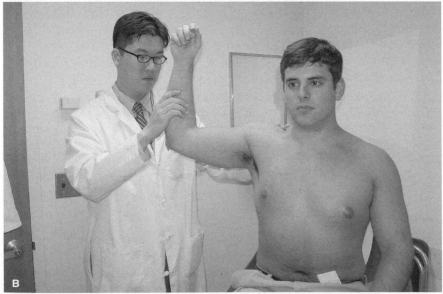

FIGURE 12-39. Passive range-of-motion exam. **(A)** External rotation at the side; **(B)** external rotation in abduction; **(C)** internal rotation in abduction; **(D)** internal rotation behind the back.

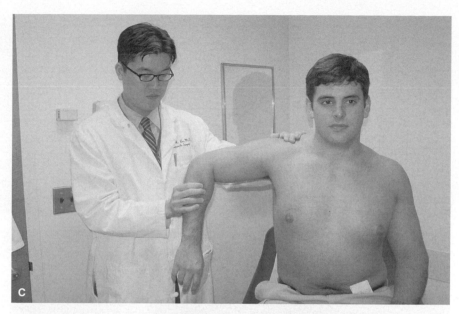

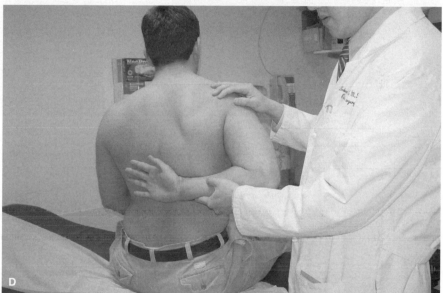

FIGURE 12-39. (*Continued*)

Treatment

The natural history of adhesive capsulitis has been described as self-limiting with resolution of symptoms occurring over 1 year. However, most patients are unwilling to endure the discomfort for this period of time without intervention. The initial management of most cases of frozen shoulder consists of physical therapy emphasizing range of motion and gentle stretching every day with the majority of patients responding to nonoperative treatment (Figure 12-40).

For those refractory cases demonstrating little or no improvement in symptoms over several months of therapy, manipulation and arthroscopic capsular release should be considered. Traditionally, manipulation alone with anesthesia has been performed to rupture the adhesions. The role of arthroscopy as an adjunct to manipulation in the treatment of frozen shoulder has been recently described. Some authors have adamantly discouraged its use in the treatment of this disorder although others have had encouraging results, noting the additional benefits of being able to release rather than tear the capsule, treat coexisting pathology, and document the results of manipulation. Nonetheless, essential to any operative form of intervention is the use of adequate postoperative analgesia and aggressive therapy. Use of interscalene brachial plexus block regional anesthesia has

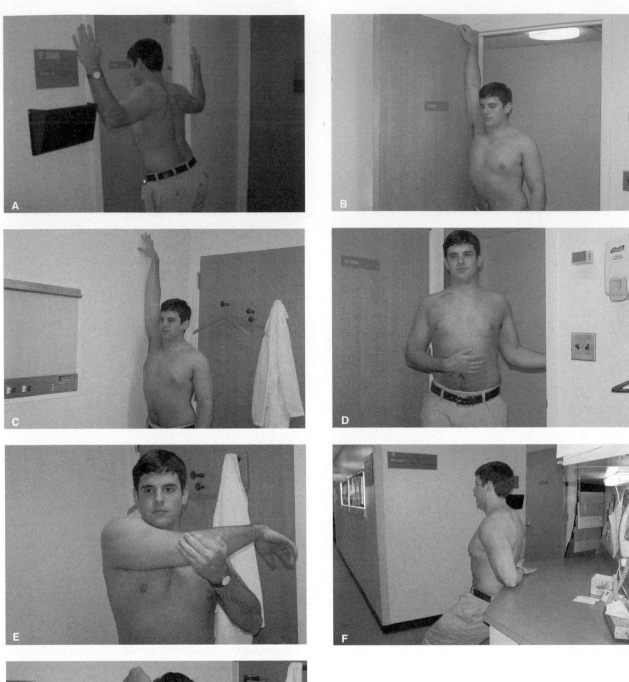

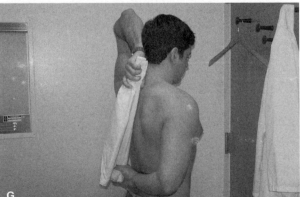

FIGURE 12-40. Stretching exercises. **(A)** External rotation and abduction; **(B)** forward elevation using a door or **(C)** against the wall; **(D)** external rotation at the side; **(E)** internal rotation with cross-body adduction, **(F)** behind the back against a counter and **(G)** with a towel.

been used to facilitate motion in the immediate post-operative period.

Patients with severe osteopenia, those who have undergone tendon or fracture repair in the previous 3 to 6 months, or have suspected or known extra-articular contractures (such as after previous Putti-Platt or Bristow procedures for instability) should undergo open release.

Crucial to all forms of treatment is early recognition and realization that several months may elapse before observing significant gains in motion.

GLENOHUMERAL INSTABILITY

Glenohumeral instability is a common problem encountered by the orthopaedic surgeon, particularly in young, active individuals. Better understanding of glenohumeral joint biomechanics and the role of various anatomic structures has led to increased recognition and advances in the treatment of instability.

Anatomy and Biomechanics

Multiple structures are involved in maintaining stability of the shoulder. The balance between stability and permitting a wide range of motion is provided by the interaction of dynamic and static factors. The static stabilizers include the glenoid, labrum, capsule, glenohumeral ligaments, and the rotator interval. The role of the biceps tendon as a static stabilizer is unclear but is also thought to contribute to glenohumeral joint stability.

The glenoid provides a small, shallow surface to articulate with the humeral head and provides little constraint for the glenohumeral joint. The fibrocartilaginous labrum attaches to the glenoid rim and increases its effective depth and surface area. Isolated labral deficiency has been shown not to allow glenohumeral dislocation without associated injury to the capsule, emphasizing the crucial role of the capsuloligamentous structures in maintaining stability.

The three major glenohumeral ligaments function as "check-reins" toward the extremes of motion while remaining relatively lax in the midrange to allow normal joint translation. The superior glenohumeral ligament, coracohumeral ligament, and the rotator interval (between the leading edge of the supraspinatus and the superior edge of the subscapularis) restrain anterior humeral head translation in 0° of abduction and external rotation. With

increasing abduction to 45°, the middle glenohumeral ligament provides the primary anterior restraint. Finally, the inferior glenohumeral ligament tightens and becomes the prime anterior stabilizer at 90° of abduction and 90° of external rotation.

The rotator cuff and scapular stabilizers serve as dynamic restraints in normal shoulder biomechanics. A primary role of the rotator cuff is to resist translational forces on the joint through compression of the humeral head into the glenoid cavity. Scapular winging—an imbalance of the scapular stabilizing musculature—has been implicated in pain and instability of the glenohumeral joint. Operative intervention addressing scapulothoracic dysfunction may lead to elimination of symptoms in select cases.

Clinical Features

Critical to the evaluation of glenohumeral instability is a careful history and physical examination. The nature of the injury surrounding the onset of symptoms should be determined and are particularly useful in identifying the type of instability. Position of the arm at the time of injury or circumstances that provoke symptoms often indicates the direction of instability. Reproduction of a patient's symptoms in a position of abduction, external rotation, and extension suggests anterior instability. Flexion, internal rotation, and adduction, in contrast, would more likely point to posterior instability. Voluntary control of instability must be carefully sought out as this may change the ultimate course of treatment. Patients with psychiatric disorders may utilize a concomitant ability to dislocate the shoulder for secondary gain. Although operative intervention in this situation would likely fail, treatment options exist for other forms of voluntary subluxation. Surgery may benefit patients who can subluxate the shoulder by placing the arm in provocative positions. Biofeedback techniques, however, may help those patients who sublux through selective muscular activation.

In determining the degree of instability, the history should ascertain whether the initial and any subsequent episodes of instability were elicited by high-energy trauma (such as violent twisting or fall), minimal repeated trauma (such as throwing a ball), or no trauma (such as reaching a high shelf). The type of reduction required (i.e., was the shoulder self-reduced or did it require manipulation by another person?) may also provide additional information about the extent of joint laxity.

Detailed record of prior treatment should also be obtained, including the type and duration of immobilization, rehabilitative efforts, and previous surgeries. Knowledge of failed interventions will help guide future treatment in the recurrent dislocator.

Pain as an isolated symptom will not typically reveal much useful information. Anterior shoulder pain may indicate anterior instability as well as other common disorders including subacromial impingement. Similarly, posterior shoulder pain is nonspecific and may represent a range of pathology from instability to cervical spine disorders. Location of the pain in combination with provoking arm positions and activities, however, may aid in making a diagnosis of instability. Altered glenohumeral kinematics in throwers, for example, may result in posterior shoulder pain during late cocking (posterior internal impingement). Patients may also report other symptoms consistent with subtle shoulder instability. Rowe and Zarins

described a phenomenon termed the "dead-arm syndrome," in which paralyzing pain and loss of control of the extremity occurs with abduction and external rotation of the shoulder.

Finally, determining the patient's level of impairment and activity level is important prior to formulating a therapeutic plan. The different expectations of a sedentary patient with minimal functional loss versus the high-performance athlete with pain and apprehension may affect the type of prescribed treatment.

A thorough physical examination is equally essential in making an accurate diagnosis and recommending the appropriate intervention. Both shoulders should be adequately exposed and examined for deformity, range of motion, strength, and laxity. Unreduced dislocations may produce an abnormal contour to the shoulder in addition to restricting active and passive motion (Figure 12-41). Demonstration of scapular winging may accompany

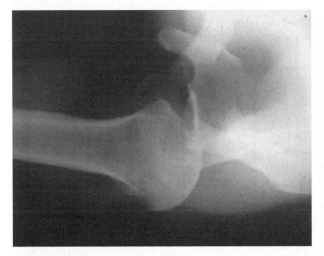

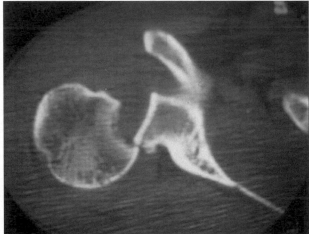

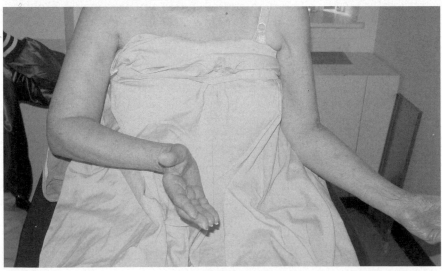

FIGURE 12-41. Posterior glenohumeral dislocation (*right side*). Clinical photo demonstrating block to external rotation.

instability, particularly of the posterior type, and should be considered a potential cause of symptoms. Generalized ligamentous laxity may also contribute to instability and can be easily elicited with the thumb-to-forearm and metacarpophalangeal hyperextension tests (Figure 12-42). Operative reports and evidence of healed anterior or posterior scars from previous instability repairs indicate what has been done and may provide a rationale for the patient's current symptoms. Limitation of external rotation may accompany a prior anterior tightening procedure (i.e., Putti-Platt or Magnuson-Stack).

Typically, there is a full range of motion with the exception of guarding at the extremes as the shoulder approaches unstable positions. Clinical suspicion should be raised, however, in the patient older than 40 years of age who is unable to actively abduct the arm after a primary anterior dislocation. It has been shown that a high percentage of these patients have a concurrent rupture of the rotator cuff with restoration of stability following repair.

Various basic provocative tests can be used to reproduce the patient's symptoms and confirm the diagnosis. In order to minimize the effects of muscle guarding, these maneuvers should be performed first on the unaffected side and then in succession of increasing discomfort. The sulcus test evaluates inferior translation of the humeral head with the arm at the side in neutral and in external rotation. The scapula is stabilized with one hand while the other applies a mild compressive force to

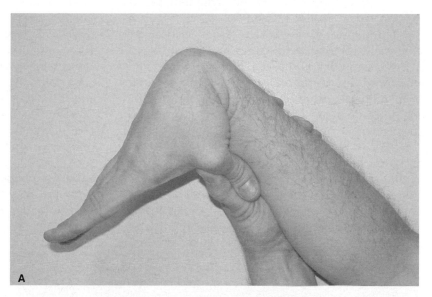

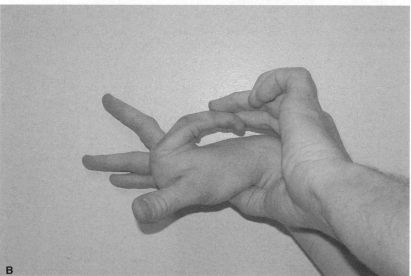

FIGURE 12-42. Ligamentous laxity. **(A)** Thumb-to-forearm; **(B)** metacarpophalangeal hyperextension.

the head in conjunction with a downward force to the arm. Significant findings would include an increased palpable gap between the acromion and humeral head compared to the opposite side as well as translation below the glenoid rim. Performing the test in external rotation will not reduce the gap when there is incompetence of the rotator interval (Figure 12-43).

Laxity can be further evaluated by anterior and posterior drawer or load-and-shift tests. The proximal humerus is shifted in each direction while grasped between the thumb and index fingers. Alternatively, with the patient supine, the scapula is stabilized while the humeral head is axially loaded and translated anteriorly and posteriorly. Translation greater than the opposite shoulder or translation over the glenoid rim indicates significant laxity (Figure 12-44). Only translations that reproduce the patient's symptoms are considered to demonstrate instability.

The anterior apprehension test is performed by externally rotating, abducting, and extending the affected shoulder while stabilizing the scapula or providing an anteriorly directed force to the humeral head with the other hand. Significant findings include a sense of impending subluxation or dislocation, or guarding and resistance to further rotation secondary to apprehension. Pain as an isolated finding is nonspecific and may indicate other pathology such as rotator cuff disease. Jobe's relocation test is done in the supine position, usually accompanying the apprehension test. As symptoms are elicited with progressive external rotation, the examiner applies a posteriorly directed force to the humeral head. A positive test is signified by alleviation of symptoms (Figure 12-45).

Posterior instability can be elicited with the posterior stress test. As one hand stabilizes the scapula, a posteriorly directed axial force is applied to the arm with the shoulder in 90° of flexion, abduction, and internal rotation. Positive findings produce posterior subluxation or symptoms of instability experienced by the patient.

Radiographic Features

Though the history and physical examination are the key elements in patient evaluation, a series of radiographic studies may be helpful in confirming the diagnosis and defining associated pathology. AP radiographs in internal and external rotation, a lateral view in the scapular plane (scapular-Y view), and an axillary view should be obtained in the initial evaluation. A Hill-Sachs lesion (posterolateral impression fracture) of the humeral head is best seen on the AP radiograph in internal rotation (Figure 12-46) or on specialized views such as the Stryker Notch or West Point Axillary. Fractures or erosions of the glenoid rim can be detected on an axillary or apical oblique view (Garth).

Other more specialized imaging studies are not routinely obtained in the initial evaluation of instability but may be useful in a preoperative workup. Computed tomography can assist in further assessment of fractures and glenoid defects as well as detect subtle subluxation of the humeral head. MRI and

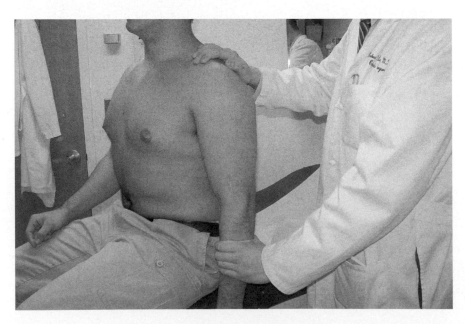

FIGURE 12-43. Sulcus sign. Downward traction of the arm will create a gap between the acromion and the humeral head.

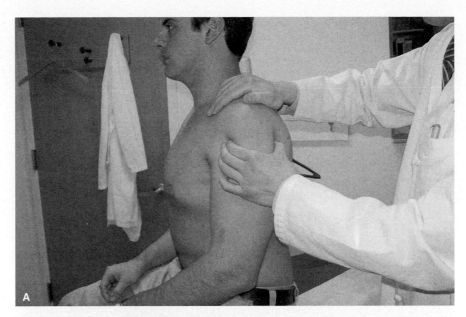

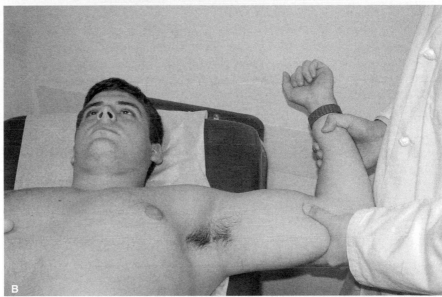

FIGURE 12-44. (A) Anterior-posterior drawer: translation of the humeral head held between the thumb and index finger and stabilization of the scapula with the other hand. **(B)** Load-and-shift: simultaneous axial loading and translation of the humeral head.

MR arthrography can identify associated pathology of the labrum, glenohumeral ligaments, and the rotator cuff (Figure 12-47). More recent radiographic modalities such as dynamic MR-imaging currently have no defined indications but may become a useful adjunct in evaluating glenohumeral instability.

Treatment

Although the results vary with age and associated bone and soft tissue injury, nonoperative treatment consisting of a period of immobilization followed by rehabilitation is typically successful in managing the majority of patients with glenohumeral instability. Early studies of young (less than 20 years old), athletic patients, however, found a recurrence rate as high as 90% after a primary dislocation. Although subsequent studies have reported lower numbers, clearly the risk for subsequent dislocations is higher with earlier onset of instability.

The length and type of immobilization remains a matter of debate. Several published series have advocated immobilization for a few days to several weeks. However, studies by Hovelius and Simonet and Cofield have found no difference in

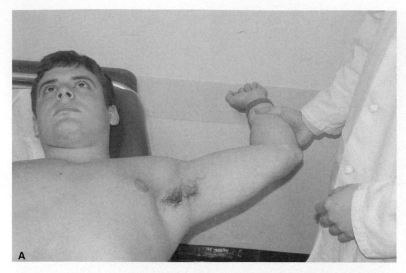

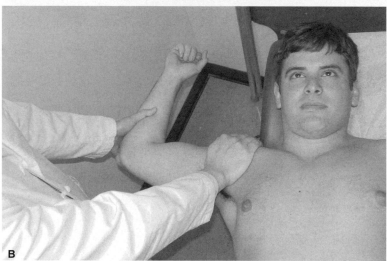

FIGURE 12-45. (A) Apprehension test: abduction and external rotation will produce sense of impending subluxation or dislocation with anterior glenohumeral instability; **(B)** relocation test: posterior-directed force on the humeral head will alleviate symptoms.

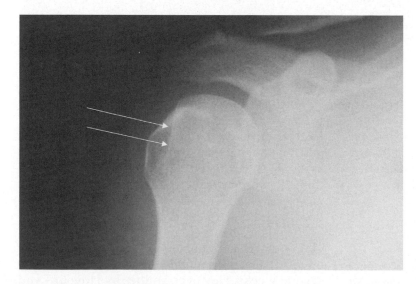

FIGURE 12-46. Hill-Sachs lesion. An impaction fracture of the posterolateral humeral head associated with an anterior glenohumeral dislocation is depicted by the small white arrows on this internally rotated anteroposterior radiograph.

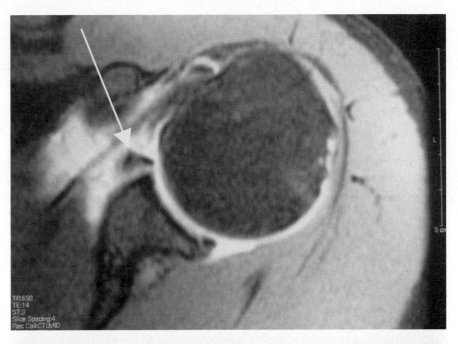

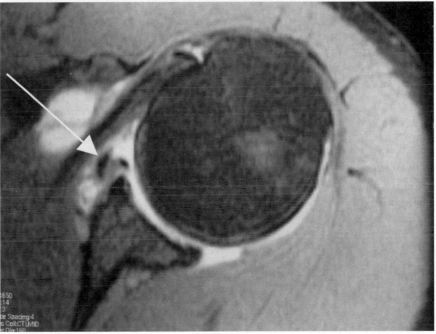

FIGURE 12-47. (A) and **(B)** Axial MRI images of a Bankart lesion (*white arrows*).

outcome from either the type or length of immobilization. In general, younger patients (less than 30 years of age) sustaining a primary dislocation are preferably immobilized for approximately 3 to 4 weeks. Older patients, who have a smaller risk of recurrent instability but a higher susceptibility to stiffness, may be immobilized for shorter periods.

Rehabilitation efforts are aimed at strengthening the dynamic stabilizers and regaining motion. Progressive resistive exercises of the rotator cuff, deltoid, and scapular stabilizers are recommended. Stress on the static restraints (i.e., capsuloligamentous structures) should be prevented in the immediate postinjury period by avoidance of vigorous stretching and provocative arm positions.

Failure of conservative management for glenohumeral instability is an indication for proceeding with operative intervention. Open procedures are currently the gold standard for repair of the disrupted soft tissue shoulder stabilizers. Historically, many of these procedures treated anterior instability through nonphysiologic shortening or transfer of muscle or bone resulting in significant loss of motion, postoperative glenohumeral arthritis, and complications of loose or prominent hardware in the joint.

Modern techniques emphasize anatomic restoration of the soft tissue structures. Based on the work of Perthes in 1906, Bankart in 1923 popularized repair of the capsule to the anterior glenoid without shortening of the overlying subscapularis. After modifications to his original description, reconstruction of the avulsed capsule and labrum to the glenoid lip is commonly referred to today as the Bankart repair. Several capsulorrhaphy procedures have also been described to address capsular laxity and the increase in joint volume. These procedures allow tightening of the anterior capsule in combination with reattachment of a capsulolabral avulsion.

Open treatment of posterior instability most commonly addresses the capsular laxity seen with this problem. Similar to the anterior procedure, a posterior capsulorrhaphy functions to reduce capsular laxity and address associated posterior labral injury. Difficulty in treatment of multidirectional instability of the shoulder is, in part, due to improper recognition. Procedures involving anterior capsular tightening fail to address the inferior and posterior components of instability seen in this disorder. The inferior capsular shift procedure, described by Neer and Foster, treats multidirectional instability by simultaneously reducing volume in the anterior, posterior, and inferior capsule.

Good results have been achieved with most open techniques to treat these various problems. Successful outcomes greater than 80 to 90% can be expected; however, results have been generally less predictable for posterior and multidirectional instability compared to anterior instability procedures.

In selected cases, current trends are moving toward arthroscopic intervention. The goals of restoring the capsulolabral anatomy and reduction of capsular volume remain the same as in open procedures. Reduced morbidity from smaller incisions,

elimination of subscapularis detachment, avoidance of scarred and distorted tissue planes in revision situations, and the ability to simultaneously address multiple factors contributing to instability have made these minimally invasive techniques more appealing.

Arthroscopic anterior instability repairs remain controversial with high (up to 70%) failure rates reported for transglenoid suture fixation. Improvements in patient selection, technique, and implant and equipment design have decreased the recurrence rate. Contraindications to arthroscopic repair include patients with glenoid bone defects, engaging Hill-Sachs lesions, and attenuated capsulolabral tissue. Athletes involved in contact sports have been a relative contraindication, although some surgeons have modified the exclusion criteria to include this subset of patients. Improved surgeon technique with bone preparation and soft tissue tensioning and the use of suture anchors have led to improved results (Figure 12-48).

Thermal energy has been used in arthroscopic instability repairs, in part, due to its easy application. Thermal capsulorrhaphy may be done alone or to tighten residual capsular laxity following capsulolabral repair or capsular plication with sutures. Complications following its use have included neurologic injury to the axillary nerve, capsular necrosis and loss of capsular and glenohumeral ligament integrity, and stiffness and loss of motion. Although proponents of thermal capsulorrhaphy have found this technique a useful adjunct for treating instability of the shoulder, long-term follow-up studies advocating its routine use are not yet available. Rehabilitation following open and arthroscopic instability repairs is identical. The shoulder is generally protected with 4 to 6 weeks of sling immobilization in internal rotation for anterior repairs and in slight abduction and neutral rotation following posterior and multidirectional instability procedures. Active hand, wrist, and elbow motion is permitted followed by progressive range of motion exercises. Resistive exercises are started between 6 to 8 weeks with return to sports at up to 9 to 12 months postoperatively. Although there are no strict guidelines, the postoperative therapy regimen must be tailored to each particular patient accounting for the quality of the tissues, the durability of the repair, patient reliability, and future demands on the shoulder.

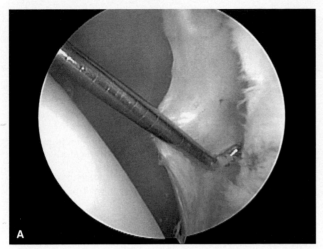 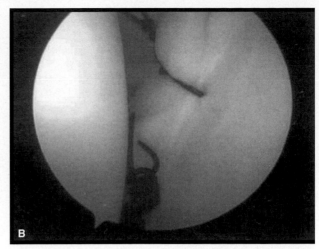

FIGURE 12-48. Arthroscopic images demonstrating **(A)** an avulsion of the anterior-inferior labrum (Bankart lesion) and **(B)** suture repair.

ANNOTATED BIBLIOGRAPHY

Birth Palsy

Hardy AE. Birth injuries of the brachial plexus: incidence and prognosis. J Bone Joint Surg 1981;63B:98–101.
This article estimated an incidence of 0.87 birth injuries to the brachial plexus per 1,000 live births at a New Zealand hospital. Nearly 80% of these children had made a complete recovery by the age of 13 months, although none of those with significant residual defects has severe sensory or motor deficit of the hand.

Kawai H, Tsuyuguchi Y, Masada K et al. Identification of the lesion in brachial plexus injuries with root avulsion: a comprehensive assessment by means of preoperative findings, myelography, surgical exploration and intraoperative electrodiagnosis. Neuro-Orthop 1989;7:15–23.
The authors compared the results of myelography, myelography-CT, and MRI, with operative findings. They found an 84% true-positive rate, 4% false-positive rate, and a 12% false-negative rate for myelography. Results improved with addition of CT. MRI had similar accuracy as myelography-CT with the additional benefit of allowing more distal visualization of the plexus.

Michelow BJ, Clarke HM, Curtis CG et al. The natural history of obstetrical brachial plexus palsy. Plast Reconstr Surg 1994; 93:675–681.
Sixty-one of 66 patients (92%) with a brachial plexus palsy recovered spontaneously and five patients (8%) required primary brachial plexus exploration and reconstruction (median age 12 months), demonstrating that most patients do well. Additional analysis was undertaken to examine ways in which outcome might be predicted. They determined that when elbow flexion and elbow, wrist, thumb, and finger extension at 3 months were combined into a test score, the proportion of patients whose recovery was incorrectly predicted was reduced to 5.2% compared to 12.8% when elbow flexion alone was used.

Rühmann O, Gossé F, Wirth CJ et al. Reconstructive operations for the paralyzed shoulder in brachial plexus palsy: concept of treatment. Injury 1999;30:609–618.
In this study, 63 patients with persistent brachial plexus palsy underwent a transfer of the trapezius muscle and 14 patients underwent a shoulder arthrodesis. In patients with brachial plexus palsy, trapezius transfer resulted in an improvement of shoulder function and stability. The increase in function was, however, less pronounced in comparison with shoulder arthrodesis. They state that the advantages of muscle transfer are regaining of normal passive function and the shorter duration of surgery. However, shoulder fusion is more suitable for those patients who require the best possible extent of function and strength in the shoulder.

Strecker B, McAllister JW, Manske PR et al. Sever-L'Episcopo transfers in obstetrical palsy: a retrospective review of twenty cases. J Pediatr Orthop 1990;10:442–444.
The authors retrospectively studied 25 patients who underwent Sever-L'Episcopo transfers for obstetrical birth palsy. A follow-up of 2 to 6 years was possible with a retrospective review of 16 patients. Substantial improvement in shoulder external rotation as well as subjective functional improvement was obtained by all patients. Three transient and one permanent axillary nerve palsies resulting from this procedure were reported.

Degenerative and Painful Conditions of the Acromioclavicular Joint

Cahill BR. Osteolysis of the distal part of the clavicle in male athletes. J Bone Joint Surg 1982;64:1053–1058.
The author reported osteolysis of the distal part of the clavicle in 46 men, none of whom had a history of acute injury to the acromioclavicular area. All patients were athletes and 45 lifted weights as part of their training. Pain and tenderness at the acromioclavicular joint associated with radiographic signs of osteoporosis, loss of subchondral bone detail, and cystic changes in the distal part of the clavicle were present. Resection of the distal end of the clavicle in 21 patients, 4 with bilateral procedures, resulted in relief of symptoms in the 19 who were followed. The 25 patients who were not operated on also had improvement, but only after activity modification with avoidance of weight training.

Esch JC, Ozerkis LR, Helgager JA et al. Arthroscopic subacromial decompression: results according to the degree of rotator cuff tear. Arthroscopy 1988;4:241–249.
In this article, the authors describe their technique of arthroscopic distal clavicle resection from a subacromial (indirect) approach performed in patients undergoing an arthroscopic subacromial decompression.

Flatow EL. The biomechanics of the acromioclavicular, sternoclavicular, and scapulothoracic joints. Instr Course Lect 1993;42:237–245.

The anatomy and biomechanics of the acromioclavicular, sternoclavicular, and scapulothoracic joints are discussed.

Flatow EL, Cordasco FA, Bigliani LU. Arthroscopic resection of the outer end of the clavicle from a superior approach: a critical, quantitative, radiographic assessment of bone removal. Arthroscopy 1992;8:55–64.

The technique of arthroscopic resection of the outer end of the clavicle through a superior approach was evaluated to determine whether adequate bone removal could be achieved. These results were compared with open resection. The authors determined that satisfactory bone removal was possible arthroscopically. Comparable pain relief and function were achieved in both groups. However, hospital stay was shortened and pain relief was achieved on average 3.4 months earlier in the arthroscopic group.

Fukuda K, Craig EV, An KN et al. Biomechanical study of the ligamentous system of the acromioclavicular joint. J Bone Joint Surg 1986;68A:434–440.

The ligamentous structures of the acromioclavicular joint were studied by gross examination and quantitative measurement in 12 human cadaver specimens. Twelve modes of joint displacement were examined. The acromioclavicular ligament acted as a primary constraint for posterior displacement of the clavicle and posterior axial rotation. The conoid ligament played a primary role in constraining anterior and superior rotation as well as anterior and superior displacement of the clavicle. The trapezoid ligament contributed less constraint to movement of the clavicle in both the horizontal and the vertical plane except when the clavicle moved in axial compression toward the acromion process. The various contributions of different ligaments to constraint changed not only with the direction of joint displacement but also with the amount of loading and displacement.

Gartsman GM. Arthroscopic resection of the acromioclavicular joint. Am J Sports Med 1993;21:71–77.

Arthroscopic resection of the distal clavicle was used to treat 26 patients who had osteoarthritis of the acromioclavicular joint and were followed for a minimum of 2 years. The preoperative ratings for pain, activities of daily living, work, and sports improved markedly in 17 patients. The author concluded that arthroscopic resection was effective in the treatment of isolated acromioclavicular joint arthritis.

Mumford EB. Acromioclavicular dislocation: a new operative treatment. J Bone Joint Surg 1941;23:799–802.

This is one of two simultaneous descriptions of distal clavicle excision as surgical treatment for acromioclavicular dislocation.

Degenerative Osteoarthritis of the Glenohumeral Joint

Cameron BD, Galatz LM, Ramsey ML et al. Nonprosthetic management of grade IV osteochondral lesions of the glenohumeral joint. J Shoulder Elbow Surg 2002;11:25–32.

The authors examined their results following arthroscopic debridement and capsular release in patients with limited osteoarthritic changes of the glenohumeral joint. They concluded that in well-selected patients with grade IV osteochondral lesions, arthroscopic debridement can provide significant improvements in pain relief and function. Furthermore, arthroscopic capsular release can be added in patients with a loss of passive arcs of shoulder motion. Osteochondral lesions greater than 2 cm², however, were associated with failure of this procedure.

Levine WN, Djurasovic M, Glasson JM et al. Hemiarthroplasty for glenohumeral osteoarthritis: results correlated to degree of glenoid wear. J Shoulder Elbow Surg 1997;6:449–454.

Thirty patients (31 shoulders) were retrospectively reviewed after hemiarthroplasty for glenohumeral osteoarthritis. Outcome correlated most significantly with the status of posterior glenoid wear. They concluded that hemiarthroplasty can be an effective treatment for both primary and secondary arthritis but should be reserved for patients with a concentric glenoid, which affords a better fulcrum for glenohumeral motion.

Neer CS II, Watson KC, Stanton FJ. Recent experience in total shoulder replacement. J Bone Joint Surg 1982;64A:319–337.

The authors expand on their earlier experience with shoulder arthroplasty for arthritis, elaborating on indications, operative findings, and technique.

Norris TR, Iannotti JP. Functional outcome after shoulder arthroplasty for primary osteoarthritis: a multicenter study. J Shoulder Elbow Surg 2002;11:130–135.

A prospective, multicenter clinical outcome study evaluated 176 shoulders in 160 patients with primary osteoarthritis. The authors concluded that total shoulder arthroplasty and hemiarthroplasty for treatment of primary osteoarthritis result in good or excellent pain relief, improvement in function, and patient satisfaction in 95% of cases.

Weinstein DM, Bucchieri JS, Pollock RG et al. Arthroscopic debridement of the shoulder for osteoarthritis. Arthroscopy 2000;16:471–476.

Twenty-five patients underwent arthroscopic debridement to treat early glenohumeral osteoarthritis. The operative procedure consisted of lavage of the glenohumeral joint, debridement of labral tears and chondral lesions, loose body removal, and partial synovectomy and subacromial bursectomy. Overall, results were rated as excellent in 2 patients (8%), good in 19 patients (72%), and unsatisfactory in 5 (20%). The authors found this as a reasonable procedure for treating early glenohumeral osteoarthritis that has failed to respond to nonoperative treatment, in which the humeral head and glenoid remain concentric, and where there is still a visible joint space on an axillary radiograph. They did not recommend this technique when there was severe joint incongruity or large osteophytes.

Osteonecrosis of the Humeral Head

Cruess RL. Steroid-induced avascular necrosis of the head of the humerus: natural history and management. J Bone Joint Surg 1976;58B:313–317.

Ninety-five patients with steroid-induced avascular necrosis of the humeral head were followed in this study. Conservative treatment consisted of pendulum exercises and avoidance of abduction, particularly against resistance. This led to satisfactory function with only intermittent symptoms in 14 patients. Five humeral heads in 4 patients required prosthetic replacement. After 1 to 7 years, the results of all 5 were classified as excellent in terms of motion and symptoms.

David HG, Bridgman SA, Davies SC et al. The shoulder in sickle-cell disease. J Bone Joint Surg 1993;75B:538–545.

This article reviewed 138 patients with sickle cell disease for clinical, radiological, and functional abnormalities of the shoulder. Radiographic lesions, frequently bilateral, were found in 28% and only 53% of patients had normal shoulder function.

Hattrup SJ, Cofield RH. Osteonecrosis of the humeral head: results of replacement. J Shoulder Elbow Surg 2000;9:177–182.

Eighty-eight shoulders treated with prosthetic replacement for osteonecrosis with average follow-up of 8.9 years were examined in this study. Inferior functional results were noted in posttraumatic osteonecrosis compared to those in steroid-induced osteonecrosis. The most common postoperative complication was rotator cuff tearing, which was more common in shoulders with a history of any surgery.

LaPorte DM, Mont MA, Mohan V et al. Osteonecrosis of the humeral head treated by core decompression. Clin Orthop 1998;355:254–260.

Sixty-three shoulders in 43 patients who underwent a core decompression for humeral head osteonecrosis were followed up from 2 to 20 years (mean 10 years). Results of core decompression according to preoperative Ficat and Arlet stage revealed stage I disease had 15 of 16 (94%) successful outcomes and stage II had 15 of 17 (88%) successful outcomes. stage III had 16 of 23 (70%) successful results and stage IV had 1 of 7 (14%) successful result. They concluded that this procedure could be successful for stages I, II, and III osteonecrosis in terms of early relief of pain and increased function.

Rheumatoid Arthritis

Cuomo F, Greller MJ, Zuckerman JD. The rheumatoid shoulder. Rheum Dis Clin North Am 1998;24:67–82.
The authors discuss the epidemiology of rheumatoid arthritis, the disease as it affects the shoulder, the differential diagnosis, clinical and radiographic manifestations, and treatment approaches.

McCoy SR, Warren RF, Bade HA III et al. Total shoulder arthroplasty in rheumatoid arthritis. J Arthroplasty 1989;4:105–113.
Twenty-nine Neer-type total shoulder arthroplasties were performed in 26 patients with rheumatoid arthritis. The most significant improvement was noted in pain relief (93% of patients). Follow-up study demonstrated poorer results for patients with rotator cuff tears.

Petersson CJ. Painful shoulders in patients with rheumatoid arthritis: prevalence, clinical and radiological features. Scand J Rheumatol 1986;15:275–279.
The shoulders of 105 patients with rheumatoid arthritis were examined. Ninety-six patients (91%) reported shoulder problems with progression of destructive changes and a decrease in the range of motion with increasing duration of the disease.

Posttraumatic Arthritis

Connor PM, Flatow EL. Complications of internal fixation of proximal humerus fractures. Instr Course Lect 1997;46:25–37.
The authors present the complications that can occur with open reduction and internal fixation of proximal humerus fractures.

Green A, Norris TR. Shoulder arthroplasty for advanced glenohumeral arthritis after anterior instability repair. J Shoulder Elbow Surg 2001;10:539–545.
Seventeen of 19 shoulders with advanced glenohumeral arthritis after anterior instability repair were treated with arthroplasty. Prior surgeries included four Bristow, four Putti-Platt (two in combination with other procedures), four Magnuson-Stack, two Bankart, and five other anterior capsulorrhaphies. Common findings included severe internal rotation contracture and posterior glenoid wear. There was improvement in functional use of the upper extremity in all cases except one.

MacDonald PB, Hawkins RJ, Fowler PJ et al. Release of the subscapularis for internal rotation contracture and pain after anterior repair for recurrent anterior dislocation of the shoulder. J Bone Joint Surg 1992;74A:734–737.
Ten patients who had an internal rotation contracture and pain after an anterior repair for recurrent dislocation of the shoulder were treated by release of the subscapularis muscle. Six patients demonstrated severe arthritic radiographic changes in the shoulder. Following release, each patient had less pain in the shoulder and an average increase of 27° of external rotation.

Sperling JW, Antuña SA, Sanchez-Sotelo J et al. Shoulder arthroplasty for arthritis after instability surgery. J Bone Joint Surg 2002;84A:1775–1781.
Thirty-one patients with glenohumeral arthritis after instability surgery were treated with shoulder arthroplasty (total shoulder or hemiarthroplasty). The group was followed for a minimum of 2 years (mean, 7 years) or until the time of any subsequent revision surgery. Shoulder arthroplasty was associated with significant pain relief as well as significant improvement in external rotation and active abduction. However, 3 patients in the hemiarthroplasty group and 8 patients in the total shoulder arthroplasty group underwent revision surgery. Their data suggest that shoulder arthroplasty for osteoarthritis following instability surgery provides pain relief and improved motion but is associated with high rates of revision surgery and unsatisfactory results due to component failure, instability, and pain due to glenoid arthritis.

Wiater JM, Flatow EL. Posttraumatic arthritis. Orthop Clin North Am 2000;31:63–76.
The authors discuss etiology, preoperative evaluation, treatment, complications, and outcomes of treatment of posttraumatic glenohumeral arthritis.

Rotator Cuff Tear Arthropathy

Franklin JL, Barrett WP, Jackins SE et al. Glenoid loosening in total shoulder arthroplasty: association with rotator cuff deficiency. J Arthroplasty 1988;3:39–46.
Seven cases of total shoulder arthroplasty exhibiting loosening of the glenoid component were evaluated to identify causative factors. Six of the patients had severe, incompletely reconstructable rotator cuff tears present at the time of surgery, and 1 patient developed a cuff tear within 1 year of surgery. The amount of superior migration of the humeral component was closely correlated with the degree of glenoid loosening. Superior displacement of the humeral component was associated with superior tipping of the glenoid component (a "rocking horse" glenoid). The authors concluded that upward riding of the prosthetic humeral head in patients with rotator cuff deficiency may contribute to loosening of the glenoid component in total shoulder arthroplasty.

Grammont PM, Baulot E. Delta shoulder prosthesis for rotator cuff rupture. Orthopedics 1993;16:65–68.
The authors describe the reverse shoulder prosthesis and its use in glenohumeral arthritis with associated rotator cuff tear.

McCarty DJ, Halverson PB, Carrera GF et al. "Milwaukee shoulder"—association of microspheroids containing hydroxyapatite crystals, active collagenase, and neutral protease with rotator cuff defects. I. Clinical aspects. Arthritis Rheum 1981;24:464–473.
Four women, aged 63 to 90 years old, presented with mildly painful shoulders and decreased mobility or stability. Radiographic evidence of a complete tear of the rotator cuff was present in 7 of 8 shoulders. Hydroxyapatite crystals were seen by scanning electron microscopy in 12 of 13 synovial fluid samples. All synovial fluids showed activated collagenase and neutral protease activity. The authors designated this constellation of findings as the "Milwaukee shoulder."

Neer CS II, Craig EV, Fukuda H. Cuff-tear arthropathy. J Bone Joint Surg 1983;65A:1232–1244.
This study described the clinical and pathological findings, differential diagnosis, and pathomechanics of cuff-tear arthropathy in 26 patients. The authors hypothesized that nutritional and mechanical factors cause atrophy of the glenohumeral articular cartilage and osteoporosis of the subchondral bone of the humeral head in a minority of patients with a massive rotator cuff tear. Their preferred method of treatment was total shoulder replacement with rotator cuff reconstruction and special rehabilitation.

Sanchez-Sotelo J, Cofield RH, Rowland CM. Shoulder hemiarthroplasty for glenohumeral arthritis associated with severe rotator cuff deficiency. J Bone Joint Surg 2001;83A:1814–1822.
In this study of 33 shoulders with glenohumeral arthritis and a massive, irreparable rotator cuff tear, the authors found that hemiarthroplasty provided marked pain relief in three-quarters of the patients. They cautioned, however, that outcomes may be complicated by instability and progressive bone loss.

Rotator Cuff Disease

Carpenter JE, Thomopoulos S, Flanagan CL et al. Rotator cuff defect healing: a biomechanical and histologic analysis in an animal model. J Shoulder Elbow Surg 1998;7:599–605.
This study examined healing of rotator cuff defects in rats. Seventy-eight percent of the specimens had persistent defects after 12 weeks. There was some evidence of healing and improved biomechanical properties; however, the response was inadequate.

Gartsman GM, Khan M, Hammerman SM. Arthroscopic repair of full-thickness tears of the rotator cuff. J Bone Joint Surg 1998;80A:832–840.
In this study of arthroscopic repair of full-thickness tears of the rotator cuff in 73 patients, the authors state the arthroscopic method offers several advantages, including smaller incisions, access to the glenohumeral joint for the inspection and treatment of intra-articular lesions, no need for detachment of the deltoid, and less soft tissue dissection. They caution, however, that these advantages must be considered against the technical difficulty of the method, limiting its application to experienced shoulder surgeons.

Iannotti JP, Bernot MP, Kuhlman JR et al. Postoperative assessment of shoulder function: a prospective study of full-thickness rotator cuff tears. J Shoulder Elbow Surg 1996;5:449–457.
Forty patients underwent surgery for chronic, symptomatic, full-thickness rotator cuff defects. The study evaluated preoperative and intraoperative factors that influence postoperative outcome. Outcome measurements correlated most closely with preoperative tear size.

Jobe CM. Superior glenoid impingement. Current concepts. Clin Orthop 1996;330:98–107.
This article is a review of superior glenoid impingement including the clinical picture and recommended treatment.

Nakajima T, Rokuuma N, Hamada K et al. Histologic and biomechanical characteristics of the supraspinatus tendon: reference to rotator cuff tearing. J Shoulder Elbow Surg 1994:3:79–87.
Histologic studies were performed on clinical rotator cuff specimens to define the cuff microstructure demonstrating that the articular surface side has an ultimate failing stress only half that of the bursal side.

Weber SC. Arthroscopic debridement and acromioplasty versus mini-open repair in the management of significant partial-thickness tears of the rotator cuff. Orthop Clin North Am 1997;28:79–82.
A comparison between patients with partial-thickness tears treated with acromioplasty and debridement were compared to patients treated with mini-open repair. Functional results were significantly better in the repair group. Healing of the partial-tear was not observed.

Lesions of the Biceps Tendon/Biceps Orgin

Becker DA, Cofield RH. Tenodesis of the long head of the biceps brachii for chronic bicipital tendinitis: long-term results. J Bone Joint Surg 1989;71A:376–381.
The authors studied 54 shoulders at an average follow-up of 13 years treated with isolated biceps tenodesis of the long head of the biceps. Short-term results were encouraging with all but 3 patients with satisfactory outcomes. However, after longer follow-up, a satisfactory result was achieved in only approximately 50% of patients.

Boileau P, Krishnan SG, Coste JS et al. Arthroscopic biceps tenodesis: a new technique using bioabsorbable interference screw fixation. Arthroscopy 2002;18:1002–1012.
Forty-three patients were treated with the technique of arthroscopic biceps tenodesis using a bioabsorbable interference screw and followed for at least 1 year. There was no loss of elbow movement and biceps strength was 90% of the strength of the other side. The ab-solute constant score improved from 43 points preoperatively to 79 points at review. Two patients, operated on early in the series, presented with a rupture of the tenodesis. The authors concluded that arthroscopic biceps tenodesis using bioabsorbable screw fixation is technically possible and gives good clinical results.

Mariani EM, Cofield RH, Askew LJ et al. Rupture of the tendon of the long head of the biceps brachii: surgical versus nonsurgical treatment. Clin Orthop 1988;228:233–239.
In this comparison of surgical versus nonsurgical treatment of proximal biceps tendon ruptures, conservatively treated shoulders demonstrated no differences in arm pain or shoulder range of motion. The authors did find 21% less supination strength and 8% loss of elbow flexion strength in the nonoperative group.

Post M, Benca P. Primary tendinitis of the long head of the biceps. Clin Orthop 1989;246:117–125.
The authors reported satisfactory results in 16 of 17 patients diagnosed with isolated biceps pathology treated with biceps tenodesis.

Snyder SJ, Karzel RP, Del Pizzo W et al. SLAP lesions of the shoulder. Arthroscopy 1990;6:274–279.
This retrospective review described a specific pattern of injury to the superior labrum of the shoulder identified arthroscopically in 27 patients. Mechanism, clinical picture, classification, and recommended treatment are described for this entity the authors termed a SLAP lesion (superior labrum anterior and posterior).

Warner JJP, McMahon PJ. The role of the long head of the biceps brachii in superior stability of the glenohumeral joint. J Bone Joint Surg 1995;77A:366–372.
The authors studied seven patients who had isolated loss of the proximal attachment of the tendon of the long head of the biceps brachii, documented operatively or with magnetic resonance imaging, in order to identify and measure superior translation of the humeral head on the glenoid. Results showed superior migration of the humeral head relative to the contralateral (control) shoulder supporting the role of the tendon of the long head of the biceps brachii as a stabilizer of the humeral head in the glenoid during abduction of the shoulder in the scapular plane.

Frozen Shoulder

Kinnard P, Truchon R, St-Pierre A et al. Interscalene block for pain relief after shoulder surgery: a prospective randomized study. Clin Orthop 1994;304:22–24.
This prospective randomized study of 30 patients who underwent outpatient acromioplasty demonstrated the efficacy and safety of interscalene block postoperatively.

Neviaser RJ, Neviaser TJ. The frozen shoulder: diagnosis and management. Clin Orthop 1987;223:59–64.
The authors define and differentiate the stiff and painful shoulder from true adhesive capsulitis and describe their recommended treatment for these distinct entities.

Pollock RG, Duralde XA, Flatow EL et al. The use of arthroscopy in the treatment of resistant frozen shoulder. Clin Orthop 1994;304:30–36.
This study describes the authors' technique for managing resistant frozen shoulder. A treatment regimen consisting of interscalene regional anesthesia, manipulation, and arthroscopic release, yielded overall satisfactory results in 25 (83%) of 30 shoulders in their series. The subgroup with diabetes mellitus fared less well than the other groups, with only 64% satisfactory results.

Scarlat MM, Harryman DT II. Management of the diabetic stiff shoulder. Instr Course Lect 2000;49:283–294.
This review describes the diabetic stiff shoulder, treatment, and outcomes. The authors detail their surgical technique, which includes manipulation followed by careful resection of capsule utilizing special release forceps.

Glenohumeral Instability

Bigliani LU, Pollock RG, McIlveen SJ et al. Shift of the posteroinferior aspect of the capsule for recurrent posterior glenohumeral instability. J Bone Joint Surg 1995;77A:1011–1020.
Thirty-five shoulders in 34 patients in this study were treated with a superior shift of the posteroinferior aspect of the capsule because of recurrent posterior glenohumeral subluxation and dislocation. Overall, the result for 17 of the 35 shoulders was rated as excellent; 11, as good; 1, as fair; and 6, as poor. Four shoulders became unstable again. Six of the 7 unsatisfactory results were in shoulders that had had previous attempts at stabilization.

Gartsman GM, Roddey TS, Hammerman SM. Arthroscopic treatment of anterior-inferior glenohumeral instability: two- to five-year follow-up. J Bone Joint Surg 2000;82A:991–1003.
This study examined 53 patients who underwent arthroscopic treatment of anterior-inferior glenohumeral instability with soft tissue sutures, suture anchors, and thermal capsulorrhaphy in select patients. Ninety-two percent (49) of the 53 patients had a rating of good or excellent at the time of the final follow-up. Thirty-four of 38 patients returned to their desired level of sports activity following the operation. The authors concluded that arthroscopic treatment of anterior-inferior glenohumeral instability is better than previous arthroscopic techniques and is equivalent to open repair.

Hovelius L, Augustini BG, Fredin H et al. Primary anterior dislocation of the shoulder in young patients: a ten-year prospective study. J Bone Joint Surg 1996;78A:1677–1684.
Two hundred and forty-five patients who had had 247 primary anterior dislocations of the shoulder were followed for 10 years. The ages of the patients at the time of the dislocation ranged from 12 to 40 years. The patients were assigned to one of three various conservative treatment groups. At the 10-year follow-up evaluation, no additional dislocation had occurred in 129 shoulders (52%). Recurrent dislocation necessitating operative treatment had developed in 58 shoulders (23%): 34 (34%) of the 99 shoulders in patients who were 12 to 22 years old, 16 (28%) of the 57 shoulders in patients who were 23 to 29 years old, and 8 (9%) of the 91 shoulders in patients who were 30 to 40 years old. The type and duration of the initial treatment had no effect on the rate of recurrence.

Sekiya JK, Ong BC, Bradley JP. Thermal capsulorrhaphy for shoulder instability. Instr Course Lect 2003;52:65–80.
This review provides an overview of current applications of thermal capsulorrhaphy for the various types of glenohumeral instability. The authors emphasize that the use of thermal capsulorrhaphy is to enhance other arthroscopically-performed stabilization procedures.

Simonet WT, Cofield RH. Prognosis in anterior shoulder dislocation. Am J Sports Med 1984;12:19–24.
Thirty-five shoulders were treated with posterior-inferior capsular shift for recurrent instability. At follow-up averaging 5 years, 80% satisfactory results were obtained overall. In cases of primary repair, the success rate was 96%.

13

Peter M. Murray

The Forearm and Elbow

CONGENITAL CONDITIONS
  Arthrogryposis Multiplex
    Congenita
  Congenital Radial Head
    Dislocation
  Congenital Radioulnar
    Synostosis
NERVE ENTRAPMENT
  SYNDROMES
  Anterior Interosseous Nerve
    Syndrome and Pronator
    Syndrome

Radial Nerve Entrapment
  Syndromes
  Ulnar Neuropathy
OLECRANON BURSITIS
DEGENERATIVE
  ARTHRITIS
OSTEOCHONDRITIS
  DISSECANS

PANNER'S DISEASE
RHEUMATOID ARTHRITIS
TENDONOPATHIES
  Intersection Syndrome
  Lateral Epicondylitis
    (Tennis Elbow)
  Medial Epicondylitis
    (Golfer's Elbow)

CONGENITAL CONDITIONS

Arthrogryposis Multiplex Congenita

Arthrogryposis is a congenital condition of uncertain origin but believed to involve nerve and muscle, possibly anterior horn cells, occurring in approximately 1/3,000 live births. These children have a predictable pattern of muscle weakness and joint contracture. Although the elbow may present in a 90° flexed position, a typical clinical presentation is shoulder girdle wasting, stiff extended elbows, pronated forearms, and flexed wrists. The primary goal is to provide these children with one elbow that will allow hand to mouth while maintaining one arm extended, facilitating lower extremity or perineal care.

Shortly after birth, the parents of the child are instructed on manual stretching exercises in an attempt to achieve some element of a supple elbow. Later during this initial treatment phase, static elbow splints are worn to maintain passive range of elbow motion. Once improved passive elbow motion is achieved, tendon transfers about the elbow are considered following posterior elbow joint release. Some prefer a two-staged operative approach while others will perform

401

both procedures at once. Muscle transfers accomplishing elbow flex can include triceps transfer, pectoralis major muscle transfer, or a free gracilis muscle transfer. Although surgical results are not ideal, these children are typically of normal intelligence, respond well to physical therapy, and can become independent.

Congenital Radial Head Dislocation

The actual cause of the infantile dislocated elbow remains speculative. Suggested origins include congenital, developmental or posttraumatic. A commonly considered traumatic cause is the "nursemaid's elbow" or the pulled elbow of infancy. Developmental causation can result from an ulnar aplasia, multiple exostosis, and multiple enchondromatosis. Radiographic evidence of a true congenital cause is hypoplasia of the capitellum, a rounded appearance of the radial head articular surface and a thin radial neck. Clinical evidence of a congenital origin for this condition is the presence of bilateral involvement.

Many patients never receive treatment of this condition. Disability from degenerative arthritis is seldom seen in patients having congenital dislocation of the radial head. If degenerative arthritis is seen, radial head resection in the adult patient is the preferred treatment option. In a recent study, Sacher and Mih have reported encouraging results in children having surgery for radial head dislocation, but the long-term efficacy of such a procedure is unknown. As many patients do well with this

condition, supportive care may be all that is necessary for congenital radial head dislocation, irrespective of the cause.

Congenital Radioulnar Synostosis

Congenital radioulnar synostosis occurs early on in fetal development when the longitudinal separation of the forearm anlage does not completely occur. The most common presentation is a failure of proximal separation of the radius and ulna leaving a coalition between these bones (Figure 13-1). Other presentations of congenital elbow synostosis include radiohumeral synostosis, ulnohumeral synostosis, or synostosis involving all three bones about the elbow. Radioulnar synostosis is seen in patients with fetal alcohol syndrome and is also seen in association with hip dysplasia, clubfoot, and a variety of congenital hand anomalies.

Diagnosis is often delayed and frequently does not become apparent until the child has difficulty with a simple task that requires forearm rotation. Physical examination often finds a forearm fixed in a midrange pronated position, which is often a functional position. Patients with a forearm in the completely pronated position likely suffer from notable functional disability. Fortunately, this condition is unusual and patients generally adapt, through wrist hypermobility, to the degree that little functional disability persists. In the patients with disability, treatment can consist of a derotational osteotomy either in the midforearm or at the level of the synostosis. When extreme forearm positions are

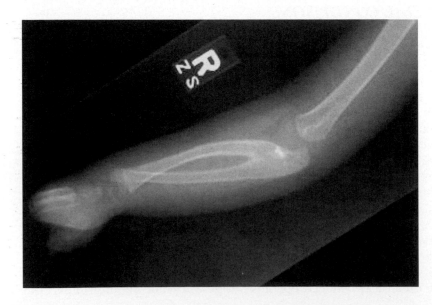

FIGURE 13-1. Congenital radioulnar synostosis involving proximal aspect of the radius and the ulna.

corrected, injury to nerve and arterial structures can occur as the forearm is derotated to a more neutral position. Such injury can result in hand ischemia or even compartment syndrome. Careful postoperative monitoring is necessary following these procedures. Fortunately, most children with congenital radioulnar synostosis are left with a forearm in a functional position and surgery is not necessary.

NERVE ENTRAPMENT SYNDROMES

Anterior Interosseous Nerve Syndrome and Pronator Syndrome

Entrapment neuropathies of the median nerve about the elbow are much less common than carpal tunnel syndrome. Some have reported that median nerve neuropathies about the proximal forearm and elbow account for less than 1% of all entrapment neuropathies. Anterior interosseous syndrome occurs due to fascial bands or aberrant blood vessels compressing the anterior branch of the median nerve. Pronator syndrome is caused from direct compression of the median nerve by the pronator teres muscle. The site of compression is distal to the branch of the anterior interosseous nerve.

Patients with anterior interosseous syndrome present with weakness of the flexor pollicis longus muscle and the flexor digitorum profundus to the index. Characteristic hyperextension posturing of the distal interphalangeal joints of the index finger and thumb are seen. Patients cannot make an "OK" sign due to FPL and FDPI weakness. Sensory examination is normal and pain, paresthesias absent. The diagnosis of anterior interosseous syndrome should be distinguished from Parsonage-Turner syndrome, or brachial neuritis. In Parsonage-Turner syndrome, a painful shoulder and arm prodrome exists with paralysis of the anterior interosseous nerve occurring later. Trauma, surgery, flu, or a vaccination may precede the diagnosis of Parsonage-Turner syndrome. The cause of this peculiar syndrome is uncertain.

Electromyographic studies are often helpful in diagnosing advanced anterior interosseous lesions, although electrodiagnostic testing is often unreliable in the earlier stages of the condition. Neurodiagnostic studies are not helpful for 6 weeks following the onset of symptoms due to neurophysiologic equilibration of the nerve.

Initial treatment is nonoperative with patients instructed to avoid repetitive gripping and lifting. Long-arm splinting and nonsteroidal antiinflammatory drugs (NSAIDs) may prove helpful. If no improvement in FPL and FDPI is seen in 3 to 4 months, surgical exploration and decompression of the anterior interosseous nerve is indicated. This decompression is accomplished through a generous incision over the volar aspect of the proximal forearm, which often leaves a rather unsightly scar. Treatment for Parsonage-Turner syndrome is nonsurgical with return of function seen up to 2 years following the onset of symptoms.

In contrast to anterior interosseous syndrome, patients with pronator syndrome present with vague anterior forearm pain and unpredictable sensory changes of the hand. The forearm pain is exacerbated by repetitive activities such as hammering and forced gripping. Decreased sensation may be found in the thumb, index finger, long finger, and the radial aspect of the ring finger. The pattern of sensory change can be distinguished from carpal tunnel syndrome by the loss of sensation in the palm of the hand caused by involvement of the palmar cutaneous branch of the median nerve. Patients with pronator syndrome typically do not experience night paresthesias, further distinguishing the condition from carpal tunnel syndrome. Electrodiagnostic studies are helpful only in 40 to 50% of cases. The diagnostic acumen of neurodiagnostic studies for pronator syndrome is limited due to the proximal forearm median nerve conduction velocity delays often seen in carpal tunnel syndrome. The diagnosis, then, is clinical. Physical examination findings include tenderness over the course of the median nerve in the forearm, a Tinel's sign in the proximal forearm, and a positive nerve compression test in the proximal forearm. Much like the carpal tunnel compression test in the wrist, the proximal forearm compression test is performed by applying firm, direct pressure over the median nerve at the pronator arcade. The pressure is held for 30 seconds. A positive test is elicited by pain in the forearm or paresthesias in the median nerve distribution of the hand. Hyperflexion of the elbow and pronation of the forearms may also elicit symptoms.

Similar to anterior interosseous syndrome, the initial treatment of pronator syndrome is nonoperative. Activity restriction with goal-directed recovery under the supervision of a certified hand therapist is, perhaps, the most effective nonoperative measure. NSAIDs and removable long-arm splinting with the elbow in 90° flexion and the forearm in neutral may prove useful. Failure to improve following 6 months of nonoperative therapy is an indication for surgical exploration and decompression of the median nerve in the forearm. Sites of compression can not only include the interval between the two heads of the pronator teres, the fibrous elements of the lacertus fibrosis, or the proximal arch of the flexor digitorum sublimus muscle.

also the ligament of Struthers

Radial Nerve Entrapment Syndromes

Proximal to the elbow joint, the radial nerve branches into the superficial radial nerve and the posterior interosseous nerve (PIN). The superficial radial nerve courses distally beneath the brachioradialis muscle over the dorsal radial aspect of the forearm before emerging to a subcutaneous position at the junction of its distal third and middle third. The posterior interosseous nerve travels around the radial neck and through the interval between the two heads of the supinator muscle. This opening, which often has an overlying, compressive fibrous arch, is known as the arcade of Frosche. The space beneath the supinator muscle belly and where the PIN travels is known as the radial tunnel. The sites of potential radial nerve compression are the entrance to the radial tunnel (arcade of Frosche) and the exit of the superficial radial nerve from beneath the brachioradialis muscle.

sites

Compressive neuropathy of the superficial radial nerve as it exits the brachioradialis muscle can result in Wartenberg's syndrome. This condition can occur following direct trauma along the course of the superficial radial nerve or, possibly, as a result

Sup. Radial n.

of repetitive forearm movements as might be sustained in certain occupations. Patients with compressive neuropathy of the superficial radial nerve present with pain, paresthesias, or anesthesia over the dorsum of the hand. Clinical examination may find tenderness over the course of the nerve or a Tinel's sign where the nerve lies in a subcutaneous position. Initial treatment is nonoperative, including splinting, NSAIDs, and activity avoidance or modification. In rare instances, surgical decompression of the nerve may be necessary.

Compressive neuropathy of the PIN can occur at the arcade of Frosche, potentially resulting in one of two different syndromes. Posterior interosseous nerve syndrome causes a painless paralysis of digital and wrist extension. External compression of the PIN may also occur due to ganglion cyst formation from the elbow joint or the development of other neoplasms. PIN syndrome may also result from proliferative synovitis from the radiocapitellar joint in the patient with rheumatoid arthritis. Electrodiagnostic testing may localize the site of compression. A brief period of observation and nonoperative treatment is indicated initially following the onset of symptoms, but surgical exploration and PIN decompression is indicated if symptoms do not resolve promptly (Figure 13-2).

Radial tunnel syndrome is a curious PIN compressive condition characterized by volar forearm pain without muscle weakness. Thought to occur as a result of PIN compression within the radial tunnel, the condition is often confused with chronic lateral epicondylitis. Some have suggested that lateral

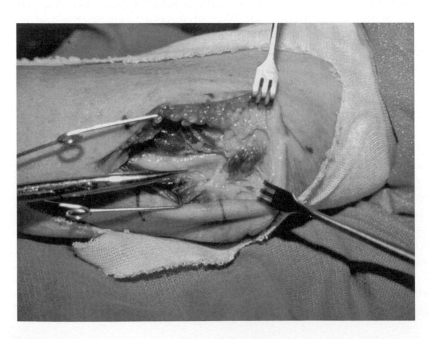

FIGURE 13-2. Dorsal aspect of the posterior forearm with posterior interosseous nerve (PIN) exposed following release of the supinator. Notice flattening and discoloration of the PIN.

epicondylitis and radial tunnel syndrome may co-exist, further complicating the clinical picture. Others, however, have questioned the existence of the condition altogether. Most patients respond to nonoperative treatment of activity modification, splinting, NSAIDs, and rest. Surgical decompression may be indicated in recalcitrant cases and is often combined with lateral epicondylar release. Electrodiagnostic testing is often of little diagnostic benefit in patients with radial tunnel syndrome.

Ulnar Neuropathy

Ulnar nerve compression most commonly occurs at the elbow within the fibro-osseous groove known as the cubital tunnel. Other sites of potential ulnar nerve compression at the elbow or ulnar include the arcade of Struthers, the medial intermuscular septum, and the ligament of Osborne. The arcade of Struthers is a constrictive condensation of fibrous tissue adjacent to the medial intermuscular septum, located approximately 12 cm proximal to the cubital tunnel. The intermuscular septum is a sheet of fibrous tissue separating the triceps from the brachialis muscle. The ulnar nerve lies immediately posterior to this structure and can be a source of impingement to the ulnar nerve when treatment calls for anterior transposition of the nerve. The ligament of Osborne is the fibrous tendinous arch of the proximal origin of the two heads of the flexor carpi ulnaris tendon. Ulnar neuropathy may develop idiopathically or as a late result of trauma. The later is known as tardy ulnar nerve palsy and results from a malunited distal humerus fracture or from posttraumatic growth arrest of the distal humerus.

Patients with ulnar neuropathy complain of paresthesias (abnormal sensations) and dysesthesias (lack of feeling) in the small finger and the ulnar portion of the ring finger. Burning ring and small finger pain as well as hand weakness and clumsiness are also common complaints. Physical examination may reveal exacerbation of the paresthesias with light percussion over the ulnar nerve within the cubital tunnel (Tinel's sign). Additionally, the ulnar nerve may be tender to touch in this region. In more active patients or patients with a history of sporting activities, the ulnar nerve may be found to slip in and out of the cubital groove (translocation) during flexion and extension of the elbow.

In more advanced cases of ulnar neuropathy, motor weakness of the ulnarly innervated muscles may result. This most notably manifests itself by clawing of the ring and small fingers (Figure 13-3). Other signs of ulnar nerve paralysis include interosseous muscle wasting, Wartenberg's sign (inability to abduct the small finger in against the ring finger due to weakness of the palmar interosseous muscles), and Froment's sign (substituting thumb IP joint flexion for thumb adduction due to weakness of the adductor pollicis muscle) (Figure 13-4). Findings can vary due to aberrations in ulnar nerve anatomy. For instance, the intrinsic muscles in the hand are innervated by the median nerve through the Martin-Gruber anastomosis in 7.5% of people. Electrodiagnostic studies are helpful in confirming the diagnosis and following recovery.

In its early stages, treatment of ulnar neuropathy is nonoperative. Queries are first made to identify in occupational or activities of daily life that may have become an irritant to the ulnar nerve at the elbow. Avoidance of these activities may be all

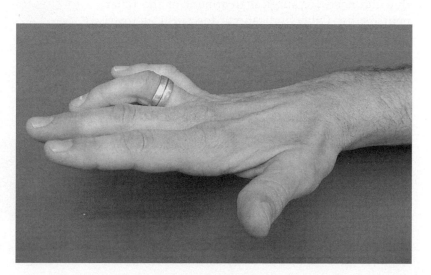

FIGURE 13-3. Clawing of the ring and small finger due to ulnar nerve dysfunction.

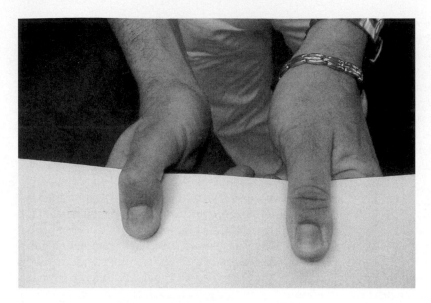

FIGURE 13-4. Froment's sign showing thumb IP joint flexion substituting for adductor pollicis weakness.

that is necessary in some patients. Further nonoperative measures include immobilization of the elbow in 30° of extension, followed by periods of mobilization with elbow padding. An often-used protocol is the fabrication of an orthoplast, anteriorly based nighttime splint with the elbow at 30° flexion. The patient is instructed to remove the pad during the day and wear an elbow pad in an effort to prevent direct trauma to the nerve and to prevent the patient from applying direct pressure on the ulnar nerve. A lack of response to these measures by 3 months is generally considered a failure of conservative treatment.

Fibrillations, sharp waves, polyphasic complexes, and insertional activity on the electromyographic portion of the neurodiagnostic studies are indicative of advanced ulnar neuropathy and indicate the need for surgical treatment of the ulnar neuropathy. Other indications for surgical treatment of ulnar neuropathy are clinical signs of ulnar nerve paralysis and failure of nonoperative management. Opinions vary on the best surgical procedure for treating ulnar neuropathy. Options include in situ release, anterior ulnar nerve transposition (either subcutaneous, submuscular, or intramuscular) and medial epicondylectomy. The in situ release is decompression of the ulnar nerve by release of the cubital tunnel retinaculum and the ligament of Osborne connecting the two muscle heads of the flexor carpi ulnaris (FCU). Anterior transposition of the ulnar nerve requires release of ulnar nerve compression sites and restraints as mentioned earlier. The transposed ulnar nerve can be placed subcutaneous, submuscular beneath the

flexor-pronator mass, or intramuscular (Figure 13-5). Medial epicondylectomy removes the anterior bony barrier to nerve anterior translation. Proponents of this procedure cite the advantage of less

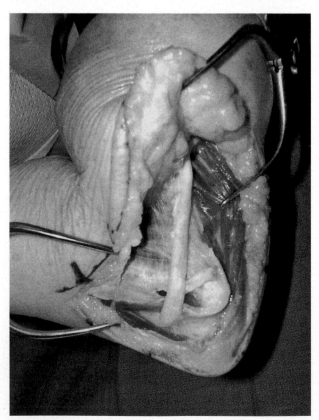

FIGURE 13-5. Anterior transposition of the ulnar nerve. Constraints of the ulnar nerve have been released and the ulnar nerve is prepared for subcutaneous placement.

dissection about the nerve and, therefore, less interruption of ulnar nerve blood supply.

For minimal or mild ulnar neuropathy, all forms of treatment are successful with a high degree of patient satisfaction including nonoperative measures. In one Kaplan-Meier analysis, 80% of patients with mild ulnar neuropathy were improved with nonoperative treatment. For the more advanced lesions, submuscular transposition has a higher patient satisfaction rate compared to the other methods of treatment.

OLECRANON BURSITIS

The olecranon bursa is a synovial-lined structure located between the olecranon process and the skin. This normal structure may become inflamed and accumulate fluid once injured from blunt or repetitive trauma. Other causes of olecranon bursitis include gout, calcium pyrophosphate deposition, and rheumatoid arthritis. Patients may or may not reveal a history of blunt trauma but repetitive trauma is often identified with careful history taking. Patients typically present with a notably swollen and fluctuant posterior elbow. For nonseptic conditions pain and warmth are generally not elicited. The diagnosis of the nonseptic olecranon bursitis is clinical and treatment is conservative. The condition usually responds to a brief period of activity modification and elbow protection. The elbow may be protected with a posterior orthoplast splint or alternatively with a pad. The condition should respond to nonoperative management in 3 to 4 weeks. If the condition does not respond and the bursitis becomes chronic, infection must be considered and the bursa aspirated for culture. Culture analysis should include aerobic, anaerobic, fungus, and mycobacterium analysis. Nonseptic, chronic, long-standing olecranon bursa unresponsive to conservative management occasionally requires surgery. However, bursectomy is often complicated by wound-healing problems and should only be considered after extensive nonoperative therapy.

Septic olecranon bursitis can occur from rather innocuous injury and must always be considered in immunocompromised patients. These infections can progress insidiously leading to devastating consequences. Abscesses can track proximally and distally in the arm along fascial planes leading to a necritizing fasciitis, particularly in the immunocompromised host. The most common organism is *Staphylococcus aureus*. The isolation of methicillin-resistant *S. aureus* is becoming increasingly more common.

The treatment for septic olecranon bursitis is incision, drainage, and debridement, leaving the wound open to heal by secondary intention. Wound care of the open olecranon wound following incision and drainage can be facilitated by use of a negative pressure wound closure assist device. The negative pressure wound healing assist device removes fluid, including proteolytic enzymes responsible for inhibiting tissue angiogenesis. Healing by secondary intention can be prolonged in these patients. Soft tissue pedicled muscle or fasciocutaneous transfer can be considered in recalcitrant cases.

DEGENERATIVE ARTHRITIS

By comparison, degenerative arthritis of the elbow is uncommon, accounting for fewer than 5% of patients receiving a total elbow replacement. Additionally, primary degenerative arthritis of the elbow has been reported to affect less than 2% of the population. Males are more commonly affected than females. Patients complain of pain on terminal extension of the elbow and less frequently pain with flexion. On occasion, patients may be bothered by pain that awakens them from sleep or locking of the elbow during daytime activities. The dominant extremity is involved in greater than 80% of patients with bilateral involvement occurring in up to 60% of patients. Characteristically, these patients lose terminal extension, but elbow flexion and forearm rotation may also be limited. Routine elbow radiographs often reveal osteophytes of the sigmoid notch of the ulna as well as osteophytes of the coronoid process (Figure 13-6A). Loose bodies may also be present.

Nonoperative treatment includes NSAIDs and a trial of intra-articular corticosteroid injections. The time from symptoms onset until surgery may be several years. Operative procedures include arthroscopic joint debridement, ulnohumeral arthroplasty (Outerbridge procedure), and total elbow arthroplasty. Relief of pain and modest improvement in motion can be anticipated following arthroscopic debridement. Long-term results of this procedure are not known. Ulnohumeral arthroplasty is an open procedure where osteophytes are debrided from the ulnar and humeral periarticular surfaces. Through a posterior approach to the olecranon, a trephine is used to remove osteophytes from the olecranon fossa. Also through this approach, the anterior aspect of the distal humerus can be reached and osteophytes removed. Pain relief can

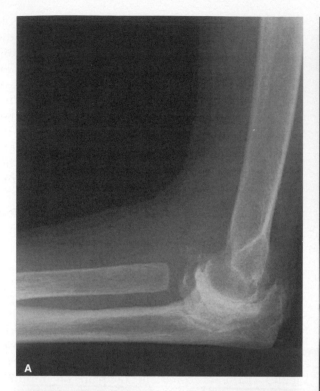

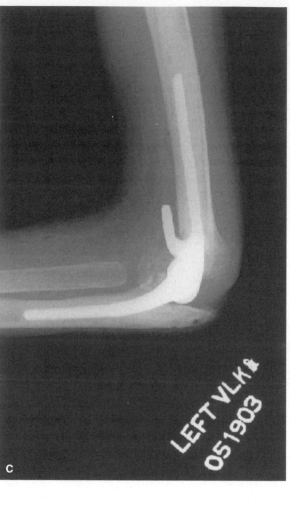

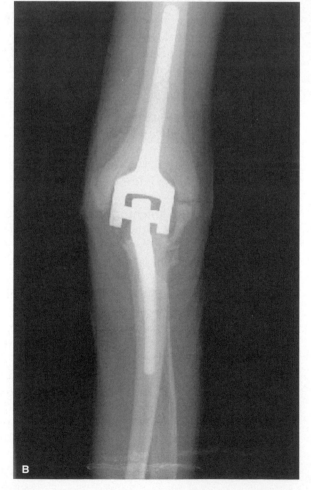

FIGURE 13-6. (A) Primary degenerative arthritis of the elbow. **(B)** and **(C)** PA and lateral elbow films showing total elbow arthroplasty for degenerative arthritis of the elbow.

be expected in 90% of patients. Modest improvements in flexion and extension can also be expected. Approximately 20% of patients experience recurrence of symptoms at 10 years postoperative.

Total elbow arthroplasty is rarely indicated for patients with primary degenerative arthritis of the elbow (Figure 13-6B and C). Patients with degenerative arthritis of the elbow joint are often relatively young and active. The combination of youth and higher activity level often makes the patient with degenerative arthritis of the elbow a poor total elbow arthroplasty candidate. Limited information exists on the treatment of primary degenerative arthritis of the elbow. Only small series have been published on the results of total elbow arthroplasty in these patients and a higher rate of complication has been reported. The semiconstrained, nonhinged surface replacement variety of total elbow arthroplasty may theoretically be better suited for the degenerative elbow because hinged components are at risk for loosening due to stress imparted at the bone cement interface. Ligament incompetence seen in the RA patient precludes the use of surface replacement components in these patients. However, the degenerative elbow would be expected to have ligamentous and capsular integrity as well as intact subchondral humeral and ulnar bone stock, thereby making surface replacement an option. Long-term results of surface replacement arthroplasty in the degenerative elbow, however, are lacking.

OSTEOCHONDRITIS DISSECANS

Osteochondritis dissecans is a condition that most frequently affects adolescent boys in which elbow articular cartilage and underlying bone separates from the articular surface. It is more common in males than females, is more common in the dominant arm, and appears in both elbows in 15% of patients. The most common presenting complaint is pain and limited motion. Osteochondritis dissecans (OCD) is a common cause of "Little League elbow." Physical examination finds loss of elbow extension and tenderness over the lateral aspect of the elbow. Irregular ossification of the capitellum, or a discrete crater, can be seen on plain radiography that should include PA, lateral, and oblique projections. Loose bodies may also develop and may be best visualized with CT scan. The actual cause of the condition remains unknown although trauma is believed to be an important factor as well as possibly ischemia and genetics.

Treatment of OCD of the elbow is based on the radiographic stability of the fragment. Intact lesions generally respond to nonoperative management, including rest, splinting, and NSAIDs. Partially detached or unstable lesions can be reattached in situ, but the ultimate outcome is unknown. Completely detached lesions are best treated with simple removal. The role of arthroscopic debridement of remaining craters following removal of unstable or detached lesions remains unknown, but some successes have been reported. An association between OCDs and the development of degenerative arthritis may exist. In the skeletally mature OCD patient with advanced capitellar irregularities, radial head resection may be an option for treatment.

PANNER'S DISEASE

Panner's disease is osteochondrosis of the capitellum. Osteochondrosis is a growth disturbance involving a center of ossification. The condition generally affects boys from the ages of 7 to 12 years, during the years of ossification of the capitellar epiphysis. Patients usually present with a painful elbow, particularly aggravated by throwing sports. Physical examination yields tenderness over the lateral aspect of the elbow and limited motion of the elbow. Radiographically, the capitellar epiphysis becomes fragmented in a fashion similar to Perthes disease of the femoral head. In time as growth progresses, the capitellar epiphysis reconstitutes. Treatment is usually symptomatic as the symptoms and limitations of motion resolve.

RHEUMATOID ARTHRITIS

Rheumatoid arthritis (RA) is an inflammatory condition of uncertain origin, although genetics is thought to play a role. The prevalence of the condition is approximately 2%, affecting females twice as commonly as males. Synovial biopsies of recently diagnosed patients with RA show macrophages, T-cell and B-cell lymphocytes, plasma cells, and polymorphonuclear lymphocytes. The resulting inflammatory response invades normal tissue causing periarticular bony erosions, cartilage destruction, and eventually joint destruction. Patients generally experience pain and stiffness in multiple joints; however, monoarticular involvement is recognized. Elbow involvement affects approximately 50% of patients with RA. The hand and wrist are the most commonly affected joints. Patients with RA affecting the elbow may experience loss of both flexion and extension range of motion. Inspection of the posterior surface of the elbow often finds loss of the normal bony contours due to synovitis. This is perhaps most easily appreciated along the medial border of the elbow, beneath the ulnar groove of the humerus or along the lateral aspect of the elbow. Radiography will show periarticular erosions as well as concentric cartilage shadow narrowing. The joint is often warm to the touch during periods of active disease.

The medical management of RA is discussed in Chapter 14 on the hand and wrist. Early nonoperative management can include a corticosteroid injection, although relief of symptoms may be temporary. It should also be remembered that the immunosuppressed status of these patients puts them at a slightly increased risk of developing an infection from a needle injection when compared to other patients. Initial surgical management for RA affecting the elbow may include synovectomy. Synovectomy combined with radial head excision is indicated in patients with pain and stiffness following failure of medical management. Radiographically, the ideal elbow synovectomy candidate shows little if any alteration in subchondral architecture despite cartilage shadow narrowing. Patients with gross deformity and marked loss of motion are contraindicated for synovectomy. Elbow synovectomy can be performed using an open technique or arthroscopically. The later technique is demanding. Gendi et al. has reported an 81% success rate at one year in 113 patients but noted that this deteriorated over time with only 54% having pain relief at a mean follow-up of $6\frac{1}{2}$ years.

The primary indication for total elbow arthroplasty is the patients with advanced, symptomatic RA of the elbow and are beyond being considered for a synovectomy (Figure 13-7A–D). These patients often seek medical attention due to constant pain and profound functional limitations from compromised elbow motion. Surgery is indicated in the patient older than 60 years who is relatively inactive. These patients have failed medical management for their elbow RA and understand that vigorous activity is not permitted once they receive an elbow replacement. Contraindications include patients who are mentally unstable or unreliable, patients with open elbow wounds, or patients with prior or active elbow joint infection. Additionally patients who are medically unstable or patients having current active infections elsewhere are considered poor candidates for the procedure.

The hinged or constrained total elbow replacement arthroplasty is the design most suitable for the RA patient. This design does not rely on the capsuloligamentous structures nor subchondral bone for elbow stability. In fact, generous portions of the medial or lateral humeral condyles can be resected to facilitate component placement, without compromising the overall result of the elbow replacement surgery. The prosthesis lends immediate stability to an otherwise unstable joint. Most constrained total elbow prosthetic designs offer 5 to 10° of out-of-plane laxity of the ulnar component, thereby unloading stress at the bone-cement interface. Otherwise, stress at this location causes premature loosening and ultimate implant failure. In one design, an anterior flange has been added to provide rotational stability (Figure 13-8). The procedure is performed through a triceps-sparing posterior approach that facilitates early rehabilitation. Unlike other joint replacement procedures, a major nerve must routinely be identified, mobilized, and transferred to a new location. During the initial surgical exposure, the ulnar nerve is identified, mobilized, and transposed anteriorly. Immediately postoperative, the patients are placed in a sling and encouraged to begin activities of daily living. Formal physical therapy is not generally needed. The patients are instructed to never lift more than 10 lbs with the operative elbow and to henceforth consider it a "helper arm."

Gill and Morrey have reviewed a population of 78 total elbow arthroplasties (TEA) at 10 years finding that 97% are not painful and calculated a 92% survival with an 86% having good or excellent results. Traditionally thought to have infection rates of 7% or greater, the infection rate in this series was 2.6%. Ulnar neuritis is one of the more common postoperative problems. In selected RA patients, TEA can be a life-altering procedure.

TENDONOPATHIES

Intersection Syndrome

The abductor pollicis longus (APL) muscle and the extensor pollicis brevis muscle (EPB)—the outcropper muscles of the thumb—cross the extensor carpi radialis brevis (ECRB) and the extensor carpi radialis longus (ECRL) in the distal forearm. At the point of contact of these crossing structures, a bursa is present that may become inflamed following repetitive wrist activities. This condition is known

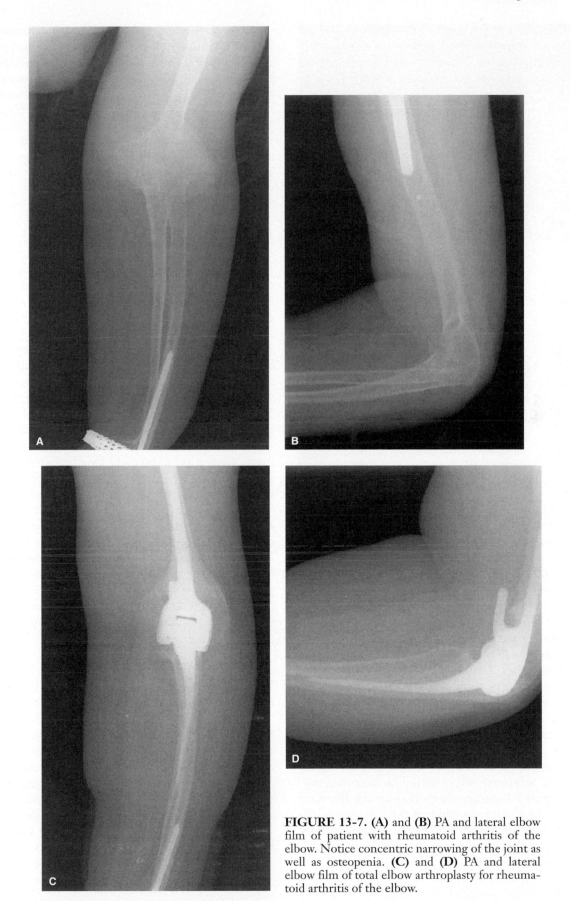

FIGURE 13-7. (A) and **(B)** PA and lateral elbow film of patient with rheumatoid arthritis of the elbow. Notice concentric narrowing of the joint as well as osteopenia. **(C)** and **(D)** PA and lateral elbow film of total elbow arthroplasty for rheumatoid arthritis of the elbow.

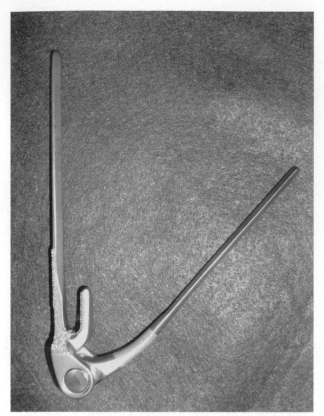

FIGURE 13-8. Coonrad-Morrey Total Elbow arthroplasty demonstrating the anterior flange of the humeral component, offering rotational stability.

as intersection syndrome of the forearm. Patients with intersection syndrome of the forearm will complain of swelling and acute pain with gripping and wrist extension. Also pain may be elicited with isolated thumb movements. On physical examination, patients will have point tenderness directly over the bursa and swelling will be identified. In more advanced cases, warmth and erythema may be present. Under certain circumstances, squeaking can be heard with wrist movements.

Treatment of intersection is largely nonoperative. Generally, a specific activity can be identified that has incited the condition. Restriction from this activity is the mainstay of initial treatment. Patients also typically respond to static splinting of the wrist in 15° for a period of 3 weeks combined with daily active, gentle wrist range of motion exercises. NSAIDs, if tolerated, are included in the nonoperative treatment regimen. A corticosteroid injection directly into the intersection of tendons (approximately 4 cm proximal to the radial styloid) can be performed if the condition proves refractory to initial treatments.

Rarely, operative intervention is performed following a failure of nonoperative treatment. The surgical approach is through a longitudinal incision over the radial aspect of the dorsal surface of the distal forearm. The APL and EPB tendons are elevated and the underlying ECRB and ECRL are released from within their investing fascia. Extensor tenosynovium is also debrided if identified. Postoperatively, the wrist is splinted in extension and aggravating activities are avoided for 4 weeks. After 4 weeks, patients resume normal activities.

Lateral Epicondylitis (Tennis Elbow)

Pain, which is activity related, along the lateral aspect of the elbow is often a result of the lateral epicondylitis. This relatively common overuse injury may stem from a variety of sporting activities that require repetitive use of the wrist and forearm, or from occupational activities requiring similar movements. The common age of onset is 35 to 50 years of age with an equal male to female ratio. The common extensor origin consists of the tendons of origin of the ECRB, ECRL, ECU, EDC, and EDQM. The pathologic process begins with the microscopic disruption of the tendon fibers, which is a degenerative process. Next, the tendon is invaded by fibroblasts, vascular granulation tissue, and myofibroblasts. This degeneration and repair process is termed *angiofibroblastic hyperplasia*. The ordinary arrangement of the tendon fibers is disrupted. Of interest is the absence of acute or chronic inflammatory tissues. Because of this absence of inflammatory tissue, several authors have referred to the condition as a "tendinosis" as opposed to "tendonitis." The arcade of Frohse is located just beneath the extensor carpi radialis brevis (ECRB) tendon and radial tunnel syndrome may be associated with chronic lateral epicondylitis.

Patients with lateral epicondylitis present due to functional limitations from lateral elbow pain. Patients complain of a sharp pain localized to the lateral aspect of the elbow, exacerbated by activities such as lifting, heavy gripping, or forearm supination and pronation. Chronic conditions may find associated tenderness over the arcade of Frohse, located two fingerbreadths distal to the lateral epicondyle. This may indicate the presence of associated radial tunnel syndrome, often confused with chronic lateral epicondylitis. Physical examination may reveal one of several positive provocative maneuvers for lateral epicondylitis. The resisted longer finger extension test is the most commonly used test for lateral epicondylitis. Other tests include resisted wrist extension test and the resisted supination test (also a test for associated radial tunnel syndrome). Patients with long-standing symptoms may show a decrease in grip strength.

Treatment of lateral epicondylitis is largely nonoperative. Initial activity restriction is perhaps the most effective, especially as it relates to racquet sports. For tennis enthusiasts, careful evaluation of the size and weight of the racquet should be evaluated and, most importantly, the the racquet's string pressure. A weight of 55 to 60 lb of pressure is preferred for most amateurs. Greater string pressure may result in injury. Other issues relate to proper tennis technique. For instance, greater reliance on elbow and forearm motion to increase racquet speed (as opposed to more proximal shoulder girdle muscles) may also result in injury. The reliance on forearm and elbow motion for racquet speed is often caused by deconditioned scapular stabilizer muscles, resulting in scapular dyskinesis. Open chain shoulder rehabilitation is an effective means of rehabilitating the tennis player following lateral epicondylitis. Other rehabilitation includes forearm stretching exercises and gradual strengthening. In the early phase, NSAIDs, wrist cock-up bracing, elbow contour force bracing (Figure 13-9), and steroid phonophoresis may prove beneficial for symptom relief. In most instances, strict immobilization and repeated corticosteroid injections are avoided. The use of corticosteroid injections in the absence of inflammation seems counterintuitive. Some have suggested that the use of corticosteroid on lateral epicondylitis may enhance the tendinosis aspect of the condition.

Surgical treatment is reserved for those patients with refractory symptoms following a year of nonoperative management. Many surgical options exist. The most popular choice is accomplished through a longitudinal incision over the lateral epicondyle, exposing the ECRB tendon of origin. Devitalized, degenerative tissue is excised from the tendon. Incomplete tears of the ECRB tendon of origin occur in approximately 35% of patients according to Nirschl.

Controversy exists regarding direct repair or advancement of the ECRB tendon versus release. Some feel that repair or advancement of the ECRB tendon may predispose to recurrence due to applied tension. Others have recommended release of the entire extensor origin with drilling of the lateral epicondyle to promote healing. More recently described alternative techniques include percutaneous and arthroscopic extensor origin release.

Generally nonoperative therapy is sufficient for lateral epicondylitis. However, when necessary, debridement with or without repair of the ECRB tendon provides a good alternative. In one study, 85.3% of patients obtained good or excellent results with open surgery. Similar results have been reported with arthroscopic and percutaneous techniques. Surgical treatment should be reserved for a select patients.

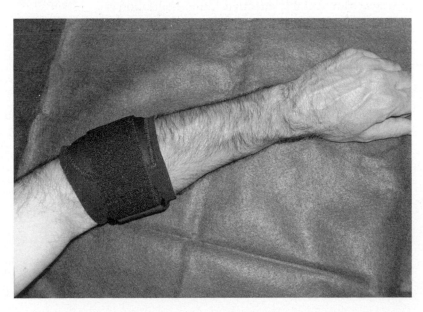

FIGURE 13-9. Counterforce bracing for the treatment of lateral epicondylitis.

Medial Epicondylitis (Golfer's Elbow)

Medial epicondylitis is one of the more common causes of medial elbow pain. Approximately one-third of patients with medial epicondylitis develop the condition subsequent to an injury. The medial condyle of the humerus gives origin to the flexor-pronator origin, including the pronator teres, the flexor carpi radialis, the humeral head of the flexor ulnaris, the palmaris longus, and the ulnar head of the flexor digitorum superficialis. The pronator teres and the flexor carpi radialis share a conjoined tendon that is regarded as the primary site of origin of this condition. With repetitive stress loading of this conjoined tendon, degenerative changes occur in the tendon leading to pain.

Patients with medial epicondylitis present due to activity-related medial elbow pain. Patients are more commonly males, presenting in the third through the fifth decades. In over one-half of cases, patients complain of associated ulnar neuropathy. This most likely relates to localized inflammation about the ulnar nerve or direct compression from the bulk of the flexor-pronator tendinopathy. Tenderness over the medial humeral condyle can be elicited on physical examination. Pain with resistive forearm pronation is also variably present. Elbow range of motion is usually preserved but grip strength may wane.

Most patients with medial epicondylitis respond to nonoperative management including activity restrictions, NSAIDs, and active hand therapy. A forearm splint with the wrist is slight extension may also prove helpful. Counterforce proximal forearm straps are variably effective. If immobilization is chosen, daily active and passive range of motion exercises of the wrist and elbow are encouraged. Corticosteroid injections to the medial epicondyle may provide temporary relief of symptoms. Injections can, however, cause subcutaneous fat atrophy and localized skin depigmentation. Medial epicondylar injections are best preformed with the elbow extended in order to avoid injection into a potentially subluxed or dislocated ulnar nerve.

Patients with greater than 6 months of persisting medial epicondylitis can be considered for surgery. Surgical options include debridement, repair, and reattachment (if needed) of the flexor-pronator tendon origin, or medial epicondylectomy. Flexor origin debridement, and repair and reattachment, is performed through a longitudinal incision over the medial epicondyle. Branches of the medial antibrachial cutaneous nerve are identified and must be carefully protected. Some authors recommend detachment of the flexor-pronator origin with debridement of the devitalized portions of the tendon followed by reattachment. Others recommend simple debridement. Less clear is the optimal treatment for associated ulnar neuropathy. Patients with mild associated ulnar neuropathy generally respond to simple ulnar nerve decompression while more advanced cases of ulnar neuropathy are best treated with anterior submuscular transposition. Results from surgical treatment of medial epicondylitis are highly favorable unless moderate or severe ulnar nerve symptoms exist. In one study, patients with more advanced ulnar nerve symptoms achieved good results in only 40% of cases.

Annotated Bibliography

Congenital Conditions

Bell SN, Morrey BF, Bianco AJ Jr. Chronic posterior subluxation and dislocation of the radial head. J Bone Joint Surg 1991;73A:392–396.
Thirty-four chronic posterior elbow dislocations in 27 patients were reviewed. Follow-up consisted of examining 18 of the patients, 10 of whom received treatment and 8 of whom did not. The authors conclude that posterior displacement did not cause serious functional impairment, although loss of forearm rotation was found. Deformity was noted as a cosmetic problem.

Cleary JE, Omer GE Jr. Congenital proximal radioulnar synostosis. Natural history and functional assessment. J Bone Joint Surg 1985;67A:539–545.
Thirty-six proximal radioulnar synostoses were evaluated in 23 patients. The patients were reevaluated at a mean age of 23 years and were found to be fixed in a mean position of 30° pronation. The patients had few if any functional complaints and the position of the forearm was not found to affect employment status. The authors conclude that operative treatment is rarely indicated in the treatment of congenital proximal radioulnar synostosis.

Mennen U. Early corrective surgery of the wrist and elbow in arthrogryposis multiplex congenita. J Hand Surg 1993;18B:304–307.
Drawing on an experience of 47 patients, the authors evaluated their results and recommend early corrective surgery for arthrogryposis multiplex congenita of the hand and wrist. Included in their surgery are a proximal row carpectomy, wrist tendon transfers, and triceps to radius transfer to improve elbow flexion. The authors conclude that the optimum age for surgery is 3 to 6 months of age.

Sachar K, Mih AD. Congenital radial head dislocations. Hand Clin 1998;14:39–47.
This article reviews the topic of radial head dislocations. The authors conclude that in their experience, early open reduction and ligament reconstruction offers advantages over late radial head resection.

Nerve Entrapment Syndromes

Dellon AL, Chiu DTW. Cubital tunnel and radial tunnel syndromes. In: Trumble TE, ed. Hand Surgery Update. 3rd Ed. Chicago: American Society for Surgery of the Hand, 2003:313–323.

This is an update and review on the subjects of cubital tunnel syndrome and radial tunnel syndrome. Included in the book are data on the results of treatment from the authors' practice. Using a Kaplan-Meier analysis, they report an 80% improvement rate in patients treated nonoperatively for mild ulnar neuropathy.

Mowlavi A, Andrews K, Lille S et al. The management of cubital tunnel syndrome: a meta-analysis of clinical studies. Plast Reconstr Surg 2000;106:327–334.
This analysis of previous clinical series of cubital tunnel treatment reports that the success of surgery is related to the initial degree of ulnar nerve compression. The authors report that the best results for more advanced cubital tunnel syndrome were found in patients who had anterior submuscular transposition.

O'Driscoll SW, Horii E, Carmichael SW et al. The cubital tunnel and ulnar neuropathy. J Bone Joint Surg 1991;73B:613–617.
In this study, the authors examine the anatomic relationships of the cubital tunnel in 27 cadaver elbows. Variations in the anatomy of the cubital tunnel at the elbow were classified into four types: type 0 = no cubital tunnel retinaculum; type 1a = cubital tunnel retinaculum taut in flexion; type 1b = cubital tunnel retinaculum was taut in a position short of full elbow flexion; type 2 = the retinaculum was replaced by an anomalous muscle, the anconeus epitrochlearis. The authors conclude that the variations in cubital tunnel retinacular anatomy may account for the development of ulnar neuropathy in some patients.

Olehnik WK, Manske PR, Szerzinski J. Median nerve compression in the proximal forearm. J Hand Surg 1994;19A:121–126.
The authors review 39 limbs in 36 patients in which surgical decompression of the median nerve was performed in the proximal forearm. Electrodiagnostic testing was abnormal in 12 of the 37 patients who received the studies. The nerve was found compressed at the flexor digitorum superficialis in 22 arms and at the pronator teres in 13 arms. Overall 30 patients had partial or complete relief of their symptoms.

Ritts GD, Wood MB, Linscheid RL. Radial tunnel syndrome. a ten-year surgical experience. Clin Orthop 1987;219:201–205.
In a review of 42 patients surgically treated for radial tunnel syndrome, 37 were followed up at an average of 24 months. Seventy-four percent had improvement following surgery but one-third still had symptoms. Electrodiagnostic studies were not helpful in making the diagnosis. Radial tunnel block was helpful in establishing diagnosis.

Szabo R. Entrapment and compression neuropathies. In: Green DP, Pedersen W, Hotchkiss RN, eds. Operative Hand Surgery, 4th Ed. St. Louis: Churchill Livingstone 1998;1417–1446.
This is a comprehensive review on the subject of compression neuropathies of the forearm and elbow. Included are detailed discussions on pronator syndrome, anterior interosseous nerve entrapment syndrome, ulnar neuropathy, posterior interosseous nerve syndrome, and radial nerve syndrome.

Osteoarthritis

Morrey BF. Primary degenerative arthritis of the elbow. Treatment by ulnohumeral arthroplasty. J Bone Joint Surg 1992;74B:409–413.
Fifteen patients were reviewed at an average of 33 months follow-up after ulnohumeral arthroplasty. Fourteen of the 15 patients had good relief of pain. Elbow extension and flexion had improved 11° and 10° respectively. Overall, 87% of patients felt they had been improved by the operation.

Osteochondritis Dissecans

Baumgarten TE, Andrews JR, Satterwhite YE. The arthroscopic classification and treatment of osteochondritis dissecans of the capitellum. Am J Sports Med 1998;26:520–523.

Seventeen elbows in 16 patients were evaluated with an average follow-up of 48 months. Each patient underwent arthroscopic abrasion arthroplasty and removal of loose bodies. The average flexion and extension contracture decreases following treatment. Six of the 9 patients active in sports returned to their preoperative level of activity. The authors conclude that arthroscopic abrasion chondroplasty is an effective form of treatment for osteochondritis dissecans.

Rheumatoid Arthritis

Gendi NS, Axon JM, Carr AJ et al. Synovectomy of the elbow and radial head excision in rheumatoid arthritis. Predictive factors and long-term outcome. J Bone Joint Surg 1997;79B:918–923.
Synovectomy with radial head resection was performed in 171 patients. Eighty-three percent of the patients were satisfied at one year. These results deteriorated with time at a rate of 2.6% per year. Poor preoperative elbow range of motion was a predictor of failure. The authors conclude that the long-term results of this procedure are poor.

Gill DR, Morrey BF. The Coonrad-Morrey total elbow arthroplasty in patients who have rheumatoid arthritis. A ten- to fifteen-year follow-up study. J Bone Joint Surg 1998;80A:1327–1335.
Seventy-eight original total elbow replacements in 69 patients were followed. At follow-up 46 total elbow replacements in 41 patients were still alive and had at least 10 years of follow-up. At follow-up, 97% of the elbows were not painful. The mean arc of flexion and extension was 28 to 131°, an improvement in 13° over preoperative. Complications included infections, ulnar fractures, and triceps avulsion. Calculated survival rate of the implanted prostheses was 92%. At final follow-up, 86% of the patients had a good or excellent result.

Tendonopathies

Gabel GT, Morrey BF. Operative treatment of medial epicondylitis. Influence of concomitant ulnar neuropathy at the elbow. J Bone Joint Surg 1995;77A:1065–1069.
The results of operative treatment of medial epicondylitis in 30 elbows were reviewed. At an average of 7 years follow-up, debridement and ulnar nerve decompression/transposition resulted in good or excellent results in 87% of patients. The patients that had moderate or advanced preoperative ulnar neuropathy had a significantly worse surgical result.

Grundberg AB, Reagan DS. Pathologic anatomy of the forearm: intersection syndrome. J Hand Surg 1985;10A:299–302.
The basic anatomy and pathoanatomy of intersection syndrome is discussed. Thirteen patients received operative treatment for the condition. The authors conclude that the basic pathologic abnormality is stenosing tenosynovitis of the radial wrist extensor tendons.

Kraushaar BS, Nirschl RP. Tendinosis of the elbow (tennis elbow). Clinical features and findings of histological, immunohistochemical, and electron microscopy studies. J Bone Joint Surg 1999;81A:259–278.

Nirschl RP, Pettrone FA. Tennis elbow. The surgical treatment of lateral epicondylitis. J Bone Joint Surg 1979;61A:832–839.
Of 1,213 elbows with lateral epicondylitis treated nonoperatively, seven percent failed and underwent operative treatment. At the time of surgery, 93% of the elbows (82 of the 88 operatively treated patients) were observed to have gross involvement of the ECRB tendon of origin. Seventy-five of the 88 operatively treated patients obtained good or excellent results with tendon debridement and ECRB repair.

14

Peter M. Murray

The Wrist and Hand

BOUTONNIÈRE DEFORMITY

central slip is responsible for extending the PIP joint.

The boutonnière deformity is a functionally compromising posturing of the digit. The deformity may follow trauma to the central slip portion of the extensor mechanism. It may occur from a laceration involving the proximal interphalangeal (PIP) joint or from a closed, axial force applied to the digit resulting in a rupture of the central slip. More commonly, the boutonnière deformity is caused by central slip attenuation due to PIP joint destruction from rheumatoid arthritis. Much like a small bouquet of flowers protruding through a buttonhole in the lapel of a suit, the proximal interphalangeal joint protrudes through the attenuated extensor mechanism of the digit.

The essential features of a boutonnière deformity include hyperextension of the metacarpal phalangeal (MCP) joint, flexion contracture of the proximal interphalangeal (PIP) joint, hyperextension of the distal interphalangeal (DIP) joint, and incompetence or attenuation of the central portion of the extensor mechanism (Figure 14-1). The deformity can be classified as either mild, moderate, or severe. The PIP joint contracture in the mild or moderate varieties is considered passively correctable, while the PIP joint contracture in the severe boutonnière deformity is rigid or fixed and is not passively correctable.

Treatment of boutonnière deformity is more or less prophylactic in the case of open or closed trauma of the extensor mechanism. Lacerations of the central slip demand careful scrutiny and prompt attention to prevent flexion posturing of the PIP joint and ultimate failure of the extensor mechanism. In the event of a closed rupture, the central slip is treated by splinting. Alternatively, the boutonniere deformity seen in rheumatoid arthritis may be treated with PIP joint synovectomy or reconstruction of the extensor mechanism when the deformity is mild or moderate. In advanced cases, PIP joint arthrodesis (fusion) or joint replacement arthroplasty is needed. In general, soft tissue reconstruction of the boutonnière deformity has been disappointing. The results from treatment with arthrodesis have been more predictable.

CARPAL TUNNEL SYNDROME

Carpal tunnel syndrome is the most common clinical entity seen by the hand surgeon, with some reporting that the condition affects up to 10% of the general population—an estimated cost to the U.S. medical system well beyond $1,000,000,000. When considering time lost from work, the cost to society as a whole is substantial. Risk factors for the condition include female, diabetes, hypothyroidism, obesity, pregnancy, rheumatoid arthritis, gout, precious trauma, acromegaly, smoking, old age, peripheral neuropathy, occupational vibrational exposure, and renal disease.

It has been established that venous blood flow and axonal transport within the median nerve is compromised with carpal tunnel pressures of 30 mm Hg. This is a carpal canal pressure clinically achievable in the carpal tunnel patient. Pressures in excess of 30 m Hg have been shown in the patient who frequently flexes and extends the wrist, pronates and supinates the forearm, or repeatedly grasps objects. The consequence of chronic compression is damage to the epineural covering of the median nerve resulting in diminished conduction velocity.

The diagnosis of carpal tunnel syndrome is based on information gathered from the history, physical examination, and electrodiagnostic studies. The classic complaint from the patient bothered by carpal tunnel syndrome is paresthesias at night. Paresthesias are typically tingling or numbness in the median nerve distribution of the hand. However, paresthesias can be characterized by some patients as "pins and needles," burning, or simply pain. Secondary symptoms include paresthesias encountered while holding a book or newspaper ("reading paresthesias") or paresthesias encountered while driving ("driving paresthesias"). Other complaints vary from "clumsiness" of the hands, such that objects are often dropped and fine digital tasks are difficult, to

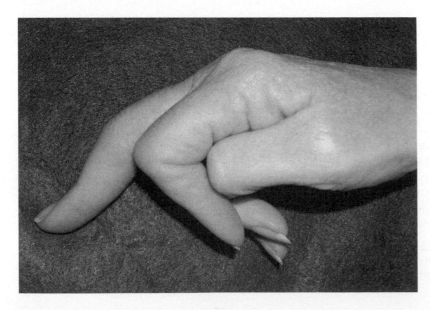

FIGURE 14-1. Posttraumatic Boutonnière deformity.

generalized hand weakness. In the elderly complaints of "constant numbness" are often heard.

Provocative testing includes Phalen's test, Tinel's test at the wrist, or the carpal tunnel compression test (Durkan's test). The carpal tunnel compression test is generally regarded as the most sensitive. This test is administered by holding pressure directly over the median nerve at the wrist. A positive test is acknowledged when the patient experiences paresthesias in the median nerve distribution within 30 seconds of the onset of the test. The most predictable sensory test to evaluate carpal tunnel syndrome is the Semmes-Weinstein monofilament test, where threshold testing of sensation is performed using various sizes of nylon filaments. Vibrometry has also been shown to be a useful sensory test for carpal tunnel syndrome.

Although recommended by most, efficacy of the electrodiagnostic testing for diagnosing carpal tunnel syndrome is debated by some. Finsen et al. reported in one series that 22% of patients who had normal nerve electrodiagnostic studies had a good outcome following carpal tunnel release surgery, indicating a substantial false-positive rate for the testing. Electrodiagnostic tests include the nerve conduction velocity (NCV) measurements and the electromyogram (EMG). The NCV is considered positive for carpal tunnel syndrome when the median motor distal latency is ≥ 4.5 ms or the distal sensory latency is >3.5 ms. In more advanced cases, diminished action potential may also be seen. On the EMG portion of the study, the presence of positive sharp waves, increased insertional activity, decreased muscle recruitment, or polyphasic activity is indicative of substantial nerve dysfunction.

The mainstay of nonoperative management is nocturnal splinting, particularly for mild or moderate carpal tunnel syndrome. When consistently used for a period of 4 to 6 weeks, permanent relief of symptoms can ensue. Other nonoperative measures include nonsteroidal anti-inflammatory agents (NSAIDs), carpal tunnel injections, ultrasound, phonophoresis, nerve gliding or stretching, and vitamin B_6. No data shows any clear advantage of adding these measures with or instead of splinting. Corticosteroid injections have been shown to have long-term efficacy in only 22% of patients with symptoms longer than 1 year. Relief of symptoms following injections has been shown to correlate as a predictor of surgical success. Work modifications to prevent sustained wrist movements or provocative wrist positioning may play a greater role than any of the nonoperative measures except splinting.

Some studies have suggested the preventative effect of wrist and hand exercises in certain occupational environments.

Surgical treatment of carpal tunnel syndrome is considered when two of the following criteria are meet following at least a 3-month course of nonoperative care: persisting symptoms, positive physical examination, and positive electrodiagnostic testing. Absolute indications for surgery are constant paresthesias, thenar atrophy, and markedly delayed median motor nerve conduction velocity or abnormal EMG testing. The surgical procedure consists of increasing the volume of the carpal canal by transecting the transverse carpal ligament. An MRI study has shown that division of the transverse carpal ligament expands the volume of the carpal canal by as much as 25%. In some instances, such as in rheumatoid arthritis, the addition of a flexor tenosynovectomy is needed. The surgical procedure is most commonly performed through a small longitudinal incision at the base of the palm, in line with the ring finger. Care must be taken to avoid injury to the thenar motor branch of the median nerve, which has variable anatomy. Misplaced or transverse incisions about the wrist may jeopardize the palmar cutaneous branch of the median nerve. Other reported complications with open carpal tunnel decompression include ulnar nerve and artery injury.

An alternative technique to the open carpal tunnel decompression is the endoscopic carpal tunnel release. Various authors have reported success rates equal to the open carpal tunnel release with less scar tenderness and quicker return to work. Concerns still, however, remain regarding the safety and efficacy of the endoscopic technique. Van Heest et al., Lee et al., and Schwartz et al., have reported incomplete release of the transverse carpal ligament using the endoscopic technique in cadaver models. Devastating complications such as median nerve transection and flexor tendon transection have been reported causing some to carefully scrutinize the routine use of the endoscopic technique.

Irrespective of the method of surgical decompression chosen, it has been well established that success from carpal tunnel surgery can approach 98% when only subjective complaints are considered. It has been generally held that these results diminish with age. It has been shown that workers applying for worker's compensation can be anticipated to have worse overall results and a slower recovery compared to a similar group of patients not submitting worker's compensation claims.

COMPLEX REGIONAL PAIN SYNDROME

In 1766, Hunter introduced the term *algodystrophy* in describing pain of uncertain origin. In 1864 Mitchell introduced the term *causalgia* to describe nerve pain following an amputation. More recently Evans forwarded the term *reflex sympathetic dystrophy* (RSD) to identify a condition that included pain, swelling, hyperhydrosis, skin color changes, skin temperature changes, stiffness, and underlying osteoporosis, with all symptoms potentially reversible with stellate ganglion blockade. Other terms often used in place of RSD include *Sudeck's atrophy*, *shoulder-hand syndrome*, or "*allodynia.*" These complex and often confusing terms for pain of uncertain origin has lead to the classification system of complex regional pain syndrome (CRPS) typed I and II. Simply stated, CRPS type I is a condition whereby pain had developed following an inciting painful circumstance. In this condition the pain, however, seems to develop out of proportion to the clinical situation. Associated findings include edema, skin blood flow changes, and abnormal sudomotor activity such as hyperhydrosis. CRPS type II has a similar clinical presentation but is associated with a known nerve injury. The predominant symptoms and findings of the initial stage are constant pain, hyperhydrosis, and a hypersensitivity to touch. The second stage of the condition is characterized more by stiffness and pain, while in stage III patients experience diminished pain but overall disuse of the extremity. The pathophysiology of CRPS is still unknown.

To date the most reliable tool for the diagnosis of CRPS is the physical examination. Other less reliable tests include the three-phase bone scan, thermography, the quantitative sudomotor axon reflex test (QSART), and plain radiography. Increased uptake is anticipated in the later phases of the bone scan while osteopenia is a later finding in the CRPS patient. CRPS I has been reported to occur following as many as 25% of all distal radius fractures. A risk factor is displacement requiring reduction. It is generally regarded that those patients experiencing CRPS of an extremity are at greater risk of recurrent symptoms following a surgical procedure.

The initial treatment of CRPS requires prompt recognition and diagnosis. Most patients diagnosed within the first 6 to 8 weeks respond favorably to treatment. Initially, hand therapy plays an important role in the treatment of CRPS. Such techniques as massage, edema control, gentle passive motion (to prevent contracture), contrast baths, and use of the transelectrical stimulator unit (TENS) have proven effective. The key concept to remember when embarking on hand therapy is the patient must be exercised within the limits of pain, otherwise a flare-up of the condition may result. Initial drug therapies have included the use of β-blocker medication (propranolol), calcium channel blockers medication (nifedipine), guanethidine, neurontin (anticonvulsant medication), nasal calcitonin, and 6-day medrol dose packs—all with some limited success. The role of NSAIDs, although theoretically attractive, has shown limited benefit.

In patients with CRPS I or II, pain may be sympathetically mediated or sympathetically independent. In those with sympathetically mediated pain, stellate ganglion blocks may be diagnostic as well as curative for the condition. Multiple such injections may be necessary to realize a benefit and are indicated when other above-mentioned measures are not effective. Surgical stellate ganglion ablation is yet another treatment alternative.

CONGENITAL HAND ANOMALIES

Congentital anomalies of the upper limb account for over 10% of all birth defects. The limb bud forms adjacent to the fifth through seventh cervical somites and can be visualized at day 25 following fertilization. During the ensuing 25 days the limb develops rapidly with individual digits and web spaces well defined. It is during this period of embryogenesis that anomalies occur due to either malformation, deformation, disruption, or dysplasia. Syndactyly (incompletely separated digits) and polydactyly (extra digits) are generally considered the most common forms of congenital hand anomalies. Certain anomalies may be associated with midline congenital defects such as those affecting the heart, lungs, or kidneys, while other congenital hand anomalies may appear as isolated events. Appropriate pediatric and medical genetic workup is recommended in all patients with upper extremity congenital anomalies. Surgery is often necessary in these children with a goal of completing all hand reconstruction by the time hand preference is established, which is approximately 2 years of age.

Radial Club Hand

Radial aplasia or radial club hand is a condition where the radius is incompletely formed or even completely absent (Figure 14-2). The condition

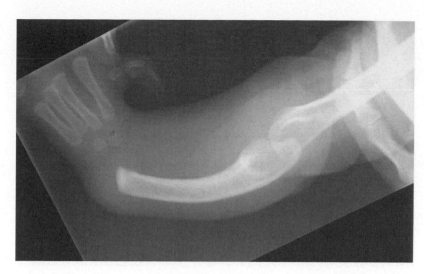

FIGURE 14-2. Radial aplasia with absence of entire radius.

may be classified as type 1—short radius, type 2—hypoplastic radius (radius growth substantially retarded), type 3—partial absence of the radius (miniature radius), or type 4—completely absent radius. Type 4 is the most common variant. The condition is frequently associated with thumb hypoplasia or complete thumb absence. In types 2–4 hypoplastic or absent radial-sided structures—including the radial artery, flexor carpi radialis tendon, or the radial wrist extensors—may contribute to the condition. Radial aplasia often associated with other conditions such as Holt-Oram syndrome, TAR syndrome (thrombocytopenia absent radius), VATER (vertebral defects, anal atresia, tracheo-esophageal atresia, esophageal atresia, and renal defects), and Fanconi's anemia. The condition occurs in 1/100,000 live births and is bilateral in 50% of children affected.

Type 1 and some type 2 deformities do not require surgery. More severe radial inclination of the hand is seen in the type 3 and type 4 radial aplasia patients, resulting in a hand that is poorly functioning and cosmetically objectionable. Contraindication to surgical correction includes poor general health, severely compromised overall functional ability, or ipsilateral elbow extension contracture. In the situation of the elbow extension contracture, the radial club hand allows the patient to reach the mouth.

Treatment consists of two stages. The first is correction of the soft tissue contractures by either closed manipulation and serial casting, or by ring external fixator application. The second stage consists of centralization of the carpus on the ulna with pin stabilization and sometimes ulnar osteotomy.

At the same time, radial extensor tendon releases and transfers to the ulnar side of the wrist is frequently needed. Thumb hypoplasia surgery is also commonly needed in the patients requiring surgical correction of the radial club hand. The failure of correction or recurrent deformity is the most common problem following reconstruction of radial aplasia.

Thumb Hypoplasia

Thumb hypoplasia occurs most commonly in the context of radial aplasia (Figure 14-3). The hypoplastic thumb may have varying degrees of intrinsic muscle deficiency, first web space narrowing, ulnar collateral ligament instability, generalized short bones, or instability of the thumb carpometacarpal (CMC) joint. In general, those hypoplastic thumbs with an unstable thumb CMC joint are not reconstructable and require ablation. Reconstructive procedures for salvageable hypoplastic thumbs include web space deepening, ulnar collateral ligament reconstruction, and tendon transfers. For the unreconstructable thumb, the index finger may be transposed to create a stable, opposable thumb. This procedure is known as pollicization.

Madelung's Deformity

Madelung's deformity occurs due to a growth disturbance of the ulnar and palmar portions of the distal radial metaphysis resulting in relative overgrowth and dorsal subluxation of the ulna (Figure 14-4). Patients present some time during

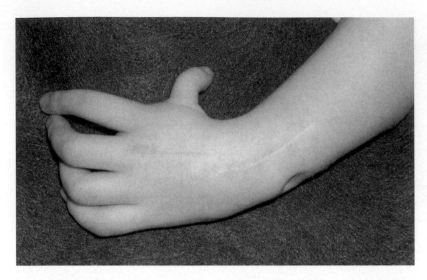

FIGURE 14-3. Unstable, hypoplastic thumb in patient with radial aplasia.

adolescence due to wrist deformity and sometimes due to pain. Radiographically, a steep ulnar slope with a deficient ulnar margin of the radius characterizes the condition. The carpus translates volar and ulnar resulting in the lunate being relatively "uncovered." If the condition is identified early in

adolescence, a distal radius physiolysis can restore a relatively normal growth pattern, correcting the deformity. Traditionally, the treatment for Madelung's deformity has commenced at the end of growth and has included a distal radius joint leveling procedure along with an ulnar shortening procedure.

Syndactyly

Syndactyly comes from the Greek words "syn" (fused) and "dactylos" (digit). The condition may occur as frequently as <u>1 in 2,000 live birth</u>s. The syndactyly may be <u>simple</u> (skin webbing only) or <u>complex</u> (skin webbing plus bony fusion); and <u>incomplete</u> (digits with partial separation) or <u>complete</u> (digits with no areas of separation). The most common digits involved are the long and ring fingers (Figure 14-5). Surgery is indicated to separate the syndactalized digits. This procedure involves a complex incision with dorsal and volar limbs that interdigitate. Skin is invariably deficient and full thickness skin grafting from the ipsilateral groin is typically needed. Surgery is performed at or around 18 months of age. The exception in syndactyly is the patient with syndactyly of the thumb/index or the ring/small. In these situations, surgery is indicated by 6 months in order to prevent deformity due to differential bone lengths of these digits.

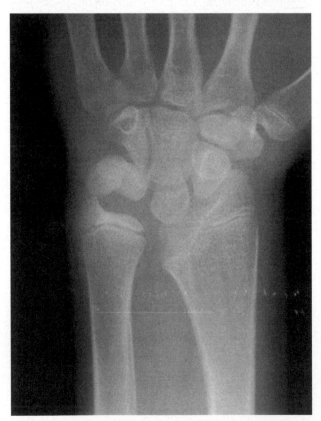

FIGURE 14-4. Madelung's deformity with growth arrest of ulnar and volar aspect of the distal radial physis and relative overgrowth of the ulna.

Polydactyly

Polydactyly, or extra digits, may occur on the thumb side of the hand, on the small finger side of the hand or in the center portion of the hand. Thumb

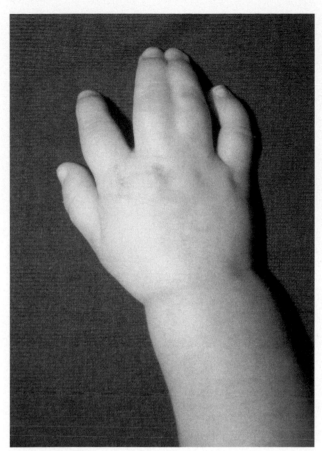

FIGURE 14-5. Complete, simple syndactyly of the long and ring fingers.

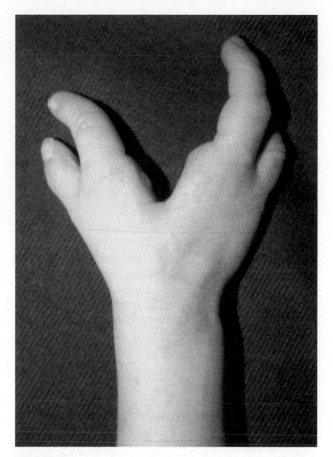

FIGURE 14-6. Cleft hand.

polydactyly may occur as several different types with the goal of treatment being the creation of one stable and cosmetically normal appearing thumb. The more ulnar of the two thumbs is the more robust digit and elements from the radial-most thumb are harvested to supplement it. Common post-reconstruction problems can include MCP joint instability. Small finger polydactyly is more common in black newborns. In these babies the duplicate digit may be well developed with a bony skeleton or a vestigial skin tag. The well-formed digit requires a formal surgical ablation at a later age. Vestigial polydactylous digits may simply be tied off in the nursery. Central polydactyly is an extra digit that affects the index, long, or more commonly, the ring finger. It is often associated with syndactyly or the cleft hand.

Cleft Hand

The untreated cleft hand has been described by Adrian Flatt as "a functional triumph and a social disaster." This congenital defect is characterized by a V-shaped cleft in the central portion of the hand associated with the absence of one or more digital rays (Figure 14-6). The cause is not known but most likely suppression of the growth of the central rays occurring at or about the seventh week of fetal development. Additional anomalies seen with this condition include polydactyly, syndactyly, and cleft palate. The principles of treatment include closure of the cleft, reconstruction of any syndactylous digits, and deepening of the first web space.

CRYSTALLINE ARTHROPATHY OF THE HAND AND WRIST

Gout is most commonly a result of an underexcretion of uric acid that leads to the deposition of monosodium urate crystals and intermittent acute articular swelling, which is termed acute gouty arthritis. Occasionally the syndrome can also occur due to the overproduction of uric acid. Gout is approximately 10 times more common in men than women and has a predilection for middle-aged males. The attacks often occur suddenly and are characterized by severe pain, warmth, and erythema. The consumption of alcohol, trauma, or acute medical illnesses can cause an attack. Attacks often also occur following a surgical procedure. Monosodium urate crystals have a lower solubility quotient at colder temperatures; therefore some have speculated that this is the cause for the gout commonly affecting the distal aspects of the extremities. Gout can affect the wrist, MCP, PIP, and DIP joints. In fact, its sudden onset can lure the unsuspecting medical student toward acute septic arthritis. The diagnosis of acute gouty arthritis is made by joint aspiration of negative birefringent, monosodium urate crystals. The treatment of gout generally does not require surgery. Colchicine, NSAIDS, or corticosteroid medication is used in the treatment of acute gout. Chronic tophaceous gout is treated with allopurinol. Occasionally, gouty tophi require surgical debridement, particularly from the carpal tunnel following the development of secondary carpal tunnel syndrome.

Calcium pyrophosphate dihydrate deposition (CPPD), or pseudogout, occurs due to the deposition of birefringent CPPD crystals into the joint, activating an inflammatory cascade. In these patients, sudden swelling, pain, and warmth occur. The wrist and the MCP joints are the most commonly affected joints of the upper extremity. And like gout, it can be misdiagnosed as infection. The condition more frequently occurs in the older age groups, particularly females. In these patients, chondrocalcinosis is frequently seen on plain radiographs, particularly in the triangular fibrocartilage of the wrist (Figure 14-7). Trauma and acute

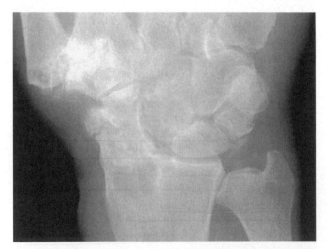

FIGURE 14-7. PA wrist radiograph showing chondrocalcinosis within the fibrocartilage of the triangular fibrocartilage complex (TFCC) of the wrist.

medical illnesses can trigger attacks. Similar to gout, treatment is primarily nonsurgical. For the wrist, joint aspiration with injection of 10 mg of Kenalog is generally successful in minimizing an acute attack. For other joints in the hand, NSAIDS may be useful.

DEGENERATIVE ARTHRITIS OF THE HAND AND WRIST

Degenerative arthritis or osteoarthritis of the hand and wrist is one of the more common afflictions seen in society. Causes include posttraumatic, post–repetitive stress, or idiopathic, and may be symmetrical or bilateral. This condition distinguishes itself from the systemic and symmetrical inflammatory arthropathies. Patients often complain of localized pain following certain provocative activities. There may be swelling and pain with passive range of motion, which are hallmarks of arthritis in general. A history of fracture may be related but this is not always the case. Scapholunate advanced collapse (SLAC) wrist is a type of degenerative arthritis of the wrist that primarily affects the radio-scaphoid articulation and spares the radiolunate articulation (Figure 14-8). Advanced cases have midcarpal joint involvement with resulting loss of carpal height and migration of the capitate proximally between the scaphoid and lunate articulation. This is easily identifiable on plain wrist radiographs. Patients may relate a history of wrist ligamentous injury, such as a scapholunate ligament disruption, or radiographs may reveal an old scaphoid nonunion. Most of these patients display weak grip and diminished range of motion. In a study of over 200 wrists with primary osteoarthritis of the wrist, the SLAC wrist pattern was identified as the most common pattern. Initial nonoperative measures include activity restriction, splinting, NSAIDs, and injections. Although many patients may remain without symptoms for years, some patients require operative intervention for relief of pain. Temporizing operative treatment includes wrist debridement and de-innervation procedures where the radiocarpal articular branches of the anterior and posterior interosseous are cut in an effort to relieve pain. Salvage procedures for SLAC wrist include removal of the scaphoid with midcarpal fusion (scaphoidectomy with four-corner fusion); removal of the scaphoid, lunate, and triquetrum thus shortening the carpus and allowing the head of the capitate to articulate in the lunate fossa (proximal

STT fusion. Problems with this operation have included persistant pain and nonunion of the fusion mass. This outcome has prompted some authors to recommend the same treatment that will be discussed for degenerative arthritis of the thumb: removal of the trapezium and tendon reconstruction of the ligaments of the base of the thumb.

Thumb carpometacarpal joint osteoarthritis is one of the most common forms of arthritis in the body. Females in the sixth and seventh decade of life are approximately eight times more likely to develop the condition than males. Patients complain of pain at the base of the thumb with most activities of daily living, such as turning keys or pinching objects between the thumb and index finger. The thumb axis itself may be misshapen with the first web space narrowed and the thumb MCP joint hyperextended to aid in grasping objects. Radiographs show narrowing of the carpometacarpal joint of the thumb (Figure 14-9). Initial nonoperative treatment includes thumb-spica splinting,

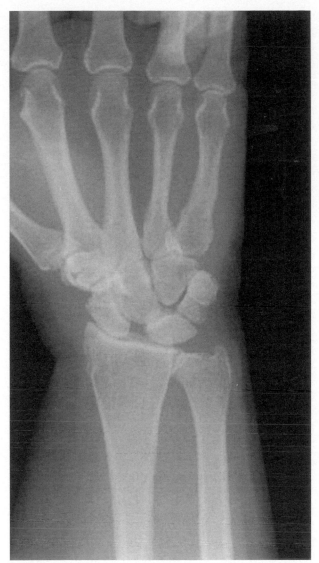

FIGURE 14-8. Scapholunate advanced collapse of the wrist (SLAC), the most common pattern of primary degenerative arthritis of the wrist.

row carpectomy); and complete wrist fusion. The choice of operative treatment is individualized.

Scapho-trapezial-trapezoidal arthritis (STT arthritis) is a form of thumb base arthritis. In these patients articulation involving the scaphoid, the trapezium, and the trapezoid degenerates. These patients may localize their discomfort at the base of the thumb joint or in the wrist in general. This form of degenerative arthritis is less common than SLAC wrist but is also recognized as either posttraumatic or idiopathic. Patients will experience difficulties with pinch tasks in particular. Initial treatment is also nonoperative similar to the treatment for SLAC wrist. Operative treatment has classically been the

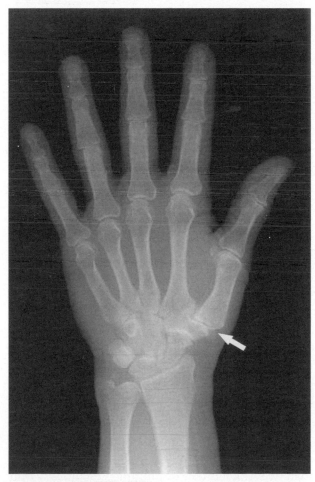

FIGURE 14-9. Thumb carpometacarpal degenerative arthritis of the wrist (white arrow).

NSAIDs, and injections. If patients fail to respond to these nonoperative measures, surgery may prove helpful. Surgery entails removal of the arthritic CMC joint by complete trapezium removal and harvest of the flexor carpi radialis (FCR) tendon. The FCR tendon is used to reconstruct the primary ligamentous stabilizer of the basilar thumb joint—the anterior oblique retinacular ligament. One long-term study showed high patient satisfaction at 10 years average follow-up. Although initial success was reported, long-term failures with the Silastic trapezial implant has been well recognized, due primarily to wear debris from the implant and subsequent fracture. The use of the Silastic trapezial implant is no longer recommended.

Ulnar impaction syndrome occurs when a mismatch in lengths occurs between the ulna and the radius such that the ulna is longer than the radius. The result is that the ulna impales the lunate or possibly the triquetrum during ulnar deviation of the wrist. Coincident with ulnar impaction, the triangular fibrocartilage complex (TFCC) is generally torn or frayed due to the impaction process. The patients complain of ulnar-sided wrist pain with strong grip, which results in ulnar deviation of the wrist. Causes of ulnar impaction syndrome may be posttraumatic or developmental. Initial treatment is nonoperative and includes long arm splinting and NSAIDs. Failure of nonoperative treatment may indicate the patient for operative intervention. The principle of surgical treatment is ulnar shortening. This joint-leveling procedure requires an osteotomy of the ulna at the metaphyseal or diaphyseal junction, necessitating internal fixation with plates and screws. Another less desirable option is distal ulnar resection, also referred to as Darrach procedure. The Darrach procedure is more appropriately performed in the elderly, debilitated individual, as it is not as well tolerated in the young active patient.

DEQUERVAIN'S SYNDROME

The extensor pollicis brevis (EPB) tendon and two abductor pollicis longus (APL) tendons are generally contained within the most radial condensation of the extensor retinaculum system, the first dorsal compartment. DeQuervain's syndrome generally occurs following certain repetitive wrist movements that cause friction within the first dorsal compartment. Anatomic variations such as more than two APL tendons or multiple septations within the first dorsal compartment may predispose to

development of the syndrome. In cadaver studies, first dorsal compartment septations have been found in approximately one-third of individuals. In one study, Jackson et al., reported 67% incidence in patients undergoing surgical treatment for DeQuervain's syndrome. Space occupying lesions such as ganglion cysts also contribute to narrowing of the first dorsal compartment.

Repetitive friction then leads to swelling and narrowing of the compartment resulting in radial-sided wrist pain. Patients will complain of soreness and tenderness at the base of the thumb exacerbated by ulnar deviation of the wrist, strong grasp, or thumb pinch. Inspection will find swelling of the radial side of the wrist in most cases. Physical examination will find tenderness and often warmth directly over the first dorsal compartment. In certain advanced cases, audible squeaking occurs with active thumb movements. The classic test confirming the diagnosis of DeQuervain's syndrome is Finklestein's test. This test is performed with the thumb slightly flexed and abducted into the palm and the wrist ulnarly deviated. A positive test is one where pain is reproduced compared to the contralateral, unaffected side. Often the test is performed incorrectly with the patient clasping the thumb into the palm and the wrist ulnarly deviated. This maneuver, if done vigorously, causes pain in most anyone. If the reader doubts this, he is encouraged to try the maneuver on himself.

Initial treatment for DeQuervain's syndrome is nonoperative. The patient is fitted with a volar forearm-based, thumb-spica splint for nighttime use. A small, lower profile, hand-based splint may be used for daily activities if suited to the patient's lifestyle. NSAIDS may also be of value and should be considered if not contraindicated due to GI intolerance. Additionally, a corticosteriod injection into the first dorsal compartment may provide sustained relief. In one study, Weiss et al. reported that injection was just as effective in DeQuervain's syndrome as splinting alone or splinting combined with injection. In another study of 63 patients, 71% of patients had sustained relief of their symptoms with one first dorsal compartment injection. Skin depigmentation and fat atrophy are known complications of corticosteroid injections of the wrist.

If a 6 to 8 month period of nonoperative treatment fails, then operative intervention can be considered. Surgical treatment is release of the first dorsal compartment under local anesthesia. This is performed through a longitudinal incision directly overlaying the first dorsal compartment. Branches of the superficial radial nerve are particularly vulnerable with this procedure. Care must be exercised in protecting these branches as injury to them can cause substantial disability. Other reported complications of this procedure include volar subluxation of the first dorsal compartment contents and hypertrophic scar formation. It is for these reasons most prefer a prolonged trial of nonoperative therapy.

DUPUYTREN'S CONTRACTURE

Dupuytren's contracture is a thickening and subsequent contraction of the palmar aponeurotic fascia (Figure 14-10). Due to factors that are poorly understood, fibroblasts transform to myofibroblasts with contractile elements (smooth muscle actin) and attach to the cells of the palmar aponeurosis. Trauma has also been mentioned as a possible cause. As the disease progresses, the affected tissues shorten as a unit, ultimately resulting in digital contractures. Along with the digital contracture, skin dimpling

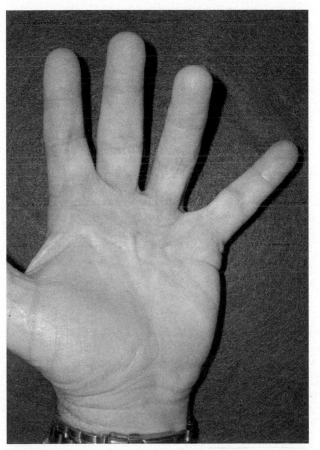

FIGURE 14-10. Dupuytren's disease involving the ring finger.

may occur. Dupuytren's diathesis generally implies a more advanced form of the disease, including "knuckle pads" (thickening over the extensor surfaces of the PIP joints), plantar fibromas (lederhosen disease), and fasciitis of the penis (Peyronie's disease). The disease has a genetic predisposition, as males of Northern European descent are more commonly affected. Incidence among affected families has been reported to approach 70%. Although the genetic predisposition in Dupuytren's disease has been well established, the condition is seen more commonly in patients with seizures, patients who use alcohol and tobacco, and patients with diabetes. Also, the combination of carpal tunnel syndrome, trigger finger, and Dupuytren's contracture has been appreciated in the diabetic population. The most commonly affected digit is the ring finger, but any finger can be affected. The prodrome of Dupuytren's contracture is inflammation with tenderness in the palm. Later, contracture ensues on an unpredictable course. The bands of palmar fascia are termed *cords* when affected by Dupuytren's disease. The most common pattern of cord development is the pretendinous cord in the palm, which progresses to cause a MCP joint contracture. The pretendinous cord develops directly over the flexor tendon system in the palm. Secondarily, a PIP joint contracture may develop due to the formation of a spiral cord that is the condensation of several diseased fascial bands in the finger. The most notable is Grayson's ligament that is a digital aponeurotic element attaching to skin volar to the digital nerve and artery. The spiral cord is so named because it often entraps the digital nerve and the digital artery along the radial or ulnar borders of the finger. Following the acute inflammatory prodrome stage of the disease, pain is usually not encountered as the contracture progresses. At some point, patients seek medical attention due to the inability to straighten their hands, making tasks such as shaking hands or donning gloves difficult. In extreme cases, the contracture can become so severe that palmar maceration develops, posing a hygiene problem.

In 1831, Dupuytren outlined the first treatment for the disease that came to bear his name, although the nature of this disease had been described years earlier by Felix Plater, Henry Cline, and Sir Ashley Cooper. For many years a variety of nonoperative treatments have been tried, all without success but, as Dupuytren first described, surgery is the preferred treatment for this condition. Although simple transection of the pretendinous cords is a viable option in the elderly or the debilitated patient, the surgery for symptomatic Dupuytren's contracture has evolved into a formal fasciectomy of the involved palmar tissue. The indications for surgery are debilitating contracture of the MCP joints or any contracture of the PIP joint. Contractures of the MCP joints are easily corrected under most circumstances. In contrast, contractures of the PIP joints are often incompletely corrected and are fraught with recurrence.

Dupuytren's fasciectomy can be performed through the standard zigzag Bruner incisions, unless the deformity is severe. With severe contracture, the fundamental problem becomes one of skin coverage after the fascia is removed and the contracture corrected. In severe cases of Dupuytren's contracture, a longitudinal incision with multiple opposing Z-plasties can be utilized to expand the coverage potential of the existing skin. Alternatively, McCash described a technique whereby fasciectomy skin incisions can be made in the transverse skin creases of the palm and the digits, without closure. The wounds then heal by secondary intention so motion is not inhibited following complex wound coverage procedures. Another alternative is performing the standard Bruner incision and leaving portions of that wound open following fasciectomy, either in the palm or in the digit. Yet another option is dermofasciectomy where diseased fascial elements are excised along with overlying skin and the resulting defect skin grafted. Whatever the surgical technique employed, the dissection of the palmar fascial can be tedious, particularly in advanced or recurrent cases. Extreme care must be exercised in dissecting the diseased fascial cords from the digital nerves and arteries because nerve injury or even nerve division can result.

One of the greatest challenges for the patient and the hand surgeon is maintaining the improvements in MCP and PIP motion following fasciectomy. Maintaining motion improvements requires close postoperative supervision by a hand therapist. Within the first 3 to 5 days the dressing is changed, and the patient is placed in an extension splint. Care is taken to not cause ischemia of the palmar skin flaps. It is important to also start active flexion exercises of the MCP and PIP joints. The patient's progress must be closely monitored and the exercise protocol modified as necessary to achieve the optimal balance between achieving digital extension and maintaining composite finger flexion.

Most patients are satisfied with the surgical outcome of palmar fasciectomy, although complete corrections of PIP joint contractures are rarely achieved. Recurrence of Dupuytren's contracture following fasciectomy has been well recognized with the incidence approaching 50% in some series. Complications of fasciectomy surgery for Dupuytren's contracture include digital nerve neuropraxia and digital sensory compromise, digital nerve division, digital ischemia, wound healing problems, and complex regional pain syndrome type 1 or type 2. Surgery for recurrent disease can be challenging even for the most experienced surgeons, with complications such as amputation having been reported.

INFECTIONS OF THE HAND AND WRIST

Felons and Paronychia

Felons and paronychial infections are the most common infections of the hand. These infections are localized in the digit. The felon is an abscess of the pulp on the pad of the fingertip. Due to the multiple septa present within the pad of the finger, an infection in this region can gain substantial pressure and become quite painful. The most commonly encountered organism is *Staphylococcus aureus*. The infection occurs secondary to direct inoculation, such as might occur following the introduction of a foreign body. Like the treatment of any other abscess, incision and drainage is the most effective treatment. The surgical decompression is best done through straight lateral incisions. Incisions directly over the finger pad are often painful and should be avoided. When the pulp is decompressed, care should be taken to break up all the septae within the pulp of the fingertip to assure that no loculation is missed. The treatment is originally supplemented with oral *S. aureus* coverage, and antibiotics should be changed if cultures show a different infection organism. Generally antibiotics are continued for 7 to 10 days. In severe infections with ascending lymphangitis, IV antibiotics may be necessary.

Paronychial infections are digital infections that occur about the nail fold (eponychium). Bacteria colonize underneath the nail fold and adhere to the nailplate. The most common organism is *S. aureus*. Causes of the paronychial infection include direct trauma, nail biting, artificial nails, and manicures. Patients with diabetes mellitus are more susceptible to developing these infections. Most paronychial infections respond to warm soaks and oral *S. aureus*

[handwritten margin note: • incision on lateral aspect of digits should be done on: • Radial asp of thumb • Ulnar asp of other digits (so, not to affect tactile sensation & pinching).]

coverage. Surgical drainage about the eponychial fold is indicated if an abscess is identified. Chronic or recurrent infections typically require removal of the nailplate because bacteria or fugal elements notoriously adhere to the nailplate beneath the nail fold. Candida albicans is one of the more common causes of recurrent of chronic paronychial infections. In patients not responsive to incision and drainage, nail removal, and culture-specific antibiotic therapy, eponychial marsupialization (wide debridement) leaving the wound open may be necessary.

Septic Flexor Tenosynovitis

If not treated early, septic flexor tenosynovitis is often devastating, leaving scar within the flexor tendon sheath and leading to substantial digital dysfunction. Septic flexor tenosynovitis often occurs secondary to a puncture wound or a deep digital cut that never receives proper attention. The diagnosis is made on clinical grounds. Patients typically present with one or more Kanaval signs: <u>tenderness along the flexor tendon sheath</u>, <u>flexed digital posture</u>, <u>fusiform swelling of the digit</u>, and <u>pain with passive stretching of the digit.</u> There is generally a history of trauma, particularly a puncture wound. Treatment must be initiated early if scarring of the flexor tendon sheath and ultimate disability is to be avoided. Infrequently, symptoms may be identified within 24 hours of onset; these patients will occasionally respond promptly to IV antibiotic therapy. Patients, however, must be carefully observed for recurrence. Those patients not promptly responding to IV antibiotics or those patients who have had symptoms longer than 24 hours are indicated for emergent surgical drainage. Surgical treatment consists of closed flexor tendon sheath irrigation using a small catheter inserted in the palm at the A1 pulley and the sheath drained at the level of the A5 pulley through an midaxial incision along the lateral aspect of the finger. No clear advantage has been shown with open tendon sheath irrigation or from postoperative tendon sheath irrigation accomplished by leaving the catheter in place.

Palmar Abscess

The deep spaces of the hand may also be subject to abscess formation. The deep spaces of the hand are actually "potential spaces" and consist of the thenar space (located deep to the flexor pollicis longus tendon), hypothenar space (containing the hypothenar muscles), the adductor space (located posterior to the adductor pollicis muscle), and the midpalmar space (located deep to the flexor tendons). Palmar abscesses are the result of a deep puncture wound. Patients often present 2 to 3 days after the event, complaining of pain, warmth, tenderness, and redness. Surgical drainage is indicated followed by culture-specific antibiotics. These infections can endanger the entire upper extremity and, especially in the immunocompromised host, are surgical emergencies.

Human and Other Animal Bites

Animal bites occur frequently. In general, the resultant bacterial infections and ultimate complications are less severe than the bacterial infections from human bites. From dog and cat bites, the most common organisms are streptococcus. *Pasturella multocida* is also a common infecting organism. Due to the sharp nature of the cat tooth, cat bites tend to become infected more often than dog bites. The initial treatment for any animal bite is prophylactic with cleansing of the wound and broad spectrum oral antibiotic coverage. Any bite developing a local abscess with or without ascending lymphangitis is indicated for emergent surgical debridement. Patients with ascending lymphangitis following a cat or dog bite should be admitted to the hospital for IV antibiotic therapy and close observation.

Typically, human bite wounds have a greater potential for infection, are colonized by more virulent organisms, and have a greater number of potential pathogens than animal bite wounds. The most common bacteria are streptococcus and staphylococcus. Eikenella is another common human oral flora that is notorious for causing infection following a clinched fist injury that strikes an opponent's tooth. Uncomplicated human bite wounds, which do not involve a joint, tendon, or nerve, may be treated with local wound care. Alternatively, a penetrating bite wound, such as occurs following a clinched fist injury, demands surgical exploration and debridement to inspect for extensor tendon injury, metacarpal phalangeal joint capsule penetration, and articular surface abrasions or defects. The wound is left open. Obvious infections seen following human bite injuries require surgical debridement and culture-specific antibiotics. While cultures are maturing following initial debridement, broad empiric antibiotic coverage should begin, covering staph, strep, and anaerobic bacteria. Eikenella infections are usually sensitive to penicillin G.

Osteomyelitis

Fortunately, due to extensive blood supply, osteomyelitis of the hand is rare, representing less than 5% of all cases of infection in the hand. Of the bones of the hand and wrist, the distal phalanx is the most commonly affected. The origin of osteomyelitis of the hand is often related to trauma with open fractures of the hand the most common situation. Penetrating wounds such as bites or puncture wounds are other common vehicles. But osteomyelitis can also be seen following elective hand surgery. Patients with diabetes or who are immunocompromised are the most susceptible to developing osteomyelitis. The most common infecting organism is *S. aureus*. Methicillin-resistant *S. aureus* is seen with increasing frequency. Clinical signs include pain, swelling, and often an open draining wound. Radiographic signs include a lucency with a sclerotic rim (Figure 14-11). Extensive surgical debridement and sustained use with culture-specific antibiotic therapy under the direction of an infectious disease specialist is the necessary treatment of this condition.

imp → it may be useful to prescribe a short course of oral Abx for diabetics

Atypical Mycobacterium Infections

The mycobacterium species are aerobic Gram-positive bacilli. Infections from the atypical mycobacterial organisms are often slow growing and underappreciated. The most widely recognized among these bacteria is the *Mycobacterium marinum* species. These bacteria are most commonly harbored on fresh or particularly saltwater environments. Infection usually requires some penetrating injury from aquatic equipment or marine organisms. Clinically the patients present with or are sent in referral due to painless cutaneous lesions. Draining skin lesions may also be present. The slow-growing nature of these bacteria makes their culturing difficult. Therefore, the bacteria should be cultured on Lowenstein-Jensen plates incubated at a cooler temperature (31°C). A culture time of 6 weeks is sometimes necessary to demonstrate growth. An exception to this is the *Mycobacterium fortuitum* species that is a more rapid growing variety that typically can be isolated within 1 week of

N.B: Remember always to send swabs for C&S and include atypical organism & fungi.

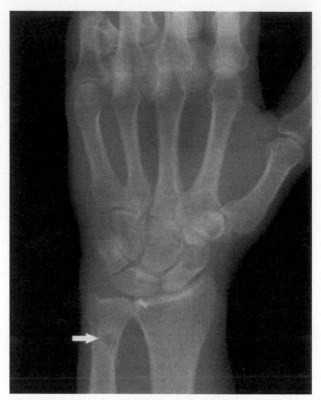

FIGURE 14-11. Osteomyelitis of the ulna following a pin-tract infection (lytic lesion depicted by white arrow).

culture. Surgical debridement is necessary for the subdermal infections. Complete surgical debridement is rarely accomplished as the infection can be very infiltrating. Combination therapy is the preferred antibiotic treatment. Empiric drug therapy must be started following biopsy and culture because the time needed to grow the organism is long. Antibiotic therapy may include a combination of minocycline, clarithromycin, rifampin, ethambutol, or trimethoprim-sulfamethoxazole. Alternatively, single drug therapy may be used. Duration of antibiotic therapy can last 1 year. Recurrence is common.

Necrotizing Fasciitis and Clostridial Myonecrosis

Necrotizing fasciitis is a serious, potentially life-threatening infection involving the fascia and subcutaneous tissues. As the name implies, the affected fascia and fat becomes necrotic. Consequently, the nutrient blood supply to the skin is compromised, and skin blistering and sloughing can also occur. The most common causative organism is β-hemolytic streptococcus. Patients may present with a localized area of erythema or an abscess that rapidly progresses as the infection dissects along superficial and deep fascial planes (Figure 14-12). The situation can occur following relatively innocuous wounds or trauma in otherwise healthy individuals. However, the infection is more common among those patients with immunocompromising conditions such as diabetes, IV drug abuse, and inflammatory arthritic disorders. Severe pain and edema may ensue and gas may be present on plain film radiography. Patients may become critically ill, requiring resuscitative measures due to septic shock, respiratory distress, and multisystem organ failure. Nearly one-third of all patients who develop necrotizing fasciitis die. The mortality rate may approach 75% where the infection spreads to the chest wall.

Treatment requires emergent, aggressive surgical debridement and early multimodal antibiotic therapy. Specifically, clindamycin may be considered for strep and staph species, penicillin for anaerobic bacteria, and gentamycin to cover Gram-negative bacteria. Multiple debridements are frequently needed to remove all necrotic tissue. Above elbow amputation, shoulder disarticulation, or four-quarter amputation is often necessary to control the infection and prevent death.

Clostridial myonecrosis (or "gas gangrene") is an aerobic infection caused by *Clostridium perfringens*, a toxin-producing, Gram-positive bacteria. As the name implies, toxins cause necrosis of muscle as well as subcutaneous tissue and fat. The infection then "snow balls" as local nutrient vessels are destroyed and relative local tissue hypoxia occurs. Culture of the clostridia species is difficult and requires sodium glycolate agar and an anaerobic environment. Predisposing factors for development of clostridial myonecrosis include crush injuries with open fractures and devitalized muscle, foreign contamination, immunosuppression, and hypovolemic shock. Patients develop massive edema and skin discoloration. Plain radiographs show gas formation within the soft tissue shadow of the muscle. Septic shock often ensues. In patients suspected of clostridial myonecrosis, aggressive surgical debridement is necessary with particular attention to the removal of any devitalized muscle. If Gram's stain shows Gram-positive rods, high dose penicillin therapy is started. Amputation is performed for life threatening situations. Several authors have reported success with the use of hyperbaric oxygen (HBO) treatment in patients with clostridial myonecrosis. Randomized, controlled studies, however, are lacking. With aggressive surgical debridement, antibiotic therapy, and HBO, mortality in the range of 20% can be expected. Fortunately, the incidence of clostridial myonecrosis is rare.

Septic Arthritis

Septic arthritis of the wrist and hand is unusual. The most common inciting event is penetrating trauma, however, hematogenous spread may also be the cause, especially in the immunocompromised host. Like most other infections of the hand and wrist, predisposing factors include diabetes, alcoholism, IV drug abuse, chronic renal failure, advanced age, enteral corticosteroid usage, and inflammatory arthritis.

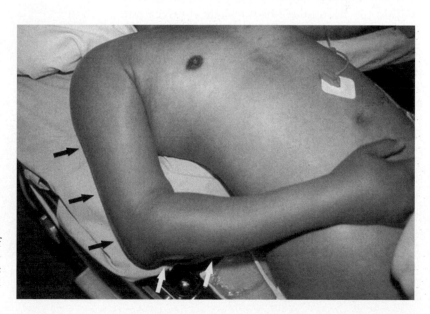

FIGURE 14-12. The rapid progression of necrotizing fasciitis of the arm (black arrows) following the development of a septic olecranon bursa in an immunocompromised patient.

- Mean Variance = 0.9mm (4.2 – 2.3 mm) → Neutral Variance ↓ 80% of loads by Radius
20% of load by Ulna

When the bacterial count within a synovial joint exceeds $100,000/cm^3$ a clinical infection will develop. Once infection develops, bacterial toxins and proteolytic enzymes are released that destroy cartilage. As the articular proteolytic enzymes are broken down the host mounts an inflammatory response, which consists of polymorphonuclear lymphocytes, lymphocytes, and macrophages. The end result of this process is the production of pus. As pus collects, pressure increases causing further articular damage due to inhibition of slowed articular blood flow and ultimate articular oxygen exchange. Ultimately joint ankylosis and contiguous osteomyelitis result if the condition is left untreated. *Staphylococcus aureus* is the most common cause of septic arthritis of the joints of the hand and wrist. Physical examination reveals warmth, swelling, and joint tenderness. The patient may complain of pain and a recent febrile illness. Laboratory examination reveals an elevated white blood cell (WBC) count in only half of the cases. The sedimentation rate and the C-reactive protein levels, however, are consistently elevated. Diagnosis is confirmed by joint aspiration with a WBC above $50,000/mm^3$. Additionally, cloudy synovial fluid aspirate also suggests the diagnosis of a septic arthritis.

imp

Treatment consists of prompt surgical drainage and culture-specific antibiotics. Empiric therapy for *S. aureus* should be initiated immediately after cultures are obtained. The differential diagnosis of the acutely swollen wrist should include CPPD. CPPD of the wrist is often misdiagnosed as a septic wrist. Patients with CPPD of the wrist will likewise have a painful, swollen, and warm wrist joint. These patients will often have notable calcifications within the triangular fibrocartilage complex and a normal WBC count. Joint aspiration will demonstrate positive birefringent crystal and a WBC well less than the $50,000/mm^3$ expected for a septic wrist. Patients with an acute attack of CPPD of the wrist will respond quite promptly to immobilization and NSAIDs.

KEINBOCK'S DISEASE

Keinbock's disease is osteonecrosis of the lunate. By a mechanism that still is not entirely understood, the blood flow to the lunate bone of the wrist is compromised to such an extent that osteonecrosis ensues and collapse and fragmentation of the bone occurs over time. The end result can be degenerative arthritis of the radiocarpal joint and

pain. Various predisposing factors exist. Approximately 75% of wrists with Keinbock's disease have a shorter ulna compared to the radius, as measured at the wrist (ulnar negative variance). Also, the → leads to ↓ load across Rad carpal j. slope of the distal radius articular surface has been shown to be more horizontal in patients with Keinbock's disease. Approximately one-fourth of lunate are thought to have a single vessel blood supply. Some believe that osteonecrosis of the lunate occurs subsequent to a single fracture although others have suggested repetitive microfracture of the bone. In reality, cause of Keinbock's is most likely multifactorial.

Keinbock's is more common in males that females. Approximately 50% of patients relate a history of trauma. Most complain of dorsal wrist pain and stiffness. Physical examination may reveal diminished range of motion, grip weakness, and tenderness over the radiocarpal joint. Some patients present with symptoms of carpal tunnel syndrome. ← imp Keinbock's can be staged radiographically into one of six categories. Stage 0: normal plain radiographs of the wrist with abnormal MRI scan of the lunate. Stage 1: fracture of the lunate without collapse of the bone. Stage 2: sclerosis of the lunate without collapse of the bone. Stage 3a: lunate collapse without loss of height of the wrist (Figure 14-13). Stage 3b: Collapse of the wrist. Stage 4: degenerative changes of the wrist joint secondary to Keinbock's disease.

The natural history of Keinbock's disease is not entirely known. In patients with stage 0 and stage 1 disease, immobilization and nonoperative support may suffice. Patients with stage 2 and stage 3a disease

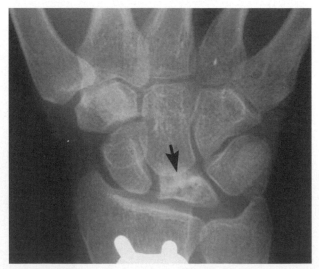

FIGURE 14-13. Stage 3a, osteonecrosis of the lunate (Keinbock's disease).

who continue with symptoms are generally indicated for surgery. The surgical procedures for patients with stage 2 and stage 3a Keinbock's disease can be divided into two broad categories: joint-leveling procedures and revascularization procedures. The most commonly performed among these procedures is the radial shortening osteotomy. This procedure is indicated in patients who have a short ulna and the goal of surgery is to shorten the radius to "level" it with the ulna. The exact reason why this procedure is effective is still unknown. The most commonly performed revascularization procedures for Keinbock's disease is a pedicled vascularized bone graft harvested from the dorsal, distal radius. For patients with symptomatic stage 4 disease and some patients with stage 3b disease, reconstructive salvage surgery of the wrist is indicated. This salvage surgery may include a partial (maintains some element of wrist range of motion), or a complete wrist fusion or a proximal row carpectomy (removal of the lunate bone along with the scaphoid and triquetral bone). Proximal row carpectomy allows the capitate to articulate in the lunate fossa. A prerequisite for this operation is maintenance of a good distal radius articular surface.

NERVE PALSY

Few injuries are as devastating functionally to the hand and wrist as median, ulnar, or radial nerve palsies. The vast majority of radial nerve palsy is posttraumatic, but can also occur as a complication of elective surgery of the upper extremity, a residual of birth palsy, or the consequence of cervical spine disc disease. Tendon transfers provide an option to restore lost motor function. The ideal tendon transfer is one in which the tendon's muscle has normal strength, has a straight line of pull, and provides adequate excursion. Additionally, the tendon should originally have a function synergistic or "opposite" to the tendon function for which it is substituted. Naturally, the tendon to be transferred must be expendable.

Loss of median nerve function at or above the elbow results in a high median nerve palsy. The consequences of a high median nerve palsy is loss of palmar sensation along the volar aspect of the thumb, index, long, and radial border of the ring finger. Motor strength deficits include loss of thumb opposition (loss of abductor pollicis brevis), loss of thumb interphalangeal (IP) joint flexion (loss of flexor pollicis longus muscle function), and loss of index distal interphalangeal joint flexion

(flexor digitorum profundus function). Restoration of thumb IP joint flexion can be restored using a transferred brachioradialis muscle (radial nerve innervated) to the FPL tendon. Restoration of FDP function of the index finger can be accomplished using the extensor carpi radialis longus (radial nerve innervated) tendon rerouted to the index FDP tendon in the mid forearm. Lastly, thumb opposition can be restored with transfer of the abductor digiti minimi muscle (ulnar nerve innervated).

Radial nerve palsy is particularly compromising to the function of the hand because extension posturing of the wrist (the prehensile position) is lost. This positioning of the hand increases grip power as well as the all-important hand function of grasp and release. The radial nerve is particularly vulnerable as it spirals around the humerus midshaft, against which it is closely applied. The radial nerve palsy is most often caused by injuries following a spiral fracture of the humerus. The sharp bony ends of the fracture can impale the radial nerve along its course. Loss of radial nerve function at this level results in loss of wrist and finger extension. This is known as "wrist drop." Tendon transfers for radial nerve palsy include flexor carpi radialis (FCR) transfer to extensor digitorum communus (EDC) tendons, pronator teres to extensor carpi radialis brevis tendon, and palmaris longus to the rerouted extensor pollicis longus (EPL) tendon. These transfers are then subsequently fired by flexion of the wrist causing tension on the transferred tendons (tenodesis) of the wrist.

Without question, the most devastating injury to the hand is the ulnar nerve palsy. The ulnar nerve supplies sensation to the volar aspect of the small finger as well as the small finger side of the ring finger. Motor function deficits following ulnar nerve palsy include loss of hand muscle function (intrinsic muscle function), which includes digital side-to-side movements as well as "thumb pinch" function. This results in substantial impairment in hand strength and digital mobility. Ulnar nerve injuries higher (more proximal) in the arm result in the loss of DIP joint flexion. Profound hand wasting accompanies ulnar nerve dysfunction.

Various signs of ulnar nerve palsy have been described. The classic "clawhand" of ulnar nerve palsy is known as Duchenne's sign. Wartenberg's sign is the inability to pull in (adduct) the small finger against the ring finger. Froment's sign is the hyperflexion of the thumb IP joint to substitute for the lack of thumb-pinch power against the index finger. Weakness of DIP joint flexion due to loss of FDP function of the ring and small finger is known as Pollock's sign. The flattening of the natural metacarpal arch of the hand seen in association with hand muscle wasting is known as Masse's sign.

Tendon transfers for ulnar nerve palsy are limited in their ability to restore hand strength. The ECRB tendon can be transferred to the thumb proximal phalanx to provide thumb pinch (adduction) while the extensor pollicis brevis (EPB) tendon is transferred to the index interosseous muscle. Additionally, the thumb MCP joint may be fused to prevent thumb hyperextension and instability. The combination of these surgeries has been reported to restore approximately 50% of the lost pinch strength.

RHEUMATOID ARTHRITIS OF THE HAND AND WRIST

Rheumatoid arthritis affects approximately 1% of the population with females affected twice as often as males. It is a systemic condition that causes a symmetrical polyarthritis. In the hand and the wrist joint, the distal radioulnar joint and the metacarpophalangeal joints are commonly affected. Patients usually present between ages 40 and 60 with joint pain and stiffness and occasionally fever. In the hand, synovial swelling is first seen followed by ligamentous failure, joint subluxation, and ultimately joint erosions and destruction. Initial treatment of rheumatoid arthritis in the hand includes medical therapy and resting night splints. Early on, medical therapy may consist of NSAIDs and rest splints but potential remittive therapy is usually necessary. Aggressive medical management often includes low dose oral corticosteroids and immunosuppressive agents such as methotrexate, Imuran (azathioprine), or Arava (leflunomide). Newer biological agents include Enbrel (etanercept), Humira (adalimumab), and Remicade (infliximab), which act by inhibiting tumor necrosis factor. These biologic response modifiers may be combined with more traditional agents such as methotrexate. Whether or not these treatments will make surgery less necessary has been suggested but not yet established.

If synovitis persists following at least 3 months of medical management, then surgical synovectomy is indicated to prevent extensor tendon rupture. Similarly, synovitis of the wrist joint or the metacarpophalangeal joints may not respond to medical management and surgical synovectomy may be indicated. The indications for MCP and wrist joint synovectomy are less clear but in the absence of joint destruction, most agree that joint surgery can be delayed. MCP joint synovectomy should be considered in those patients with recalcitrant synovitis who have no radiographic evidence of joint destruction.

The distal radioulnar joint (DJUJ) may be the first joint affected in patients with rheumatoid arthritis. DRUJ subluxation is often observed and as the distal ulna becomes eroded, rupture of the overlying extensor digiti quinti minimi (EDQM) tendon can occur. The result is the Vaughan-Jackson sign, which is a prominent distal ulna with the inability to extend the small finger. In these patients, extensor tenosynovectomy is indicated with EDQM reconstruction. A side-to-side tendon repair to the adjacent EDC to ring finger can accomplish EDQM reconstruction. In these patients it is also incumbent to stabilize the distal radioulnar joint. This is most commonly done with a distal radioulnar joint fusion with the creation of a more proximal pseudoarthrosis (Suave-Kapandji procedure). As disease progresses, the remainder of the wrist joint becomes involved, further destruction of the wrist may occur, and wrist arthrodesis may be necessary. Wrist arthrodesis is a reliable procedure well suited for providing pain relief. Alternatively, a total wrist replacement can be considered in low demand individuals with bilateral disease. Total wrist arthroplasty is contraindicated in patients with previous infection. The failure rate with total wrist replacement approaches 25% at intermediate-term follow-up in one recent series. The most common mode of failure is distal component loosening.

Progression of the rheumatoid hand deformity includes MCP joint destruction with subluxation of the joint and drift of the digits toward the small finger side of the hand (ulnar drift). Tightness of the surrounding soft tissue structures ultimately prevents correction of this deformity (intrinsic muscle tightness). Wrist involvement may also occur with sliding of the carpal bones toward the ulna (ulnar translation of the carpus) as ligamentous destruction occurs (Figure 14-14). These patients also commonly have pain and have noticed a recent decline in overall hand performance. These patients are reasonable candidates for MCP joint arthroplasties. The Swanson flexible silicone implant that has been in service for well over 35 years functions as a spacer following resection of the destroyed MCP joint. It has been well recognized that these implants typically fracture but remain in service for

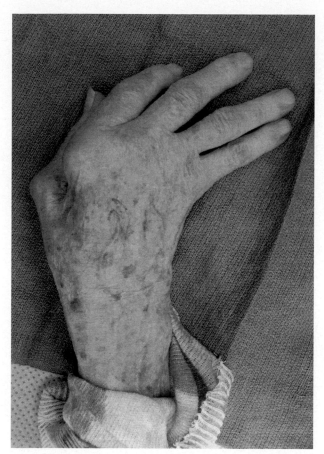

FIGURE 14-14. Ulnar deviation deformity of the wrist and digits in a patient with advanced rheumatoid arthritis.

years, continuing to function as a spacer. Hansraj et al. has reported a 90% 10-year survival rate with this spacer. The biomechanical shortfall of the Swanson Silastic implant is the amount of bone and soft tissue resection needed for implantation of the device. Current alternatives to the Silastic implants are surface replacement arthroplasties that attempt to recreate the normal articular surface anatomy while requiring less soft tissue resection for implantation of the device. Further follow-up data on these newer generation devices are needed.

STENOSING TENOSYNOVITIS (TRIGGER FINGER)

Stenosing tenosynovitis condition is a mechanical problem of a mismatch in size of the flexor tendons within their flexor tendon sheath. The result is a bunching or catching of the tendons as they pass through the orifice of the A1 pulley. This mismatch in size results in the mechanical problem of triggering that is the clinical hallmark of the condition. A fibrocartilagenous dysplasia develops at the A1 pulley, leading to a similar lesion on the corresponding surface of the flexor tendon. This results in degenerative tendinopathy over time. The process can occur at any digit but more commonly affects the ring finger. Patients usually present with a complaint of a painful catching of the finger with gripping. In more advanced cases, the finger may be locked in flexion and very painful to reduce. The patients may complain of the occurrence more in the morning hours than later in the day. Prior to experiencing the triggering or catching symptoms, patients may just have a tender and sore flexor tendon sheath that is aggravated by activities. On physical examination, actual triggering may not be elicited but tenderness directly over the A1 pulley usually is. The condition is more frequently seen in patients with rheumatoid arthritis, gout, diabetes, and degenerative arthritis. Patients usually present in the fifth to seventh decade of life.

Initial treatment is nonoperative. Simple splinting with the use of NSAIDs has been shown to be effective in some patients. Injection of corticosteroid into the flexor tendon sheath has been shown to be effective in 70% of patients. Another study has shown the percentage to increase to 84% when a regimen of two injections is used. Alternatively, reports of splint therapy alone have yielded improvement in 66% of patients. The trigger finger injection is performed using a 25-gauge needle and 1 cc of lidocaine and 10 mg of Kenalog solution or an equivalent of another water insoluble steroid preparation. Water insoluble steroid preparations are longer acting. The lidocaine steroid preparation is injected into the flexor tendon sheath at the level of the A2 pulley, and the examiner palpates the filling of the sheath. Flexor tendon sheath release or trigger finger release is indicated when nonoperative management fails. This is done at the opening of the flexor tendon sheath, or at the level of the A1 pulley. Results approaching 100% in appropriately indicated patients were recently reported by Turowski et al. An alternative to open trigger finger release is percutaneous flexor tendon sheath release. This technique employs a 20-gauge needle placed percutaneously at the level of the A1 pulley. The needle is manipulated such that the A1 pulley is cut by the bevel of the needle. Complications of this technique include scoring of the tendon.

SWAN-NECK DEFORMITY

Similar to the boutonnière deformity of the digit, the swan-neck deformity may cause substantial functional limitation. It can arise following trauma but more typically is seen in the context of the rheumatoid hand. The essential features of the digital swan-neck deformity include hyperextension of the PIP joint and flexion of the DIP joint subsequent to incompetence of the PIP joint volar plate (Figure 14-15). The swan-neck deformity is often accompanied by the presence of intrinsic tightness. In this condition the interosseous muscles of the hand become contracted, which causes tightness of the lateral band portion of the extensor mechanism. With the metacarpal phalangeal (MCP) joint extended, the lateral band portion of the extensor mechanism is placed on stretch, causing tightness of the terminal tendon. This imbalance then causes restriction in the passive or active flexion of the PIP joint. A simple test for intrinsic tightness involves hyperextending the PIP joint and then examining the passive range of motion (ROM) of the PIP joint. Patients with intrinsic tightness of a digit experience diminished passive range of motion at the PIP joint when the test is performed.

Digits with a swan-neck deformity may be classified into four stages. Stage 1 is a finger with a swan-neck deformity and no limitation of PIP joint ROM. Stage 2 is a swan-neck digit with limitation of ROM with certain positions of the MCP joint. Stage 3 is a digit with limitations of PIP ROM in any MCP position. Stage 4 is fixed and rigid swan-neck deformity. The stage 4 swan-neck deformity in the rheumatoid is characterized by advance PIP joint destruction.

Treatment for the swan-neck deformity includes splinting for the stage 1 deformity, and extensor mechanism reconstruction or release of tight intrinsic muscles for the stage 2 and 3 deformities. Arthrodesis or arthroplasty is required for the stage 4 condition. In general, results for soft tissue reconstruction of the rheumatoid swan-neck deformity has been disappointing while treatment with arthrodesis has been more predictable.

TUMORS AND TUMOR-LIKE CONDITIONS OF THE HAND AND WRIST

Ganglion Cyst

The most common soft tissue lesion of the hand and wrist is the ganglion cyst. The most common location is the dorsal aspect of the wrist (originating from the scapholunate interosseous ligament. One study found MRI-associated pathology in 30% of wrist ganglia imaged, suggesting a traumatic origin for this lesion. The pathogenesis of ganglions remains unclear. Recent series have documented enhanced success rates using serial aspiration treatments. However, recurrence rates with aspiration exceed 40%. Definitive management is open surgical excision. Recurrence rates with surgical removal are as low as 5%. Arthroscopic ganglion removal is gaining increasing popularity for dorsal wrist ganglions. When treating ganglion cysts it is important to consider the patients perspective. In one study, 28% of patients sought medical attention for their ganglion over concern of malignancy.

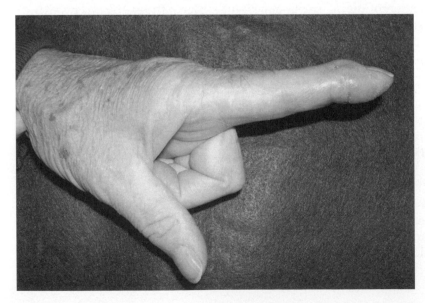

FIGURE 14-15. Swan-neck deformity of the index finger following trauma.

Giant Cell Tumor of Bone

Giant cell tumor of bone can be locally aggressive (Figure 14-16), and even metastasize causing death, but are regarded as benign. Eighty-five percent of giant cell tumors are diagnosed in patients older than 20 years in age, occurring slightly more often in females. Only 2% of giant cell tumors arise in the hand bones while approximately 14% originate in wrist. The patient with a giant cell tumor of the hand or wrist presents with pain and localized swelling. The tumor is lytic radiographically with cortical expansion and indistinct borders. Mitotic activity is quite common.

Giant cell tumors of the bones of the hand and wrist should be treated with wide excision and reconstruction. A recurrence rate of 79% has been reported with curettage within the margins of the lesion (intralesional). Curettage beyond the limits of the lesion is permissible when the giant cell tumor has not violated the cortex of the bone and extended into the soft tissue. No recurrences were reported in 10 patients treated with wide excision

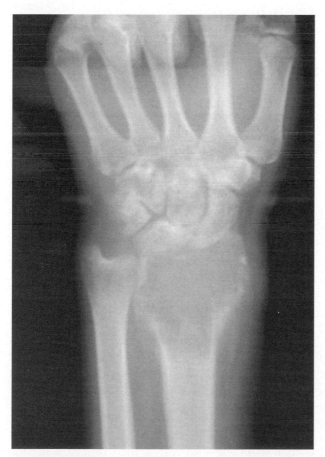

FIGURE 14-16. Giant cell tumor of bone.

and arthrodesis of the wrist. Other than arthrodesis, other reconstructive surgeries about the wrist that can be considered are vascularized or nonvascularized bone grafting and composite osteo-articular allograft reconstruction of the distal radius joint surface. Cementation and cryosurgery can also be considered in place of bone grafting when curettage is chosen as a primary treatment.

Giant Cell Tumor of Tendon Sheath

The giant cell tumor of tendon sheath is among the more common soft tissue tumors of the hand. It is a slowly progressive, painless, rubbery mass predominating on the radial three digits of the hand and is typically identified adherent to the digital flexor tendon sheath of the hand. The histology is variable but the tumors consistently contain multinucleated giant cells and xanthoma cells. Some lesions possess increased cellularity and mitotic activity. Recurrence rates as high as 44 to 50% have been reported in series with extended follow-up. A recent study of 43 patients found that following surgical excision, the only lesions that recurred were those that originally had multiple discrete tumors. Tumors composed of single masses did not recur following surgical excision. MRI may be helpful in determining the anatomic extent of the lesion.

Epidermal Inclusion Cyst

Epidermal inclusion cysts are also among the more common soft tissue lesions of the hand. This tumor-like condition results from the puncture of epithelium beneath the skin. The resulting growth of epithelial cells is typically painless and seldom functionally limiting. The fingertip is the most common location for epidermal inclusion cysts. Marginal surgical excision is curative and indicated when the lesion is bothersome to the patient. Involvement of the distal phalanx has been mistaken for malignancy.

Enchondroma

Enchondroma is the most common bone tumor in the hand and wrist. It is seen in all age groups and has an equal male and female distribution. These benign tumors may present due to a pathologic fracture or may be observed incidentally on routine hand radiographs. Analysis of over 5,500 bone tumors from Bauer et al., found that nearly 90% of all primary hand tumors were enchondromas. The most common location of the enchondroma is the proximal phalanx, followed by the metacarpal and the middle phalanx.

Radiographically, these lesions are often expansile with distortion of the cortex and punctate calcification. Multiple enchondromas in the same extremity is known as the nonhereditary condition, Ollier's disease. In Ollier's disease the enchondromas are larger, causing notable cosmetic and functional problems. Growth of enchondromas usually stops after skeletal maturity. Enchondroma growth after skeletal maturity, particularly when associated with radiographic progression and pain, raises the question of malignancy. Malignant transformation of enchondromas to chondrosarcoma in Ollier's disease is much more likely than solitary enchondroma transformation and is considered to be approximately 30%. Maffucci's syndrome is an extremely rare nonhereditary condition composed of multiple enchondromas and associated hemangiomatas.

Small, asymptomatic enchondromas require no specific treatment. If lesions grow and become painful, biopsy should be obtained. Pathologic fractures (fractures through tumor) occurring through enchondromas are treated as fractures first. Once fracture healing has occurred, formal treatment of the enchondroma is initiated. Enchondromas that reach substantial size are excised to prevent pathologic fracture. Enchondroma removal involves thorough curettage (intralesional scrapping of the tumor) followed by packing of the defect with bone graft. The recurrence rate with this method is approximately 4.5%.

MALIGNANT TUMORS OF THE HAND AND WRIST

Fortunately, malignancy of the hand and wrist is rare. The most common primary malignant bone tumor of the hand and wrist is the chondrosarcoma. The chondrosarcoma often develops in relationship to a preexisting enchondroma, particularly enchondromas associated with Ollier's disease. Osteosarcoma is seen less frequently in the hand by comparison to the lower extremities and is typically seen in an older population than the classic young adult presentation. Radiation exposure has been suggested as a possible cause for osteosarcoma development in the hand. Metastatic tumors to the hand may present as the original presentation of a previously undiagnosed cancer. The most common

metastatic tumor to the hand is lung and the most common site is the distal phalanx. Other reported primary sites include the esophagus, colon, breast, ovary, prostate, bladder, uterus, and thyroid. In one study, there was only a 6-month average life expectancy of patients with tumors metastatic to the hand. The most common soft tissue sarcomas of the hand and upper extremity is the epithelioid sarcoma, the malignant fibrous histiocytoma (MFH), and the synovial cell sarcoma. The epithelioid sarcoma is often misdiagnosed at original presentation leading to delays in treatment. Synovial cell sarcoma presents associated with the synovial joints of the wrist. They are slow growing and may go undiagnosed for years. MFH is becoming increasingly more recognized in the hand, particularly in older adults. It is often painless, also leading to original misdiagnosis and treatment delays. Treatment for bone and soft tissue sarcomas are wide tumor resection and limb salvage reconstruction. Adjuvant chemotherapy and external beam radiation may prolong survival, depending on the histologic diagnosis and grade of the tumor.

VASCULAR INSUFFICIENCY OF THE HAND AND WRIST

Vascular insufficiency of the hand and wrist may arise as result of penetrating trauma, repetitive trauma, primary vasospastic disease (Raynaud's disease), or vasospastic disease secondary to another disorder (Raynaud's phenomena). Whatever the cause, patients complain of color changes of the digits anywhere from pale white to bluish purple. They often experience pain and particularly cold intolerance. In some advanced conditions, fingertip soft tissue necrosis may result. Important information to be gained from the patient is any history of smoking, penetrating or blunt trauma, repetitive trauma, or excessive occupational vibration exposure. Also, the examiner should query the patient for a history of malignancy, blood dyscrasias, or any other hypercoagulable condition. Physical examination should include an Allen's test, which assesses the patency of both the radial and ulnar arteries. In this test, the examiner occludes both arteries at the wrist and then has the patient repetitively make a fist in an effort to remove blood from the palm. Sequentially, the examiner releases pressure from one of the arteries while continuing to occlude the other. The return of capillary refill to the palm of the hand is then assessed. The test is then repeated for the other artery. The test can also be performed using a Doppler probe. Symptomatic, chronic vascular insufficiency of the hand warrants a workup that includes an upper extremity arteriogram and includes images of the aortic arch and subclavian arteries. The arteriogram is obtained to rule out the presence of vascular occlusion anywhere in the vascular system of the upper extremity. Additionally, an echocardiogram is obtained to rule out mural thombi in the ventricles of the heart. Other testing includes the use of noninvasive vascular studies such as color-duplex imaging, cold immersion testing, and magnetic resonance angiography.

A primary vasospastic disorder of the digits in which symmetric discoloration of the digits occur, primarily in females under the age of 40 is known as Raynaud's disease. These patients seldom experience any trophic changes of the digits and have no clinical evidence of occlusive arterial disease or connective tissue disorder. The diagnosis is established following 2 years of symptoms. Alternatively, secondary vasospastic conditions resulting from such conditions as connective tissue disorders (including scleroderma, rheumatoid arthritis, systemic lupus erythematosus, vasculitis, and CREST syndrome), occlusive arterial disease, hematologic disorders, and occupational trauma is referred to as Raynaud's phenomena. Patients developing Raynaud's phenomena, are typically over age 40, have some underlying disease, and often experience progressive trophic changes of the digits. Raynaud's phenomena is seen in approximately 80% of patients with scleroderma, 25% of patients with systemic lupus erythematosus, and 10% of patients with rheumatoid arthritis. Initial nonoperative treatment of Raynaud's phenomena includes oral calcium channel blockers and axillary sympathetic blocks. Anticoagulation therapy may also have some merit. Patients with continued symptoms but a favorable response to axillary sympathetic blocks may be good candidates for peripheral arterial sympathectomy.

Buerger's disease (thromboangiitis obliterans) is an inflammatory vascular occlusive disorder related to the use of nicotine. The condition is more common in men. In these patients, narrowing of the digital arteries generally occurs resulting in ischemic finger pain and Raynaud's phenomena. Smoking cessation arrests the progression of the disease in most instances.

Hypothenar hammer syndrome is the result of chronic repetitive trauma to the ulnar side of the wrist, resulting in thrombosis of the ulnar artery and Raynaud's phenomena. These patients often have

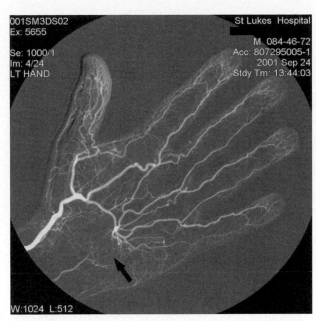

FIGURE 14-17. Posttraumatic ulnar artery occlusion (hypothenar hammer syndrome).

engaged in activities such as drywall hanging, carpentry, or other construction activities. In some instances, patients will give a dramatic history of how they have used the ulnar border of the wrist as a "hammer" to secure or stabilize objects. These patients often complain of coldness in the digits, color changes, or frank pain while engaged in certain occupational maneuvers. Arteriogram shows an ulnar artery devoid of flow and in many instances markedly diminished or absent blood flow to the ring and small digits (Figure 14-17). Treatment in symptomatic individuals requires resection of the thrombosed ulnar artery segment and superficial palmar arch reconstruction using a reverse flow vein graft, normally harvested from a dorsal foot vein. Following ulnar artery reconstruction, symptoms of ring and small finger ischemia can be expected to improve.

Annotated Bibliography

Boutonnière Deformity and Swan-Neck Deformity

Kiefhaber TR, Strickland JW. Soft tissue reconstruction for rheumatoid swan-neck and boutonnière deformities: long-term results. J Hand Surg 1993;18A:984–989.
Ninety-two digits were treated with soft tissue reconstruction for rheumatoid swan-neck deformity and 19 digits for boutonnière deformity. Overall the results were mediocre and unpredictable leading the authors to conclude that arthrodesis is the best treatment of advanced rheumatoid digital deformities.

Smith RJ. Intrinsic Contracture. In: Green, DP, Hotchkiss, RN, Pederson WC, eds. Green's Operative Hand Surgery. 4th ed. New York: Churchill Livingstone, 1999:604–618.
This chapter has been included in every edition of this textbook and has been left unaltered from the author's original version. Digital contractures of the hand are outlines with an emphasis on pathologic anatomy and treatment.

Smith RJ. Intrinsic muscles of the fingers: Function, dysfunction and surgical reconstruction. In: AAOS Instr Course Lect, vol. 24. St. Louis: CV Mosby, 1975:200–220.
This is a classic review defining the anatomy and pathologic anatomy of the intrinsic muscle system of the hand. The specific characteristic of boutonnière and swan neck deformities are discussed and illustrated.

Carpal Tunnel Syndrome

Brown RA, Gelberman RH, Seiler JG III et al. Carpal tunnel release: a prospective, randomized assessment of open and endoscopic methods. J Bone Joint Surg 1993;75A:1265–1275.
In a prospective, randomized fashion, this study examined the results in 169 hands having either open or endoscopic carpal tunnel release surgery. Overall, 90 to 98% of patients experienced relief of paresthesias. There was no significant difference in objective outcome measures. The open method resulted in more scar tenderness and a longer return to work than did the endoscopic method. A greater complication rate was found with the endoscopic carpal tunnel release surgery.

Finsen V, Russwurm H. Neurophysiology not required before surgery for typical carpal tunnel syndrome. J Hand Surg 2001;26B:61–64.
In this study, 14 of 63 patients who had successful carpal tunnel release surgery had preoperative electrodiagnostic testing that were normal.

Gelberman RH, Aronson D, Weisman MH. Carpal tunnel syndrome: results of a prospective trial of steroid injection and splinting. J Bone Joint Surg 1980;62A:1181–1184.
In patients with carpal tunnel syndrome, 80% of patients receiving a carpal tunnel steroid injection experience relief of their symptoms but only 22% will still be symptom free at 1 year. Patients who had symptoms for less than 1 year were likely to have sustained relief.

Szabo PM, Gelberman RH, Dimick MP. Sensibility testing in patients with carpal tunnel syndrome. J Bone and Joint Surg 1984;66A:60–64.
Clinical threshold testing, such as Semmes-Weinstein monofilament testing and vibrational testing, are more sensitive in detecting abnormalities in hand sensory dysfunction. Overall, the Semmes-Weinstein monofilament testing was found to provide the most reliable sensory test.

Szabo RM, Slater RR II, Farver TB et al. The value of diagnostic testing in carpal tunnel syndrome. J Hand Surg 1999;24A:704–714.
The authors evaluated a variety of diagnostic tests for carpal tunnel syndrome. They concluded that there is an 86% chance of patients having carpal tunnel syndrome when there is the combination of a positive carpal tunnel compression test, abnormal monofilament testing, subjective night pain, and a positive hand diagram. The results of electrodiagnostic studies did not add to the diagnostic accuracy.

Complex Regional Pain Syndrome

Brown DL. Somatic or sympathetic block for reflex sympathetic dystrophy. Which is indicated? Hand Clin 1997;13:485–497.
The rationale for the use of nerve blocks is discussed as well as the nerve block options available for complex regional pain syndrome. The techniques for various nerve blocks are discussed and illustration provided.

MacKinnon SE, Holder LE. The use of three-phase radionuclide bone scanning in the diagnosis of reflex sympathetic dystrophy. J Hand Surg 1984;9A:556–563.
In 145 patients, the three-phase bone scan was used to diagnose RSD. The authors found that increased radiotracer uptake in phase III of the scan was diagnostic for RSD with a sensitivity of 96% and specificity of 98%.

Stanton-Hicks M, Janig W, Hassenbusch S et al. Reflex sympathetic dystrophy: changing concepts and taxonomy. Pain 1995;63:127–133.
This article discusses the various terms associated with pain of uncertain origin and redefines pain as either complex regional pain syndrome type I or type II. The term sympathetic mediated pain is also explained.

Congenital Hand Anomalies

Buck-Gramcko D. Pollicization of the index finger: methods and results in aplasia and hypoplasia of the thumb. J Bone Joint Surg 1971;53A:1605–1617.
This article provides the original technical description of index finger pollicization for thumb hypoplasia along with early results.

Buck-Gramcko D. Radialization as a new treatment for radial club hand. J Hand Surg 1985;10A:964–968.
Thirty hands in 23 patients that were treated with a radialization technique are presented with the need for overcorrection stressed as well as soft tissue balancing from releases and tendon transfers. The indications for ulnar osteotomy are also discussed.

Damore E, Kozin SH, Thoder JJ, Porter S. The recurrence of deformity after surgical centralization for radial club hand. J Hand Surg 2000;25A:745–751.
The authors review the results of centralization of 19 radial club hands in 14 patients treated over an 18-year period. The follow-up averaged 6.5 years. Sixteen of the cases have radial aplasia. On average the patients lost a 38° of the correction obtained at surgery. A correlation was found between the preoperative angle and the final angle achieved. Better results were obtained when complete correction could be obtained at initial surgery.

Flatt AE. Cleft hand and central defects. In: Flatt AE, ed. The Care of Congenital Hand Anomalies. 2nd Ed. St. Louis: Quality Medical Publishing, 1994:337–365.
This chapter provides a comprehensive and detailed discussion of all aspects of cleft hand and is considered a classic. The etiology, classification, and operative treatment are discussed. The primary surgical procedures are illustrated.

Kozin SH. Syndactyly. J Am Soc Surg Hand 2001;1:1–13.
This article reviews the genetics and etiology of the condition as well as the classification and indications for surgical treatment. Surgical decision making is also discussed with emphasis on the technique of syndactyly release. Associated conditions such as Poland's syndrome, constriction band syndrome, central deficiency, and Apert's syndrome are discussed. Complications of treatment are also discussed.

Manske PR, Rotman MB, Dailey LA. Long-term functional results after pollicization for the congenitally deficient thumb. J Hand Surg 1992;17A:1064–1072.
This is a review of 28 index finger pollicizations following correction of congenital hypoplastic thumb. The final total active range of motion was approximately 50% of the contralateral normal thumb and the average grip 21%. The pollicized digit was used as a thumb in 84% of cases with a 22% prolonged time period to accomplish standard tasks. Patients having radial club hand had significantly poorer results. Age at the time of surgery did not correlate with final results.

Crystalline Arthropathy of the Hand and Wrist

Ali Y. Crystalline arthritis and other arthritides. In: Berger RA, Weiss APC, eds. Hand Surgery, vol. II, ch. 70. Philadelphia: Lippincott Williams & Wilkins, 2004:1241–1252.

This chapter provides a complete overview of the crystalline arthropathy conditions of the wrist. The pathogenesis, epidemiology, natural history, and treatment are outlined.

Degenerative Arthritis of the Hand and Wrist

Tomaino MM. Pellegrini VD, Burton RI. Arthroplasty of the basal joint of the thumb: long-term follow-up after ligament reconstruction with tendon interposition. J Bone Joint Surg 1995;77A:346–355.
Twenty-four thumbs in 22 patients were reviewed at an average follow-up of 9 years. Over 95% of the patients had relief of their pain. Grip strength and pinch strength both improved. Follow-up radiographs showed loss of carpal height compared to preoperative evaluation but this did not portend a poor outcome.

Watson HK, Ballet FL. The SLAC wrist: scapholunate advanced collapse pattern of degenerative arthritis. J Hand Surg 1984; 9A:358–365.
This is a review of over 200 patients presenting to the authors' clinic with a primary degenerative arthritis of the wrist. One of the more common patterns of degenerative arthritis observed was the scapholunate advanced collapse pattern whereby the scaphoid-distal radius articulation becomes primarily involved. In the more advance condition, the midcarpal joint becomes involved with proximal migration of the capitate and diastasis of the scaphoid and lunate. This condition results in a loss of carpal height.

DeQuervain's Syndrome

Harvey FJ, Harvey PM, Horsley MN. De Quervain's disease: surgical or nonsurgical treatment. J Hand Surg 1990;15A:83–87.
Sixty-three wrists treated for De Quervain's disease were retrospectively reviewed. Seventy-one percent of the wrists treated with one wrist corticosteroid injection achieved sustained relief of symptoms. An additional 11% of the wrists gained relief with a second injection. Of the 11 wrists that ultimately underwent first dorsal compartment release, 10 had septations within the first dorsal compartment.

Jackson WT, Viegas SF, Coon TM et al. Anatomical variations in the first extensor compartment of the wrist. J Bone Joint Surg 1986;68A:923–926.
Three hundred cadaver wrists were examined for anatomic variations in the first dorsal compartment. In 40% of the wrists, a septum divided the first dorsal compartment. In a separate clinical series, patients undergoing release of the first dorsal compartment for DeQuervain's syndrome, there was a 67% incidence of septations within the first dorsal compartment.

Weiss APC, Akelman E, Tabatabai M. Initial treatment of DeQuervain's disorder. J Hand Surg, 1994; 9A:595-598.
Eighty-seven patients with DeQuervain's disease were treated with either injection alone, injection plus splinting, or splinting alone. The results from injection alone were superior to splinting alone and not significantly different from the combination of splinting and injection.

Dupuytren's Contracture

McFarlane RM. On the origin and spread of Dupuytren's disease. J Hand Surg 2002;27A:385–390.
This review examines the history of Dupuytren's disease and dating its origin somewhere between 1200 BC–200 BC. The author concludes that the disease is probably not due to a single gene but is most likely multifactorial.

Badalamente MA, Hurst LC, Grandia SK et al. Platelet-derived growth factor in Dupuytren's disease. J Hand Surg 1992;17A: 317–323.
Palmar facia obtained from surgical release of Dupuytren's contracture release was analyzed in 28 patients. An association between platelet-derived growth factor (PDGF) and myofibroblasts found in the proliferative stages of Dupuytren's disease. The results of the

study suggest that the PDGF is bound to a cell membrane. The authors conclude that PGDF may play a role in the proliferative events of myofibroblasts.

Roush TF, Stern PJ. Results following surgery for recurrent Dupuytren's disease. J Hand Surg 2000;25A:291–296.
Twenty-eight digits in 19 patients were treated surgically for recurrent Dupuytren's contracture and followed up at a median of 4 years. Dermatofasciectomy and full-thickness skin grafting did not prevent recurrent contracture. Three of the digits were anesthetic at follow-up. At follow-up, 18 of 19 patients were pleased with their results. There were no vascular injuries, infections, flap, or graft losses.

Tomasek J, Rayan GM. Correlation of alpha-smooth muscle actin expression and contraction in Dupuytren's disease fibroblasts. J Hand Surg 1995;20A:450–455.
Eleven specimens from the palmar fascia from patients with Dupuytren's disease where analyzed for smooth muscle actin. The results of the study show that fibroblasts in patients with Dupuytren's disease can acquire contractile characteristics and the increased presence of smooth muscle actin in these fibroblasts correlates with increased contractile activity.

Infections of the Hand and Wrist

Gonzalez MH, Kay T, Weinzweig N et al. Necrotizing fasciitis of the upper extremity. J Hand Surg 1996;21A:689–692.
This retrospective study reviewed the results of 12 patients with necrotizing fasciitis of the upper extremity. Eleven of the 12 infections were caused by β-hemolytic strep organisms. Ten of the patients had a history of IV drug abuse and 2 patients were diabetic. An average of 3 surgical debridements were necessary to control the infection. Two patients required shoulder disarticulation and all patients resolved their infection. The authors stress the importance of early recognition of this condition as well as the need for aggressive surgical debridement and appropriate antibiotic therapy.

Jebson PJ. Infections of the fingertip. Paronychias and felons. Hand Clin 1998;14:547–555.
This review article discusses the anatomy of the nailbed and the distal fingertip as well as the various infection forms seen in this area including the acute paronychial infection, the chronic paronychial infection, and the felon.

Reilly KE, Linz JC, Stern PJ et al. Osteomyelitis of the tubular bones of the hand. J Hand Surg 1997;22A:644–649.
The review of 700 patients with hand infections found 6% with osteomyelitis of the hand bones. Fifty-seven percent were caused by trauma while 13% were hematogenous. Twenty-two percent were immunocompromised or had peripheral vascular disease. Cultures were positive in 74% with 35% having multiple organisms and 35% Gram-positive organisms. The overall amputation rate was 39%.

Synder CC. Animal bite infections of the hand. Hand Clin, 1998;14:691–711.
This comprehensive review of the spectrum of animal bite injuries covers such common bite wounds as dogs and cats as well as more obscure bite wounds such as those from wolves, badgers, bears, skunks, snakes, spiders, scorpions, and various marine species.

Keinbock's Disease

Bonzar M, Firrell JC, Hainer M et al. Keinbock disease and negative ulnar variance. J Bone Joint Surg 1998;80(A):1154–1157.
Forty-four patients with Keinbock's disease were examined to determine the relationship if any with the presence of ulnar negative variance. The patients were compared to a group of 99 control patients and the authors determined that an association did exist between Keinbock's and the presence of ulnar negative variance.

Salmon J, Stanley JK, Trail IA. Keinbock's disease: conservative management versus radial shortening. J Bone Joint Surg 2000;82(B):820–823.

The results of 18 patients with stage 2 or 3 Keinbock's treated conservatively were compared with 15 patients treated operatively. The mean follow-up was 3.6 years. The patients treated with radial shortening had better pain relief and a stronger grip than patients treated conservatively. Some patients treated conservatively rapidly progressed to carpal collapse. Patients treated with radial shortening osteotomy had a slower progression to carpal collapse.

Shin AY, Bishop AT. Pedicled vascularized bone grafts for disorders of the carpus: scaphoid nonunion and Keinbock's disease. J Am Acad Orthop Surg 2002;10:210–216.
This article reviews the anatomy and indications of the reverse flow, pedicled vascularized bone graft options of the dorsal aspect of the distal radius. These vascularized bone grafts can be adapted for revascularization of the lunate in patients with Keinbock's disease.

Nerve Palsy

Green DP. Radial nerve palsy. In: Green DP, Hotchkiss RN, Pederson WC, eds. Green's Operative Hand Surgery, 4th Ed., vol. 2. New York: Churchill Livingstone, 1999:1481–1496.
Extensive review of the subject with detailed discussion of the techniques for transfer.

Omer G. Ulnar nerve palsy. In: Green DP, Hotchkiss RN, Pederson WC, eds., Green's Operative Hand Surgery, 4th Ed., vol. 2. New York: Churchill Livingstone, 1999:1526–1541.
Comprehensive review of the ulnar nerve palsy condition, including a detailed discussion of physical examination findings and techniques for restoring function.

Rheumatoid Arthritis of the Hand and Wrist

Barbier O, Saels P, Rombouts JJ et al. Long-term functional results of wrist arthrodesis in rheumatoid arthritis. J Hand Surg 1999;24(B):27–31.
Eighteen patients were reviewed at an average of years following wrist arthrodesis. All patients were pleased with the procedure and had satisfactory pain relief.

Cobb SD, Beckenbaugh RD. Biaxial total-wrist arthroplasty. J Hand Surg 1996;21A:1011–1021.
Forty-six patients followed-up at an average of 6.5 years with the biaxial total wrist arthroplasty. Ninety-two percent of the patients rated themselves as better. Eleven cases had failures, 8 of these at the distal implant. Survival analysis determined an 83% probability of survival at last follow-up.

Cook SD, Beckenbaugh RD, Redondo J et al. Long-term follow-up of pyrolytic carbon metacarpophalangeal implants. J Bone Joint Surg 1999;81(A):635–648.
Twenty-six patients were followed up at an average of 11.7 years after placement of pyrolytic carbon MCP implants. Ninety-four of the implants showed osteointegration. The 16-year survival rate was 70.3%. Ulnar drift was unchanged from preoperative and digital range of motion was improved to a relatively extended position.

Hansraj KK, Ashworth CR, Ebramzadeh E et al. Swanson metacarpophalangeal joint arthroplasty in patients with rheumatoid arthritis. Clin Orthop 1997;342:11–15.
The results of 170 Swanson Silastic MCP implants were evaluated at a mean of 5.2 years. No pain was reported in 54% of the joints. Mean postoperative range of motion was 27° compared to 38° preoperatively. Prosthesis survivorship at 10 years was 90%.

Stenosing Tenosynovitis

Patel M, Bassini L. Trigger fingers and thumb: when to splint, inject or operate. J Hand Surg 1992;17A:110–113.
Fifty patients with trigger finger were treated with MCP joint splinting, and another 50 trigger fingers were treated with injection. All patients were followed up at one year. Treatment was successful in 66% of the splinted patients and 84% of the injected patients. Patients with multiple trigger fingers and symptoms greater than 6 months had worse results in both groups.

Turowski G, Zdankiewicz T, Thompson J. The results of the surgical treatment of trigger finger. J Hand Surg 1997;22A:145–149.
Fifty-nine patients were assessed after open release of A1 pulley for trigger finger. One hundred percent of patients had either complete relief or substantial relief of their symptoms. Only 3% had recurrence.

Tumors and Tumor-Like Conditions of the Hand and Wrist

Amadio PC, Lombardi RM. Metastatic tumors of the hand. J Hand Surg 1987;12:311–316.
Twenty-two metastatic lesions in 18 patients were reviewed. The most common location was the distal phalanx while the most common primary tumors were in the lung and kidney. Over 50% of the patients in this series died within 6 months of hand metastasis diagnosis.

Murray P. Primary bone tumors. In: Berger RA, Weiss A-PC, eds. Hand Surgery. Philadelphia: Lippincott Williams & Wilkins; 2004.
Comprehensive review of the most common benign and malignant bone tumors of the hand and wrist. The chapter also reviews the important features of the tumor workup and staging. An algorithm is provided for malignant bone tumor decision making.

Thornburg LE. Ganglions of the hand and wrist. J Am Acad Orthop Surg 1999;7:231–238.
Although observation is an acceptable form of treatment, aspiration or surgical excision is indicated for lesions causing pain, skin ulcerations, functional limitations, or nerve compression. Recurrence rates of greater then 50% are common following aspiration and puncture of most ganglions. Aspiration is most successful for ganglion of the flexor tendon sheath. When performed properly, the recurrence rate following surgical excision is less than 5%.

Vander Griend RA, Funderburk CH. The treatment of giant-cell tumors of the distal part of the radius. J Bone Joint Surg 1993;75A:899–908.
The results of treatment for giant cell tumor of the distal radius were studied in 23 patients. Extended curettage and cementation was performed in 5 patients who had limited or no extraosseous tumor extension. Eighteen patients having extraosseous tumor extension were treated by distal radius resection and arthrodesis. At a follow-up there were no recurrences.

Vascular Insufficiency of the Hand

Koman LA, Smith BP, Pollock FE et al. The microcirculatory effects of peripheral sympathectomy. J Hand Surg 1995;20A:709–717.
Seven patients with Raynaud's phenomena due to a systemic process had refractory pain and digital tip ulcerations. Following microvascular peripheral sympathectomy, all patients had improved pain, and improvement in the digital ulcerations. Although total blood flow was not appreciably improved, the sympathectomy increased overall nutritional flow to the digit.

Miller LM, Morgan RF. Vasospastic disorders. Hand Clin 1993;9:171–187.
This review article discusses Raynaud's phenomenon and Raynaud's disease including the pathophysiology of each condition. Various vasospastic disorders causing secondary Raynaud's phenomenon are categorized and listed. Treatment options including digital sympathectomy are discussed. A digital algorithm is provided.

15

Stuart L. Weinstein

The Pediatric Hip

DEVELOPMENTAL HIP
   DYSPLASIA AND
   DISLOCATION
LEGG-CALVÉ-PERTHES DISEASE
TRANSIENT SYNOVITIS

DEVELOPMENTAL COXA VARA
SLIPPED CAPITAL FEMORAL
   EPIPHYSIS

DEVELOPMENTAL HIP DYSPLASIA AND DISLOCATION

The diagnosis of developmental hip dysplasia and dislocation is difficult to make in a newborn. The diagnosis is based on the subtleties of the physical examination. The consequences of not making the diagnosis may be disastrous to the patient. A confusing area in the literature is the terminology used to discuss this condition. Various authors use the terms *instability, dysplasia, subluxation,* and *dislocation* interchangeably. We prefer to use the term *developmental hip dysplasia* (or developmental dysplasia of the hip, DDH) to refer to any hip in which the normal relation between the femoral head and the acetabulum is altered.

In normal embryonic development, the hip joint components—the femoral head and acetabulum—develop from the same primitive mesenchymal cells. In the seventh week of gestation, a cleft develops in these precartilaginous cells, defining the femoral head and acetabulum. By 11 weeks of gestation, the hip joint is fully formed. Although rare, this is theoretically the earliest point in development that a hip dislocation could occur. At birth, the femoral head is deeply seated in the acetabulum and held there by the surface tension of the synovial fluid. A normal infant's hip is extremely difficult to dislocate even after division of the hip joint capsule. In hips with dysplasia, however, this tight fit between the femoral head and the acetabulum is lost, and the head can be easily displaced from the acetabulum. The femoral head displacement is usually in a posterosuperior direction. Pathologic specimens of this condition show varying degrees of hip joint malformation from mild capsular laxity to severe acetabular, femoral head, and neck malformations. Therefore, *developmental hip dysplasia* probably appropriately refers to the many stages of this complex deformity.

443

We use the term *DDH* clinically for any hip that may be provoked to subluxate (partial contact between the femoral head and the acetabulum) or dislocate (no contact between the femoral head and acetabulum) or for any hip in which the femoral head is either subluxated or dislocated in relation to the acetabulum but that can be reduced into the acetabulum. We prefer to use the term *developmental hip dislocation* when there is no contact between the femoral head and the acetabulum and the femoral head is not reducible. True dislocations in the newborn are rare and are usually associated with generalized conditions or anomalies such as arthrogryposis or myelodysplasia. These antenatal teratologic dislocations are at the extreme end of the DDH pathologic spectrum and account for only 2% of the cases seen in most series. The diagnosis and prognosis of these two separate conditions (dysplasia versus dislocation) are quite different.

The incidence of DDH varies considerably and is influenced by geographic and ethnic factors as well as the diagnostic criteria used, the acumen of the examiner, and the age of the patient at diagnosis. The results of newborn screening programs estimate that 1 in 100 newborns have some evidence of hip instability but that the true incidence of dislocation is between 1 and 1.5 per 1,000 live births.

The cause of DDH remains unknown. Ethnic and genetic factors no doubt play a key role. The incidence of DDH has been reported to be as high as 25 to 50 cases per 1,000 live births in Lapps and North American Indians and to be almost nonexistent among Chinese and blacks. Up to one-third of patients may give a positive family history for DDH. The genetic effects of the condition may be manifest primarily by acetabular dysplasia, joint laxity, or a combination of both. The role of excessive femoral neck anteversion or acetabular anteversion in the development of DDH remains controversial. Intrauterine mechanical and neuromuscular mechanisms can profoundly affect the intrauterine development of the hip.

In white infants, there is an increased incidence of DDH in firstborn children. It has been postulated that the prima gravida uterus and abdominal muscles are unstretched and subject the fetus to prolonged periods of abnormal positioning. This positioning tends to force the fetus against the mother's spine, limiting motions of the hip, particularly hip abduction. This "crowding phenomenon" may also be manifested by the association of other abnormalities thought to be due to the intrauterine compression, such as torticollis (up to

20% of patients with torticollis may have associated DDH) and metatarsus adductus. DDH is also manifested in patients with oligohydramnios, another condition that causes limited fetal mobility. The left hip is more frequently involved; in the uterus, it is the left side that is most often forced into the adducted position against the mother's sacrum.

Breech presentation is another strong associative feature. About 60% of children with DDH are firstborn children. Firstborn children have a high association of breech presentation. About 30 to 50% of patients with DDH are delivered in the breech presentation. About 60% of breech presentations are in firstborn children, and most breech-born infants have leg-folding mechanism arrests. Children born frank breech (knees in the extended position) are at an even greater risk of developing hip instability. This is evidenced by the higher incidence of DDH in children born with congenital recurvatum or dislocation of the knee. Eighty percent of the cases of DDH occur in girls. A contributory factor is that twice as many girls are born breech as boys. The extrauterine environment may also have a profound effect on the development of DDH. Societies in which swaddling is used postnatally (hips kept extended and adducted), for example, in many native North American tribes, the incidence of DDH is considerably higher than expected.

Hip joint laxity, either genetically determined or secondary to maternal estrogens and those hormones necessary for pelvic relaxation at delivery, may have an effect on the development of DDH. These hormones have been thought to cause temporary laxity of the hip joint capsule in the newborn, particularly the newborn girl. Hip joint laxity, however, is seen often in newborn infants. This may allow for some instability in the absence of a positive Ortolani sign. DDH is extremely rare in conditions characterized by excessive laxity such as Down, Ehlers-Danlos, and Marfan syndromes.

Most DDH cases are detectable at birth; however, despite newborn screening programs, some cases are missed. The diagnostic test for DDH is caused by the femoral head gliding in and out of the acetabulum over a ridge of abnormal acetabular cartilage. This test was originally described by LeDamany. He referred to the sensation palpated as *signe de ressaut*. The Italian pediatrician, Ortolani, in 1936 described the pathogenesis of this diagnostic sign and referred to the sensation palpated as the *segno dello scotto*. This palpable sensation has been likened to the femoral head gliding in and out of the acetabulum over a ridge. This ridge

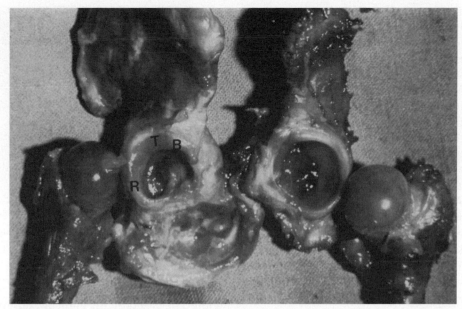

FIGURE 15-1. In this full-term female infant with fairly severe dysplasia of the right hip, the acetabulum and femoral head are smaller on the right than on the left. Extending along the posterosuperior margin of the articular surface of the right dysplastic acetabulum is a shallow trough (T). At the anterior end of this trough is a bulge (B), and extending posteriorly along the inferior and anterior margin of the trough down to the inferior margin of the acetabulum is a ridge (R) that separates the primary acetabulum inferiorly and anteriorly from the trough and the rest of the secondary acetabulum superiorly and posteriorly. (Ponseti IV. Morphology of the acetabulum in congenital dislocation of the hip: gross, histological and roentgenographic studies. J Bone Joint Surg 1978;60A:586–599)

of hypertrophied acetabular cartilage (Figure 15-1) was called the *neolimbus* by Ortolani. Unfortunately, inadequate translation of both LeDamany's and Ortolani's work into English has resulted into the use of the term *click* to describe this diagnostic sign. Experienced evaluators of hips in newborns realize that many high-pitched soft tissue clicks are often elicited in the hip examination of newborns that have no diagnostic significance. Unfortunately, this poor understanding of the pathology of the diagnostic sign in DDH has led to the misdiagnosis and overtreatment of infants. This diagnostic maneuver must be done gently. In the newborn period, such findings as asymmetry of the gluteal, thigh, or labial folds (asymmetric thigh and skin folds occur in a significant percentage of normal infants); limitation of abduction; or asymmetry of range of motion may make the physician suspect the presence of hip dysplasia, but the most reliable diagnostic sign is the Ortolani sign. The Ortolani test is performed with the infant in the supine position and the hips and knees flexed at 90°. The middle finger is placed over the greater trochanter, while the thumb is placed on the lesser trochanter bilaterally. The hips are then slowly abducted with pressure

over the greater trochanter. A palpable sensation indicates reduction of a dislocated or subluxated hip. Also with the legs in mid–abduction-adduction, posterior pressure can be applied to the lesser trochanters with the thumbs, and a similar sensation can be palpated, indicating whether the hip is subluxating or dislocating. (The provocation portion of the diagnostic test is often referred to as the Barlow maneuver.) It is essential that this test be performed with the infant relaxed.

Some evidence suggests that a small number of cases of DDH may occur late. It is therefore extremely important to continually look for this condition after the newborn period when the disorder is manifested by the secondary adaptive signs. It is especially important to look for DDH in high-risk infants. The high-risk group of infants includes those who have a combination of any of the following risk factors: breech position, female, positive family history, lower limb deformity, torticollis, metatarsus adductus, significant persistent asymmetric thigh folds, excessive ligamentous laxity, any other significant musculoskeletal abnormality, and ethnic background associated with an increased incidence of DDH.

The longer after the newborn period, the greater is the likelihood of the patient exhibiting physical findings secondary to adaptive changes. With persistent subluxation or dislocation, the patient develops secondary contractures of the adductor muscles on the involved side. This leads to limited abduction (Figure 15-2), the key late diagnostic finding in DDH. In addition, after the newborn period, the incidence of a positive Ortolani sign decreases markedly, particularly after 1 to 2 months of age. The disturbed relation between the proximal femur and the acetabulum may, in addition to limitation of abduction, lead to the presence of asymmetry of the gluteal, thigh, buttock, or labial folds. The patient may manifest apparent shortening of the femur (Allis sign) in comparison to the opposite side (Figure 15-3) or "pistoning" or "telescoping" of the involved extremity, depending on the laxity of the hip joint capsule. In a child of walking age with unilateral DDH, the apparent limb length inequality may result in a limp secondary to the apparent shortening of the extremity. This also may lead to a secondary equinus deformity of the ankle. Clinically, bilateral dislocations are much more difficult to detect because the physical findings may be symmetric. Also in bilateral DDH, the child may walk with a waddling gait and hyperlordosis of the lumbar spine. Any gait abnormality in a child should not be dismissed without a careful clinical and radiographic evaluation of the hips.

The diagnosis of DDH in the newborn period is a clinical one. The femoral ossific nucleus is not present in the newborn, and a great portion of the pelvis of an infant is cartilaginous. Thus, normal relations are difficult to interpret radiographically,

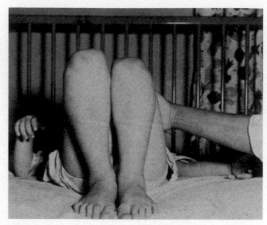

FIGURE 15-3. The Allis or Galeazzi sign. The knee is lower on the dislocated side.

and all treatment decisions in the newborn nursery should be based on the clinical examination. Routine radiographs are generally unnecessary. A normal-appearing radiograph does not rule out the presence of DDH. Complete dislocations may be missed, and mild degrees of dysplasia are not easily detected. Ultrasonography, while routinely used as a screening tool for DDH in Europe, has not been shown to be cost effective in the United States as a screening device. It is very operator and position dependent and has resulted in the overdiagnosis and overtreatment of infants. With increasing age and lack of the normal relation between the proximal femur and the acetabulum, the anatomic changes of this abnormal relation become increasingly evident. The femoral ossific nucleus, which normally appears between 4 and 7 months of age, may be delayed in its appearance and its general overall development stunted. The proximal femur is seen to lie laterally with varying degrees of proximal migration compared with the ilium. The Shenton line is disrupted. The acetabulum fails to develop, as manifested by an increase in the slope of the acetabular roof (Figure 15-4). Most important in assessing radiographic measurements is the accurate positioning of the child for the radiograph. The lower extremities must be aligned and in neutral rotation. Unless radiographic positioning is standardized, measurement differences between patient visits may not be reliable.

In the newborn, the primary pathoanatomy consists of varying degrees of capsular laxity and the thickening of the acetabular cartilage in the superior, posterior, and inferior aspects of the acetabulum. This thickening in the cartilage was called *neolimbus* by Ortolani (see Figure 15-1). It is the

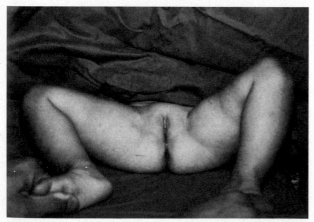

FIGURE 15-2. Eighteen-month-old girl with left congenital hip dysplasia. Note the limited abduction of left hip compared with the right.

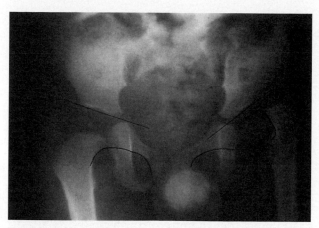

FIGURE 15-4. Eleven-month-old boy with left congenital hip dysplasia. Note the delayed appearance of left femoral ossific nucleus, disruption of the Shenton line with proximal migration of the femur, and lack of development of the acetabulum manifested by an increased slope of the acetabular roof.

sensation of the femoral head gliding in and out of the acetabulum over this thickened ridge that produces the Ortolani sign. Without treatment, this ridge of hypertrophied acetabular cartilage may become more prominent, and within a few weeks or months after birth, the femoral head may remain dislocated into a secondary acetabulum. The child manifests the secondary adaptive physical findings mentioned previously. Pathologically, the anatomic obstacles to reduction change and become more difficult to overcome. The extra-articular and intra-articular pathologic changes may prevent concentric reduction. Extra-articular obstacles may include contraction of the adductor longus and the iliopsoas muscles as a consequence of the dislocation. The most common secondary intra-articular change is varying degrees of anteromedial capsular constriction. The ligamentum teres may become thickened and hypertrophied or elongated, and in some cases, its sheer bulk precludes reduction. In the crawling or walking child, the constant pull of ligamentum teres on its attachment at the base of the acetabulum may cause hypertrophy of the transverse acetabular ligament, which secondarily decreases the diameter of the acetabulum. A true inverted labrum or limbus (hypertrophied labrum) may also be an obstacle reduction in the late diagnosed DDH. This, however, is a rare finding and is seen only in teratologic dislocations (2%) and in previously failed closed reductions, in which case it is an iatrogenic condition.

To understand the natural history of untreated DDH, it is important to appreciate that the normal concave shape of the acetabulum develops in response to the presence of a spherical femoral head. Experimental studies in animals as well as observations in humans with unreduced congenital hip dislocations show that the acetabulum does not develop its normal concave shape. Instead, with a complete dislocation, the triradiate cartilage grows normally, and hence the innominate bone reaches its normal length (Figure 15-5); but the acetabular cartilage atrophies and degenerates, and the acetabulum appears flattened. The depth of the acetabulum increases normally as a result of continued interstitial growth within the acetabular cartilage, oppositional growth at the periphery of this cartilage, and periosteal new bone growth at the edge of the acetabulum along the ilium. The depth of the acetabulum is further increased at puberty by the development of secondary centers of ossification in the three pelvic bones. For this normal growth and development to occur, a concentric relation must be maintained between the femoral head and the acetabulum throughout growth.

Most unstable hips at birth stabilize in a short time. A certain percentage of untreated hips, however, go on to subluxation (partial contact with the acetabulum) or dislocation (no contact between the femoral head and acetabulum), and some hips may remain located but retain dysplastic features. Unfortunately, the means to determine which of the unstable hips will attain spontaneous stability are

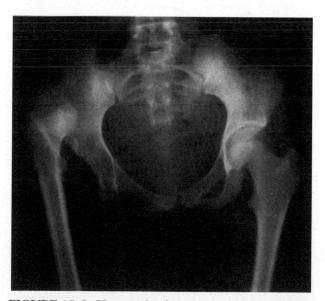

FIGURE 15-5. Untreated right congenital hip dysplasia in an adult. Note the lack of development of acetabular shape and depth. No secondary acetabulum exists. The left hip is normal.

not available, and hence all unstable hips in the newborn period must be treated to ensure the proper environment for hip joint development.

It is important to make the diagnosis early and institute treatment so that normal development may occur. If the hip remains completely dislocated, its natural history depends on two factors: the presence or absence of a false acetabulum and bilateralness.

In the absence of a false acetabulum, most patients with complete dislocations do well, maintaining a good range of motion and little functional disability. Completely dislocated hips with well-developed false acetabuli, however, are more likely to develop degenerative joint disease in the false acetabulum and have a poor clinical result (Figure 15-6). Degenerative joint disease in the false acetabulum usually occurs in the fourth and fifth decades of life. In bilateral complete dislocations, lower-back pain may occur. This may be secondary to the hyperlordosis of the lumbar spine associated with the hip flexion adduction deformities caused by the dislocations.

In unilateral complete dislocations, the natural history is affected by the secondary problems of limb length inequality, ipsilateral knee deformity, pain (usually on the lateral side of the knee), secondary scoliosis, and gait disturbances. In these patients, the same factors concerning the development of secondary degenerative changes in any false acetabulum that may occur are also applicable.

After the neonatal period, *dysplasia* refers to inadequate development of the acetabulum, femoral head, or both. All subluxated hips are by definition dysplastic. Radiographically, however, the major difference between dysplasia and subluxation is the intactness of the Shenton line (Figure 15-7). In subluxation, the Shenton line is disrupted, and the femoral head is superiorly or laterally displaced from the medial wall of the acetabulum. In dysplasia, the normal Shenton line relation is intact. Unfortunately, in the DDH natural history literature, these two radiographic and clinical entities are often not separated. In addition, the development of secondary degenerative arthritis in the dysplastic hip may convert it to a subluxated hip. Because the physical signs of hip dysplasia are usually lacking, cases are often diagnosed only incidentally on radiographs taken for other reasons or not until the patient develops symptoms.

The natural history of hip subluxation clearly indicates that this condition leads to the development of radiographic degenerative joint disease and clinical disability. The more severe the subluxation, the earlier is the symptom onset. Those patients with the most severe subluxations usually develop symptoms of degenerative joint disease during the second decade of life. The symptoms of degenerative joint disease and hip subluxation and dysplasia often predate radiographic changes of degenerative joint disease (decreased joint space, cyst formation, double acetabular floor, inferomedial femoral head osteophyte) by as much as 10 years. Often, the only

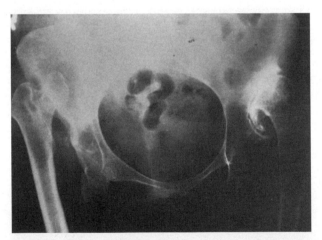

FIGURE 15-6. Radiograph of a 43-year-old woman with complete dislocation of both hips. She has no symptoms on the right but has disabling symptoms from the left hip. She has no false acetabulum on the right but has a well-developed false acetabulum on the left with secondary degenerative changes present. (Weinstein SL. Natural history of congenital hip dislocation [DDH] and hip dysplasia. Clin Orthop 1987;225:62–76)

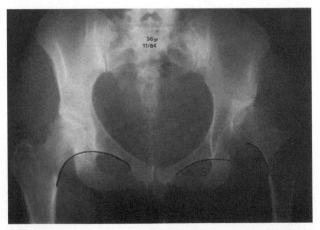

FIGURE 15-7. Radiographically, the major difference between dysplasia and subluxation is the intactness of the Shenton line. The right hip is dysplastic (Shenton line intact). The left hip is subluxated (Shenton line disrupted). All subluxated hips are, by definition, dysplastic. (Weinstein SL. Natural history of congenital hip dislocation [DDH] and hip dysplasia. Clin Orthop 1987;225:62–76)

radiographic feature present at symptom onset may be increased sclerosis in the weight-bearing area. In the absence of subluxation, the natural history of dysplasia cannot accurately be predicted, but hip dysplasia is definitely associated with radiographic degenerative joint disease, especially in female patients.

Once the diagnosis of DDH is made, treatment should be initiated immediately. The use of triple diapers in the treatment of DDH in the newborn should be condemned. It is ineffective and gives the family a false sense of security. Pathologic changes seen in the newborn with DDH are reversible in 95% of cases with simple, appropriately applied treatment methods. The most widely used device in North America is the Pavlik harness (Figure 15-8). The Pavlik harness prevents adduction and extension while allowing further flexion, abduction, and rotation. This position allows for gentle spontaneous reduction of dislocated hips. Stretching of tight adductors is also achieved with the Pavlik harness. The device is worn full time until hip stability is achieved. The physician must provide extensive parent education in addition to the use of the Pavlik harness. Patient noncompliance is the main cause of failure of this device. Appropriate application of the device is essential. Careful follow-up at weekly intervals is extremely important. Adjustments in the flexion and abduction straps of the Pavlik harness must be made to accommodate the hip stability assessed by physical examination of the patient. Clinical hip stability is usually obtained within 2 to 4 weeks of treatment by this method. Most physicians use the harness for a period of 6 to 12 weeks on a full-time basis. Initial radiographs or sono-grams should be obtained in the harness to document adequate flexion and redirection of the femoral shaft toward the triradiate cartilage in the harness. Once clinical stability is obtained, a radiograph is not indicated until about 3 months of age to determine acetabular development. The Pavlik harness may be used in dysplasia and subluxation up to 6 months of age. Once the child begins to crawl, use of the Pavlik harness is extremely difficult, and the success rate with the harness decreases to less than 50%.

If hip stability is not achieved in the previously mentioned time frame, treatment with the Pavlik harness should be discontinued and alternative methods of treatment employed. The Pavlik harness is contraindicated in the patient who has DDH in association with conditions of muscle imbalance (e.g., upper-level meningomyelocele), joint stiffness (e.g., arthrogryposis), or excess ligamentous laxity, (e.g., Ehlers-Danlos syndrome). Applied correctly and used for the appropriate indications, the Pavlik harness may achieve 95% successful results in treatment of DDH. Inappropriately applied and poorly monitored use of the harness is associated with problems such as inferior hip dislocations from prolonged excess flexion of the hip in the harness. This hyperflexion may also be associated with femoral nerve palsies, which are usually transient. Brachial plexus palsies from pressure of the shoulder straps have also been reported. The parent must pay attention to skin care in the groin folds and the popliteal fossa area to prevent skin maceration and breakdown. The most devastating complication of the Pavlik harness is aseptic necrosis of the femoral head. Reported incidence of this complication ranges from 9 to 15%. This is generally produced by excess

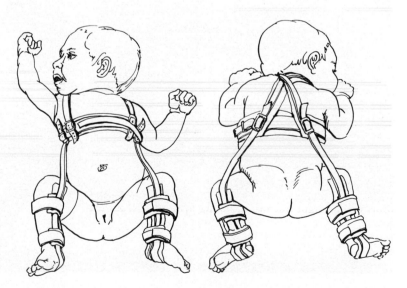

FIGURE 15-8. Pavlik harness. The posterior strap acts as a check rein against adduction to prevent redislocation.

of tightening of the abduction strap. It has been well documented that the hyperabduction position of the hip compromises the vascular supply to the proximal femur.

In a child with dysplasia or subluxation who is older than 6 months of age, a fixed-abduction orthosis may be used to achieve hip stability and allow for growth and development of the hip joint. It can be used only if the hip is well reduced on a radiograph taken in the orthoses. The complications of fixed-abduction orthoses include skin problems and aseptic necrosis. It is important in positioning the fixed-abduction orthoses that the hip not be placed in extreme positions of abduction to avoid aseptic necrosis.

In the late diagnosed case (over 6 months of age) or the case that fails treatment with a Pavlik harness and is not amenable to a fixed-abduction orthosis, the obstacles to reduction are different, treatment has greater risks, and the results are less predictable. The general goals of treatment in the late diagnosed case are to obtain and maintain a reduction, to allow for femoral head and acetabular development, and to avoid a development of aseptic necrosis.

In these cases or in those that have failed Pavlik harness treatment, closed reduction is indicated. Closed reduction is generally preceded by a 1- to 2-week period of traction (Figure 15-9). Although the use of prereduction traction is somewhat controversial, the purpose of the traction is, in theory, to allow gradual stretching of the soft tissue structures impeding reduction as well as of the neurovascular bundle. The primary purpose of traction is the avoidance of aseptic necrosis, the most devastating complication of the treatment of DDH. The traction can be applied in the hospital or at home. Generally, 1 to 2 weeks is sufficient. Skin traction is usually adequate; skeletal traction is rarely necessary. The skin tapes should be applied above the knee to distribute the traction over a large area. Complications of traction include skin loss and ischemia of the lower extremities due to inappropriate application. Neurocirculatory checks must be done frequently and traction applied in a carefully supervised fashion. Home traction has become popular because of the decreased cost and convenience. Home traction should follow a 24-hour hospitalization to familiarize the parents with application of the traction and how to look for problems. It can only be used with cooperative, informed parents.

Closed reductions are usually performed in the operating room setting. Under general anesthesia, the hip is gently manipulated into the acetabulum. Arthrography is extremely helpful in assessing the adequacy of reduction (Figure 15-10). Because a large portion of the acetabulum is cartilaginous, the relations of the femoral head and acetabulum are nicely visualized on arthrography. The use of arthrography can help to assess any obstacles to reduction and also the quality of reduction. Reduction is then maintained by a well-molded cast (Figure 15-11) for a variable amount of time (range, 6 weeks to 4 months), depending on the child's age.

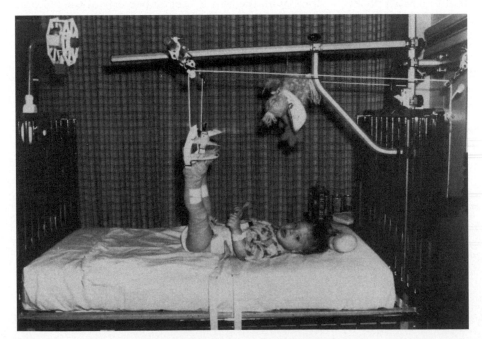

FIGURE 15-9. Preliminary traction. Bryant traction was used before attempted closed reduction to stretch soft tissue structures about the hip.

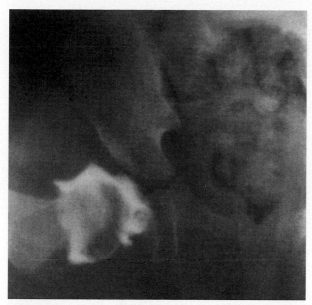

FIGURE 15-10. Attempted closed reduction under arthrographic control. Note pooling of dye medially. The hip cannot be reduced.

The so-called human position of hyperflexion and limited abduction should be used in closed reductions. Extreme positions of abduction, as well as abduction and internal rotation, should be avoided because of their association with the development of aseptic necrosis. After removal of the cast, a fixed-abduction orthosis is applied and worn at night and during napping hours until acetabular development has returned to normal. The postoperative reduction can be confirmed by the use of computed tomographic (CT) scanning or ultrasound.

Open reductions are indicated for failure to obtain a closed reduction, failure to maintain a closed

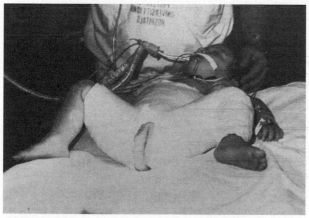

FIGURE 15-11. Reduction of left congenital hip dysplasia is maintained by a well-molded 1½ hip spica cast.

reduction, or an unstable reduction. If an open reduction is necessary, it can be done through a variety of surgical approaches. During the open reduction, each obstacle to reduction must be addressed. The most common obstacle is the tight anteromedial joint capsule, which must be released. The transverse acetabular ligament often requires sectioning, and the ligamentum teres may need to be removed. A true inverted labrum or limbus should never be excised but only radially incised because excision of this tissue may interfere with the normal growth and development of the acetabulum.

After the age of 2 years, there is a high likelihood of a patient's requiring an open reduction to obtain and maintain a reduction. By the age of 3 years, preliminary traction should not be used, but open reduction should be accompanied by a femoral shortening (removal of a section of the proximal femur) to decrease the incidence of aseptic necrosis. Between the ages of 2 and 4 years, the question of whether to use femoral shortening versus traction before open reduction remains unanswered. The trend today however for pediatric orthopaedic surgeons treating the over 2-year-of-age group is to accompany open reduction by a femoral shortening procedure.

The acetabulum has potential for growth for many years once a closed or open reduction has been obtained. If, however, the acetabulum does not make adequate progress toward normal development after a closed or open reduction, one of several types of innominate osteotomy should be performed to increase femoral head coverage (Figure 15-12).

All children with DDH have associated femoral neck anteversion. In general, children reduced before they are 2 years of age rarely require derotation osteotomies to correct the anteversion. Anteversion usually corrects once the reduction is obtained. Aseptic necrosis is the most devastating complication associated with the treatment of DDH. Aseptic necrosis may be caused by many errors in treatment, as mentioned previously. In the newborn, excessive use of abduction or the abduction internal rotation position can cause aseptic necrosis. In the older child, aseptic necrosis may be caused by insufficient use of prereduction traction, failure to perform an adductor tenotomy, injuries to the blood vessels during surgery, failure to do femoral shortening, or persistence of closed techniques in the face of obstacles to reduction.

In adolescent patients with residual dysplasia, deformity may be present in the femoral head, acetabulum, or both. In these cases, normal anatomy

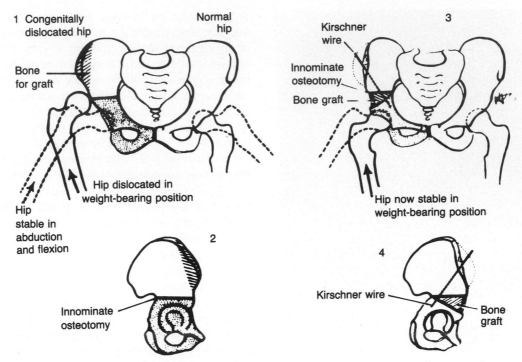

FIGURE 15-12. Technique of Salter innominate osteotomy. Diagram of principle involved. (Salter RB. Innominate osteotomy in the treatment of congenital dislocation and subluxation of the hip. J Bone Joint Surg 1961;43B:518.

and relation must be restored. In many cases, osteotomies are necessary on both the femoral and pelvic sides of the hip joint.

LEGG-CALVÉ-PERTHES DISEASE

Legg-Calvé-Perthes disease (LCPD) is a disorder of the hip in young children. The disease is characterized by varying degrees of necrosis of the femoral ossific nucleus. It is most common in the age range of 4 to 8 years, but has been reported in children as young as 2 years of age and also in the late teenage years. It is more common in boys than girls by a ratio of 4:1, and the incidence of bilateralness is about 10 to 12%.

Epidemiologic studies of patients with Legg-Calvé-Perthes disease reveal an incidence of a positive family history of about 10%. There is a high association of abnormal birth presentation, such as breech or transverse lie, in affected patients. There are also racial and ethnic factors, with LCPD being more common in Japanese, Eskimos, and Central Europeans and uncommon in native Australians, Polynesians, American Indians, and blacks.

Other epidemiologic factors include lower birth weights and delay in skeletal maturation as evidenced by retarded bone age. Affected children are shorter than nonaffected children. Anthropometric studies have confirmed this growth delay, with affected children being smaller in all dimensions except head circumference and with the distal portion of the extremities affected more than the proximal. The short stature of the patients affected with the disorder at a young age tends to correct during adolescence, while those affected at an older age tend to be small throughout life. An abnormality of growth hormone-dependent somatomedin in males with LCPD has recently been demonstrated.

An increased incidence of LCPD is seen in later born children, particularly the third to the sixth child, and in lower socioeconomic groups.

LCPD is more common in certain geographic areas, particularly in urban rather than rural communities. Parental age of affected patients is higher than in the general population. Affected children have an increased association of genital urinary tract abnormalities, inguinal hernia, and minor congenital abnormalities.

The cause of LCPD remains unknown. LCPD has been thought to be an inflammatory disease, secondary to trauma or a developmental disorder. Toxic synovitis is thought by some authors to be a precursor to LCPD; however, a literature review of patients with toxic synovitis revealed that only about 3% subsequently develop LCPD. The most widely accepted etiologic theories are those involving interruption of the vascular supply to the femoral head. It has been well demonstrated in animal studies and confirmed by human pathologic material that LCPD is caused by repetitive episodes of infarction. Recent studies have postulated that the cause of the vascular embarrassment may be disturbed venous drainage, intraosseous venous hypertension, or increased blood viscosity leading to decreased blood flow.

Some evidence suggests that LCPD may be a generalized disorder of epiphyseal hyaline cartilage and thus should be called Legg-Calvé-Perthes syndrome. This may account for the delayed skeletal maturation and for the disease's manifestation in the hip because of the unusual and precarious blood supply of the proximal femur, which makes the femoral head especially vulnerable.

Skeletal surveys in patients with LCPD demonstrate irregularities of ossification in other epiphyses and abnormalities in the contralateral, so-called unaffected capital epiphysis compared with matched controls.

Histologic changes of the epiphyseal and physeal cartilage of patients with LCPD were described as early as 1913 by Perthes. The superficial zone of the cartilage covering the affected femoral head is normal but thickened (Figure 15-13). In the middle layer of the epiphyseal cartilage, however, two types of abnormalities are seen: areas of extreme hypercellularity, with the cells varying in size and shape and often arranged in clusters; and in other areas, a loose, fibrocartilaginous-like matrix. These abnormal areas in the epiphyseal cartilage have different histochemical and ultrastructural properties than normal cartilage or fibrocartilage. Areas of small secondary ossification centers are evident, with bony trabeculae of uneven thickness forming directly on the abnormal cartilage matrix.

The physeal plate in LCPD shows evidence of cleft formation with amorphous debris and extravasation of blood. In the metaphyseal region, enchondral ossification is normal in some areas; but in other areas, the proliferating cells are separated by a fibrillated cartilaginous matrix that does not calcify. The cells in these areas do not degenerate but continue to proliferate without enchondral ossification. This is evidenced by "tongues" of cartilage extending into the metaphysis as bone growth proceeds in adjoining areas (Figure 15-14).

Catterall demonstrated thickening, abnormal staining, sporadic calcification, and diminished evidence of ossification in the deep zone of the articular cartilage of the unaffected hip. He also demonstrated the physeal plate in these unaffected hips to be thinner than normal, with irregular cell columns and cartilage masses remaining unossified in the primary spongiosa. Similar histologic changes have been seen in the acetabular cartilage and other epiphyses. Thus, the epidemiologic, anthropometric, radiographic, and histologic data lend support to the concept of the susceptible child. LCPD may thus represent a localized manifestation of the generalized transient disorder of the epiphyseal hyaline cartilage, clinically manifested in the proximal femur because of its unusual and precarious blood supply. The persistence of the abnormally soft cartilage through which blood vessels have to penetrate into the femoral head could cause repeated episodes of infarction and prolong the disease.

LCPD must not be thought of as simply aseptic necrosis similar to that seen in the adult or child after a femoral neck fracture or a traumatic dislocation of the hip. After a fracture at the femoral neck or a traumatic dislocation of the hip in a child, the vascular insult usually heals rapidly without going through the prolonged stages of fragmentation and repair that are seen in LCPD.

Patients with LCPD most commonly present with a history of the insidious onset of a limp. Most patients do not complain of much discomfort unless

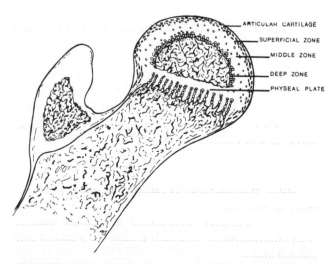

FIGURE 15-13. Anatomic regions of the proximal femur in a growing child. (Weinstein SL. Legg-Calvé-Perthes disease. In: Morrissy RT, Weinstein SL, eds. Lovell and Winter's Pediatric Orthopaedics, 5th Ed. Philadelphia: Lippincott Williams & Wilkins, 2001:962)

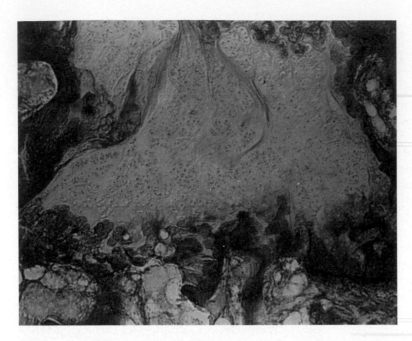

FIGURE 15-14. Photomicrograph (×80) showing a large area of cartilage in between the bone trabeculae of the femoral neck (case 1). (Ponseti IV. Legg-Perthes disease: observations on pathological changes in two cases. J Bone Joint Surg 1956;38A:739)

specifically questioned about this aspect. Pain when present is usually activity related and relieved by rest. Because of its mild nature, most patients do not present for medical attention until weeks or months after the clinical onset of disease. The pain that patients experience is generally localized to the groin or referred to the anteromedial thigh or knee region. Failure to recognize that thigh or knee pain in the child may be secondary to hip pathology may cause further delay in the diagnosis. Some children present with more acute symptom onset. As with most childhood musculoskeletal disorders, patients with LCPD usually present with limited hip motion, particularly abduction and medial rotation. Early in the course of the disease, the limited abduction is secondary to muscle spasm of the adductor muscles; however, with time, subsequent deformities may develop, and limitation of abduction may become permanent. Occasionally, long-standing adductor spasm leads to adductor contracture. The Trendelenburg test in patients with LCPD is often positive. These children most commonly have evidence of thigh, calf, and buttock atrophy from inactivity secondary to pain. This is further evidence of the longstanding nature of the condition before detection. Limb length should be measured; inequality is indicative of significant head collapse and a poor prognosis. Evaluation of the patient's overall height, weight, and bone age may be helpful in the differential diagnosis and may provide confirmatory evidence of the disorder. Laboratory studies are generally not helpful in LCPD, although they may be necessary to rule out other conditions.

The diagnosis is made and the condition followed by plain radiographs taken in the anteroposterior (AP) and frog-leg lateral positions. These radiographs are generally sufficient for the assessment of the patient and for subsequent follow-up evaluations. From the plain radiographs, the physician can determine the stage of the disease and the extent of epiphyseal involvement. Additional radiographic or imaging studies may be helpful in the initial assessment or follow-up of the condition.

Radionuclide bone scanning with technetium and pin-hole collimation may be helpful in the early stages of the disease when the diagnosis is in question, but this is rarely necessary. Some investigators consider scanning helpful in determining the extent of the epiphyseal involvement and hence prognosis.

Magnetic resonance imaging (MRI) is sensitive in detecting infarction, but as of yet cannot accurately portray the stages of healing. Its role in the management of LCPD is yet to be defined.

There are four radiographic stages of LCPD. In the initial stage, the earliest radiographic signs of LCPD are failure of the ossific nucleus to grow compared with the unaffected hip and widening of the medial joint space caused by hypertrophy of the articular cartilage of the femoral head (Figure 15-15). The physician may also see a relative increase in radiodensity of the femoral ossific nucleus in relation to the femoral neck. Radiolucencies may be present in the metaphysis with thinning and irregularity of

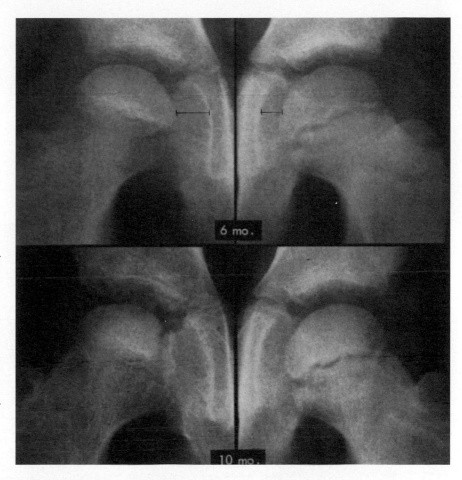

FIGURE 15-15. AP radiographs of the hip in a patient who developed Legg-Calvé-Perthes disease. On the initial film taken 6 months after onset of symptoms, the right ossific nucleus is smaller than the left, and the medial joint space is widened. Note also the retained density of the ossific nucleus compared with that of the normal hip and the relative osteopenia of the viable bone of the proximal femur and pelvis. Ten months after onset of symptoms, the evolution of the radiographic changes is seen. (Weinstein SL. Legg-Calvé-Perthes disease. Instr Course Lect 1983;32:272)

the physeal plate (Figures 15-16 and 15-17). A subchondral radiolucent zone (crescent sign) may also be present. This radiolucent zone generally corresponds to the extent of the necrotic portion of the ossific nucleus (Figure 15-18).

The second radiographic stage is the fragmentation phase. In this phase, the physician sees resorption of the necrotic portion of the ossific nucleus (Figure 15-19). This is followed by a reparative or reossification phase, in which the physician sees return to normal radiodensities of the ossific nucleus until the lesion is completely healed (see Figure 15-19).

The femoral head and neck may become deformed as a result of the disease, the repair process, or premature physeal plate closure. The actual deformity that develops is profoundly influenced by the duration of the disease. This in turn is proportional to the extent of the epiphyseal involvement, the age of disease onset, the remodeling potential of the patient, and the stage of disease when treatment is initiated. An additional factor may be the type of treatment.

Prognostic factors must be gleaned from series of long-term follow-ups. In the 20- to 40-year postsymptom-onset follow-ups, most patients (70 to 90%) are active and free of pain. Most patients maintain a good range of motion despite the fact that few patients have normal-appearing radiographs. Clinical deterioration, increasing pain, decreasing range of motion, and loss of function are observed in only those patients with flattened irregular femoral heads at the time of primary healing and in those with evidence of premature physeal closure. The follow-up studies beyond 40 years, however, demonstrate marked reduction in function, with most patients developing degenerative joint disease by the sixth or seventh decade.

Reviews of long-term series of patients with LCPD identify certain clinical and radiographic features that have prognostic value. These interrelated factors include deformity of the femoral head and hip joint incongruence, age of disease onset, extent of epiphyseal involvement, growth disturbance secondary to premature physeal closure, protracted disease course, acetabular and femoral

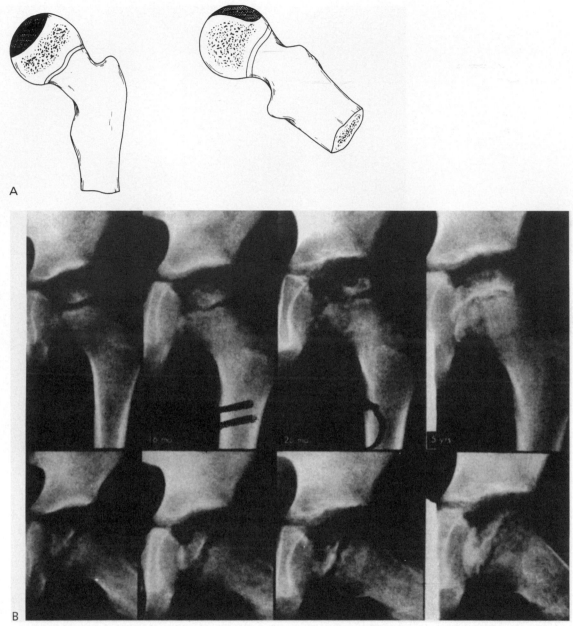

FIGURE 15-16. **(A)** Catterall group 1 disease: anterior head involvement, with no evidence of sequestrum or of a subchondral fracture line or metaphyseal abnormalities. **(B)** Catterall group 1 disease 1 week to 5 years after onset of symptoms. (Weinstein SL. Legg-Calvé-Perthes disease. In: Morrissy RT and Weinstein SL, eds. Lovell and Winter's Pediatric Orthopaedics, 5th Ed. Philadelphia: Lippincott Williams & Wilkins, 2001:964)

head remodeling potential, type of treatment, and stage during which treatment is initiated.

Partial or anterior head involvement leads to a more favorable prognosis than whole femoral head involvement. Catterall demonstrated the importance of the extent of epiphyseal involvement relating to prognosis and proposed four groups based on the presence or absence of seven radiographic signs

in 97 untreated hips (Table 15-1; see Figures 15-16 and 15-19). He reported that 90% of the good results in untreated patients were in groups 1 and 2, while 90% of the poor results were in groups 3 and 4.

Salter and Thompson proposed a simplified, two-group classification based on prognosis: group A had less than 50% femoral head involvement (Catterall groups 1 and 2); and group B had more

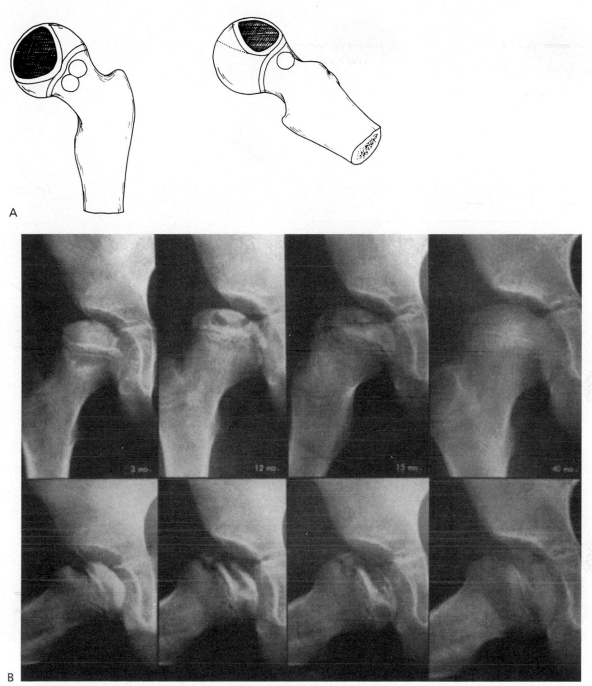

FIGURE 15-17. (A) Catterall group 2 disease: anterolateral involvement, sequestrum formation, and a clear junction between the involved and uninvolved areas. There are anterolateral metaphyseal lesions, and the subchondral fracture line is in the anterior half of the head. The lateral column is intact. **(B)** Catterall group 2 disease 3 to 40 months after onset of symptoms. Note the intact lateral pillar. (Weinstein SL. Legg-Calvé-Perthes disease. In: Morrissy RT, Weinstein SL, eds. Lovell and Winter's Pediatric Orthopaedics, 5th Ed. Philadelphia: Lippincott Williams and Wilkins, 2001:975)

than 50% femoral head involvement (Catterall groups 3 and 4). The major determining factor between groups A and B is the presence or absence of a viable lateral pillar of the epiphysis. This intact lateral column (Catterall group 2, Salter-Thompson group A) may thus shield the epiphysis from collapse and subsequent deformity (see Figures 15-17 and 15-18).

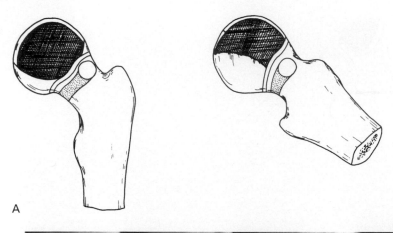

A

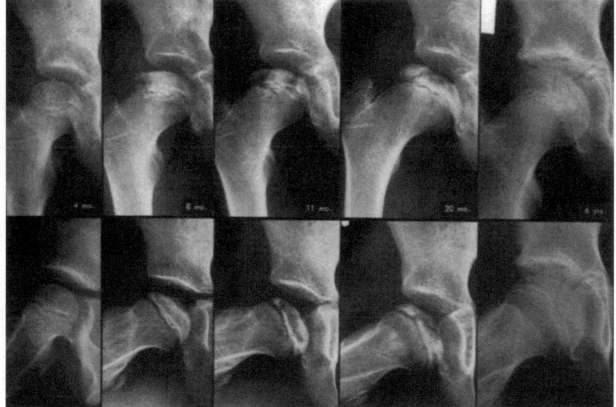

B

FIGURE 15-18. (A) Catterall group 3 disease: large sequestrum involving three-quarters of the head. The junction between the involved and uninvolved portions is sclerotic. Metaphyseal lesions are diffuse, particularly anterolaterally, and the subchondral fracture line extends to the posterior half of the epiphysis. The lateral column is involved. **(B)** Catterall group 3 disease 4 months to 6 years after onset of symptoms. Note involvement of the lateral pillar as well as the subchondral radiolucent zone on the radiograph taken 8 months after onset of symptoms. (Weinstein SL. Legg-Calvé-Perthes disease. In: Morrissy RT, Weinstein SL, eds. Lovell and Winter's Pediatric Orthopaedics, 5th Ed. Philadelphia: Lippincott Williams & Wilkins, 2001:967–968)

Another classification scheme, the lateral pillar classification, depends on the radiographic appearance of the lateral pillar (lateral 15 to 30% of the femoral head) on an AP radiograph (Figure 15-20 and Table 15-2). The more the lateral pillar height is maintained in the maximal fragmentation phase of the disease, the better the outcome.

Catterall identified other radiographic signs of prognostic value (Figure 15-22). These at-risk signs include the Gage sign (radiolucency in the lateral

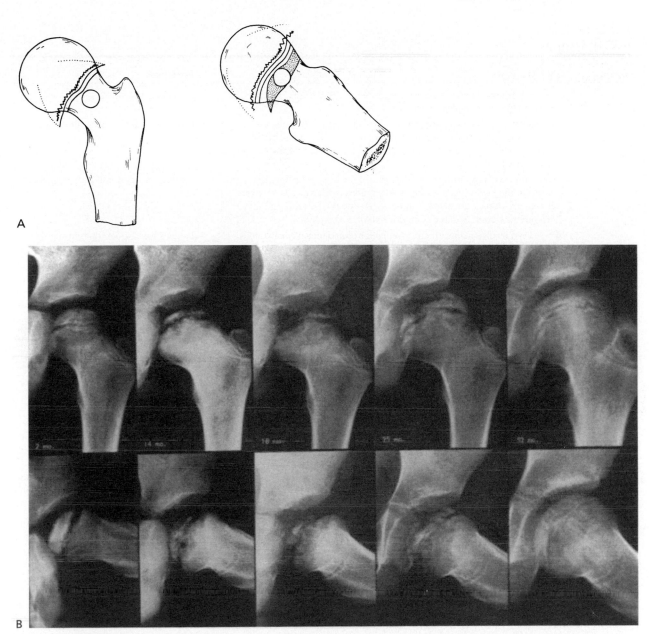

FIGURE 15-19. **(A)** Catterall group 4 disease: whole head involvement with either diffuse or central metaphyseal lesions and posterior remodeling of the epiphysis. **(B)** Catterall group 4 disease 2 to 52 months after onset of symptoms. Note the stage: 14 months—fragmentation; 18 months—early reossification; 25 months—late reossification; 52 months—healed. Note also the growth arrest line and evidence of reactivation of the growth plate along the femoral neck. (Weinstein SL. Legg-Calvé-Perthes disease. In: Morrissy RT, Weinstein SL, eds. Lovell and Winter's Pediatric Orthopaedics, 5th Ed. Philadelphia: Lippincott Williams & Wilkins, 2001:966–967)

epiphysis and metaphysis) and calcification lateral to the epiphysis. These two signs indicate early ossification in the enlarged epiphysis and are therefore present only when the head is deformed but at a stage when the changes are reversible. Another at-risk sign is metaphyseal lesions. These radiolucencies may herald the potential for growth disturbance of the physeal plate. The final two at-risk signs are lateral subluxation and a horizontal growth plate. Lateral subluxation indicates a widened femoral head. The horizontal growth plate indicates a developing deformity that, if left untreated, leads to a fixed deformity, hinge abduction, and further deformity. These radiographic at-risk signs are

TABLE 15-1.
Catterall Groups

Group	Characteristics	Prognosis
1	Anterior head involvement, no evidence of sequestrum or of a subchondral fracture line or metaphyseal abnormalities.	Patients uniformly do well.
2	Anterolateral involvement, sequestrum formation and a clear junction between the involved and uninvolved areas. There are anterolateral metaphyseal lesions, and the subchondral fracture line is in the anterior half of the head.	Clinical results are generally good.
3	Large sequestrum involving three-quarters of the head. The junction between the involved and uninvolved portions is sclerotic. Metaphyseal lesions are diffuse, particularly anterolaterally, and the subchondral fracture line extends to the posterior half of the epiphysis.	Healing is slower and less complete.
4	Whole head involvement with either diffuse or central metaphyseal lesions and posterior remodeling of the epiphysis.	Patients have a poor long-term prognosis.

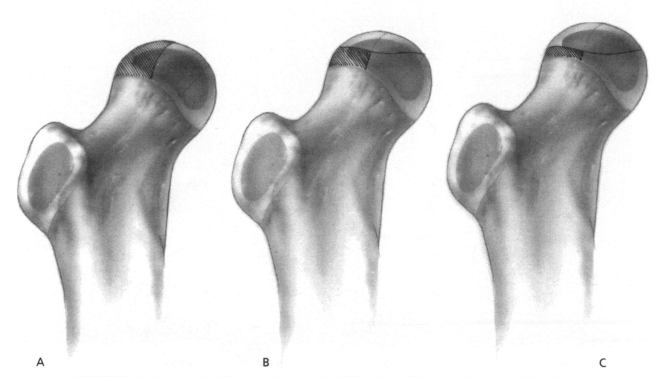

A   B   C

FIGURE 15-20. Lateral pillar classification. See Table 15-2. (Weinstein SL. Legg-Calvé-Perthes disease. In: Morrissy RT, Weinstein SL, eds. Lovell and Winter's Pediatric Orthopaedics, 5th Ed. Philadelphia: Lippincott Williams & Wilkins, 2001:976)

TABLE 15-2.
Lateral Pillar Classification

Type A	No involvement of the lateral pillar; lateral pillar is radiographically normal; possible lucency and collapse in the central and medial pillars, but full height of the lateral pillar is maintained.
Type B	Greater than 50% of the lateral pillar height is maintained; lateral pillar has some radiolucency, with maintenance of bone density at a height between 50 and 100% of the original height of the lateral head.
Type C	Less than 50% of lateral pillar height is maintained; lateral pillar becomes more radiolucent than in type B, and any preserved bone is at a height of <50% of the original height of the lateral pillar.

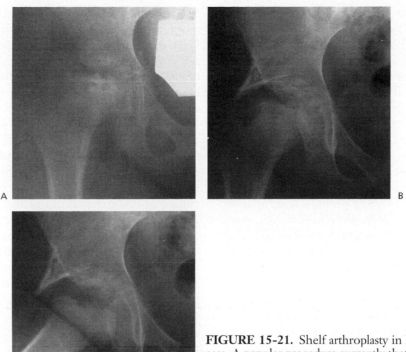

FIGURE 15-21. Shelf arthroplasty in Legg-Calvé-Perthes disease. A popular procedure currently that will have to await long-term results to know if it improves prognosis. (Weinstein SL. Legg-Calvé-Perthes disease. In: Morrissy RT, Weinstein SL, eds. Lovell and Winter's Pediatric Orthopaedics, 5th Ed. Philadelphia: Lippincott Williams & Wilkins, 2001—Fig. 24-27)

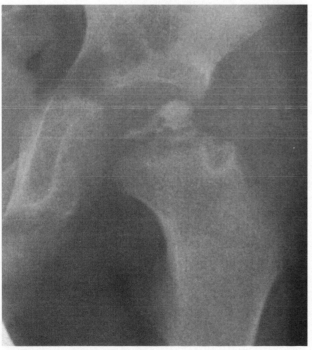

FIGURE 15-22. A 6-year, 5-month-old boy with Catterall group 4 disease and all the at-risk signs. (Weinstein SL. Legg-Calvé-Perthes disease. In: Morrissy RT, Weinstein SL, eds. Lovell and Winter's Pediatric Orthopaedics, 5th Ed. Philadelphia: Lippincott Williams & Wilkins, 2001:978)

manifested clinically by loss of motion and adduction contracture. Catterall reported no poor results in patients not manifesting two or more at risk signs.

The extent of epiphyseal involvement is related to the duration of the disease. In general, the greater the extent of epiphyseal involvement, the longer the duration and course of the disease. End results are worse with prolonged disease duration.

Age of disease onset is a significant factor in relation to outcome. The younger the patient at disease onset, the better is the prognosis. Eight years of age appears to be the watershed age in most long-term series. Age at healing, however, is probably a more important factor. Because of the overall skeletal maturation delay and the knowledge that this is usually compensated for during the adolescent growth spurt, patients affected at a younger age have an enhanced potential for femoral head and acetabular remodeling. Femoral head at-risk signs are also less likely to occur in younger patients, particularly those younger than 5 years of age.

The development of the acetabulum depends on the geometric pattern within it during growth, and because the acetabulum continues to have significant development potential up to age 8 or 9 years of age, if a young patient does develop deformity, the immature acetabulum conforms to the altered femoral head shape. This leads to aspheric congruency, which may be compatible with normal function for many years.

The patient history, physical examination, and plain radiographs are usually sufficient to make a diagnosis of LCPD. Diagnosis early in the initial phase of the disease, however, must be differentiated from conditions such as transient synovitis (Table 15-3) and septic arthritis (primary or secondary to proximal femoral osteomyelitis). A complete blood count, including white blood cell differential, erythrocyte sedimentation rate, C-reactive protein, and hip joint aspiration, and analysis of the fluid may be necessary to rule out infection. All laboratory studies of LCPD are generally normal, although the erythrocyte sedimentation rate and or the C-reactive protein may be slightly elevated. In early cases, if all the laboratory studies are normal, and doubt as to the diagnosis persists, radionuclide scanning may be helpful.

In patients with bilateral hip involvement, generalized disorders, such as multiple epiphyseal dysplasia and hypothyroidism, must be considered. Patients with bilateral involvement, particularly those with atypical radiographic features, must have a careful family history obtained as well as a bone survey to rule out a metabolic or a genetic condition. In children younger than 4 years of age, Meyer dysplasia, a benign-resolving condition, must be considered.

Most patients with LCPD (60%) do not need treatment. Treatment modalities have evolved from the earliest treatments of weight relief until the

TABLE 15-3.
Differential Diagnosis of Legg-Calvé-Perthes Disease

Chondrolysis
Gaucher disease
Hemophilia
Hypothyroidism
Juvenile rheumatoid arthritis
Lymphoma
Mucopolysaccharidosis
Multiple epiphyseal dysplasia
Meyer dysplasia
Neoplasm
Old congenital hip dysplasia residuals
Osteomyelitis of proximal femur with secondary septic arthritis
Septic arthritis
Sickle cell disease
Spondyloepiphyseal dysplasia
Toxic synovitis
Traumatic aseptic necrosis

head was reossified to the present day containment methods. The essence of containment is that, to prevent deformities of the diseased epiphysis, the femoral head must be contained within the depths of the acetabulum to equalize the pressure on the head and subject it to the molding action of the acetabulum. Containment is an attempt to reduce the forces through the hip joint by establishing an actual or relative varus relation between the femoral head and the acetabulum. Considering all methods of containment, the physician must realize that the femoral head represents over three-fourths of a sphere and the acetabulum only half of a sphere. Therefore, no method of containment can provide a totally contained femoral head within the acetabulum during all portions of the gait cycle.

The primary goals in the treatment of LCPD are to prevent deformity, alter growth disturbance, and prevent degenerative joint disease. To attain these goals, the patient must be assessed clinically and radiographically. Clinically, the patient is evaluated for at-risk signs of pain and loss of motion. AP and lateral radiographs are evaluated to determine the radiographic stage of the disease, the extent of epiphyseal involvement, and the presence of any at-risk signs. The optimal time for treatment is during the radiographic initial or fragmentation stage of the disease. Once the head is in the reossification stage, little further deformity occurs; thus, to influence deformity, treatment must be initiated earlier. Some difficulties may be encountered in determining the extent of epiphyseal involvement, especially early in the disease process, and radionuclide scanning or MRI may be helpful.

Treatment is *not* indicated if the child demonstrates none of the clinical or radiographic at-risk signs, if the patients has Catterall group 1 disease, lateral pillar A (Salter-Thompson group A), or if the disease is already in the reossification stage. A child who demonstrates clinical or radiographic at-risk signs, regardless of the extent of epiphyseal involvement, should receive treatment. Even patients with Catterall group 2 disease or lateral pillar B who are at risk may end up with a poor result without treatment.

The first principle of treatment is restoration of motion. Motion enhances synovial nutrition and thus cartilage nutrition. Restoration of motion can be accomplished by putting the patient at rest with skin traction and progressive abduction to relieve the adductor spasm. Occasionally, surgical release of the contracted adductors may be necessary. Restoration of motion allows abduction of the hip, which reduces the force on the hip joint and allows positioning of the uncovered anterolateral aspect of the femoral

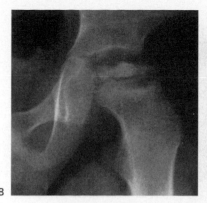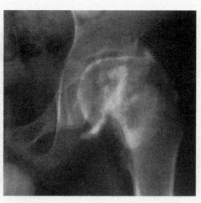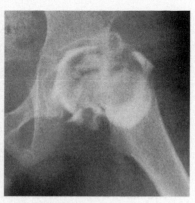

A,B   C

FIGURE 15-23. A 4-year, 9-month-old boy with Catterall group 4 disease and at-risk status. **(A)** Plain film. **(B)** Arthrogram in neutral abduction, adduction, and rotation. Note enlargement and flattening of the cartilaginous femoral head and how the lateral margin of the acetabulum is deformed by the femoral head. **(C)** Arthrogram in abduction and slight external rotation. Note how the femoral head hinges on the lateral edge of the acetabulum, further deforming the lateral acetabulum. Also note the slight pooling of dye medially. (Weinstein SL. Legg-Calvé-Perthes disease. In: Morrissy RT, Weinstein SL, eds. Lovell and Winter's Pediatric Orthopaedics, 5th Ed. Philadelphia: Lippincott Williams & Wilkins, 2001:966)

head in the acetabulum (containment). Mobilization of the hip joint may also be obtained by use of progressive abduction casts. Treatment appears to give superior results in severely involved patients (Catterall groups 3 and 4, or Salter-Thompson group B, lateral pillar B, C) compared with no treatment.

Arthrography is a useful adjunct in determining whether the head actually can be contained and, if so, in what position this is best accomplished. Arthrography demonstrates any flattening of the femoral head that may not be seen on plain film. More important, it may demonstrate the hinge abduction phenomenon, which is a contraindication to any type of containment treatment. Once the femoral head becomes deformed and is no longer containable within the acetabulum, the only motion that is allowed is in the flexion and extension plane, with abduction leading to hinging on the lateral edge of the acetabulum. This hinge abduction causes acetabular and secondary femoral head deformity (Figure 15-23).

The two most commonly advocated methods of containment treatment are femoral osteotomy and innominate osteotomy. Abduction bracing, which was the most commonly used method of treatment for many years, is now rarely used. Most abduction braces were modifications of the Atlanta Scottish Rite orthosis (Figure 15-24). Several studies, however, questioned the efficacy of brace treatment in LCPD, and in recent years braces are rarely used.

Surgical methods of providing and maintaining containment offer the advantage of early mobilization and avoidance of prolonged brace or cast treatment. Varus osteotomy with or without rotation offers the advantage of deep seating of the femoral head and positioning of the vulnerable anterolateral portion of the head away from the deforming influences of the acetabular margin (Figure 15-25). It has been reported that this procedure improves disturbed venous drainage and relieves interosseous venous hypertension, thus accelerating the healing process. This, however, has not been conclusively confirmed. Prerequisites for the procedure include full range of motion, congruency between the head and the acetabulum, and the ability to seat the head in abduction and internal rotation. As with all containment treatment modalities, to have any effect, treatment must be instituted in the initial or fragmentation stage of the disease. The negative aspects of this treatment include the associated risks and costs of the surgical procedure in addition to a second surgical procedure necessary for any hardware removal. The affected limb is also shortened by the procedure. The varus angulation normally decreases with growth, but if there has been physeal plate damage by the disease, this remodeling potential may be lost, leaving the patient with a permanent varus deformity and limb shortening.

Innominate osteotomy (see Figure 15-12) provides for containment by redirection of the acetabular roof, providing better coverage for the anterolateral portion of the head. It places the head in relative flexion, abduction, and internal rotation with respect to the acetabulum in the weight-bearing position. Any shortening caused by the disease process is corrected. Prerequisites for innominate osteotomy include a full range of hip joint motion, joint congruency with the

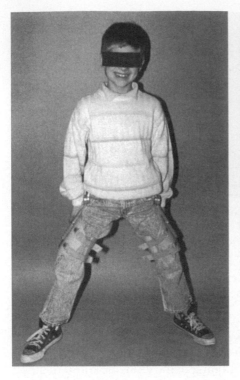
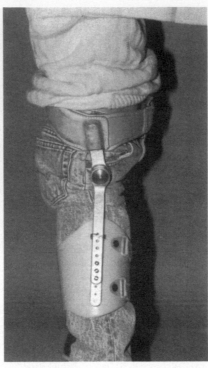

FIGURE 15-24. An abduction orthosis. (Weinstein SL. Legg-Calvé-Perthes disease. In: Morrissy RT, Weinstein SL, eds. Lovell and Winter's Pediatric Orthopaedics, 5th Ed. Philadelphia: Lippincott Williams & Wilkins, 2001:986)

ability to seat the head in flexion, abduction, and internal rotation. The procedure must be done in the initial or fragmentation stage of the disease. The disadvantages of innominate osteotomy are the inherent risks of the surgical procedure, the fact that the operation is being performed on the normal side of the joint, and the suggestion that the procedure may increase the forces on the femoral head by lateralizing the acetabulum and increasing the lever arm of the abductors. Satisfactory anatomic results have been reported for all these containment methods in carefully selected patients.

In recent years, the shelf arthroplasty (Figure 15-21) has been gaining in popularity in the patient with a poor prognosis (Catterall 3, 4, lateral pillar B, C, children > 8 years of age). This procedure is aimed at providing coverage for a femoral head that is certain to enlarge because of the disease process. Long-term outcomes of this procedure will determine its role in LCPD treatment.

Regardless of the method of containment treatment chosen, any episode indicative of loss of containment (i.e., recurrent pain and loss of range of motion) must be treated aggressively by rest and traction or casting to restore lost motion.

For noncontainable hips, particularly those that demonstrate the hinge abduction phenomenon on arthrography, the physician must consider other alternatives. These salvage procedures include Chiari osteotomy, cheilectomy, abduction extension osteotomy, and acetabular shelf procedures alone or in combination with femoral osteotomies. These procedures in an already deformed head must be viewed as salvage procedures with the limited aims of pain relief, correction of limb length inequality, and improvement of movement and abductor weakness. Cheilectomy removes the anterolateral portion of the head that is impinging on the acetabulum in abduction. This procedure must only be done after the physis is closed; otherwise, a slipped capital femoral epiphysis (SCFE) may ensue. This procedure does not correct any residual shortening or abductor weakness. The Chiari osteotomy improves the lateral coverage of the deformed femoral head but does not reduce the lateral impingement in abduction and may exacerbate any existing abductor weakness. Its role in LCPD is yet to be defined. Abduction extension osteotomy of the femur is indicated when arthrography demonstrates joint congruency improved by the extended, adducted position. Preliminary results indicate improvement in limb length, decrease in limp, and improvement in function and range of motion. This osteotomy is gaining many advocates because of its early promising results. Long-term results will be necessary to determine its role in the treatment of LCPD.

Long-term series of patients with uniform treatment matched for age and degree of epiphyseal involvement are needed to determine the

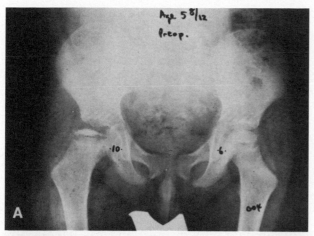

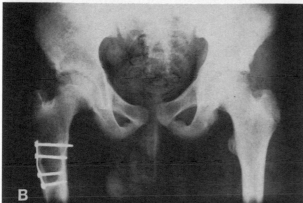

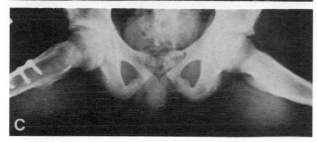

FIGURE 15-25. Varus/derotation osteotomy of Axer. This embodies the principle of containment of the diseased femoral head in the treatment of Legg-Calvé-Perthes disease, which is achieved by surgical means. Postoperatively, the child is permitted to walk with no restrictions, and the range of motion is full, so that the molding effect of the acetabulum on the femoral head is attained. (A) Severe involvement of femoral epiphysis in a boy 5 years 8 months of age, 9 months after onset of limp and pain in the left hip. (B) and (C) Ten years after varus/derotation osteotomy, excellent development of the femoral head is seen. (Courtesy of Dr. A. Axer)

most effective treatment of LCPD. As our fundamental understanding of LCPD increases, so too will our understanding of how various treatment modalities influence this complex growth disturbance.

TRANSIENT SYNOVITIS

Transient synovitis is the most common source of hip pain in the young child. This condition is often referred to in the literature by other terms, including *irritable hip, toxic synovitis, observation hip, coxitis serosa,* and *coxalgia fugax,* to name a few.

The cause of the condition is unknown. Because a high percentage of the children have a recent history of an upper respiratory tract infection, a viral origin has been suspected, as has an allergic reaction to an infectious agent. A history of trauma can sometimes be associated with symptom onset, but no causal relation has been established. Biopsy material from patients with transient synovitis demonstrates nonspecific inflammatory changes and synovial hypertrophy.

Transient synovitis is the most common cause of hip pain and limp in children under 10 years of age. Affected children range in age from 3 to 12 years, with the average patient being between 5 and 6 years of age. Boys are affected two to three times as often as girls. Right and left hips are affected equally. Ninety-five percent of cases are unilateral.

Children with transient synovitis traditionally present with a history of hip pain or limp. The pain onset is acute in about half of cases, with symptoms being present for 1 to 3 days before presentation. In the other half of patients, the symptoms of limp or pain are more chronic in nature, often being present for weeks to months. The pain in most cases is mild, but in some children, it may be severe enough to awaken the child at night. In some cases, the patient may not admit to pain. When present, pain is usually localized to the groin region but may be referred to the medial thigh or knee region. Take a careful medical history, looking for any history of antecedent infection, such as an upper respiratory infection, otitis media, strep throat, trauma, or other precipitating factors.

Physical examination is characterized by guarded rotation of the hip joint. Pain can usually be elicited at the extremes of motion, especially abduction and medial rotation. In some children, guarding may be evident by gently trying to roll the leg into internal rotation while the hip is extended. Patients may have evidence of thigh atrophy, depending on the duration of symptoms. There may also be tenderness to palpation in the groin. The gait of an affected child is usually antalgic. The child may walk with the hip in slight flexion, external rotation, and abduction.

The child may have a low grade fever on presentation. The sedimentation rate and C-reactive protein are usually normal but may be mildly elevated. The white blood cell count is generally normal with a normal differential.

Radiographs may demonstrate slightly widened joint space medially (Figure 15-26). Bone density is normal in all cases; if alteration in normal densities is present, another source of the hip pain should be sought. Loss of the hip capsular shadow outline has been reported in cases of toxic synovitis; this sign, however, is a radiologic artifact related to holding the hip in abduction and external rotation. Bone scanning may reveal normal or increased uptake in the proximal femoral epiphysis. Ultrasonography may demonstrate the presence of a mild effusion.

The differential diagnosis of this condition is important in that certain of these conditions can have devastating consequences if not diagnosed. Septic arthritis must be ruled out. Children with septic arthritis generally present with pain, elevated temperature, elevated white blood cell count, and elevated sedimentation rate and C-reactive protein. Septic arthritis of the hip may be accompanied by osteomyelitis of the proximal femur (Chapter 5). Aspiration of the joint must be done when the diagnosis is uncertain. An arthrogram should be done at the same time as the aspiration to make sure that the hip joint has been entered. Rheumatic fever must also be excluded. The hip may be the first joint involved before the development of migratory polyarthralgia. These patients usually give a history of a *β-hemolytic* streptococcal infection 1 to 3 weeks before the onset of hip pain. Other major or minor manifestations of this disorder should be sought.

LCPD often presents in a similar manner. It occurs in the same age range as transient synovitis but has a slightly greater male predominance. Most LCPD patients have retardation of bone age. Bone scans in the early stages of LCPD may show decreased uptake in the femoral head. MRI scans may prove to be helpful to differentiate transient synovitis from LCPD. Many studies in the literature suggest that transient synovitis is a precursor to LCPD disease. The literature, however, suggests that only 1 to 3% of cases of transient synovitis are associated with the later development of LPCD.

Juvenile rheumatoid arthritis, SCFE, and tumors, particularly osteoid osteoma of the proximal femur, must be included in the differential diagnosis of any child with hip pain. Osteoid osteoma usually is accompanied by a history of night pain relieved by aspirin. SCFE is usually seen in the obese adolescent during a growth spurt and has typical radiographic features.

Long-term follow-up studies of patients with transient synovitis reveal that many of the patients have secondary coxa magna and a widened femoral neck as a residual of the condition. The question of whether these patients will develop degenerative arthritis over the long-term remains to be answered.

Rest is the primary method of treatment for this condition. When the diagnosis is in question or the patient is particularly uncomfortable, hospitalization is often necessary. Light skin traction may be applied for comfort. Anti-inflammatory agents may be used for a short time to relieve pain. As symptoms resolve, crutch-protected weight bearing may begin, with gradual resumption of full weight bearing as symptoms abate. Most patients have resolution of symptoms in 3 to 7 days, but in many patients, symptoms may persist for weeks to months. The condition is self-limiting; most children have only a single episode of hip pain, and recurrences are uncommon unless the child is returned to full activity before symptoms resolve.

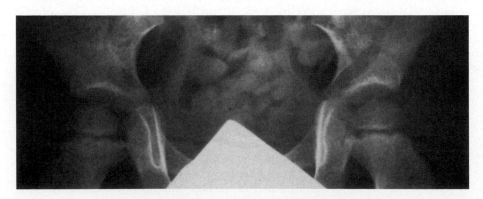

FIGURE 15-26. AP radiograph of a child with transient synovitis of the right hip. Note the slightly widened medial joint space in the right hip.

DEVELOPMENTAL COXA VARA

The term *coxa vara* is a descriptive term referring to the angular relation between the femoral head or neck, or both, and the femoral shaft, which is less than the normal value for the patient's age. This abnormal relation may be congenital, developmental, or acquired. It is most important to distinguish between these three etiologic groups because each has its own natural history. This section deals only with developmental coxa vara.

Developmental coxa vara refers to defects localized to the cervical region of the proximal femur that are accompanied by a widened and vertically oriented physeal plate (Figure 15-27). The shaft of the femur is normal. Clinical and radiographic features are not present at birth. Developmental coxa vara is an extremely rare condition equally affecting boys and girls. About 30% of the cases are bilateral. A familial tendency has been reported, but the exact mode of inheritance is unknown. The cause of developmental coxa vara is unknown, but many theories have been postulated, including an embryonic vascular disturbance and regional dysplasia of the proximal femur.

Clinically, most patients present to the physician for a limb length inequality or abnormal gait. Although the gait abnormality may be evident when the child starts to walk, patients generally do not seek medical attention until the child is 3 to 7 years of age. The limp or waddling gait (in bilateral cases) is painless and usually progressive. Older children may complain of easy fatigability. Limb shortening is usually evident.

On physical examination, patients have short stature. Examination of the involved extremity reveals limited abduction and internal rotation, a positive Trendelenburg test, limb shortening, and trochanteric elevation. In bilateral cases, hyperlordosis of the lumbar spine is present, and the patient may have genu valgum. Limb length inequalities in developmental coxa vara rarely exceed 2 cm. In bilateral cases, the amount of shortening may be asymmetric.

The diagnosis can be made by an AP radiograph of the femurs and hips. The diagnosis is made by the presence of anatomic coxa vara, widened vertically oriented physeal plate, shortened neck, normal straight femoral shaft, and separate triangular ossification center on the inferior part of the femoral neck. This triangular ossification center may appear irregular and fragmented. A vertically oriented physeal plate borders the triangular fragment medially, while lateral to it is a vertical defect in the femoral neck. The femoral head is spherical and the acetabulum generally normal, although mild dysplasia may be apparent in comparison to the opposite, normal side.

Various measurements have been made to quantify the relations in the proximal femur (see Figure 15-27). These measurements include the head-shaft angle, the neck-shaft angle, and the Hilgenreiner epiphyseal angle. The head-shaft angle has been found best to follow progression of deformity in that the neck-shaft angle remains fairly constant even in the face of progressive deformity. The Hilgenreiner epiphyseal angle has been found to be a method of evaluation and prognostication for patients with developmental coxa vara.

Developmental coxa vara must be differentiated from congenital coxa vara and coxa vara acquired secondary to other conditions. Congenital coxa vara is detectable at birth and is accompanied by shortening of the proximal femur. Congenital coxa vara with a short femur is part of the spectrum of proximal femoral focal deficiency. The varus in this condition is generally in the subtrochanteric region or in the upper femur, and varying degrees of femoral shortening are seen. The head is abnormal in appearance, and acetabular dysplasia is generally present. The varus relation in this condition generally does not worsen with time and in general need not to be addressed. Anatomic coxa vara can also be seen in patients with metabolic bone disease such as

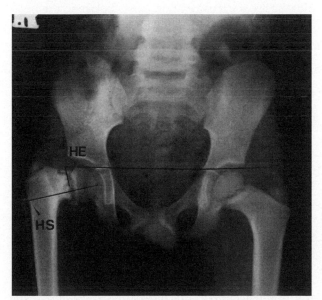

FIGURE 15-27. Coxa vara development. Note head-shaft angle (HS) and Hilgenreiner epiphyseal angle (HE).

rickets, fibrous dysplasia, osteogenesis imperfecta, Ollier's disease, SCFE, and sepsis. A radiographic appearance similar to developmental coxa vara is seen in patients with coxa vara secondary to metaphyseal chondrodysplasia and in patients with coxa vara and cleidocranial dysostosis. Coxa vara associated with cleidocranial dysostosis is usually present at birth, and patients have clavicular abnormalities, wormian bones, and abnormal dentition. In metaphyseal chondrodysplasia, there is generalized widening of the physeal plates. The hip radiographic abnormalities are bilateral and symmetric, and the femoral shafts are bowed. In bilateral cases of developmental coxa vara, the deformity may not be symmetric.

The goals of treatment in developmental coxa vara are to promote ossification of the defect and to correct the varus deformity, allowing restoration of the mechanical advantage of the hip abductors to improve gait and to equalize limb lengths. In progressive coxa vara, the natural history suggests increasing deformity (Figure 15-28), decreasing function, and early degenerative joint disease.

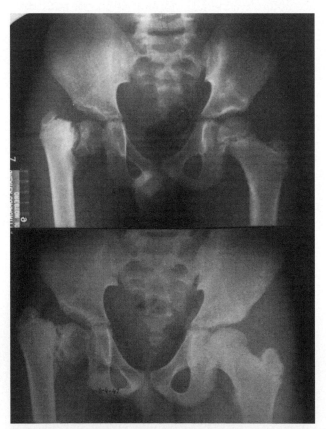

FIGURE 15-28. Coxa vara development. Note triangular fragment and worsening of condition over a 2-year period (*bottom*).

The general indications for surgical treatment include increasing coxa vara and a neck-shaft angle of less than 100°. In mild, nonprogressive cases with a neck-shaft angle of greater than 100° and a Hilgenreiner epiphyseal angle of less than 45°, resolution of the defect may occur, and observation of the patient with serial follow-up radiographs is indicated. In patients with a limp, progressive deformity, and a Hilgenreiner epiphyseal angle of greater than 60°, intertrochanteric or subtrochanteric abduction osteotomy is the treatment of choice (Figure 15-29). In these patients, the neck-shaft angle should be restored to decrease the shear stress across the vertical defect. With surgery, the defect generally heals, but growth plate arrest may be seen in a significant number of patients, leading to limb length inequality. Generally, patients older than 5 years of age at the time of surgery maintain their correction.

SLIPPED CAPITAL FEMORAL EPIPHYSIS

Slipped capital femoral epiphysis (SCFE) is a disorder in which the capital femoral epiphysis is displaced from the metaphysis through the physeal plate (Figure 15-30). The term *slipped capital femoral epiphysis* is actually a misnomer in that the head is held in the acetabulum by the ligamentum teres, and thus it is actually the neck that comes upward and outward while the head remains posterior and downward in the acetabulum (Figure 15-31). In most cases, a varus relation exists between the head and neck, but occasionally the slip is into valgus, with the head displaced superiorly and posteriorly in relation to the neck.

The overall incidence of SCFE in the general population is about 2 cases per 100,000. The incidence of SCFE is higher in all blacks, but especially black girls. The disorder generally occurs in the age range of 10 to 14 years in girls (mean, 11.5 years) and 10 to 16 years in boys (mean, 13.5 years). Seventy percent of affected patients have delayed skeletal maturation. Skeletal age may lag behind chronologic age by as much as 20 months. There is a male predominance of 2.5:1. The left hip is twice as often affected as the right hip. Other epidemiologic factors may include seasonal variations and social class.

Affected patients have a tendency toward obesity. Almost half of affected patients are above the 95th percentile in weight for their age. Three-fourths of affected boys and half of affected girls are

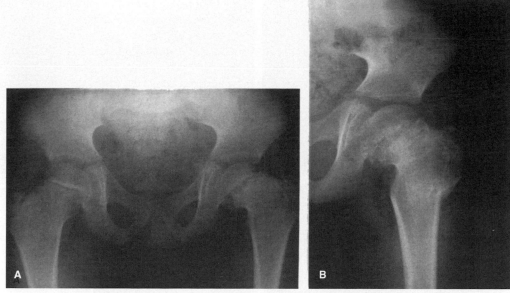

FIGURE 15-29. (A) Eight-year-old boy with coxa vara. **(B)** Eighteen months after abduction osteotomy.

above the 90th percentile in weight for their height. It has been disproved that tall thin people are predisposed to this condition.

The incidence of bilateralness of SCFE is generally accepted as being 25%. This figure may be low in that about half of bilateral slips are asymptomatic. This factor becomes important when considering the natural history of the disease.

Pathologically, the synovium from patients with SCFE generally exhibits changes characteristic of synovitis, with hypertrophy and hyperplasia of the synovial cells, villus formation, increased vascularity, and round cell infiltration. Light microscopic studies reveal that the physis is widened and irregular, sometimes reaching 12 mm in width (normal is 2.6 to 6 mm). Normally, the resting zone accounts for 60 to 70% of the width of the physis, whereas the hypertrophic zone accounts for only 15 to 30% of the width. In SCFE, the hypertrophic zone may constitute up to 80% of the physis width. Light microscopic studies also document that the actual slip takes place through the zone of hypertrophy, with occasional extension into the calcifying cartilage (Figure 15-32). On the basis of histologic studies, it is apparent that the slip occurs through the weakest structural area of the plate, the hypertrophic zone.

The origin of SCFE is unknown. All etiologic agents probably act either by altering the strength of the zone of hypertrophy or by affecting the shear stress to which the plate is exposed. Although trauma may be a contributing factor, it is certainly not the sole cause; the pathology of SCFE differs from that seen in physeal fractures.

Hormonal and endocrine abnormalities have long been implicated in the cause of SCFE. Although there have been no specific endocrine abnormalities detected in patients with SCFE, there are numerous reports of SCFE associated with specific endocrine abnormalities, such as primary hypothyroidism, hypothyroidism secondary to panhypopituitarism, intracranial tumors, hypogonadism, treatment with chorionic gonadotropin, and treatment of hypothyroidism and growth hormone deficiency with growth hormone. SCFE has also been reported in patients undergoing radiation to the pelvis, patients with rickets, and patients with renal osteodystrophy.

Experimentally, the administration of growth hormone in castrated rats leads to increased thickness of the zone of hypertrophy and decreased shear strength. Estrogen, on the other hand, given to otherwise normal rats, leads to thinning of the growth plate and increased shear strength in similar experiments (Figure 15-33).

Hormonal factors have been repudiated as contributing to the slippage because 78% of slips occur during the adolescent growth spurt, and in girls, slips occur before menarche. Hormonal theories have been used to account for many of the epidemiologic factors. For example, the age range of occurrence corresponds to the adolescent growth spurt for boys and girls. The gender prevalence of boys

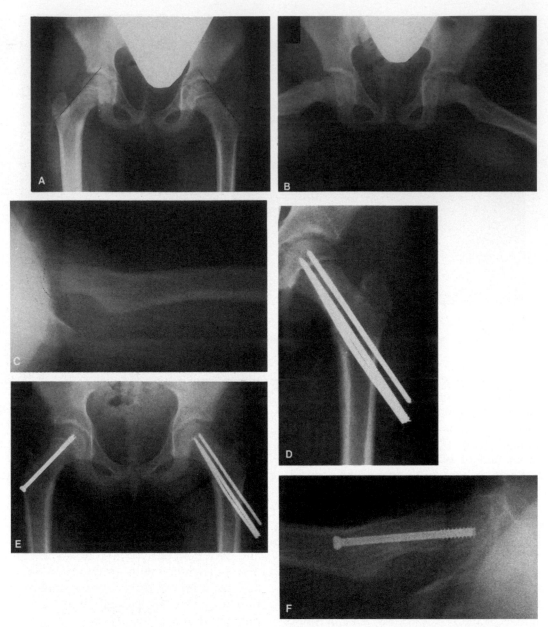

FIGURE 15-30. Ten-year-old girl with left hip pain for 3 months. **(A)** AP radiograph of pelvis. Note the Klein line. It should normally intersect at least 20% of the femoral head. **(B)** Lauenstein view demonstrates mild slip on left side. **(C)** True lateral view of left hip demonstrating mild slip. **(D)** The slip was treated with multiple threaded pins. **(E)** One year later, the patient complained of pain in the right groin and had a minimal slip. The right-sided slip was treated with a single screw (AP view). **(F)** Lateral view of postoperative pinning. Note central position of screw in epiphysis. With the advent of cannulated screws, threaded pins are rarely used unless cannulated screws are unavailable. Threaded pins often cause soft tissue irritation and later removal.

may be accounted for by boys having a longer and more rapid growth spurt. The high percentage of obesity (adiposogenital syndrome patients) has been attributed to an abnormal relation between growth hormone and sex hormone, giving a relative predominance to the growth effect. Thus, hormonal imbalance may lead to a structural weakening of the growth plate, leaving it more susceptible to slipping.

Other etiologic theories include SCFE being a localized manifestation of a generalized systemic disorder, secondary to a biochemical abnormality in cartilage collagen production or secondary to a

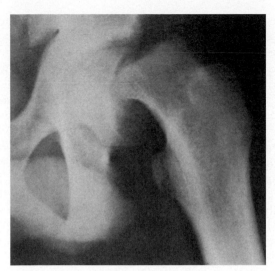

FIGURE 15-31. Complete slipped upper femoral epiphysis. Commonly termed *acute slipped epiphysis*, in reality, it is a form of fracture displacement that can also occur at other epiphyseal sites.

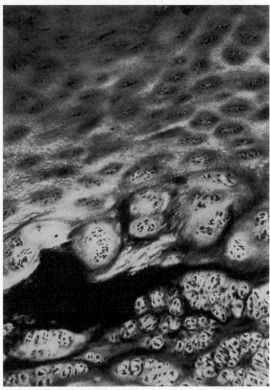

FIGURE 15-32. Physeal plate from a patient with slipped capital femoral epiphysis. Note slip (cleft) in zone of hypertrophy. Also note the abnormal architecture of the physeal plate. The zone of hypertrophy is increased in width, and the cells are in clusters and clumps.

mechanical disturbance caused by shear forces applied to a retroverted proximal femoral epiphysis. Genetic factors may contribute but have thus far not been identified. SCFE is probably a multifactorial disorder, with the slip representing the final manifestation of one of several predisposing factors.

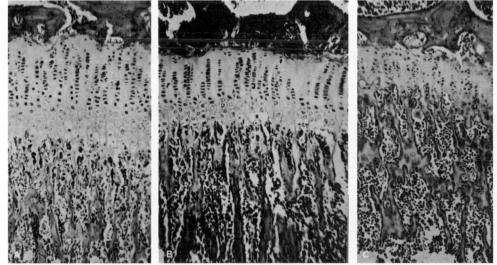

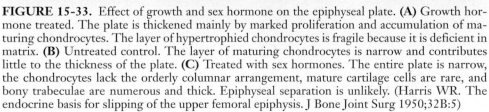

FIGURE 15-33. Effect of growth and sex hormone on the epiphyseal plate. **(A)** Growth hormone treated. The plate is thickened mainly by marked proliferation and accumulation of maturing chondrocytes. The layer of hypertrophied chondrocytes is fragile because it is deficient in matrix. **(B)** Untreated control. The layer of maturing chondrocytes is narrow and contributes little to the thickness of the plate. **(C)** Treated with sex hormones. The entire plate is narrow, the chondrocytes lack the orderly columnar arrangement, mature cartilage cells are rare, and bony trabeculae are numerous and thick. Epiphyseal separation is unlikely. (Harris WR. The endocrine basis for slipping of the upper femoral epiphysis. J Bone Joint Surg 1950;32B:5)

On the basis of the patient's history, physical examination, and radiographs, SCFE can be classified into four categories—preslip, acute, acute on chronic, and chronic. This traditional classification is being superceded by a more clinically relevant two group scheme (stable versus unstable), which is dependent on stability of the hip and relates well to outcome.

In the preslip phase, patients complain initially of weakness in the leg or limping on exertion; pain may occur in the groin, adductor region, or knee with prolonged standing or walking. On physical examination in this phase, the most consistent positive finding is lack of medial rotation of the hip in extension. When the affected leg is fixed, the thigh goes into abduction and external rotation, a sign pathopneumonic for SCFE. Radiographically, there is generalized bone atrophy and disuse osteopenia of the hemipelvis and upper femur only in those patients who limped or limited their activity. There is widening, irregularity, and blurring to the physeal plate (Figure 15-34). The preslip may in actuality be a minimal slip that is not seen on standard radiograph but may possibly be seen on CT or MRI scans.

An acute slip is the abrupt displacement through the proximal epiphyseal cartilage plate in which there was a preexisting epiphysiolysis. Acute slips account for about 10% of the slips in most large reported series (see Figure 15-31). The clinical criterion of having the acute onset of symptoms for less than 2 weeks is generally accepted as the clinical definition of an acute slip. A review of the literature, however, reveals that 76% of patients with acute slips give a history of mild prodromal symptoms for 1 to 3 months before their acute episode, thus indicating that they probably had a preslip or mild slip preceding their acute symptom onset. These prodromal symptoms of mild weakness, limp, and intermittent groin, medial thigh, or knee pain are usually followed by some history of minor trauma or of direct trauma, with immediate increase in pain and inability to use the extremity. The pain is usually severe enough to prevent weight bearing. If the patient can walk, it is with difficulty and with a limp. SCFE in the patient with a history of mild prodromal symptoms may better be classified as an acute-on-chronic slip.

If the patient with an acute SCFE can walk, it is with an antalgic gait. These patients have an external rotation deformity, shortening, and marked limitation of motion. Any attempted motion is painful because of the marked spasm of the hip muscles. In general, the greater the amount of slip, the greater is the restriction of motion. The physical examination must be performed gently so as not to cause further displacement. In the acute slip, because of pain, the physician may not be able to elicit the classic sign of SCFE (thigh abduction and external rotation as the thigh is flexed). Generally thigh or calf atrophy is present, except in those few patients without any prior symptoms.

Patients with chronic SCFE generally have a history of groin or medial thigh pain for months to years. A high percentage have knee or lower medial thigh pain as their initial symptom. They may give a history of exacerbations and remissions of the pain or limp. On physical examination, all these patients have limitation of motion (particularly medial rotation) and shortening, and most have thigh or calf atrophy.

The patient with an *unstable slip* presents much like an acute trauma patient with the inability to walk even with crutches. This slip encompasses many patients who would fall into the old classification as acute or acute on chronic. This unstable group has a significant risk of developing aseptic necrosis of the epiphysis, which generally leads to a poor long-term outcome. *Stable slips* are all others that present with nonacute fracture-like symptoms—that is, the patient is able to walk on the hip even with crutches. Outcomes of treatment of this group are related to the amount of displacement and the avoidance of complications of treatment.

Radiographs must be taken in two planes: AP and true lateral. Because of the unstable nature of the hip, the frog-leg lateral view may accentuate the deformity in the unstable, acute, or acute-on-chronic slip.

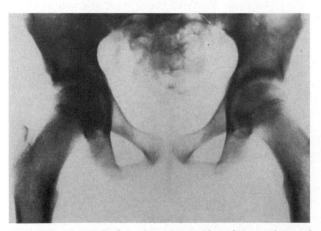

FIGURE 15-34. Before slip. Note widened, irregular, and blurry physeal plate on left hip. Left hemipelvis is relatively osteopenic.

The diagnosis of SCFE can be made on the AP radiograph by drawing a line along the superior basal margin of the neck. Normally, it should transect 20% or more of the epiphyses (see Figure 15-28). Widening and irregularity of the physeal growth plate and decreased height of the epiphyses in the central acetabulum are also seen, and the medial junction of the epiphyses and the metaphyses fall outside the acetabulum. The lateral view is probably the best to detect the slip because the head is posterior in relation to the neck at first and thus may be missed on the AP view. In minimal slips, the displacement is initially posterior and may only be seen on the lateral radiograph.

Radiographically, slips are classified by the maximal anatomic displacement either on the AP or lateral radiograph. This classification is important as long-term outcome in the absence of surgical complications is totally related to the amount of displacement. One classification of displacement is as follows:

Minimal slip: maximal displacement is less than one-third the diameter of the neck

Moderate slip: greater than 1 cm of displacement but less than half the diameter of the neck

Severe slip: displacement greater than half the diameter of the neck

CT and MRI scans have been done to demonstrate predisposing factors such as retroversion or a widened physeal plate in the radiographically normal hip to try and predict a propensity to slip. The role of these modalities must await further investigation.

Review of the literature on natural history is at best controversial because there are very few studies. There are few long-term studies of patients with SCFE, and included in these are few untreated patients. What is clear however is that SCFE should be considered an orthopaedic emergency and patients treated immediately. Any delay in management runs the risk of further displacement and worse long-term outcome.

In large series of patients with degenerative joint disease, the percentage of patients with known SCFE is small, averaging about 5%. The actual incidence may be higher because controversy exists about whether a higher percentage of patients with so-called primary degenerative arthritis had unrecognized slips or whether these radiographic features are merely secondary to primary degenerative joint disease.

The amount of deformity appears to be related to long-term prognosis, with degenerative joint disease and function being related to the severity of deformity. Those with moderate slips retain good function for many years, whereas those with severe slips have early degenerative joint disease and poor function. Poor results are occasionally seen even in minimal slips, usually as a result of a complication of treatment. The radiographic changes, however, do not always correlate with clinical symptoms over time.

Specific goals in the treatment of SCFE are to prevent further displacement of the epiphysis and to promote closure of the physeal plate. Treatment of SCFE should be considered an emergency. Once the diagnosis is made, the patient should not be allowed to bear weight. Treatment should be initiated immediately. Delay in treatment as mentioned above may result in further displacement of the femoral epiphysis with compromise of the remaining intact blood supply to the epiphysis. Further displacement also leads to increasing deformity and secondary increased risk of degenerative joint disease over time. Long-term goals of treatment include restoration of a functional range of motion, freedom from pain, and avoidance of aseptic necrosis and chondrolysis. Treatment considerations are based on the clinical classification (preslip, acute, acute on chronic, chronic; stable versus unstable) and the radiographic classification (mild, moderate, severe).

General principles of treatment of SCFE include reduction of the *unstable* acute slips and the acute component of acute-on-chronic slips if displaced more than mildly, followed by stabilization of the epiphysis. Stable slips or chronic slips and the chronic component of acute-on-chronic slips should never be reduced but only stabilized. Any attempt at reduction of chronic components (or of a stable slip) runs the risk of aseptic necrosis (the most common cause of a poor result) and long-term disability.

In acute or unstable slips, aseptic necrosis may occur with the sudden acute displacement of the epiphysis by interruption of blood supply to the capital femoral epiphysis. Reduction attempts of the slip must be gentle. The use of skeletal traction to reduce the acute or unstable slip remains controversial. Most pediatric orthopaedic surgeons do not use traction, but treat the unstable slip as an orthopaedic emergency; taking the patient to the operating room as soon as is feasible. Skin traction may be used while waiting for the patient to be ready to go to the operating room. In the operating room, reduction is obtained of the moderate or severely displaced unstable slip by gentle traction on the fracture table with a gentle internal rotation moment—the goal being to reduce a moderate or severe displacement to a mild one so as to improve the long-term prognosis. If displacement is mild, no attempt at reduction is done.

Stabilization of the acute, unstable slip is accomplished by epiphysis pinning. The most widely used method of stabilization is pinning with large cannulated bone screws or multiple large threaded pins (see Figure 15-30). These techniques require the use of image intensification in the operating room. Radiographic control intraoperatively must include the ability to obtain images at 90° to each other to minimize the risk of pin penetration, which is thought to be associated with chondrolysis. The fixation device must enter the epiphysis perpendicular to the physeal plate of the femoral head. The fixation device must cross the physis into the head but must be well short of the subchondral cortex. The pins or screws should be in the center of the epiphysis on the AP and lateral views of the hip (see Figure 15-30). Pins or screws should also avoid the superior quadrant of the femoral head to avoid the lateral epiphyseal vessels. Pins in this quadrant are associated with a higher incidence of aseptic necrosis. Although many authors recommend two screws for unstable slips, a single, large diameter centrally placed screw is generally adequate.

Postoperatively, patients are kept to light weight bearing until they are pain free and have a comfortable range of motion (generally 4 to 6 weeks). Rapid advance to full weight bearing may then begin.

All patients must be followed closely until the physeal plate closes. Loss of range of motion after treatment may be the first sign of chondrolysis. Pain in the other hip (groin, medial thigh, or knee) warrants careful investigation. Most bilateral slips are diagnosed within 1 year of the diagnosis of the initial slip. Pins are generally not removed, but if for some reason removal is considered, it should be delayed until physeal closure.

Stable or chronic slips should not have attempts at reduction but should be treated by stabilization procedures primarily, regardless of their degree of displacement. Stable slips pinned in situ may rapidly advance postoperatively to full weight bearing. Long-term results of mild and moderate slips are generally good concerning function and range of motion. A certain amount of remodeling of the proximal femur can be expected.

Severe slips can also be treated by stabilization procedures primarily. Debate exists about whether these slips should be treated by realignment procedures in addition to stabilization to improve joint kinematics and hence long-term outcome. Long-term follow-up studies indicate that the greatest risk to the long-term outcome of patients with SCFE is the development of aseptic necrosis or chondrolysis, not malalignment. The use of realignment procedures (neck, intertrochanteric, or subtrochanteric osteotomy or manipulative reductions in chronic slips) is associated with significantly higher complication rates than pinning in situ alone. Realignment procedures should therefore be reserved for those situations in which restricted range of motion impairs function after plate physeal closure.

Aseptic necrosis is the most devastating complication of SCFE. It is most commonly associated—in acute slips and unstable slips—with the abrupt displacement of the epiphysis disrupting retinacular vessels. In chronic stable slips, aseptic necrosis can occur as a result of treatment. As mentioned previously, attempts at reduction of stable or chronic slips, over-reduction of unstable, acute slips, improper pin placement, and femoral neck osteotomies are associated with this complication.

Chondrolysis or cartilage necrosis is often associated with SCFE. Chondrolysis is manifest clinically by loss of range of motion, pain, limp, and joint contracture. Radiographically, the condition is manifest by loss of joint space, irregularity of the subchondral bone of the femoral head and the acetabulum, and disuse osteopenia. It can occur in untreated slips, but this is unusual (it can also occur as an isolated disorder). The cause of this condition remains unknown, but it is associated with prolonged immobilization, unrecognized pin penetration, severe slips, and a long duration of symptoms before treatment. Whether the condition represents an autoimmune phenomenon or other source of interference with cartilage nutrition remains to be proved. Treatment of chondrolysis is difficult. Symptomatic treatment should begin immediately and should include anti-inflammatory agents and bed rest in skeletal traction to relieve pain and contractures. The role of continuous passive motion with or without a surgical capsulectomy is yet to be defined.

The key to the management of SCFE is prompt diagnosis and management by accepted techniques that have a high rate of success with minimal risk of complications.

Annotated Bibliography

Congenital Hip Dysplasia and Dislocation

Malvitz TA, Weinstein SL. Closed reduction for congenital dysplasia of the hip: functional and radiographic results after an average of thirty years. J Bone Joint Surg 1994;76A:1777.
The functional and radiographic results of closed reduction in 152 congenitally dislocated hips of 119 patients who had been managed between 1938 and 1969 were reviewed retrospectively. The average age of the patients at the time of reduction was 21 months (range, 1 to 96 months). The average duration of follow up was 30 years (range, 15 to 53 years). At the latest follow-up evaluation, the Iowa hip rating averaged 91 points. Sixty-five hips (43%) had radiographic evidence of degenerative joint disease. Function tended to deteriorate with time, even in the absence of disturbance of growth in the proximal end of the femur. Despite generally good function at the latest follow-up evaluation, the prognosis for those patients remained guarded.

Mubarak SJ, Garfin S, Vance R et al. Pitfalls in the use of the Pavlik harness for treatment of congenital dysplasia, subluxation and dislocation of the hip. J Bone Joint Surg 1981; 63A:1239.
The authors review 18 cases of failure of management of DDH with the Pavlik harness. They describe the pitfalls in the use of the most common device employed in the management of DDH. The appropriate protocol for use of the Pavlik harness is described.

Ponseti IV. Growth and development of the acetabulum in the normal child: anatomical, histological and roentgenographic studies. J Bone Joint Surg 1978;60A:575.
This classic article deals with normal acetabular development based on anatomic, histologic, and radiologic evaluation of the normal hip. Information in this article is essential to the management of DDH.

Ponseti IV. Morphology of the acetabulum in congenital dislocation of the hip: gross, histological and roentgenographic studies. J Bone Joint Surg 1978;60A:586.
The author describes acetabular development in DDH in contrast to previous studies of normal development. Alteration in ossification of acetabulum is described in late, reduced DDH by the development of accessory ossification centers. The pathology of the "neolimbus" is described.

Weinstein SL. Developmental hip dislocation and dysplasia. Lovell and Winters' Pediatric Orthopaedics, 5th Ed. Philadelphia: Lippincott Williams & Wilkins, 2001:905.
Textbook chapter reviewing in detail all aspects of DDH.

Weinstein SL, Mubarak SJ, Wenger DR. Developmental hip dysplasia and dislocation: Part I. J Bone Joint Surg 2003;85A: 1824–1832.
Part I of an instructional course lecture from American Academy of Orthopaedic surgeons course on DDH.

Weinstein SL, Mubarak SJ, Wenger DR. Developmental hip dysplasia and dislocation: Part II. J Bone Joint Surg 2003;85A: 2024.
Part II of an instructional course lecture from American Academy of Orthopaedic surgeons course on DDH.

Legg-Calvé-Perthes Disease

Catterall A. The natural history of Perthes disease. J Bone Joint Surg 1971;53B:37.
This classic article describes the radiographic extent of epiphyseal involvement and prognosis based on natural history in a large group of untreated patients.

Catterall A. Legg-Calvé-Perthes disease: current problems in orthopaedics. New York, Churchill Livingstone, 1982.
This is a superb monograph on the subject by the leading authority. The author addresses all aspects of the disease. The monograph is beautifully illustrated and well referenced.

Herring JA, ed. Legg-Calvé-Perthes Disease. Rosemont, IL: American Academy of Orthopaedic Surgeons, 1996.
This monograph provides an overview of the clinical knowledge base and treatment options of LCPD.

Herring JA, Neustadt JB, Williams JJ et al. The lateral pillar classification of Legg-Calvé-Perthes disease. J Pediatr Orthop 1992;12:143.
Description of the Lateral Pillar classification which is widely used in making treatment decisions.

Martinez AG, Weinstein SL, Dietz FR. The weight-bearing abduction brace for the treatment of Legg-Perthes disease. J Bone Joint Surg 1992;74A:12.
This study reviewed 34 hips in 31 patients, who had severe LCPD (5 hips with Catterall group 3 disease and 29 hips with Catterall group 4 disease). These patients were treated with weight-bearing abduction orthoses. The mean duration of follow-up was 7 years. The authors concluded that, although containment is the most widely accepted principle of treatment for patients who have LPCD, and the Atlanta Scottish Rite orthosis is the most commonly used orthosis for this condition, there are few clinical data supporting the effectiveness of this device. On the basis of the results of their studies, the authors did not recommend the use of a weight-bearing abduction brace for the treatment of severely involved hips. These results were also confirmed by another study in the same issue of the journal from the Atlanta Scottish Rite Hospital.

McAndrew MP, Weinstein SL. A long-term follow-up of Legg-Calvé-Perthes disease. J Bone Joint Surg 1984;66A:860.
The authors describe a longitudinal 48-year average follow-up of a group of patients with Perthes disease. Marked deterioration of function was seen between 36 and 48 years of follow-up. By an average age of 56 years, 40% of patients had undergone arthroplasty, and an additional 10% had disabling osteoarthritis.

Stulberg SD, Cooperman DR, Wallensten R. The natural history of Legg-Calvé-Perthes disease. J Bone Joint Surg 1981; 63A:1095.
This article describes a long-term follow-up study of a large number of patients from three hospitals. The authors describe five radiographic classes of deformity at maturity and discuss the long-term prognosis of each class.

Weinstein SL. Legg-Calvé-Perthes disease. In: Morrissy RT, Weinstein SL, eds. Lovell and Winter's Pediatric Orthopaedics 5th Ed. Philadelphia: Lippincott Williams & Wilkins, 2001:957.
This textbook chapter covers all aspects of Legg-Calvé-Perthes disease in detail and has an extensive bibliography.

Weinstein SL. Long-term follow up of pediatric orthopaedic conditions: natural history and outcomes of treatment. J Bone Joint Surg 2000;82A:980.
The author summarized long-term follow up to maturity of patients with CPD who have had either no treatment or brace treatment. Generally favorable results are found at 20 to 40 years follow-up, unless the femoral head is flattened and irregular, the neck is deformed, or the trochanter is overgrown.

Transient Synovitis

De Valderrama JAF. The "observation hip" syndrome and its late sequelae. J Bone Joint Surg 1963;45B:462.
This article describes a follow-up study of 23 patients with an average 21-year follow-up (range, 15 to 30 years). Twelve patients had evidence of coxa magna, osteoarthritis, and widening of the femoral neck. The author discusses possible mechanisms for causation of coxa magna.

Haueisen DC, Weiner DS, Weiner SD. The characterization of "transient synovitis of the hip" in children. J Pediatr Orthop 1986;6:11.
This is an excellent, well-referenced review of the topic and includes a 30-year retrospective review of 497 cases. The authors report a detailed radiographic and clinical follow-up of 147 cases.

Nachemson A, Scheller S. A clinical and radiological follow-up study of transient synovitis of the hip. Acta Orthop Scand 1969;40:479.

The study described is a 20- or 22-year follow-up of 73 cases of transient synovitis. Of the original pool, 6% (102 patients) subsequently developed Perthes disease. There was a statistically significant difference in the incidence of coxa magna, cysts, and radiodensity in the femoral heads of affected patients, but these were of no clinical significance. The paper documents the benign natural history of this condition.

Sharwood PF. The irritable hip syndrome in children: a long-term follow-up. Acta Orthop Scand 1981;52:633.

The author reviews 101 children with irritable hip syndrome who were followed an average of 8.2 years (range, 5 to 15 years). Most patients had prompt resolution of symptoms (within 16 days). Only one subsequent case of Perthes disease and one of coxa magna were seen, both in patients who had prolonged symptoms and radiologic abnormalities on presentation.

Wingstrand H, Egund N, Carlin NO et al. Intracapsular pressure in transient synovitis of the hip. Acta Orthop Scand 1985;56:204.

The authors evaluated 14 patients with sonography, scintigraphy, and intracapsular pressure recording and aspiration. They found an effusion in all cases and increased intracapsular pressure with the hip in extension. The authors recommended treatment with rest with the hip joint in about 45° flexion to reduce intracapsular pressure and decrease the risk of ischemia to the femoral head from vascular tamponade.

Developmental Coxa Vara

Amstutz HC. Developmental (infantile) coxa vara—a distinct entity: report of 2 patients with previously normal roentgenograms. Clin Orthop 1970;72:242.

The author distinguishes between developmental coxa vara and proximal femoral focal deficiency. Two patients are reported who had normal hip radiographs obtained incidentally during the first year of life and later developed developmental coxa vara. The author further refines a classification previously presented.

Amstutz HC, Wilson PD Jr. Dysgenesis of the proximal femur (coxa vara) and its surgical management. J Bone Joint Surg 1962;44A:1.

This classic article includes classification of coxa vara into the categories of congenital and acquired. The authors discuss in detail the general characteristics and treatment of patients with congenital short femur with coxa vara, congenital bowed femur with coxa vara, and congenital coxa vara.

Schmidt TL, Kalamchi A. The fate of the capital femoral physis and acetabular development in developmental coxa vara. J Pediatr Orthop 1982;2:534.

A retrospective review of 22 hips in 15 children with developmental coxa vara. The authors found that acetabular depth did not improve if the neck-shaft angle was not corrected to at least 140 degrees. Premature physeal plate closure was a frequent sequelae (89%) of valgus osteotomy, leading to relatively greater trochanteric overgrowth and the development of limb length inequality.

Weinstein JN, Kuo KN, Millar EA. Congenital coxa vara: a retrospective review. J Pediatr Orthop 1984;4:70.

This article describes a retrospective long-term review of 22 cases of congenital coxa vara. This study presents the Hilgenreiner epiphyseal angle and the natural history and surgical indications based on this angle.

Slipped Capital Femoral Epiphysis

Aronsson DD, Loder RT. Treatment of the unstable (acute) slipped capital femoral epiphysis. Clin Orthop 1996;322:99.

Good general discussion of newer classification of SCFE into stable and unstable with treatment recommendations.

Carney BT, Weinstein SL, Noble J. Long-term follow-up of slipped capital femoral epiphysis. J Bone Joint Surg 1991;73A:667.

This article describes a long-term follow-up study of 155 hips in 124 patients, with a mean follow-up of 41 years after onset of symptoms. The authors determined that the natural history of the malunited slip is mild deterioration related to the severity of the slip and complications. Techniques of realignment are associated with a risk of appreciable complications and adversely affect the natural history of the disease. Regardless of the severity of the slip, pinning in situ provides the best long-term function and delay of degenerative arthritis, with a low risk of complications.

Carney BT, Weinstein SL. Natural history of untreated chronic slipped capital femoral epiphysis. CORR 1996;322:43.

From 1915 to 1952, 31 hips in 28 patients with slipped capital femoral epiphysis were observed without interventional treatment. The mean duration of patient follow-up from the onset of symptoms was 41 years. Untreated slipped capital femoral epiphysis can progress to a severe degree. The natural history of chronic slipped capital femoral epiphysis is favorable provided that displacement is minimal and remains so.

Jerre R, Billing L, Hansson G et al. Bilaterality in slipped capital femoral epiphysis: importance of a reliable radiographic method. J Pediatr Orthop 1996;5B:80.

This retrospective radiographic study of 100 patients with SCFE assessed the incidence of bilaterality. Evidence of bilateral SCFE was found in 59% of patients; 71% of these patients were asymptomatic. There was no evidence of a second slip during adolescence in 18% of patients. A standard radiographic view improved measurement.

Loder RT. The demographics of slipped capital femoral epiphysis: an international multicenter study. Clin Orthop 1996;322:8.

In this retrospective multicenter analysis of 1,630 children with SCFE, the high prevalence of SCFE in Polynesian children and low prevalence in Indo-Mediterranean children were identified. Age, gender, and physical characteristics were similar throughout the world. More than 60% of children with SCFE were above the 90th percentile for weight.

Matava MJ, Patton CM, Luhmann S et al. Knee pain as the initial symptom of slipped capital femoral epiphysis: an analysis of initial presentation and treatment. J Pediatr Orthop 1999;19:455.

This retrospective review analyzed the presenting complaint of 106 patients with SCFE. A primary report of knee pain, a longer delay to diagnosis, and a more severe femoral deformity were seen in 15% of children. The presence of knee pain alone may delay the diagnosis because the knee might be investigated before the hip.

Schai PA, Exner GU, Hansch O. Prevention of secondary coxarthrosis in slipped capital femoral epiphysis: a long-term follow-up study after corrective intertrochanteric osteotomy. J Pediatr Orthop 1996;5B:135.

This is a retrospective study of 51 hips treated with early intertrochanteric osteotomy for severe SCFE. Good results at an average follow up of 24 years were seen in 55% of patients; 45% of patients had decreased motion and degenerative arthritis. The complication rate was low. The average age at review was 37 years for women and 39 years for men.

Stasikelis PJ, Sullivan CM, Phillips WA et al. Slipped capital femoral epiphysis: prediction of contralateral involvement. J Bone Joint Surg 1996;78A:1149.

In a retrospective review of 50 children with unilateral SCFE, the characteristics of those in whom a contralateral slip developed were evaluated. The authors found that, for boys, younger age at presentation of the first slip was predictive of bilateral involvement.

16

Stuart L. Weinstein

The Thoracolumbar Spine

SPINAL DEFORMITY

Deformities of the spine may occur either in the coronal or sagittal plane. All deformities of the spine are classified according to the magnitude and the direction of the curvature, the location of its apex, and the origin. Curvature of the spine may be associated with many conditions (Table 16-1). The language used to describe the various aspects of spinal deformity is often confusing (Table 16-2).

General Considerations

In any patient presenting with a spinal deformity, it is incumbent on the examining physician to try to ascertain the origin because this has bearing on the natural history of the condition and implications for treatment. The cause may be determined on the basis of a careful history, complete physical examination, and appropriate imaging studies. The patient and family should be asked how the curve was detected (e.g., school screening, observation by a friend or health care worker, apparent body asymmetry) and their impression about whether the curve is static or progressive. Idiopathic scoliosis in children is not a painful condition. If the patient gives a history of back pain associated with the deformity,

477

TABLE 16-1.
SRS Classification of Spine Deformity

SCOLIOSIS

Idiopathic
  Infantile (0-3 years)
    Resolving
    Progressive
  Juvenile (4 years to puberty onset)
  Adolescent (puberty onset to
    epiphyseal closure)
  Adult (epiphyses closed)
Neuromuscular
Neuropathic
  Upper motor neuron lesion
    Cerebral palsy
    Spinocerebellar degeneration
      Friedreich
        Charcot-Marie-Tooth
        Roussy-Levy
    Syringomyelia
    Spinal cord tumor
    Spinal cord trauma
    Other
  Lower motor neuron lesion
    Poliomyelitis
    Traumatic
      Spinal muscular atrophy
      Myelomeningocele (paralytic)
    Dysautonomia (Riley-Day)
    Other
  Myopathic
  Arthrogryposis
  Muscular dystrophy
    Duchenne (pseudohypertrophic)
    Limb-girdle
    Facioscapulohumeral

Congenital hypotonia
Myotonia dystrophica
Other
Congenital
  Failure of formation
    Partial unilateral (wedge vertebra)
    Complete unilateral
      (hemivertebra)
      Fully segmented
      Semisegmented
      Nonsegmented
  Failure of segmentation
    Unilateral (unilateral unsegmented
      bar)
    Bilateral (bloc vertebrae)
  Mixed
  Associated with neural tissue defect
    Myelomeningocele
    Meningocele
    Spinal dysraphism
      Diastematomyelia
      Other
Neurofibromatosis
Mesenchymal
  Marfan
  Homocystinuria
  Ehlers-Danlos
  Other
Traumatic
  Fracture or dislocation (nonparalytic)
  Postradiation
  Other

Soft tissue contractures
  Postempyema
  Burns
  Other
Osteochondrodystrophies
  Achondroplasia
  Spondyloepiphyseal dysplasia
  Diastrophic dwarfism
  Mucopolysaccharidoses
  Other
Tumor
  Benign
  Malignant
Rheumatoid disease
Metabolic
  Rickets
  Juvenile osteoporosis
  Osteogenesis imperfecta
Related to lumbosacral area
  Spondylolysis
  Spondylolisthesis
  Other
Thoracogenic
  Postthoracoplasty
  Postthoracotomy
  Other
Hysterical
Functional
  Postural
  Secondary to short leg
  Due to muscle spasm
  Other

KYPHOSIS

Postural
Scheuermann disease
Congenital
  Defect of segmentation
  Defect of formation
  Mixed
Paralytic
  Poliomyelitis
  Anterior horn cell
  Upper motor neuron
Myelomeningocele
Posttraumatic
  Acute

  Chronic
Inflammatory
  Tuberculosis
  Other infections
  Ankylosing spondylitis
Postsurgical
  Postlaminectomy
  Postexcision (eg, tumor)
Postradiation
Metabolic
  Osteoporosis
  Senile

  Juvenile
  Osteogenesis imperfecta
  Other
Developmental
  Achondroplasia
  Mucopolysaccharidoses
  Other
Tumor
  Benign
  Malignant
    Primary
    Metastatic

(continued)

TABLE 16-1.
(Continued)

> LORDOSIS
> Postural
> Congenital
> Paralytic
> Neuropathic
> Myopathic
> Contracture of hip flexors
> Secondary to shunts

(Winter RB. Spinal problems in pediatric orthopaedics. In: Morrissy RT, ed. Lovell and Winter's pediatric orthopaedics. Philadelphia, JB Lippincott, 1990:697–698)

other sources should be considered; Scheuermann kyphosis, spondylolysis, spondylolisthesis, and spinal or spinal cord tumor must be ruled out. Symptoms of shortness of breath, physical limitations, and psychosocial effects possibly caused by the curvature should be noted. The timing of reaching developmental milestones should be recorded. A careful family history must be obtained seeking any history of neurologic or congenital conditions that may be associated with the curvature.

TABLE 16-2.
Glossary of Scoliosis-Related Terms

Adolescent scoliosis: spinal curvature developing after onset of puberty and before maturity

Adult scoliosis: spinal curvature existing after skeletal maturity (closure or epiphyses)

Apical vertebra: vertebra most deviated from the vertical axis of the patient

Cervical curve: spinal curvature that has its apex between C2 and C6

Cervicothoracic curve: spinal curvature that has its apex at C7 and T1

Compensation: accurate alignment of the midline of the skull over the midline of the sacrum

Compensatory curve: curve (which can be structural) above or below a major curve that tends to maintain normal body alignment

Congenital scoliosis: scoliosis due to congenital anomalous vertebral development

Double structural curve (scoliosis): two structural curves in the same spine, one balancing the other

Double thoracic curve (scoliosis): two structural curves, both having their apex within the thoracic spine

End vertebra: the most cephalad vertebra of a curve whose superior surface or the most caudad vertebra whose inferior surface tilts maximally toward the concavity of the curve

Fractional curve: curve that is incomplete because it returns to the erect position; its only horizontal vertebra is its caudad or cephalad one

Full curve: curve in which the only horizontal vertebra is at the apex

Gibbus: sharply angular kyphos

Infantile scoliosis: spinal curvature developing during the first 3 years of life

Juvenile scoliosis: spinal curvature developing between the skeletal ages of 4 years and the onset of puberty

Kyphos: abnormal kyphosis

Kyphoscoliosis: lateral curvature of the spine associated with either increased posterior or decreased anterior angulation in the sagittal plane in excess of the accepted normal for that area

Lordoscoliosis: lateral curvature of the spine associated with an increase in anterior curvature or a decrease in posterior angulation in the sagittal plane in excess of normal for that area

Lumbar curve: spinal curvature that has its apex from L2 to L4

Lumbosacral curve: spinal curvature that has its apex at L5 or below

Major curve: most apparent curve and usually the most structural curve

Nonstructural scoliosis: spinal curvature without structural characteristics (see *Structural curve*)

Pelvic obliquity: deviation of the pelvis from the horizontal in the frontal plane

Primary curve: the first or earliest of several curves to appear; usually, but not necessarily, the most structural curve

Structural curve: segment of spine with a fixed lateral curvature; not necessarily the major or primary curve; identified radiographically in supine lateral side-bending or traction films by the failure to demonstrate normal flexibility

Thoracic curve (scoliosis): curve with the apex between T2 and T11

Thoracolumbar curve: spinal curvature that has its apex at T12 and L1 or at the interspace between these vertebrae

(Winter RB. Spinal problems in pediatric orthopaedics. In: Morrissy RT, ed. Lovell and Winter's pediatric orthopaedics. Philadelphia, JB Lippincott, 1990:697)

Treatment decisions and probabilities of curve progression depend on the patient's growth potential, so it is important to assess maturity historically. The age at onset of pubic hair, axillary hair, breast budding, and menarche should be noted (Figure 16-1). Finally, details of any previous treatment for the condition should be noted.

Each patient should have a general physical examination, paying particular attention to the patient's body habitus and any evidence of congenital abnormalities in the face, palate, ears, upper extremities, and heart. The skin should be inspected for neurofibromas or café-au-lait spots indicative of neurofibromatosis. The skin over the sacral area should be examined for evidence of hair patches, dimpling, pigmentation changes, nevi, and lipomas, which may be associated with spinal dysraphism. Secondary sex characteristics, including breast development and the presence of pubic and axillary hair (graded according to the Tanner scale), must be noted. Limb lengths should be measured to rule out limb length inequality. Sitting and standing height should also be measured. A complete neurologic examination including gag and abdominal reflexes must also be performed. Any abnormality indicative of an associated neurologic condition should be further investigated by a neurologist, and possible further diagnostic studies—such as a spinal cord magnetic resonance imaging (MRI), electromyography (EMG), and nerve conduction velocities—should be considered. Abnormalities detected that suggest a syndrome may require genetic consultation.

Spinal deformity is suspected by the presence of body asymmetry (Figure 16-2). The patient should be examined from both the front and the back, looking for asymmetry in shoulder height, waistline, chest, scapular height, and prominence. The relation of the thorax to the pelvis should be noted. Spinal compensation can be measured by dropping a plumb line from the spinous process of C7 and measuring the distance it falls from the midgluteal cleft.

Rotational asymmetry is best detected on the Adams forward bend test. The test is performed by having the patient stand with the feet together and the knees straight. The patient bends forward at the waist with the arms dependent and the hands held with palms opposed (Figure 16-3). The rotational asymmetry is best assessed by viewing the patient from in front. Any leg length inequality should be compensated for by placing an appropriate-sized block underneath the short leg. The patient should be assessed in three positions to observe the thoracic, thoracolumbar, and lumbar spine (Figure 16-4). The patient should also be viewed from the side to assess any abnormal increases in thoracic or thoracolumbar kyphosis and any evidence of failure to reverse the normal lumbar lordosis.

If on physical examination the patient has evidence of a structural scoliosis, a standing posteroanterior (PA) unshielded upright radiograph of the spine is ordered. The entire spine, as well as iliac crests, must be included on the radiograph so that no curves are missed and skeletal maturity can be assessed. If the patient has complaints of pain or signs

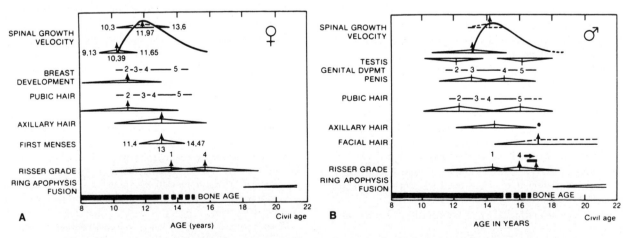

FIGURE 16-1. (A) The relation of spinal growth velocity to maturity landmarks and the events of puberty in girls. **(B)** The relation of spinal growth velocity to maturity landmarks and the events of puberty in boys. (Modified from Trever S, Kleinman R, Bleck EE. Growth landmarks and the evolution of scoliosis: a review of pertinent studies on their usefulness. Dev Med Child Neurol 1980;22: 675–684)

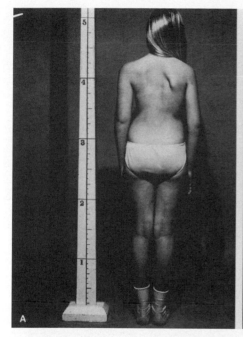

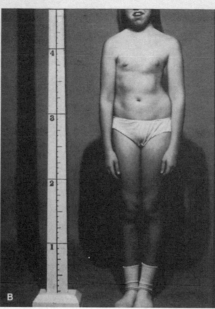

FIGURE 16-2. (A) A patient with a typical right thoracic curve as viewed from the back. The left shoulder is lower, and the right scapula is more prominent. The thorax is shifted to the right with a decreased distance between the right arm and the thorax. Because of the shift in the thorax to the right, the waistline is altered with the left iliac crest appearing higher. This crest asymmetry is apparent, not real. **(B)** A patient with a typical right thoracic curve as viewed from the front. The left shoulder appears lower. The thorax is shifted to the right with a decreased distance between the right arm and the thorax. The left hip appears more prominent secondary to the rightward shift of the thorax.

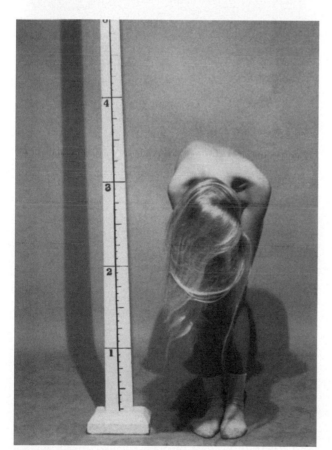

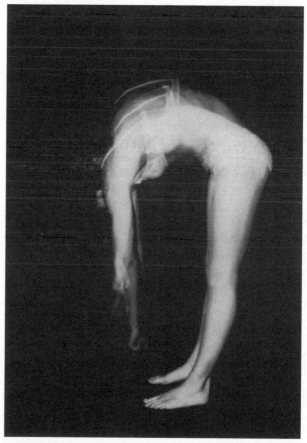

FIGURE 16-3. A patient with atypical right thoracic curve as viewed from the front on the forward bend test. Note the right thoracic prominence.

FIGURE 16-4. Forward bend test: three positions are required to observe the thoracic, thoracolumbar, and lumbar levels of the spine.

of a sagittal spinal deformity, a standing, full-length lateral radiograph of the spine is also ordered.

The radiographs are assessed for any congenital abnormalities in the vertebral bodies, ribs, and pelvis. All curves are assessed for magnitude (Cobb measurements), direction (direction of the curve convexity), location (e.g., thoracic lumbar, thoracolumbar, double major, double thoracic), and pedicle rotation (Figure 16-5). Maturity is assessed by the Risser sign (Figure 16-6). Additional diagnostic and radiographic studies may be indicated if other than idiopathic scoliosis is suspected.

Assessment of patients with spinal curvature depends on the probabilities of curve progression. These probabilities are based on the natural history of the specific curve, which depends on its origin, pattern, magnitude, and associated sagittal plane deformity. This natural history must be considered in relation to the patient's growth potential as determined by history, physical assessment of skeletal maturity, plotting of a growth chart and radiographic assessment of maturity (i.e., Risser sign, ossification of vertebral apophyses, wrist film for bone age assessment, or a combination of these tests).

Scoliosis

Scoliosis is a descriptive term that refers to a lateral curvature of the spine. The scoliosis may be structural or nonstructural. A nonstructural scoliosis corrects or overcorrects on supine side-bending radiographs or traction films. A structural scoliosis is a fixed lateral curvature with rotation. On a radiograph, the spinous processes in a structural curve rotate to the curve concavity. On a supine side-bending radiograph or a traction radiograph, a structural curve lacks normal flexibility. Many conditions are associated with structural scoliosis (see Table 16-1). The most common structural curvature has no known cause and is referred to as *idiopathic scoliosis*. Examples of nonstructural curvatures include scoliosis secondary to limb length inequality or scoliosis secondary to a herniated nucleus pulposus with nerve root irritation causing a list. If the primary problem is corrected (e.g., the limb length inequality), the scoliosis resolves.

The various causes of scoliosis are related to different natural histories. These varying natural histories profoundly influence the effect of the curvature on the patient's life and the indications for treatment.

Idiopathic scoliosis is the most common type of structural scoliosis. This type of scoliosis has a genetic

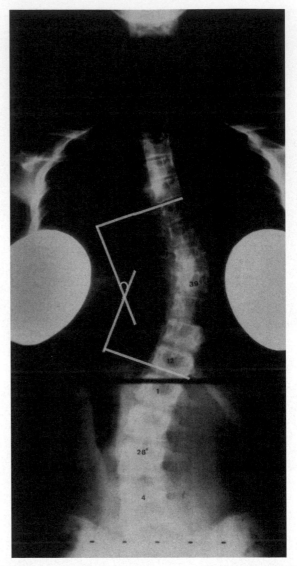

FIGURE 16-5. Curve measurements (Cobb method). (1) Apparent perpendicular is erected from the endplate of the most caudal vertebrae, whose inferior endplate tilts maximally to the concavity of the curve (inferior end vertebrae). (2) A perpendicular is erected from the end-plate of the most cephalad vertebrae, whose superior end-plate tilts maximally to the concavity of the curve (superior end vertebrae). The curve value is the number of degrees formed by the angle of intersection of these perpendiculars, in this case 39°.

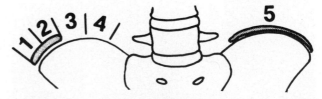

FIGURE 16-6. Ossification of the epiphysis usually starts at the anterosuperior iliac spine and progresses posteriorly. The iliac crest is divided into four quarters, and the excursion or stage of maturity is designated as the amount of progression.

predisposition, and although many etiologic theories have been proposed, the cause remains unknown.

Idiopathic scoliosis is subclassified into three groups by age at onset of the conditions: infantile (0 to 3 years of age), juvenile (3 to 10 years of age), and adolescent (older than 10 years of age but before maturity). Although these subtypes may represent a continuum of the same condition, their natural histories differ. Therefore, these three subtypes of idiopathic scoliosis are considered separately. An alternative classification puts patients into two main categories: early onset (under 10 years of age) and late onset (over 10 years of age). This classification is more reflective of outcome; with early onset cases having more severe effects on outcome measurements (pulmonary function compromise; deformity; mortality) than those with the late onset variety.

Infantile Idiopathic Scoliosis

Infantile idiopathic scoliosis is a structural spinal deformity detected during the first 3 years of life. It accounts for less than 1% of all cases of idiopathic scoliosis in the United States. It is more commonly seen in Europe, especially Great Britain. Most of these curves develop within the first 6 months of life, with the left lumbar curve pattern being the most common. Epidemiologic and associated problems include older maternal age, increased incidence of inguinal hernias among relatives, and association with congenital heart disease (2.5%), congenital hip dysplasia (3.5%), and developmental problems, particularly mental retardation (13%). Intrauterine molding is thought to be a cause because 83% of patients have plagiocephaly, and more than half have evidence of rib-molding deformities. Natural history studies indicate that 85% of the curves regress spontaneously, particularly if the curve onset was before 12 months of age. Fifteen percent of the curves may progress, often leading to severe deformities. Compensatory curves are generally not seen in patients with infantile idiopathic scoliosis. Because of the early onset of the spinal curvature and its effect on pulmonary parenchyma development, patients with progressive untreated infantile, early onset scoliosis may develop severe restrictive pulmonary disease, cor pulmonale, and early death.

The differential diagnosis in this age group (0 to 3 years) includes congenital scoliosis and scoliosis of a neuromuscular origin or intraspinal pathology (e.g., Chiari malformations; syringomyelia). Careful neurological examination is imperative. Radiographs rule out congenital spinal abnormalities. In this age group, MRI of the brain and spinal cord is warranted because of the increased association with intraspinal pathology (Chiari malformation and syrinx) with early onset scoliosis.

If the patient can sit or stand, upright PA and lateral radiographs should be obtained. The Cobb angle and the rib-vertebral angle difference should be measured (Figure 16-7). If the rib-vertebral angle difference is greater than 20°, the curvature is likely progressive. With measurements of less than 20°, the curve is likely to resolve. All patients must be followed by serial radiographic examination, calculating the Cobb angle and the rib-vertebral angle difference at each visit. In progressive curves, the convex side rib head is overlapped by the shadow of the vertebral body. This radiographic sign indicates a progressive curve. Curves that maintain a Cobb angle of less than 35° have a high likelihood of

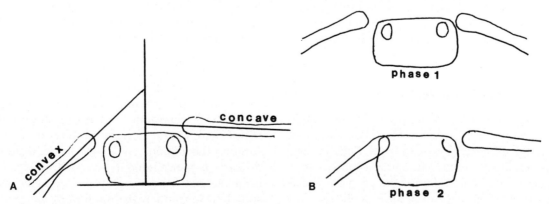

FIGURE 16-7. (A) The rib-vertebral angle difference is calculated by subtracting the convex value from the concave value at the thoracic curve apical vertebra. **(B)** Phase changes at apical vertebra. Phase 2 appearance denotes probable progression.

resolution. Compensatory curves are not common in patients with infantile idiopathic scoliosis. The development of a compensatory curve is a bad prognostic sign that indicates a probable curve progression (Figure 16-8).

Observation is indicated for curves with less than a 25° Cobb angle and less than a 20° rib-vertebral angle difference. The patient should be reevaluated in 4 to 6 months with a repeat standing radiograph of the spine. With resolution of the curvature, the patient can be followed at 1- to 2-year intervals. In curves with a 25 to 35° Cobb angle and with a rib-vertebral angle difference of 25°, repeat clinical and radiographic evaluation at 4- to 6-month intervals is warranted. If the Cobb angle increases by 5 to 10° with or without changes in the rib-vertebral angle difference, treatment is indicated.

Initial treatment for a progressive curve may consist of serial casting to correct the deformity followed by the use of a Milwaukee brace (cervical-thoracic-lumbar-sacral orthosis) or another spinal orthotic to maintain correction. In the infantile patient, the corrective cast usually needs to be applied with sedation or under general anesthesia. The casts are worn for 6 to 12 weeks and are serially changed until maximal correction is obtained. An orthotic is then fabricated and worn full time (22 to 23 hours per day) for 2 to 3 years to maintain the correction obtained by casting. If correction is maintained, the patient may be gradually weaned from the brace. If progression occurs, full-time orthotic use must be reinstituted.

If curve progression continues despite the use of an orthotic, subcutaneous "growing rods"—spinal instrumentation without fusion—followed by bracing is indicated. The rod can then be lengthened periodically to allow for growth with a formal posterior spinal fusion and instrumentation at maturity. Recent studies have questioned the success of these "growing rod" techniques, and thus in certain cases, even at a very young age (over 5 years of age), definitive surgical intervention may need to be considered.

Juvenile Idiopathic Scoliosis

Juvenile idiopathic scoliosis is a lateral curvature of the spine that presents after 3 years of age but before the adolescent growth spurt. Patients classified as having juvenile idiopathic scoliosis may actually have late-onset infantile idiopathic scoliosis or early-onset adolescent idiopathic scoliosis. This group of patients accounts for about 20% of all idiopathic scoliosis patients.

Juvenile idiopathic scoliosis occurs more commonly in girls, with right thoracic curves accounting for about two-thirds of all curve patterns. Double major curves (right thoracic and left lumbar) and thoracolumbar curves follow in frequency.

Juvenile adolescent idiopathic curvatures may progress and cause severe deformity. Some may progress relentlessly from onset, but others may be stable or progress slowly until the adolescent growth spurt when rapid progression ensues. Unlike some infantile curves, juvenile idiopathic scoliosis curvatures do not resolve spontaneously. This group of patients should also have routine brain and spine MRI studies to rule out intraspinal pathology.

The indication for treatment is a progressive curve of 25° or more. The rib-vertebral angle difference has not been shown to be prognostic in these patients. Curves rarely progress more than 1° per month. Therefore, if the patient has a curve of less than 20°, follow-up evaluation in 6 to 8 months is appropriate. Treatment is indicated for progression of at least 10°.

If the curve is between 20 and 25° at detection, follow-up evaluation clinically and radiographically should be obtained in 5 to 6 months, with treatment indicated for a greater than 5° increase in curve. For curves greater than 25°, because of the high probability of progression, treatment should begin immediately.

If the curve is flexible, as determined by clinical evaluation and in some cases by supine side-bending radiographs, orthotic treatment is indicated in an attempt to prevent further progression. If the curve is rigid, serial cast correction, much like that recommended for infantile idiopathic scoliosis, is warranted before fitting the patient with a spinal orthotic. The orthosis is worn on a full-time basis (although protocols for brace wear may vary) for several years until curve correction is achieved. Then, weaning may begin and continue as long as curve correction is maintained. The brace is then worn at night only until the patient reaches skeletal maturity (i.e., Risser grade 4 or 5, or no spinal growth for the previous 18 months).

If curve progression continues despite casting or bracing, distraction instrumentation without fusion should be considered (Figure 16-9). After surgery, the patient continues in an orthosis. The distraction device is lengthened with skeletal growth until the patient reaches puberty, when posterior spinal fusion and instrumentation are performed. In this age group, however, the worry about loss of growth potential associated with definitive surgical

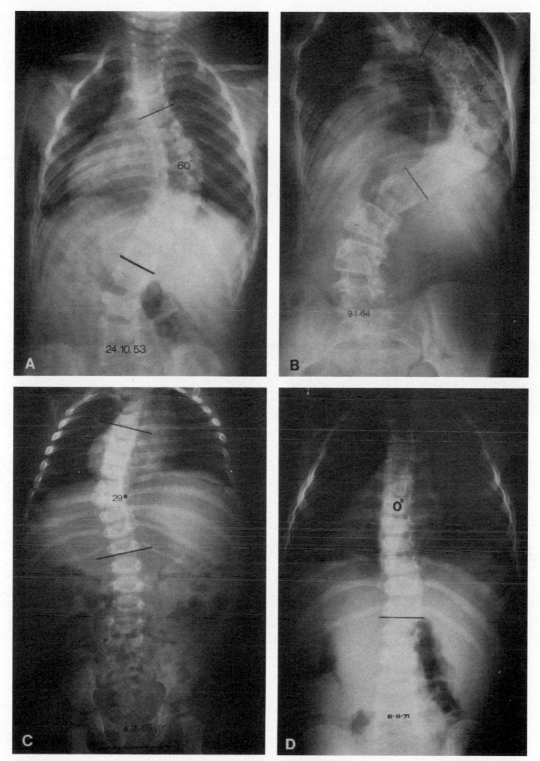

FIGURE 16-8. **(A)** Progressive type of infantile idiopathic scoliosis, early radiograph. Curve measures 60°. **(B)** Late radiograph showing marked increase of primary curve and developing secondary curves. **(C)** Resolving type, early radiograph. Curve measures 29°. No secondary curve. **(D)** Resolving type, later radiograph. Curve reduced to zero. (Courtesy of Dr. J. I. P. James)

fusion of the spine is less concerning than in the very early onset group (infantile) and hence definitive fusion and instrumentation may need to be considered in this group if progression occurs despite bracing (Figure 16-9).

Adolescent Idiopathic Scoliosis

Adolescent idiopathic scoliosis is structural curvature of the spine presenting at or about the onset of puberty and before maturity. Adolescent idiopathic scoliosis accounts for about 80% of cases of idiopathic scoliosis. Its origin is unknown. The prevalence (i.e., occurrence in the at-risk population, children 10 to 16 years of age) of adolescent idiopathic scoliosis is about 2 to 3%. Although there is an overall female predominance for the condition (3.6:1); the prevalence in males and females is equal in small-magnitude curves (10°). With increasing curve magnitude, there is an overwhelming female predominance (curves greater than 30°; female predominance 10:1).

Four major curve patterns are seen in adolescent idiopathic scoliosis (Figure 16-10). Because most thoracic curve patterns are convex to the right, a child presenting with a left convex thoracic curve should be examined carefully for a neurologic deficit. In this situation, neurologic consultation and MRI scanning should be considered because of the high association of intraspinal pathology with this curve pattern. Also, a history of rapid progression of an adolescent curvature should alert the physician to consider similar diagnostic evaluations.

Initial radiographic evaluation includes PA and lateral radiographs of the entire spine taken in the standing position. At follow-up visits, only PA radiographs are usually necessary. It is important to minimize the radiation that the patient receives

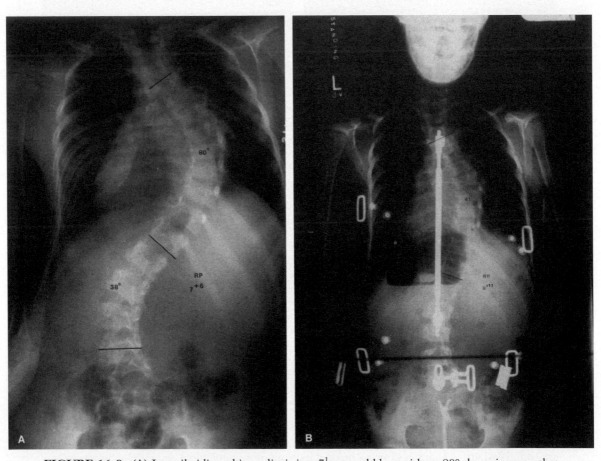

FIGURE 16-9. (A) Juvenile idiopathic scoliosis in a $7\frac{1}{2}$-year-old boy with an 80° thoracic curve that progressed despite bracing. **(B)** Same patient at age 8 years and 11 months. Curve is maintained at 41° with distraction instrumentation and fusion at hook sites. Patient is wearing TLSO external support. Definite surgery is planned at puberty. **(C)** A $7\frac{1}{2}$-year-old girl with juvenile onset scoliosis; she was initially treated in a brace but her curve progressed **(D)**, necessitating anterior and posterior fusion **(E)**.

(continued)

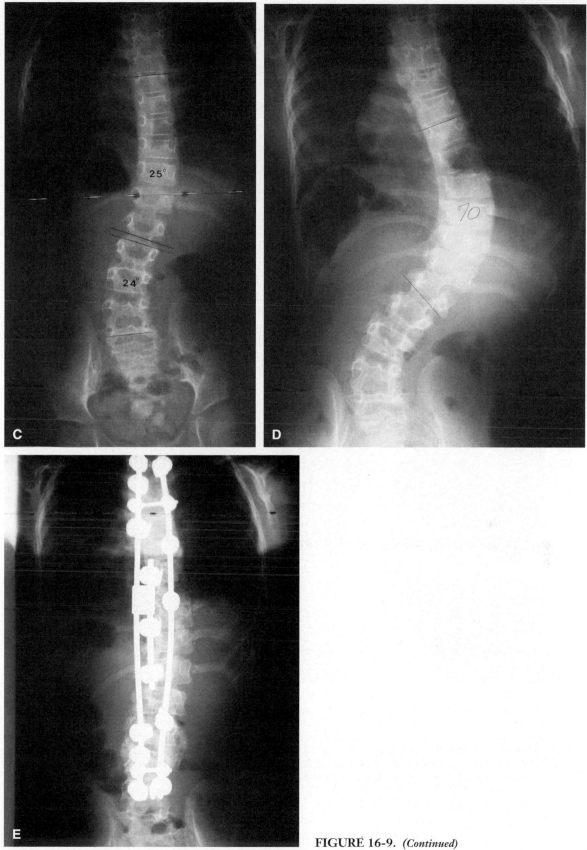

FIGURE 16-9. *(Continued)*

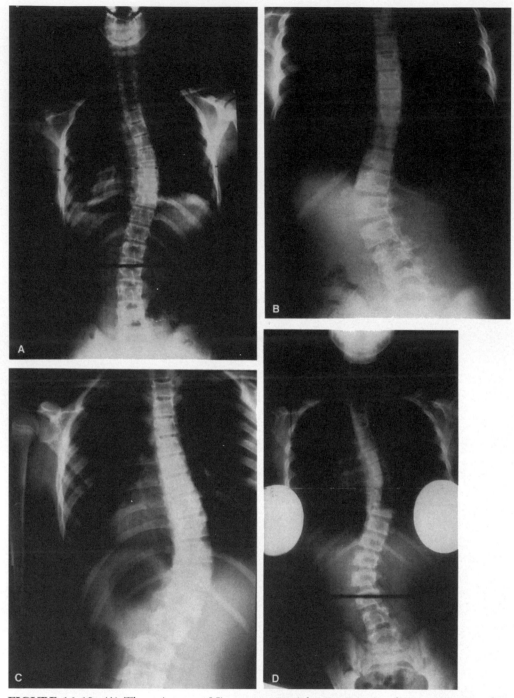

FIGURE 16-10. (A) Thoracic curve. Ninety percent right convexity involving an average of six vertebrae: apex—T8, T9; upper end vertebrae—T5, T6; lower end vertebrae—T11, T12. **(B)** Lumbar curve. Seventy percent left convexity involving an average of five vertebrae: apex—L1, L2; upper end vertebrae—T11, T12; lower end vertebrae—L3, L4. **(C)** Thoracolumbar curve. Eighty percent right convexity involving an average of six to eight vertebrae: apex—T11, T12; upper end vertebrae—T6, T7; lower end vertebrae—L1, L2. **(D)** Double curve. Ninety percent right thoracic convexity and left lumbar convexity. Thoracic component, average five vertebrae: apex—T7; upper end vertebrae—T5, T6; lower end vertebrae—T10. Lumbar component, average five vertebrae: apex—T2; upper end vertebra—T11; lower end vertebra—L4.

over time. Radiographs should be taken only when necessary for treatment decisions. Appropriate technique should be used to avoid the need for repeat films. Other radiation protection measures include beam collimation, antiscatter grids, beam filtration, high-speed film, intensifying screens, gonadal and breast shields, and PA as opposed to anteroposterior (AP) projections. The use of the PA projection avoids radiation to the developing breast tissue, which is radiosensitive. Special radiographic views, such as side-bending radiographs, are rarely indicated unless the patient is being considered for surgical management. Each radiograph is measured for the Cobb angle, rotation, and ossification of the iliac apophysis (Risser sign).

Treatment of any condition is an attempt to alter the natural history of that condition. It is important to understand the natural history of untreated adolescent idiopathic scoliosis with regard to curve progression, effect on pulmonary function, back pain, mortality, psychosocial problems, and effect of on pregnancy.

Most treatment decisions are based on curve progression or the probability of curve progression. Most information available on curve progression is from studies of girls, particularly those with thoracic curves. The factors that influence the probability of curve progression in the immature patient include growth potential factors, such as age, gender, and maturity, and curve factors, such as type and magnitude. Double-curve patterns have a greater tendency for progression than single-curve patterns. Curves detected before menarche have a much greater chance of progression than those detected after menarche. With increasing age at detection, there is a decreasing risk of curve progression. The larger the curve magnitude at detection, the greater the chance of progression; the lower the Risser grade at curve detection, the greater the risk of progression. The risk of progression for boys is about one-tenth that of girls with comparable curves.

The risk of curve progression decreases with increasing skeletal maturity. Large-magnitude curves, however, may continue to progress after maturity (Table 16-3). Many curves continue to progress throughout the patient's life. In general, curves less than 30° at maturity tend not to progress regardless of the curve pattern. Many curves greater than 30°, and particularly thoracic curves greater than 50°, continue to progress.

The generally accepted incidence of backache in the general population is about 60 to 80%, although the incidence varies considerably. The incidence of

TABLE 16-3.
Probabilities of Progression Based on Curve Magnitude and Age

Curve Magnitude at Detection (Degrees)	Age		
	10–12 y	13–15 y	16 y
<19	25%	10%	0%
20–29	60%	40%	10%
30–59	90%	70%	30%
>60	100%	90%	70%

(Nachemson A, Lonstein JE, Weinstein SL. Prevalence and natural history: committee report. Scoliosis Reasearch Society, 1982)

back pain in patients with scoliosis is comparable to that in the general population. Scoliosis patients, however, often have an increased incidence of frequent or daily backache compared with the general population. Patients with lumbar and thoracolumbar curves, particularly those with lateral listhesis or translatory shifts (Figure 16-11) at the lower end of their curves, tend to have a slightly greater incidence of backache than patients with other curve patterns. Back pain in adult patients with scoliosis is not always related to the curvature; it may emanate from the counter-curve below, or it may be discogenic, neurogenic, or facet joint related.

With regard to pulmonary function, only in thoracic curves is there a direct correlation between decreasing vital capacity and FEV1 with increasing curve severity. In all other curve patterns in idiopathic scoliosis, there is no direct correlation between curve magnitude and limitation in pulmonary function. Most patients with adolescent idiopathic scoliosis have loss of the normal thoracic kyphosis. This loss of thoracic kyphosis (hypokyphosis) further diminishes pulmonary function associated with increasing curve severity.

Patients do not die from adolescent idiopathic scoliosis. The only patients at risk are those with high-angled (greater than 100°) thoracic curvatures. In these patients, mortality rates are significantly increased because of secondary cor pulmonale and right ventricular failure.

The cosmetic deformity of scoliosis may be associated with psychosocial concerns. There is, however, no correlation between the location or degree of the curvature and the extent of the psychosocial effects. Some adults with moderate to severe deformity may have severe psychosocial problems.

Scoliosis has no adverse effects on pregnancy. The reproductive experiences of scoliotic women

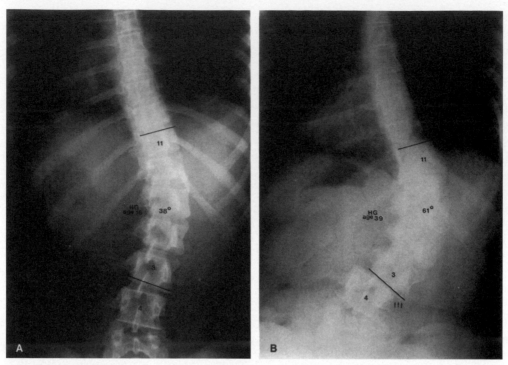

FIGURE 16-11. (A) Sixteen-year-old girl with a 38° right lumbar curve from T11 to L3. Her skeletal maturity is assessed as grade 5 on the Risser scale. **(B)** At 39 years of age, her right lumbar curve has increased to 61°. Note the translatory shift of L3 on L4 (*arrows*). (Weinstein SL. The natural history of scoliosis in the skeletally mature patient. In: Dickson JH, ed. Spinal deformities, vol 1. Philadelphia: Hanley & Belfus, 1987:199)

are the same as those of nonscoliotic women. Whether pregnancy causes curve progression is unknown, with evidence being present on both sides of the issue.

Few patients with adolescent idiopathic scoliosis ever require active treatment (less than 10%). It is important to individualize all treatment decisions, taking into consideration the probabilities of progression based on the curve magnitude, skeletal and sexual maturity of the patient, and age of the patient. The general indications for treatment are a progressive curve of 25° or more in a skeletally immature patient. In a skeletally immature patient with a curve of less than 19°, curve progression of 10° should be documented before instituting treatment. If the curve is between 20 and 29°, progression of least 5° should be documented before instituting treatment. If a curve on initial evaluation is over 30°, because of the high probability (over 90%) of progression, no documentation of progression is necessary, and treatment should be initiated immediately. Because curves rarely progress at more than 1° per month, follow-up appointments can be scheduled accordingly (i.e., for a 15° curve in a skeletally immature girl, follow-up reevaluation is in 10 months).

The gold standard of nonoperative treatment for adolescent idiopathic scoliosis has been the Milwaukee brace. Despite widespread use, few long-term studies have evaluated the results of treatment with the Milwaukee brace (Figure 16-12). In most of the studies performed, curve progression was not documented; thus, it is uncertain whether those patients braced would have had continued progression had they not been braced.

No controlled, prospective, randomized trial of bracing for scoliosis has been done to date. Reviews of the few studies that are available demonstrate conflicting results. The general feeling among physicians treating scoliosis is that bracing appears to alter the natural history of curve progression. It is generally accepted that the curve progression can be arrested in 85 to 90% of at-risk patients. The most common response to bracing is a moderate amount of correction while the brace is worn, with slow, steady progression of the curve back to the original magnitude after weaning from the brace. Occasionally, maintenance of correction obtained in the brace occurs in some patients who achieve at least a 50% reduction in their curvature during the course of treatment. The brace is worn 22 to 23 hours a day

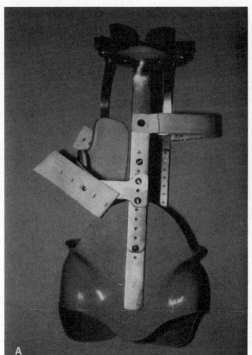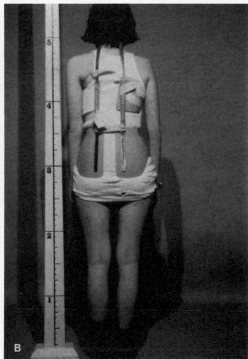

FIGURE 16-12. Milwaukee brace (CTLSO). The brace was developed in the late 1940s (**A,** frontal view of bone). Despite its widespread use, few long-term studies are available that evaluate the results of treatment (**B,** view from behind with patient wearing brace). In addition, most studies fail to document curve progression; thus, it is uncertain whether those patients braced would have had continued progression had they not been braced. This type of brace was the "gold standard" for bracing but is rarely used today. It has been replaced by various models of underarm low profile braces such as seen in Figure 16-13. There arc no published prospective controlled studies on bracing.

and is removed only for bathing or sporting activities. When the patient reaches skeletal maturity (i.e., Risser grade 4, or no spinal growth over an 18-month period), the patient is gradually weaned out of the brace. The brace is used on a part-time basis followed by nighttime use only so long as no increases in curvature are noted. Bracing is reported to be ineffective in curves greater than 40°.

Although full-time bracing has been the standard, many physicians are choosing part-time bracing programs and using underarm orthoses (Figure 16-13) because of compliance problems. An underarm brace (thoracic-lumbar-sacral orthoses, TLSO) is generally acceptable for use in curves with an apex of T8 or below. Electrical stimulation was used in the past but has been shown to be ineffective. Although bracing for scoliosis remains in common usage, as mentioned earlier, final determination as to the success of bracing in adolescent (late onset) idiopathic scoliosis must await a randomized, prospective, controlled clinical trial.

Surgical treatment is indicated if the patient has evidence of curve progression despite bracing or has a curve magnitude that would be unsuccessfully treated by a brace (i.e., greater than 45 to 50° and skeletally immature). In the adult patient with adolescent idiopathic scoliosis, indications for surgical treatment include pain unresponsive to nonsurgical treatment and documented curve progression.

Surgical treatment of adolescent idiopathic scoliosis involves a posterior spinal fusion in combination with one of the various forms of spinal instrumentation (Figure 16-14). The purpose of the procedure is to obtain a spinal fusion. Instrumentation is used to correct the deformity and prevent bending of the fusion mass (Figure 16-15). Over the past few years, many implant devices have been introduced for the correction of spinal curvatures. These devices allow for correction of the sagittal in addition to the coronal plane deformity (see Figure 16-14). Some of these devices allow for decreasing the number of segments of the spine that need to be fused by doing the procedure from the front of the spine.

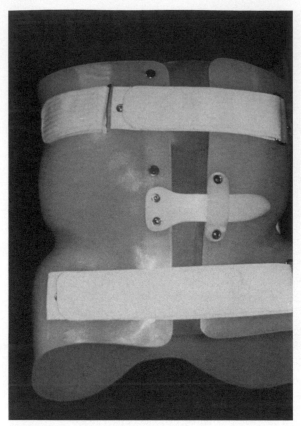

FIGURE 16-13. Underarm brace (TLSO): frontal view of one model.

CONGENITAL SPINAL DEFORMITY

Congenital spinal deformities are due to abnormalities of vertebral development. These abnormalities may result in scoliosis, kyphosis, lordosis, or combinations of these. Deformities may be of three structural types: failure of formation (e.g., hemivertebrae); failure of segmentation (e.g., unilateral unsegmented bar); or combinations of defects of segmentation and formation (Figures 16-16 and 16-17). The resultant deformity is related to the location and type of the congenital anomaly and to the growth potential of the unaffected segments; for example, a lateral segmentation defect causes a pure scoliosis, a posterolateral segmentation defect causes a lordoscoliosis, and an anterior failure of segmentation causes a kyphosis. With defects of formation, any portion of the vertebrae may be hypoplastic or absent. Absence of a vertebral body causes a pure kyphosis, and presence of the posterolateral portion of the vertebrae causes a kyphoscoliosis. Failure of formation of various portions of the posterior elements results in spina bifida.

Isolated congenital vertebral abnormalities are not thought to have genetic implications. Patients with congenital scoliosis may, however, have other associated congenital abnormalities. The most frequently affected systems are the genitourinary, cardiac, and spinal cord. Some syndromes (e.g., VATER

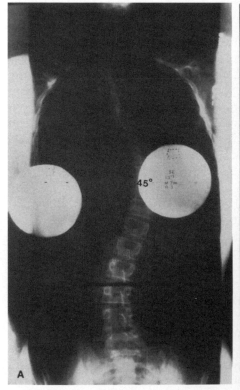
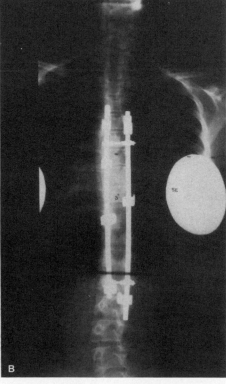

FIGURE 16-14. (A) Thirteen-year, 1-month-old girl with a curve that progressed from 23 to 45° despite bracing. (B) After spinal fusion and Cotrel-Dubousset instrumentation, the same patient's curve measures 3°.

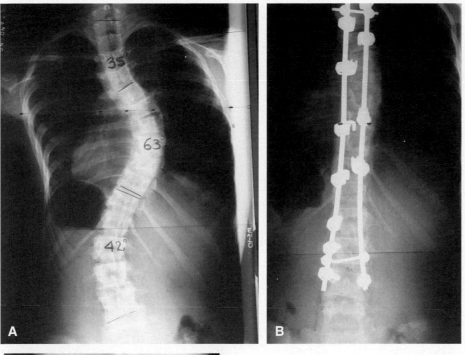

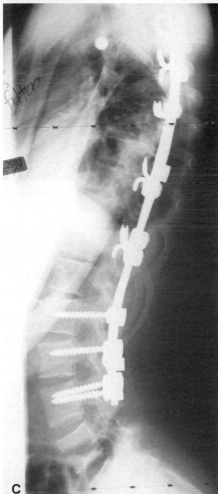

FIGURE 16-15. Spinal fusion for progressive idiopathic scoliosis using a hybrid system of rods, hooks, and pedicle screws. **(A)** preoperative PA view; **(B)** postoperative PA; and **(C)** lateral view.

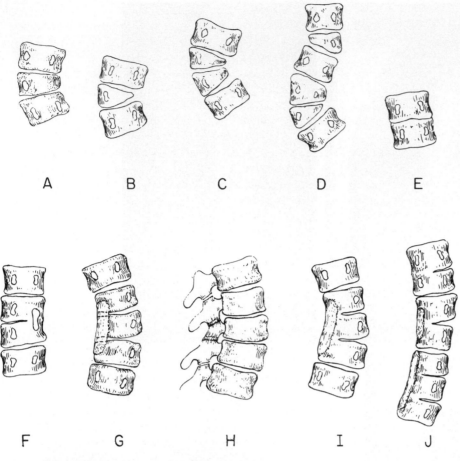

A   B   C   D   E

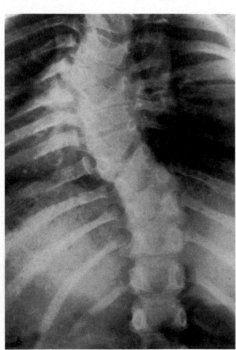

F   G   H   I   J

FIGURE 16-16. Scoliosis anomalies. **(A)** Unilateral failure of vertebral formation, partial (wedged vertebra). **(B)** Unilateral failure of vertebral formation, complete (hemivertebra). **(C)** Double hemivertebrae, unbalanced. **(D)** Double hemivertebrae, balanced. **(E)** Symmetric failure of segmentation (congenital fusion). **(F)** Asymmetric failure of segmentation (unsegmented bar). **(G)** Asymmetric failure of segmentation (unsegmented bar involving posterior elements only, anteroposterior view). **(H)** Asymmetric failure of segmentation, oblique view showing intact disc space and lack of segmentation confined to the posterior elements (surgically easy to divide). **(I)** Unsegmented bar involving both the disc area and posterior elements (a very difficult surgical problem to divide this). **(J)** Multiple unsegmented bars, unbalanced. (Winter RB, Moe JH, Eilers VE. Congenital scoliosis: a study of 234 patients treated and untreated. J Bone Joint Surg 1968;50A:1)

FIGURE 16-17. Congenital scoliosis. The ribs on the concave side are misshapen and fused. The seventh thoracic vertebra is wedged.

syndrome) are also associated with congenital vertebral abnormalities. Many congenital spine deformities are discovered only incidentally on radiographs taken for other reasons, and some are associated with severe deformities noted at birth.

Progressive, untreated congenital spinal anomalies may produce severe functional and cosmetic deformities. If the deformity is associated with kyphosis, spinal cord compression and paralysis may occur. Early detection and careful follow-up of these patients is imperative.

All patients with congenital spinal deformity must have a careful and detailed neurologic examination. Five to 20% of patients have associated spinal dysraphism (e.g., tethered cord, diastematomyelia, dural lipoma). Subtle physical findings, such as limb atrophy or mild foot abnormalities, may be the only evidence of spinal dysraphism. The skin should be inspected over the spine, looking for hair patches, dimpling, cyst formation, and hemangiomas, which are often associated with a spinal dysraphic condition. The chest wall should be examined for any evidence of defects or asymmetry.

About 15% of patients with congenital scoliosis have associated cardiac abnormalities. A cardiologist should evaluate any cardiac abnormality detected.

All patients with congenital spinal deformity should have a urologic evaluation. Twenty to 40% of patients with congenital spinal abnormalities have an associated abnormality in the genitourinary tract. Six percent of these genitourinary tract abnormalities are potentially life threatening. Renal ultrasound is generally sufficient to provide a screening test for genitourinary tract abnormalities. Evaluation of the lower tracts, however, may require excretory or retrograde urograms. The kidneys are also seen well on the MRI.

Spinal abnormalities are best demonstrated in infancy on supine AP and lateral radiographs. These films provide the best detail of the congenital abnormalities (Figure 16-18). It is important to pay attention to the sagittal plane deformity because many patients with congenital scoliosis may have accompanying kyphosis or lordosis. A baseline lateral radiograph should be obtained to assess any associated lordosis or kyphosis. Sagittal plane deformity may progress without progression of the scoliosis as the patient matures. Follow-up radiographs can be taken in the standing position (when possible) and measured by the Cobb angle to follow curve progression.

Each radiograph should be evaluated for gross abnormalities, such as hemivertebrae or nonsegmented vertebrae. The ribs should be examined for congenital abnormalities, and all pedicles should be counted, disc spaces examined, and growth potential assessed. The prognosis for congenital deformities depends on the presence of asymmetric growth. Pedicular widening may be a sign of diastematomyelia, especially in patients with cutaneous or clinical manifestations of spinal dysraphism. CT scanning may be helpful in defining some congenital lesions, particularly in older patients. MRI is indicated if the patient has any evidence of spinal dysraphism or prior to any corrective surgery.

The natural history of congenital spinal deformities relates specifically to the location of the abnormality (e.g., thoracic, thoracolumbar, lumbar spine), the type of abnormality (e.g., unilateral unsegmented bar, hemivertebrae), and the patient's spinal growth potential. In general, about half of all congenital spine anomalies have significant enough progression to require treatment. By counting the number of growth centers, as represented by the pedicles on the concave and convex sides of the curve, as well as examining the quality of the disc spaces between vertebrae, the physician can estimate the probability of curve progression. If there is greater growth potential in the convexity of the curve than the concavity, progression is certain. The

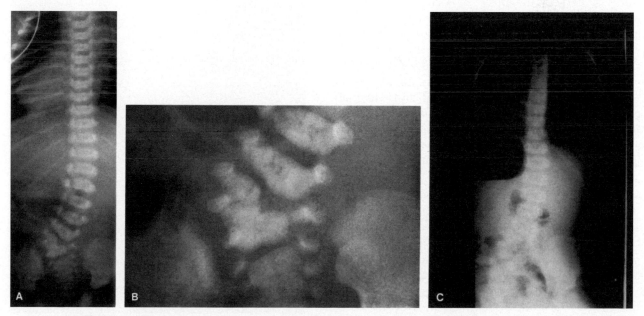

FIGURE 16-18. Eight-day-old boy with lumbosacral hemivertebrae. Radiographs of newborns generally provide the best detail of congenital spine abnormalities. **(A)** Spine film. **(B)** Coned-down view of lumbosacral junction. **(C)** Standing film at 2 years of age; because of progression of curve and pelvic obliquity, patient underwent excision of hemivertebra.

worst prognosis for progression of congenital anomalies is the unilateral unsegmented bar opposite to a convex hemivertebrae, followed by the unilateral unsegmented bar and the double-convex hemivertebrae (see Figure 16-16).

The prognosis for progression in patients with hemivertebrae is difficult to predict in that there are three types of hemivertebrae: fully segmented (worst prognosis), semisegmented, and nonsegmented (most benign). The younger the patient at the age of detection, the more likely the patient is to have a progressive deformity. If a congenital anomaly is detected at an older age or only incidentally, it rarely causes significant problems.

Stable, nonprogressive curves require only observation until skeletal maturity. Patients with congenital spinal deformity should be followed with radiographs every 6 months during the first 3 years of life. If the curve remains stable, follow-up can be on a yearly basis until the adolescent growth spurt, when repeat evaluations every 6 months may be warranted.

Congenital spinal deformities tend to be rigid; therefore, bracing is generally not a treatment option. Bracing, however, can be used in certain situations, particularly in long, flexible curves or compensatory curves above or below congenital abnormalities.

Progression of the curve regardless of the patient's age is an indication for surgical stabilization. In certain instances in which the natural history is well known (e.g., unilateral unsegmented bar opposite a convex hemivertebrae), surgical stabilization is indicated without documentation of progression. The standard method of surgical stabilization is posterior spinal fusion without instrumentation. The deformity is then corrected by a plaster cast. This type of treatment is at times (particularly in the young patient) associated with bending of the fusion mass and continued rotational curve progression (often referred to as the "crankshaft phenomenon"). Promising results have been reported with combination anterior hemiepiphysiodesis and posterior hemiarthrodesis, even demonstrating correction for some curves by growth on the unfused concave side in very young patients with significant growth potential and with certain types of congenital deformities.

Distraction instrumentation may be used in certain cases. This mode of treatment, however, is associated with an increased risk of neurologic deficit. If correction of the congenital spinal deformity is contemplated, thorough investigation for intraspinal pathology (MRI) must be done before operation. The presence of a diastematomyelia without neurologic deficit does not require treatment. If correction of the spinal deformity is contemplated, however, then the diastematomyelia must be addressed surgically. Hemivertebrae excision may be considered in cases of a lumbosacral hemivertebrae with spinal decompensation (see Figure 16-18).

Treatment of congenital kyphotic deformities is surgical. Patients with failure of formation causing either pure kyphosis or kyphoscoliosis are at high risk for spinal cord compression. Posterior hemivertebrae or failure of formation of a vertebral body should be treated by immediate surgical stabilization. These patients generally benefit from a combined anterior and posterior surgical spinal fusion (Figure 16-19).

With failures of segmentation, a progressive kyphosis may ensue, although this rarely leads to neurologic deficit. A short, posterior fusion arrests spinal growth and halts progression of the deformity.

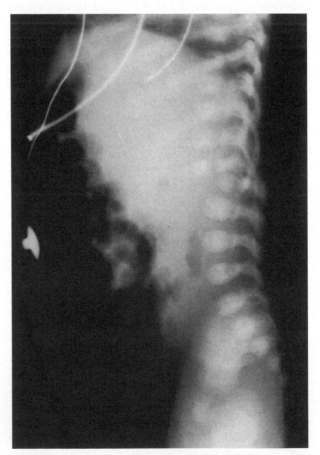

FIGURE 16-19. Six-week-old boy with hypoplasia of L1 with kyphosis. At 14 months of age, the patient underwent AP spinal fusion to prevent progression.

If the deformity exceeds 50°, anterior fusion must be done in conjunction with the posterior spinal fusion; otherwise progression may occur by bending of the fusion mass. Any neurologic deficit associated with congenital kyphosis or congenital kyphoscoliosis must be treated by spinal cord decompression and stabilization.

BACK PAIN IN CHILDREN

The child presenting with a chief complaint of back pain warrants careful evaluation because, although back pain is a common complaint in adults, back pain in children is uncommon. The younger the child is the more worrisome the complaint.

The normal child may have occasional complaints of back pain after strenuous physical activity, prolonged sitting or standing, or repetitive heavy lifting. Back pain may also accompany a viral illness. Repetitive or chronic backache symptoms should be carefully investigated. There are many causes of backache in children (Table 16-4), and the cause can be established in about 85% of cases.

The child and family should be questioned to quantitate and characterize the pain. The pain should be characterized as to nature, intensity, location, and time of occurrence. Was the onset of the pain acute or insidious? Is it associated with any other illnesses? Is it activity related? Is it relieved by rest? Does it occur in the morning, the afternoon, or with repeated stress? Are there any associated bowel or bladder symptoms? What makes the pain better? What makes it worse? Is there associated night pain? Does aspirin or NSAIDs relieve the pain? Are there associated radicular symptoms, leg pains, or paresthesia? Does the child have any complaints of a systemic illness, such as fever, weight loss, or general malaise? Is there a history of injury? Is the pain associated with repetitive trauma, such as gymnastic activities or other sports?

By taking a careful history, the physician should be able to narrow down the possible sources of the back pain. For example, if the patient is complaining of back pain usually at night with symptoms relieved by aspirin, an osteoid osteoma or osteoblastoma should be suspected. Pain during athletic events, such as gymnastics or blocking in a football lineman, is suggestive of spondylolysis or spondylolisthesis. Leg pain with or without associated back pain may be radicular pain associated with a herniated nucleus pulposus or may be secondary to hamstring tightness because of cauda equina irritation from a spondylolysis or spondylolisthesis. Back pain in children with or without neurologic deficits may also be a manifestation of intraspinal pathology.

Physical examination of the child presenting with the chief complaint of back pain should consist of a general overall evaluation, including examination of the head and neck, the upper and lower extremities, gait, and spine. A careful, detailed neurologic examination, including muscle, reflex, and sensory testing, is mandatory. The presence of normal or abnormal contours of the spine in either the coronal or sagittal plane should be noted. Skin lesions, such as nevi, sinuses, hair patches, or abnormal pigmentation over the lumbosacral area may indicate spinal dysraphism. The Adams forward-bend test should be performed, looking for evidence of scoliosis or an exaggerated kyphosis. Spinal motion should be assessed to be certain that the patient reverses the normal lumbar lordosis. Any loss of normal spinal motion or failure to reverse lumbar lordosis on forward flexion is suggestive of a pathologic condition and should be investigated.

The back should be palpated for any areas of tenderness over the spine or paraspinous region. The flank should be percussed, looking for areas of tenderness that may indicate a visceral abnormality. The abdomen should be palpated for masses. Limb lengths should be measured. Thighs and calves should be measured for any evidence of atrophy. Straight-leg raising tests are performed looking for signs of nerve root irritation or excessive hamstring tightness. The sacroiliac region, particularly the sacroiliac joints, should be examined for any signs of joint pathology. Signs of meningeal irritation should be sought.

TABLE 16-4.
Causes of Back Pain in Children

Tumors
  Spine
  Spinal cord
Herniated nucleus pulposus
Spondylolysis
Spondylolisthesis
Scheuermann kyphosis
Postural kyphosis
Vertebral osteomyelitis
Diskitis
Overuse syndromes
Rheumatologic condition

In the child presenting with the chief complaint of back pain, a supine AP and lateral radiograph of the involved area of the spine is taken to assess bony detail. Standing PA and lateral radiographs can be ordered if the patient is being assessed for scoliosis or kyphosis associated with the pain. If spondylolisthesis or spondylolysis is suspected, a cone-down lateral view of the L3 to S1 region should be ordered. Oblique views may also be helpful.

If plain films are negative, special studies may be warranted. Bone scanning is useful in the face of a negative radiograph in diagnosing stress fractures, bone tumors, or infections of the spine. CT scanning may be helpful in documenting the anatomic details of lesions seen on plain films. For soft tissue lesions around the spine or for evaluating the spinal cord, MRI is the diagnostic procedure of choice.

Depending on the patient's clinical history, physical examination, and radiographic findings, certain laboratory studies may be helpful. A complete blood count and an erythrocyte sedimentation rate or C-reactive protein, although nonspecific, may be abnormal in infections, tumors, or rheumatologic conditions. If a collagen disease is suspected, HLA-B27 and rheumatoid factors may help in the diagnosis.

Some of the common causes of back pain in children are covered in the remainder of this section. Other causes, such as vertebral osteomyelitis, diskitis, and neoplastic lesions, are discussed elsewhere in the book.

Scheuermann Kyphosis

Scheuermann kyphosis is a structural sagittal plane deformity in the thoracic or the thoracolumbar spine. Patients have an increased kyphosis in the thoracic or thoracolumbar spine with associated diagnostic radiographic changes. Normal thoracic kyphosis is generally accepted to be between 20 and 45°. The degree of kyphosis in the thoracic spine increases with age. Kyphosis should never be present at the thoracolumbar junction. Any kyphotic deformity present at this level is considered abnormal.

The incidence of Scheuermann kyphosis is thought to be between 0.4 and 8%, with a slight male predominance. The diagnosis is usually made during the adolescent growth spurt and is rarely made in patients younger than 10 years of age. An increased incidence of spondylolysis and spondylolisthesis is reported in patients with Scheuermann kyphosis (this fact has been refuted by a more recent study) as well as a 20 to 30% incidence of an associated scoliosis in the region of the kyphosis.

The origin of Scheuermann disease is unknown. Many theories have been advanced, including mechanical, metabolic, and endocrinologic. There is a definite hereditary component, but no mode of inheritance is known. Patients with Scheuermann kyphosis are generally taller than comparably aged patients, and their skeletal age is advanced over their chronologic age.

Histologic changes demonstrate that vertebral growth endplate cartilage is abnormal, with a decreased collagen–proteoglycan ratio on electron microscopic examination. Enchondral ossification is profoundly altered in affected segments, and proteoglycan levels are increased. The matrix of the endplates is abnormal, thus interfering with normal vertebral growth.

The two types of thoracic Scheuermann kyphosis are kyphosis with the apex at the T7-T9 level and kyphosis with the apex in the lower thoracic spine at the thoracolumbar junction (T11-T12). There is generally an associated secondary increased lumbar lordosis. The so-called lumbar Scheuermann kyphosis has the apex at L1-L2. This condition is generally more common in boys and in young athletes. It is thought to have a traumatic origin.

Clinically, most patients with thoracic Scheuermann kyphosis present with a history of deformity. The child is often brought in by the parent because of poor posture or is referred from a school screening program. The incidence of pain in the adolescent is low, although about 20% of patients present with a history of discomfort in the region of the kyphosis. In patients with lumbar Scheuermann kyphosis, the chief complaint is generally that of pain (80%). The pain is usually intermittent in nature. It is characterized as dull and aching and is generally activity related and relieved by rest.

On physical examination, patients with upper thoracic Scheuermann disease present with a kyphotic deformity. This is best demonstrated in the forward flexed position (Figure 16-20). The flexibility of the kyphosis can be demonstrated by having the patient either hyperextend from a prone position or sit on a chair with the hands held behind the head and hyperextend. Lack of flexibility indicates the structural nature of the kyphotic deformity in contrast to patients with flexible postural kyphosis. These patients also have a hyperlordosis in the lumbar spine. In lower thoracic Scheuermann disease, the kyphosis is at the thoracolumbar junction. There

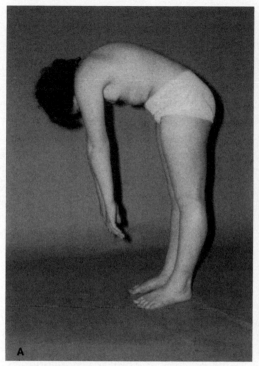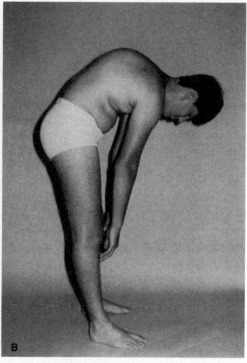

FIGURE 16-20. (A) Thirteen-year-old patient with normal sagittal plane spine contours on forward flexion. **(B)** Thirteen-year-old patient with Scheuermann kyphosis. Note the sharp angular thoracic spine kyphosis on forward flexion.

may also be hypokyphosis above the thoracolumbar junction and hypolordosis in the lumbar spine.

Hamstring tightness may be present in these patients. Because of the high association of scoliosis with Scheuermann kyphosis, scoliosis too must be assessed. The thoracic Scheuermann patient may have tenderness to palpation above or below the apex of the kyphosis. In the lumbar variety, tenderness to palpation is generally in the region of the curve apex.

Each patient should have a careful neurologic examination. Although rare, with extreme degrees of kyphosis, neurologic deficit can ensue. In addition, there is an association of epidural cyst, causing spastic paraparesis in patients with Scheuermann kyphosis.

A paucity of natural history data are available on Scheuermann kyphosis. Many authors think that, in the thoracic variety, if pain is present, it subsides with growth and that there are few adverse long-term sequelae of the condition. Others postulate that the incidence of pain with Scheuermann kyphosis increases throughout life, as may the deformity. The pain in adults with Scheuermann disease is generally described as the feeling of tiredness in the back. These patients may have pain

in the hyperlordotic lumbar spine or at the apex of the kyphosis because of ankylosis.

The diagnosis of Scheuermann kyphosis is confirmed on a standing lateral radiograph of the spine. Standard radiographic technique is important. The radiograph should be taken with the arms parallel to the floor and resting on a support (Figure 16-21). An alternative method is to curl the fingers and to put the pip finger joints in the supraclavicular notch on each side. It is important to see the entire spine to measure the thoracic kyphosis, lumbar lordosis, and any secondary cervicothoracic curves that may accompany the kyphosis. The kyphosis is measured by determining the angle between the maximally tilted end vertebrae (similar to the Cobb method for measuring scoliosis). A PA scoliosis film should be obtained to detect the presence and magnitude of any associated scoliosis.

The radiographic diagnosis of Scheuermann kyphosis is made by the presence of irregularities of the vertebral endplates, anterior vertebral body wedging, Schmorl nodes, and decreased intervertebral disc space height. In older patients, degenerative changes may be evident. The endplate irregularity, Schmorl nodes, and disc space narrowing are often but not always seen. There is some discrepancy in the literature regarding the number of consecutive vertebrae that need to be wedged to make the diagnosis of Scheuermann kyphosis. By one criterion (Sorenson criterion), there should be wedging in three or more adjacent vertebrae of more than 5°. In other studies, the diagnosis is made by the presence of only one wedged vertebrae of more than 5°. Discrepancies compound the problem of determining the natural history.

On the PA radiograph, any evidence of interpedicular widening should be noted because of the association of epidural cysts with Scheuermann kyphosis. Any scoliosis present should be assessed; curves rarely exceed 20 to 25°. The flexibility of the kyphosis is best demonstrated in a supine hyperextension lateral view with a "bump" under the apex of the kyphosis.

In lumbar Scheuermann disease, irregularities of the vertebral endplates are usually present, as are Schmorl nodes. The intervertebral disc spaces are normal, and there is no evidence of vertebral wedging.

In a patient with an apparent exaggerated kyphosis, the differential diagnosis includes postural round back. In postural round back, there is a slight increase in the thoracic kyphosis. The kyphosis, however, is flexible, as demonstrated on the prone or sitting hyperextension tests. On the standing lateral radiograph, there are no structural changes as noted for Scheuermann kyphosis. The kyphosis in postural kyphosis patients is usually in the range of 45 to 60°. On the supine hyperextension lateral view, the deformity is totally flexible. The question remains whether a postural kyphosis left untreated may progress and get secondary bony changes resembling Scheuermann disease. Postural kyphosis, if flexible, should be treated by exercising.

Thoracic hyperkyphosis is also seen in patients with various types of skeletal dysplasia, such as spondyloepiphyseal dysplasia congenita and Morquio disease. These conditions can usually be diagnosed by the clinical examination and other radiographic features. Ankylosing spondylitis may present a similar picture, but 97% of these patients are HLA-B27-positive. Kyphosis may also be present in patients who had a laminectomy before skeletal maturity and in patients who had radiation to the spine for a regional tumor, such as Wilms, tumor or neuroblastoma. Kyphosis may also been seen with eosinophilic granuloma. Type II congenital kyphosis (failure of segmentation) may be confused with Scheuermann disease. It may be necessary to use CT scanning to identify the anterior failure of segmentation seen in this condition to differentiate it from Scheuermann kyphosis.

The treatment of Scheuermann kyphosis is controversial. Lumbar Scheuermann disease generally responds well to nonoperative measures, such as nonsteroidal anti-inflammatory agents and temporary activity restriction. There are no adverse long-term sequelae from lumbar Scheuermann disease.

Some authors think that the natural history of thoracic Scheuermann kyphosis is benign and therefore needs no treatment. Others report increasing pain with progression of the deformity. It is uncertain whether treatment prevents any of the consequences that may occur without treatment. Treatment of Scheuermann kyphosis in the skeletally immature patient is recommended in the hope of preventing excessive deformity that may cause pain and cosmetic concerns. Exercises alone are not beneficial. Hyperextension body casts changed at monthly intervals to correct the curvature may be used in the skeletally immature patient with a rigid Scheuermann kyphosis (i.e., less than 10 or 15° of correction on hyperextension lateral radiograph) followed by bracing; this technique is rarely used today. In those patients with a somewhat flexible Scheuermann kyphosis, the Milwaukee brace is prescribed, although some orthopaedists prefer to use a hyperextension underarm orthosis to hopefully improve brace wear compliance. In some centers, particularly in Europe, casting alone is used as a treatment for this condition. Treatment is generally continued until the patient reaches skeletal maturity. In immature patients, some of the anterior wedging associated with Scheuermann kyphosis may be corrected by treatment. Follow-up studies of patients treated for Scheuermann kyphosis demonstrate increase of the kyphosis over time even after brace treatment.

Surgery is rarely indicated in patients with Scheuermann kyphosis. In patients with curves greater than 75° and with pain unresponsive to nonoperative measures, spinal fusion can be considered. Treatment of kyphosis of this magnitude requires anterior and posterior spinal fusion throughout the length of the kyphosis. Cord decompression is indicated for the rare patient who has neurologic deficits secondary to epidural cysts or increased kyphotic angulation.

Spondylolysis and Spondylolisthesis

Spondylolysis is a descriptive term referring to a defect in the pars interarticularis. The defect may be unilateral or bilateral and may be associated with spondylolisthesis. *Spondylolisthesis* refers to the anterior displacement (translation) of a vertebra with

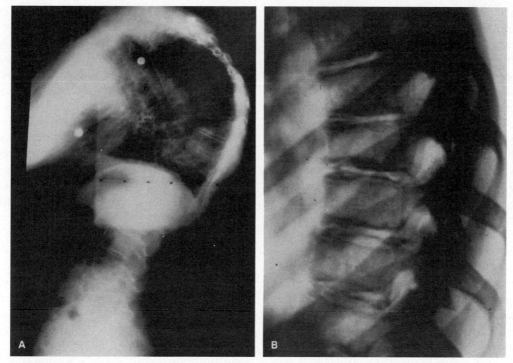

FIGURE 16-21. (A) Standing lateral radiograph of patient with Scheuermann disease (94°). Note the marked vertebral wedging at the curve apex. **(B)** Coned-down views of spine in another patient with Scheuermann disease. Note the vertebral wedging, endplate irregularity, and disc space narrowing.

respect to the vertebra caudal to it. This translation may also be accompanied by an angular deformity (kyphosis). These two topics are considered together in that the most common cause of spondylolisthesis in children is spondylolysis.

Spondylolysis occurs most commonly at the L5 to S1 level and less frequently at the L4-L5 region. Spondylolytic lesions may occur at other lumbar levels or at multiple levels. Spondylolytic lesions are found in about 5% of the general population. Spondylolysis is an acquired condition. It has not been reported in infants and is rarely present before 5 years of age. There is an increased incidence of spondylolysis and spondylolisthesis up to the age of 20 years, after which the incidence remains stable.

Spondylolisthesis is classified into five types (Table 16-5). It is further classified by the degree of angular and translational displacement. The diagnosis and treatment of the condition depends on the type.

TABLE 16-5.
Classification of Spondylolisthesis

Type	Description
I	Dysplastic
IIA	Fracture in pars interarticularis (stress fracture)
B	Elongated intact pars interarticularis
C	Acute fracture
III	Degenerative
IV	Traumatic (fracture in other than pars interarticularis)
V	Pathologic

(Adapted from Wiltse LL, Newman PH, MacNab I. Classification of spondylolysis and spondylolisthesis. Clin Orthop 1976;117:23–29.

Spondylolysis is thought to be an acquired condition secondary to a stress fracture at the pars interarticularis. Experimental studies showed that extension movements of the spine, particularly in combination with lateral flexion, increase the shear stress at the pars interarticularis. Clinical evidence for this theory includes the high association (four times more than normal) in female gymnasts, football linemen, and soldiers carrying backpacks. This etiologic theory is also supported by a reported higher association in patients with Scheuermann kyphosis with secondary excessive lumbar lordosis. In contrast, spondylolysis has never been seen in patients who have never walked.

Evidence supports the concept the spondylolysis and spondylolisthesis may be inherited conditions. There is a high association of the condition in family members of affected patients. There are racial and gender differences, with the lowest incidence in black females and the highest incidence in white males. Most patients with type I spondylolisthesis have abnormalities at the lumbosacral junction with poor development of the superior aspect of the sacrum and superior sacral facets and with associated sacral spina bifida. Similar congenital changes have also been reported in about one-third of patients with type II spondylolisthesis. Thus, these conditions may be genetic, acquired, or both.

The presenting complaints of patients with spondylolysis and spondylolisthesis are determined primarily by the age of the patient and, in spondylolisthesis, by the type. Although pain is the most common presenting complaint in the adult, it is relatively uncommon in children or the symptomatology is usually mild. Children most commonly present with gait abnormalities, postural deformity, and hamstring tightness. Back pain is usually localized to the lower-back region, with occasional radiation to the buttocks and the thighs. Occasional L5 radiculopathies are present, although this is not common in children.

The adult patient with type III degenerative spondylolisthesis generally is older than 40 years of age, and women are more commonly affected than men. Pain in degenerative spondylolisthesis is often similar to the pain patterns in patients with a herniated nucleus pulposus (i.e., the patient has pain radiating down the leg and complaints of sciatica). Patients may complain of pain similar to spinal stenosis and have claudication-type symptoms (i.e., pain and cramping in the calves and back brought on by walking and relieved by sitting in a flexed spinal posture). In most cases of spondylolysis and spondylolisthesis, pain is precipitated by activity, especially flexion and extension on a repetitive basis, and relieved by rest or lowered activity levels.

Each patient must have a complete physical examination, including detailed neurologic examination. About 80% of children with spondylolysis and accompanying spondylolisthesis have evidence of hamstring tightness. The cause for this is unknown but is thought to be instability in the area of the spondylolysis and spondylolisthesis resulting in cauda equina irritation. Hamstring tightness is responsible for the postural abnormalities often seen as the presenting complaint of the patients with spondylolisthesis. Restrictive flexion secondary to the hamstring tightness and the pelvic tilt gives the patient a stiff-legged gait with a short stride length. The pelvis rotates as the child takes a step, and often the child walks on tiptoes with the knees slightly flexed. The hamstring tightness may be so severe in some children that, in performing a straight-leg raising test in a supine position, the leg can only be lifted several inches off the table.

The physical findings referable to the back depend on the type and degree of the slip. Patients may present with mild tenderness to palpation in the area of the spondylolysis or spondylolisthesis. In severe grades of slip, a "step-off" may be palpated. There may be an apparent increase in lumbar lordosis with a backward tilting of the pelvis (Figure 16-22). The patient may present with protrusion of the lower abdomen, and in severe cases of spondylolisthesis, a deep transverse abdominal crease may be noted. A detailed neurologic examination, including deep tendon reflexes, sensory examination, and motor strength, should be performed on each patient with particular attention to any dysesthesia near the sacrum and rectum. A history of bowel or bladder dysfunction may be indicative of cauda equina syndrome.

About one-third of patients with symptomatic spondylolisthesis have evidence of scoliosis. The scoliosis most commonly seen in association with symptomatic spondylolisthesis is generally not structural. It is more commonly seen in patients with high-degree slips. The curve is usually in the lumbar region and resolves with the resolution of the symptoms of the spondylolisthesis. Some patients have a characteristic idiopathic scoliosis that is unaffected by the spondylolisthesis or its treatment.

Spondylolisthesis in patients with isthmic spondylolysis may occur any time after the pars fractures. Most slippage occurs during the adolescent growth spurt. Rarely are significant increases

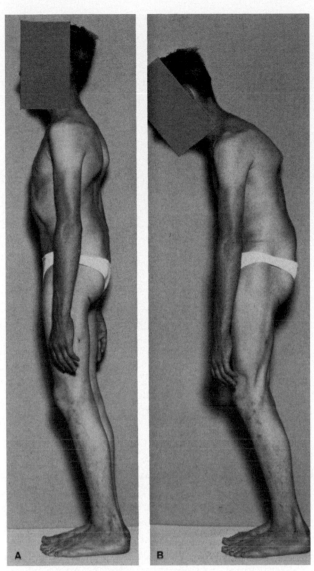

FIGURE 16-22. High grade spondylolisthesis, physical findings. **(A)** Note the flattening of the buttock, anterior protrusion of the pelvis, visible lumbar slip-off, and apparent shortening of the trunk. **(B)** Displaying characteristic hamstring tightness, limiting his ability to touch his toes without flexing the knees. (Turner RH, Bianco AJ. Spondylolysis and spondylolisthesis in children and teenagers. J Bone Joint Surg 1971;53A:1298)

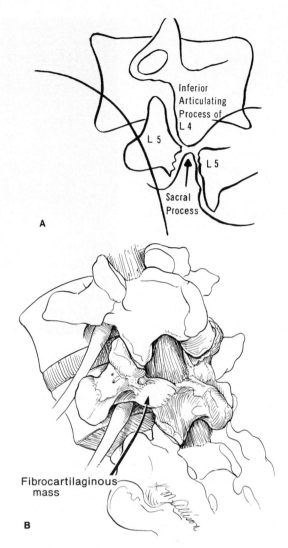

FIGURE 16-23. (A) Diagram of oblique radiograph of lumbosacral junction, showing cleft in isthmus of the fifth lumbar vertebra. The articular process of the sacrum projects upward and penetrates the cleft, meeting the inferior articular process of the fourth lumbar vertebra. **(B)** Pathology of spondylolisthesis showing the relation of the nerve root as it courses through the intervertebral foramen. The continuity of the pars interarticularis is bridged at the defect by a fibrous or fibrocartilaginous mass that rarely may encroach on the nerve root of L5.

in the degree of spondylolisthesis seen after skeletal maturity.

If spondylolysis or spondylolisthesis is clinically suspected, standing PA and standing lateral radiographs of the spine with a cone-down lateral view of L3 to the sacrum are indicated. In most cases, the pars interarticular defect can be seen on the spot lateral views. The defect is usually at the L5 to S1 level. Defects at the L4 level are more common in patients who have complete or partial sacraliza-

tion of the L5 vertebra. If the defect is not visualized on the lateral film and the condition is suspected, an oblique view may be helpful. On this view, one can see what has been described as a Scotty dog with a broken neck or wearing a collar (Figure 16-23). In about 20% of patients, the lytic defect is unilateral and may be accompanied by reactive sclerosis in the opposite pedicle, lamina, or both. This situation often presents a difficult diagnostic dilemma in that the sclerotic region can be confused with lesions

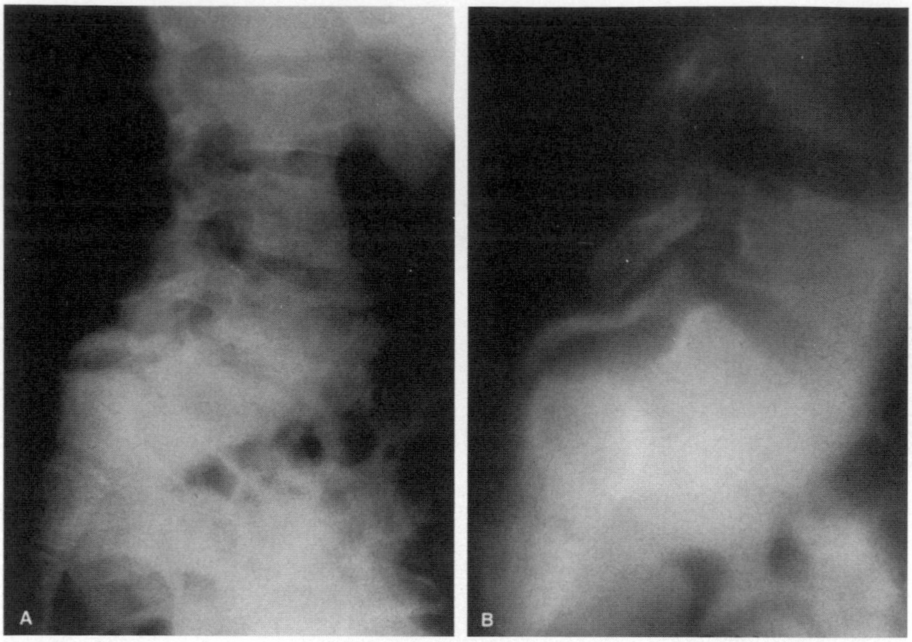

FIGURE 16-24. (A) Nine-year-old girl with type I spondylolisthesis. Note how pars interarticularis has become attenuated, allowing for severe slippage (translation and angulation). The entire posterior arch has slipped forward. (B) Polytome demonstrating the elongation of pars interarticularis.

such as osteoid osteoma and osteoblastoma. If the lesion is not visualized on plain radiograph, technetium bone scanning, Spect scan, or CT scan may be helpful in identifying the lesion. In an acute injury, a "hot" bone scan may allow for early detection. Bone scanning is also used to assess whether an established lesion has the potential to heal. If the lesion is "cold," there is an established nonunion, and hence immobilization would probably not result in healing of the stress fracture.

In type I spondylolisthesis, the entire posterior arch slips forward (Figure 16-24). There is dysplasia of the superior articular facets of the sacrum and inferior articular facets of L5. Type I slips are generally limited to 25 to 30% slippage unless the pars becomes attenuated or fractures, allowing for severe degrees of slippage to occur.

In type II spondylolisthesis, the spinous process and posterior elements remain behind (Figure 16-25). Other changes should be noted, including the shape of the sacrum (i.e., whether it is flattened or dome-shaped; Figure 16-26) and the amount of wedging of L5 (Figure 16-27). In the adult disc space, narrowing and degenerative changes at the intervertebral disc and posterior elements should be noted. Patients with a more rounded S1 and a more wedged-shaped L5 have a greater risk of progression.

Spondylolisthesis is graded on a scale of 1 to 4 depending on the percentage of anterior translation of L5 on S1, with grade 1 being a 25% slip; grade 2, a 50% slip; grade 3, a 75% slip; and grade 4, a complete slip (Figures 16-28 and 16-29). The term *spondyloptosis* is used to describe complete displacement of L5 in front of S1. It is important in assessing spondylolisthetic patients to have standing lateral radiographs of the lumbosacral junction because instability is not uncommon, particularly in childhood (Figure 16-28). Several standard methods of measurements are used to quantitate spondylolisthesis; these include the percentage of translation, sagittal roll, and slip angle (Figures 16-30 and 16-31). These measurements of angulation or lumbosacral kyphosis are important prognostic indicators.

Additional radiographic studies may be in order, especially in the adult patient with degenerative spondylolisthesis. These studies include flexion-extension lateral views to detect instability and CT scanning with or without myelographic enhancement to assess the integrity of the disc and to look for other potential sources of the discomfort. They are also useful to ascertain the specific pathology in spondylolisthesis associated with or causing spinal stenosis and to rule out intraspinal pathology in patients who do not have resolution of symptoms by nonoperative measures. Myelography is rarely indicated in the child or adolescent with spondylolisthesis; MRI may be used if the patient has signs or symptoms of nerve root compression or cauda equina syndrome. In the adult patient, other diagnostic tests, such as EMG, motor nerve condition studies, and psychological testing, may be considered.

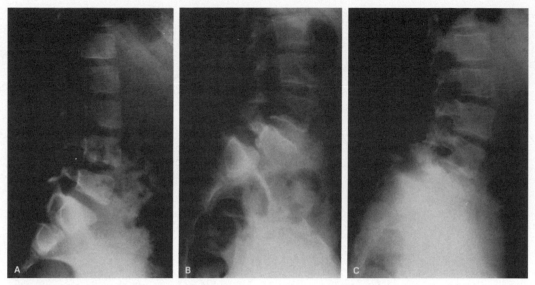

FIGURE 16-25. (**A**) Six-year-old female gymnast who complained of mild backache. Narrowing of pars interarticularis noted in radiograph. (**B**) At age 11, she had increasing pain. Radiograph demonstrates a lytic defect (type IIA) of the pars interarticularis and significant translation; surgery was recommended but refused. (**C**) Because of increasing pain, surgery was performed at age 12. The preoperative radiograph demonstrates increasing anterior translation and lumbosacral angulation (kyphosis).

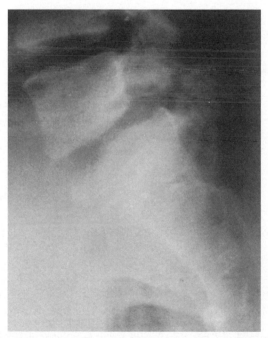

FIGURE 16-26. Spondylolisthesis. Note the attempt at formation of a supporting ledge at the anterior edge of the sacrum.

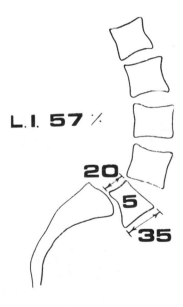

L.I. 57 ⅟.

20
5
35

LUMBAR INDEX

FIGURE 16-27. The lumbar index represents the degree of trapezoidal deformation of the fifth lumbar vertebral body. Although a decreased lumbar index is secondary to increased slipping, when considered in conjunction with other factors, such as the adolescent growth spurt, a dome-shaped first sacral vertebra, and female gender, it indicates that the patient is at risk for progression of slipping. (Boxall D, Bradford DS, Winter RB et al. Management of severe spondylolisthesis in children and adolescents. J Bone Joint Surg 1979;61A:479)

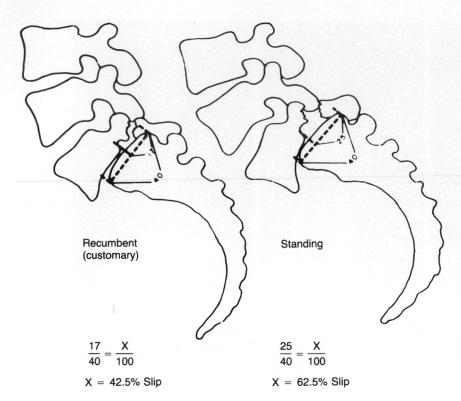

Recumbent
(customary)

Standing

$$\frac{17}{40} = \frac{X}{100}$$

X = 42.5% Slip

$$\frac{25}{40} = \frac{X}{100}$$

X = 62.5% Slip

FIGURE 16-28. Spondylolisthesis, demonstrating the accuracy of the standing radiograph. The displacement is measured as a percentage of the width of the adjacent vertebral body. The standing and recumbent views are compared. (Lowe RW, Hayes TD, Kaye J, et al. Standing roentgenograms in spondylolisthesis. Clin Orthop 1976;117:80)

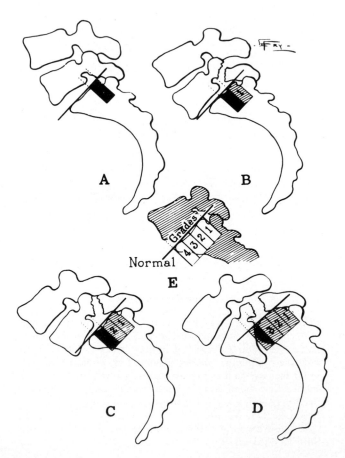

FIGURE 16-29. Meyerding grading system for spondylolisthesis, demonstrating the degrees of slipping of the fifth lumbar vertebra on the sacrum. (Meyerding HW. Spondylolisthesis. Surg Gynecol Obstet 1932;54:374)

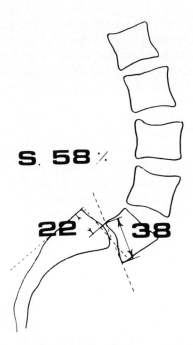

FIGURE 16-30. Percentage of slipping. A line is extended upward from the posterior surface of the first sacral vertebral body, and a second line is drawn downward from the posterior surface of the fifth lumbar vertebral body. The extent of slip is the distance between these two lines. This measurement is expressed as a percentage of the AP dimension of the fifth lumbar vertebral body. (Boxall D, Bradford DS, Winter RB et al. Management of severe spondylolisthesis in children and adolescents. J Bone Joint Surg 1979;61A:479)

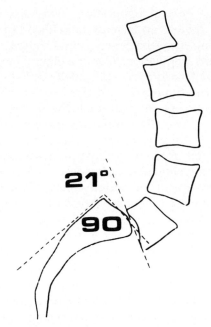

FIGURE 16-31. The slip angle measures the degree of forward tilting of the fifth lumbar vertebral body over the first sacral vertebral body, or the kyphosis at the level of slipping. The angle is formed by a line drawn perpendicular to the posterior aspect of the first sacral body and one drawn parallel to the inferior aspect of the fifth lumbar vertebral body. It represents the degree of instability and potential for progression, particularly when the slip angle is high and a significant increase is noted in the standing roentgenogram as compared with the supine roentgenogram. (Boxall D, Bradford DS, Winter RB et al. Management of severe spondylolisthesis in children and adolescents. J Bone Joint Surg 1979;61A:479)

Most children with spondylolysis can be treated successfully without surgery. If the diagnosis is made as an incidental finding, no activity restrictions are necessary. The patient should, however, be followed through skeletal maturity with standing spot lateral radiographs of the lumbosacral spine every 6 to 8 months to watch for the development of spondylolisthesis.

In a patient with spondylolysis with acute onset of symptoms, bone scanning is helpful to assess the lesion and to follow healing. In such patients, particularly athletes, some evidence suggests that immobilization in a cast or brace allows for healing of the lesion. There are some differences of opinion about whether the cast should extend from the nipple line to include one or both legs or if the same results may be achieved in a TLSO. If this treatment is attempted, the patient can be followed by serial radiographs and bone scans to assess healing.

Most patients with nonacute lesions can be successfully treated by activity restriction and exercises, including hamstring stretching. If symptoms are more severe, a short period of bed rest may be tried

before immobilization in a TLSO. Exercises should be prescribed. Nonsteroidal anti-inflammatory medications are a useful adjuvant to treatment.

If the patient does not respond to conservative management, other conditions, including neurologic conditions and tumors of the spine and spinal cord, must be ruled out before instituting surgical treatment. In patients whose symptoms do not respond to nonoperative treatment, lumbosacral intertransverse process fusion of L5 to S1 has a 90% chance of obtaining a solid fusion with relief of symptomatology, including resolution of hamstring tightness. In patients with isolated or multiple defects in the L1 to L4 region, surgical repair of the defect by one of many available techniques is often recommended to allow for sparing of lumbar motion segments.

In asymptomatic patients who have spondylolisthesis with less than a 25% slip, no treatment is indicated. Natural history indicates that the likelihood of having future problems is essentially the same as that of the general population. With slips greater than 25%, there is an increased likelihood of the patient having lower-back symptoms compared with the general population. Certain clinical and radiographic risk factors have been determined to be associated with future pain, progressive deformity and increasing degree of spondylolisthesis (Table 16-6).

In the skeletally immature patient with less than a 50% slip, nonoperative measures should be tried in attempt to control symptomatology. These measures are similar to those described previously for the treatment of spondylolysis. About two-thirds of these patients have resolution of symptomatology with nonoperative treatment.

Indications for surgery in the skeletally immature patient are failure of relief of symptoms by nonoperative measures or a slip of greater than 50%. L4-sacrum intertransverse process fusion is recommended in those patients with a greater than 50% slip, and L5-sacrum fusion is recommended for those patients with a less than 50% slip. By this method, 90% of children can expect to have a solid fusion within 1 year of surgery and gain resolution of any mild neurologic symptoms, including hamstring tightness, over the ensuing 12 to 18 months. Nonunions and curve progression despite a solid fusion, however, have been reported in children undergoing in situ fusion. Because of these problems, particularly with high grade slips, many authors advocate fusion and closed reduction, followed by pantaloon casting for about 3 months to decrease the sagittal rotation and improve the cosmetic deformity. Although sagittal role or slip angle can be changed by closed methods, vertebral translation is generally unaltered or is changed little by these techniques. The use of instrumentation accompanying fusion with or without reduction is being done more commonly to increase the rates of union and decrease the prolonged immobilization necessary with other techniques. Decompression is rarely necessary in childhood spondylolisthesis and must be accompanied by a fusion to prevent further progression.

In the adult being treated for type I or type II spondylolisthesis, careful assessment must be done to rule out other associated conditions (e.g., herniated nucleus pulposus) and to evaluate disc degeneration and nerve compression. In the adult, the symptomatology is generally confined to back pain. In situ fusion may be all that is necessary. If the patient has leg pain, however, decompression and fusion may be warranted. In the adult patient with spondylolisthesis with or without radiculopathy, it is incumbent on the surgeon to obtain a solid fusion. Many surgeons advocate internal fixation along with a spinal fusion. Internal fixation is most commonly attained by means of pedicle screws, plates, or rods. In the adult, because the risk of further displacement is minimal, pantaloon cast immobilization as advocated by some in children as unnecessary.

In the adult with degenerative spondylolisthesis (type III), the source of the pain must be sought before recommending surgical treatment. These patients rarely develop spondylolisthesis greater than 25%. Radiographs show evidence of degenerative disc disease as well as degeneration of the facet joints. Some patients develop retrolisthesis, and others may develop intraspinal synovial cysts. A complete diagnostic evaluation must be done in these patients, including diskography to ascertain the source of the pain. Adult patients require a much more extensive workup, including the possibility of EMG, motor nerve conduction studies,

TABLE 16-6.
Risk Factors in Spondylolisthesis for Pain, Progression, and Deformity

CLINICAL RISK FACTORS

Younger age

Female patient

Recurrent symptoms

Hamstring tightness, if associated with gait abnormalities or postural deformity

RADIOGRAPHIC RISK FACTORS

Type I greater risk than type II

Greater than 50% slip

Increased risk with increased slip angle

L5-S1 instability with rounded sacral dome and vertical sacrum

(Adapted from Heinsinger RN. Spondylolysis and spondylolisthesis in children and adolescents. J Bone Joint Surg 1989; 71A:1098–1107)

psychological testing, diskography, epidural steroid injections, or nerve root blocks, to ascertain the cause of pain and prognosticate the effectiveness of treatment. Most patients with degenerative spondylolisthesis can also be treated nonoperatively. In those who fail conservative treatment, exhaustive diagnostic measures must be undertaken to determine the source of pain.

Herniated Nucleus Pulposus

Of all cases of herniated nucleus pulposus reported, less than 3% occur in children. An estimated 30 to 60% of cases reported have an associated history of trauma. There is a male predominance. Herniated nucleus pulposus in children is associated with additional vertebral disease, including sacralized L5, lumbarized S1 (either complete or incomplete), asymmetric articular facets, and spina bifida.

Symptoms of a herniated nucleus pulposus in the child may be minimal or they may be characteristic of the adult condition. In children, however, there is occasionally an associated scoliosis secondary to muscle spasm. The neurologic symptoms in children are less common and less severe. Herniated nucleus pulposus may also occur in association with a slipped vertebral apophysis or fracture of the vertebral apophysis. The most common levels involved in children are L4 to L5 and L5 to S1. Treatment recommendations are the same as those in the adult.

BACK PAIN IN ADULTS

Back pain in the adult is one of the most common and costly medical problems. About 80 to 90% of the adult population suffers from back pain during their life. Most cases of back pain resolve spontaneously. Half of patients who complain of back pain are generally asymptomatic within 2 weeks, and 90% are asymptomatic after 3 months. It is estimated that 1 year after symptom onset, only 2% of all adults with back pain have persistent pain.

Back pain is the most common cause of disability for patients under 45 years of age. Although back pain is a common complaint, in 80 to 90% of cases, a pathologic cause cannot be determined. Epidemiologic studies determined that risk factors related to the development of back pain include job dissatisfaction, repetitive lifting, low-frequency vibration, low educational level, smoking, and social problems.

In the adult patient who presents with backache, the history, careful physical examination of the musculoskeletal system, and complete neurologic examination generally allow the physician to make the diagnosis. Diagnostic tests are only used to confirm the suspected diagnosis. Most causes of back pain are self-limiting. Over half of patients with back pain recover within 7 days. Patients who have back pain-associated sciatica (pain down the distribution of the nerve roots contributing to the sciatic nerve) generally recover within 4 weeks.

Historically, the onset of the patient's pain should be assessed in terms of whether it is acute or chronic and whether it had an insidious onset or whether it can be related to a traumatic event. Risk factors should be sought. Pain should be characterized regarding location and whether it is confined to the back or the leg. It is important to determine the pattern of the pain. In patients with sciatica, the pain (and sometimes numbness or tingling) characteristically radiates down the distribution of one of the nerve roots that contributes to the sciatic nerve, characteristically L4, L5, or S1. If the pain does not radiate below the knee but is localized primarily to the back, buttock, hip, and distal thigh, it is likely to be referred pain rather than pain caused by compressive irritation of one of the nerve roots of the sciatic nerve.

The patient should be asked about the effect of position and activity on the pain. The patient should also be queried about muscle weakness or numbness and its location. Medications taken by the patient and their effect on pain should be noted. The effect of previous treatments should also be assessed. A necessary line of questions includes whether or not there is workman's compensation or litigation involved. Job description and satisfaction should also be assessed. The patient must also be questioned about the symptoms impact activities of daily living. Swelling, erythema, and pain in other joints should be noted because they may be indicative of a generalized condition, such as metabolic bone disease or rheumatoid spondylitis.

The patient should specifically be asked about urinary incontinence or retention or change in pattern of stream, which may indicate bowel or bladder dysfunction. Complaints of nonanatomic sensory loss (e.g., stocking-glove anesthesia or nonspecific motor loss throughout the entire lower extremities) should alert the physician to the possibility of a neuropathy or a nonorganic cause of the symptoms. Psychosocial factors can contribute to back pain or response to treatment in patients with chronic back pain. It is important to use additional studies, including psychological inventories such as the Minnesota Multiphasic Personality Inventory, to assess these patients.

In most cases, the pathologic condition causing the patient's symptoms can be ruled in or out by the history alone. Careful physical examination, however, must be done. The patient should be evaluated in a standing position to assess the presence or absence of the normal sagittal and coronal plane contours. The spine should be assessed in flexion, extension, and lateral bending. Restriction of motion or abnormality in any of these motions should be noted. The effect of various motions on the patient's back or leg pain should be noted. The spine should be examined in the prone position. The entire spine should be palpated, assessing both the soft tissues and bone elements for tenderness. The effect of palpation on the patient's symptomatology should also be noted. The sacroiliac joint should be examined, as should the hips. Pathology in these areas may be confused with pain of spinal origin. Each dermatomic region must be assessed for all sensory modalities (Figure 16-32). Motor function in each muscle group must be graded. Reflexes should be tested and any asymmetry noted (Table 16-7). A positive Babinski sign may indicate an upper motor neuron lesion. Assessment of rectal tone and perianal sensation is imperative in any patient complaining of back pain. The straight-leg raising test should be performed both in the supine and prone (femoral stretch) positions. In the supine position, the test is performed by passively elevating the patient's leg with the knee extended and pelvis

TABLE 16-7.
Reflexes

DEEP TENDON REFLEXES
Biceps: C5
Brachioradialis: C5, C6
Triceps: C7, C8
Patella: L3, L4
Achilles: L5–S1
SUPERFICIAL REFLEXES
Upper abdominal: T5–T10
Lower abdominal: T10–T12
Cremasteric: L1, L2
SPHINCTERIC REFLEXES
Bladder: S3–S4
Anus: S3–S4

stable. The test is positive if this maneuver reproduces sciatic pain (radiating below the knee). If the patient only complains of back pain or tightness of the hamstring muscles behind the thigh, the test is considered negative.

The straight-leg raising test is one of the so-called tension signs indicative of neural irritability. This specific test should be done on both legs. If the patient's asymptomatic straight-leg raising test elicits sciatic pain down the contralateral leg, this is called a positive contralateral straight-leg raising test and indicates nerve root irritation.

Another tension sign is the bow-string test; this is a straight-leg raise performed with the knee flexed. With the leg held in this position, the popliteal fossa is palpated. A positive bow-string test occurs

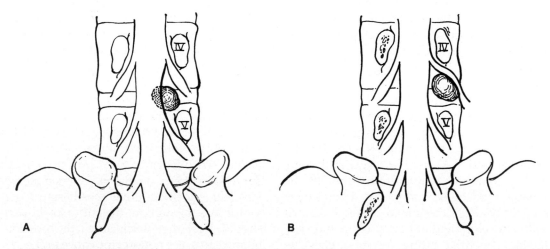

FIGURE 16-32. (A) The usual relation of the protruded disc at the fourth lumbar interspace. The fifth lumbar nerve root is compressed. **(B)** An uncommon relation of the protruded disc at the fourth lumbar interspace. The fourth lumbar nerve root is compressed.

if, during the compression of the tibial nerve in the popliteal fossa, the patient complains of radiating pain both proximally and distally or of paraesthesia in the distribution of any particular branch of the sciatic nerve.

The reverse straight-leg raising test (femoral stretch test) is performed with the patient in the prone position. The leg is extended from the hip, stretching the femoral nerve. Any pain along the distribution of the femoral nerve is considered a positive stretch test.

Pulses should be evaluated in the lower extremity. Patients with spinal stenosis have symptoms of claudication. The presence of palpable pulses in the extremities is helpful in ruling out a vascular cause of the claudication symptoms.

It is important during the physical examination to look for inconsistencies. The Wadell tests for nonorganic causes of lower-back pain are useful in evaluating patients with chronic backache (Table 16-8).

The urgency with which the physician must proceed with further diagnostic workup depends on whether the patient has a history or physical examination compatible with lumbar radiculopathy, keeping in mind the natural history. The remainder of the diagnostic tests and treatment alternatives depend on whether the patient has acute or chronic back pain and whether there is an associated radiculopathy.

Acute Back Pain With Lumbar Radiculopathy

The most common cause of lumbar radiculopathy in patients younger than 40 years of age is a herniated nucleus pulposus. The nucleus pulposus may bulge into the canal. Tears of the fibers of the annulus fibrosis may allow the disc to extrude through the annulus, or the disc may sequester through the annulus and lie free in the spinal canal or neural foramina. Nerve root compression may cause secondary inflammation of the nerve root, giving the patient subjective symptoms of pain, numbness, or tingling along the distribution of the particular nerve root. The most commonly affected nerve roots are L5 and S1. In the lumbar spine, the exiting nerve root is named for the vertebra about which it exits. Therefore, the L5 nerve root exits before the L5 to S1 disc space below the L5 pedicle. Thus, L5 to S1 disc herniation usually causes irritation of the S1 nerve root (Figure 16-33). Herniations occur less frequently at higher levels. Pain associated with a herniated nucleus pulposus varies from mild pain along the distribution of the nerve to severe incapacitating pain.

TABLE 16-8.
Nonorganic Physical Signs in Lower-Back Pain

Category	Test	Comment
Tenderness	Superficial palpation	Inordinate, widespread sensitivity to light touch of the superficial soft tissues over the lumbar spine is nonanatomic and suggests amplified symptoms.
	Nonanatomic testing	Tenderness is poorly localized.
Simulation (to assess patient cooperation and reliability)	Axial loading	Light pressure to the skull of standing patient should not significantly increase symptoms.
	Rotation	Physician should rotate the standing patient's pelvis and shoulders in the same plane; this does not move the lumbar spine and should not increase pain.
Distraction	Straight-leg raising	Physician asks the seated patient to straighten the knee. Patients with true sciatic tension arch backward and complain. These results should closely match those of the traditional, recumbent straight-leg raising test.
Regional		Diffuse motor weakness or bizarre sensory deficits suggest functional regional disturbance if they involve multiple muscle groups and cannot be explained by neuroanatomy principles.
Overreaction		Excessive and inappropriate grimacing, groaning, or collapse during a simple request is disproportionate.

(Adapted from Waddell G, McCulloch JA, Kummel E, Venner RM. Nonorganic physical signs in low back pain. Spine 1980;5:117–125)

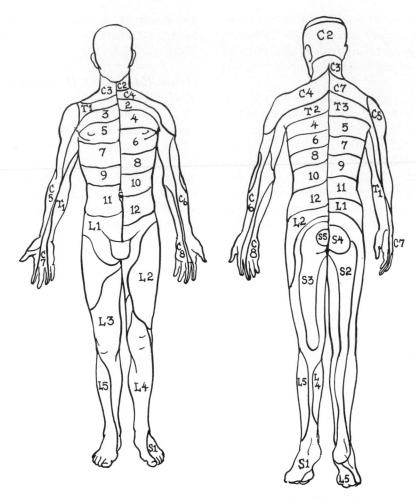

FIGURE 16-33. Distribution of spinal dermatomes. Considerable overlap occurs; consequently, involvement of a single spinal segment may not be evident.

Physical examination of the patient with a herniated nucleus pulposus generally reveals restricted range of motion with forward flexion increasing the pain. The patient may list to one side. Sensory and motor examination may show evidence of nerve root compression with decrease in sensation, muscle weakness, or both and diminished reflexes in the region of the affected nerve (see Table 16-7 and Figure 16-32). Circumference of extremities should be measured to detect any evidence of atrophy. Acute nerve root irritation is evidenced by positive tension signs and straight-leg raising, contralateral straight-leg raising, and bow-string stretch tests. A contralateral straight-leg raising test is the most specific sign of herniated nucleus pulposus.

The natural history of acute lumbar radiculopathy shows about half resolve within 4 weeks. Diagnostic studies thus are not indicated initially. The patient should be treated with a short period of bed rest (1 to 2 days), limitation or modification of activities, and in some cases, anti-inflammatory drugs (aspirin or nonsteroidal anti-inflammatory agents). Epidural steroid injections may provide short-term relief for patients with a herniated nucleus pulposus. Treatment modalities advocated in the past (traction, spinal manipulation, corsets or braces, and physical therapy) have little scientific validity. As the adult symptoms resolve, it is important to get the patient on a rehabilitation program to prevent recurrent episodes of back pain and disability. Patients should be encouraged to increase their activity level and begin a conditioning and physical fitness program.

Because it is unusual for an acute herniated nucleus pulposus to cause bilateral sciatica, the presence of bilateral lower-extremity neurologic signs and symptoms should alert the physician to the possibility of a central disc herniation or, rarely, intraspinal pathology other than disc herniation. The presence of back pain, sciatica, and bowel or bladder dysfunction associated with motor weakness is referred to as *cauda equina syndrome* and is generally caused by extrinsic compression of the thecal sac in the area of the cauda equina. Cauda equina syndrome often requires immediate surgical intervention. Only patients with acute cauda equina syndrome should undergo immediate diagnostic evaluation. These patients should have immediate MRI, myelography, or both to determine the cause of the cauda equina syndrome before surgical intervention.

In patients with persistent symptomatology despite nonoperative treatment or progressive neurologic deficit, further diagnostic evaluation is often necessary. Plain lumbosacral radiographs rarely provide diagnostic information. With aging, normal degenerative changes occur in the lumbar spine that often confuse the diagnostic picture. Changes of spine degeneration are seen in as many of 70% of radiographs. These radiographic changes have little effect on management outcomes. Plain radiographs, however, may be taken to rule out other pathologic conditions, such as infection or tumor.

The ideal diagnostic confirmatory test for herniated nucleus pulposus is MRI. MRI is both sensitive and specific. CT scanning can act as an alternative if MRI is not available. Patients who have CT scans should have a myelogram to assess the thecal sac both proximal and distal to the suspected level so that abnormalities simulating radiculopathies are not missed. If radiographic studies correlate with the patient history and physical findings, treatment outcomes are generally favorable. If the patient's symptomatology persists despite nonoperative measures, then operative intervention can be considered. Discrepancies between the radiographic findings and the patient's clinical picture require further investigation.

In the face of a static neurologic deficit, there is no evidence to suggest that surgical intervention offers any improvement in weakness or sensory deficit over continued nonoperative treatment. In the short term, however, most surgically treated patients with acute lumbar radiculopathy are pain free in a relatively shorter time. Limited surgical disc excision has a success rate of 90% in patients who have good correlation between history, physical examination, and diagnostic studies. Laminectomy is often the procedure of choice when surgery is indicated. If half or more of both or all of one facet joint is injured causing secondary instability, fusion across the segment may be necessary. In the absence of facet joint injury, fusion in conjunction with diskectomy is unnecessary.

Procedures such as chemonucleolysis, percutaneous diskectomy, and microsurgical diskectomy have been advocated to decrease hospitalization, minimize perineural scarring associated with laminectomy, and speed rehabilitation. Chemonucleolysis has the potential complications of anaphylactic shock and neurologic deficit secondary to acute transverse myelitis. It is contraindicated in patients who previously underwent operative treatment or have evidence of spinal stenosis. Transverse myelitis has been reported in patients undergoing chemonucleolysis using chymopapain and having concomitant diskography. Percutaneous diskectomy may not be used in patients with sequestered fragments or in the presence of spinal stenosis. With microdiskectomy, sequestered fragments can be missed, and the lateral recess may not be adequately decompressed.

Chronic Back Pain

Assessment of the patient with chronic lower-back pain with or without radicular pain is much more difficult than that of the patient with acute pain. Chronic back pain is usually defined as back pain present for at least 6 months and not responsive to nonoperative interventions. This is the most difficult group of patients facing the clinician. As with the patient with acute onset of back pain, the chronic pain must be characterized regarding onset location, radiation, pattern, effect of positions, associated weakness, bowel or bladder symptomatology, and effect of medications. Most important, however, a psychosocial history needs to be taken. How the pain affects the patient's lifestyle is important; any litigation or workman's compensation involved must be noted. Previous treatment modalities and their effects must be carefully documented because many patients with chronic lower-back pain previously had either surgical or nonoperative treatment. Each patient must have a complete and thorough physical examination, including neurologic examination. It is important to test the patient for nonorganic physical signs. Many patients have been seen by multiple physicians. Psychosocial evaluation of these patients is often necessary.

The establishment of special centers devoted to the assessment and treatment of patients with chronic back disorders use the multidisciplinary approach. These clinics employ physicians, surgeons, psychologists, social workers, occupational therapists, vocational rehabilitation counselors, and others to evaluate these difficult and often complex patients.

In the evaluation of a patient with chronic back pain, plain films are not often helpful. Degenerative changes may be seen on plain radiographs in a high percentage of normal patients. This is secondary to the normal aging process. Spina bifida occulta, Schmorl nodes, vacuum discs, mild scoliosis, transitional vertebrae (sacralization of L5 or lumbarization of S1, partially or completely) occur as frequently in asymptomatic patients as in patients with lower-back pain.

Plain radiographs may be helpful when the diagnosis of metabolic bone disease, tumor, fracture, or traumatic injury of the spine is suspected. As mentioned in the section on spondylolisthesis, degenerative spondylolisthesis may be evident on plain radiographs secondary to facet joint degeneration with subsequent subluxation. Subluxation may occur in a posterior direction (retrolisthesis). These conditions in some cases cause nerve root compression and radicular symptoms. Inflammatory disease may also be detected on plain radiographs. If the patient has any other joint complaints in association with spinal pain, radiographs of the sacroiliac joint may help to make the diagnosis of ankylosing spondylitis.

In the patient with chronic back pain, MRI is useful in determining the presence of recurrent disc herniation. MRI is especially helpful in patients who have had previous lumbar spine surgery and continue to have chronic back pain to differentiate recurrent disc herniation from dural scarring. Gadolinium-enhanced MRI increases diagnostic accuracy for identifying recurrent disc herniation. MRI has the ability to reveal early degenerative changes in the disc. The MRI is, however, overly sensitive in that about 40% of asymptomatic people older than 50 years of age have an abnormal signal on MRI. It is also difficult to visualize the lateral recesses with MRI.

Myelography, once the most common diagnostic tests in the evaluation of a patient with back pain, has limited use because of the increased diagnostic sensitivity and specificity of MRI and CT scanning. Myelography complications include seizures, arachnoiditis, and induction of nausea and vomiting. It is also inadequate for evaluating pathology in the lateral recesses. Myelography with water-soluble dye is most commonly used in conjunction with CT scanning to evaluate the thecal sac proximally and distally to the suspected level.

CT scanning is useful in revealing the anatomic parameters of spinal stenosis and lateral recess stenosis as well as foraminal stenosis. CT scanning is also useful in patients suspected of having vertebral osteomyelitis, tumors of the spine, and unrecognized trauma. In patients with chronic back pain and radiculopathy, electromyography may be useful in documenting a radiculopathy and in differentiating a neuropathy from a myelopathy. Motor nerve conduction velocity and sensory nerve conduction velocity testing may also help in differentiating neuropathies. Electrodiagnostic studies help differentiate patients with peripheral neuropathy or generalized or demyelinating disorders from patients with compressive neuropathy.

The various diagnostic evaluations must be used in conjunction with the patient's history and physical findings to help the physician arrive at a diagnosis and appropriate plan of management. Few patients with chronic back pain require surgical intervention. The most common conditions requiring back surgery in the adult are recurrent disc herniation, spinal stenosis, and segmental lumbar instability. Patients with chronic back pain without evidence of any of the above conditions should be treated nonoperatively. Patients who do not improve with symptomatic treatment (i.e. limited periods of rest, anti-inflammatory agents, exercise and muscle strengthening programs) should be evaluated in a comprehensive back pain clinic. These patients generally need the multidisciplinary approach to provide for lifestyle modification and rehabilitation. Otherwise, this limited group of patients continues to be a financial, social, and economic burden on society.

Spinal Stenosis

Spinal stenosis is a generic term that refers to any narrowing of the spinal canal or intervertebral foramen. Stenosis of the spinal canal occurs primarily, as in congenital spinal stenosis, or it can be a developmental condition, such as in achondroplasia. Most often, it occurs secondary to degenerative changes in the lumbar disc and facet joints, leading to compression of the dural sac by the ligamentum flavum disc or bony hypertrophy of the facet joints. Spinal stenosis can also occur after an infectious process or a traumatic injury to the spine. Men and women in the seventh and eighth decades of life are the group primarily affected by degenerative spinal stenosis.

The clinical presentation of spinal stenosis is variable. The most common symptom scenario is that of either unilateral or bilateral leg pain precipitated by walking and relieved by rest. Other patients complain of pain or paresthesia in the buttocks, thighs, or groin or in various distributions near the lower extremity.

Physical findings are variable. Tension signs are often absent. Neurologic deficits may or may not be present. Most patients, however, have aggravations of symptomatology by extension of the lumbar spine with relief of symptoms by forward flexion. Because of the claudication-type symptoms, the main differential diagnostic disorder is vascular claudication. All peripheral pulses should be checked; vascular consultation may be needed. Plain radiographs generally reveal degenerative changes of the spine consistent with aging changes. Patients may show evidence of degenerative spondylolisthesis or retrolisthesis. The diagnosis of spinal stenosis can best be made by myelography followed by CT scanning.

Nonoperative management may be tried, including anti-inflammatory agents and epidural steroid injections, but these methods are generally unsuccessful. The treatment of choice for spinal stenosis is often surgical decompression of the stenosed area. All bone and soft tissues compressing the thecal sac or roots should be removed, with care taken when possible to preserve the facet joints to avoid creating segmental instability and the need for a fusion. About 70 to 85% of patients have good results from this procedure.

Annotated Bibliography

Spinal Deformity

Dickson RA, Weinstein SL. Bracing (and screening): yes or no? J Bone Joint Surg Br 1999;81B:193.
This review article raises the key issues about nonsurgical scoliosis treatment.

Dobbs MB, Weinstein SL. Infantile and juvenile scoliosis. Orthop Clin North Am 1999;30:331.
This review article on early onset types of scoliosis outlines fundamental aspects of diagnosis and management of these entities.

Lenke LG, Bridwell KH, Blanke K et al. Radiographic results of arthrodesis with Cotrel-Dubousset instrumentation for the treatment of adolescent idiopathic scoliosis: a five- to ten-year follow-up study. J Bone Joint Surg 1998;80A:807.
The radiographic results of posterior spinal arthrodesis using Cotrel-Dubousset instrumentation in 76 patients with adolescent idiopathic scoliosis were evaluated. At an average of 6 years postoperatively, the fusion appeared to be solid in all patients.

Lonstein JE, Carlson M. Prognostication in idiopathic scoliosis. J Bone Joint Surg 1984;66A:1061.
The authors studied the risk of progression in 727 patients with idiopathic scoliosis. The risk of progression versus skeletal maturity, as well as other risk factors in progression, are discussed.

Morrissy RT. School screening for scoliosis. Spine 1999;24: 2584.
This is an in-depth analysis of the issues related to school screening for scoliosis, the pertinent aspects of screening programs, and the controversy surrounding them.

Nachemson AL, Peterson LE. Effectiveness of treatment with a brace in girls who have adolescent idiopathic scoliosis: a prospective controlled study based on data from the brace study of the Scoliosis Research Society. J Bone Joint Surg 1995;77A:815.
In a prospective study, 286 girls with adolescent idiopathic scoliosis, a thoracic/thoracolumbar curve of 25 to 35°, and a mean age of 12.6 years were followed. Brace treatment was successful in 74%; observation only in 34%; and electrical stimulation in 33%.

Noonan KJ, Weinstein SL, Jacobson WC et al. Use of the Milwaukee brace for progressive idiopathic scoliosis. J Bone Joint Surg 1996;78A:557.
Immature patients with idiopathic scoliosis who were treated with a Milwaukee brace were evaluated. This study raises questions about whether the natural history of progressive idiopathic scoliosis is truly altered by use of the Milwaukee brace.

Tolo VT, Gillespie R. The characteristics of juvenile idiopathic scoliosis and results of its treatment. J Bone Joint Surg 1978;60B:181.
This is a review article of 59 patients with juvenile idiopathic scoliosis. The prognostic value of the rib-vertebral angle is discussed.

U.S. Preventive Services Task Force. Screening for Idiopathic Scoliosis in Adolescents: Recommendation Statement. June 2004. Agency for Healthcare Research and Quality, Rockville, MD. http://www.ahrq.gov/clinic/3rduspstf/scoliosis/scoliors.htm

Weinstein SL, ed. The Pediatric Spine. 2nd Ed. Philadelphia: Lippincott Williams & Wilkins, 2001.
Classic reference textbook on all pediatric spine conditions; detailed bibliography included and surgical techniques are discussed.

Weinstein SL, ed. Pediatric Spine Surgery. 2nd Ed. Philadelphia: Lippincott Williams & Wilkins, 2001.
Second part of classic reference textbook that concentrates on surgical treatment of spinal disorders.

Weinstein SL, Dolan LA, Spratt KF et al. Health and function of patients with untreated idiopathic scoliosis: a 50-year natural history study. JAMA 2003;289:559.
Fifty-one year long-term follow up of 117 patients with untreated adolescent idiopathic scoliosis evaluating outcomes related to health and function. They were compared with 62 age- and sex-matched volunteers. The main outcome measures were mortality, back pain, pulmonary symptoms, general function, depression, and body image. The article concluded that untreated adults with adolescent idiopathic scoliosis are productive and functional at a high level at 50-year follow-up. Untreated adolescent idiopathic scoliosis causes little physical impairment other than back pain and cosmetic concerns.

Weinstein SL, Ponseti IV. Curve progression in idiopathic scoliosis. J Bone Joint Surg 1983;65A:447.
The authors discuss the factors in curve progression after skeletal maturity in a group of 102 untreated patients followed for an average of 40 years.

Weinstein SL, Zavala DC, Ponseti IV. Idiopathic scoliosis: long-term follow-up and prognosis in untreated patients. J Bone Joint Surg 1981;63A:702.
The authors followed 194 patients with untreated adolescent idiopathic scoliosis for an average of 39.3 years. The authors studied the effects on pulmonary function, psychological effects, mortality, morbidity, and backache in this large, untreated population.

Congenital Spinal Deformity

McMaster MJ, David CV. Hemivertebra as a cause of scoliosis: a study of 104 patients. J Bone Joint Surg 1986;68B:588.
The authors reviewed the natural history of 154 hemivertebrae in 104 patients. The authors determined the various risk factors, including the type of hemivertebrae, location, age of the patient, and number of hemivertebrae as well as their relation to each other.

McMaster MJ. Congenital scoliosis caused by unilateral failure of vertebral segmentation with contralateral hemivertebrae. Spine 1998;23:998.
This article examines the behavior of congenital scoliosis caused by this particular anomaly. The combination of growth on one side of the spine and complete absence of longitudinal growth on the opposite side inevitably results in severe deformity. The author also reports the presence of intraspinal and neurologic anomalies, as well as anomalies in other organ systems.

McMaster MJ, Ohtsuka K. The natural history of congenital scoliosis: a study of 251 patients. J Bone Joint Surg 1982;64A:1128.
The authors reviewed the natural history of 251 patient with congenital scoliosis. Abnormalities are classified in regard to prognosis for each pattern and curve location.

McMaster MJ, Singh H. Natural history of congenital kyphosis and kyphoscoliosis: a study of one hundred and twelve patients. J Bone Joint Surg 1999;81A:1367.
This study examines congenital vertebral anomalies that result in deformity in the sagittal plane. The authors expand the existing classification system and emphasize that this pattern of congenital vertebral malformation has the highest risk of neurologic defect, including paraplegia.

Winter RB, Moe JH, Lonstein JE. The surgical treatment of congenital kyphosis: a review of 94 patients 5 years or older, with 2 years or more follow-up of 77 patients. Spine 1985;10:224.
The authors reported on a 7-year average follow-up of 94 patients with congenital kyphosis. The results of posterior fusion alone versus combined anterior and posterior fusion are presented.

Winter RB, Moe JH, Lonstein JE. Posterior spinal arthrodesis for congenital scoliosis: an analysis of the cases of 290 patients, 5 to 19 years old. J Bone Joint Surg 1984;66A:1188.
This article reports on a 6-year average follow-up of 290 patients between 5 and 19 years of age who were treated by posterior spinal arthrodesis with or without Harrington instrumentation. The authors report that the most common problem was bending of the fusion mass.

Back Pain in Children

Burton AK, Clarke RD, McClune TD et al. The natural history of low back pain in adolescents. Spine 1996;21:2323.
Back pain occurs in more than half of children by age of 15 years, but an orthopaedic evaluation is rarely sought.

Fredrickson BE, Baker D, McHolick WJ et al. The natural history of spondylolysis and spondylolisthesis. J Bone Joint Surg 1984;66A:699.
This article describes a prospective study of 500 unselected first-grade children and their families, discussing the incidence, relation of listhesis to lysis, and cause of disease.

Freeman BL III, Donati NL. Spinal arthrodesis for severe spondylolisthesis in children and adolescents. J Bone Joint Surg 1989;71A:594.
The authors report on a 12-year follow-up of 12 patients with grade III or IV (over 50%) spondylolisthesis. The article demonstrated that posterior in situ arthrodesis is effective, reliable, and safe for treatment of severe spondylolisthesis.

Ginsburg GM, Bassett GS. Back pain in children and adolescents: evaluation and differential diagnosis. JAAOS 1997;5:67.
Back pain in children and adolescents usually has a recognizable organic origin. The most common entities seen are spondylolysis, spondylolisthesis, Scheuermann's kyphosis, disc herniations, infections, and tumors. Early recognition and treatment can provide patients the best chance at relief of symptoms and eradication of the underlying disease process.

Harris IE, Weinstein SL. Long-term follow-up of patients with grade-III and IV spondylolisthesis: treatment with and without posterior fusion. J Bone Joint Surg 1987;69A:960.
This article compares an 18-year follow-up of 11 patients with grade-III and IV spondylolisthesis treated nonoperatively with a 24-year follow-up of 21 surgically treated patients. The surgical group was less symptomatic and less restricted in their activities than the nonsurgical group. In situ fusion gave good functional long-term results in grade-III and IV spondylolisthesis.

Hensinger RN. Current concepts review: spondylolysis and spondylolisthesis in children and adolescents. J Bone Joint Surg 1989;71A:1098.
This superb review article covers all aspects of the topic and has an extensive bibliography.

King HA. Evaluating the child with back pain. Pediatr Clin North Am 1986;33:1489.
This review article covers the history, physical examination, radiographic examination, and differential diagnosis of the child presenting with the chief complaint of back pain.

Lowe TG. Scheuermann's disease and postural round back. J Bone Joint Surg 1990;72A:940.
This is an excellent review article on the topic of Scheuermann's disease with a complete bibliography.

Morita T, Ikata T, Katoh S et al. Lumbar spondylolysis in children and adolescents. J Bone Joint Surg 1995;77B:620.
These authors investigated 185 adolescents younger than age 19 years with spondylolysis. The authors suggest that spondylolysis is caused by repetitive microtrauma during growth and can be successfully treated nonsurgically if treatment is started in the early stage.

Muschik M, Hahnel H, Robinson PN et al. Competitive sports and the progression of spondylolisthesis. J Pediatr Orthop 1996;16:364.
The authors investigated the effects of several yeas of competitive sports training on children and adolescents with spondylolisthesis. The authors conclude that there is no justification for generally advising children and adolescents with limited spondylolytic spondylolisthesis not to take part in competitive sports.

Murray PM, Weinstein SL, Spratt KF. Natural history and long term follow-up of Scheuermann kyphosis. J Bone Joint Surg 1993;75A:236.
The authors report on a 31-year follow-up of 81 patients with Scheuermann's kyphosis. Pulmonary function, pain, work attendance, and disability are evaluated.

Peek RD, Wiltse L, Reynolds JB et al. In situ arthrodesis without decompression for grade-III or IV isthmic spondylolisthesis in adults who have severe sciatica. J Bone Joint Surg 1989;71A:62.
The authors report on in situ fusions in 8 patients who had back pain and sciatica caused by grade-III or IV isthmic spondylolisthesis of the lumbar vertebrae and the sacrum. All patients achieved a solid fusion with excellent relief of back pain and sciatica at 5.5 year average follow-up.

Pizzutillo PD, Hummer CD III. Nonoperative treatment for painful adolescent spondylolysis or spondylolisthesis. J Pediatr Orthop 1989;9:538.
The authors demonstrate symptomatic relief of pain in two-thirds of patients with spondylolysis and grade-I and II spondylolisthesis treated nonoperatively. Adolescents with symptomatic grade-III and IV spondylolisthesis are appropriately treated surgically.

Ramirez N, Johnston CE, Browne RH. The prevalence of back pain in children who have idiopathic scoliosis. J Bone Joint Surg 1997;79A:364.
Although back pain was noted in 32% of 2,442 patients with presumed idiopathic scoliosis, only 9% of the patients with pain had an underlying pathologic condition. If the neurologic examination was normal and plain radiographs did not reveal lesions, MRI and bone scans were not helpful.

Sachs B, Bradford D, Winter R et al. Scheuermann kyphosis: follow-up of Milwaukee brace treatment. J Bone Joint Surg 1987;69A:50.
This article describes the long-term follow-up of 120 patients treated for Scheuermann kyphosis with a Milwaukee brace, with a minimum follow-up of 5 years after treatment. The authors demonstrate that the Milwaukee brace is an effective method of treating patients with Scheuermann kyphosis.

Saraste H. Long-term clinical and radiological follow-up of spondylolysis and spondylolisthesis. J Pediatr Orthop 1987;7:631.
The author reports on a long-term (mean, 29 years) clinical and radiographic follow-up of 255 patients with spondylolisthesis and spondylolysis. Half of these patients were treated for lower-back symptoms.

Back Pain in Adults

Allan D, Wadell G. An historical perspective on low back pain and disability. Acta Orthop Scand Suppl 1989;234:1.
This is a superb monograph that reviews the history of lower-back pain and sciatica for the past 3,500 years. The authors also discuss the problem of chronic disability screening.

Booth KC, Bridwell KH, Eisenberg BA et al. Minimum 5-year results of degenerative spondylolisthesis treated with decompression and instrumented posterior fusion. Spine 1999;24:1721.
This study evaluated outcome and complication rate in 49 patients who had undergone no prior surgery for degenerative spondylolisthesis. Eighty-three percent reported satisfaction with the procedure. Radiographic transition syndromes were common (12 patients) with 5 of 12 patients being symptomatic. Major complications (2%), implant failures (2%), and symptomatic pseudoarthrosis (0) were low.

Deyo RA, Phillips WR. Low back pain: a primary care challenge. Spine 1996;21:2826.
Most patients come to the physician with uncomplicated low back pain. Identifying the rare patient with significant pathology is challenging. Assessment must be rapid with limited extensive investigation, a rational pragmatic approach is outlined.

Eismont FJ, Currier B. Current concepts review: surgical management of lumbar intervertebral-disc disease. J Bone Joint Surg 1989;71A:1266.
This is an excellent review article on management of the lumbar spine intervertebral-disc disease. The authors discuss treatment by various modalities and the status of imaging techniques.

Frymoyer JW, Newberg A, Pope MH et al. Spine radiographs in patients with low-back pain: an epidemiologic study in men. J Bone Joint Surg 1984;66A:1048.
The authors demonstrate that degenerative changes of the lumbar spine increase with age. They report that congenital and developmental changes and aging changes of the spine occur in frequencies that do not support the use of radiographs in back pain as a predictive tool for individual cases.

Gordon SL, Weinstein JN. A review of basic science issues in low back pain. Phys Med Rehabil Clin North Am 1998;9:323.
A comprehensive, well-referenced review of the current state of knowledge of the science of back pain and future directions of research is presented.

Katz JN, Stucki G, Lipson SJ et al. Predictors of surgical outcome in degenerative lumbar spinal stenosis. Spine 1999;24:2229.
This prospective study evaluated predictors of outcome, including sociodemographic factors, physical examination, radiographic, psychological, social, and clinical history variables. The patients' assessments of their own health and co-morbidity are the most important outcome predictors of surgery for spinal stenosis.

Kelsey JL, White AA III. Epidemiology and impact of low back pain. Spine 1980;5:133.
This article reports that back pain is the most common cause of disability for people under 45 years of age. A herniated disc is the most common problem in the age group of 30 to 39 years and is associated more with sedentary occupations than active occupations. Degenerative changes seen on spinal radiographs are more closely linked to the natural aging process.

Loupasis GA, Stamos K, Katonis PG et al. Seven- to 20-year outcome of lumbar discectomy. Spine 1999;24:2313.
The long-term result of standard lumbar diskectomy is not very satisfying. More than one-third of the patients had unsatisfactory results and more than one-fourth complained of significant residual pain. Heavy manual work, particularly agricultural work, and low educational level were negative predictors of a good outcome.

Weber H. Lumbar disc herniation: a controlled, prospective study with 10 years of observations. Spine 1983;8:131.
In this study, between 85 and 90% of surgically treated and non-surgically treated patients with disc hernias were asymptomatic after 4 years. Only 2% of subjects in both groups were symptomatic after 10 years. After 1 year, the surgical group had less pain, but after 4 years there was no statistically significant difference in relief of symptoms between the two groups.

Weinstein JN, Wiesel SW. The Lumbar Spine. Philadelphia: WB Saunders, 1990.
This textbook, from the International Society for the Study of the Lumbar Spine, covers all aspects of adult lumbar spine disease in great detail and has a superb bibliography.

17

Peter Devane
Geoffrey Horne

The Adult Hip

Assessment and treatment of adult patients with hip problems, whether pain, deformity, gait disturbance, or radiological abnormality in the absence of clinical symptoms and signs, has altered significantly in the last 50 years. Before that time, treatment of most hip conditions arose as a sequel of infection leading to stiffness, or posttraumatic deformity. Options for treating arthritic conditions were limited. The advent of total hip joint arthroplasty has dramatically increased treatment options and represents the greatest orthopaedic advance of this century. Indications for total hip arthroplasty (THA) are continually widening to include a multitude of other conditions in progressively younger patients. This chapter gives a clinically oriented view of the assessment and treatment of adult hip conditions. Emphasis has been placed not only on the practicalities of a particular surgical procedure but its indications. It commences with a review of relevant anatomy and embryology.

APPLIED SURGICAL ANATOMY

Surface Anatomy

Accurate location of landmarks around the hip joint aids greatly in the proper placement of skin incisions during hip surgery. Identifiable landmarks include the anterosuperior spine, crest of ilium, greater trochanter, and shaft of femur. The tip of the greater trochanter is a reliable marker to the center of the femoral head and acetabulum (Figure 17-1). Soft tissue identifiable beneath the skin includes the tensor fascia lata muscle, which originates from the external lip of the iliac crest below the anterior iliac spine and inserts into the iliotibial tract, and the gluteus maximus, which originates from the posterior half of the ilium behind the posterior gluteal line and inserts three-quarters of its fibers into the iliotibial tract and one-quarter into the posterior shaft of the femur below the greater trochanter. These two muscles are often termed the deltoid of the hip joint, and most surgical approaches to the hip joint split them in some way.

Gluteal Muscles

Gluteus medius and gluteus minimus originate in different planes from the side of the pelvis, with medius lying superficial to minimus. What is not well illustrated in anatomy drawings is that their tendons converge into a single layer that is inserted into the greater trochanter. The original Hardinge approach for total hip arthroplasty split these two muscles in one layer, but separate identification of each and suturing of the split in gluteus minimus

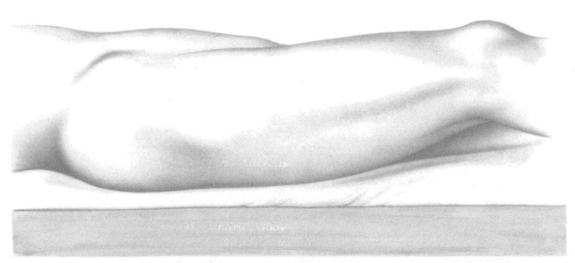

FIGURE 17-1. Surface anatomy of the hip and thigh as patient lies on operating table. Important landmarks include anteroposterior spine, crest of ilium, greater trochanter, and iliotibial track. There is a prominent tensor fascia lata, and a depression between gluteus medius and the tensor fascia lata muscle. These surface landmarks assist in proper placement of skin incisions at the time of surgery. (Eftekhar NS. Total Hip Arthroplasty, vol 1. St. Louis:Mosby-Year Book 1993)

as a separate repair will reduce potential dead space, which may decrease the subsequent risk of postoperative dislocation. Care should be taken during the lateral approach to protect the superior gluteal nerve that lies between gluteus medius and minimus. Dissection should not be taken beyond 5 cm from the tip of the greater trochanter to avoid damage to this structure. A small bursa often lies under the most anterior fibers of gluteus medius tendon. This bursa can often be confused with hip capsule during the direct lateral surgical approach. During this exposure, a reliable indicator of the outer surface of hip capsule is the insertion of the anterior fibers of vastus intermedius. The undersurface of the gluteus minimus may be adherent to the hip capsule in osteoarthritis and must be dissected free from it prior to a capsulectomy being performed.

Femoral Anatomy

The greater trochanter may have an altered shape due to underlying disease or previous surgery, and care should be taken to avoid its fracture. The femoral neck may not be easily identified from the femoral head if there is extensive osteophyte formation. During THA, orientation of the femoral neck osteotomy in the correct anteversion should always be assessed after hip dislocation by reference to the shaft of the femur with the knee flexed at 90°, because there is a wide variation in anteversion of the femoral neck. If the femoral neck osteotomy is made with reference to femoral neck anteversion, an inaccurate cut may result, and subsequent malpositioning of the prosthesis may occur.

Acetabular Anatomy

The acetabulum is made up of three walls and a floor to form a spherical receptacle for the femoral head. The ischium, which makes up the posterior column, is the most substantial wall. The ilium contributes to the superior wall or dome, and a thin contribution from the pubis completes the anterior column. Medially, the floor of the acetabulum receives contributions from all three bones. Screws placed through cementless acetabular cups to aid fixation should be placed between the 10 and 2 o'clock positions when the acetabulum is viewed from the side, to avoid damage to the internal iliac vessels anteriorly, and the sciatic nerve posteriorly. Revision surgery of the acetabulum often involves bony defects in one or more of the columns, putting neurovascular structures even more at risk.

A medial defect will often be covered by a pseudomembrane, which overlies the iliacus muscle. Directly medial to this lies the obturator nerve and artery, the ureter, and the bladder. Great care should be taken when preparing the acetabulum to avoid damage to any of these structures, which may have catastrophic consequences (Figure 17-2).

EMBRYOLOGY

The skeleton develops from condensed mesenchyme (embryonic connective tissue), which undergoes chondrification to form hyaline cartilage models of the bones. The limb buds appear toward the end of the fourth week as slight elevations of the venterolateral body wall. The apical ectodermal ridge, a thickening of ectoderm at the distal end of the limb bud, exerts an inductive influence on the mesenchyme in the limb buds that promotes growth and development of the limbs. Nerves grow into the limb buds during the fifth week (Figure 17-3). The upper and lower limbs rotate in opposite directions and to different degrees.

Between 24 and 36 weeks after fertilization—a critical period of limb development, formation of synovial mesenchyme occurs as the synovium differentiates and is responsible for the development of the synovial lining, the joint capsule, and the intracapsular ligaments of the future hip joint. Cavitation begins in the central part of these areas, with small multiple spaces that eventually coalesce to form the joint cavity. At about the same time, a synovial membrane develops that undergoes vascular invasion with accompanying macrophages and other cell types. This sequence of differentiation suggests that development of congenital hip dislocation must occur after the hip joint has formed.

At birth, the acetabulum has formed from the ilium, ischium, and pubis as they join at the triradiate cartilage. The proximal femur consists of the femoral head and neck and the greater and lesser trochanters. Secondary ossification centers form in the femoral head and greater trochanter. The triradiate cartilage fuses in boys on average at 15 years of age and in girls on average at 13 years of age. The femoral head growth plate fuses on average at 17 years of age in boys and at 14 years of age in girls. The greater trochanteric physis fuses on average at 16 years of age in boys and at 14 years of age in girls.

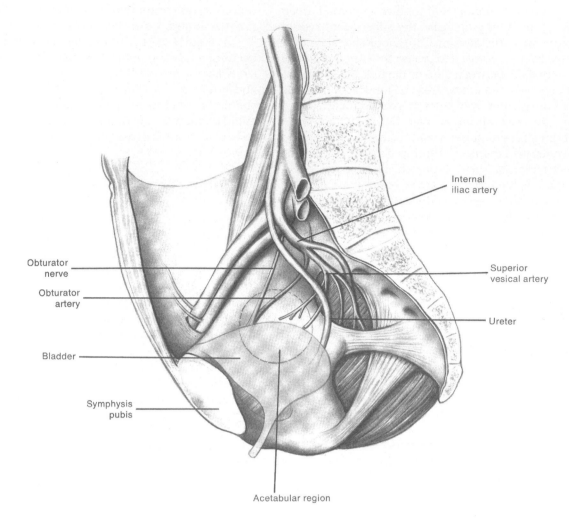

FIGURE 17-2. Site of origin of gluteal muscles on the ilium is indicated. Relationship of the sciatic nerve to the acetabulum, acetabular branch of the obturator artery, femoral artery and vein, femoral nerve, and iliopsoas in relation to the acetabulum should be noted. The acetabular floor is marked by a horseshoe articulating zone and acetabular fossa. The ligamentum teres and its synovial folds are supplied by the acetabular branch of the obturator artery. (Eftekhar NS. Total Hip Arthroplasty, vol 1. St. Louis: Mosby-Year Book, 1993)

SURGICAL APPROACHES TO THE HIP

The surgical approach to the hip depends on the condition being treated, the surgeon's experience, and underlying pathology. Surgeons should have a sound working knowledge of the appropriate anatomy and be aware of the pitfalls of each approach when applied to specific patients. There are four commonly used approaches to the hip: the anterior or Smith-Peterson; the anterolateral or Watson-Jones; the direct lateral or Hardinge; and the posterior or Southern approach. There are many descriptions of these approaches, most with a variation to meet a certain need. The principles, however, are the same.

Anterior (Smith-Peterson) Approach

This approach is commonly used to access the hip in cases of suspected septic arthritis. The patient is placed supine on the operating table. The skin incision runs along the anterior aspect of the iliac crest, and as the anterior-superior iliac spine is

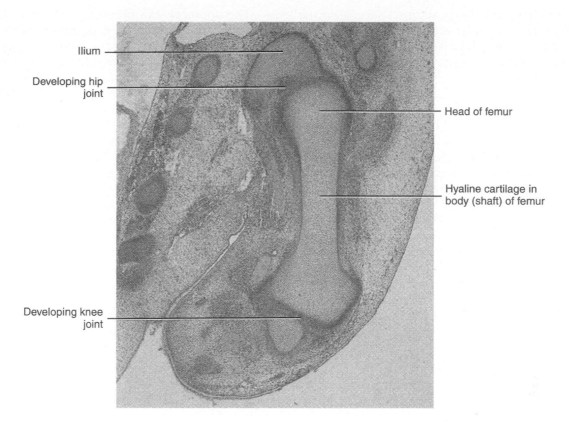

FIGURE 17-3. Longitudinal section of the lower limb of an embryo at about 48 days. Chondrofication has begun in the bone and occurs in a proximodistal sequence. (Moore KL, Persaud TV, Shiota K. Color Atlas of Clinical Embryology, 2nd Ed. Philadelphia:W. B. Saunders, 2000)

reached, extends distally for approximately 10 to 15 cm. The incision extends through the skin and subcutaneous tissue to the tensor fascia lata muscle. Care is taken to identify and protect the lateral cutaneous nerve of the thigh as it penetrates the fascia just below and medial to the anterior superior iliac spine. The medial edge of tensor fascia lata is easily seen laterally and the fascia is incised just medial to this edge. The interval between tensor fascia lata and sartorious is developed directly down to the tendinous portion of the rectus femoris muscle.

The reflected head of rectus femoris may need to be elevated off the edge of the pelvis to allow visualization of the hip joint capsule. The hip capsule can then be incised over the front of the femoral neck. This approach allows drainage of the hip in cases of suspected infection. If a wider exposure is required, then the tensor fascia lata muscle, and a varying amount of gluteus medius muscle, can be reflected off the outer aspect of the ilium, and the interval between tensor fascia lata and sartorious

developed further distally. This distal extension often results in disruption of the lateral cutaneous nerve of the thigh and extensive dissection proximally may be followed by the development of heterotopic ossification in the gluteus medius.

Anterolateral (Watson-Jones) Approach

This approach is used for hemiarthroplasty and total hip arthroplasty. The approach's major disadvantage is the potential for damage to the anterior edge of gluteus medius while exposing the femoral shaft. It should be used with caution in obese patients, as access to the femur is very restricted. Also, as the approach places considerable torsional stress on the femur, it should be used with caution in patients with osteoporosis or other diseases likely to weaken the femur. This approach does have the advantage of minimal muscle disruption if performed well and maximum stability of the joint postoperatively.

The patient may be positioned supine on the operating table, with the buttock elevated on a bolster, or they may be placed in the lateral position. The skin incision begins at the iliac crest 5 cm posterior to the anterior superior iliac spine, runs obliquely down to the tip of the greater trochanter, and extends posteriorly from the tip for 3 cm. It then curves anteriorly and distally for a further 10 to 15 cm. The incision is deepened to the fascia lata, and the anterior edge of gluteus medius is identified beneath the fascia. The fascia is incised longitudinally just distal to the anterior edge of gluteus medius, and over the greater trochanter follows the skin incision. This incision allows the interval between tensor fascia lata muscle and gluteus medius to be developed. Be aware that the terminal branch of the superior gluteal nerve crosses this interval in its proximal third and is susceptible to injury in this area. Clear the fibro-fatty tissue off the front of the hip joint capsule and identify the reflected head of rectus femoris crossing the capsule proximally. Place a Holman retractor around the medial side of the capsule, one around the lateral side, and one under the reflected head of rectus femoris.

The whole of the anterior capsule should now be clearly visible. The capsule can be opened and the medial and lateral Holman retractors placed around the neck of the femur within the joint. The femoral neck can be transected and the head removed. Access to the acetabulum is excellent, with the femur retracted posteriorly by a Holman retractor placed immediately behind the acetabulum. Access to the femoral canal is obtained by adduction and external rotation of the leg, and a Holman retractor placed deep to the tip of the greater trochanter. If the lower end of gluteus medius is attached more distally on the anterior aspect of the greater trochanter, it may need to be detached to improve access to the proximal femur.

Direct Lateral (Hardinge) Approach

The direct lateral approach allows excellent access to the acetabulum and proximal femur. It has the potential disadvantage that it may weaken the abductors with a subsequent limp, and it may not be extensile enough to allow surgeons complete visualization of the anterior and posterior acetabular columns during revision hip surgery. Its major advantage is that dislocation following total hip replacement is uncommon.

The approach can be performed with the patient supine or in the lateral decubitus position. If the lateral decubitus position is used, care should be taken that the pelvis is correctly aligned to ensure that component positioning is not compromised. The skin incision begins in the midlateral line approximately 6 cm proximal to the tip of the greater trochanter and runs distally for 10 cm. The incision is deepened to the fascia lata, which is incised along the line of the skin incision. A large self-retaining retractor is placed under the fascia lata anteriorly and posteriorly, exposing the gluteus medius proximally and vastus lateralis distally.

The anterior edge of gluteus medius forms a consistent landmark where it inserts into the most distal aspect of the greater trochanter. The tip of the greater trochanter is palpated, and beginning proximally the gluteus medius is split along the line of its fibers for approximately 3 to 4 cm, toward the anterior superior iliac spine. This incision is then curved distally over the anterior third of the greater trochanter, and beyond the trochanter into the vastus lateralis muscle (Figure 17-4). Avoid splitting the gluteus medius more than 5 cm proximal to the tip of the greater trochanter to avoid damage to the superior gluteal nerve. A small amount of sharp dissection (cutting diathermy) proximal to the greater trochanter allows the gluteus muscle to be split along the line of its fibers. Blunt dissection can be used to sweep the fat deep to gluteus medius superiorly, thus protecting the superior gluteal neurovascular bundle. The exposed gluteus minimus muscle can then be split along the same line, giving access to hip capsule. Dissection superiorly up this line allows placement of a Holman retractor deep to the reflected head of rectus femoris, thus exposing the capsule up to the anterior acetabular edge. Hip capsule is most easily identified at the inferior extent of the greater trochanter, where sharp dissection combined with external rotation of the leg will eventually expose muscle fibers that are the capsular insertion of vastus intermedius. The bursa under gluteus medius is often mistaken for hip capsule and is a much less reliable indicator.

A complete capsular exposure, extending medially onto the acetabular margin, proximally under the free edge of the previously split gluteus minimus tendon (which is often adherent to, and requires dissection off, the superior hip capsule), and distally under the vastus intermedius muscle (often a vascular area), allows good visualization of the femoral neck and head. The remainder of the exposure is similar to the anterolateral approach. The lateral approach may be

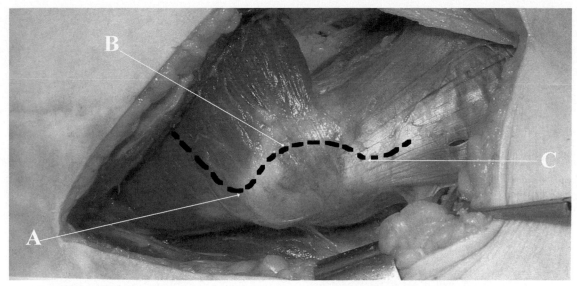

FIGURE 17-4. Modification of the Hardinge direct lateral approach to the right hip. The fascia lata has been split along the line of the skin incision, allowing good exposure of the lateral deeper structures. **(A)** Tip of greater trochanter forms the initial landmark. **(B)** Incision is curved over anterior third of greater trochanter approximately 1 mm posterior to musculotendinous junction of gluteus minimus muscle. **(C)** Incision is extended for 2 to 4 cm into vastus lateralis muscle. Note the well-defined anterior edge of gluteus medius muscle inserting into the most distal extent of the greater trochanter.

combined with trochanteric osteotomy, which allows wide exposure of the acetabulum and improves access to the proximal femur. Many techniques of osteotomy have been described, and when using this technique surgeons should be aware that nonunion of the greater trochanter can be a particular problem in total hip replacement.

Posterior Approach

The posterior approach gives excellent exposure of the proximal femur and acetabulum, is extensile for revision surgery and involves minimal muscle disruption. However, when used for hemiarthroplasty or total hip replacement, dislocation is more common. Careful attention to closure of the deep layers of the incision is essential to minimize this risk.

The patient is placed in the lateral decubitus position, with the pelvis appropriately positioned for correct orientation of the components. The incision begins 3 cm distal to the tip of the greater trochanter and is centered over it. The incision passes posteriorly and proximally at 45° to the long axis of the femur for 8 to 10 cm. The incision is deepened to the fascia lata, and beginning distally the fascia is incised over the trochanter and then proximally over gluteus maximus along the line of the skin incision. The gluteus maximus muscle is split along the line of its fibers. A large self-retaining retractor retracts the gluteus maximus. The leg should then be internally rotated 20° so as to better expose the fatty layer over the external rotators. This fat is swept posteriorly off the short rotators by blunt dissection, allowing visualization of the muscles and the sciatic nerve. The tendon of piriformis is identified and an incision is made along the proximal edge of piriformis distally, to the posterior margin of the greater trochanter. It then turns distally along the posterior margin of the greater trochanter as far as the proximal margin of quadratus femoris. This incision extends through the capsule and thus forms an L-shaped flap that is retracted to protect the sciatic nerve (Figure 17-5). The hip can then be dislocated. Proximal and distal extension of the exposure is possible to improve access to the acetabulum and femur as necessary. The relatively high rate of postoperative dislocation (when compared to other recognized surgical approaches for THA) has been dramatically improved by repair of the external rotators (Figure 17-6).

EXAMINATION OF THE HIP

Patients presenting with hip pain may have a disease affecting other parts of the body, and doctors taking a history and examining patients whose main

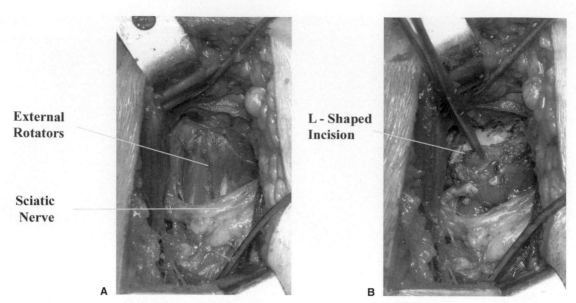

FIGURE 17-5. (A) Posterior approach to the hip joint for THA. Gluteus maximus has been split along the line of its fibers, exposing piriformis and the external rotators. **(B)** An L-shaped incision in the external rotators allows good exposure of the hip joint while the soft tissue flap is reflected posteriorly to protect the sciatic nerve.

complaint is "hip" pain must not forget to examine other regions to exclude pathology in those areas. Disorders of the spine and abdomen often present with pain in the hip or proximal thigh and a thorough assessment of these areas is essential if diagnostic errors are to be avoided.

Examination begins with an assessment of gait. Gait abnormalities such as a short leg, Trendelenburg, or antalgic should be easily identified. More complex patterns such as those seen in patients with ankylosed hips or hips that have had multiple surgical procedures can be difficult to analyze, but each abnormality identified should be documented. An assessment of leg length is performed by assessing the level of the iliac crests with the patient standing evenly on both feet with the knees straight. During

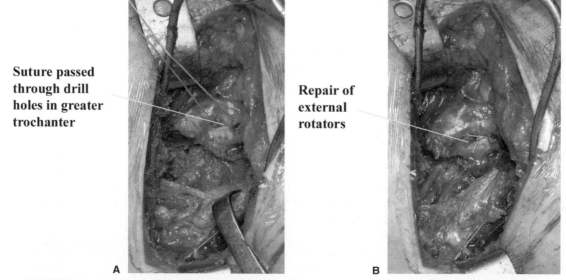

FIGURE 17-6. (A) At the end of a THA procedure, a drill hole is passed through the greater trochanter. **(B)** Strong suture material (5 Ticron) is used to repair the defect in the external rotator (which in the past has led to posterior dislocation).

this maneuver, a Trendelenburg sign is sought. The range of spinal movement should be recorded, with particular attention to lateral flexion, as this can be adversely influenced by long-standing hip disease or leg length inequality. Patients with long-standing hip disease may also have a marked increase in lumbar lordosis.

With the patient supine, the real and apparent leg length should be assessed. Particular care is necessary in patients who have had surgery that might influence pelvic geometry, and in these cases leg length assessment using computerized tomography scanning may be appropriate. If the patient has long-standing hip disease such as dysplasia or frank dislocation, there may be secondary changes in the lumbar spine. If this is suspected leg lengths should be equalized using blocks and then the range of lumbar spine movement, particularly lateral flexion, noted. The hip and pelvis are checked for surgical scars and if any are present these should be noted as they may influence future surgery and also may be an indicator of underlying muscle damage that will influence the outcome of further surgery. Muscle wasting around the hip is assessed. This is often seen in the quadriceps and less commonly the buttock. Palpation of the hip area for local tenderness can be helpful in identifying disorders such as gluteus medius tendinosis, but as the hip itself is a deep joint, palpation is of limited value.

Assessment of range of movement of the hip is best carried out passively rather than actively. The presence of a fixed flexion deformity is tested with the Thomas test. The maximum flexion, abduction, and adduction should be measured taking care to immobilize the pelvis to prevent pelvic motion giving a false sense of motion at the hip. Rotation of the hip should be assessed with the patient prone and supine. Assessment with the patient prone allows more accurate measurement of rotation in the position of function. In young patients an impingement test, done by flexing the hip to 90° and then adducting and internally rotating the leg, may illicit pain if there is labral pathology.

A brief neurological examination of the lower extremity is performed to exclude disorders such as meralgia paresthetica that may masquerade as hip disease. The remaining joints of the affected extremity should be assessed, checking for any fixed or paralytic deformity that may influence the outcome of any proposed hip surgery. Where appropriate, the contralateral leg and the upper extremities should be assessed. This is particularly important in patients with multijoint disease such as rheumatoid arthritis. The vascular supply of the affected leg should also be assessed. Functional assessment of the hip joint and the patient as a whole may be appropriate in patients who have had multiple surgical procedures or who have polyarthritis.

CLINICAL PRESENTATION OF HIP PATHOLOGY

Disorders of the hip most often present with pain and or stiffness. However, the pattern of symptoms varies with the pathology and the pathology varies with age. Thus, an elderly patient most often presents with primary or secondary osteoarthritis whereas a young patient may have acetabular dysplasia or labral pathology. Thus, it is logical to divide patients presenting with hip symptoms into three age bands although, of course, there may be considerable overlap.

The Young Adult

Hip dysplasia, labral pathology, pigmented villonodular synovitis, and loose bodies may present in the young adult. Dysplastic hips are associated with intermittent postexercise pain, which becomes more frequent with time. The pain is usually felt in the groin or proximal thigh, but as with all patients with hip pain it may be felt in the knee and occasionally even further down the leg. Stiffness is rarely an early complaint, but as the condition progresses, reduction in abduction and rotation is common.

The patient may have noted a limp. Labral pathology causes pain and this may be positional, such that there is pain associated with extreme flexion and adduction but not with other positions. The patient may have a feeling of a "catch" in the hip with certain movements. There is often a history of minor trauma preceding the onset of pain. Loose bodies cause pain and occasional "catching" in the hip, although frank locking of the hip is unusual.

Middle Age

At this age, dysplasia of the hip may have developed into early osteoarthritis. Pain, which may have been a relatively mild problem in early adulthood, is now a much greater problem. Stiffness and the development of a leg length discrepancy are not uncommon, particularly if the acetabular dysplasia is severe. Other causes of secondary osteoarthritis, such as gout and pseudogout may also present at this age. Ankylosing spondylitis and avascular necrosis of the femoral head commonly present with hip pain in middle age. In the case of the former there may be a history of back stiffness but this is not always the case. Patients with avascular necrosis may have some identifiable risk factors such as alcohol abuse or corticosteroid ingestion but in many cases no risk factors are evident. Transient osteoporosis of the femoral head is a recently recognized condition whose onset is sudden, with rapidly developing pain and apparently normal radiographs. The diagnosis can only be confirmed on MRI.

The Elderly

Primary and secondary osteoarthritis are common in the aging population. Hip, thigh, and knee pain are common and stiffness influences simple activities such as cutting toenails and putting on underwear. The history and physical findings are usually diagnostic, but other diseases such as spinal stenosis and metastatic neoplasm should always be considered.

THE DYSPLASTIC HIP

Hip dysplasia is a consequence of failure of normal development of the acetabulum, proximal femur, or both. Symptoms of dysplasia vary in both site and severity, but commonly appear in patients of 20 to 30 years.

Clinical Assessment

Aspects of the history are important and include any prior treatment of the hip, especially surgery, for this may alter the already abnormal anatomy. Special aspects of examination include the Trendelenburg sign, the presence or absence of a fixed flexion deformity, and the range of internal and external rotation measured with the patient prone. Signs of labral pathology should be sought with the impingement test.

Radiographic Assessment

Radiographs should include a standard anterior-posterior (AP) pelvic radiograph, a lateral of the hip, a false profile view to assess anterior acetabular coverage, and AP views with the hip in abduction and adduction, and internal and external rotation. From the radiographs, a number of measurements to determine the type and severity of the dysplasia can be made. The center-edge angle, the acetabular index, the teardrop to head distance, and the anterior head coverage as determined from the false profile view allow accurate assessment of the pelvic contribution to hip dysplasia. The abduction-adduction and internal-external rotation views, together with measurement of the neck shaft angle allow the surgeon to assess the contribution by the femur to hip dysplasia. The position of the greater trochanter relative to the center of the femoral head should be assessed. Occasionally CT scanning of the hip is advisable if there has been prior surgery as the anatomy of the acetabulum, in particular, may be hard to define with standard radiographs.

The Role of Osteotomies

If the patient has pain that cannot be reduced by a 3- to 6-month program of nonoperative treatment including analgesia, anti-inflammatory medication, and physiotherapy, then surgery should be considered. Surgery can take several forms from acetabular redirection to acetabular supplementation and femoral osteotomy.

There is considerable variation in the approach to surgery for hip dysplasia. The shape of the femoral head and acetabulum need to be considered. If the femoral head is nonspherical, a repositioning osteotomy of the femur or pelvis is generally contraindicated. If the patient has a fixed deformity of the hip, however, a repositioning osteotomy of femur may improve hip function and reduce pain. If the hip joint is congruous, then the site of the "maximum" dysplasia needs to be identified. In many cases dysplasia is most marked on one side of the hip and correction of that abnormality is sufficient to alleviate symptoms.

If there is radiographic evidence on the false profile view of reduced anterior femoral head coverage, the acetabular index is at least 15°, and there are no or minimal degenerative changes, then an acetabular redirecting osteotomy is indicated. Many redirection osteotomies have been described but ones in contemporary use include the Ganz, Tonnis, and Ninomiya. The type chosen depends on the experience and philosophy of the surgeon. The Ganz osteotomy is performed through a single Smith-Peterson type incision and is a periacetabular osteotomy, which preserves the posterior column of the pelvis allows correction of deficient anterior coverage, and may allow alteration in the position of the center of rotation of the hip (Figure 17-7). The Tonnis osteotomy uses two incisions and divides the pelvis into two, achieving a similar degree of correction to that of the Ganz. Both osteotomies have a number of potentially serious complications, including nerve palsies, nonunion, heterotopic ossification, and fractures extending into the joint. If these are avoided, however, the short- to medium-term results are excellent. If there are advanced degenerative changes then the results tend to be less satisfactory. The long-term results of periacetabular osteotomies of the Ganz and Tonnis types have yet to be determined. The long-term (10–23 years) results of a different type of periacetabular osteotomy, described by Ninomiya, have been reported as very good, providing that there was little evidence of osteoarthritis at the time of surgery. If the radiographs show evidence of advanced degenerative change, then a Chiari supra-acetabular osteotomy may be considered as a pain relieving procedure.

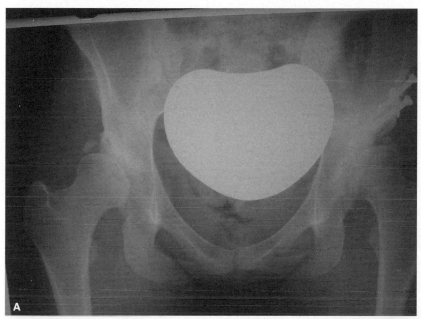

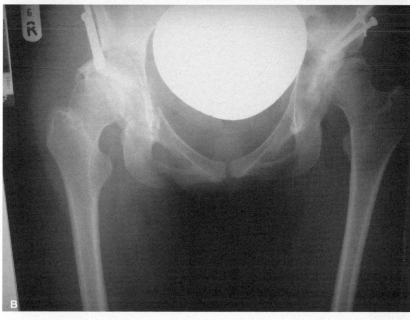

FIGURE 17-7. (A) Radiograph of a 27-year-old female with severe acetabular dysplasia of the right hip. **(B)** Post-operative radiograph after undergoing a right periacetabular osteotomy of the Ganz type.

adv

Requirements

Proximal femoral varus–varus plus rotation osteotomy is a more straightforward procedure, which is indicated if the radiographs show that proximal femoral dysplasia is the predominant dysplasia. Another requirement for proximal femoral osteotomy to be considered is whether the femoral head can be better covered, if the head can be better centered in the acetabulum, and if the hip is either abducted, or rotated or both. Careful preoperative planning is necessary to provide the optimal femoral head coverage. The degree of varus angulation seldom exceeds 15°. If greater than 15° is planned, then advancement of the greater trochanter is necessary to avoid a Trendelenburg gait. Varus femoral

osteotomy has the advantage that the recovery is reasonably short and the risk of serious complications is low. All varus femoral osteotomies, however, have the potential to shorten the leg, and this should be explained to the patient preoperatively. The results in appropriately selected patients are excellent, although pain over the internal fixation device often necessitates its removal (Figure 17-8).

The results of osteotomy for the treatment of early osteoarthritis in other joints strongly suggests that even in ideal circumstances, osteotomies for the treatment of hip dysplasia can only be expected to give satisfactory results for 10 to 12 years before pain becomes a significant problem again.

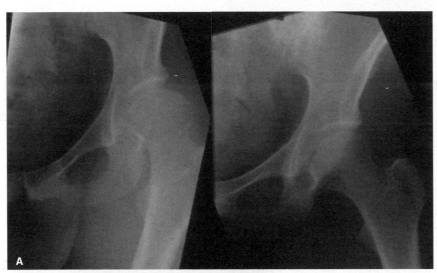

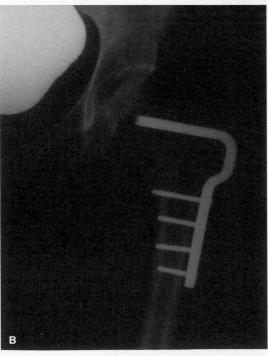

FIGURE 17-8. (A) Adduction and abduction radiographs of a 29-year-old female with moderate left hip dysplasia. Her pain was severe enough that surgery was considered necessary. The adduction view shows that there is good coverage of the femoral head when the femur is placed in that position. **(B)** A varus intertrochanteric osteotomy gave her good pain relief without subjecting her to the risks of THA at a young age.

Total Hip Replacement in Hip Dysplasia

When preoperatively planning a THR in a patient with a dysplastic hip, the two components of the hip, the acetabulum and the femur, should be considered individually and then together. Dealing first with the acetabulum, it may be present in its normal position, in a more proximal position, or absent (with or without a false acetabulum). When it is present in its normal position, it may be relatively small—in which case the surgeon requires small diameter acetabular components. Depending on the degree of femoral dysplasia, the anterior, or less commonly posterior, wall of the acetabulum may be dysplastic or absent, compromising acetabular fixation. If the surgeon has any doubts about the geometry of the acetabulum, then preoperative Judet views or a CT scan should be obtained. If the acetabulum is present but has migrated proximally, the shape of the ilium causes it to become progressively more shallow. Also, as previously indicated, the anterior or posterior walls may be deficient, and the roof may slope. In these circumstances, a CT scan of the pelvis with appropriate reconstructions allows the surgeon to plan the surgery.

In cases where a high false acetabulum is present, there is little or no anterior or posterior columns to aid with cup fixation. Restoration of the center of the rotation to the anatomical position in this situation not only improves the biomechanics of the THA but also improves the amount of host bone available into which an acetabular cup can be placed (Figure 17-9). Location of the true acetabular position may be difficult in a high-riding DDH, but can be achieved in one of three ways: (1) an intact ligamentum teres that runs from the femoral head down into the

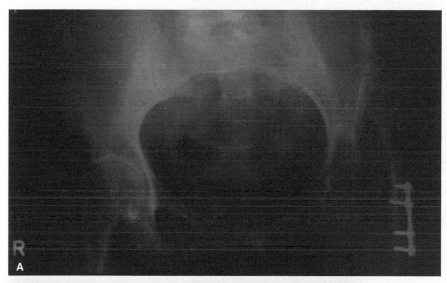

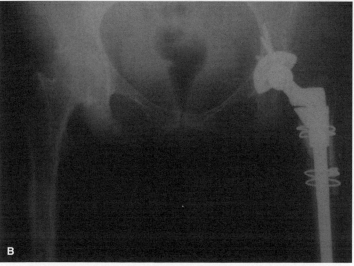

FIGURE 17-9. (A) Radiograph of a 57-year-old woman with high-riding congenital dislocation of the left hip. Her major symptom was back pain and fatigue with exercise, not hip pain. **(B)** Careful preoperative planning was required to restore her center of rotation to the anatomic position. Use of a small diameter (46 mm) acetabular shell prevented a structural graft being required. A subtrochanteric femoral shortening was required to prevent lengthening the leg more than 5 cm.

acetabular fossa; (2) identification of the greater sciatic notch posteriorly and the anterior column, which runs down and converges at the teardrop; (3) if neither of these anatomic landmarks is easily identified, an intraoperative AP radiograph may be performed. Most surgeons prefer cementless fixation of the acetabular implant with supplemental screw fixation.

Factors such as leg length, bone deficiency, previous surgery, and the femoral anatomy need to be taken into consideration. When the roof is sloping, the femoral head may be used as a graft to support the acetabular component (Figure 17-10). When there is a high dislocation, there is at best a false acetabulum, which generally plays no part in the reconstruction. Many of these hips do not cause pain until later life, and THR is not indicated. If surgery is considered desirable, then a CT scan of the true acetabulum usually reveals a small acetabulum with relatively osteoporotic bone. This situation requires small diameter acetabular components, and because of the osteoporosis, great care should be taken to prevent reaming through the floor.

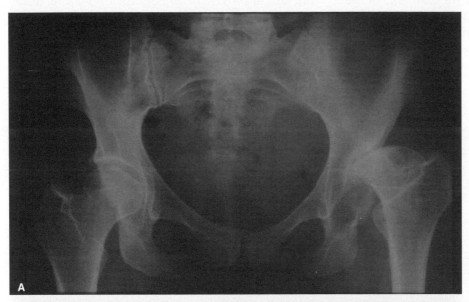

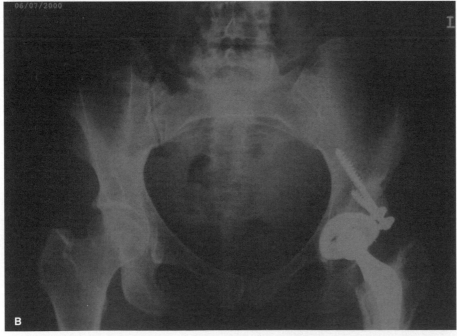

FIGURE 17-10. (A) This 38-year-old woman with severe acetabular dysplasia of the left hip, developed severe pain from secondary osteoarthritis of the femoral head articulating against a false acetabulum. **(B)** The patient's own femoral head was required as a structural bone graft to support the acetabular cup. Note that screws used to hold the graft should be directed superiorly into the pelvis to prevent collapse of the graft before bone ingrowth of the acetabular cup has occurred.

With regard to the femur, the size and shape of the femoral canal should be considered, as it is often small or distorted. It will be necessary to have available a number of small implants, including micro implants for some patients. Choice of femoral fixation is still controversial, but surgeons should be aware that cemented femoral components in the small femora may give an inadequate cement mantle. In cases of femoral dysplasia there is frequently a marked increase in the femoral anteversion. This possibility should be assessed preoperatively with CT scanning. If the anteversion is greater than 15°, then there are several different strategies available. A small femoral component may be used in association with a low neck cut to correct the anteversion. If using uncemented components of a tapered design, then cutting out a piece of the back of the femoral neck allows the component to be inserted in the correct degree of anteversion. The anterior neck may have to be trimmed to prevent impingement. If the anteversion is severe, then a modular prosthesis that allows the femoral component to be rotated within a proximal metaphyseal sleeve may be used. If a femoral shortening needs to be performed, then the proximal fragment can be rotated back to its correct position.

Finally, the issue of leg length needs to be addressed. If the leg is short, do not consider lengthening of over 5 cm. However, to work within this limit and to achieve the appropriate acetabular and femoral component positioning, it may be necessary to shorten the femur through a subtrochanteric osteotomy. This requires special prostheses, and should not be undertaken without appropriate training. If there is bilateral high riding DDH, but only one side is symptomatic and requires THA, consideration has to be given to resulting leg length inequality and the functional disturbance to gait this might cause. In this situation, the contralateral hip occasionally requires THA to maintain function (Figure 17-11).

Often dysplastic hips have had previous surgery and this always makes hip replacement more difficult. The old incisions may make access difficult. There may be extensive scarring on the lateral side of the pelvis and femur, making dissection, access, and restoring leg length more difficult. The bony anatomy may be quite abnormal, and preoperative CT scanning is very useful to delineate the features of the pelvis and proximal femur. The surgical approach adopted for THR in dysplasia depends on the experience of the surgeon, but as a general rule the posterior approach is more extensile and allows better visualization of the acetabulum than the direct lateral. Also dealing with severe femoral abnormalities may be facilitated through the posterior approach.

AVASCULAR NECROSIS OF THE HIP

Avascular necrosis (AVN) of the femoral head is a disorder whose incidence shows great international variation, and thus its origin varies from region to region. Generally trauma is the major cause of AVN. Avascular necrosis has also been associated with steroid use, alcohol abuse, Gaucher's disease, hemoglobinopathies, and in patients subject to severe changes in barometric pressure, such as deep sea divers. The common pathway in the latter conditions is likely to be alteration in the fat content or composition of the bone marrow, with a consequent increase in the intraosseous pressure and a reduction in blood flow to bone trabeculae. The exception to this pathway is in trauma, where the blood supply to the femoral head is disrupted when the retinacular vessels crossing the surface of the femoral neck are torn as a result of displacement of the femoral head following a fracture, or stretched when the femoral head dislocates from the acetabulum. Thus, AVN is common following femoral neck fractures in the elderly, and its incidence is related to the degree of head displacement.

Clinical Assessment

The clinical presentation of AVN depends on the age of the patient. In the elderly who have sustained a subcapital fracture, AVN is often heralded by increasing pain and a radiograph that shows fixation failure, collapse of the femoral head, or both. In younger patients with idiopathic AVN, pain is the most common presenting feature. An associated feature is synovitis of the hip, which manifests clinically with a decrease in the range of movement, and the hip is irritable (there is pain throughout the range of motion). If the patient presents late in the evolution of the disease, then the symptoms and signs will be indistinguishable from advanced osteoarthritis.

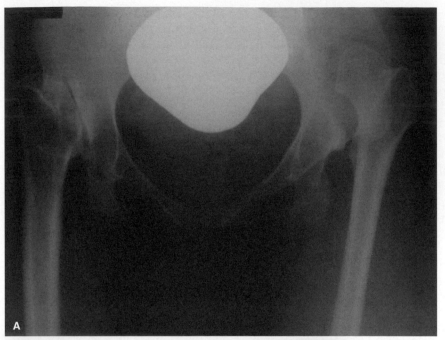

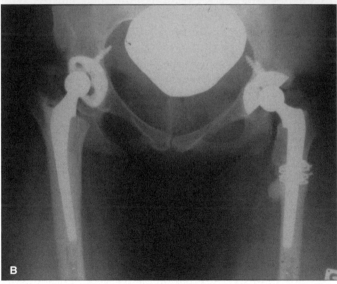

FIGURE 17-11. (A) Twenty-nine-year-old female who used a motor scooter outside the house for mobility, and was unable to get up or down stairs. She developed pain in her right hip that threatened her independence. **(B)** A right THA was performed. Despite no complications and good relief of her pain, her functional status and mobility were not improved. Seven months later a left THA with femoral shortening was performed. She now lives independently, does not require walking aids, and can manage three flights of stairs. Her leg lengths are equal.

Radiographic Assessment

Radiographic investigation begins with plain anteroposterior and lateral radiographs of the hip. Early in the disease, radiographs may be normal, but as the disease progresses it goes through several stages. A number of authors have classified the stages, the most commonly used classification being that described by Ficat. Ficat's classes divide the disease into four stages. Stage 1 refers to a hip that on plain radiographs appears normal. The diagnosis is made by measuring a raised intraosseous pressure, histologic examination of biopsy specimens, or an abnormal magnetic resonance imaging (MRI) examination. Stage 2 avascular necrosis may show patchy osteoporosis but an otherwise normal radiographic examination. Clinically, however, the hip is painful, and there may be a reduced range of motion. Stage 3 shows some change in the contour of the femoral head, and there may be a subchondral fracture. Stage 4 shows a loss of joint space and collapse of the femoral head. Radiographs may be indistinguishable from advanced osteoarthritis of the hip joint.

MRI is the best radiological modality to diagnose AVN early in the evolution of the disease. Care must be taken, however, not to misdiagnose transient osteoporosis of the hip as AVN. The former condition involves the whole of the femoral head and lacks the focal changes seen in AVN. Transient osteoporosis is a self-limiting condition with symptoms and MRI findings clearing in 6 to 8 months.

Treatment of AVN

Management of AVN depends on the age of the patient, size of the lesion, and stage of the disease. In the elderly who develop AVN following a hip fracture, total hip arthroplasty is the treatment of choice. In younger patients with idiopathic AVN, determining the size of the lesion is important as this has a direct influence on the prognosis. The size is best determined by MRI. Small lesions (less than 15% of the femoral head) may resolve without treatment. Large lesions (greater than 50% of the femoral head) tend to progress to collapse of the head and secondary osteoarthritis, despite treatment. For intermediate-sized lesions, a number of treatment options have been proposed. A classification based on the location of the lesion also has prognostic significance. If the lesion is medial in the head, then progression is rare; if it is lateral in the head the prognosis is worst.

There is a paucity of well-conducted trials that show conclusively that any one treatment is superior. Treatments range from simple decompression of the femoral head to lower the intraosseous pressure, to bone grafting of the involved area either directly after dislocating the hip and elevating the involved segment, or by using a vascularized fibular graft placed up the center of the femoral neck. There have been a number of osteotomies described whose purpose is to remove the affected area of the femoral head from the weight-bearing axis of the hip. These include varus and valgus osteotomies and more complex rotational osteotomies. The choice of osteotomy depends on the location of the lesion and the ability of the proposed procedure to remove the affected segment from the weight-bearing axis of the hip. Osteotomies are generally contraindicated for those patients who remain on corticosteroids or have untreated metabolic bone disease. They are generally only effective when a small area of the femoral head is involved.

When considering surgery designed to save the femoral head and prevent progression of the disease to degenerative arthritis, surgeons should be aware that, ultimately, conversion to THA is common following these procedures and the risks and potential benefits of such surgery should be very carefully weighed in each case. Hemiarthroplasty or bipolar prostheses should be avoided in AVN of the femoral head, as histologic assessment of the acetabular cartilage shows abnormalities in the majority of cases, which may adversely influence the outcome of such surgery. Idiopathic AVN is frequently bilateral with a reported incidence of 50 to 80%, and thus MRI should be performed in all cases.

RHEUMATOID ARTHRITIS

Rheumatoid arthritis is a chronic, systemic, inflammatory disorder with a predilection for articular cartilage. The hip joint is less frequently afflicted in the adult form of rheumatoid arthritis than other joints; however, its involvement may result in disabling symptoms and significant diminishment of function. Likewise, juvenile rheumatoid arthritis also more frequently involves larger, more rapidly growing joints, including the knees, wrists, elbows, and ankles and less commonly affects the hip joints. It has been estimated that about 1% of the U.S. adult population has rheumatoid arthritis. Therefore, it is reasonable to estimate that between 4 and 6 million cases of rheumatoid arthritis are found in the United States.

The disease affects women more frequently, with a female–male ratio of between 2:1 and 4:1. The disease affects all ages but generally increases in incidence with advancing age. In women, the peak incidence is between the fourth and sixth decades.

Origins and Pathology

Extensive research continues to be done, but the exact cause of rheumatoid arthritis remains obscure. Regardless of its cause, it may be described as an inflammatory process that somehow is triggered and centers in the joints with articular cartilage. The inflammation manifests as a stimulus for synovium to hypertrophy and becomes increasingly hyperplastic and hypervascular with increasing cellularity. This hypertrophic synovial tissue invades and degrades articular cartilage. The actual destruction of articular cartilage is done in large part by rheumatoid pannus, a fibrovascular granulation tissue that protrudes from the inflamed synovium into articular cartilage. It contains fibroblasts, small vessels, and multiple inflammatory cells that are responsible for the destruction of articular cartilage and its underlying bone.

Pathology within the hip joint generally involves varying degrees of articular cartilage loss secondary to the inflammatory process. This loss usually involves the entire femoral head, resulting in concentric loss of cartilage and subsequent concentric joint space narrowing. There may also be varying amounts of bone loss and even femoral head collapse. Varying degrees of cyst formation occur, and in about 5% of patients, significant protrusio acetabuli develops.

Clinical Assessment

A full history and physical examination should be performed in someone presenting for consideration of surgical treatment of a rheumatoid hip. Special attention should be taken of what medications the patient is taking. Prior to any joint replacement, a review with a rheumatologist to minimize or stop steroids or antimetabolic drugs should occur, because these medications compromise fixation of the implant and predispose the patient to an increased risk of infection. Careful attention to the state of the cervical spine and jaw for ease of anesthesia, and the state of the upper limbs and contralateral leg for ease of postoperative mobilization, should be made.

Radiography of the hip joint shows varying degrees of osteopenia and loss of joint space. The loss of joint space, in contrast to that seen in osteoarthritis, is generally concentric, and varying degrees of protrusio acetabuli may be present (Figure 17-12). Osteophyte formation is rare, and subchondral sclerosis is not a prominent feature. Cysts may develop within both the femoral head and the acetabulum. These changes may culminate in varying degrees of femoral head collapse, and in severely advanced cases, spontaneous bony fusion may occur with no range of motion.

Treatment

Conservative measures are usually the domain of the rheumatologist and include analgesics, nonsteroidal anti-inflammatories, steroids, and antimetabolite drugs such as methotrexate.

Total hip arthroplasty remains the mainstay in the treatment of end-stage rheumatoid arthritis of the

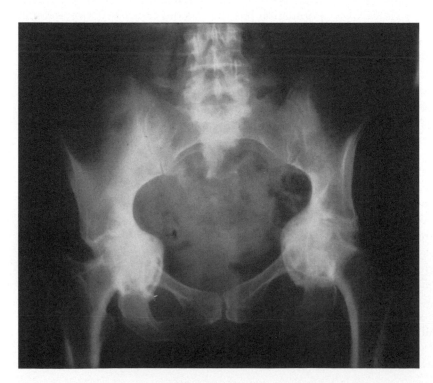

FIGURE 17-12. Severe protrusio of both hips in a 35-year-old female with juvenile rheumatoid arthritis. At the time of THA, an in situ femoral neck osteotomy prior to dislocation of the femoral head.

hip. In mature adults with rheumatoid arthritis, care should be taken during dislocation to prevent fracture in osteoporotic bone, and reaming of soft acetabular bone. Large cysts should be bone grafted with reamings from the femoral head or acetabulum.

THA in juvenile rheumatoid arthritis may present an array of technical complexity because of the small size of the patient and deficiencies in the femoral and acetabular bone stock. These problems may require customized or miniature components. Additionally, although the early result of cemented total hip arthroplasty may be good, these patients are young, and the total hip replacement must withstand many years of function.

HEMOPHILIA

Hemophilic arthropathy of the hip occurs four times less commonly than that of the knee in patients with severe hemophilia A (less than 1% of factor VIII levels). Management of the hemophilic patient uses a dedicated multidisciplinary clinic, involving hematologists, physiotherapists, occupational therapists, and orthopaedic surgeons.

THA in Hemophilia

The indication for THA in young patients who have hemophiliac arthropathy of the hip should be severe, disabling pain with activity and at rest that is unresponsive to nonoperative treatment. Careful preoperative planning to overcome deformities of the proximal femur, resulting from growth arrests from multiple childhood bleeds, is often needed. Osteoporosis is common and care should be taken to avoid fracture of the femur. Full factor VIII replacement is required not only during the surgery but until the stitches have been removed. A serious problem affecting the complication rate is a high prevalence of seropositivity for HIV and the eventual development of AIDS.

In one multicenter study of 34 THAs performed in 27 patients, at a mean follow-up of 8 years, 3 patients (11%) had developed a deep infection necessitating prosthesis removal, 7 hips (21%) had required revision for aseptic loosening, and 9 patients (33%) had died. Almost all the deaths were related to AIDS.

This relatively high complication rate illustrates the problems surgeons face when performing THA in young immunocompromised patients.

MANAGEMENT OF THE YOUNG PATIENT WITH A PAINFUL HIP

Pain and restricted joint movement are the most common complaints in young patients presenting with hip problems, but other clinical complaints can include locking, crepitus, loss of muscle strength, instability, and feeling of a mass lesion. Recent advancements in both hip arthroscopy and MRI have elucidated several sources of intra-articular abnormalities that result in chronic and disabling hip symptoms. Many of these conditions were previously unrecognized and, thus, left untreated.

Diagnosis

The diagnosis of hip pain in young patients has evolved significantly in the past few years. Referred pain and common hip pathologies, such as stress fractures of the femoral neck of pelvis avascular necrosis and early osteoarthritis, can usually be diagnosed by a combination of careful history and physical examination, followed up by AP and lateral radiographs and possibly a Technetium-99 isotope bone scan. If a diagnosis has still not been obtained, an MRI can be requested.

The MRI diagnosis may include symptomatic acetabular labral tears, hip capsule laxity and instability, chondral lesions, osteochondritis dissecans, ligamentum teres injuries, snapping hip syndrome, iliopsoas bursitis, loose bodies (for example, synovial chondromatosis), bony impingement, synovial abnormalities, crystalline hip arthropathy (gout and pseudogout), infection, and posttraumatic intra-articular debris. Occasionally, MRI arthrography can be a particularly useful technique for dedicated assessment of hip joint internal derangements.

Once a diagnosis has been obtained, the correct treatment can be instituted.

Hip Arthroscopy

Current indications for hip arthroscopy include the presence of symptomatic acetabular labral tears, hip capsule laxity and instability, chondral lesions, osteochondritis dissecans, ligamentum teres injuries, snapping hip syndrome, iliopsoas bursitis, and loose bodies (for example, synovial chondromatosis). Less common indications include management of osteonecrosis of the femoral head, bony impingement, synovial abnormalities, crystalline hip arthropathy (gout and pseudogout), infection, and posttraumatic intra-articular debris. In rare cases, hip arthroscopy can be used to temporize the symptoms of mild-to-moderate hip osteoarthritis with associated mechanical symptoms.

Technique for hip arthroscopy usually involves distraction of the joint, usually with a dedicated fracture table, and image intensification to ensure the portal placement is accurate. The patient may be positioned supine or in the lateral decubitus position. Anterior and peritrochanteric portals are most commonly used, giving good access and working space, to the lateral and superior part of the hip joint (Figure 17-13).

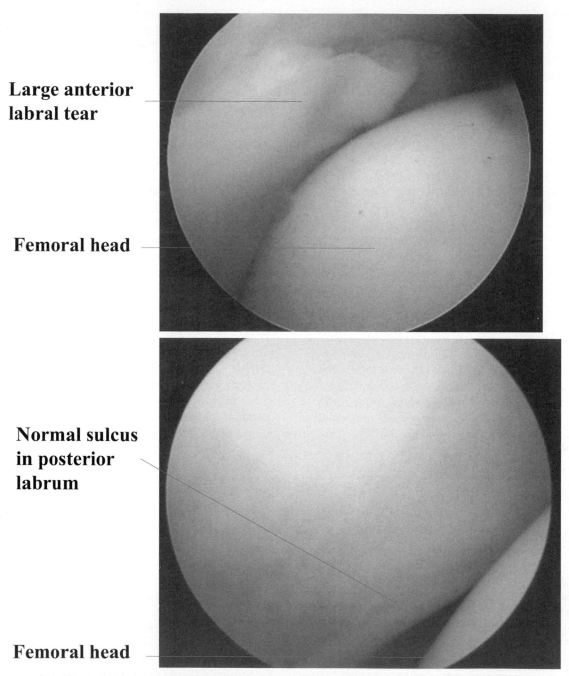

Large anterior labral tear

Femoral head

Normal sulcus in posterior labrum

Femoral head

FIGURE 17-13. Intraoperative photographs made during arthroscopy of the hip. Distraction of the femoral head out of the acetabulum is important to prevent inadvertent damage to the articular cartilage by intra-articular surgical instruments.

Surgical Dislocation

Recently, Ganz from Bern, Switzerland, has developed a new technique for surgical dislocation of the hip, based on detailed anatomical studies of the blood supply. It combines aspects of approaches that have been reported previously and consists of an anterior dislocation through a posterior approach with a "trochanteric flip" osteotomy. The external rotator muscles are not divided and the medial femoral circumflex artery is protected by the intact obturator externus. He reported his experience using this approach in 213 hips over a period of 7 years. Perfusion of the femoral head was verified intraoperatively and none subsequently developed avascular necrosis. It allows the treatment of a variety of conditions, which may not respond well to other methods, including arthroscopy. The most common conditions treated with this technique include impingement of the femoral neck on the bony acetabulum, and debridement of osteophytes and osteochondral lesions in patients with early osteoarthritis of the hip who are not suitable candidates for THA.

PRIMARY TOTAL HIP ARTHROPLASTY

History of Total Hip Arthroplasty

In order to understand how some modern concepts surrounding total hip arthroplasty have evolved to their current form, it is important to review the history of hip arthroplasty. This history can be broken down into three distinct eras based around the innovations of the man considered to be the father of total hip arthroplasty, Sir John Charnley.

Charnley's contributions to THA between 1954 and 1974 represent this century's most significant developments in orthopaedic surgery.

Pre-Charnley Hip Arthroplasty

The prevalence of tuberculosis causing ankylosis of the hip joint generated many innovative solutions to restore movement in the 1700 and 1800s. The first osteotomy of the femur below a stiff hip was credited to John Rhea Barton in 1826, who then manipulated the osteotomy site for 20 days following surgery to maintain motion. The patient was said to have enjoyed a pain-free functional "joint," until his death 10 years later of pulmonary tuberculosis.

From the 1840s, interest turned to the positioning of a material between the two bone ends forming a joint, so-called interposition arthroplasty. As well as tissue from the patient, such as the tensor fascia lata muscle and skin, a variety of foreign material was used, including gold foil, pigs' bladder, silver plates, wooden blocks, and rubber sheets. In 1923, Smith-Peterson placed a glass mould in a patient's hip. It turned out to be too fragile, but in 1938, at the suggestion of his dentist, Smith-Peterson used Vitallium, a cobalt-chrome alloy, as an interpositioning material (Figure 17-14). This method was probably the first clinically successful precursor to the modern THA and proved that the acetabulum

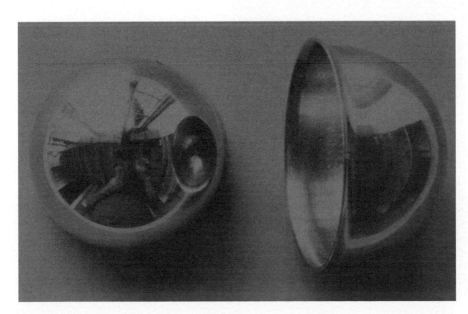

FIGURE 17-14. Smith-Peterson Vitallium mold arthroplasty.

could tolerate a foreign body performing a weight-bearing function.

In 1831, James Syme, an Edinburgh surgeon, is credited with the first publication of resection of the femoral head for ankylosis. This procedure was made popular in 1928 by an Oxford surgeon, Girdlestone, and the procedure still bears his name today. In 1940, Bohlman and Moore removed a tumor from the upper end of a femur and inserted the first metallic prosthesis. They performed this case in South Carolina through a posterior surgical approach, and because they came from the southern United States, their approach became known as the Southern approach, a name it still bears today. In 1948, the Judet brothers in France replaced the femoral head with a plastic (methyl methacrylate) prosthesis, but breakage and loosening caused early failure and the procedure fell into disrepute (Figure 17-15).

Throughout the 1950s, more than 50 types of prosthesis were introduced. The short-stem type was replaced by the intramedullary long-stem type, which gave more stability, and the nonmetallic type was replaced by the metallic type, which provided greater durability. Most shared similar design features to those prostheses developed by F. R. Thompson in 1950 and Moore in 1952. These procedures never became popular for osteoarthritis because of ongoing pain from movement of the prosthesis within the femur, as well as ongoing disease in the acetabulum.

Charnley's Contributions

In 1954, John Charnley began to investigate the phenomenon of lubrication that produces low friction in normal joints. He had previously observed that squeaking, which occurs in artificial joints, does not occur in normal joints. A previous investigator had suggested this was due to hydrodynamic lubrication (fluid enters the zone of contact and lubricates it) by synovial fluid. Charnley speculated this could not occur because of the unique situation in the hip joint of weight bearing, which would prevent synovial fluid from performing this function.

After observing that articular cartilage remained smooth, even after having been being wiped clean (boundary lubrication), he concluded that boundary lubrication was responsible for the low frictional resistance of the hip joint. He then assumed that a material such as polytetrafluoroethylene (Teflon), which was self-lubricating, would be an appropriate substitute for the damaged cartilage, and pursued its use with spectacular (early) results.

Initially, both sliding surfaces were made of Teflon, which replaced the damaged articular cartilage. After 12 months, however, there was evidence of mechanical loosening and failure when the stump of the femoral neck lost its blood supply and became necrotic, and the two Teflon surfaces lost their frictional properties and became bound together, thereby causing movement and wear between the plastic socket and the native bone of the acetabulum.

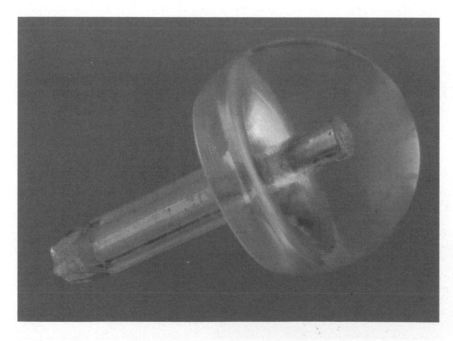

FIGURE 17-15. Judet glass mold of a patient's hip. This was secured to the patient by a pin inserted down the stump of the femoral neck. It never gained widespread acceptance due to premature failure of the base material.

Torque: is a force that
causes rotation

In order that low frictional resistance be maintained within an artificial joint, torque transmitted from a metal femoral head to a plastic socket can be minimized by reduction of femoral head size. Likewise, for a plastic socket to be stable within an acetabulum, torque should be maximized, achievable by maximizing the outer diameter of the acetabular cup. These principles led Charnley to begin work with a smaller diameter metal femoral head and method of bonding implants to bone. He began by rejecting the premise of using small amounts of acrylic cement as an adjuvant to a tight mechanical fit, instead using cement as a grout (rather than an adhesive) with the components achieving a loose mechanical fit. Results with Teflon had been disappointing, and an alternative was required. Although initially rejected in favor of Teflon's self-lubricating properties, high-density polyethylene had been tested in Charnley's laboratory, and proved to be remarkably wear resistant. The first high-density acetabular prosthesis was inserted into a human hip joint in November 1962.

A 90% success rate in his early series prompted Charnley to continue the procedure, but he continued to search for the cause of the 10% failure. Chemical rejection of the cement was initially suspected, but this was reduced to 5% by introduction of the clean air enclosure, suggesting infection was the major culprit (Figure 17-16).

The "Modern" Era of THA

Although Charnley's new operation, based on sound principles, was an astonishing success for sufferers of hip arthritis, its use was limited to surgeons who had been trained directly by Charnley himself. Other surgeons throughout the world also developed total hip arthroplasty prostheses. Maurice Muller from Switzerland developed a plastic acetabular cup with a 32 mm diameter chromium-cobalt-molybdenum femoral head, which he used extensively between 1966 and the early 1980s (Figure 17-17). Peter Ring began using metal-to-metal components without cement in 1964, but its use never became popular because poor tolerances between the components led to binding of the articular surfaces and eventual failure.

Charnley's original prosthesis tended to dominate into the early 1970s, but with rigorous follow-up of patients, a problem with radiological loosening of the component at the bone cement interface was identified. Continuing follow-up showed this was a progressive problem, with massive resorption of bone around the prosthesis, limiting options for treatment. This loss of bone was initially attributed to the acrylic cement and became known as cement disease.

Search for an alternate method of fixation led researchers to the concept of cementless fixation of the prosthesis to bone. Prostheses were designed allowing solid initial fixation to bone during the

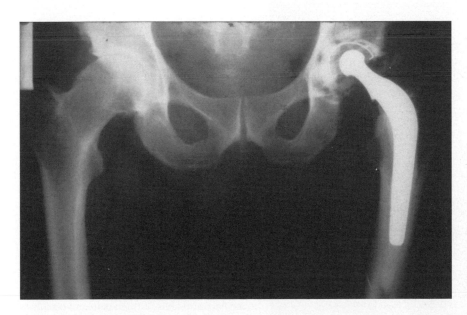

FIGURE 17-16. Radiograph of a left Charnley THA. This patient had his original operation in 1978. The hip was still functioning well 22 years postoperatively. Many of the original surgical principles, as promoted by Charnley, are evident: all-polyethylene acetabular cup with wire marker (showing evidence of loosening and wear), well-fixed monoblock femoral stem with 22.225 mm diameter femoral head, and absence of distal plug.

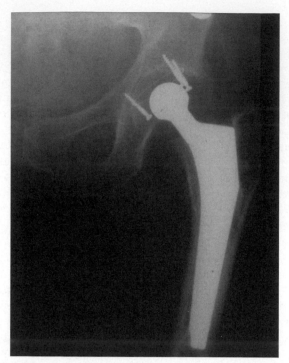

FIGURE 17-17. The SLS femoral stem and the Morscher cup. This combination of design features is very commonly used in Europe.

operation. A porous-coated surface finish of the prosthesis then allowed bone to grow onto the prosthesis, and in some cases, into it. Initially, two types of porous coating became popular, a titanium fiber-metal composite wire mesh developed by Harris, Galante, and coworkers, and cobalt-chrome beads developed by Engh, Bobyn, Hungerford, and coworkers (Figure 17-18). Later, plasma-sprayed titanium was used.

During the 1970s, a concept of prosthesis modularity developed. The femoral component now came as two distinct parts, assembled by the surgeon during the operation. A femoral stem could be individually sized to a patients femoral canal, to which was attached a separate femoral head using a morse taper. This gave the surgeon flexibility to alter femoral head diameter to match the chosen acetabular cup, and femoral neck length to restore correct offset and length of the patient's leg. The acetabular component also came as two parts—a metal shell, which was fixed to the patient's acetabular bone (often supplemented with spikes, lugs, or screws), and a high-density polyethylene liner, which was fixed to the shell using some form of locking mechanism. Even the original Charnley prosthesis adopted this trend with the development of the Charnley Elite prosthesis, which had a modular femoral head.

Concurrently, there was a movement toward increasing the size of the femoral head from the 22.225 mm of Charnley's original work, to 32 mm, in order to increase the range of hip movement and decrease the rate of dislocation. This increase in head size coupled with modularity of the acetabular cup was to have a dramatic effect that was not foreseen.

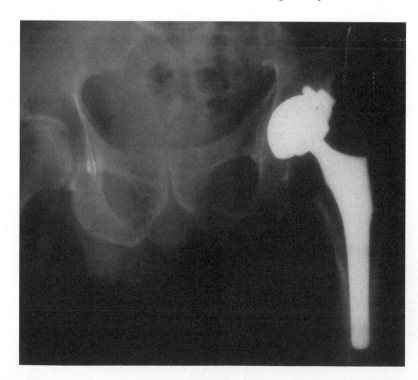

FIGURE 17-18. Porous-coated anatomic (PCA) THA. The first major cementless femoral and acetabular components. Many are still functioning well today, nearly 20 years after their introduction. They did, however, introduce new problems of thigh pain and osteolysis not commonly seen with cemented THA.

The three most popular cementless prostheses, at least in the United States, were the porous-coated anatomic prosthesis from Howmedica (associated with Hungerford and Headley), the AML prosthesis from DePuy (associated with Engh), and the Harris–Galante prosthesis from Zimmer. These were the so-called first generation cementless THA. By the mid 1980s, it became apparent using these components to eliminate cement did not eliminate cement disease. Indeed, the massive resorption of bone around these components continued to occur at an even more alarming incidence and volume than had occurred with the original Charnley components.

Longer-term (over 15 years) failure of cemented acetabular cups during that period led to the concept of the so-called hybrid hip, which incorporated cementless acetabular fixation and a cemented femoral stem. Some cementless femoral stems had introduced a new problem, thigh pain, which did not seem to occur with cemented prostheses. This pain was attributed to the tip of a stiff femoral stem rubbing on the femoral cortex and generated some dissatisfaction among surgeons with cementless femoral stems.

Enormous research was directed toward analysis of this bone loss from both physiologic and histologic perspectives. It rapidly became apparent that this so called cement disease was actually particle disease. Any foreign material, if broken into small enough particles, when introduced into the prosthesis bone interface, caused resorption of bone by the body, leading to the radiological findings of bone loss and clinical signs of pain caused by loosening. This particulate material could be generated from cement or prosthesis substrate, but the most common source was high-density polyethylene.

By the late 1980s, polyethylene wear from the bearing surface was identified as the major cause of loosening and late failure of total hip replacement. Decrease of polyethylene thickness below a critical level was found to increase polyethylene wear debris, and many first generation prostheses had inadvertently contributed to this by increasing femoral head size, and decreasing liner thickness to accommodate for the metal shell and locking mechanism.

With identification of high-density polyethylene as the major contributor to prosthetic loosening and clinical failure, researchers in the 1990s turned to identification of alternate bearing surfaces to reduce or eliminate generation of particulate debris. Improved machining-processes and prosthesis-manufacturing techniques have seen a reemergence of metal-on-metal articulations. Although there have been concerns raised about metal ion levels in blood and tissues, to date there has been no recorded incidence of problems in patients from these metals.

Ceramics may reduce particulate debris, as they have the property of self-polishing, which diminishes surface disparities caused by third body wear (damage to the bearing surface caused by a material getting "caught" between the two articulations). Ceramics can articulate with either themselves or with high-density polyethylene. The major concern with ceramic use is the risk of fracture. This was illustrated in a 2001 worldwide recall of all zirconia ceramic femoral heads, after a defect was found in the manufacturing process.

Although changes in the mechanical properties appear with laboratory testing to be promising, clinical results were disappointing. Poly-Two was an attempt to strengthen high-density polyethylene with carbon fiber but was a spectacular clinical failure. Hylamer was an attempt to stiffen polyethylene, but clinical results suggest a 15% increase in wear, not a 15% decrease as first believed. Methods of sterilization and the shelf life after manufacture are also known to have an effect on wear, but to date have not been used to successfully improve wear.

The most promising avenue currently for alteration of polyethylene to improve its wear is cross-linking the polyethylene by subjecting it to ionizing radiation during the manufacturing process. This process produces cross-linked polyethylene, which is currently in extensive use worldwide since its approval in 2000. Laboratory simulator testing shows a 90 to 99% reduction in wear, but clinical results in patients are not yet available.

Cost of Primary THA

The aging population with a higher incidence of hip osteoarthritis, combined with a decreasing patient acceptance of disability, is leading to increasing strain on a the health care budget, accounting for up to 1 to 2.5% of a county's gross national product. In the last 15 years, surgeons have been asked to evaluate the success of a THA not only for prosthesis longevity, but also cost effectiveness. Health economists can now create models for comparing the cost effectiveness of a THA with coronary bypass and renal transplantation. These models measure cost-benefit analysis using a Health Related Quality of Life Index, and for patients in their fifth and sixth decade of life, THA comes out significantly ahead of these other more complex procedures. Governments use these economic indicators and other outcome measures to allocate health budgets more appropriately.

One of the most important variables in cost-benefit analysis (CBA) of THA is the age of the patient. Despite an increase of cost over benefit with increasing age, THA has been shown to be beneficial in the octogenarian population. The benefit of THA can now be accurately measured, and none would argue that it is a huge success, leading politicians and health providers to look more closely at cost containment. With the advent of new design, materials and surface finishes over the last 20 years, nowhere is this more applicable than implant costs. The original Charnley cemented stem and cemented cup costs approximately 30% of a cementless porous-coated femoral and acetabular component. In young active total hip recipients, a new prosthetic design, which offered a 90% improvement in survivorship over 15 years and a 15% reduction in the cost of revision surgery, could be sold at a price of 2 to $2\frac{1}{2}$ times that of conventional cemented components such as the Charnley prosthesis and still remain cost effective. Using more likely estimates of the improved performance of new technology, however, the upper limit of cost effectiveness is an increase of $1\frac{1}{2}$ to 1. Only a very small increase in the cost of a prosthesis could ever be justified for older patients of either sex.

In many institutions cost concerns have led to the concept of implant matching, where cementless porous-coated prostheses are reserved for younger more active patients, and cemented THA reserved for elderly more sedentary patients. Another area that is being evaluated for cost savings is length of hospitalization. The time a patient spends in hospital contributes the largest proportion to the overall cost of THA. Day of surgery admission, and improved surgical technique, rehabilitation, and home services all allow patient discharge on day 3 or 4.

Perhaps the most extreme expression of improved length of stay is the newly emerging mini-incision surgery (MIS) techniques. Although promising from a surgical perspective, length of hospitalization is probably more influenced by age, patient co-morbidities, patient expectations, and home circumstances. The potential benefits of MIS have yet to be proven and careful analysis of the long-term results will be needed.

Measurement of Outcomes in Primary THA

Specific scoring systems have been widely used to assess the clinical results following primary THA. Most studies attempt to measure the outcomes of technique and procedure, and do not assess the effect on general function and the satisfaction of the patient. Measurement of outcome in THA is usually achieved using two different systems, one that measures health-related quality of life (HRQOL), and the second group that contain joint-specific tools. Only validated outcome measures should be used for assessment.

Health Related Quality of Life

The Medical Outcomes Study Short Form 36 (SF-36) Health Status Survey is widely used for measuring the HRQOL. The patient responds to 36 questions regarding their physical and social functioning and mental health, with no physician input to bias the results. It has the sensitivity to document improvement in HRQOL following surgery and to reveal differences in THA.

The Western Ontario and McMaster Universities (WOMAC) Osteoarthritis Index is a tested questionnaire to assess symptoms and physical functional disability in patients with osteoarthritis of the hip and knee. The three domains assessed include pain, stiffness, and function.

Joint-Specific Instruments

A 12-item Oxford Hip Score is hip specific and is more able to distinguish between symptoms and functional impairment produced by the index joint, as compared with other joints and conditions. The Merle d'Aubigne and Harris hip scores are widely used to grade improvement after THA.

Numerous studies measure patient satisfaction with THA and evaluate the relationships of expectations and outcome to patient satisfaction. Patients' different expectations can be grouped into five categories reflecting improvement in pain, walking, psychological state, essential activities, and nonessential activities. Approximately 90% of patients will be satisfied with the results of surgery. Lower rates of satisfaction can be expected in patients who have a better preoperative condition.

CEMENTED ACETABULAR COMPONENTS

Cemented acetabular components currently comprise a very small percentage of acetabular components implanted in the United States, but continue to be popular in many parts of Europe. Long-term data on cemented THA continues to show that acetabular component loosening is generally more of a problem than femoral stem loosening beyond 10 years. For a group of patients whose prosthesis remains in place at 25 years postoperatively, the prevalence of acetabular revision is approximately 15%, compared with a prevalence of 7% for revision of the femoral stem. These figures are magnified when patients receive a THA under the age of 50 years. In a group of patients under the age of 50 with an average 18-year follow-up, 50% of the acetabular components were radiologically or clinically loose, compared with only 8% of the femoral stems. Modern consensus is that failure of a cemented femoral component is nontime dependent, reaching a failure rate of approximately 8% by 15 years, and maintaining this rate beyond that time. Conversely, rate of failure of a cemented acetabular component is time dependent and may increase in a nonlinear manner after 10 years.

This situation caused many surgeons to convert their practice to the use of porous-coated cementless acetabular components during the early 1980s. The concept of the hybrid hip—a cemented femoral stem articulating with a press-fit porous-coated modular acetabular component—became increasingly popular during this period.

In an effort to improve performance of all-polyethylene acetabular cups, metal-backing was introduced during the mid 1980s. This backing was thought to distribute stress more evenly through the cement mantle, leading to improved longevity. Follow-up of these implants has revealed the converse situation, with a higher incidence of radiological lucent lines at the cement bone interface, and a higher incidence of clinical failure than was documented for all-polyethylene acetabular cups. These poorer results were attributed to reduced polyethylene thickness and the introduction of another interface for ingress of wear debris.

The greatest development with cemented all-polyethylene cup implantation has occurred not with cup design but with cementing technique. Since 1962, cement has been hand-mixed and then finger packed into the femur. This is now termed *first generation cement technique*, and has been superceded by mixing of cement in a gun that is used to deliver cement, under pressure, into the femoral canal in a retrograde fashion. A distal plug below the tip of the prosthesis prevents cement from being pushed too far down the canal. These alterations in cement delivery are now called *second generation*

cement technique. Although developed mainly for the femoral component, similar principles are applied to cementing of the acetabular component.

When a cemented all-polyethylene acetabular cup is implanted, surgical technique is very important in achieving a good postoperative radiograph appearance. Preparation of the acetabular bone, clearance of soft tissue from the acetabular margins, and careful drying of the acetabular bone bed are all essential to eliminating the appearance of lucent lines at the cement bone interface. When the early postoperative radiograph shows radiolucency in the lateral margin of acetabulum, the incidence of subsequent acetabular loosening increases dramatically. In a recent long-term follow-up study, additional drilling of peripheral holes around the acetabular margin for anchorage of the cement was shown to increase longevity of the acetabular component.

The evolution from first to second generation cement technique has been largely developed for the femoral component, making its impact on the cemented all-polyethylene acetabular component difficult to assess. Femoral components implanted with the use of second-generation cementing techniques appear to have fared much better than acetabular components inserted with second generation cement techniques in most series. Recent matched-pair studies comparing cemented acetabular components to cementless porous-coated components, have shown a lower revision rate and lower incidence of radiographic loosening for porous-coated components compared with cemented components.

The place of cemented all-polyethylene cups currently continues to be defined. They seem to function best over the long term in older, less active patients. A recent study of 132 THA in 112 patients over 75 years of age showed that, at a mean 14.6 year follow-up, no acetabular component in those patients still living had required revision for aseptic loosening.

Cementless Acetabular Components

The clinical results of the so-called first-generation porous-coated cementless acetabular components with a minimum 10-year follow-up have now been reported by a number of centers, independent of their developers. From a clinical and radiologic perspective, reliable fixation to the acetabular socket is reported in the range 95 to 99% of cases. During the development of titanium fiber mesh, plasma spray, or sintered cobalt-chrome beads as a surface finish applied to the outer diameter of metal shells, animal models suggested that only 20 to 40% of the roughened surface achieved histologic bony ingrowth (Figure 17-19). Time has proven that this figure seems to give satisfactory stability for prolonged loading, and the results do not appear to deteriorate over time.

The noningrown areas of the acetabular cup have, however, produced a new problem. Access of particulate debris, especially polyethylene from the bearing surface to these noningrown areas, gives rise to large areas of bone resorption that we now term *osteolysis*. Although this phenomena of bone resorption was seen with cemented acetabular cups and femoral stems, it was present at a much lower rate, size of the lesions were much less, and perhaps most importantly, their increase in size over time was much less than is seen with cementless metal-backed acetabular components.

This increase in osteolysis rate is thought to be due to design alterations in the porous-coated

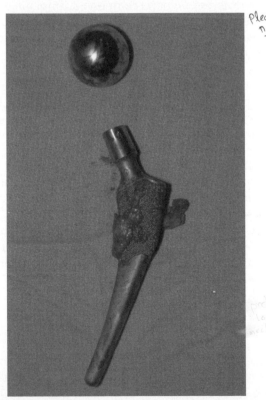

FIGURE 17-19. This PCA femoral component was removed for intractable thigh pain in a 49-year-old male. It had been implanted $2\frac{1}{2}$ years previously. Radiological appearances suggested no evidence of loosening, and at the time of revision it was found to be quite stable. Despite this, after explantation, only 25% of the proximally coated porous surface was found to be bony ingrown.

acetabular components. Increased thickness of the metal shell to increase its stiffness, and increase in femoral head size to 32 mm to improve range of hip movement and joint stability led to a large decrease in thickness in the polyethylene insert. In many cases, thickness of the insert fell below the critical level of 6 mm, which is now known to cause a dramatic increase in polyethylene wear at the bearing surface. Two other factors played a part in this early problem: introduction of a secondary bearing surface between the polyethylene liner and the inner surface of the metal shell, and poorly designed locking mechanisms.

In many early designs, little attention was given to congruity between the inner surface of the metal shell and the outer surface of the polyethylene liner, and in some cases, there was up to 2 mm of gap between the two surfaces. Subsequent loading of the liner by the femoral head transmitted the force through the polyethylene in a nonuniform manner, leading to stress concentration, liner deformation, and high wear not only at the primary bearing surface but also on the outer surface of the liner, so-called back-side wear. An additional problem with this lack of conformity also occurred. Any fluid in the gap between the shell and liner is hydraulically forced out by the bottoming out of the liner during weight bearing. This fluid, laden with polyethylene particles, follows the path of least resistance through screw holes in the shell, and so gains access to the prosthesis–bone interface and leads to osteolysis (Figure 17-20). Fluid can also be forced, under this hydraulic pressure, into other areas of the prosthesis bone interface of both the femoral and acetabular component where bone ingrowth has not occurred, again causing osteolysis. This process has led to the concept of the "effective joint space," where surfaces of the prosthesis that are not bony ingrown can potentially be bathed in joint fluid rich in debris particles that cause osteolysis.

Locking mechanisms between the metal shell and polyethylene liner involve the use of peripheral mechanisms around the opening of the shell that capture the polyethylene liner. Incorporation of this locking mechanism often involved additional sacrifice of polyethylene thickness in an area that often was subjected to the high stress and subsequent polyethylene wear. With time, these locking mechanisms often lost their rigid grip on the liner, allowing movement that further aggravated back-side polyethylene wear.

Despite these shortcomings, a prospective report was conducted of 100 hips with a porous-coated

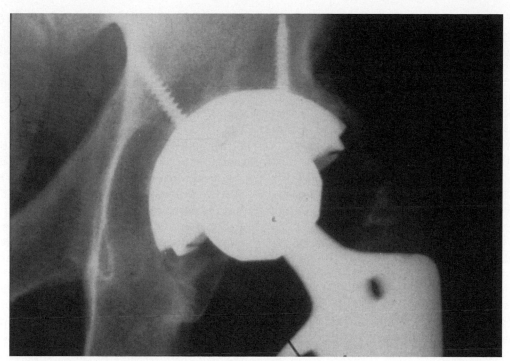

FIGURE 17-20. The Harris-Galante I titanium fiber mesh acetabular component has proved to be the most durable first generation acetabular component. Thin polyethylene and a suboptimal locking mechanism, however, led to the concept of the "effective joint space." Particle-laden joint fluid is forced through the screw holes into the areas of nonbone ingrowth, leading to screw osteolysis, as seen in this radiograph. The component has been implanted for $4\frac{1}{2}$ years, but required revision because of this appearance.

anatomic (PCA) THA (Howmedica, Rutherford, NJ) with a mean age of 58 years. At 15-year follow-up, 17% (17 hips) of the entire cohort and 23% (15 hips) of the living cohort (64 hips in 55 patients) had undergone revision due to loosening of the acetabular component or osteolysis. These results compare favorably with a study of cemented acetabular components with a 25-year follow-up reported by the same author. Patients still alive 25 years after surgery had a mean age of 56 years at the time of operation. These patients received a cemented Charnley THA with first generation cementing techniques. There was a 15% revision rate for acetabular loosening, and a further 36% that demonstrated definite or probable radiographic loosening.

The component that has been studied most extensively is the Harris-Galante I (Zimmer, Inc, Warsaw, IN). This component comprises a titanium fiber mesh coating that was usually implanted with line-to-line reaming (last acetabular reamer used is exactly the same diameter as prosthesis to be implanted) and screw fixation. A 9- to 14-year follow-up study of 71 hips in 56 patients less than 50 years old at the time of surgery, revealed no revision or

radiological loosening of the components, but a 23% incidence of pelvic osteolysis.

Contemporary acetabular cup design trends now minimize the number of screw holes through the acetabular metal shell to prevent fluid gaining access to the prosthesis bone interface. The central hole, present to allow the surgeon to ensure the cup is fully seated in the acetabular bed after cup insertion, can now be blocked with a plug. The locking mechanism has been redesigned to ensure the polyethylene shell is solidly fixed to the metal shell, congruity between the inner surface of the metal shell and outer surface of the polyethylene liner has improved, and that the inner surface of the shell is smooth to reduce abrasive wear against the liner. The minimum thickness of the polyethylene (even with incorporation of the locking mechanism) is 8 mm. This has necessitated a return to smaller femoral head size when smaller cups are used. The use of 32 mm metal femoral heads articulating against conventional polyethylene has disappeared.

There are two principles of cementless acetabular fixation. The first involves implantation of the component using a technique that ensures initial stability of the metal shell against the acetabular bone. Supplemental fixation, such as screws through the cup, spikes, lugs, or fins in the periphery, may be used to achieve stability. Another ② method is to under-ream the acetabular bone bed by 1 to 2 mm, and then use the roughness of the outer surface of the metal shell to achieve a "scratch fit." Other initial fixation modes include an expansion cup, where the cup diameter is reduced with a special instrument, the cup is implanted, and then allowed to return to its initial diameter; and screw in designs, where the cup has a thread incorporated into its outer surface, and is screwed into the acetabular bone.

Achieving initial stability allows the second principle to occur, that of bony ingrowth onto and into the metal shell. Different surface finishes of the cup, including titanium fiber mesh, cobalt-chromium beads, titanium plasma spray, tantalinium fiber metal, and grit-blasting of the surface, are currently used by manufacturers to obtain bony ingrowth. Hydroxyapatite may be used as supplemental fixation and to improve initial stability, but unless used in conjunction with a porous ingrowth surface, it does not appear to maintain long-term fixation on its own.

Although acetabular cup modularity (separate acetabular shell and polyethylene liner assembled at the time of surgery) was introduced to reduce surgical inventory, increase surgical options, and allow future liner exchanges, a disadvantage is that it introduces a further interface from which wear debris can be generated. This has lead surgeons back toward using a single piece acetabular cup, where the bony ingrowth surface and polyethylene come as one piece. Disadvantages of this design, however, are that visualization of the medial acetabular margin during implantation is not possible (ensuring the cup is fully seated), and also that few options exist for additional fixation with screws through the metal shell if initial stability is not achieved with a scratch fit.

Reports of increased rates of polyethylene wear with use of cementless acetabular components is a major concern. Surgeon selection of a porous ingrowth acetabular cup should balance wear issues with concerns of initial stability (i.e., unusual acetabular anatomy requiring additional fixation) and bony ingrowth (previously damaged bone from irradiation or fracture seems to reduce the amount of bony ingrowth) for each patient.

ALTERNATE BEARING SURFACES

The clinical performance of cementless porous-coated acetabular components over 10 years suggests that problems with component fixation are rare. Periprosthetic pelvic and acetabular osteolysis caused by polyethylene wear at a linear rate greater than 0.2 mm/year, has led to a search for alternative bearing surfaces to articulate on both the femoral and acetabular side. A metal femoral head articulating with conventional polyethylene has been intensively studied and has by far the longest follow-up, but the accelerated wear seen in a small number of patients with porous-coated cementless acetabular components means that there will always be a limited longevity of the prosthesis with this bearing surface.

Increasing patient expectations of a return to normal activities, including sport and heavy manual labor after THA, means an alternative must be found. Articulations can be broken into two broad groups: conventional bearing surfaces, where the acetabular side of the joint consists of conventional or cross-linked polyethylene; and hard-on-hard bearing surfaces, where both sides of the joint are made up of either alumina oxide ceramic or metal.

Ceramic on Polyethylene

Three types of ceramic, alumina, zirconia, and more recently oxinium, have been used as femoral head bearing surfaces against conventional polyethylene. Alumina oxide has also been used in a ceramic-on-ceramic (hard-on-hard) bearing surface. Early hip simulator studies have suggested a five- to tenfold reduction in polyethylene wear rate compared to metal femoral heads, but more recent simulator studies are variable with some showing a similar rate to metal on polyethylene, depending on variables such as temperature of the polyethylene, type of lubrication, and introduction of third body debris. In clinical studies of polyethylene wear rates made from clinical radiographs, there are conflicting results, with some showing that ceramic femoral heads confer an advantage and an equal number showing no difference.

The claimed material advantage of ceramic femoral heads over their metal counterparts is their self-polishing ability, making them resistant to scratches. Generation of particulate debris is a time-dependent process, meaning that the advantage of ceramics only becomes evident after a given time period (claimed to be 5 to 7 years). This phenomena might explain the variability of the clinical studies, where only those with a follow-up greater than 5 to 7 years show a difference, but this has yet to be proven.

disadv

Two major issues with ceramic femoral heads include the potential for fracture and the cost. With improved manufacturing techniques, the risk of ceramic femoral head fracture was lowered to approximately 1 in 50,000 implants. In 1999, a defect in the manufacturing process of the supplier of 80% of the world's zirconia femoral heads led to a significant number of zirconia femoral head fractures, which prompted a worldwide recall of all zirconia femoral heads. Use of zirconia femoral heads, because of this defect and recall has been limited.

When ceramic femoral heads were first released, they were approximately three times as costly as metal femoral heads, and although these costs have declined, the clinical studies to date make it difficult for surgeons to justify their use on the basis of improved prosthesis longevity.

Ceramic on Ceramic

disadv

Alumina oxide ceramic has been used in Europe for many years as a hard-on-hard bearing surface. Wear rates with this articulation have been reported as 10 times less than the lowest conventional polyethylene wear rates. An identified drawback of ceramic-on-ceramic is the limited head and neck sizes available. There is also concern about the state of the bearing surface and the rim of the acetabular component if a dislocation occurs. The elimination of polyethylene does not eliminate the problem of wear debris and osteolysis, as at least one alumina-on-alumina hip of early design had a high incidence of wear and osteolysis.

Metal on Metal

This bearing couple has been around as long as metal-on-polyethylene THA, but results from early designs were poor because of poor manufacturing tolerances between the acetabular cup and femoral head, leading to binding of the surface and eventual loosening of the prosthesis. This result was compounded by the early prostheses not being fixed to the bone, but even the introduction of acrylic cement

could not improve the results sufficiently to compete with the results of metal-on-polyethylene THA. Improved manufacturing techniques and research into lubrication methods at the interface have led to a resurgence of interest in metal-on-metal THA. There is no doubt that there is a dramatic reduction in wear rate to negligible levels, using both radiographic wear measurement techniques and retrieval specimens, but there remains major concern regarding the production of cobalt and chromium metallic debris, and its elimination from the body.

A recent randomized clinical trial comparing one type of metal-on-metal with metal-on-polyethylene had to be abandoned when very high levels of erythrocyte and urine cobalt-chromium were detected. Metallic wear particles have also been isolated in lymph nodes, livers and spleens of patients with THA, raising concerns about the long-term effects these materials might produce.

Problems with Metal-on-Metal.

Metal on Cross-Linked Polyethylene

There have been many attempts to modify the wear characteristics of polyethylene by altering its material properties. Highly crystalline polyethylene (Hylamer) and Poly-Two (carbon fiber-reinforced polyethylene) were developed to improve the wear performance of conventional polyethylene, but clinical results have been disappointing and their use has been discontinued. The most promising current area for improving the wear performance of polyethylene is by increasing the amount of cross-linking that occurs between the individual polyethylene molecules.

Several studies have demonstrated the favorable long-term results of this cross-linked polyethylene using cemented nonmetal backed all-polyethylene cups. A report on 62 ultra high molecular components gamma irradiated in air with 100 megarads of ionizing radiation and a control group of 10 nonirradiated polyethylene cups implanted between 1971 and 1978. Twenty-eight hips (45%) were available for follow-up at a mean 17.3 years after operation. At 2 years, the cross-linked group had a linear wear rate of 0.15 mm/year and the control group a linear wear rate of 0.39 mm/year. This high initial wear rate was attributed to a highly oxidized surface layer. After 2 years, the rates decreased to a steady state of 0.06 mm/year for the cross-liked group and 0.29 mm/year for the nonirradiated cups. These figures suggest a 79%

reduction in linear wear when using cross-linked polyethylene.

In 1999, a report on 14 chemically cross-linked all-polyethylene acetabular cups articulating with a 22 mm diameter zirconia femoral head. There were four non–cross-linked all-polyethylene cemented acetabular cups with a 22 mm diameter zirconia femoral head used as a control group. Follow-up ranged between 10 and 11.3 years. Rate of linear wear in the cross-linked polyethylene group was 0.04 mm/year, while rate of wear in the control group was 0.16 mm/year—a 75% reduction in wear rate using cross-linked polyethylene. Historical studies of THJR polyethylene wear using the same implants, similar follow-up, and same wear measurement technique gave a wear rate of 0.07 mm/year, demonstrating a 45% reduction in wear when cross-linked polyethylene is used.

Results of these two important studies should be interpreted with caution, however, because the method of cross-linking was radically different from that currently used by manufacturers, resulting in a material so brittle that a locking mechanism for use in modular acetabular components could not be machined. Careful attention to heating and cooling temperatures as well as cooling times by manufacturers, has reduced this problem, and the material stiffness is now much closer to traditional polyethylene.

The cross-linking process involves the bonding together of carbon atoms in adjacent molecular chains, achieved by replacing carbon-hydrogen bonds with carbon-carbon bonds. An unwanted side effect of this process is the generation of free hydrogen atoms, charged particles known as free radicals. Free radicals are known to cause surface oxidation, which in turn increases polyethylene wear, and so their reduction is critical during the manufacturing process.

Each of the THJR implant manufacturing companies uses its own proprietary process for cross-linked polyethylene manufacture. This process involves four steps, and each surgeon who uses a particular brand of cross-linked polyethylene should be aware of the steps used in its manufacture. There are choices available at each step in the manufacture of cross-linked polyethylene.

1. Consolidation—either compression molding or ram extrusion
2. Cross-linking—either electron beam or gamma irradiation
3. Free radical reduction—either heat anneal or remelt in oven
4. Sterilization—either ethylene oxide or gas plasma or gamma in nitrogen

Each choice has advantages and disadvantages, and may result in differences in the wear performance and material properties of cross-linked polyethylene from the different manufacturers. To date, all wear testing of cross-linked polyethylene has been performed using multidirectional wear simulators. Crossing path wear tracts are used in an attempt to reproduce in vivo THJR conditions. Depending on the degree of cross-linking (determined mainly by the dosage of radiation of strength of chemical cross-linking), a 70 to 90% reduction in polyethylene wear using a hip simulator can be achieved.

Since 1999, the Food and Drug Administration has approved a number of highly cross-linked polyethylene components for clinical use. The 2-year results of many clinical studies comparing conventional and highly cross-linked polyethylene are expected in the near future, but it will be some years before the true benefits of cross-linked polyethylene (if any!) are known.

Cemented Femoral Stems

Charnley Type Cemented Femoral Stems

The Charnley cemented femoral stem has the most extensively documented results in the literature, including several published studies with 25-year follow-up. The femoral stem, as developed by Charnley, was designed to overcome mechanical failures resulting from the use of earlier prostheses. The original flat-back design derived from the Austin Moore and Thompson prosthesis was modified to a round-back design, and then further altered with an additional flange design (Cobra) to enhance load transfer to the cement.

By the early 1980s, most total hip prosthesis designs had adopted a straight tapered configuration for the stem. Larger caliber prostheses were introduced to reduce the incidence of stem fracture, but this problem was virtually eliminated by improved metallurgical processes and a better choice of metals accompanied by improvements in design. The various types of Charnley prosthesis have been developed over a period of 30 years and have been based on clinical experience demonstrating the need for modifications. Whether design modifications will be an improvement over the original has not been proven, because so many other variables such as improved surgical technique and cement technique also play a role. All of the modifications have retained the original monoblock Charnley principle of even stress distribution to the cement mantle, but have included increases in prosthesis diameter and length, modularity of the femoral head using a morse taper, and increases in offset that may be selected by the surgeon. The current system is called the Charnley Elite Plus.

Twenty-five year follow-up results are available from several dedicated hip centers. The most widely quoted is that from the Iowa group and were from Charnley THAs implanted during the early 1970s. Of 330 Charnley THAs performed between 1970 and 1972, 62 hips (51 patients) were available for follow-up. Mean age at surgery of these 51 patients was 56 years. Fourteen of these hips (23%) had been revised at a minimum 25-year follow-up, and the prevalence of revision due to aseptic loosening of the femoral component was only 7% (4 hips). This demonstrates the durability of the Charnley femoral component when implanted by a single dedicated surgeon.

In a recent study, results of the Charnley cemented stem were evaluated across an entire health region rather than from a single dedicated total joint center. Results were dramatically different from those of a dedicated hip center, with a known rate of aseptic loosening of 2.3% at 5 years, infection rate of 1.4%, dislocation rate of 5%, revision rate of 3.2%, and a radiographic impending failure rate of 5.2%. These results suggest an overall failure rate of 10% within 5 years and may be more representative of the true situation.

The Swedish National Hip Arthroplasty Register, initiated in 1979 by Dr. Peter Herberts et al., has given invaluable information on the comparison of different prostheses and surgical techniques across an entire population. Although the Charnley cemented stem is frequently referred to as the gold standard, the Swedish Hip Register has reported higher stem survival rates with other cemented stems. Across the entire country during a similar time period (which assumes the use of similar cementing technique), the Charnley cemented hip had a 92% 10-year survival rate compared to a Stanmore at 91.9%, Exeter at 94.9%, and Spectron at 98.4%.

Surface Finish of Cemented Femoral Stems

Perhaps the greatest design change as an alternative to the original Charnley stem has come with the manufacturing of prostheses with different surface finishes. These surface finishes are described in terms of "roughness," as measured by a profilometer. The average roughness (R_a) is the average distance between peaks and valleys across the surface of the prosthesis, and can vary by a factor of 40 from the polished Exeter femoral stem ($R_a < 2\,\mu$ inch) to the Precoat femoral stem ($R_a = 80\,\mu$ inch). The smoother implants used initially, including the Charnley stem ($R_a = 2\,\mu$ inch), had lower cement-metal interface fixation strength, whereas rougher surfaces have greater fixation strength. This greater fixation strength has a lower probability of interface motion, but at the same time, due to its greater abrasiveness, a higher debris generation consequence if motion does occur.

The highly polished Exeter femoral stem, designed by Dr. Robin Ling, actively discourages fixation between the metal surface and the cement. The consequence of this is distal migration under loading conditions, but the double wedge taper design of the prosthesis transfers only compression stress to the cement mantle when this occurs. Cement is strongest under compression and the Exeter femoral stem ues this principle to obtain outstanding long-term results.

There has been a move toward smoother cemented femoral stems due to high rates of wear and osteolysis from the debris products generated by abrasive wear of some femoral stem designs employing a rough surface finish. Rough surfaces, in themselves, are not necessarily associated with a high incidence of osteolysis or loosening. The Spectron (Smith & Nephew, Memphis, TN) femoral stem has a grit-blast surface in its proximal third, yet enjoys the highest 10-year survivorship of any prosthesis (98.4%) reported by the Swedish National Arthroplasty Register. Excellent results with the Spectron are attributed mainly to stem geometry being a rectangular cross-section to enhance rotational stability and smoothing of the rectangular edges to decrease stress concentration within the cement mantle.

Roughening the surface finish of a smooth prosthesis, such as occurred with the Exeter, Iowa and T-28 stems, has a higher incidence of loosening and osteolysis. Other considerations such as length, substrate material, cross-sectional shape, and incorporation of a collar, all contribute to the successful long-term results of a cemented femoral stem.

Cementing Technique

Arguably the greatest improvement in the long-term results of cemented femoral stems has occurred through improvement in surgical technique, specifically at the time of cement and prosthesis insertion into the femur. Cementing technique has been broken into three distinct generations by many authors, but the evolution of cementing technique essentially represents a continuum over time, with various components of each generation being introduced at different times.

First generation cementing technique, dating back to 1962, involved limited sizes of femoral stem, finger packing of the cement in an antegrade fashion, no femoral canal preparation, no intramedullary cement restrictor, and no pressurization of the cement with a gun. Second generation cementing technique, first used as a term in 1975 (although cement guns had been available since 1971!), involved a greater number of femoral stem sizes, broaching the canal to obtain a uniform thickness of cement around the femoral stem, insertion of an intramedullary cement restrictor, pulsatile lavage followed by brushing and drying of the canal, use of a venting tube to remove fluid, and retrograde filling of the femoral canal using cement pressurized into the canal with a cement gun.

Third generation cement technique, a term used from 1985, involved porosity reduction of the cement using vacuum mixing and a centralizer on the tip of the femoral component to ensure it remained in the center of the cement during insertion. Each of the generations have been described using specific femoral component designs (e.g., third generation is usually associated with roughened femoral stems), but strictly speaking, each of the three techniques has been applied to all femoral stem designs during the time of their use.

Strongest evidence suggesting that second generation cementing technique improves implant survival when compared to first generation cementing technique comes from the Swedish National Arthroplasty Register. Cemented implants used during the period 1979–1989 (first generation cementing technique) have a 91.5% 10-year survival with index diagnosis osteoarthritis and endpoint revision due to aseptic loosening. The same implants used during the period 1990–2000 (second generation cementing technique) had a 94.8% 10-year survival. Evidence of third generation cementing technique further improving prosthesis survival is not (yet!) available.

Cementless Femoral Stems

The use of cementless fixation for the femoral component is a popular approach. Most early failures of cementless components occurred on the acetabular side associated with accelerated polyethylene wear and osteolysis. Porous-coated femoral stems have been relatively successful in achieving constant fixation with a minimum of unwanted problems. Assuming good initial fixation and a porous-surface that encouraged bony ingrowth, the major problems have been with thigh pain and stress shielding. Clinical results with the first generation cementless stems are now out to 15 years, and assuming a good initial femoral stem design is used with a good acetabular component, porous-coated stems do not appear to show the deteriorating results with time that have been reported with cemented components.

Circumferential Porous Coating

A major flaw with one of the first generation cementless femoral stems, the Harris-Galante I, was that titanium fiber-metal pads were attached to the proximal $\frac{3}{4}$ sides of the implant in a noncircumferential fashion. This design left areas of smooth titanium proximally with no bony ingrowth, allowing a channel through which polyethylene wear debris could gain access from the articulating surface to the prosthesis-bone interface distally, leading to osteolysis around the femoral stem. The problem has since been addressed and all current cementless femoral stems have circumferential porous coating, but there is still considerable controversy regarding the length of proximal porous coating required to give durable long-term clinical results.

Extensively Coated Stems

Most cylindrical prostheses, designed for achieving initial stability through a tight fit in the isthmus of the femoral canal, use porous coating at least $\frac{5}{8}$ of the proximal length down the prosthesis. These components are fabricated from cobalt-chrome because notch sensitivity of titanium (weakening of material in areas of high stress concentration, such as where porous coating is applied) does not allow extensively coated femoral stems at diameters used in primary THJR. Results of the anatomic medullary locking stem (AML, DePuy, Warsaw, IN) have reported a 97% stem survival at 12 years. Approximately 9% of patients with this stem, however, have pain that limits activity, but only 3% localized this to the thigh. A recent study reported that a proximally coated stem had twice the incidence of thigh pain compared to a fully porous-coated stem. The incidence of thigh pain with a fully coated stem is similar to that reported using a cemented femoral stem. In another study of 174 hips followed for more than 2 years, 26% showed radiological evidence of stress shielding. This same group, however, when followed to 5 years, showed no progression of stress shielding. The long-term consequences of stress shielding are not known.

The major disadvantage to extensively coated femoral stems is their difficulty of removal at revision surgery for reasons other than aseptic loosening, such as infection or dislocation. Techniques for removing an extensively porous-coated femoral component that is solidly fixed include an extended femoral osteotomy, use of a Gigli saw to free the prosthesis from calcar bone, cutting the prosthesis transversely with a diamond saw, and trephining the remaining stem with a dedicated mill slightly larger than the diameter of the prosthesis.

Removal concerns with solidly fixed, extensively coated femoral stems have led many surgeons to only use these components in a revision situation when there is poor quality proximal bone.

Proximally Coated Stems

A recent study on the porous-coated anatomic hip (PCA, Howmedica, Rutherford, NJ), which has a cobalt-chrome, proximally circumferentially porous-coated femoral stem, reported that of 64 hips in 55 patients still alive at 15 years, only 4 femoral stems (4.0%) had been revised for isolated loosening (without osteolysis, which is attributed to accelerated polyethylene wear from factors unrelated to the stem). In another proximally coated implant system, the Omnifit cementless total hip (Osteonics Corporation, Allendale, NJ), with an average 10-year follow-up, there was a 2.6% incidence of femoral stem revision. The incidence of thigh pain in this series was 4.5%.

Concerns with thigh pain in all of the proximally coated first generation porous-coated femoral prostheses have led to modifications of design. The PCA E stem is modified by widening of the proximal flare as well as modification of the curve of the tip to reduce the incidence of stem tip abutment on the anterior cortex of the femur, which was thought to be responsible for thigh pain with the original PCA prosthesis. A study comparing the PCA E series with a matched group of patients who received the original PCA component, showed significant improvement in all areas, with 98% versus 81% good or excellent clinical results, 2% versus 19% revision rate, and 19% versus 50% incidence of femoral radiolucencies.

Tapered Femoral Stems

Another approach to cementless stem fixation has involved use of a stem with a tapered geometry to achieve mechanical stability in the proximal portion of the femur, achieved by wedging the component into place rather than using a cylindrical reamer. This design, with a porous coating or a roughened titanium surface, has been popular in Europe for many years. In one series of 100 hips, using a plasma spray proximally coated tapered titanium stem (Taperloc, Biomet, Warsaw, IN), with a 10-year follow-up, there were no instances of femoral loosening and only seven cases of femoral osteolysis. Similar results have been obtained with a cobalt-chrome hip (Trilock, DePuy, Warsaw, IN) where only 1 in 66 femoral components were revised at 10 years, and no cases of distal osteolysis were reported.

One study compared the results of a cobalt-chrome versus a titanium tapered stem, using the same type of acetabular component and polyethylene. Although clinical results were equivalent in both groups, the linear wear rate was significantly higher for the titanium stems with a plasma spray surface (0.22 mm/year) compared with the cobalt-chrome stems with a sintered bead surface (0.07 mm/year). Prevalence of osteolysis was 16% in the titanium group and 0% in the cobalt-chrome group. One potential cause for the higher wear rate and higher incidence of osteolysis is accelerated polyethylene wear secondary to third body particulates from either the modular head-neck junction or the titanium plasma spray surface.

Hydroxyapatite Coatings in Primary THA

Hydroxyapatite is the most popular osteoinductive calcium phosphate coating used in total hip arthroplasty. It was originally used as the sole coating on the surface of a prosthesis to obtain initial stability. Although early clinical results were good, over time it appears to resorb leading to loosening and failure necessitating revision. In one study comparing the same cup design with either hydroxyapatite coating or porous coating, at a minimum follow-up of 5 years, the aseptic loosening rate was 11% (21 in 188) for the hydroxyapatite component versus 2% (2 in 109) for the porous-coated component.

There is also concern that hydroxyapatite could increase polyethylene wear and increase the incidence of osteolysis. This is not shown, however, in one study of 314 hips (274 patients) in which a tapered hydroxyapatite-coated titanium femoral stem (ABG, Howmedica, Rutherford, NJ) was assessed at a minimum 10-year follow-up. No stems showed aseptic loosening and there were no cases of distal endosteal femoral osteolysis. In another study of the same prosthesis, a mean 6-year follow-up (4–10 years) of 97 patients showed that although there were very good clinical results and 100% survivorship of the femoral stem, there was an alarmingly high rate of polyethylene wear, 0.24 mm/year (range, 0.05–0.76 mm/year).

The place of hydroxyapatite as a femoral stem coating has not been established in the literature at this time.

Surface Hip Replacement

Surface hip replacement consists of resurfacing the acetabulum with a thin layer of bearing surface, and replacement of only the femoral head (not neck) with a metal ball. Historical failure of surface replacement has been due to the production of wear debris with subsequent bone resorption, loosening, and failure. Recently, to avoid these problems a surface replacement using a metal-on-metal bearing, allowing thin components and femoral design and instrumentation to avoid varus alignment, has been designed. McMinn, the designer of this prosthesis, reported on his experience with 235 joints over a 5-year period. There were no femoral neck fractures and no dislocations. Over that time, problems with premature failure of component fixation necessitated changes in fixation technique from press-fit, to cemented, to the current system that uses a peripherally expanded hydroxyapatite coated acetabular cup and a cemented metal head. Potential advantages of this system over conventional THA include conservation of bone for later revision surgery if necessary, improvement in range of motion, and reduction in dislocation rate. The major concern is early femoral neck fracture, which seems to occur more commonly in females where osteoporosis might be a factor.

Minimally Invasive THA

Although there has been a recent resurgence of interest in performing THA through very small incisions by both the public and implant companies, there are several reports in the literature of using small incisions 15 years or more ago. Interest in this as a technique for performing THA has probably followed from a resurgence of interest in performing unicompartment total knee replacement approximately 5 to 7 years ago.

There are two types of minimally invasive THA: the single-incision technique and the two-incision technique. Almost all THA done in this manner are press-fit using porous-coated femoral and acetabular components because of difficulty cementing through a small incision. The single-incision technique can be performed as a limited anterior approach as described by Hardinge, where a very limited splitting of gluteus medius occurs through a 5 cm incision, or a posterior approach through a 5 cm incision based over the femoral neck posteriorly.

The two-incision technique employs an incision 1 cm greater than the femoral head diameter, based over the femoral neck anteriorly. Through this, the hip is dislocated anteriorly and a femoral neck osteotomy performed. Acetabular preparation is performed with the aid of an image intensifier, which is also used to ensure correct positioning of a press-fit acetabular cup. A separate 4 cm incision is made over the tip of the greater trochanter, and femoral canal preparation and stem insertion are again aided by an image intensifier.

Potential advantages of performing less tissue dissection include quicker postoperative mobilization and a shorter hospital stay. Studies that have attempted to demonstrate an improvement in these outcome measures have found that patient comorbidities and domestic circumstances have a greater impact on these than the length of the surgical incision. Long-term results of prosthesis survival using current minimally invasive surgical techniques are not available.

COMPLICATIONS OF TOTAL HIP ARTHROPLASTY

Death

Death associated with THA may be broken into several categories: intraoperative, in-hospital but postoperative, 30-day rates, and 90-day rates. Intraoperative rates in one study from the Mayo Clinic database on 38,488 THAs in 29,431 patients between 1969 and 1997 showed 23 deaths during surgery. Predisposing factors included elderly patients with preexisting cardiovascular conditions with acute hip fractures or pathological fractures (17 of

23). The strongest predictor of sudden death was use of cement for fixation in all 23 cases. The authors recommend avoidance of cement if possible in predisposed patients with acute fracture or malignancy.

The postoperative in-hospital mortality after primary THA is in the range 0.1 to 0.8%, 30-day mortality between 0.15 to 1.42%, and 90-day mortality between 0.2 to 0.74%. Ninety-day mortality after revision surgery is approximately the same as for primary THA (0.6 to 0.9%).

Nerve Palsy

Nerve palsy following a THA is an uncommon (prevalence 1%) but concerning outcome for both the surgeon and the patient. Informed consent should include this complication as a possible outcome. Predisposing factors include female gender, revision surgery, lengthening of the limb, and bleeding tendencies. The most common nerve injured is the sciatic (78%), followed by the femoral (13.2%) and the obturator (1.6%).

The sciatic nerve is composed of independent tibial (medial) and common peroneal (lateral) divisions that usually (90%) are united as a single nerve down to the lower border of the thigh. Although grossly united, the funicular bundles of the two are separate and there is no exchange of bundles between them. In 10% of cases the two divisions exit the pelvis as distinct nerves. In these situations the tibial nerve always passes below the piriformis muscle while the common peroneal component can pass above or through piriformis. The common peroneal nerve is more prone to mechanical injury than the tibial nerve because it has larger and more tightly packed funiculi with less protective connective tissue, and because of its more lateral position and tethering in the sciatic notch and head of fibula.

Nerve palsy can occur after THA from one of three reasons: direct physical damage from dissection, poor retractor placement, or entrapment during cerclage femoral wiring from excessive traction or from compression usually by postoperative hematoma associated with anticoagulation. During surgery attention should always be given to sharp retractor placement over the anterior of posterior columns. Formal dissection of the sciatic nerve is not usually considered necessary, but its position should always be kept in mind during surgery. If cerclage wiring of the femur is required, care should be taken to split the posterior linea apsera as close to the femoral shaft as possible. The wire should always be passed from posterior and lateral to anterior and medial, and the leg should be placed in the anatomic, not dislocated position during passing of the wire.

If a nerve palsy is noted in the recovery room, an attempt should be made to identify its origin. After checking that it is not anesthesia related (patient received a partial spinal or epidural anesthetic), the operative procedure should be reexamined. If there is any chance of the nerve being trapped by a cerclage wire, or the limb has been lengthened more than 3 cm, the patient should be returned immediately to the operating room for either removal of the wire or shortening of the leg (femoral head exchange if possible). Hematoma compressing the nerve may give clinical signs of ongoing bleeding and buttock pain. Discontinuation of anticoagulation may be considered, but there is no absolute indication for reoperation to evacuate a hematoma. Good outcomes have been reported with conservative management.

During preoperative planning for THA, if there is the possibility of the leg being lengthened more than 2 to 3 cm (such as commonly occurs with reconstruction of a congenital hip dislocation), a wake-up test can be discussed with the patient. This involves telling the patient he or she will be asked to "wriggle their toes" on both feet before extubation. The anesthetist must ensure no motor block or muscle relaxant, and the ability to increase the patient's level of consciousness to allow understanding of commands. If the patient is able to dorsiflex his or her toes on the contralateral foot but not the toes on the operated leg, the patient is assumed to have a sciatic nerve palsy, and consideration should be given to reoperation.

If the nerve palsy is treated nonoperatively, there is a 41% chance of complete recovery, a 44% chance of partial recovery, and 15% of patients will have a poor outcome. Prognosis is good if limited motor function is present immediately after surgery or if some motor function returns in the first 2 weeks postoperatively. Femoral nerve injury generally has a better outcome than sciatic nerve injury.

Leg Length Inequality

One of the commonest findings noted by the patient after primary THA is a leg-length inequality (approximately 25%). Most studies of large groups of people show that approximately 30% of the population have a discrepancy between 1 and 2 centimeters, however, and often the patients' complaint of a longer leg after operation is not borne out with clinical or radiologic measurement. This functional leg-length difference is caused by contractures around the hip that create a pelvic obliquity. Commonly, this is caused by tightness of the gluteus medius muscle in a hip that has been short and has had a decreased offset and then is corrected to the normal hip length and offset. Over time, the feeling of a "long leg" will become less obvious, but it is important to warn the patient of this preoperatively so they are not worried that something was done incorrectly at the time of surgery.

A true lengthening of the leg at the time of surgery can be avoided by accurate preoperative planning, anatomic component geometry, and intra-operative assessment (including use of outrigger jigs, center of head to lesser trochanter distance, and relationship of knees and heels before and after reconstruction as well as intraoperative radiographs if there is still uncertainty. Correct restoration of offset and leg length in a diseased hip is always balanced against risk of dislocation by making the soft tissues too loose, but both goals can always be achieved with careful surgical technique.

Dislocation

A recent large study of 58,521 elective primary THA (excluding acute fractures) in the United States reported a 3.9% dislocation rate during the first 6 months after surgery, and for 12,956 revision THAs, a 14.4% dislocation rate. These figures are much higher than are generally quoted for single surgeon series of THA, which are approximately 0.5 to 2%. Factors that influence rate of dislocation include patient factors (including cerebral dysfunction and alcoholism), surgical approach (traditional posterior approach has a fourfold greater risk of dislocation compared to Hardinge approach), surgical factors (correct positioning of acetabular and femoral component, trimming of marginal osteophytes from the acetabulum), and implant factors (head size, head–neck ratio, elevated rim acetabular liner, choice of neck length, choice of offset).

Recent techniques designed to repair the posterior capsule and external rotators to the hip have reduced dislocations with the posterior approach to 0.5%. A large study from the Mayo Clinic demonstrated no benefit in dislocation rates with a larger head, but a definite benefit with use of an elevated rim liner (2.2% incidence if elevated rim used,

3.85% if no rim). Laboratory data suggests decreased impingement between the femoral neck and acetabular rim with a 28mm femoral head compared to a 22 mm femoral head, but no additional benefit is gained by using a 32 mm femoral head for this purpose.

An important recent study has shown a large increase in dislocation rate when the acetabular cup diameter was 32 mm or greater than the femoral head diameter. The authors postulated that site of attachment of pseudocapsule is moved further from the femoral head, potentially allowing greater laxity, and they recommended use of a 22 mm diameter femoral head for acetabular cups less than 50 mm diameter, and a 32 mm femoral head for acetabular cups greater than 62 mm outer diameter.

Treatment of a dislocation depends on the suspected cause and the number of previous dislocations. Most first-time dislocations where there is no obvious cause such as osteophyte impingement or component malposition are treated by closed reduction and gradual mobilization (Figure 17-21). There is no evidence that prolonged immobilization or physiotherapy after closed reduction decreases the likelihood of recurrence. If an obvious cause is identified, then operative treatment is indicated. The late dislocation (occurring at least 2 to 5 years after surgery) raises the possibility of wear of the acetabular component, which may require revision.

Multiple dislocations are of great concern to the patient because they cannot be sure of the circumstances when they will occur. Often these patients request surgery. If the anteroposterior and lateral radiograph fail to show acetabular malposition that can be corrected by revision surgery, a decision must be made as to the best form of treatment. Most recurrent dislocations are posterior, and in the majority of these cases the original THA was performed through a posterior approach. There is little guidance in the literature as to which surgical approach should be performed in this situation, but the authors prefer a Hardinge type approach through nonscarred tissue.

The least complicated option is to increase tissue tension by increasing the length (and offset) of the femoral neck and performing a careful soft tissue repair. A further option is augmentation of the cup with a custom-made wedge of polyethylene (often a liner cut into thirds), held to the existing cup with screws, placed in the position where the dislocation was occurring. Trochanteric advancements have not been reported as useful in the literature. Complete revision of both components is a

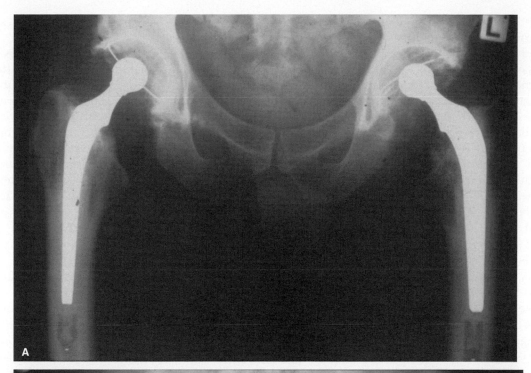

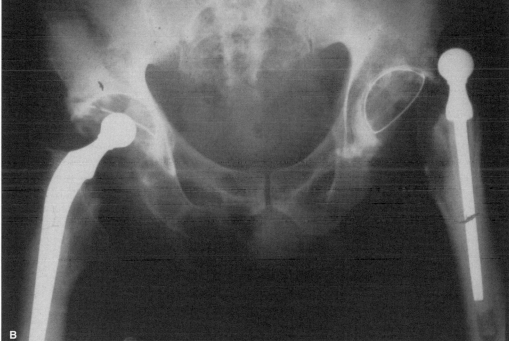

FIGURE 17-21. (A) This 47-year-old male underwent bilateral simultaneous cemented THA through a direct lateral approach for severe idiopathic osteoarthritis. His postoperative radiographs appeared satisfactory and he was discharged from hospital 6 days after surgery. **(B)** He was readmitted with an anterior dislocation of the left hip $3\frac{1}{2}$ weeks after surgery. He claimed that he fell forward out of a chair, causing the dislocation. The hip was reduced with sedation, and he was discharged the following day. No splint was used. He made an uneventful recovery, and at latest follow-up (9 years) has not had any further instances of dislocation.

drastic option if both are well-fixed and there is no obvious component malposition.

A study on the operative treatment of 116 recurrently dislocating hips using one of the above operations, showed only a 61% success rate. An increasingly popular alternative is revision of the acetabular cup with a constrained liner. A constrained liner is one that "captures" the femoral head and prevents it from dissociating from the acetabulum. A 5-year follow-up of 56 patients who were treated with a constrained acetabular component showed a 97% success rate at preventing further dislocation. The potential disadvantage of decreased range of movement and component loosening (because the internal surface of the polyethylene is greater than a hemisphere causing impingement and greater stress transmission to the prosthesis-bone interface) has not been seen in medium-term follow-up studies of this component. It remains the most effective solution to date for this distressing and very difficult problem.

Heterotopic Ossification

Those patients at risk of heterotopic ossification (HO), the laying down of bone in tissues, should be identified preoperatively and some form of prophylaxis instituted. Risk factors include ankylosing spondylitis, previous acetabular or pelvic fracture, or previous problems with heterotopic ossification during THA on the contralateral hip.

Prophylaxis for this problem can be given with pharmacological means or radiation. Aspirin has been shown to be not effective in preventing HO, and most surgeons would now recommend indomethacin, which is the most studied nonsteroidal anti-inflammatory drug used for this purpose. One study showed that in 123 male patients undergoing primary THA, given a 10-day course of 25 mg Indomethacin three times daily, there was a 7.6% incidence of mild HO and no cases of Brooker grade III or IV compared to the normal quoted prevalence of 3 to 10% of patients who experience functional impairment in the form of diminished range of motion due to HO.

A randomized prospective study directly comparing 3×3.3 Gy of radiation with 150 mg of diclofenac for 3 weeks showed that radiation was slightly more effective than nonsteroidal anti-inflammatory tablets in reducing the incidence of HO, but that both were very effective. The dose of radiation that is effective at preventing HO has steadily decreased over the last 20 years, and now 0.7 Gy is shown to be effective.

If HO does occur after THA and it is symptomatic, with decreased range of motion after maturity (as determined by isotopic bone scan usually 6 months after surgery), the HO may be excised and the patient treated with postoperative radiation. Often a preoperative CT scan is helpful to document exactly where the HO is located, and an appropriate surgical approach can be used. With this regime an average increase of 45° flexion and 25° of abduction can be anticipated (Figure 17-22).

Infection

Treatment of an acute periprosthetic infection depends on the elapsed time since surgery. Acute infections occurring within 4 to 6 weeks of surgery, where the components are judged to be stable and there is no reaction in the surrounding bone, can be treated with thorough debridement of infected material, pulsatile lavage, and prolonged IV antibiotics, yielding a very high prosthesis retention rate (>95% depending on the infecting organism). The majority of organisms in early infection are staphylococcus, and the antibiotics of choice here are flucloxacillin combined with rifampicin.

In patients who sustain an infected THA more than 6 weeks after surgery, there is a greater chance of infected material having gained access to the prosthesis patient interface. This does not always equate with prosthetic loosening, but almost always necessitates removal of the prosthesis. Removal of the prosthetic components can be performed as a one- or two-stage revision procedure. The two-stage exchange remains the standard for treatment, with the first stage consisting of removal of all components and foreign material such as cement, cement restrictors and wires, meticulous extensive debridement, and accurate identification of the infecting organism. Use of an articulating spacer containing antibiotic to maintain tissue tension is becoming more popular, but even if not used, some form of antibiotic impregnated cement should be placed in the acetabulum and upper femoral canal.

Postoperative management consists of IV antibiotics for 2 to 4 weeks, followed by 2 to 4 weeks of oral antibiotics. Debate exists about whether the patient should undergo a period without antibiotic cover before reimplantation, and the value of hip aspiration to ensure no organisms are present prior to reimplantation. The patient's erythrocyte

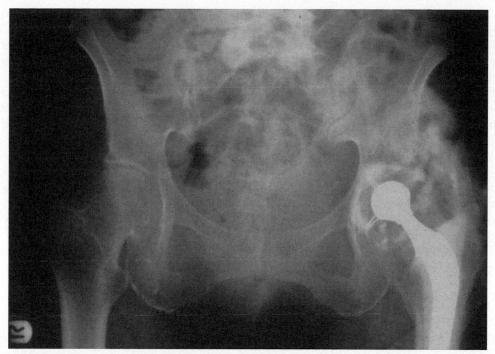

FIGURE 17-22. Anteroposterior radiograph of a 52-year-old patient involved in a motor vehicle accident. He sustained a displaced left femoral neck fracture and a severe head injury. Although admitted in an unconscious state with a Glasgow Coma Scale of 12, a CT scan of his head revealed no intracerebral lesion. A THA was performed on the night of admission to hospital. He remained intubated and unconscious in the intensive care unit for 13 days. Despite making a full neurological recovery, he developed severe heterotopic ossification around the left THA.

sedimentation rate and C-reactive protein should be close to normal before reimplantation, and this usually occurs 6 to 10 weeks following prosthesis removal. Reimplantation is usually performed with a cemented femoral component to allow further direct antibiotic delivery to the bone. Acetabular revision may be performed with a cemented or cementless component. Success rates for this procedure with a nonresistant organism exceed 95%.

Recent studies have supported selective use of a one-stage exchange, where the organism is considered of low virulence and responsive to antibiotic therapy, an adequate debridement can be achieved, and the patient's medical condition contraindicates further major surgery. Success rates in excess of 80% can be achieved when this approach is used in carefully selected cases.

Periprosthetic Fractures

The incidence of fractures around the femoral component of a THA, both intraoperative and postoperative, has been increasing over the last 20 years.

Intraoperative fractures are generally caused by the need to achieve good initial stability of porous-coated components. They are usually stable, involving a split in the femoral cortex, and can be treated by keeping the patient from weight bearing in the early post operative period. If an intraoperative fracture is identified as unstable, cerclage wires can be passed around the femur. Postoperative fractures are occurring due to an increase in the number of THAs, younger patients, increasing survival of the prosthesis in patients who are simultaneously loosing bone mass, and fractures through osteolytic lesions.

The Vancouver classification (A, B, C) for these fractures is based on the level of the fracture and stability of the femoral component. Type A_G is a fracture of the greater trochanter. Type A_L is a fracture of the lesser trochanter. Type A fractures are treated conservatively if stable and operatively if unstable. Type B fractures occur around the lower stem or tip of the prosthesis. Type B_1 includes fractures where the femoral component is solidly fixed. They are treated with plating or strut allografts. Type B_2 includes fractures where the femoral component is loose and are treated with revision of the loose femoral component to a long-stemmed prostheses, usually cementless, to bypass the fracture, and fixation of the fracture with wires or plates (Figure 17-23). Type B_3 fractures occur when there is severe underlying bone stock loss, and the femoral component is almost always loose (Figure 17-24). They are treated in a similar fashion to Type B_2 fractures, often with additional allograft. Type C fractures occur below the tip of the femoral stem and are treated independently of the prosthesis.

Nonunion of periprosthetic fractures is usually treated by revision to a long-stemmed porous-coated component, but treatment is difficult with a high rate of complications and a poor functional outcome.

Fractures of the acetabulum are less common than of the femur, and usually occur during insertion of a porous-coated component into an acetabulum that has been under-reamed by 1 to 2 mm to gain good initial stability. Fractures occur more frequently in women with osteopenic bone. If an intraoperative acetabular fracture is recognized, assessment of stability of both the fracture and the component is required. An unstable component requires removal. If the medial wall has been breached, over-reaming and a larger component with rim fit can achieve a good result. If a column fracture has occurred, it will need to be exposed and plated, followed by implantation of an acetabular cage or a larger diameter cup. If a fracture occurs but the cup appears stable, the situation can be accepted, and the fracture will usually heal, but the component has a higher chance of not achieving bony ingrowth, and thus requiring revision at a later date.

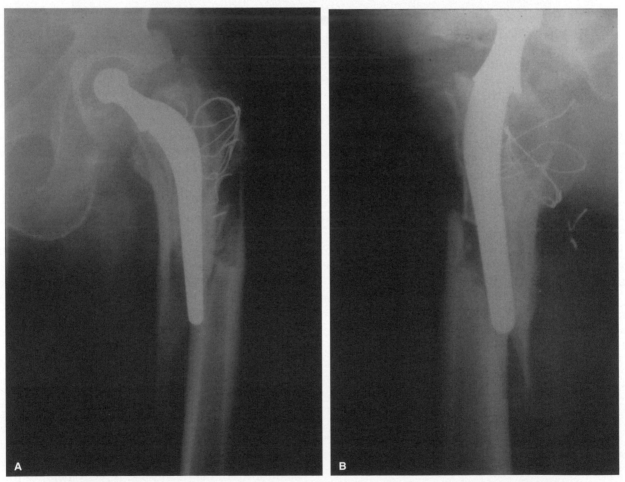

FIGURE 17-23. (A) Anteroposterior radiograph of a 61-year-old male who fell in the shower. This Charnley type THA had been in place for 18 years. **(B)** Lateral radiograph of the same patient. A loose prosthesis, associated with extensive osteolysis required revision of both the femoral stem and acetabular cup.

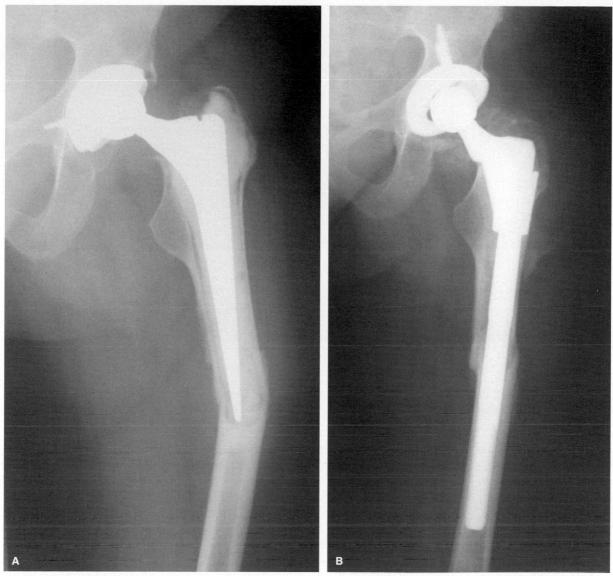

FIGURE 17-24. (A) Distal femoral fracture around a radiologically loose cemented THA that had been in place for 7 years. **(B)** At the time of operation, the cement was able to be easily removed from the proximal femur without disturbing the fracture site with any soft tissue exposure. A modular cementless stem bypassed the fracture and led to radiological healing at 10 weeks postoperatively.

Wear and Osteolysis

Improved fixation has led to emergence of other modes of failure in THA. Wear is the removal of material, with the generation of wear particles that occurs as the result of relative motion between two opposing surfaces under load. The mechanical consequences (mechanical thinning) of polyethylene wear have been recognized since the early 1970s when the first wear studies on THA suggested a limited life span of the polyethylene bearing. This concept was partly responsible for the development of modular acetabular components, which allowed exchange of the plastic liner without disturbance of the bone prosthesis interface (Figure 17-25).

Since the 1980s, it has been recognized that the clinical consequences of wear—the release of excessive wear particles into the biological environment—is the predominant cause of late failure of THA, and this still remains the case today. When particles within a certain size range are phagocytized in sufficient amounts by macrophages, they enter a state of activated metabolism, with the release of cytokines that result in periprosthetic bone

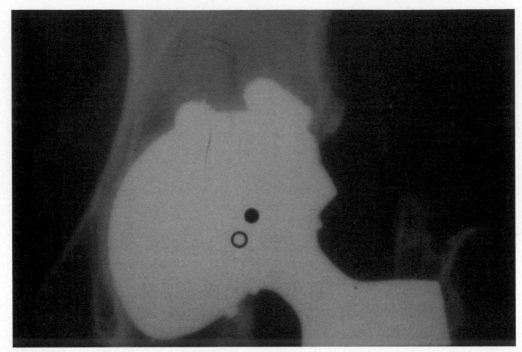

FIGURE 17-25. A marker has been placed on this radiograph of a PCA total hip arthroplasty to indicate both the initial and final position of the center of the femoral head. The prosthesis had been implanted $4\frac{1}{2}$ years previously. Most of this femoral head penetration was attributed to a small cup combined with a 32 mm femoral head leading to a polyethylene thickness of 7mm, and a suboptimal locking mechanism.

loss leading to eventual loosening and necessitating component revision (Figure 17-26). The concept of the effective joint space includes all areas of the joint that can be accessed by synovial fluid laden with wear particles. This includes all areas of the bone and prosthesis (cementless implants) and bone and cement (cemented implants) interfaces, which often extend far beyond the areas of capsular attachment associated with a nonreplaced hip. Synovial fluid can excite this response, leading to areas of osteolysis (focal areas of progressive periprosthetic bone loss) in locations removed from the primary articular surface (Figure 17-27).

Wear can be classified into two areas: wear mechanisms (adhesion, abrasion, and fatigue) and wear modes (conditions under which the prosthesis was functioning when the wear occurred). Adhesive wear occurs when two surfaces are bonded together under load, and material is pulled away from one or more surfaces when movement occurs between them. Abrasive wear is a mechanical process wherein asperities on the harder surface removes material form the softer surface. Fatigue occurs when local stresses exceed the strength of the material, causing it to fail, usually after a particular number of cycles. Bearing surfaces are designated

primary (intended to articulate) or secondary (not intended to move against any other material, whether this is the patient's bone or another component of the THA prosthesis).

Mode 1 wear occurs as a result of motion (which is intended to occur) between two primary bearing surfaces. Mode 2 wear occurs when a primary bearing surface moves against a secondary surface (dislocation). Mode 3 wear takes place when a third substance gains access between two primary bearing surfaces (often referred to as third body wear). Mode 4 wear occurs when two secondary bearing surfaces rub together, such as impingement of the femoral neck on the rim of the acetabular cup, motion of the prosthesis in the bone, or motion between modular connections of the femoral stem (morse taper fretting) or acetabular cup (back-side wear).

Surgeons choosing a particular primary THA system for implantation should evaluate all of these areas for that system carefully, because the type and incidence of wear modes for that prosthesis vary widely, a well as variation in when they occur over the service life of that prosthesis. In most primary THA, the greatest contribution to wear is from mode 1 wear—polyethylene particles generated from the primary bearing surface (Figure 17-28). Two types of

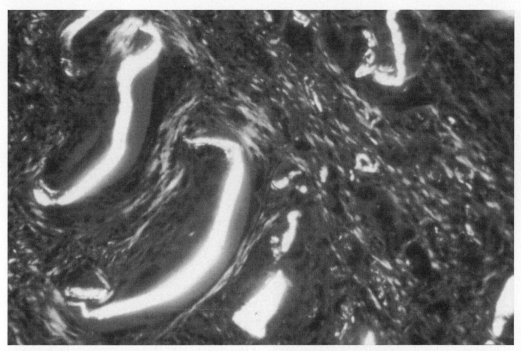

FIGURE 17-26. Low power microscopy (×250) of the tissue retrieved from an osteolytic granuloma at the time of revision surgery. The polyethylene particles in the tissues are easily identified under polarized light by their birefringence.

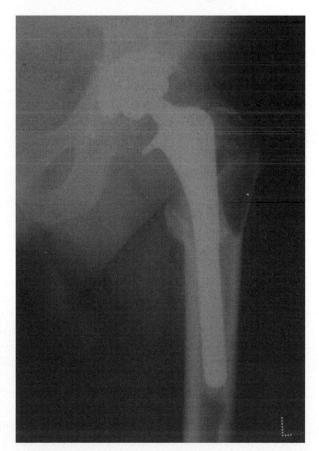

FIGURE 17-27. Despite very little visible wear appearing in the articulating surface of this Harris-Galante I total hip arthroplasty which had been implanted 5 years previously, a massive osteolytic lesion is seen extending from the greater trochanter down the lateral side of the femur. At the time of surgery, there was an impingement of the titanium femoral neck on the acetabular cup, which had generated much of the wear debris causing the osteolysis. Another source of wear in this case was titanium debris generated from a loose femoral component. There was no visible wear of the acetabular liner.

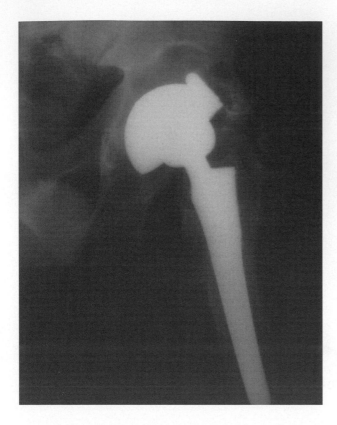

FIGURE 17-28. Wear from the primary bearing surface of this PCA total hip arthroplasty has contributed to the large osteolytic lesion seen in the superior quadrant of the acetabular component.

assessment for this are available: simulator studies and measurement from clinical radiographs.

Modern simulator studies of polyethylene wear now incorporate the critical fact that, in the hip as opposed to the knee, the path that a point on the femoral head makes within the polyethylene is multidirectional, and there are often crossing paths. Although this allows comparison of two bearing surfaces within the same simulator, many surgeons are skeptical that simulator wear studies can truly reproduce the in vivo situation under which a THA functions. Variables still to be fully understood include lubrication medium, presence of third body particles, temperature of the primary bearing surface, and loading (there is some recent radiologic evidence that the primary bearing surfaces of a THA dissociate by up to 1 mm during a normal gait cycle). Wear simulator results vary greatly but tend to show polyethylene wearing at a rate of 0.06–0.10 mm/million cycles. Historically one million cycles were taken to represent one year's wear, but a recent pedometer study shows variation between 0.4 to 4 million cycles/year among study patients.

Measurement from clinical radiographs assumes that a change in displacement of the femoral head between two radiographs taken at different times represents polyethylene wear. Calculation of volumetric polyethylene wear is then made on the basis of femoral head diameter and direction of displacement. Measurements are based on locating the center of the femoral head, and either measuring the shortest distance to the edge of the acetabular cup, or locating the center of the cup and measuring the difference between head and cup center. Radiostereometric analysis (RSA), originally developed for measurement of component migration, can be used if beads are prospectively implanted in the pelvis at the time of surgery, the acetabular cup has beads implanted, and a dedicated RSA setup for taking radiographs is available. It can only be used prospectively, and expense usually constrains numbers of subjects that can be recruited.

Retrospective measurements from clinical radiographs can be made by placing radiographs on a tablet and using a stylus to digitize points (manual method) or by taking points directly from the digital image of an radiograph (usually automated). Recent studies have shown good correlation between radiologic measurements and retrieved prostheses. Hips with linear wear rates of greater than 0.2 mm/year have been associated with an increased prevalence of osteolysis, while hips with linear wear less than 0.1 mm/year have infrequently been associated with osteolysis.

REVISION TOTAL HIP ARTHROPLASTY

There are multiple steps that need to be considered when performing the revision of a THA.

Step 1. Reason for Failure

The historical mode of failure of cemented femoral acetabular and femoral components was by aseptic loosening associated with mild or moderate osteolysis, and moderate or severe component migration. With the advent of modularity, hybrid THA, multiple revisions, porous-coated femoral and acetabular components, and alternate problems (fractured ceramic femoral heads), different modes of failure require different solutions to be applied. The primary philosophy is to achieve a solidly fixed, stable component with minimal bone loss (or bone restoration where necessary). The minimum surgery, carrying with it the minimum risk of complications to achieve this aim, is often the best solution.

Step 2. Which Components Need Revising

If a well-designed component with a good clinical track record is found to be solidly fixed at the time of revision surgery, and there is minimal evidence of wear of its primary bearing surface (or it can be replaced, as with a modular femoral head or modular acetabular cup), then consider retaining the component at the time of revision. This decision must also take into account ease of exposure (exposure of an acetabular defect around a solidly fixed femoral stem), leg length and tissue tension issues (increased risk of postoperative dislocation if neck length options are limited), and head size (a monoblock femoral stem with a femoral head diameter that cannot be matched to options available for the acetabular revision).

Revision for progressive periprosthetic osteolytic defects in the presence of well-fixed components often involves grafting of the defect with allograft, removal of screws from the cup, and downsizing the diameter of the primary bearing surface from 32 to 28 or less millimeters (to increase polyethylene thickness) by replacing the polyethylene liner (Figure 17-29). Increasing the neck length,

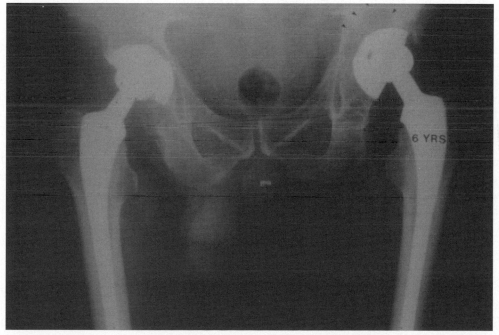

FIGURE 17-29. A large osteolytic lesion in the superior acetabulum, around a titanium grit-blasted acetabular component, caused by excessive mode 1 wear from a titanium femoral head articulating against polyethylene. Despite this cup having a reasonable track record and being stable at revision, the locking mechanism was nonfunctional after removal of the polyethylene liner. An intraoperative decision was made to revise the acetabular component, because cementing an appropriate sized polyethylene liner into the metal shell would have given a polyethylene thickness less than 8 mm.

to rectify poor tissue tension caused by the exposure (which can lead to an increased risk of dislocation), is often necessary.

Step 3. Assessment of Bony Defects

Bony defects of the femoral shaft can be assessed by good quality anteroposterior and lateral radiographs of the hip, as well as proximal femur beyond the tip of the femoral prosthesis. Defects are always more extensive than they appear on radiograph. Acetabular defects often require additional imaging, such as Judet views to assess the anterior and posterior columns, and occasionally CT if a pelvic dissociation (loss of bony continuity through both anterior and posterior columns) is suspected. If there is intrapelvic migration of the acetabular component, pelvic angiography to document the proximity of the iliac vessels is often required.

Step 4. What Acetabular Revision Components Are Required

Choice of acetabular revision components is often dictated by the experience, training and philosophy of the operating surgeon, and tempered by the extent of any bony defect (or other major structural consideration, such as pelvic dissociation) present. The most commonly used grading system for acetabular bone loss emphasizes the presence or absence of the acetabular rim, deficiencies of the acetabular dome and walls, and integrity of the anterior and posterior columns. Type I defects, with intact rims, walls, and columns, may be dealt with using cementless components with or without supplemental screw fixation, or cemented components using impaction grafting techniques. Twelve-year results of the Harris-Galante titanium fiber mesh socket used for revision of type I defects approach the 95% good or excellent results they enjoy in primary THA.

Type II defects have a distorted rim and wall, but an intact anterior and posterior column, and may be treated with a cementless acetabular component with supplementary screw fixation. Defects are filled with compacted allograft bone chips. If the major acetabular deficiency is superior, with minimal anterior or posterior column bone loss, a slightly higher hip center may be accepted to prevent over-reaming and sacrifice of good bone from the anterior and posterior columns.

Type III defects have a missing rim, the walls are severely compromised, and the columns offer no support. Two choices are present here—a very large ("jumbo") acetabular component (outer diameter greater than 66 mm) or an antiprotrusio cage. The guarded long-term prognosis of structural acetabular allografts (failure rates up to 50% at 10 years have been reported), and the difficulty and expense of supporting a dedicated structural allograft bone bank, have limited their use outside of dedicated hospital units. For most patients (elderly with a multiply revised hip and component migration) with a type III defect, the component of choice is either a jumbo or bilobed cup. Jumbo cups are a good option when there is a large central defect. The acetabular margin is reamed down to create a horseshoe-shaped lateral acetabular margin, and an oversized acetabular cup is then placed on this margin and held with multiple screws. The central defect can be allografted. Alternatively, if an oval defect is present and the surgeon wishes to restore the hip center to normal, a bilobed cup may be used.

In a younger patient with a type III defect, where bone stock preservation and restoration must be maximized to allow future procedures during that patient's lifetime, compacted allograft bone chips can be packed into defects (including structural allograft supplementation to prevent bone chip migration). If there is likely to be less than 50% contact between host bone and the acetabular prosthesis, an antiprotrusio cage should be used. This is attached to the ilium ischium and pubis, overcoming problems with column or medial wall deficiency. Bypassing of the acetabulum allows load sharing to occur with underlying allograft, encouraging its incorporation for restoration of bone stock. A polyethylene acetabular socket is then cemented into the cage. Care should be taken with component orientation, because bony landmarks that can usually be identified will no longer be available (Figure 17-30).

Pelvic discontinuity cannot always be predicted preoperatively, but where there are major column defects and acetabular component migration, it should be suspected, and appropriate component inventory for intraoperative treatment of discontinuity should be available. Three choices are available:

1. Stabilization with a pelvic reconstruction plate along the posterior column, followed by a cementless acetabular component. This is most commonly used where a posterior column fracture has occurred (often during

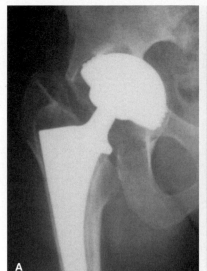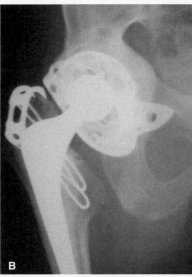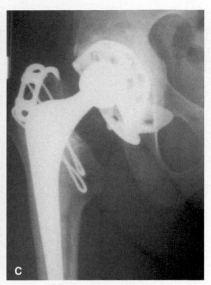

FIGURE 17-30. (A) Radiograph of the right hip of a 31-year-old female patient with rheumatoid arthritis who had a THA with a threaded type acetabular component 6 years previously. She presented with increasing groin pain after a minor stumble. A pelvic dissociation was assumed. **(B)** At the time of revision, the radiological diagnosis of a pelvic dissociation was confirmed. When a young patient is being treated for revision THA, the emphasis is always on bone stock preservation. For this reason, an acetabular cage into which was cemented a polyethylene component was chosen as the implant of choice. This allowed a large amount of morselized bone allograft (two femoral heads) to be placed medial to the cage. **(C)** An 8-year postoperative radiograph shows incorporation of the medial morselized allograft. Currently the patient is pain free with a stable construct. If this reconstruction fails, a press-fit acetabular cup will be the procedure of first choice.

extraction of a well-fixed component), but there is sufficient posterior column bone to obtain stable fixation.

2. Bypassing the discontinuity using an antiprotrusio cage with stable fixation proximally into the ilium and distally into the ischium.

3. Use of a jumbo cup. If the metal shell of the cup is thick enough in the acetabular system chosen, the screws placed through the cup will only travel in one direction, perpendicularly away from the cup center. This greatly enhances fixation of the two mobile pelvic bones by the cup, and if careful screw placement is selected, allows a very stable construct without a supplemental posterior column plate (Figure 17-31).

Step 5. What Femoral Revision Components Are Required

Selection of an appropriate revision femoral component should take into account any difficulties with potential femoral fractures, cortical windows, or extended femoral osteotomies that might be encountered during extraction of the existing implant. Well-fixed cemented and cementless stems may be difficult to remove, and vigorous extraction attempts that might lead to bony fracture should be avoided (Figure 17-32). Cemented implants should be initially removed from the cement mantle. A decision can then be made as to whether the cement can be removed from the canal proximally, or whether a distal cortical window will be required. An extended femoral osteotomy may be performed if there is varus femoral remodeling. Most well-fixed cementless femoral implants have to be removed using thin power instruments to divide the areas of bone where ingrowth has occurred into the porous-coated surfaces of the prosthesis.

Cemented femoral revision relies on interdigitation between the cement and the bone for a mechanically durable interface. The loss of cancellous bone seen at revision surgery compromises this interdigitation. Although the 10-year results of cemented femoral revisions have an 80 to 85% prosthesis survival, improved cementless prosthesis design has decreased the role of cemented femoral revision.

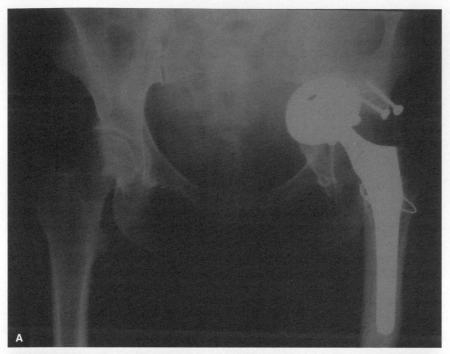

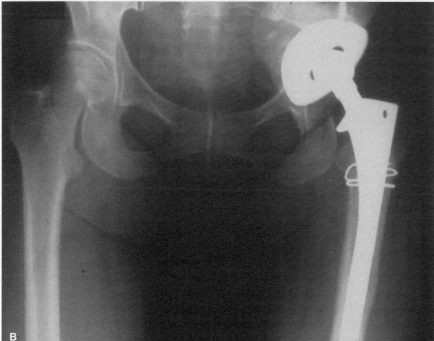

FIGURE 17-31. (A) This loose uncemented acetabular component has eroded through into the pelvis, and caused disruption of both anterior and posterior acetabular columns. **(B)** Morselized allograft femoral head is used to fill the lesion. A 70 mm diameter acetabular cup with multiple screws (inferior screws placed into ischium are hidden by the bulk of the cup) was then used to stabilize the pelvic dissociation.

Occasionally, it will be necessary to change a well-fixed cemented femoral component due to unusual head size, or leg length issues. If the cement mantle is radiologically intact, another component may be cemented into the intact cement mantle without its removal, with good medium-term (5 to 7 year) results.

Cementless femoral revision has become increasingly popular as it provides a stable initial construct and has good long-term results. Proximal porous-coated implants provide the theoretical advantage of biologic fixation with a minimum of stress shielding (loss of bone from the proximal femur when it is not loaded). This benefit is outweighed by the

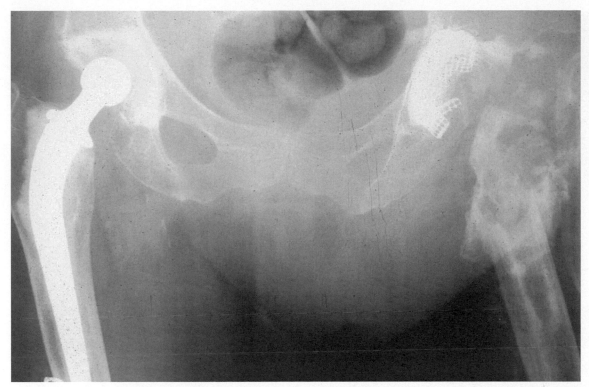

FIGURE 17-32. Severe destruction of the proximal femur and pelvis, following removal of a cemented THA. The patient had undergone six previous THAs.

disadvantage of obtaining initial stability and long-term fixation in the damaged proximal femur, and their use in the revision setting is limited.

The most popular method for femoral revision is bypassing the damaged proximal bone using diaphyseal fixation. Most femoral stems designed for diaphyseal fixation are either extensively porous-coated devices with a cylindrical distal shape, or grit-blasted fluted devices with a conical distal shape. Titanium stems have a lower modulus of elasticity to potentially reduce stress shielding, but cannot be fully porous coated because notch sensitivity reduces their strength, increasing the risk of stem fracture. The stress shielding associated with diaphyseal fixation has not yet become a major clinical problem, but concern remains about extraction of an extensively porous-coated device.

Step 6. Which Surgical Approach Should Be Used

There is little literature suggesting the best surgical approach to employ in revision surgery. The posterior approach makes an extensile exposure of the femoral shaft easier, but, as in primary THA, suffers from a higher dislocation rate. If an anterior approach has been used previously, there is no contraindication to using a posterior approach for revision, and the converse also applies.

A trochanteric osteotomy may be required if extensive exposure of an anterior or posterior column deficiency is required, such as when an antiprotrusio cage is used. A recent advance in revision surgery has been the extended greater trochanteric osteotomy, where in the greater trochanter and the lateral third of the circumference of the femur are raised as a flap, with their soft tissues still attached, for approximately 10 cm down the femoral shaft (Figure 17-33). As well as good acetabular exposure, it has the advantage of facilitating removal of well-fixed cemented and cementless implants in a bone sparing manner. Indications include:

1. Trochanteric overhang above the prosthesis, increasing the risk of fracture during device extraction.
2. Removal of a well-fixed large amount cement in the femoral canal.

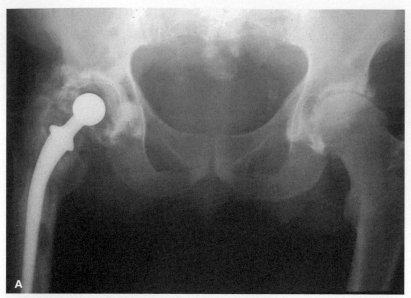

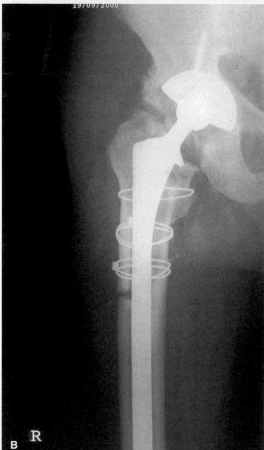

FIGURE 17-33. (A) This Stanmore THA had been implanted 16 years previously. The patient presented with pain, severe stiffness, and a limp. He weighed 270 pounds. **(B)** An extended trochanteric osteotomy through a direct lateral approach gave excellent exposure of the acetabulum, and allowed easy cement removal from the shaft. It was repaired with three cables, and the patient kept touch weight bearing for 6 weeks postoperatively.

3. Removal of extensively porous-coated solidly fixed cementless femoral stem.
4. Varus remodeling of the proximal femur such that placement of a long straight stemmed femoral component would predispose a fracture.

Step 7. What Fixation Method Should Be Used

The vast majority of femoral and acetabular revisions currently use cementless fixation of both the acetabular and femoral components. A technique popularized by the Exeter group has used an alternative for many years with good medium-term clinical results—impaction grafting with cement. This method seeks to restore cancellous structure to the femoral canal using densely packing cancellous bone chips. These bone chips are packed tightly enough to provide axial and rotational stability to a femoral stem when it is cemented into them. Technical difficulty has limited its use, however, with many centers reporting a high incidence of femoral fracture and component subsidence. Ten-year results from the center that initiated the technique have recently been published, but until long-term results show a definite improvement over cementless femoral revision with regards to restoration of bone stock, its use will remain limited to a few dedicated revision centers.

Step 8. What Is the Role of Allograft and Tumor Prostheses in Femoral Revision

These constructs are required if there is severe segmental proximal femoral bone loss that is inadequate to provide initial stability for conventional revision femoral stems. Allograft prosthetic composites, where the prosthesis is cemented into the allograft and has a porous-coated surface for bony ingrowth of host bone where available, allows better soft tissue attachment than does an all-metal tumor prosthesis. A tumor prosthesis is reserved for the older low-demand patients who need a faster operation and earlier weight-bearing mobilization.

Allograft prosthetic composite results in the medium term have been good, but there remains a high rate of dislocation and infection. Healing of the allograft-host bone junction usually requires 3 to 6 months of protected weight bearing. Segmental allografts remain largely avascular, with a zone of revascularization only extending for 1 to 2 cm into the allograft from the junction with host bone. Greater trochanteric union to an allograft with a stable fibrous or bony interface occurs in approximately 70% of cases.

Annotated Bibliography

Alberton GM, High WA, Morrey BF. Dislocation after revision total hip arthroplasty: an analysis of risk factors and treatment options. J Bone Joint Surg 2002;84A(10):1788–1792.
A database of 1,548 patients was evaluated for the risk factors leading to instability after revision THA. The expected outcome of various treatment strategies is discussed.

Amstutz HC, Grigoris P. Metal on metal bearings in hip arthroplasty. Clin Orthop 1996;329(Suppl):S11–34.
Very comprehensive overview of the current state of metal-on-metal bearings, including a historical review.

Amstutz HC, Grigoris P, Dorey FJ. Evolution and future of surface replacement of the hip. J Orthop Sci 1998;3(3):169–186.
Surface replacement is now much improved with instrumentation for nontrochanteric osteotomy approaches and off-the-shelf components in 1 mm increments. For arthritic hips, a new era of surface replacement has emerged. With metal-on-metal bearings, the volumetric wear has been reduced 20–100 times from those with polyethylene, and there is no penalty for the large ball size. The devices are now conservative on the acetabular as well as femoral side. Hybrid or all-cementless fixation is superior to earlier all-cemented devices.

Aydingoz U, Ozturk MH. MR imaging of the acetabular labrum: a comparative study of both hips in 180 asymptomatic volunteers. Eur Radiol 2001;11(4)567–574.
The aim of this study was to determine the MR imaging characteristics of normal acetabular labra on both hips. The most common labrum shape was triangular, whereas absence of labrum was the least common condition. A difference of labral shapes between both hips was present in approximately 15% of volunteers. A size difference of over 25% between each labrum was noted in approximately one-fourth of 180 volunteers.

Baber YF, Robinson AH, Villar RN. Is diagnostic arthroscopy of the hip worthwhile? a prospective review of 328 adults investigated for hip pain. J Bone Joint Surg 1999;81B(4):600–603.
Arthroscopy altered the diagnosis in 176 hips (53%). The new primary diagnoses were osteoarthritis (75 patients), osteochondral defects (34), torn labra (23), synovitis (11), and loose bodies (9). In 172 hips (52%), an operative procedure was undertaken.

Barrack RL, Paprosky W, Butler RA et al. Patients' perception of pain after total hip arthroplasty. J Arthroplasty 2000;15(5): 590–596.
Type of stem fixation was the only parameter statistically correlated with a higher incidence of thigh pain. Patients with proximally-coated stems were more than twice as likely to complain of pain than patients with fully coated or cemented hips.

Berger RA, Jacobs JJ, Quigley LR et al. Primary cementless acetabular reconstruction in patients younger than 50 years old. 7- to 11-year results. Clin Orthop 1997;344:216–226.
During this study, two stable acetabular reconstructions were revised during femoral revision. Two excessively worn polyethylene liners were exchanged and one acetabular osteolytic area was debrided and grafted; these procedures retained the metal shell. At final follow-up, all 72 acetabular reconstructions were radiographically stable. Acetabular osteolysis occurred in five cases (7.4%), from 84 to 104 months.

Berry DJ. Unstable total hip arthroplasty: detailed overview. Instr Course Lect 2001;50:265–274.
Early postoperative dislocations and first or second dislocations usually are treated with closed reduction and a hip guide brace or hip spica cast, but when dislocation becomes recurrent, surgical treatment usually is needed. When possible, surgical treatment is based on identifying and treating a specific problem leading to the dislocation,

Berry DJ, Lewallen DG, Hanssen AD et al. Pelvic discontinuity in revision total hip arthroplasty. J Bone Joint Surg 1999; 81A(12):1692–1702.
Twenty-seven patients (31 hips) with a pelvic discontinuity are described. Twenty-seven were reconstructed in an attempt to obtain a stable construct, often supplemental plate fixation of the posterior column. Nine of the 27 reconstructions required a further operation, showing just what a difficult problem this can be to treat.

Bobyn JD, Jacobs JJ, Tanzer M et al. The susceptibility of smooth implant surfaces to periimplant fibrosis and migration of polyethylene wear debris. Clin Orthop 1995;311:21–39.
A landmark paper where an animal model of a femoral stem implant showed that non circumferentially coated implants allow access of wear debris to the distal femur, causing osteolysis.

Bourne RB, Rorabeck CH, Skutek M et al. The Harris Design-2 total hip replacement fixed with so-called second-generation cementing techniques: a ten to fifteen-year follow-up. J Bone Joint Surg 1998;80A(12):1775–1780.

Excellent results were achieved with second generation cementing technique, where 186 of 195 acetabular cups were still in situ at 12 years.

Brand RA, Yack HJ. Effects of leg length discrepancies on the forces at the hip joint. Clin Orthop 1996;333:172–180.
An experimental study to determine if the slight lengthening (<2cm) often associated with THA altered forces across a replaced hip. On the side of the replaced hip, mean peak intersegmental resultant hip forces were actually decreased by 6 to 12%.

Callaghan JJ, Forest EE, Olejniczak JP et al. Charnley total hip arthroplasty in patients less than fifty years old: a twenty to twenty-five-year follow-up note. J Bone Joint Surg 1998; 80A(5):704–714.
Seventy of the 72 hips in the living patients were followed radiographically for at least 20 years. Twenty-seven hips (29%) had a revision or a resection of the prosthesis during the follow-up period. Eighteen acetabular components (19%) and 5 femoral components (5%) were revised because of aseptic loosening, and an additional 14 acetabular components (15%) and 7 femoral components (8%) demonstrated definite or probable radiographic loosening. This landmark study demonstrates the long-term durability of total hip arthroplasty performed with cement in an active population of patients, but demonstrated that long-term fixation of a cemented acetabular prosthesis remains the weak link.

Clohisy JC, Harris WH. The Harris-Galante porous-coated acetabular component with screw fixation: an average ten-year follow-up study. J Bone Joint Surg 1999;81A(1):66–73.
One hundred and ninety-six hips in 177 patients were followed up at a mean of 122 months (range, 84 to 155 months). The average age of these 177 patients at the time of the operation was 59 years (range, 23 to 87 years). Eight well-fixed acetabular shells (4%) were revised: 3 were revised because of dissociation of the liner in association with fractures of the tines, 3 were revised during revision of the femoral component, and 2 were revised because of retroacetabular osteolysis. In 8 other hips, the acetabular liner was exchanged during revision of a loose femoral component. These 10-year results of a cementless acetabular component equal or better those of a cemented acetabular component.

Dearborn JT, Harris WH. Postoperative mortality after total hip arthroplasty: an analysis of deaths after two thousand seven hundred and thirty-six procedures. J Bone Joint Surg 1998; 80A(9):1291–1294.
A retrospective review of mortality as many as 90 days after 2,736 primary and revision total hip arthroplasties performed in 2,002 patients by one surgeon at a teaching hospital. All but 71 of the patients had received prophylaxis against venous thromboembolic disease. There were no intra-operative deaths, and no events during the operation could be linked directly to postoperative mortality. Eight deaths (mortality rate, 0.3%) occurred within 90 days after the 2,736 procedures. Four deaths (mortality rate, 0.15%) occurred during the initial hospitalization.

Demos HA, Rorabeck CH, Bourne RB et al. Instability in primary total hip arthroplasty with the direct lateral approach. Clin Orthop 2001;393:168–180.
One thousand five hundred and fifteen primary total hip arthroplasties done via a direct lateral approach were reviewed. At the most recent examination, 11.6% of the patients had a moderate or severe limp and 2.5% had severe heterotopic ossification. Only six hips (0.4%) had a dislocation or episode of instability. Three patients had more than one dislocation and required revision surgery.

Dowd JE, Sychterz CJ, Young AM et al. Characterization of long-term femoral-head-penetration rates: association with and prediction of osteolysis. J Bone Joint Surg 2000;82A(8):1102–1107.
Polyethylene wear of 48 hips was measured. The true wear rate averaged 0.18 mm per year (range, 0.01 to 0.44 mm per year). Osteolysis at 10 years was strongly associated with increasing true wear rates (p < 0.001). Osteolysis did not develop in any of the nine hips with a true wear rate of less than 0.1 millimeter per year. However,

osteolysis developed in 9 (43%) of 21 hips with a rate between 0.1 and less than 0.2 millimeter per year, in 8 of 10 hips with a rate between 0.2 and 0.3 millimeter per year, and in all 8 hips with a rate of greater than 0.3 millimeter per year.

Eggli S, Hankemayer S, Muller ME. Nerve palsy after leg lengthening in total replacement arthroplasty for developmental dysplasia of the hip. J Bone Joint Surg 1999;81B(5):843–845.
In 508 THA for dysplasia, there were 8 nerve palsy's (2 femoral, 6 sciatic), 2 complete and 6 incomplete. No statistical correlation between the amount of lengthening and the incidence of nerve damage was found (p = 0.47), but in 7 of the 8 hips, the surgeon had rated the intervention as difficult because of previous surgery, severe deformity, a defect of the acetabular roof, or considerable flexion deformity.

Engh CA, Hooten JP, Zettl-Schaffer KF et al. Evaluation of bone ingrowth in proximally and extensively porous-coated anatomic medullary locking prostheses retrieved at autopsy. J Bone Joint Surg 1995;77A(6):903–910.
Three proximally (40%) and 5 extensively (80%) porous-coated anatomic medullary locking femoral components were retrieved from 7 cadavers at autopsy. All 8 components had some bone growth into the porous space. A mean of 35% of the surface of the implants had bone ingrowth. In the areas where bone was present, 67% of the available porous space on the extensively coated stems and 74% on the proximally coated stems contained bone.

Ganz R, Gill TJ, Gautier E et al. Surgical dislocation of the adult hip a technique with full access to the femoral head and acetabulum without the risk of avascular necrosis. J Bone Joint Surg 2001;83B(8):1119–1124.
A technique is described for operative dislocation of the hip, based on detailed anatomical studies of the blood supply. It combines aspects of approaches that have been reported previously and consists of an anterior dislocation through a posterior approach with a "trochanteric flip" osteotomy. The external rotator muscles are not divided and the medial femoral circumflex artery is protected by the intact obturator externus. It allows the treatment of a variety of conditions, which may not respond well to other methods including arthroscopy.

Gross AE. Revision arthroplasty of the acetabulum with restoration of bone stock. Clin Orthop 1999;369:198–207.
A detailed discussion of acetabular defects and their treatment with allografts. Surgical technique is evaluated, and the results of the author's vast clinical experience in this area is presented.

Haddad FS, Garbuz DS, Masri BA, et al. Structural proximal femoral allografts for failed total hip replacements: a minimum review of five years. J Bone Joint Surg 2000;82B(6):830–836.
A series of 40 proximal femoral allografts performed for failed total hip replacements with a minimum follow-up of 5 years is analyzed. In all cases the stem was cemented into both the allograft and the host femur. The proximal femur of the host was resected in 37 cases. There were four early revisions (10%), two for infection, one for nonunion of the allograft-host junction, and one for allograft resorption noted at the time of revision of a failed acetabular reconstruction. Junctional nonunion was seen in three patients (8%), two of whom were managed successfully by bone grafting, and bone grafting and plating respectively. Instability was observed in four (10%). Trochanteric nonunion was seen in 18 patients (46%) and trochanteric escape in 10 of these (27%). Although a high radiological complication rate, these results are good when severity of the cases is considered.

Jacobs JJ, Skipor AK, Patterson LM et al. M etal release in patients who have had a primary total hip arthroplasty: a prospective, controlled, longitudinal study. J Bone Joint Surg 1998;80A(10):1447–1458.
This study showed that, 36 months postoperatively, patients who have a well functioning prosthesis with components containing titanium have as much as a threefold increase in the concentration of titanium in the serum and those who have a well functioning prosthesis with cobalt-alloy components have as much as a fivefold and

an eightfold increase in the concentrations of chromium in the serum and urine, respectively. The predominant source of the disseminated chromium-degradation products is probably the modular head-neck junction and may be a function of the geometry of the coupling. Passive dissolution of extensively porous-coated cobalt-alloy stems was not found to be a dominant mode of metal release.

Katz RP, Callaghan JJ, Sullivan PM et al. Long-term results of revision total hip arthroplasty with improved cementing technique. J Bone Joint Surg1997;79B(2):322–326.
Eighty one consecutive cemented revision THA using improved cementing techniques were analyzed. The average age of the patients at revision was 63.7 years. At the final follow-up 18 hips (22%) had had a reoperation, two (2.5%) for sepsis, three (4%) for dislocation and 13 (16%) for aseptic loosening. The incidence of rerevision for aseptic femoral loosening was 5.4% and for aseptic acetabular loosening 16%. These results confirm that cemented femoral revision is a durable option in revision hip surgery when improved cementing techniques are used, but that cemented acetabular revision is unsatisfactory.

Kelley, SS, Lachiewicz PF, Hickman JM et al. Relationship of femoral head and acetabular size to the prevalence of dislocation. Clin Orthop 1998;355:163–170.
Femoral head size (22 mm) and acetabular component outer diameter (≥56 mm) were found to increase the risk of dislocation.

Longjohn, D, Dorr LD. Soft tissue balance of the hip. J Arthroplasty 1998;13(1):97–100.
Release of static and dynamic contractures around the hip provides significant immediate benefits for the patient and accelerates postoperative rehabilitation. Knee pain is decreased, groin pain is eliminated, range of motion of the hip is increased, and functional leg length difference is reduced. This article emphasizes the importance of techniques used to ensure soft tissue balance.

Maloney WJ, Herzwurm P, Paprosky W et al. Treatment of pelvic osteolysis associated with a stable acetabular component inserted without cement as part of a total hip replacement. J Bone Joint Surg 1997;79A(11):1628–1634.
Thirty-five patients who had had a primary total hip replacement with a porous-coated acetabular component inserted without cement had a revision procedure to treat pelvic osteolysis. The metal shell was left in place and the acetabular liner was exchanged in all 35 patients. The osteolytic lesions were debrided, and 35 of the 46 lesions were filled with allograft bone chips. Evaluation at a minimum of 2 years (range, 2 to 5 years; mean, 3.3 years) after the revision operation, showed all 35 sockets were found to be radiographically stable.

Mulroy WF, Harris WH Revision total hip arthroplasty with use of so-called second-generation cementing techniques for aseptic loosening of the femoral component: a fifteen-year-average follow-up study. J Bone Joint Surg 1996;78A(3):325–330.
Thirty-five hips had revision of the femoral component with so-called second generation cementing technique. At an average duration of follow-up of 15.1 years, seven (20%) had a repeat revision of the femoral component because of aseptic loosening. These results support the concept that so-called second-generation cementing techniques have decreased the prevalence of aseptic loosening after femoral revision.

Nakamura S, Ninomiya S, Takatori Y et al. Long-term outcome of rotational acetabular osteotomy: 145 hips followed for 10-23 years. Acta Orthop Scand 1998;69(3):259–265.
The long-term outcome of rotational acetabular osteotomy in 145 dysplastic hips of 131 patients after an average follow-up of 13 (10 to 23) years is presented. The long-term outcome of rotational acetabular osteotomy was satisfactory for a dysplastic hip with little, if any, osteoarthrosis, but was unsatisfactory for a hip with more advanced osteoarthrosis.

Paprosky WG, Perona PG, Lawrence JM. Acetabular defect classification and surgical reconstruction in revision arthroplasty: a 6-year follow-up evaluation. J Arthroplasty 1994;9(1):33–44.
One hundred and forty-seven cemented acetabular components were revised with cementless hemispheric press-fit components, with an average follow-up period of 5.7 years (range, 3 to 9 years). Acetabular defects were typed from 1 to 3 and reconstructed with a bulk or support allograft. Classification of the defects allows appropriate surgical treatment. The results of treatment of each defect type are presented.

Parvizi J, Johnson BG, Rowland C, et al. Thirty-day mortality after elective total hip arthroplasty. J Bone Joint Surg 2001; 83A(10):1524–1528.
Factors that are associated with an increased risk of mortality within 30 days after elective hip arthroplasty include an older age, male gender, and a history of cardiorespiratory disease. There has been a significant decline in the 30-day mortality rate after elective hip arthroplasty in the last decade (p < 0.0002).

Pellicci PM, Bostrom M, Poss R. Posterior approach to total hip replacement using enhanced posterior soft tissue repair. Clin Orthop 1998;355:224–228.
The two senior authors independently began using an identical enhanced posterior soft tissue repair after total hip replacement through a posterior approach. In the first author's experience, a dislocation rate of 4% in 395 patients before using the enhanced closure was reduced to 0% in 395 patients in whom the enhanced closure was performed. In the second author's experience, 160 total hip replacements had a dislocation rate of 6.2% before the enhanced closure whereas 124 total hip replacements had a dislocation rate of 0.8% after the enhanced closure.

Ritter MA. The cemented acetabular component of a total hip replacement: all polyethylene versus metal backing. Clin Orthop 1995;311:69–75.
All-polyethylene total hip replacements demonstrated statistically improved survival rates as compared with the metal-backed acetabular components.

Schmalzried TP, Shepherd EF, Dorey FJ et al. The John Charnley Award: wear is a function of use, not time. Clin Orthop 2000;381:36–46.
Polyethylene wear in 37 hip replacements was measured. Patient activity was assessed with a pedometer, a step activity monitor, and a simple visual analog scale. Joint use was related to wear at the 90% confidence level. Without three recognized outliers, wear was highly correlated to use.

Schmalzried TP, Noordin S, Amstutz HC. Update on nerve palsy associated with total hip replacement. Clin Orthop 1997;344: 188–206.
Overall prevalence of nerve palsy following THA is approximately 1%. The sciatic nerve, or the peroneal division of the sciatic nerve, is involved in nearly 80% of cases. The risk of nerve palsy in association with total hip replacement is increased for female compared with male patients, with a diagnosis of developmental dysplasia, and with patients undergoing revision surgery.

Schmalzried TP, Callaghan JJ. Current concepts review wear in total hip and knee replacements. J Bone Joint Surg 1999; 81A(1):115–136.
This article is a very comprehensive review of the current literature concerning wear of the primary bearing surface in THA.

Shanbhag AS, Hasselman CT, Rubash HE. The John Charnley Award: inhibition of wear debris mediated osteolysis in a canine total hip arthroplasty model. Clin Orthop 1997;344:33–43.
Oral bisphosphonate therapy was found to significantly inhibit wear debris mediated bone resorption when evaluated in a canine total hip replacement model.

Sotereanos DG, Plakseychik AY, Rubash HE. Free vascularized fibula grafting for the treatment of osteonecrosis of the femoral head. Clin Orthop Rel Res 1997;344:243–256.
Eighty-eight hips that received free vascularized fibula grafting for treatment of osteonecrosis of the femoral head are described. The hip survival rate for subgroups at 5.5 years was 100% for stages IC and IIA, 94% for stage IIB, 50% for stage IIC, 80% for stage IIIB, 58% for stage IIIC, 72% for stage IVA, and 58% for stage IVB.

Strathy GM, Fitzgerald RHJ. Total hip arthroplasty in the anky-losed hip: a ten-year follow-up. J Bone Joint Surg 1988;70A(7): 963–966.
Failure of the total hip arthroplasty performed for an ankylosed hip was more common (p < 0.05) in the patients who had had a previous surgical attempt at arthrodesis and in the patients who were 50 years old or less at the time of the arthroplasty.

Tonnis D, Heinecke, A. Current concepts review: acetabular and femoral anteversion: relationship with osteoarthritis of the hip. J Bone Joint Surg 1999;81A(12):1747–1770.
A clinical and theoretical examination of why osteoarthritis occurs in hips of a certain geometry is presented.

Trousdale RT, Ekkernkamp A, Ganz R et al. Periacetabular and intertrochanteric osteotomy for the treatment of osteoarthrosis in dysplastic hips. J Bone Joint Surg 1995;77A(1):73–85.
Forty-two patients who underwent a periacetabular with or without an intertrochanteric femoral osteotomy for dysplastic hips. Mean age was 37 years (11 to 57 years). At mean follow-up of 4 years, six patients had a subsequent total hip arthroplasty and three patients had an additional intertrochanteric osteotomy. Five of the nine patients who had a second major operation had had grade-3 osteoarthrosis before the periacetabular osteotomy.

Urbaniak JR, Coogan PG, Gunneson EB et al. Treatment of osteonecrosis of the femoral head with free vascularized fibular grafting: a long-term follow-up study of one hundred and three hips. J Bone Joint Surg 1995;77A(5):681–694.
The results for 103 consecutive hips (89 patients) that had been treated with free vascularized fibular grafting because of symptomatic osteonecrosis of the femoral head were reviewed in a prospective study. By the time of the most recent follow-up evaluation (minimum 5 years), a total arthroplasty had been performed in 31 hips.

Wroblewski BM, Siney PD, Fleming PA. Charnley low-frictional torque arthroplasty in patients under the age of 51 years: follow-up to 33 years. J Bone Joint Surg 2002;84B(4):540–543.
A group of 1,092 patients under the age of 51 years at the time of surgery, underwent 1,434 primary Charnley low-frictional torque arthroplasties and were followed up indefinitely. The mean follow-up was 15 years (11 to 33 years). The incidence of deep infection for the whole group was 1.67%. The indication for revision was aseptic loosening of the cup (11.7%), aseptic loosening of the stem (4.9%), a fractured stem (1.7%), deep infection (1.5%), and dislocation (0.4%).

Younger TI, Bradford MS, Magnus RE et al. Extended proximal femoral osteotomy: a new technique for femoral revision arthroplasty. J Arthroplasty 1995;10(3):329–338.
An osteotomy technique for removal of distally fixed cemented and cementless femoral components is described. The anterolateral proximal femur is cut for one-third of its circumference, extended distally, and levered open on an anterolateral hinge of periosteum and muscle. This creates an intact muscle-osseous sleeve composed of the gluteus medius, greater trochanter, anterolateral femoral diaphysis, and vastus lateralis, and exposes the fixation surface as well as distal cement. The first 20 patients treated with this technique are reviewed.

18

Hyun Woo Kim
Hui Wan Park

The Pediatric Leg and Knee

CONGENITAL SUBLUXATION
AND DISLOCATION OF THE
KNEE
CONGENITAL DISLOCATION
OF THE PATELLA
PHYSIOLOGIC GENU VARUM
AND VALGUM
TIBIA VARA (BLOUNT'S
DISEASE)
CONGENITAL POSTEROMEDIAL
BOWING OF THE TIBIA

CONGENITAL
PSEUDOARTHROSIS OF THE
TIBIA
CONGENITAL FIBULAR
HEMIMELIA
DISCOID MENISCUS
OSTEOCHONDRITIS
DISSECANS OF THE KNEE
OSGOOD-SCHLATTER DISEASE
PATELLAR LESIONS

PATELLOFEMORAL PAIN
SYNDROME
RECURRENT PATELLAR
SUBLUXATION AND
DISLOCAITON
TRAUMA
LIGAMENTOUS INJURY

Problems of the leg and knee are probably the most common and obvious abnormalities to affect the child's lower extremities. Trauma is the major concern; however, the understanding of other congenital or acquired deformities is important to minimize or prevent the long-term sequelae in later life. Some of the deformities are *physiologic* and periodic observation and reassurance of the parents that the *deformity* is a variant of normal but not a disease. In this chapter, the various physiologic and pathologic conditions affecting the leg and knee are discussed, and the trauma affecting the physis and impacting on both the growth and development of the child's leg and knee are also addressed.

CONGENITAL SUBLUXATION AND DISLOCATION OF THE KNEE

Congenital subluxation or dislocation of the knee presents as recurvatum and is evident at birth. The incidence is approximately 1% of the incidence of congenital dislocation of the hip. It may be an isolated entity or may occur with associated problems, such as dislocated hips, clubfoot, myelodysplasia, Larsen's syndrome, or arthrogryposis (Figure 18-1). Special attention must be paid to the hip joint because approximately 50% of children have congenital dislocation of the hip. Several terminologies have been used in describing congenital hyperextension of the knee, a descriptive term indicating recurvatum of the knees at birth. Hyperextension of the knee in newborn infants may be caused by aberrations in intrauterine positions, such as the frank breech position, which slowly stretches the hamstrings and soft tissues of the posterior aspect of the knee. Fibrosis of the quadriceps mechanism is generally believed to be secondary to the dislocation rather than its cause. At least half of all babies presenting with this clinical appearance have some passive knee flexion at birth, and the severity of the deformity is variable.

Routine lateral radiographs identify the femoral–tibial relationship. In type I, hyperextension is minimal, and the knee can passively be flexed to 90°. In type II, or moderate type, in which there is subluxation of the tibia anteriorly on the femoral condyles, the knee can be flexed up to 45°. In type III, or severe type, there is complete anterior dislocation of the proximal tibia on the femoral condyles with no contact between the tibia and the femur. Most of type I and type II cases respond quickly to a gentle manipulation and serial casting program or Pavlik harness to maintain knee flexion for a few weeks. However, treatment of congenital dislocation of the knee or hip associated with Larsen's syndrome or myelodysplasia is difficult.

Fibrosis of the quadriceps is present in this type, and this is the change that separates congenital knee dislocations from the more easily treatable postural deformations. In patients unresponsive to nonoperative treatment and in most of type III cases, early open reduction and quadricepsplasty are required. Surgical lengthening of the quadriceps-patellar tendon complex is the first step, and then the knees can be flexed and reduced. Knee dislocation must be resolved prior to treatment of congenital hip instability. Postoperative management includes initial positioning of the knee in slight flexion to remove tension on the skin incision and then progressive flexion to obtain at least 90° of knee flexion. Long-term outlook is variable; however, lack of complete flexion is common.

CONGENITAL DISLOCATION OF THE PATELLA

Congenital dislocation of the patella is an unusual condition, where hypoplasia of the patella, lateral femoral condyle, trochlea groove, and quadriceps mechanism are seen along with lateral displacement and fixation of the patella (Figure 18-2). There is a fixed flexion contracture of the knee, and the patella is laterally displaced with genu valgum and the tibia is externally rotated. Nonoperative treatment is futile. Surgical correction includes extensive lateral release, advancement of the vastus medialis obliquus, semitendinosus tenodesis to the patella and the centralization of the patella tendon insertion.

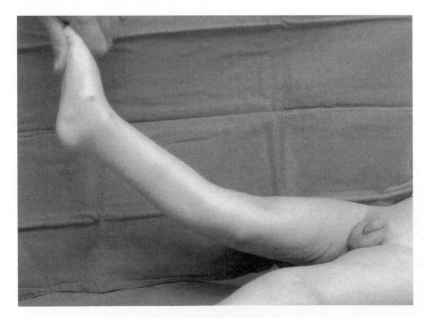

FIGURE 18-1. Clinical appearance of congenital dislocation of the right knee in a child with arthrogryposis and hyperextended knee.

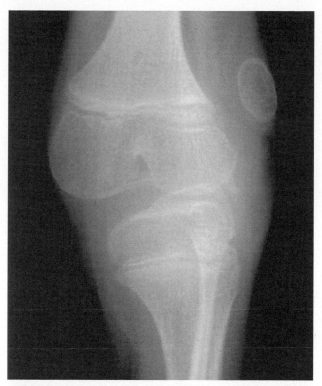

FIGURE 18-2. Anteroposterior radiograph of the congenital dislocation of the patella demonstrates lateral displacement of the patella and externally rotated tibia.

PHYSIOLOGIC GENU VARUM AND VALGUM

Bowleg (genu varum) and knock knee (genu valgum) in young children are frequent causes of anxiety in parents and a common cause of referral to the orthopaedic surgeons. In the vast majority of cases, genu varum corrects by itself with growth. Evaluating angular malalignment is simplified, if one is familiar with the normal development of the tibio-femoral angle. Normal knee alignment is approximately 10 to 15° of varus at birth, which progresses to neutral alignment at about 18 months of age. The appearance of genu varum frequently is exacerbated or accentuated by concurrent internal tibia torsion (Figures 18.3 and 18.4). Most report that persistence of genu varum beyond 2 years of age is abnormal. However, spontaneous correction of the physiologic genu varum will occasionally be delayed until 30 months of age, and even pronounced physiologic genu varum greater than 30° can correct with continuing growth. Overcorrection to excessive genu valgum is maximal at 4 years of age, and the valgus

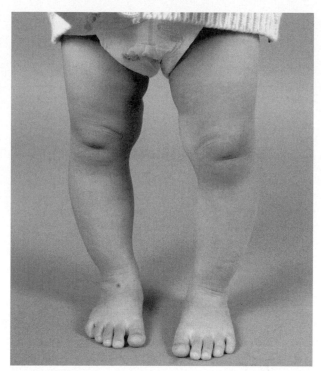

FIGURE 18-3. Clinical appearance of physiologic genu varum in a 26-month-old boy.

angulation averages 8°. Correction to physiologic valgus is usually by 5 or 6 years of age.

Genu varum is not routinely evaluated radiographically; however, if there is a concern that this falls outside the normal range in a child 18 to

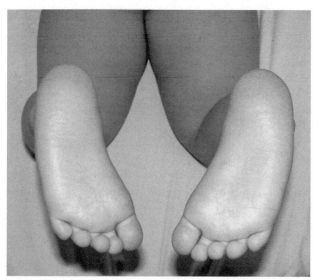

FIGURE 18-4. Thigh-foot angle. Concurrent internal tibial torsion exacerbates the clinical appearance of physiologic genu varum.

36 months old, or is associated with short stature or asymmetric involvement, standing anteroposterior radiographs should be taken to rule out any pathologic conditions. The treatment of physiologic genu varum and valgum is periodic observation and examination, together with education and reassurance of the parents that the *deformity* is a variant of normal but not a disease. Fat thighs, ligamentous laxity, and flatfoot often result in toed-out habitus, and can accentuate the knock-kneed appearance and make physiologic genu valgum appear more severe. Torsional malalignment can have a similar effect. In rare cases of uncorrected physiologic genu valgum greater than 20°, hemiepiphysiodesis or osteotomy may be indicated.

TIBIA VARA (BLOUNT'S DISEASE)

Tibia vara is the most frequent nonphysiologic cause of genu varum in children and adolescents. It is considered to be a developmental condition, which affects posteromedial aspect of the proximal medial tibial physis, resulting in a progressive varus deformity. Biopsy of the lesions reveals disorganized physeal cartilage with abnormally large groups of capillaries, densely packed hypertrophic chondrocytes, and islands of almost acellular fibrous tissue. Both fibrovascular and cartilaginous reparative tissue can be found at the physeal-metaphyseal junction. Infants affected by this condition are usually of black or Mediterranean origin, often have a history of early walking, and are in the upper percentile of weight for height. Examination of the child with tibia vara reveals an angular deformity discernable just below the knee. In contrast, young child with physiologic genu varum will have a more gentle curvature of the entire extremity. A lateral thrust, indicating laxity of the lateral ligamentous complex, may be seen in children over the age of 3 with tibia vara.

It is generally subdivided into infantile and late onset forms. Infantile Blount's disease may be difficult to diagnose in its early form until 2 years of age, when the radiographic changes suggestive of infantile tibia vara are more evident (Figure 18-5). The Langenskiöld radiographic staging classification reflects the progression of tibia vara in untreated cases. The natural history of untreated cases is to progress to complete medial physeal arrest, which can occur by the age of 6 (Figure 18-6). In such an event, subsequent treatment is difficult, because both angular deformity and tibial shortening must

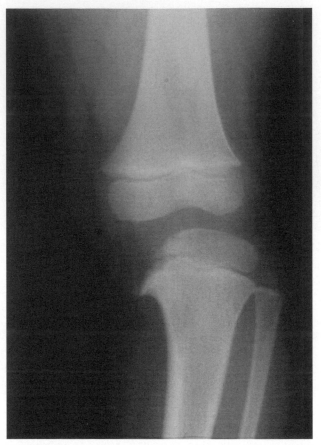

FIGURE 18-5. Anteroposterior radiograph of a 3-year-old boy with infantile tibia vara. Prominent beaking of the medial metaphysis and varus angulation at the epiphyseal-metaphyseal junction are evident.

be addressed. Other radiographic criteria have been developed, such as the metaphyseal-diaphyseal angle for the early diagnosis of Blount's disease. Some children with metaphyseal-diaphyseal angles described as compatible with infantile tibia vara (an angle of 16° is currently accepted) spontaneously improve without treatment; at the present, this differentiation continues to be very difficult in the early Langenskiöld stages.

The role of bracing remains unclear; however, brace management in patients younger than 3 years old may be successful in correcting the mild deformity. Obesity, instability, and delayed bracing are considered as risk factors for failure. Early valgus osteotomy before 4 years of age is strongly recommended to minimize deformity of the proximal medial physis. With this in mind, overcorrection into 5 to 10° valgus angulation beyond normal should be the goal. The pathology of late onset tibia vara between the ages of 6 and 13 is similar to that of

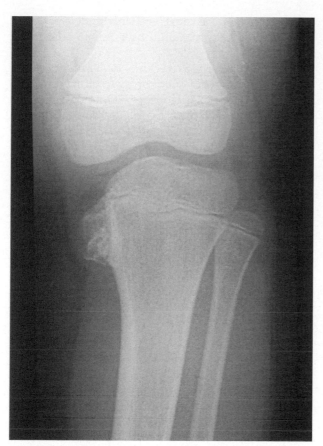

FIGURE 18-6. Anteroposterior radiograph of a 7-year-old boy with untreated infantile tibia vara demonstrates complete medial physeal arrest of the proximal tibia.

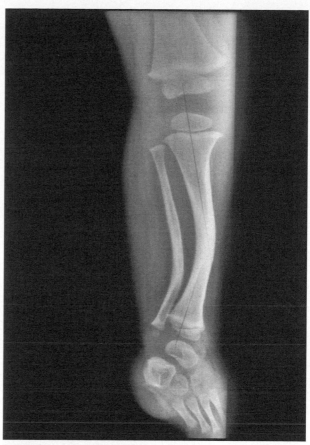

FIGURE 18-7. Anteroposterior radiograph of a 4-year-old girl with posteromedial bowing of the tibia.

infantile tibial vara; however, because growth at the tibia is closer to maturity in the adolescent, bracing is not effective. Various techniques, including plate, monolateral, or circular external fixation, have been described to maintain position after osteotomy. Use of rigid external fixation with acute or gradual correction allows accurate alignment of the lower extremity and prevents complications such as nerve palsy, compartment syndrome, overcorrection, or undercorrection. For those adolescent patients with significant growth remaining, consider selective lateral epiphysiodesis. The rate of correction following this procedure has been reported to be 4° per year.

CONGENITAL POSTEROMEDIAL BOWING OF THE TIBIA

Posteromedial bowing of the tibia is thought to be due to intrauterine position. The posture of the newborn with posteromedial bowing of the leg is characteristic (Figure 18-7), with marked calcaneovalgus

and dorsiflexion of the foot, which may even be opposed to the tibia. The natural history of this condition would be gradual resolution of the foot deformity and the tibial bowing with growth. In general, the severity of initial deformity is related to the amount of ultimate leg shortening, and final leg length discrepancies at the maturity vary from 5 to 27% relative to the contralateral normal side. No treatment for bowing is necessary or indicated. Serial documentation of discrepancy throughout childhood is advisable, and physeal arrest of the contralateral leg or lengthening of affected tibia should be performed, if the discrepancy is projected to exceed 2.5 cm at maturity.

CONGENITAL PSEUDOARTHROSIS OF THE TIBIA

Congenital anterolateral bowing of the tibia, as opposed to congenital posteromedial bowing, is not a benign condition and is the heralding physical sign of actual or impending fracture with subsequent pseudoarthrosis of the tibia (Figure 18-8). Congenital pseudoarthrosis of the tibia is relatively rare, occurring in 1 in 190,000 live births. The cause of congenital pseudoarthrosis of the tibia is unknown and appears to be the end expression of several different pathologic conditions. Neurofibromatosis is linked to about 50% of cases, and the pathology is not particularly different from other causes of pseudoarthrosis, with a cuff of harmartous tissue surrounding the lesions. Congenital pseudoarthrosis, which is not associated with neurofibromatosis, develops often after a seemingly innocuous fracture in what appears to be reasonably normal bone.

There are five forms of congenital pseudoarthrosis of the tibia: dysplastic, cystic, sclerotic, fibular, and clubfoot or congenital band type. The most common type is dysplastic, where the tibia is tapered at the defective site; an *hourglass constriction* is more often associated with neurofibromatosis. Furthermore, this type has a poor natural history with regard to fracture healing, and recurrent fracture is common even if union is achieved. In the sclerotic type, the medullary canal is absent, and the fracture

often appears transverse and incomplete initially, like a stress fracture. Late onset fractures seem to have a better prognosis.

Prophylactic bracing with a total contact ankle-foot orthosis may prevent or delay fracture, however, after the fracture has occurred, cast immobilization is generally unsuccessful. The management of established pseudoarthrosis remains controversial, and currently popular methods include excision of the lesion followed by compression with external fixator, vascularized fibular grafts, or intramedullary rodding. When treatment fails, Syme amputation and prosthetic fitting are needed for a functional limb. Treatment and follow-up through adolescence are appropriate, because a high rate of refractures often need retreatment, and delayed fracture of the tibia in late adolescence is frequent. Patients with union at skeletal maturity usually, but not necessarily, fare well in adult life.

CONGENITAL FIBULAR HEMIMELIA

This is the most common longitudinal deficiency of the lower extremity with or without a terminal deficiency at the foot. It is a paraxial deficiency, and the spectrum varies from complete absence of the fibula with missing lateral rays to a fibula that is slightly short with a ball and socket type of ankle joint (Figure 9-2). The tibia has an anterolateral bow, and the femoral shortening may accompany fibular hemimelia. If it does, the lateral femoral condyle is always deficient. The magnitude of the projected shortening usually is related to the severity of fibular and lateral ray absence. Tarsal coalition may exist with a mass representing the talus and calcaneus.

In severe deformities in which the foot cannot be rendered stable weight-bearing surface or there is excessive predicted leg length discrepancy, patient satisfaction following Syme's amputation and prosthetic fitting is high. This procedure is optimally performed before the time when children would normally ambulate. Staged limb lengthening in some cases has been demonstrated to be successful in achieving limb-length equality in children with less than 35% projected shortening of the tibia and fibula, when undertaken carefully with protection of the ankle and foot to avoid exacerbation of the valgus position of the hind foot. Complex assemblies for lengthening are required to protect the foot from further deformity during the lengthening for fibular hemimelia.

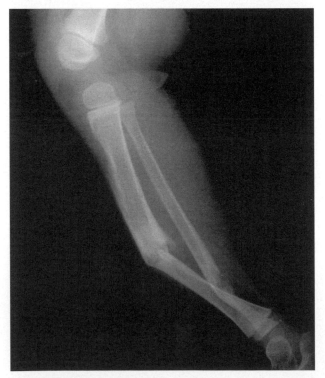

FIGURE 18-8. Lateral radiograph of a 5-year-old girl with congenital pseudoarthrosis of tibia demonstrates anterior bowing of the tibia and the fracture occurred in the cystic lesion.

DISCOID MENISCUS

Discoid meniscus is an infrequent congenital anomaly of the knee in which the lateral meniscus is discoid in shape rather than normal semilunar configuration. It is seen in 1 to 3% of normal population with a higher frequency in Asians. It can be complete, incomplete, or the Wrisberg type. The latter is characterized by the absence of a menisco-tibial attachment, and the increased mobility allows the development of a discoid configuration as a secondary event.

Mothers will describe a *clunk* in the knee in the infant, especially when the child is agitated. Most patients present in childhood and early in adolescence. The hallmark complaint in the Wrisberg type is a snap or clunk in the knee with motion. Symptoms of snapping and popping usually occur between the ages of 6 and 12 years. There may be associated pain or limp. Routine radiographs may show a widened lateral joint space and tibial eminence flattening. Three or more cuts of MRI showing a meniscus 5 mm thick from anterior to posterior are indicative of a discoid meniscus (Figure 18-9). In addition, the meniscus may extend into the notch and demonstrate intrasubstance degeneration.

No treatment is indicated if the knee is pain free, has full mobility, and no effusion. Most discoid meniscal surgery is performed by arthroscopic techniques. The first goal is to establish the presence of stability. Arthroscopy-assisted sculpturing of the meniscus to a normal configuration is attempted for the complete and incomplete types. If the meniscus is unstable, this should be repaired; however, complete meniscectomy should be avoided.

OSTEOCHONDRITIS DISSECANS OF THE KNEE

Osteochondritis dissecans is a condition in which a portion of the articular cartilage of the knee and its underlying subchondral bone becomes separated from the remaining articular cartilage. Its origin is unknown. Repetitive trauma imposed by the tibial spine on the medial femoral condyle has been suggested as a principal cause. Symptoms are related to the condition's acuity, may be present only with activity, and may be associated with recurrent effusions. Occasionally, there are symptoms of locking or catching of the knee when an osteochondritis dissecans fragment is a free loose body. Local tenderness may be present with direct pressure at the lesion, if it is unstable.

Standard radiographs, particularly the anteroposterior tunnel view, demonstrate the lesion. The most common site is in the non–weight-bearing, posterior lateral aspect of the medial femoral condyle, and the lesion is seen as an osseous fragment surrounded by a lucent defect. A portion of lateral femoral condyle or patella can also be involved. MRI or arthroscopy helps determine the fragment's articular cartilage continuity, size, and integrity of its subchondral bone (Figure 18-10).

The natural history is directly related to the patient's age, and treatment recommendations are

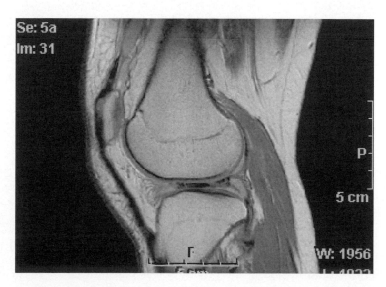

FIGURE 18-9. T2-weighted magnetic resonance image of a discoid lateral meniscus shows a continuous bow-tied or slab appearance of lateral meniscus and degenerative changes within the posterior horn of meniscus.

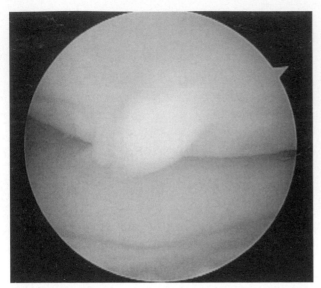

FIGURE 18-10. Arthroscopic examination of the knee in a 12-year-old boy with osteochondritis dissecans. The lesion is partially detached and a hinge of intact cartilage on one edge of the femoral condyle.

based on the age and status of the fragment. In children and adolescents in whom the lesion is not yet separated from the remaining subchondral bone, cast immobilization for a period of 6 to 12 weeks is warranted, with healing in most patients. Conversely, instability or loss of continuity of the articular surface compromise healing. When the articular surface of the condyle is disrupted, it is important to stabilize the fragment and to encourage revascularization by drilling the base of the lesion or by bone grafting of large osteochondral defects. Currently, these procedures are performed arthroscopically in most cases. Excision of irregular lesions with curettage of the underlying bone may be of value in some cases. When a large portion of the weight-bearing surface of the medial compartment of the knee is involved, degenerative arthritis of the knee with narrowing and sclerosis of the joint can be expected to occur at an early age.

OSGOOD-SCHLATTER DISEASE

Osgood-Schlatter disease is a common problem that is typically seen in athletic boys between the ages of 10 and 15. The lesion is considered secondary to unresolved, submaximal avulsion fractures at the patella tendon–tibial tubercle junction. As the apophysis of tibial tubercle matures, ossification changes from membranous to endochondral. During the endochondral phase, the physis is less resistant to

tensile stress, and failure may manifest by fragmentation of bone at this site.

The classic presentation is a painful bump at the anterior tibial tubercle, and pain with kneeling or activity involving quadriceps contraction. Symptoms may span the spectrum from pain solely with direct contact of the tibial tubercle to pain during physical activities such as running and jumping, to chronic pain associated with activities of daily living. Radiographs show fragmentation or prominence of tibial tubercle (Figure 18-11). Ossicle formation occurs in nearly 40% of patients within the patella ligament, and the radiographic findings do not necessarily correlate with clinical symptoms.

The natural history of the disease is benign, with almost all cases asymptomatic by skeletal maturity. In children who have pain merely with contact and are able to be athletically active without symptoms, no intervention is required except for provision of knee pads during sports. In patients who have pain during sports activity in the absence of direct knee contact or who have pain with

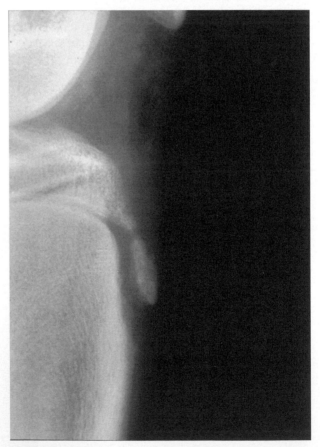

FIGURE 18-11. Lateral radiograph of a 13-year-old boy with Osgood-Schlatter disease shows fragmentary ossification of the tibial tubercle.

activities of daily living, rest from offending activities and temporary substitution of nonoffensive activities are recommended. Surgical excision of a residual loose ossicle remaining at skeletal maturity has been described with good outcome; however, skeletal maturity does not necessarily need to be reached before the ossicle is enucleated. Debulking of the tibial tubercle may be done at the time of ossicle excision in patients who are mature.

PATELLAR LESIONS

Multipartite patellae are often asymptomatic, and radiographic curiosities are noted incidentally. An incompletely ossified portion of the patella is a radiographic characteristic. Involvement of the superolateral corner of the patella occurs in 75% of cases. Symptoms may occur at the patella-fragment junction due to acute trauma or repetitive microtrauma causing separation.

Patellar cysts are usually noted as incidental radiographic findings but may present in patients with knee pain. Typically, cysts are bilateral and well circumscribed in the patella. Biopsy of patellar cysts reveals nothing more than a cyst with synovial fluid. Surgical intervention is not indicated.

Sinding-Larsen-Johansson syndrome refers to lesions at the inferior patella pole–superior patellar ligament junction and represents a sequelae of chronic tensile stresses at that site. Healthy athletic boys are commonly affected. In the adolescent, signs and symptoms occur at the proximal patella ligament, the so-called *jumper's knee*. Radiographic evaluation of the knee may be normal or may demonstrate variable changes in distal patellar pole ossification. Treatment consists of ice, massage, anti-inflammatory medication, and rest from running and jumping activities with resolution of the pain in 2 to 4 weeks. Healing of the lesion may be ascertained radiographically by increased ossification at the pole of the patella with increased longitudinal length of the patella. Surgical intervention is not indicated.

PATELLOFEMORAL PAIN SYNDROME

Patellofemoral pain syndrome is a relatively common complaint among the skeletally immature adolescents, but it is not rare in preadolescence. The symptoms are usually well localized to the peripatellar region, and giving way is a common complaint.

Knee pain in the skeletally immature patient must be considered referred hip pain until proven otherwise, and a thorough hip examination must be a part of the evaluation of knee complaints.

Typically patients complain about vague anterior knee pain and swelling associated with activities such as prolonged walking, running, or jumping. Pain gets worse by prolonged sitting, stair climbing, squatting, and inclement weather, and the patient has a sense that the involved knee will give way. Patients with anterior knee pain demonstrate full range of motion of the knee and no instability. There may be low grade synovitis, and significant muscle weakness of the lower extremity is frequently present. A comprehensive rehabilitation program is the treatment of choice with no need for bracing, arthroscopic evaluation, or other interventional modalities.

RECURRENT PATELLAR SUBLUXATION AND DISLOCATION

Recurrent subluxation and dislocation of the patella most commonly occur laterally. The loss of articular continuity occurs during a phase of patellar excursion, usually at 0 to 25° of flexion. The most common cause is lateral malalignment of the quadriceps mechanism, and ligamentous laxity in Down syndrome or Ehlers-Danlos syndrome, lateral soft tissue contractures, external tibial torsion, a shallow intercondylar notch of the femur, patella alta, or vastus medialis insufficiency may be contributing factors (Figure 18-12). In recurrent patella instability, the frequency and magnitude of precipitating events and any previous treatment need to be addressed. The patient presents with a complaint of sudden knee pain and a sensation of instability or giving way of the knee. With recurrent subluxation or dislocation, the vicious cycle of pain and reflex weakness of the dynamic stabilizers of the knee result in activity-related pain, swelling, and instability.

Physical examination should include evaluation of lower extremity alignment, joint motion, patella alta, ligamentous laxity, muscle strength, and quadriceps retinacular competence. It reveals a hypermobile patella with lateral displacement of the patella and may reveal contracture of lateral retinaculum with only minimal medial displacement of the lateral edge of the patella from the lateral femoral condyle. The quadriceps complex, patella, and femur must be thought of as a unit. The Q angle is formed by a line drawn along the quadriceps

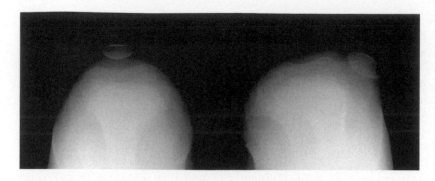

FIGURE 18-12. A skyline view of the knee shows lateral dislocation of the patella with hypoplastic lateral femoral condyle.

tendon and a line drawn along the patella liga-ment, and a large Q angle is associated with a ten-dency toward lateral subluxation of the patella. Patellofemoral sulcus incongruity may be due to anatomic maldevelopment. Four-view knee radi-ographs should be obtained. A tangential view ob-tained with the knee in 40° of flexion shows the relationship of the patella to the anterior part of the femoral intercondylar groove, and may also demon-strate loose bodies and fractures of the patella or lat-eral condyle. CT scan is helpful in assessing the relationship of the patellofemoral joint in terms of tilt or translation, or both.

Although treatment is individualized and is based on the pathology, the initial management should be nonoperative. Strengthening the vastus me-dialis is of the utmost importance and may reduce the frequency of dislocation. If conservative treatment fails, the surgical approaches to growing children should be focused on realigning the quadriceps mech-anism, usually in combination with a lateral release and the creation of a medial patella restraint. How-ever, the surgeon's options are limited by the open growth plate of the tibial tubercle, which prohibits op-erations that transfer the origin of the patellar tendon. To date, proximal realignment of the quadriceps and the transfer of the semitendinosus tendon to the patella has been the best option to recurrent dislocat-ing patella in skeletally immature children, even in cases with ligamentous laxity. Tibial tubercle rota-tional realignment, described by Elmslie and Trillat, has proven successful without drastically altering patellar realignment. After operation, an intensive physical therapy program is required.

TRAUMA

Fracture of the distal femoral physis may mimic injury of the medial collateral ligament and may require stress radiographs for definitive diagnosis.

Minimally displaced fractures of the distal femoral epiphysis may be treated by immobilization in a long-leg cast, while those fractures that are com-pletely displaced, such as in Salter-Harris type II, have unexpectedly higher incidences of physeal arrest than epiphyseal fractures in other locations (Figure 18-13). Closed reduction can often be ob-tained; however, because of inherent instability, percutaneous internal fixation with the aid of an image intensifier may be necessary to maintain re-duction of Salter-Harris types I and II fractures. Premature closure of the distal femoral physis is common due to the significant energy required to produce such a fracture. Complete cessation of growth of the distal femoral physis may occur, re-sulting in leg length discrepancy; partial closure of the physis results in progressive angular deformity of the knee.

Patella fractures are much less common in chil-dren than in adults, and usually occur in older chil-dren. Avulsion fractures may involve the superior, medial, inferior, or lateral patella. A sleeve fracture of the distal pole of patella is actually the most com-mon type in children, and often appears benign on a radiograph, because only a fleck of bone is seen. However, a rather large cartilaginous sleeve is avulsed along with the periosteum and retinacu-lum. Displaced transverse fractures are treated as in adults, with open reduction and tension band wiring.

In tibial eminence fractures (Figure 18-14), the anterior spine is fractured many times more often than the posterior. By placing the knee in exten-sion, the displaced fragment can generally be re-duced, although the medial meniscus has been found interposed with completely displaced frag-ments. If radiographs of the knee in full extension demonstrate anatomic reduction of the fracture, immobilization of the knee in this position is ex-pected to result in an excellent return of function. However, an unreduced fragment is managed either

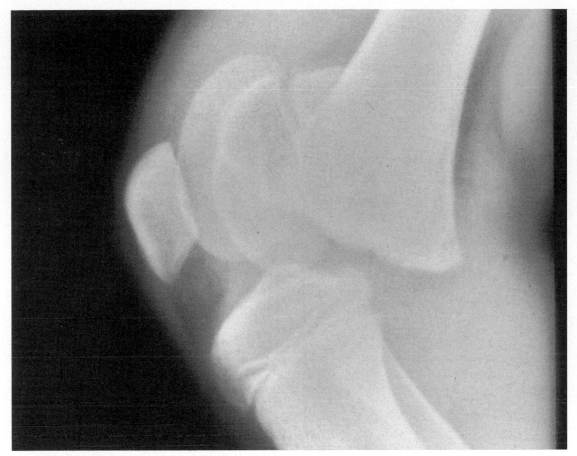

FIGURE 18-13. Lateral radiograph of the knee shows anteriorly displaced Salter-Harris type II fracture of the distal femoral physis.

arthroscopically or with open reduction. Anterior cruciate ligament laxity has often been noted on follow-up of completely displaced fractures, but complaints or subjective instability is infrequent.

Fracture of the proximal tibial physis requires a tremendous amount of energy and carries poor prognosis, because the metaphysis can be displaced posteriorly and peripheral ischemia occurs in 15% of the patients. Most Salter-Harris types I and II fractures are treated with closed means, but types III and IV injuries are usually treated with open reduction and internal fixation. Angular deformity can occur due to asymmetrical growth arrest or malunion, and this is treated with physeal bar excision if less than 50% of the physis is involved.

Tibial tubercle fracture is an injury of the adolescent knee joint, usually occurring in boys between 13 and 16 years of age (Figure 18-15). The mechanism of injury for avulsion of the tubercle is

forceful quadriceps contraction against resistance. Treatment for all but minimally displaced fractures consists of open reduction and internal fixation. Posttraumatic genu recurvatum can occur in younger children due to premature arrest of the anterior aspect of the growth plate.

Fractures of the proximal tibial metaphysis, even those nondisplaced, with or without fibular fracture, may result in a valgus angular deformity. Although exact mechanism of this phenomenon is unknown, the deformity worsens for about 2 years and then improves gradually. Osteotomy at the time of the greatest deformity is very often unrewarding, as the osteotomy can induce the same reaction as the fracture, producing recurrent valgus.

The tibia is the most commonly fractured bone of the lower extremity in children, and the shaft fractures can generally be managed with casting. Less than 10° of angulation should be the goal in older children, and varus angulation remodels better than

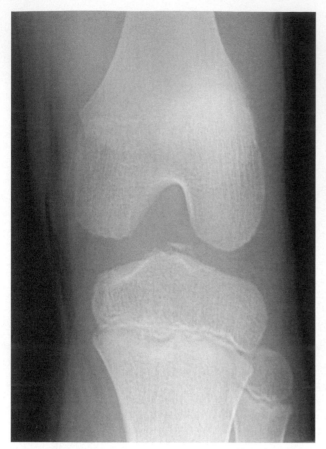

FIGURE 18-14. Anteroposterior radiograph of the knee shows displaced fracture fragment of tibial eminence.

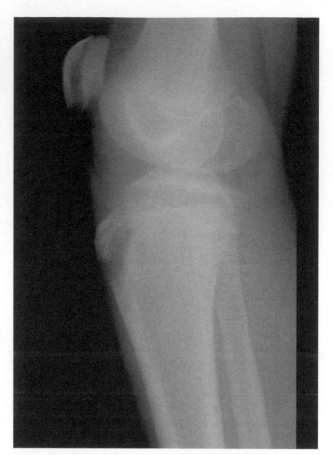

FIGURE 18-15. Lateral radiograph of the knee shows Salter-Harris type II fracture of the tibial tubercle.

valgus or posterior angulation. Reports also indicate that the incidence of compartment syndrome, vascular injury, infection, and delayed union in children is similar to that in adults.

LIGAMENTOUS INJURY

Knee ligaments injuries in children and adolescents are being recognized more frequently, and tears of both cruciate and collateral ligaments have been reported. Hemarthrosis without fracture implies significant soft tissue injuries. The natural history of anterior cruciate ligament (ACL) injuries is simply not good. There is no doubt at present regarding whether operative reconstruction is necessary; the question is rather on a technique that will not interfere with subsequent growth. Many ACL injuries in skeletally immature patients occur at the tibial insertion. The substantial series of untreated posterior cruciate injuries in children has not been reported.

Annotated Bibliography

Angel KR, Hall DJ. Anterior cruciate ligament injury in children and adolescents. Arthroscopy 1989;5:197–200.
The authors reported arthroscopically documented anterior cruciate ligament tears, and recommended arthroscopic assessment for any patient with an acute hemarthrosis.

Bell MJ, Atkins RM, Sharrard WJW. Irreducible congenital dislocation of the knee. J Bone Joint Surg 1987;69B:403–406.
This article describes congenital dislocation of the knee and its associated abnormalities and expected outcomes. The authors emphasize the need for treatment of knee dislocation before treatment of hip or foot deformities.

Drennan JC. Congenital dislocation of the knee and patella. Instr Course Lect 1993;42:517–524.
Classification and treatment of subluxation, tilt plus subluxation, and tilt alone are suggested. In addition to the author's recommended treatment of realignment of the quadriceps mechanism, a comprehensive review of the literature is presented.

Kim HW, Weinstein SL. Intramedullary fixation and bone grafting for congenital pseudarthrosis of the tibia. Clin Orthop 2002;405:250–257.
This article reports good results with intramedullary rod fixation and bone grafting, and suggests the indications and technical aspects of intramedullary fixation.

Kling TF Jr, Hensinger RN. Angular and torsional deformities of the lower limbs in children. Clin Orthop 1983;176:136–147.

This is an excellent review of the commonly encountered angular and torsional problems in early childhood and discusses presentation, differential diagnosis, and recommended treatment.

Krause BL, Williams JP, Catterall A. Natural history of Osgood-Schlatter disease. J Pediatr Orthop 1990;10:65–68.
This large series documenting the natural history of Osgood-Schlatter disease provides a valuable baseline for comparison. Results in patients with or without immobilization were the same.

Langenskiöld A. Tibia vara: osteochondrosis deformans tibiae. Blount's disease. Clin Orthop 1981;158:77–82.
The presentation, treatment, and radiographic classification of tibia vara, or Blount disease, are discussed.

Pappas AM. Congenital posteromedial bowing of the tibia and fibula. J Pediatr Orthop 1984;4:525–531.
The growth and development of 33 patients with congenital posteromedial bowing of the tibia and fibula are documented with the demonstration of progressive improvement and leg length discrepancy.

Riseborough EJ, Barrett IR, Shapiro F. Growth disturbances following distal femoral physeal fracture-separations. J Bone Joint Surg 1983;65A:885–893.
This article demonstrates the high incidence of early growth plate disorders associated with this injury.

Sponseller PD, Stanitski CL. Fractures and dislocations about the knee. In: Beaty JH, Kasser JR, eds. Fractures in Children. Philadelphia: Lippincott Williams & Wilkins 2001:981–1076.
This chapter clearly describes the pathophysiology of the fractures/dislocations around the knee and suggests the treatment guidelines.

Staheli LT, Corbett M, Wyss C et al. Lower-extremity rotational problems in children: normal values to guide management. J Bone Joint Surg 1985;67A:39–47.
This classic study of clinical changes in the rotational profile of 500 subjects presents data on individuals from infancy through the eighth decade. Graphs include changes by age in foot progression angle, tibial version, and femoral version, and provide mean ± 2 standard deviations for each parameter at each age.

Stanitski CL. Anterior knee pain syndromes in the adolescent. J Bone Joint Surg 1993;75A:1407–1416.
This article reviews potential causes of anterior knee pain in adolescents (Osgood-Schlatter disease, Sinding-Larsen Johansson disease, multipartite patellae, pathologic plica, and reflex sympathetic dystrophy). The need for a search for a specific diagnosis in idiopathic anterior knee pain is emphasized.

19

Sandeep Munjal
Kenneth A. Krackow

The Adult Knee

MENISCAL INJURIES

The menisci protect the articular cartilage by increasing both joint congruity and contact area as well as preventing focal contractions of stress. When a load is transmitted across the knee joint, the circumferentially oriented collagen fibers within the menisci generate a hoop stress, which resists extrusion of the menisci from between the femoral condyle and tibial plateau. Menisci transmit approximately 50% of weight-bearing forces across the knee joint in extension and 85% at 90° of knee flexion. In the medial compartment, the medial meniscus bears 50% of the load; whereas in the lateral compartment, the lateral meniscus carries approximately 70% of the load transmitted across the lateral compartment.

Removal of the medial meniscus results in 50 to 70% reduction in femoral condyle contact area and in a 100% increase in contact stress. Total lateral meniscectomy causes a 40 to 50% decrease in contact area and increases contact stress in the lateral compartment to 200 to 300% of normal. Along with biomechanical changes that can occur with meniscectomy, the improved joint congruity that occurs through the meniscus contact is thought to play a role in joint lubrication and cell nutrition.

The meniscus also plays a role in enhancing joint stability. Medial meniscectomy in the ACL intact knee has little effect on anteroposterior motion, but in an ACL deficient knee, it results in an increase in anterior tibial translation of up to 58% at 90° of flexion. The posterior horn of the medial meniscus provides the most significant contribution to resisting anterior tibial displacement. Although the inner two-thirds of the meniscus is important in maximizing joint contact area and increasing shock absorption, the integrity of the peripheral one-third is essential for both load transmission and stability. The meniscus also plays a role in shock absorption. Compression studies have demonstrated that meniscal tissue is approximately one-half as stiff as articular cartilage. Shock absorption capacity was reduced by 20% after meniscectomy.

Finally, it has been suggested by some, based on presence of type I and II nerve endings in the menisci, that they function in providing proprioceptive feedback for joint position sense.

Anatomy

From a gross anatomic perspective, the menisci are C-shaped or semicircular fibrocartilaginous structures with bony attachment at anterior and posterior tibial plateau. The medial meniscus is C-shaped, with a posterior horn larger than the anterior horn in the anteroposterior dimension. The anterior horn of medial meniscus has the largest insertion site surface area (61.4 mm^2) and the posterior horn of lateral meniscus, the smallest (28.5 mm^2). The capsular attachment of medial meniscus on the tibial side is referred to as the coronary ligament. A thickening of the capsular attachment in the midportion spans from the tibia to femur and is referred to as the deep medial collateral ligament. The lateral meniscus is also anchored anteriorly and posteriorly through bony attachments and has an almost semicircular configuration. It covers a larger portion of the tibial articular surface than does medial meniscus. Discoid

variants have been reported with an incidence of 3.5 to 5%, most being an incomplete type.

The fibrocartilaginous structure of the meniscus has a varied architecture of coarse collagen bundles. Scanning electron microscopy has revealed the orientation of collagen fibers to be mainly circumferential, with some radial fibers at the surface and within the midsubstance. This orientation allows compressive loads to be dispersed by the circumferential fibers while the radial fibers act as tie fibers to resist longitudinal tearing. At the surface of the meniscus, fiber orientation is more of a mesh network or random configuration, thought to be important in distribution of sheer stress. Collagen is 60 to 70% of the dry weight of meniscus. The majority of collagen (90%) is type I, with types II, III, V, and VI present in smaller amounts. At birth the entire meniscus is vascular; by age 9 months, the inner one-third has become avascular. This decrease in vascularity continues by age 10 years, when the meniscus closely resembles the adult meniscus. In adults, only 10 to 25% of the lateral meniscus and 10 to 30% of the medial meniscus is vascular. This vascularity arises from superior and inferior branches of the medial and lateral genicular arteries, which form a perimeniscal capillary plexus. Because of the avascular nature of the inner two-thirds of the meniscus, cell nutrition is believed to occur mainly through diffusion or mechanical pumping.

Diagnosis

Meniscal tears are more common in males; the male to female ratio ranges from 2.5:1 to 4:1. The peak incidence is in men 21 to 30 years old and in girls and women 11 to 20 years old. One-third of tears in this age group are associated with an ACL injury. Degenerative types of meniscal tears commonly occur in men in their fourth, fifth, and sixth decades. In patients with acute ACL injury, lateral meniscus tears occur more frequently than do medial meniscal tears. In patients with chronic ACL deficient knees, however, medial meniscal tears are more prevalent. Meniscal injury is also frequently associated with tibial plateau fracture and femoral shaft fractures. Diagnosis of meniscal injury is based primarily on a thorough history and physical examination. In athletic populations, the patient typically describes a twisting injury or hyperflexion as inciting event. Often with degenerative tears, there is no one inciting event. Complaints of locking or catching may be present but also may be secondary to other pathology, such as chondral injury or patellofemoral chondrosis. Loss of motion with a mechanical block to extension is commonly the result of a displaced bucket handle meniscal tear and usually requires acute surgical treatment.

The examiner should assess for joint effusion, quadriceps hypotrophy, and any joint line swelling that may occur with a perimeniscal cyst. Range of motion must be assessed to determine whether a meniscal block to extension or loss of flexion is present. Joint line tenderness, pain with squatting, a positive flexion McMurray test, and positive Apley compression and distraction tests are all indicative of meniscal injury. In one study, joint line tenderness was the best clinical sign of a meniscal tear, with 74% sensitivity and 50% positive predictive value.

Plain radiographs should be a part of routine evaluation and include standard views, a 45° posteroanterior weight-bearing view (also known as Rosenberg view), and lateral and axial (Merchant or sunrise) views. Although these radiographs cannot confirm the diagnosis of the meniscal tear, they are extremely important in defining bone pathology and evaluating knee for joint space narrowing. Because articular cartilage wear is often more advanced in the posterior aspect of femoral condyles, the 30 or 45° posteroanterior flexion weight-bearing view is more sensitive than standard standing views (Figure 19-1). Magnetic resonance imaging (MRI) is noninvasive and has the ability to assess the knee in multiple planes and other structures within the joint. With improved technology and increased experience, the accuracy of detecting the meniscal tear is now considered to be approximately 95% or better.

The normal appearance of meniscus on MRI is that of uniformly low signal. Meniscal tears are represented by a high signal in the meniscus, which contacts the superior or inferior articular surface. Areas of increased signal within the meniscus occur in children and increase with age in adults. These intrasubstance changes are seen frequently and are a common cause of overreading meniscal tears on MRI scans. Extension of an abnormal signal to an articular surface on only one image is often shown to be normal at arthroscopy.

Common Pitfalls in MRI of Meniscal Tears Involve the Lateral Meniscus

High signal in the region of confluence of the transverse ligament with the anterior horn of the lateral meniscus can mimic a meniscal tear. At the posterior horn of the lateral meniscus, the popliteus tendon sheath may be mistaken for grade III signal. The insertion of meniscofemoral ligament can mimic the appearance of vertical tear in the posterior horn of the lateral meniscus. Separate portions of the posterior horn can be mistaken for a bucket handle tear as the most posterior coronal images traverse both the body and the posterior horn, especially images of the lateral meniscus.

Meniscal cysts are associated with complex meniscal tears and are more likely to be degenerative in origin. These cysts are more common laterally in

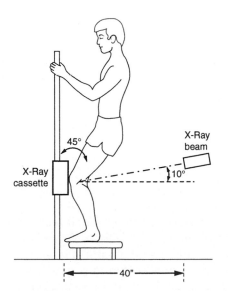
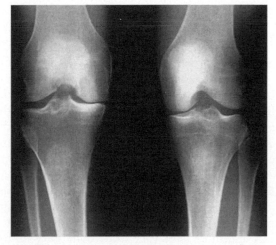

FIGURE 19-1. The Rosenberg view. PA weight-bearing view at 45° of flexion can facilitate the diagnosis if standard standing AP view is not sensitive enough.

the weak area between lateral collateral ligament (LCL) and iliotibial band. Medial meniscal cysts are usually found posteriorly in the weak area immediately posterior to the medial collateral ligament (MCL).

Treatment

Treatment for meniscal tear depends on the patient's symptoms, chronicity, age, activity, and location and length of tear. Options include no intervention, partial meniscectomy, and meniscal repair. In the setting of ACL injury, the surgical treatment of meniscal pathology is most often done concurrently with ACL reconstruction. Surgical timing is most often dictated by issues related to the ACL surgery, such as range of motion, swelling, quadriceps function, and associated ligament injuries. The final decision is made during arthroscopic examination. Thorough systematic arthroscopic inspection allows the surgeon to delineate the type of tear present. Use of 70° arthroscope allows for optimal visualization of the posterior compartment, for defining the location of tear with respect to the meniscofemoral junction, and for preparation of the meniscus for any repair. Prior to arthroscopy, the patient must consent to any possible procedure and all necessary equipment must be available during initial arthroscopy.

Commonly described patterns of meniscal tear include vertical longitudinal, oblique (flap), radial, horizontal, and complex tears (Figure 19-2). With increasing age, degenerative tears are more frequently seen, with most pathology in the posterior horns. Individuals with degenerative tears may frequently have an associated radiographic finding of joint narrowing, squaring of condyles, and osteophyte ridges. Treatment decisions regarding degenerative meniscus must be made with caution, as it can be difficult to differentiate between symptoms of degenerative meniscus and degenerative articular pathology.

Vertical longitudinal tears can be either complete (bucket handle) or incomplete. Incomplete tears usually occur in younger individuals and occur either in superior or inferior surface of meniscus. These tears have predilection for occurring in posterior horns and are frequently seen in conjunction with ACL injuries. Stable tears are those noted to be less than 1 to 1.5 cm in length and can be abraded with arthroscopic rasps that can stimulate vascular ingrowth. Larger incomplete tears greater than 1.5 cm in length or tears that show instability with probing should be treated with meniscal repair

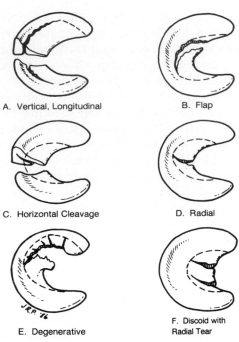

FIGURE 19-2. Types of meniscal tears with typical area of resection.

or partial meniscectomy, as the likelihood of tear propagation and secondary cartilage damage is increased. Bucket handle tears are large vertical longitudinal tears, typically occurring in young active patients often with tears of the ACL. Treatment by partial meniscectomy will most likely result in excision of large percentage of involved meniscus; therefore, more recently many surgeons are advocating repair of bucket handle tears, which can be congruently reduced. Chronically displaced tears can be permanently deformed, and congruent reduction cannot be obtained.

Radial and oblique tears result in disruption of the circumferential collagen fibers of the meniscus. *Complete radial tears result in loss of weight-bearing function of meniscus;* they are typically located at the junction of middle and posterior thirds of the medial meniscus or near the posterior attachment of the lateral meniscus. Because radial tears, as well as the traditional treatment that includes subtotal or total meniscectomy, can result in accelerated degenerative changes in the knee, some surgeons have advocated repair of large radial tears and have often used fibrin clot at the time of meniscal repair citing good results. These repairs of large radial or oblique tears can often be tenuous, and patients must be prepared for the increased surgical morbidity and possible need for further surgery.

Horizontal tears are believed to begin near the inner margin of meniscus and extend toward the capsule. They may occur in all age groups but may increase in frequency with age. They are commonly seen in the lateral menisci of runners. Meniscal cysts are often associated with horizontal tears and can be symptomatic because of localized swelling. Treatment of these tears involves partial meniscectomy with resection of flap peripherally until a stable rim is obtained.

Partial Meniscectomy

To avoid the sequelae of total meniscectomy, partial resection of meniscus is advocated when repair is not feasible. General guidelines to arthroscopic resection that apply to most respectable meniscal lesions include removal of all mobile fragments that can be pulled past the inner margin of meniscus into the center of the joint. Although a perfectly smooth rim is not necessary, the remaining rim should be smoothed to remove any sudden changes in the contour. The meniscocapsular junction and the peripheral meniscal rim should be protected; in uncertain situations, more rather than less meniscal rim should be left to avoid segmental resection, which essentially results in a total meniscectomy (Figure 19-2).

Meniscal Repair

There is relative increase in trends to preserve the meniscus as much as possible, especially when there is an associated ACL injury and need for reconstruction. Many factors need to be considered before making a decision. These factors include the patient's age, preinjury activity level and postinjury expectations, chronicity, type, location and size of tear, and associated ligament injuries. Based on vascularity, the meniscus has a red zone at the periphery indicating the presence of vascularity and white zone with the central two-thirds of the meniscus indicating avascularity. The red–white zone is the transition zone between vascular and avascular portion. The red–red tears have blood supply on both central and capsular sides and have excellent healing potential. Red–white tears have relatively good healing potential following adequate repair. White–white tears have the worst potential of healing, as they are in avascular zone. However repair of white–white tears with utilization of fibrin clot has shown somewhat better results. *The ideal candidate for meniscal repair is the young, active individual who has an acute longitudinal tear in peripheral vascularized meniscus measuring 1 to 2 cm; the ideal situation is when performed at the same time as ACL reconstruction.* Beyond this ideal situation, the treatment must be individualized.

Techniques

Four basic approaches to meniscal repair include open repair, all inside repair, inside-out repair, and outside-in repair. All share the basic principles of adequate rim preparation and stable fixation. Open repair is most useful in peripheral tears. In setting of the open collateral ligament repair or reconstruction, open repair is often necessary. Direct suturing of peripheral tear may be the most effective means of treating these injuries. The success rate is high because of acuteness of injury, peripheral tear, and associated hemarthrosis.

The *all inside arthroscopic technique* is indicated for unstable vertical longitudinal tears of the peripheral posterior horns of meniscus; tears of the anterior to posterior one-third are not amenable to this technique. This technique is performed entirely under arthroscopic control with an intra-articular method of suturing the meniscus. The vertically oriented sutures oppose the components of meniscal tear only without incorporating the joint capsule. This technique necessitates specialized setup and equipment, including 70° arthroscope and posterolateral and posteromedial portals. Advantages of this technique include the ability to place vertically placed sutures, and to achieve coaptation of the tear components without entrapping the posterior capsule and any vital structures contained within it. Disadvantages include technical difficulty in passing the 70° arthroscope anterior to posterior through the intercondylar notch as well as placing posterior operative cannula.

Inside-out repair is the most common type of repair performed. This technique uses double-armed sutures with long flexible needles positioned with arthroscopically directed cannulas. Either a single or double-barreled cannula can be used (Figure 19-3). The single barrel cannula has the advantage of allowing for vertically oriented sutures, which provide better coaptation at the tear site. A medial or lateral incision is required to retrieve the needle as it exits the knee joint. Proper positioning of the incision and appropriate dissection down to the capsule are necessary to minimize the risk of neurovascular injury. On the lateral side, peroneal nerve is at greatest risk;

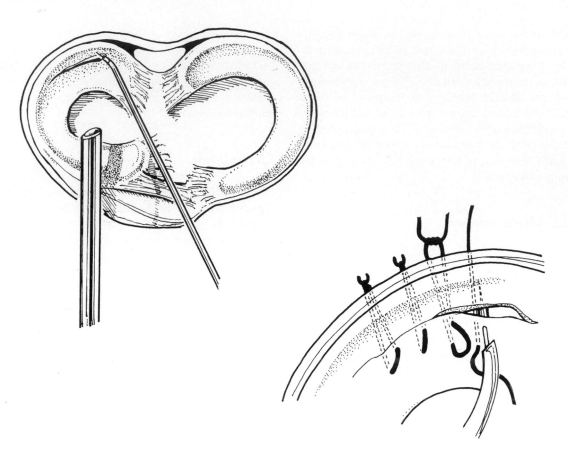

FIGURE 19-3. Inside-out technique for meniscal repair. Vertical sutures provide the strongest repair.

on the medial side, the most commonly injured structure is one of the branches of saphenous nerve.

Outside-in technique involves the passage of an 18-gauge needle across the tear from outside to inside the joint where it is grasped and brought out the anterior portal. The suture is then tied into a mulberry knot and withdrawn back abutting the meniscus. A series of sutures 3 to 4 mm apart are placed in this manner and tied to one another over the capsule, after the soft tissue is bluntly dissected to avoid possible entrapment of important neurovascular structures (Figure 19-4). This technique is most applicable for tears involving anterior and middle thirds of the meniscus.

The *nonsuture technique* involves sutureless meniscus fixation devices, which obviate the need for additional incisions. The meniscus arrow (Bionx Implants, Bluebell, PA) is made of poly-L-lactic acid, and its barbed design allows for compression of vertical tears. Numerous other sutureless implants have been designed for all inside fixation of meniscal tears. Although initial studies have shown efficacy, further studies are necessary.

Meniscal Transplant

Studies of the biomechanical consequences of meniscal transplant have demonstrated improved contact areas and decreased contact pressures after allograft placement in cadaveric models, provided both the anterior and posterior horns of meniscus are secured. Indications of meniscal transplantation continue to change as clinical experience increases. At present, the *ideal indication is the patient who has previously undergone a total or near total meniscectomy and has joint line pain, early chondral changes, normal anatomical alignment, and a stable knee.* In this setting, meniscal transplantation may decrease pain and possibly prevent progressive degeneration of articular cartilage. In addition, in patients who have complete rupture of ACL and a completely destroyed medial meniscus, it is felt that medial meniscus transplantation will provide additional joint stabilization and help protect the reconstructed ACL. The role of meniscal transplantation in asymptomatic patients who have undergone total meniscectomy is controversial.

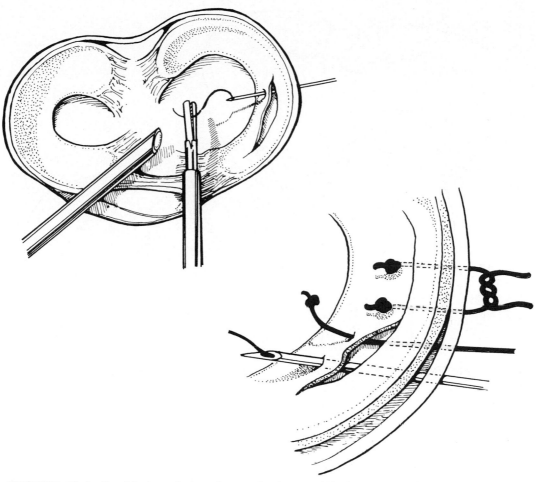

FIGURE 19-4. Outside-in technique for meniscal repair. The knot captures the meniscus being repaired.

Key surgical issues are graft selection, sizing, and technique. In general, menisci do not elicit an immune response. However, the primary concern is the transmission of diseases. Fresh frozen, and cryopreserved grafts are commonly used. Fixation of the meniscal graft has been described with soft tissue fixation alone, or in conjunction with bone plug or bone bridge fixation between the anterior and posterior horns placed into a bony trough to provide secure fixation and recreate hoop stress within the meniscus when loaded and prevent meniscus extrusion (Figure 19-5).

ACUTE LIGAMENT INJURIES

General Considerations

Complete rupture of isolated ligaments is rare without damage to other structures because the extreme joint displacement required to disrupt a ligament completely must produce at least some disruption in the other supporting structures. Single collagen fibers are not extensible and begin to fail at 7 to 8% elongation. The number of disrupted collagen fibers in the ligament determines whether it is functionally or morphologically disrupted. Complete disruption with loss of continuity requires extreme joint displacement. Although methods of treating ligamentous injuries have seen substantial improvement in recent years, there remain many questions about enhancing the rate, quality, and completeness of ligament healing.

Long-term animal studies have demonstrated that histologic and morphologic appearance of healed ligaments is different from that of noninjured ligaments. When tissue is viewed using electron microscopy after 2 years of healing, the number of collagen fibrils is increased compared with the noninjured ligament, but their diameter and masses are actually smaller. Additionally, crimping patterns within the healing ligament remain abnormal for up

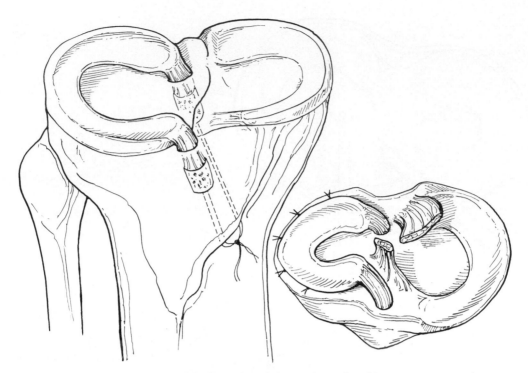

FIGURE 19-5. Meniscal allograft with bone plugs placed into osseous tunnels.

to a year and collagen fiber alignment remains poor. The number of mature collagen cross-links is only 45% of normal after one year. *If the joint is immobilized during the healing process, significant changes in the collagen synthesis and degradation can occur.* Immobilization results in disorganization of collagen fibrils, decreases the structural properties of bone-ligament-bone complex, and resorption of bone at ligament insertion sites. Intermittent passive motion has been reported to improve the longitudinal alignment of cells and collagen at 6 weeks, as well as matrix organization and collagen concentration and ultimate load.

The effects of motion, while positively affecting the ultimate load and healing of the MCL, are debated for ACL and PCL injuries. It is generally agreed that early rehabilitation is critical to prevent arthrofibrosis and restore knee function; some have supported less aggressive rehabilitation to allow vascularization and incorporation of graft.

Origins

Knee ligaments are often injured in contact athletic activities such as American football. Other sports like skiing, ice hockey, and gymnastics can also produce enough stress to disrupt knee ligaments.

Motor vehicle accidents, especially those involving motorcycles, are common causes of knee ligament disruptions. Sudden severe loading without a fall or contact, like deceleration of a running athlete can also cause ligament disruption. By far the most common mechanism is abduction, flexion, and internal rotation of femur on tibia. The medial structures MCL and medial capsular ligament are first to fail, followed by ACL tear, if the force is of sufficient magnitude. The medial meniscus may be trapped between condyles and have a peripheral tear, thus producing *unhappy triad of O'Donoghue.* The mechanism of adduction, flexion, and external rotation is less common and produces primary lateral disruption. Hyperextension force usually injures the ACL. If the force is severe, stretching and disruption of posterior capsule and PCL can occur. Anteroposterior forces, such as a tibia striking a dashboard can cause injuries to either ACL or PCL, depending on the direction of tibial displacement.

History and Physical Examination

The history of mechanism is important; information about the position of the knee, weight-bearing status, direct or indirect force, and previous injury are also important. The patient's description of knee buckling, jumping, audible pop, location of pain, ability to bear weight after injury, and rapidity of knee swelling may be valuable. Intra-articular swelling within first 2 hours of trauma suggests hemarthrosis, whereas swelling that occurs overnight usually is an indication of acute traumatic synovitis that may be caused by degenerative meniscus or a chronic process. Hemarthrosis suggests rupture of cruciate ligament, an osteochondral fracture, or peripheral meniscal tear. *Absence of hemarthrosis does not necessarily indicate a less severe ligament injury because in severe disruptions blood escapes into soft tissues of popliteal space, rather than distending the joint.* Palpation of the collateral ligament and its attachment, joint line, patellofemoral compartment should be systematically performed. Neurovascular examination should be accurate and complete. Stability of the knee is determined by stress testing. Both knees should be examined for comparison.

Abduction (valgus) and Adduction (varus) Stress Test

The valgus stress test should be performed on the normal extremity first for later comparison. The involved knee is flexed to 30°, and a gentle valgus stress is applied to the knee with one hand placed on the lateral aspect of the thigh and the other hand grasping the foot and ankle. It tests for medial ligamentous laxity. The varus stress test is similar to the valgus stress test and is carried out with the knee both in full extension and in 30° of flexion. The integrity of the lateral ligamentous structures is tested by this maneuver. Flexing the knee 30° removes the lateral stabilizing effect of the iliotibial band so that the lateral collateral ligament can be isolated for examination. Testing in extension that reveals significant varus and valgus instability suggests cruciate ligament disruption in addition to collateral ligament disruption.

Anterior Drawer Test

An anterior displacement of 6 to 8 mm greater than opposite knee indicates torn ACL. Examiner must make sure that tibia is not sagging posteriorly from a lax PCL and returning to neutral starting position indicating PCL deficiency. Small degrees of anterior translation of tibia on femur may be better detected in more extended position, to avoid

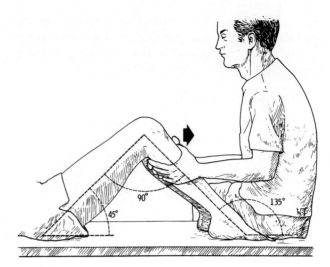

FIGURE 19-6. Anterior drawer test is performed with the patient supine and the affected knee bent 90°. The examiner applies anterior force.

doorstop effect of posterior horn of medial meniscus (Figure 19-6).

Lachman Test

The Lachman test also assesses anterior knee laxity and stiffness with the knee in about 20° of flexion and applying an anterior drawer to the proximal calf. Endpoint stiffness is assessed. A soft endpoint signifies a torn anterior cruciate ligament, whereas a firm endpoint demonstrates an intact structure (Figure 19-7).

Posterior Drawer Test

Careful attention to the neutral position of tibia prevents misinterpretation. Loss of normal 1 cm step-off of the medial tibial plateau with respect to the medial femoral condyle indicates a torn PCL (Figure 19-8). Examining the patient with hips and

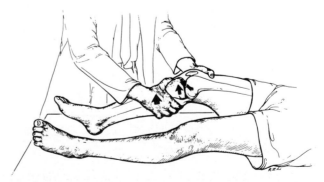

FIGURE 19-7. The Lachman test is performed with the knee flexed between 15 and 30°. The examiner applies anterior force.

knees flexed to 90° with the heel supported by examiner's hands, posterior sag can be visible when examined from the side in patients with posterior instability.

Quadriceps Active Test

With the patient in drawer test position, contraction of quadriceps muscle in a knee with PCL deficiency will result in an anterior shift of tibia of 2 mm or more.

Pivot Shift Test

With the knee extended, the foot is lifted and internally rotated, and a valgus stress is applied to the lateral side of the leg. The knee is flexed slowly while valgus and internal rotation is maintained. In ACL deficient knee, the tibia is subluxed anteriorly, as the knee is flexed past 30°, and the iliotibial band on lateral femoral condyle passes posterior to the center of rotation of knee and reduces the lateral tibial plateau on lateral femoral condyle (Figure 19-9).

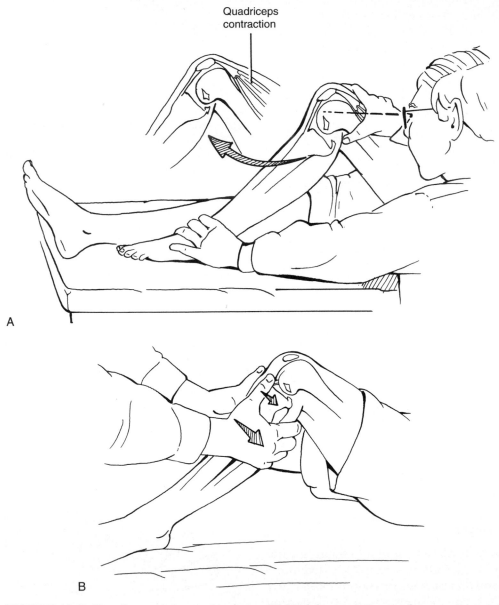

FIGURE 19-8. Tests for posterior cruciate laxity. **(A)** With knee at 90°, note the posterior sag of tibial tubercle relative to normal knee (posterior sag sign). In the PCL deficient knee, the pull of quadriceps translates tibial tubercle anteriorly toward its preinjury position. **(B)** The posterior drawer test is done with the knee flexed 90°. A posteriorly directed force is applied to the tibia.

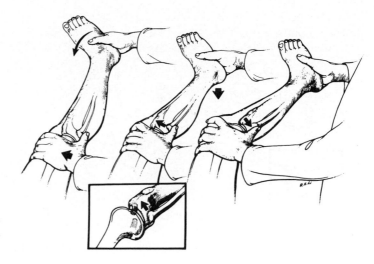

FIGURE 19-9. Pivot shift test is performed with the knee in full extension. A valgus and internal rotation stress is applied.

Tibial External Rotation Test

This is the test for posterolateral instability. External rotation of tibia on femur at 30 and 90° of flexion is measured and compared to the normal side. A 10° difference is pathological. More than 10° difference in external rotation at 30° of knee flexion but not at 90° indicates an isolated posterolateral corner injury, while increase of more than 10° external rotation at both 30 and 90° indicate injury of both PCL and posterolateral corner (Figure 19-10).

Posterior Pivot Shift Test

The posterior pivot shift test is used to diagnose injuries to the posterolateral ligament complex. The clinician supports the limb with a hand under the heel and puts the knee in full extension and neutral rotation. A valgus stress is applied, and the knee is flexed. In a positive test, at about 20 to 30° of flexion, the tibia externally rotates, and the lateral tibial plateau subluxates posteriorly and remains in this position during further flexion. When the knee is extended, the tibia reduces (Figure 19-11A).

External Rotation Recurvatum Test

The examiner grasps the great toes of both feet simultaneously and lifts the lower off the table. Positive findings indicative of posterolateral injury and instability include recurvatum of the knee, external rotation of the tibia, and increased varus deformity of the knee (Figure 19-11B).

Instability is divided into *straight* and *rotatory*. There are four types of straight instability.

Medial instability is caused by a tear of the medial ligaments combined with a tear of the anterior cruciate ligament. In full extension, the knee joint opens on the medial side with a valgus stress test with the knee in a fully extended position. This instability indicates disruption

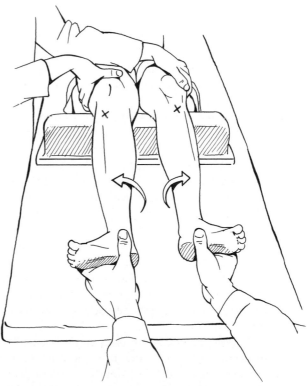

FIGURE 19-10. External rotation test or dial test. An increase in external rotation of greater than 10° relative to normal knee indicates tearing of posterolateral complex.

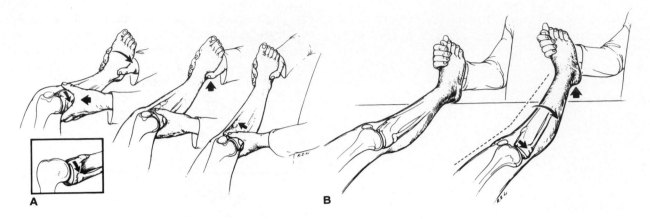

FIGURE 19-11. **(A)** Reverse pivot shift test. **(B)** External rotation recurvatum test.

of the medial collateral ligament, the medial capsular ligament, the anterior cruciate ligament, the posterior oblique ligament, and the medial portion of the posterior capsule.

Lateral instability results from a tear of lateral structures and the posterior cruciate ligament. The knee opens on the lateral side with a varus stress test with the knee in the fully extended position. It indicates disruption of the lateral capsular ligament, the lateral collateral ligament, and commonly, the posterior cruciate ligament.

Posterior instability develops after disruption of the posterior cruciate ligament, the arcuate ligament complex, and the posterior oblique ligament complex.

Anterior instabililty is caused by disruption of the anterior cruciate ligament, the lateral capsular ligament, and the medial capsular ligament.

There are four types of rotatory instability.

Anteromedial instability is manifest in tibial abduction, external tibial rotation, and anterior tibial translation and causes the medial tibial plateau to translate or subluxate anteriorly in relation to the femur. This implies disruption of the medial capsular ligament, medial collateral ligament, posterior oblique ligament, and anterior cruciate ligament. An intact medial meniscus may provide added stability in this instability.

Anterolateral instability is shown by excessive internal rotation of the tibia on the femur with the knee at 90° of flexion. This implies disruption of the lateral capsular ligament, the arcuate complex, and the anterior cruciate ligament.

Posterolateral instability is a result of the lateral tibial plateau rotating posteriorly in relation to the femur with lateral opening of the joint. This implies disruption of the popliteus tendon, the arcuate complex, and the lateral capsular ligament, and at times injury to the posterior cruciate ligament. This results in an external rotatory subluxation in which the tibia rotates around an axis in the intact posterior cruciate ligament.

Posteromedial instability is manifest by medial tibial plateau rotation posteriorly in reference to the femur with medial opening of the joint. This implies a disruption of the medial collateral ligament, the medial capsular ligament, the posterior oblique ligament, the anterior cruciate ligament, and the medial portion of the posterior capsule.

ANTERIOR CRUCIATE LIGAMENT INJURIES

Biomechanics

The ACL is a major stabilizer of the knee. It accounts for 85% of the resistance to the anterior drawer test when the knee is at 90° flexion and neutral rotation. The ACL is 31 to 35 mm in length and 31.3 mm^2 in cross-section. The primary blood supply to the ligament is from middle geniculate artery. The anteromedial band is tight in flexion, and the bulky posterolateral band is tight in extension. The posterolateral band provides the principal resistance to hyperextension. Tension in the ACL is least at 30 to 40° of knee flexion. In addition to excessive anterior translation, the ACL also resists tibial rotation and varus valgus angulation. The muscle forces around the knee can introduce large changes in the forces experienced by the knee. In general, quadriceps muscle forces induce increased tibial translation, while the hamstring has the potential of negating the increased strains in the ACL caused by quadriceps contracture and may indicate the usefulness of closed chain (cocontraction) kinetic exercises during rehabilitation following ACL reconstruction.

History and Physical Examination

Injury of the ACL is most commonly associated with valgus and external rotation, hyperextension, deceleration, and rotational knee movements. Often the history is of noncontact deceleration, jumping, or cutting action. Athletic shoes and artificial turf may play a role in ACL injury. The patient often describes the knee as having been hyperextended or popping out of joint with an audible pop. Frequently there is swelling within the next few hours of injury indicating hemarthrosis. Injury to ACL has been shown to occur in 70 to 75% of all cases of acute hemarthrosis. The Lachman test is most sensitive. The pivot shift test requires a relaxed patient and intact MCL. A side-to-side difference of more than 3 mm or maximum translation of 10 mm is highly suggestive of ACL insufficiency. MRI is very helpful; the reported accuracy of detecting tears is 70 to 100%. Because ACL crosses the knee joint at a

slightly oblique angle, MRI in an orthogonal plane that is obtained by externally rotating the knee approximately 15° will show the entire ACL in one frame (Figure 19-12). Often there is evidence of bone bruising and edema in the lateral femoral condyle associated with ACL tear.

Natural History

The ACL has limited ability to heal. Unrepaired isolated ACL rupture and resultant abnormal force distribution can lead to progressive knee deterioration. Current research also focuses on the biochemical environment of the knee after ACL injury. In chronic ACL injury, proinflammatory cytokine such as interleukin-1 and tumor necrosis factor-α are elevated whereas protective anti-inflammatory proteins such as interleukin receptor antagonist protein are significantly decreased. Recent studies have implicated gender and intercondylar notch index as factors contributing to ACL injury. The *notch index* is the ratio of width of intercondylar notch to the width of distal femur. The normal ratio is 0.231 +/− 0.044. Athletes sustaining noncontact ACL tears have statistically significant notch stenosis. Data from the National College Athletic Association Injury Surveillance system shows significantly higher ACL injury in female soccer and basketball players than in male players. Female soccer players have ACL injury rate of more than double and women's basketball players have ACL injury rate of more than four

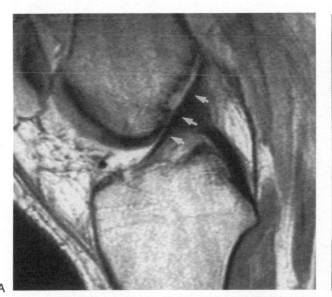
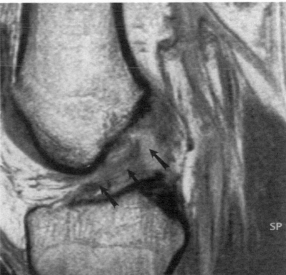

FIGURE 19-12. **(A)** Normal ACL signal. **(B)** Acute ACL tear.

times as compared to their male counterparts. Possible causative factors may be hormonal influences, limb alignment, notch dimensions, ligament size, skill level, muscle strength, and body movement.

Treatment

Acute repair is appropriate when bony avulsion occurs with the ACL attached. The avulsed bony fragment often can be replaced and fixed with transosseous sutures or screws. ACL avulsion is usually at the tibial insertion. Avulsion of femoral attachment has been reported with low velocity ski injuries. ACL tears can be treated nonoperatively with lifestyle changes—avoiding activities that cause recurrent instability—and an aggressive rehabilitation program. The use of a knee brace is controversial and has not been shown to reduce the incidence of reinjury significantly if a patient returns to high activity sports. Persistent instability and significant reinjury to the knee are potential problems of nonoperative management. There is evidence in the literature that ACL reconstruction may prevent secondary injury to the meniscus.

The factors at the time of initial evaluation that correlate with need for surgery are younger age, amount of anterior instability as measured by KT-1000 arthrometer, and preinjury hours of participation in sports. Repair of ACL is no longer advocated. Reconstruction with bone patellar tendon bone and hamstring autograft are the two most popular techniques (Figure 19-13). Timing of surgery is important. It is recommended that surgery be delayed until the swelling, pain, inflammation, and stiffness subside, and full range of motion and muscle function, especially quadriceps have returned. Waiting reduces the incidence of postoperative stiffness. The operative details are beyond the scope of this chapter; however we will discuss key issues of graft selection, placement, tension, pitfalls, and complications.

Graft Selection

The common graft choices are bone patellar tendon bone graft and quadrupled hamstring tendon graft. Bone patellar tendon bone graft has high tensile strength, and adjacent patella and tibial bone plug provide possibility of rigid fixation. The quadruple stranded tendon graft also has high tensile strength, provides multiple bundle replacement, and has minimum donor site morbidity. Recently quadriceps graft with or without patella bone plug has attracted interest.

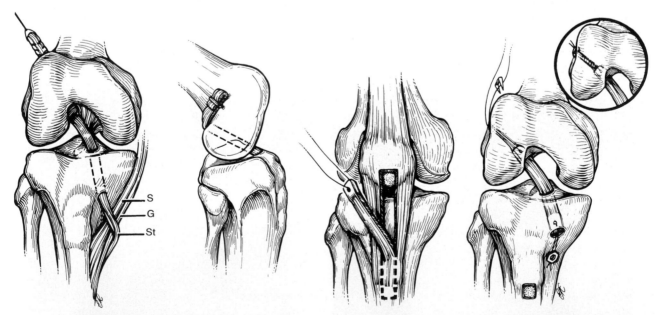

FIGURE 19-13. **(A)** Anterior cruciate ligament reconstruction using the transfer of the semitendinosis tendon secured proximally with a staple. The gracilis tendon may also be used along with the semitendinosis tendons to add strength to the overall surgical construct. **(B)** Anterior cruciate ligament reconstruction using the bone-patellar tendon-bone preparation. The middle third of the patellar tendon is used. **Direct fixation devices include interference screws (most common), staples, washers, and cross pins.**

Graft Placement and Tension

Errors on femoral side are more critical than on the tibial side because of closer proximity to the center of axis of knee motion. A femoral tunnel that is too anterior will produce lengthening of intra-articular distance between tunnel with knee flexion, resulting in loss of flexion or stretching and failure of graft. Posterior placement of femoral tunnel produces a graft that is taut in extension and lax in flexion, with acceptable clinical result as ACL deficiency occurs in full extension. However if this position is chosen, graft should be secured in full extension, as securing graft in flexion may result in loss of extension.

Anterior tibial placement can cause graft impingement by the roof of intercondylar eminence. The desired tension in the graft should be sufficient to obliterate the instability. Too much tension results in difficulty with regaining motion, or it may lead to articular degeneration from altered joint mechanics.

Graft Fixation

The weak link in the early postoperative period is the point of fixation. Fixation of replacement grafts can be classified into direct and indirect methods. Direct fixation devices include interference screws, staples, washers, and cross pins. Indirect fixation devices include polyester tape–titanium button and suture-post. Bioabsorbable screws recently have been introduced. With improvements made in the material properties as well as in screw design, the pullout strength of bioabsorbable screws is comparable to their metal counterparts. Soft tissue grafts can be secured to bone with soft tissue interference screws, screws and spiked washers, screws and fixation plates, or staples.

Posterior Cruciate Ligament

The PCL is an extrasynovial, intracapsular structure; it is composed of two parts, a large anterior portion, that forms the bulk of the ligament and a smaller posterior portion that runs obliquely to the back of tibia. It has a broad origin that forms a semicircle on the lateral aspect of the medial femoral condyle, and it inserts in a depression on fovea 1 cm inferior to the articular surface on the posterolateral aspect of the knee between medial and lateral tibial plateaus. Most authors believe that it is stronger and larger than ACL. *The anterolateral portion, which*

is 95% of the total PCL substance, is taut with knee flexion and lax with knee extension. The posteromedial portion is lax with knee flexion and taut in extension. Either the anterior or posterior meniscofemoral ligament is present in approximately 70% of all knees. The posterior meniscofemoral or ligament of Wisberg is more common and its femoral origin merges with that of PCL.

Biomechanics

The maximal failure force of the PCL is similar to ACL (1,627 +/− 491N and 1,725+/− 660N). PCL is more vertical than obliquely oriented, and it appears to guide the screw-home mechanism on internal rotation of femur during terminal extension of knee. The PCL accounts for 90% of resistance to posterior translation and checks hyperextension only after the ACL is ruptured. Selected cutting of the PCL demonstrates that it is important in flexion. Rotational stability is unchanged in extension but altered in flexion after the PCL is cut.

The natural history of the disrupted PCL is debated, whether the PCL deficient knee is at risk for the development of degenerative changes is not clear at this time. Despite the lack of prospective studies, it appears that progressive degenerative changes may occur in some PCL deficient knees. In theory, compartment degeneration could result from acute chondral injury associated with PCL injury or from increased joint forces created by the absence of the PCL. In cadaver models, increased medial and patellofemoral compartment pressures have been demonstrated after sectioning of the PCL. In chronically PCL-deficient knees, moderate to severe medial compartment changes have been reported in knees that underwent PCL reconstruction more than 4 years after original injury.

The commonly quoted criteria for nonoperative treatment include a posterior drawer of less than 10 mm with tibia in neutral rotation, rotatory laxity of less than 5°, and no significant varus valgus laxity. It is clear that not all knees treated conservatively do well; more recent longer-term studies show that knee function tends to deteriorate with time and that most patients are eventually affected by some degree of disability.

Most surgeons treat avulsion fracture of the PCL's tibial insertion surgically, with open reduction and internal fixation. In case of midsubstance tears of the PCL, there is considerable debate. For *grade I* with loss of anterior step-off, but with proximal tibial eminence remaining anterior to the distal femur, PCL is stretched with less than 5 mm laxity. In *grade II* with proximal tibial eminence flushed with the distal femur on posterior drawer and if the PCL is torn with 5 to 9 mm of laxity, there is agreement on conservative management consisting of brief mobilization and early quadriceps strengthening program. For *grade III* tears with proximal tibial eminence posterior to the distal femur PCL and meniscofemoral ligament torn with more than 10 mm laxity, reconstruction of PCL is recommended in young, active patients with greater than 10 mm of posterior drawer. For *grade IV* or combined ligamentous injuries, surgical reconstruction is recommended (Figure 19-14).

The optimal method of PCL reconstruction is not clear. Reconstruction can be performed with open or arthroscopic-assisted techniques. If an arthroscopically assisted technique is chosen, fluoroscopic control and a posteromedial portal to assist tibial preparation is helpful. This procedure is technically demanding. Because the graft is passed at a sharp angle from the tibia to femur, it may create fraying of the patella tendon graft and subsequent laxity. If the tibia is of poor bone quality, the patellar tendon graft may erode through proximal tibia, creating laxity. The arthroscopic-assisted technique requires patella tendon of 40 mm or more to maintain bone blocks within their tunnel (Figure 19-15). To circumvent the problems associated with the graft making an acute

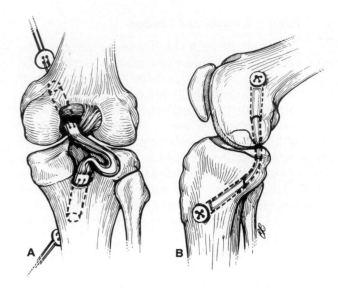

FIGURE 19-15. The Clancy technique of posterior cruciate reconstruction uses the same bone-patellar tendon-bone preparation that is seen in the anterior cruciate ligament reconstructions. However, the placement of bone tunnels is different. **Note the sharp angle ("killer turn") at posterior edge of tibia.**

turn at tibial tunnel exit with potential for graft abrasion and difficulties with graft tensioning, posterior open approaches to tibial attachment of the PCL with tibial inlay reconstruction have been described with encouraging results.

Pitfalls of PCL Reconstruction

A common problem associated with PCL reconstruction is loss of motion. Flexion loss is more common than extension loss, most likely caused by improper graft placement or inadequate rehabilitation. The position of femoral tunnel is more critical than the tibial tunnel. Femoral attachment anterior and distal to the isometric region results in increased graft tension with flexion loss. Femoral tunnel placement posterior and proximal to the most isometric region results in decreased graft tension in flexion and hence laxity. Loss of extension or flexion contracture is caused by prolonged immobilization in flexion. Graft laxity with inability to prevent posterior sag is another complication resulting in failure to obtain objective stability. Selection of improper graft material with insufficient strength like the iliotibial band or hamstring may result in failure. Improper tunnel placement can result in graft abrasion and failure.

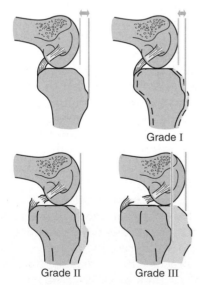

Grade I

Grade II   Grade III

FIGURE 19-14. Grades of PCL laxity.

MEDIAL COLLATERAL LIGAMENT INJURIES

The main medial stabilizer of the knee is the MCL. It contributes 78% to the restraining valgus force on the medial aspect of the knee. Because of its parallel collagen arrangement, only 5 to 8 mm of increased opening indicates a complete failure of the ligament. The MCL is attached proximally to the medial femoral condyle and distally to the metaphyseal area of the tibia, 4 to 5 cm distal to the medial joint line, beneath the pes anserinus insertion. Immediately deep to the MCL is the medial capsular ligament. Posterior to the MCL is a thickening of the capsular ligament referred to as posterior oblique ligament. The MCL complex also resists abnormal external tibial rotation and prevents an increase in anterior tibial translation in the ACL deficient knee.

The majority of injuries to the MCL are caused by contact or noncontact valgus stresses to a flexed knee. *The main test for MCL injury is a valgus stress in 30° of knee flexion.* It is important to apply this force through the foot and ankle rather than the distal tibia as applying force to distal tibia constrains the knee. In addition to joint opening, joint line crepitations or clunk would be suspicious of the medial meniscus tear, chondral injuries, or baseline medial compartment arthritis. Amount of medial opening is graded according to American Medical Association guidelines; grade I injuries would be less than 5 mm; grade II, 5 to 10 mm; grade III or complete tear, more than 10 mm. It is important to assess side-to-side difference. *In an adolescent with open physis, it is important to verify with stress radiograph that the injury is ligamentous and not a Salter-Harris fracture.*

An asymmetrical opening in full extension is indicative of combined MCL and posterior oblique ligament injury, and possible cruciate ligament injury. If the knee is stable, in full extension, there is no significant damage to posterior oblique ligament. MRI can be helpful to highlight the location and extent of ligamentous damage, as well as damage to other structures.

In general, incomplete tears of the MCL are treated with temporary immobilization, use of crutches for pain control, range of motion exercises performed within the first 24 to 48 hours, and an attempt to regain full range of motion as soon as possible. Isometric, isotonic, and eventually isokinetic progressive resistive exercises are begun within a few days of subsidence of pain and swelling. Complete MCL tears without structural damage to other ligaments can be treated in similar fashion; if the knee is not too painful, a hinged brace is used, and quadriceps strengthening exercises and straight leg raises are encouraged immediately.

POSTEROLATERAL CORNER INJURIES

Injuries involving the posterolateral corner of the knee are less common but can be disabling due to both instability and articular cartilage degeneration. A coupled relationship exists between posterolateral structures and the cruciate ligaments. As a result, a high incidence of combined injury is clinically observed. Lateral structures of the knee have been described in three layers. Layer I, or the superficial layer, consists of iliotibial band with its anterior expansion and superficial portion of biceps femoris with its expansion posteriorly. The middle layer or layer II, consists of the quadriceps retinaculum anteriorly and patellofemoral ligament posteriorly. Layer III, or deep layer, is composed of the lateral joint capsule and coronary ligaments, the popliteus tendon, the lateral collateral ligament (LCL), and the fabellofibular and arcuate ligaments. The popliteofibular ligament is the part of deep layer.

The LCL is the primary static restraint to the varus stress of the knee and also provides resistance to external rotation. Isolated injuries of the LCL are uncommon and usually occur in conjunction with injuries to other ligamentous structures. Popliteus plays a major role in both dynamic and static stabilization of the lateral tibia on the femur including restriction of posterior tibial translation, restriction of external and varus rotation of tibia, and dynamic internal rotation of tibia. The popliteofibular ligament represents a direct static attachment of popliteus tendon from the posterior aspect of the fibular head to the anterior aspect of the lateral femoral epicondyle. It provides a significant share of overall resistance to posterior tibial translation, external rotation, and varus rotation. The arcuate ligament reinforces the posterolateral capsule and spans from lateral femoral condyle to fibular styloid. The biceps femoris in conjunction with iliotibial band is a strong external rotator, as well as dynamic lateral stabilizer of the knee; it is frequently injured in posterolateral injuries.

Biomechanics

The posterolateral structures function primarily to resist posterior translation as well as external and varus rotation of tibia; they act with the PCL to provide overall stability. Selective ligament sectioning in cadaveric models has demonstrated the importance of posterolateral structures. Sectioning the posterolateral structures alone results in an increase in posterior translation of the lateral tibial plateau primarily at 30° of flexion, with a minimum increase at 90° of flexion. However when both the PCL and posterolateral structures are sectioned, increases in posterior translation are observed at both 30 and 90° of flexion. Isolated sectioning of posterolateral complex, primarily the LCL, results in increased varus rotation from 0 to 30° of flexion, with maximum increase observed at 30°. Combined sectioning of the PCL and posterolateral structures results in increased varus rotation of the knee at all angles of flexion, with maximal increase observed at 60°. Thus, the posterolateral structures appear to provide resistance to posterior translation, restraint to varus rotation, and tibial external rotation at lesser degrees of flexion. Sectioning of the PCL and posterolateral structures also results in increased medial and lateral compartment pressures and increased patellofemoral pressures secondary to a "Reverse Maquet" effect.

Clinical Presentation

Most cases of Posteolateral Rotatory Instabiliy (PLRI) are secondary to trauma, with approximately 40% occurring as a result of sports injuries. The usual mechanism is hyperextension with a varus moment combined with twisting force. Other mechanisms can be noncontact hyperextension and external rotation, sudden deceleration, with a fixed lower leg. Presenting features in addition to history of trauma can be pain, weakness, numbness, and paresthesias associated with peroneal nerve injury. Chronic PLRI patients may describe pain localized to joint line and may also report instability primarily with knee in extension, such as knee buckling in toe-off. These patients typically exhibit gait abnormalities characterized by varus thrust at the knee coupled with a knee hyperextension in the stance phase. Patients often maintain the knee in internal rotation as the knee is more unstable in external rotation. In addition, patients may exhibit overall varus alignment with increased adduction moment. In acute

situations, the examiner should have high suspicion for knee dislocations in cases of multiple ligamentous injuries. A careful neurological examination must be performed.

The most useful tests for the diagnosis of posterolateral injuries are the prone external rotation test at 30 and 90° of flexion and varus stress test at 0 and 30° of flexion. Other tests like reverse pivot shift test and external rotation recurvatum tests can be used to supplement the clinical impression.

Imaging

Plain radiographs may show abnormal widening of lateral joint space, avulsion of proximal tip of fibular head, avulsion of Gerdy's tubercle, or a Segond fracture (lateral capsular sign), which is avulsion of lateral aspect of capsule from tibial plateau. Although Segond fracture is usually associated with ACL injury, it can also occur with isolated posterolateral injury (Figure 19-16). Chronic posterolateral injury patients may have degenerative changes in the tibiofemoral and patellofemoral compartment. The lateral compartment is usually more involved. Varus stress radiographs may be helpful. In addition full-length weight-bearing radiographs of both lower extremities may be helpful in determining overall alignment. MRI is very helpful in evaluating posterolateral injuries. A bone contusion of the posteromedial femoral condyle is frequently observed. MRI can provide visualization of individual posterolateral structures. Coronal oblique T2 images provide better visualization than standard coronal and sagittal images.

Treatment

Nonoperative Treatment

The natural history of these injuries is not clearly delineated; nonoperative treatment of complete tears involving the posterolateral corner has generally led to poor results. It is believed that there is an increased degree of disability with combined injury pattern and predisposition to early degenerative joint changes. In general nonoperative treatment should be prescribed for patients with mild instability and without significant symptoms or limitations. Patients with chronic PLRI often have quadriceps atrophy and gait abnormalities, and programs consisting of gait training and muscle rehabilitation may be beneficial.

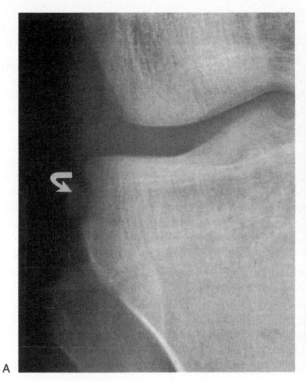
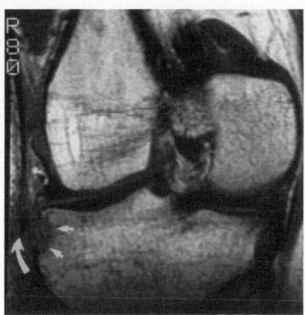

FIGURE 19-16. Segond fracture. **(A)** AP radiograph demonstrates the capsular avulsion fragment. **(B)** MRI demonstrates the defect within the lateral tibia and small adjacent avulsion fracture.

Operative Treatment

Currently, the indications of operative treatment of PLRI include symptomatic instability with functional limitations as confirmed by significant objective physical findings. Operative treatment of acute injuries is usually more successful than surgery for chronic injury. In general, surgical repair is recommended within the first 2 to 3 weeks. It is important to simultaneously evaluate and treat other injuries. In one study, the most common identifiable cause of ACL reconstruction failure was unrecognized and untreated posterolateral corner injuries. In cases of concomitant injuries, reconstruction of the ACL or PCL should be performed either prior or with the reconstruction of posterolateral structures. In chronic cases, it is also important to correct any varus knee alignment, and valgus osteotomy with distal advancement of iliotibial band with bone block may be performed.

Acute Injury

In acute injury, primary repair should be attempted initially. Major structures that should be evaluated include the iliotibial tract, biceps femoris, peroneal nerve, LCL, popliteus muscle, and tendon and popliteofemoral ligament. Treatment of posterolateral injuries should proceed from deep to superficial, with repair of structures by direct repair, suture by drill holes through bone, or suture anchors as appropriate. In acute situations where the severity of injury precludes direct repair, involved structures can be augmented with hamstring tendons, biceps tendon, iliotibial band, or allograft.

Chronic Injury

There is lack of consensus in the literature regarding the best technique of operative treatment for chronic injury. Proximal advancement of arcuate complex (lateral head of gastrocnemius, LCL, popliteus tendon, and arcuate ligament) in line with the LCL into a trough in distal femur can be performed with good results. Tensioning is performed with the knee in 30° flexion and the tibia in neutral rotation. The disadvantage of the procedure is that the insertion sites of the LCL and popliteus are drifted anterior to the center of rotation, which may lead to attenuation and eventual failure.

Biceps tenodesis as described by Clancy, has the proposed advantage of recreating the LCL as the arcuate complex is tightened. The entire biceps tendon is transferred anteriorly to the lateral femoral epicondyle leaving the distal insertion intact (Figure 19-17). However, the disadvantage is that the popliteus and popliteofemoral ligaments are not reproduced, and a fixation point other than 1 cm anterior to the LCL femoral origin results in nonisometric graft position that does not reduce external rotation or varus stress at any degree of flexion. Salvage posterolateral reconstruction after failed biceps tenodesis may be quite difficult.

Posterolateral reconstruction using autograft or allograft for reconstructing the popliteus and popliteofemoral ligament, an extracapsular sling procedures reconstructing LCL by using bone tendon bone allograft secured with interference screws in the fibular head, and lateral femoral condyle have been described with favorable results. Surgical complications of these procedures include peroneal nerve palsy, failure of reconstruction, knee stiffness, hamstring weakness (especially in biceps tenodesis), infection, and hardware irritation.

OSTEONECROSIS

The knee is second to hip as the most common area affected by osteonecrosis. Osteonecrosis of knee occurs in approximately 10% of patients with osteonecrosis of hip. Ahlbäck and associates first described the disease in 1968. *Osteonecrosis of knee represents two distinct entities—spontaneous osteonecrosis of the knee and steroid-associated osteonecrosis.*

Osteonecrosis indicates death of a segment of the weight-bearing portion of the femoral condyle or tibial plateau with associated subchondral fracture and collapse. In the typical case, the patient, who is usually older than 60 years of age, presents with an acute onset or exacerbation of pain on the medial side of the knee with or without associated minor trauma or increased activity. Patients often have a history of insidious knee pain, commonly experienced in early and mild osteoarthritis. Mechanical symptoms, such as locking, catching, and buckling, are not widespread. However, during the acute phase, the knee can appear locked because of pain, effusion, and muscle contracture. Although it

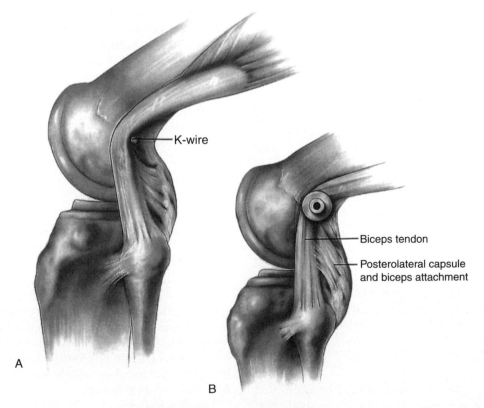

FIGURE 19-17. Biceps tenodesis.

is most common in the medial femoral condyle, osteonecrosis may also occur in the lateral femoral condyle and tibial plateau. The tibial lesions occur on the medial side. Radiographs may be normal, but bone scintigraphy is markedly abnormal. MRI also shows this lesion during the acute phase before it is clearly shown on plain radiographs. After 2 or 3 months, radiographs typically show flattening and radiolucency of the subchondral bone of the medial femoral condyle with a sclerotic line of demarcation around the lesion. Degenerative changes may also be present at this time if a large weight-bearing area of the femoral condyle is involved.

The condition may present in a similar manner to a spontaneous tear of the medial meniscus and should be differentiated from it in a patient who is older than 60 years of age. These patients often erroneously undergo arthroscopic surgery for presumed meniscal tear, based on changes observed on MRI studies that are so common in this age group, without symptomatic relief.

Most cases are idiopathic in nature. Vascular and traumatic theories also have been proposed, with the vascular theory being the most widely accepted. Fat embolism has been suggested as a possible mechanism. Bone microcirculation is contained within an expandable compartment, and an increase in bone marrow pressure can cause bone ischemia. Elevated bone marrow pressure is found in patients on steroid therapy, but it is also found in osteoarthritis of the knee.

Osteonecrosis presents radiographically in five stages. In stage 1, the radiographs are normal, but MRI is abnormal. Slight flattening of the condyle is seen in stage 2. An area of radiolucency with a distal sclerosis and a faint halo of bony reaction are found in stage 3. Stage 4 shows a calcified plate with radiolucency surrounded by a definite sclerotic halo. Stage 5 represents narrowing of the joint space with subchondral sclerosis and osteophyte formation typical of osteoarthritis.

The differential diagnosis includes osteochondritis dissecans, osteoarthritis, meniscal tears, pes anserinus bursitis, and insufficiency fracture. The area of the lesion is important in predicting which knee will develop osteoarthritis. Knees with lesions smaller than 5 cm^2 have a better clinical and radiographic prognosis.

In general, there are five basic options for the treatment of osteonecrosis: (1) conservative care, (2) core decompression of the distal femur, (3) arthroscopic debridement, (4) proximal tibial osteotomy, and (5) total or unicompartmental arthroplasty.

Conservative therapy consists of analgesia as needed, protected weight bearing, and activities to tolerance. Excellent to good results can be obtained with conservative means if lesions are relatively small, that is, less than 40% of the width of condyle. If the disease progresses, a few cases can be treated by arthrotomy, or arthroscopy and drilling of the lesion. Arthroscopy may be effective in debriding unstable or delaminating chondral fragments, particularly to resolve mechanical symptoms like catching and locking. It is more advisable to drill in an antegrade nonarticular direction, rather than retrograde through overlying intact cartilage, to stimulate revascularization of the osteonecrotic fragment. Core decompression by extra-articular drilling of the femoral condyle can relieve the initial acute pain that occurs with the onset of spontaneous osteonecrosis of the knee. The best results are reported in stage 1 lesions. If femoral flattening is already apparent, the progression cannot always be avoided. Core decompression is a really effective treatment for steroid-induced osteonecrosis because steroid-induced osteonecrosis is an entirely different entity with different anatomic involvement in the distal femur. The central factor is that steroid-induced osteonecrosis does not necessarily involve the subchondral plate. The principal involvement is metaphyseal; therefore it has different structural and mechanical ramifications for the joint surface.

High tibial osteotomy, unicompartmental arthroplasty, and total knee replacement are reserved for knees in which advanced osteoarthritis has developed. The indication of high tibial osteotomy is in stage 3 lesions where less than 50% of the condyle is involved in active patients younger than 65 years of age. There is a role of unicompartment replacement of spontaneous osteonecrosis of one condyle or plateau; however the possibility of subsequent osteonecrosis of the opposite compartment is a critical concern. Any change involving the epiphysis of metaphyseal bone on the preoperative MRI should be considered as compromised osseous structures that may predispose the subsidence and compromise long-term survivorship. Total knee arthroplasty (TKA) has provided good results in well over 90% of patients; however careful review of the literature of these results for spontaneous osteonecrosis suggests that while satisfactory results are obtainable, there is need to remain guarded in the final results. Inferior results are reported in TKA for spontaneous and steroid-induced osteonecrosis when compared with matched group of patients with osteoarthritis.

ARTICULAR CARTILAGE LESIONS

Articular cartilage has a very limited potential for healing. In adults it possesses neither a blood supply nor lymphatic drainage, and is sheltered from immunologic recognition by the surrounding extracellular matrix. Although the cells continue to produce the extracellular matrix, they are ineffective in responding to injury. Wounds that are limited to cartilage itself without injuring the subchondral bone stimulate only a slight reaction in the adjacent chondrocytes. The natural history of isolated chondral defects is not known; it is assumed that these chondral and osteochondral defects may progressively enlarge with time and play a role in the development of more generalized osteoarthritic changes. Trauma to articular cartilage beyond a critical level causes a reduction in viscoelasticity and stiffness of cartilage. As a result, more force is transmitted to the subchondral bone, with consequent thickening and eventual stiffening of the subchondral plate. The increased stiffness of subchondral bone allows more impact stresses to be transmitted to the cartilage, creating a vicious circle of cartilage degeneration and stiffening. Treatment of full thickness articular surface lesions in young and middle-aged individuals is a challenge. These lesions may be small and asymptomatic at discovery or may increase in size and may become painful. In a review of more than 31,000 arthroscopies, chondral lesions were reported in more than 60% of patients. It is proposed that 5 to 10% of all patients who present with acute hemarthrosis of the knee after work- or sport-related injury have full thickness chondral injury.

Clinical Presentation

The most common presentation of a full thickness articular cartilage lesion is a loose body. It may be associated with an acute injury with large effusion or may have insidious onset with no effusion. Some patients may have joint line pain and mechanical symptoms of locking. Injuries associated with full thickness articular surface injuries include patellar dislocation with lateral femoral condyle and medial patella facet lesions, dashboard injuries, and ligament injuries. The physical examination usually does not elicit a distinct consistent finding other than localized pain with or without an effusion. The presence of loose body is considered predictive of articular surface injury.

Plain radiographs, including standing posteroanterior flexion views, may show compartment joint space narrowing or an osteochondritis dissecans type of defect, with or without loose body. With full thickness articular cartilage lesions, plain radiographs may not reveal any changes, and MRI may be helpful. Defects in articular cartilage appear as focal areas of cartilaginous thinning in which the defect is filled with synovial fluid, which demonstrates a characteristic bright signal of T2 images. An abnormal signal in the underlying bone often aids diagnosis. On follow-up MRI or arthroscopy, the contusions in the subchondral bone are associated with high incidence of osteochondral abnormalities, such as thinning, or loss of articular cartilage and subchondral sclerosis. Proton density imaging and T2 imaging with fat saturation sequences optimize resolution of the articular chondral surface. The sensitivity of MRI in consistently analyzing changes in the articular surface has been reported to be 40 to 70%. Arthroscopy is a more accurate technique for diagnosing articular surface lesions, documenting the location, size, shape, or depth of the lesion.

Nonoperative Treatment Options

The vast majority of articular defects and degenerative articular cartilage changes do not cause symptoms of any significant disability. However, some patients may present with complaints of pain, swelling, giving way, and mechanical symptoms of locking, catching, or crepitus. The goal of nonoperative treatment is to reduce symptoms related to articular cartilage lesion. Treatment modalities include patient education, activity modification, and physical therapy for muscle strengthening, a nonaggravating fitness program.

Pharmacologic therapies include mild analgesics; anti-inflammatory drugs such as cyclooxygenase-2 (cox-2) inhibitors; local corticosteroid injections; and chondroprotective agents, such as oral glucosamine and chondroitin sulfate and injectable hyaluronic acid for viscosupplementation. In symptomatic patients for whom these treatment modalities are unsuccessful, surgical interventions can be considered. The appropriate treatment of an asymptomatic patient with an incidental finding of a full thickness articular cartilage lesion is an enigma. The natural history of this lesion is not well known. Whether these lesions if left untreated become symptomatic in short time or if the joint destruction can be prevented by treating these lesions—these questions at present remain unanswered. Also the natural history of surgically treated symptomatic patients is still evolving; until it is confirmed, surgical treatment of asymptomatic patients is not recommended, though continual observation and follow-up monitoring is warranted.

Operative Treatment Options

The operative techniques currently most widely used are arthroscopic debridement, lavage, and repair stimulation. The direct transplantation of cells or tissue into a defect and replacement of defect with biological substitutes can restore articular surface in selected patients.

Microfracture and Arthroscopic Lavage and Debridement

Using microfracture and arthroscopic lavage and debridement to remove loose flaps or edges can improve symptoms; however, the effects are temporary and there is no potential for healing. Attempts to enhance the intrinsic healing potential of articular cartilage have been focused on recruiting pluripotential cells from the bone marrow by penetrating the subchondral bone or providing mechanical, electrical, laser, or other stimulus for healing. The usual result of these penetrating techniques (drilling, abrasion arthroplasty, or microfracture) is the partial filling of articular defect with fibrocartilage that contains principally type I collagen. *Unlike the desired hyaline cartilage, this fibrocartilage has diminished resilience and stiffness, poor wear characteristics, and predilection for deterioration with time.*

The current role of these techniques is controversial, although they have some chance of helping the patient and are a reasonable first step in the management of a previously untreated cartilage defect. Because of the limited capacity of the cartilage to heal, a more attractive approach is to transplant cells or tissue with chondrogenic potential. These living cells or tissue may be directly transplanted into an articular cartilage defect. Both autologous committed chondrocytes and undifferentiated mesenchymal cells placed in articular defects survive and are capable of producing new cartilaginous matrix.

Osteochondral Autograft

An alternative to biological regeneration is to replace the defect with a substitute, either primarily or a series of small osteochondral plugs (mosaicplasty). This procedure involves the autogenous transplantation of at least one cylindrical osteochondral plug from a relatively nonweight-bearing region of the knee into an articular defect (Figure 19-18). The donor site is usually the edge of the patella groove or the area just next to intercondylar notch. The technique involves excising all injured or unstable tissue, creating cylindrical holes in the base of defect and underlying bone. These holes are filled with cylindrical plugs of healthy cartilage and bone in mosaic fashion. The goal is to fill the defect as completely as possible. Histologic evidence demonstrates that hyaline cartilage on cylindrical graft has the ability to survive in its new setting and maintain its structural integrity. Osteochondral autografts are indicated for patients less than 45 years of age, with sharply defined defect surrounded by healthy cartilage. Lesions should be unipolar and no more than 2 to 2.5 cm^2. The technique of fixation and continuous passive motion are reported to be important in obtaining optimal results.

Autologous Chondrocyte Implantation (ACI)

In this technique, the mature articular chondrocytes are harvested, expanded in cell culture, and implanted into the defect. This technique preserves the subchondral bone plate (Figure 19-19). Early results indicate a good to excellent result in more than 80% of patients. Follow-up arthroscopic examination showed good fill with repair tissue, good adherence, and hardness close to that of adjacent tissue. *ACI is indicated for the younger (20 to 50 year old) active patient with an isolated traumatic femoral chondral defect greater*

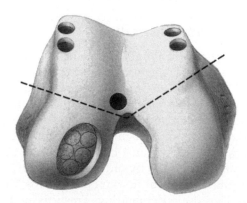

FIGURE 19-18. Location of recommended donor sites for osteochondral grafts. Osteochondral plugs 15 to 25 mm long are harvested and implanted in the prepared base of defect. Coverage of 80 to 90% of defect is recommended.

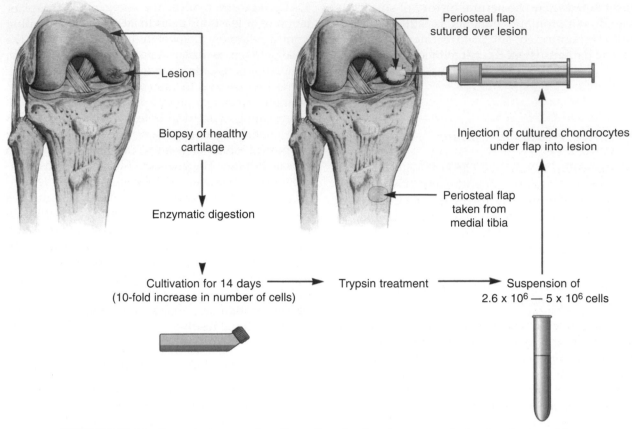

FIGURE 19-19. From the harvested cartilage slices the chondrocytes are isolated and cultured for 2 weeks before the implantation can take place.

*than 2 to 4 cm². *Accompanying ligamentous, meniscal lesions, joint malalignment, and patellofemoral instability must be corrected concurrently. Absence of meniscus, bipolar lesions, osteoarthritis, and instability may preclude such treatment.

Osteochondral Allografts

Osteochondral allografts may be used for larger (>10 cm²) full thickness lesions after failure of one or two previous surgical procedures. Fresh allografts provide the greatest likelihood of chondrocyte survivability, but also carry higher risk of immunologic and transmissible disease. Use of shell graft with less than 1 cm of subchondral bone reduces immunogenecity of the graft. The technical constraints of surgical implantation of fresh osteochondral graft are demanding. Fresh tissue from a young (<30 years) donor must be available and recipient and surgeon must be on call at all hours of day and night.

The best indications are posttraumatic defect or osteochondritis dissecans. Concern related to preservation techniques, disease transmission, tissue viability and availability, and graft host reactions limit the use of this technique. Although fresh frozen allografts have a decreased risk of immunogenic response and visual transmission, there is concern regarding viability of chondrocytes potentially decreasing the longevity of allograft.

Biologic and Synthetic Materials

Biologic and synthetic polymers can be used to cover and cushion underlying exposed bone, reestablish a congruent articulating surface, and provide physical and mechanical properties of articular cartilage. Synthetic matrices can bridge the void of the osteochondral defect and potentially delay or avoid major surgery. An example of one of these polymers is flowable in situ curable polyurethane, which is a cross-linked, segmented polyurethane that exhibits high tensile strength and excellent fatigue resistance under physiologic loads.

PATELLOFEMORAL DISORDERS

The patellofemoral joint is biomechanically complex, but the most important function of the patella is to improve the efficiency of the quadriceps by increasing the lever arm of the extensor mechanism. The thickness of the patella displaces the patellar tendon away from the femorotibial contact point throughout knee range of motion, thereby increasing the moment arm of the patellar tendon. It has been shown that 3.3 times the body weight is generated across the patellofemoral joint at 60° of knee flexion during stair climbing, and up to 7.8 times the body weight at 130° during deep knee bends. Patellofemoral contact pressures are uniformly spread over all contact areas, but peak pressures are highest between 60 and 90° of flexion. The symptoms of patellar dysfunction include anterior knee pain, giving way, locking, and swelling. Occasionally, pain may be referred to the joint lines, mimicking the symptoms associated with meniscal tears. In addition to routine radiographs, patellofemoral radiographs in the form of axial views in different degrees of extension should be obtained (Figure 19-20). There are several congenital anomalies of the patella, including bipartite patella, congenital absence of the patella (patellar aplasia), a small patella (patellar hypoplasia), and a large patella (patella magna).

Osteochondritis dissecans of the patella is best seen on a slightly overexposed lateral radiograph. An axial ("skyline") radiographic view determines whether the lesion is in the medial or lateral facet. In the patella it usually is associated with chondromalacia that extends considerably beyond the peripheral margins of the avascular bone. Residual disability after treatment usually is proportional to the size of the chondromalacia area. Treatment options include conservative management, excision of the fragment and curetting the crater, excision of the lesion followed by curettage, and drilling of the lesion. Arthroscopic treatment of a patellar osteochondritic lesion using retrograde placement of a Herbert screw or absorbable screws have also been reported. Rarely is chondromalacia so extensive as to require patellectomy; the patella should almost always be preserved.

Bipartite patella usually is asymptomatic and is noted incidentally on an anteroposterior or tunnel tangential radiograph. When present, it occurs

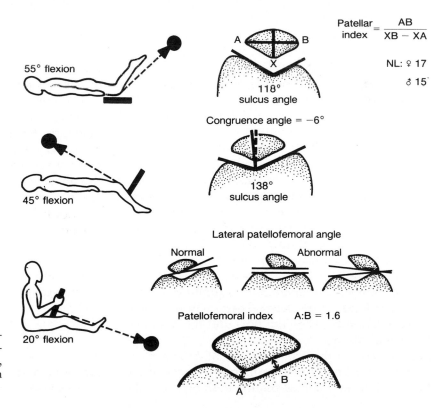

FIGURE 19-20. Schematic representations of the different radiographic evaluations of the patella: the Hughston (55°), Merchant (45°), and Laurin (20°) patella views.

bilaterally in approximately 40% of patients. Three types have been described. Type I, which accounts for 5%, occurs at the inferior pole and may be associated with Sinding-Larsen-Johannson syndrome. Type II, which accounts for 20%, occurs along the entire lateral border of the patella and may be associated with a nonunion of a patellar fracture. Type III, the most common type, occurs as an elliptical area in the superolateral portion of the patella and accounts for 75% of cases. Pain is unusual in bipartite patella, and when present it is caused by overuse. A diagnostic radiographic test to determine if pain is caused by a nonunion at the bipartite site is to obtain a normal skyline view followed by a skyline view taken with the patient in a squatting weight-bearing position. The test is considered positive if the separation is greater in the squatting weight-bearing position than on the normal skyline view. If pain occurs with a bipartite patella, treatment should include limiting and restricting activity, correcting the activity that is causing an overuse syndrome, and prescribing nonsteroidals and a short arc exercise program. Immobilization for 3 weeks or more relieves the symptoms of repetitive microtrauma of the synchondrosis. Rarely does conservative treatment fail, making operative treatment unnecessary. Excision of the bipartite fragment, especially in the superolateral quadrant can be successful in relieving symptoms if conservative measures fail.

Excessive lateral patellar compression syndrome (ELPS) is characterized by pain. Pain is characteristically dull, poorly localized, and increased by activities that overload the patellofemoral joint. Symptoms may follow a trauma. A sense of the knee buckling may occur, which makes this syndrome difficult to differentiate from patients with true patellar instability. True episodes of patellar instability, however, followed by considerable swelling that persists a few days, are lacking. An apprehension test (whereby the patient becomes apprehensive when the physician attempts to move the patella medially and laterally with the knee extended, simulating the feeling of instability) is negative, and only minor tracking abnormalities of the patella are present.

On physical examination, squinting of the patella is easily appreciated. There may be a mild varus relation between the tibia and the femur. A half-squat usually provokes pain. A quadriceps angle of greater than 20° is abnormal. This angle is formed by a line drawn through the center of the long axis of the thigh across the midportion of the

patella and a line drawn along the patellar tendon. The lateral retinaculum is considered tight if the patella is unable to be moved medially more than one-fourth of its width. Pain on compression of the patella against the femoral sulcus is usually present. Radiographically, lateral placement of the patella on an axial, skyline (Merchant) view may be evident. Radiographic clues of long-standing ELPS include lateral facet sclerosis, lateralization of trabeculae, and lateral traction spurs (Figure 19-21). The pain is thought to result from excessive lateral loading of the patellar ridge. Excessive lateral ligamentous tension may also contribute to the syndrome.

Treatment consists of rest, restriction of activity, quadriceps training, anti-inflammatory medication, rehabilitation program, and taping. Occasionally, surgical treatment is necessary and includes lateral retinacular release done by open arthrotomy or arthroscopic means.

Chondromalacia Patellae and Patellofemoral Arthritis

Chondromalacia patellae and patellofemoral arthritis are secondary to damaged or softened articular cartilage of the patellofemoral joint. The term *chondromalacia* should be used only to describe the changes that occur in the articular cartilage, if the disease has progressed to involve changes of the bone (osteophyte formation, subchondral sclerosis, and cysts) and of the synovium (synovitis), it should be classified as patellofemoral arthritis.

Observable age-related changes in chondromalacia occur commonly after the second decade and in almost all knees after the fourth decade. Unfortunately, the term *chondromalacia* has become synonymous with patellofemoral pain. Numerous other terms have been proposed to describe the syndrome, such as patellofemoral syndrome, patellofemoral arthralgia, extensor mechanism dysplasia, anterior knee pain syndrome, and others, but these are not commonly accepted. Some patients with

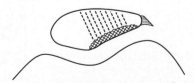

FIGURE 19-21. Radiographic clues of long-standing lateral compression syndrome.

minimal changes in the articular surface have marked patellofemoral joint symptoms, and conversely, some patients with no patellofemoral joint pain have marked changes in the articular surface of the patella. *Chondromalacia of the patella should describe a pathologic condition of the cartilage and not a clinical syndrome.* In chondromalacia of the patella, the initial lesion is a change in the ground substance and collagen fibers at the deep levels of the cartilage. It is a disorder of the deep layers of the cartilage that involves the surface layer only late in its development. In contrast, in osteoarthritis the initial changes occur on the surface of the cartilage, with loss of continuity of the transverse fibers followed by fibrillation, which usually becomes grossly visible. Changes occur most commonly at one of two sites in the deep layer of cartilage. The first is an area about 1 cm in diameter astride the ridge that separates the lateral facet from the medial facet; the second area straddles the inferior part of the central ridge that separates the medial and lateral facets.

Outerbridge classified chondromalacia in four different grades: *Grade I* included softening and swelling, *Grade II* included fragmentation and fissuring in a 0.5 inch or smaller area, *Grade III* showed fragmentation and fissuring in a 0.5 inch or larger area, *Grade IV had* cartilage erosion down to bone. The most comprehensive and specific grading system for articular cartilage lesions was published by Noyes and Stabler. They classified articular cartilage lesions by defining the surface description, the extent of the articular cartilage involvement, the diameter, location and the degree of flexion that will put the lesion in contact with the weight-bearing area. Grade 1 lesion is chondromalacia 1A: soft cartilage, 1B: softening with definite indentation; Grade 2 are open lesions, 2A: fissures/fragmentation of half thickness and 2B: full thickness; Grade 3A: bone exposed and 3B: bone cavity.

Most chondromalacia is idiopathic in nature. It may, however, result from lateral patellar compression syndrome, patellar instability, trauma, previous anterior cruciate ligament surgery, prolonged immobilization for fracture treatment, or synovial conditions affecting the articular cartilage surface. Pain is associated with increased patellar pressure and basal degeneration of the cartilage. The signs and symptoms of chondromalacia of the patella are nonspecific; there is no pathognomonic symptom. Most patients with chondromalacia describe a dull, aching discomfort that is well localized to the anterior part of the knee and that is most prominent after sitting in one position for a long time. This has been called the "movie sign." Crepitation in the patellofemoral joint also varies. The patient may describe a catching or giving way sensation with activity; pain and giving way both tend to be much more prominent while descending stairs. Puffiness or swelling may be noted, depending on the degree of synovitis present.

Articular cartilage is devoid of nerve endings and therefore cannot be the direct source of pain. The synovium and subchondral bone probably are the two areas producing pain in chondromalacia of the patella. Many authors believe, however, that pain in the patellofemoral syndrome, with or without chondromalacia, originates from the subchondral bone. It is hypothesized that the biomechanical failure of articular cartilage in chondromalacia of the patella results in an alteration of load transfer to the subchondral bone. Insall suggested that most young people with chondromalacia of the patella have an extensor mechanism malalignment and this, rather than the articular changes themselves, is responsible for the pain.

Articular cartilage breakdown occurs on different portions of patella articular surface, depending on the nature of malalignment or trauma. When there is recurrent shear stress as in patellar malalignment, the distal central portion may break down. The lateral facet is the site of breakdown in excessive lateral pressure syndrome (ELPS) with chronic patellar subluxation and tilt. The medial facet is more commonly damaged at the time of patellar dislocation and relocation. Another cause of medial facet articular cartilage breakdown is previous medial tibial tubercle transfer with posterior placement of tibial tubercle (Hauser procedure). The proximal patella is more commonly damaged as a result of a dashboard or crush type of injury in which the knee is flexed at the time of injury. This injury responds poorly to tibial tubercle anteriorization procedures as these procedures cause load shift onto more proximal patella. Diffuse articular cartilage damage more frequently occurs as a result of generalized arthritis or extensive damage following malalignment and recurrent dislocations.

Patellofemoral arthritis involves predominantly the lateral joint line in most cases. Narrowing of the joint line, with osteophytes on the lateral patellar border and trochlea, subchondral sclerosis of the lateral facet, and possibly cyst formation, may be present on axial radiographs. Most often, patellofemoral arthrosis appears to arise de novo in a structurally normal joint for which no obvious cause can be assigned. There is a frequently associated femorotibial arthrosis.

Nonoperative treatment consists of isometric quadriceps exercises, knee braces, and anti-inflammatory medications. Surgical treatment involves procedures that relieve stress on the patellofemoral joint and that directly address the pathology of the articular cartilage. Patellar cartilage shaving can be done open or arthroscopically and yields the best results (83% satisfactory) in the earlier stages of chondromalacia. Subchondral bone drilling with cortical abrasion yields more unpredictable results (60% satisfactory), as does lateral retinacular release. Elevation of the tibial tubercle, patellar resurfacing, and patellectomy show limited success (70% satisfactory) and are formidable procedures with high complication rates.

Treatment of chondromalacia of the patella depends on the underlying cause of the articular surface changes and should be directed to the cause rather than to the results. Most often, this treatment involves nonsurgical measures, such as anti-inflammatory medications, quadriceps exercises, and hamstring stretching. Prone quadriceps stretching exercises are particularly helpful, they enable the patient and physician to see the progress and reduce stiffness around the anterior knee. Strengthening of the entire kinetic chain will benefit the patient, although specific emphasis on vastus medialis obliquus (VMO) will improve support to the patella. Some patients also benefit from braces and activity modification.

Operative treatment is divided into two phases: (1) treatment directed at malalignment and other abnormalities of the extensor mechanism and patellofemoral joint and (2) treatment of the diseased cartilage. Surgery is indicated for chronic patellofemoral pain after all attempts at nonoperative management have failed.

Arthroscopy has proved extremely reliable in diagnosing chondromalacia of the patella. The degree of fibrillation and fragmentation of the surface can be probed under direct vision, and careful probing can identify areas of softness.

Malalignment of the extensor mechanism is believed to be one of the most common causes of patellofemoral pain and chondromalacia changes in the patellofemoral joint. Malalignment problems related to bony abnormalities, such as excessive femoral anteversion, excessive external tibial torsion, and severe genu valgum, may require osteotomy for skeletal realignment.

Lateral retinacular release by open, subcutaneous, or arthroscopic technique is indicated for painful arthrosis with radiographically documented incongruity, lateral tilting, or lateral orientation of the patella in the patellofemoral joint. *Surgery for chondromalacia of the patella has been unpredictable in patients with normal axial radiographic studies.*

Commonly used procedures involving the articular surface include (1) arthroscopic patellar shaving, (2) local excision of defects with drilling of the subchondral bone, (3) facetectomy, (4) mechanical decompression of the patellofemoral joint by elevating anteriorly the tibial tuberosity (Maquet procedure), and (5) patellectomy. Patellar resurfacing or patellofemoral replacements have not been sufficiently successful to indicate their use for unicompartmental patellofemoral arthritis or severe chondromalacia of the patella.

Arthroscopic shaving of the patella has become popular; the major benefit is probably from the lavage of the joint and removal of articular surface debris.

Maquet, in 1963, recommended anterior advancement or elevation of the insertion of the patellar tendon onto the tibial tuberosity to reduce the articular pressures in the patellofemoral joint. This technique has been used more often for patellofemoral arthritis than for chondromalacia of the patella. Patellectomy should be used only in advanced chondromalacia and severe patellofemoral joint degeneration. Fulkerson described slightly oblique osteotomy of the tuberosity, (Figure 19-22) that transfers the tuberosity anteriorly and medially. This procedure achieves both unloading of the patella and improved alignment in one operation and does not require bone graft or distraction of tibial tubercle.

OSTEOARTHRITIS

Osteoarthritic disease is the result of mechanical and biological events that destabilize the normal processes of degradation and synthesis of articular cartilage chondrocytes, extracellular matrix, and subchondral bone. These changes include increased water content, decreased proteoglycan content, and altered collagen matrix, all leading to the deterioration of articular cartilage. Arthritis of the knee results from a wearing away of the articular cartilage of the joint. Arthritis may be idiopathic, or it can result from trauma, rheumatoid synovitis, pigmented villonodular synovitis, and seronegative arthropathies such as gout, chondrocalcinosis, osteonecrosis, and idiopathic disorders. Osteoarthritis is predominantly a mechanical deterioration that may be associated

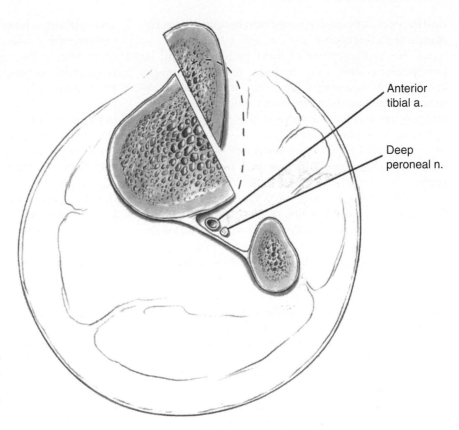

Anterior
tibial a.

Deep
peroneal n.

FIGURE 19-22. Anteromedial tibial tubercle transfer as described by Fulkerson. Note the close relationship of deep peroneal nerve and anterior tibial vessel to the oblique osteotomy.

with malalignment of the knee. Familial, genetic predisposition may exist, however, and osteoarthritis may result from and be associated with significant synovitis. Rheumatoid arthritis is associated with significant synovitis, with 80% of patients having a positive rheumatoid factor, indicating an autoimmune basis for cartilage destruction.

The knee is the most commonly affected joint with osteoarthritis. Posttraumatic causes include torn menisci with previous complete meniscectomy, fractures, patellar instability, and loose bodies caused by chondromalacia or synovial chondromatosis. Mechanical varus or valgus malalignment with obesity may cause abnormal loading of the knee over time and produce premature degeneration of the joint cartilage. Infection causes joint cartilage destruction owing to the proteolytic enzymes released by the leukocytes that enter the knee to combat infection where the enzymes are nonselective in their destructive capabilities.

Clinically, the patient with arthritis presents initially with stiffness and pain. Characteristically, the patient has stiffness on initiation of gait, which gets better as the knee "warms up." There may be an antalgic or painful gait in which the stance phase of

the walking cycle is shortened. A knee with varus malalignment may demonstrate a lateral thrust due to instability of the lateral collateral ligament. A patient with valgus malalignment may show a medial thrust due to an incompetent medial collateral ligament. The knee may show swelling caused by an effusion and synovitis. Locking may also occur as the bare bony surfaces grate against each other, causing severe pain. Osteophytes may also be palpable on clinical examination.

Radiographically, weight-bearing views should be obtained to give the appearance of the knee while it is under stress. A weight-bearing view in full extension shows most of the clinical destruction of the joint. Only the posterior condyles may be involved, however, in which case a weight-bearing view with the knee flexed 45° shows joint space narrowing, indicating significant cartilage destruction. Osteoarthritis is characterized by joint space narrowing, osteophytes, cortical sclerosis on the weight-bearing bony surfaces, and subchondral cysts. Usually, the medial or lateral joint with mechanical malalignment is seen, with or without patellofemoral involvement, on the radiograph. Rheumatoid arthritis, on the other hand, demonstrates a more symmetric joint destruction appearance without osteophytes on the standing radiographs.

Initial management of most patients should be nonoperative and may include physical therapy, bracing, orthoses, ambulatory aids, nonsteroidal anti-inflammatory medications, intra-articular steroid injections, and analgesics. After the acute pain and synovitis has calmed, gentle exercises and stretching of the joint may begin. Exercises often slow the onset of permanent stiffness and flexion contractures. Changes in daily, work, and recreational activities also may be necessary. Obesity is a known risk factor for osteoarthritis of the knee, and weight loss has been shown to slow the progression of the disease. Because of the progressive nature of the disease, many patients with osteoarthritis of the knee eventually require operative treatment. A variety of procedures have been described for treatment of the osteoarthritic knee, ranging from arthroscopic lavage and debridement to total knee arthroplasty. The choice of procedure depends on the patient's age and activity expectations, the severity of the disease, and the number of knee compartments involved.

Treatment of the arthritic knee should initially consist of a period of rest and avoidance of weight bearing if the knee is painful. Occasionally, a splint or elastic bandage is needed to allow the synovitis to calm down. Moist heat may be applied to decrease stiffness. Ice should be used if the knee becomes acutely swollen and painful. Nonsteroidal anti-inflammatory medications may be prescribed to decrease the synovitis. Prudent use of intra-articular cortisone injections may be used; however, the use of cortisone injections at frequent intervals (e.g., every month) has been shown to accelerate arthritic deterioration. After the acute pain and synovitis has calmed, gentle exercises and stretching of the joint may begin. Exercises often slow the onset of permanent stiffness and flexion contractures. Surgical intervention is indicated if the patient has persistent pain that is not relieved by rest, anti-inflammatory medications, and cortisone injections.

Joint debridement is the first surgical method of treatment. A radical resection of the synovium and removal of osteophytes with shaving of degenerated cartilage down to subchondral bone through an open arthrotomy was used in the past. However, arthroscopic debridement is now the procedure of choice. It can be redone in the future if the patient feels successful long-term pain relief was obtained. Debridement is less predictable if there is mechanical deformity of the joint. Knees with loose bodies

and cartilage tears were shown to do well with arthroscopic intervention. Arthroscopic debridement should be considered in active, older adults with mild to moderate osteoarthritis of the knee after conservative treatment has been exhausted. Response to treatment is unpredictable, and patients should be informed of this. Patient selection should be based on the history of symptoms, physical examination, and radiographic findings. Age should not be the sole criterion for selecting arthroscopic treatment. Patients with symptoms of short duration and those with mechanical symptoms tend to do well. Patients with radiographic malalignment, especially valgus deformities, tend to have poor outcomes, as do patients with pending litigation or worker's compensation claims. Several authors have reported a "placebo effect" after arthroscopy for osteoarthritis of the knee that occurs even when no specific procedure is performed, but most suggested that this effect was of short duration. None of these arthroscopic procedures can significantly alter the natural progression of osteoarthritis. In a recent study that retrospectively reviewed over 14,000 arthroscopic debridement procedures performed for osteoarthritis, almost 20% had total knee arthroplasty within 3 years of the surgery. At best, arthroscopic techniques may delay the need for a more definitive procedure, especially in younger, active patients with localized degenerative arthritis that causes pain at rest without malalignment or instability.

Advanced arthritis poses a more formidable problem for the surgeon. The surgical decision is based primarily on the age and activity of the patient, the mechanical deformity, and the type of arthritis.

Knee arthrodesis is reserved for the young, heavy, active person who has premature severe destruction of the knee due to arthritis. Most of the time, however, the patient refuses arthrodesis owing to the postoperative appearance and the inability to bend the knee after the procedure. The procedure provides permanent pain relief and allows the patient to return to durable, active work.

Medial joint osteoarthritis in a patient younger than 60 years of age can be treated by upper tibial osteotomy. This procedure alters the mechanical axis of the knee by the removal of a triangular wedge of bone based laterally from the proximal aspect of the tibia above the tibial tubercle (Figure 19-23). Success remains durable in patients who have a postoperative alignment of at least 8° of valgus and who are not obese. The correction is done on the tibial side

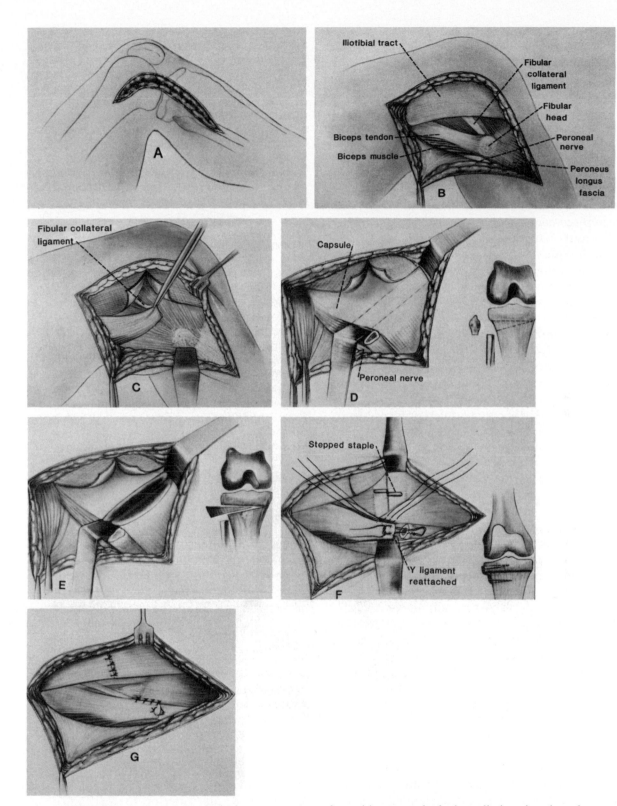

FIGURE 19-23. Proximal tibial osteotomy is performed by removal of a laterally based wedge of bone from the proximal tibia, which in turn creates a valgus alignment to restore the normal mechanical axis to the leg. The tibiofibular joint must be released or the proximal fibular head should be resected to allow closure of the osteotomy.

since most of the bone destruction is tibial. Women tolerate the postoperative valgus alignment less well than men and represent a relative contraindication for the procedure. The procedure is not indicated in grossly obese patients, unstable knees, or knees with less than 75° of motion, greater than a 15° flexion contracture, and instability. Deformities of up to 10° of varus can be treated in this manner. There are numerous techniques of fixation of the fragments after osteotomy, including staples, plates, and cylinder casts. The procedure allows the patient to remain active and delays the time when total knee replacement becomes necessary. The procedure permits participation in rigorous sports. Another technique described for high tibial osteotomy is opening wedge osteotomy with a dynamic uniplanar external fixator using hemicallotasis techniques. In this procedure, the medial osteotomy is made below the tibial tuberosity. A dynamic external fixator is applied, and beginning 7 days postoperatively the fixator is distracted 0.25 mm four times a day until correction is obtained. Most reports have shown approximately 80% satisfactory results 5 years after osteotomy. However, these results also have been shown to deteriorate over time. Nevertheless, high tibial osteotomy still is a useful procedure for some patients. Reported complications of proximal tibial osteotomy include recurrence of deformity (loss of correction), peroneal nerve palsy, nonunion, infection, knee stiffness or instability, intra-articular fracture, deep venous thrombosis, compartment syndrome, patella infera, and avascular necrosis of the proximal fragment.

For the young, active patient with a valgus arthritic deformity, supracondylar femoral osteotomy is the treatment of choice (Figure 19-24). Arthritic knees with valgus malalignment typically have bone destruction located on the lateral femoral condyle. Hence, correction of the deformity should be on the femoral side. If the valgus deformity at the knee is more than 12 to 15° or the plane of the knee joint deviates from the horizontal by more than 10°, Coventry recommended a distal femoral varus osteotomy rather than a proximal tibial varus osteotomy. Reported success rates for distal femoral osteotomies performed for osteoarthritis range from 71 to 86% good or excellent results. Poor outcomes have been noted in patients with rheumatoid arthritis or those with inadequate motion of the knee before distal femoral osteotomy.

Unicompartmental knee arthroplasty has been controversial since its introduction in the early 1970s. Early reports on the success of the procedure

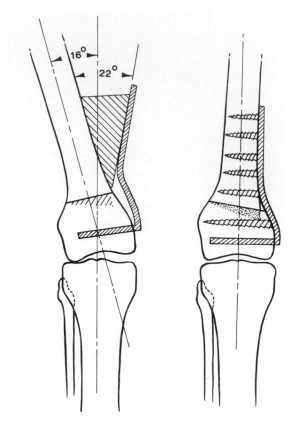

FIGURE 19-24. Distal femoral osteotomy for valgus knee.

were conflicting. However, recent long-term reports have showed success rates for unicompartmental knee arthroplasty approaching those of primary total knee arthroplasty in properly selected patients. Early reports of unicompartmental arthroplasty noted failure and revision rates of up to 40%, most related to mechanical alignment, implant design, cemented fixation, and debris from polyethylene wear. Newer implant designs that provide more adequate surface replacement with less stress concentration, thickened and metal-backed polyethylene tibial inserts, improved fixation, and less bony resection have reduced the incidence of mechanical failure dramatically. More recent reports have indicated that intermediate and long-term results of unicompartmental arthroplasty are comparable to those of total knee arthroplasty and high tibial osteotomy.

Disadvantages of unicompartmental arthroplasty include narrow indications, difficult surgical technique, results inferior to total knee arthroplasty, and complexity of revision similar to that of tricompartmental replacement. With recent design improvements unicompartmental arthroplasty is becoming a viable alternative for patients in whom osteoarthritis is limited to either the medial or lateral compartment. *Ideal candidates for unicompartmental arthroplasty are older than 60 years of age, have low activity demands, weigh less than 180 pounds, experience minimal pain at rest, and have preoperative arc of flexion of 90°, no flexion contracture of more than 5°, and no angular deformity of more than 15°.* Although we prefer proximal tibial osteotomy and total joint arthroplasty, unicompartmental arthroplasty may be appropriate in carefully selected patients.

In older patients with advanced osteoarthritis, total knee replacement is the preferred treatment. The indications for joint replacement have been stretched for younger patients with tricompartmental (medial and lateral tibiofemoral and patellofemoral) disease owing to the predictable pain relief and durability of the implants over time. Joint replacement for the young, active patient, however, ensures the need for future revision surgery, thus the operation should be delayed as long as possible for these patients. Age is not a factor in recommending total knee replacement for rheumatoid arthritic patients because the disease generally affects the patient's overall activity level significantly so that wear and loosening of the implants are of less concern.

TOTAL KNEE ARTHROPLASTY

Evolution, Types, and Constraint

A major feature of total knee arthroplasty is *constraint*, namely stability between the tibial and femoral components due to the shape and design features of each. In considering different levels of constraint, they can be appreciated by reviewing the evolution of modern TKA. The first *total* knee arthroplasties are the fixed hinges of Waldius and Shiers. These are examples of maximal constraint. Flexion-extension motion is about a fixed, single axis. There is no internal or external rotation. Early loosening and other problems led to more anatomic designs, which started with the Gunston and Geomedic knees. These bicondylar and biplateau components are four ligament knees, generally preserving the cruciates and the collaterals. While not operating about a fixed hinge, the component shapes led to nearly single axis rotation, and the interfaces between tibia and femur provided little rotation. Early failure rates led to designs with less constraint. As well, the discrete pieces, especially the four-piece nature of the polycentric Gunston knee spurned designs that were relatively monolithic.

Also, the next generation of TKAs offered resurfacing of the patellofemoral joint—patellar plastic buttons and coverage of the femoral trochlear groove.

The two-ligament condylar designs of Insall, Ranawat, P. Walker, and Townley are good examples of these less constrained knees. They relied on tibial surface dishing to create anterior posterior stability. Posterior and anterior cruciates were routinely excised. Most initially, and nearly all ultimately, provided matching patellar buttons as well as shaping of the femur component to model the trochlear groove of the biologic knee.

The Freeman-Swanson entry had certain similar features, and MAR Freeman began to emphasize ligament balancing or correction of preoperative varus and valgus deformities. Limited ranges of motion due to shapes, tightness in the collaterals, and absence of the cruciates led to less conforming tibial surfaces while preserving the PCL. This type may be called *cruciate condylar* knees. An alternative developed was the posterior substituting design. This is earliest exemplified by the Insall-Burstein prosthesis, which uses an intercondylar tibial peg to articulate inside an intercondylar femoral housing. The interaction of these two prevents posterior displacement of the tibia in relation to the femur, especially during flexion. Interaction of this post with the femoral housing also usually provides a camming relationship so that the femur is induced into a posterior roll as the knee is flexed. This kinematic pattern allows better clearance of the posterior aspect of the distal femur in its relationship to the posterior edge or the tibial surface. Various forms of posterior cruciate retain (PCR) sparing knees (derivatives of the cruciate condylars just mentioned) are, together with posterior substituting (PS) knees, the most popular implants. An interminable debate exists as to the relative merits of each, that is PS versus PCR for the routine and even difficult knee cases.

After years of debate, there are no or few established indications for one versus the other. The choices are largely due to surgeon training, experience, and taste. Most would probably agree that the postpatellectomized knee and the cruciate deficient knee with posterior tibial subluxation should be managed with PS components. A variation, reintroduced to the array has been a deep-dished PCR version. The rationale is to permit maintenance of the PCL and some of its function while enhancing posterior stability by having a deeper tibial dish, particularly at the anterior lip. This is different from the original total condylar, which relied more on a posterior lip to prevent anterior dislocation.

Anterior subluxation or dislocation seems not to have been a clinical problem.

A final design feature is the inclusion of mobile bearings (Figure 19-25). They have been in use for more than 15 years and are based on a rationale of providing complex motion with maximum contact surface area. Their use has been increasing, but the value versus cost and potential risks are not so clearly established. This is a violently debated issue.

Component Materials, Fixation, and Size

The most common component materials are titanium alloy, used now for tibial baseplates, and cobalt-chrome alloys for femoral components, as well as tibial baseplates. The softer titanium proved to be a bad choice for a bearing surface. Nearly all knees worldwide use polyethylene tibial surfaces at the articulation. The poly, as it is frequently termed, may constitute the entire baseplate so that the poly is cemented to the bone, or may be an insert fitting on a metallic baseplate. These latter are mostly modular designs supplied with separate metal baseplates. Polyethylene has also been the most consistent material for resurfacing the patella. Patellar design features have related to component thickness, general size, and overall surface shape. In the 1980s metallic features connected to thinner polyethylene structures, were provided with porous surfaces to permit bone ingrowth. The correspondingly thinner plastic frequently led to wear-through and its associated problems of metal debris, scratching of the femoral component and osteolysis. Metal-backed ingrowth patellar components exist, but they are not very popular. The overall question of whether even to use a patellar component is another hotly contested one. Clearly the vast majority of U.S. orthopaedic surgeons do resurface, while a moderate number of European and Asian surgeons do not. True experts line up enthusiastically on both sides of the topic and marshal convincing arguments for the two views. Indications for leaving the patella unresurfaced are a primary diagnosis of osteoarthritis, satisfactory patellar cartilage with no eburnated bone, congruent patellofemoral tracking, a normal anatomical patellar shape, and no evidence of crystalline or inflammatory arthropathy. Patient weight also appears to be a factor, with lighter patients tending to do well with unresurfaced patellae.

A key feature in total knee arthroplasty is component size. In general, surgeons seek to place components that are as close to equal in size as the bone removed and the aspect of bone that is covered or capped. The *finite size problem* leads to the necessity of compromise. A nearly continuous array of patient sizes has to be fit with a fixed, limited selection of prosthesis sizes. Thus, the component size may be just right, or the component will be a bit large or a bit small. Undersizing can lead to lack of maximal bone interface and therefore support. Oversize can lead to tightness—tightness of gaps, the capsule, and so on—all of which can lead to poor motion.

Fixation

A large majority of TKAs done today are fixed to bone via methyl methacrylate cement. Bone ingrowth porous surfaces were introduced in 1980. Other cobalt-chrome beads, titanium beads, fiber metal, and pseudocancellous structures, including mesh-like constructs have been used. Many of the clinical results with these materials were excellent, but failure rates on balance have been higher than with cemented implants. Surgeons in many countries remain dedicated to uncemented fixation; however the majority moved back to the use of cement in combination with many other improvements in cementation, realignment, and so on. Uncemented fixation may reappear as there is greater successful experience obtained with the use of hydroxyl-apatite-coated surfaces.

The Operation

Alignment Preop, Postop Goals

Varus, valgus, flexion contracture, and recurvatum are the four deformities that are encountered. Varus, generally in combination with mild flexion contracture, is the most common. Particularly varus and valgus are seen on radiographs, and seen most

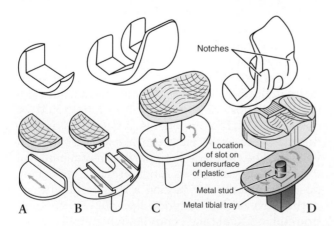

FIGURE 19-25. Schemes of mobile bearing knees.

clearly on long-standing views. Drawing a few simple lines displays the angle of deformity on these radiographs. The accepted target for normal, that is the surgeon's goal, should be clear. A line drawn from the center of the femoral head should pass through the center of the knee as it goes on through the center of the ankle. The net anatomic tibiofemoral angle equals the angle of offset between the anatomic shaft of the femur and the mechanical line of the femur—the line from the center of the femoral head to the center of the distal femur. That number is generally between 5 and 6° (Figure 19-26). Numerous studies have shown a correlation between long-term success of total knee arthroplasty and restoration of near-normal limb alignment.

Malalignment of total knee prostheses has been implicated in long-term difficulties, including tibiofemoral instability, patellofemoral instability, patellar fracture, stiffness, accelerated polyethylene wear, and implant loosening. Rotational alignment of total knee components is difficult to discern radiographically, making the assessment of rotation primarily is an intra-operative determination. The rotation of the femoral component has effects not only on the flexion space but also on the patellofemoral tracking. Because the proximal tibial cut is made perpendicular to the mechanical axis of the limb instead of in the anatomically correct 3° of varus, rotation of the femoral component also must be altered from its anatomical position to create a symmetrical flexion space (Figure 19-27). To create this rectangular flexion space, with equal tension on the medial and lateral collateral ligaments, the femoral component usually is externally rotated approximately 3° relative to the posterior condylar axis. In a normal femur, this technique rotationally places the femoral component with the posterior condylar surfaces parallel to the epicondylar axis. This technique fails when the posterior aspect of either the native femoral condyle has significant wear or when the lateral femoral condyle is hypoplastic, as is frequently seen in knees with valgus deformity.

Exposure

Most surgeons use a nearly midline to slightly anteromedial skin incision in combination with some form of medial capsulotomy. The capsulotomy

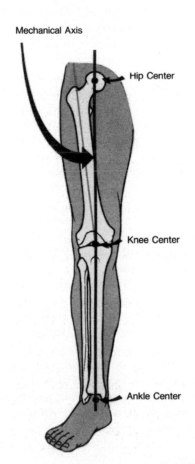

FIGURE 19-26. Mechanical and anatomical alignment.

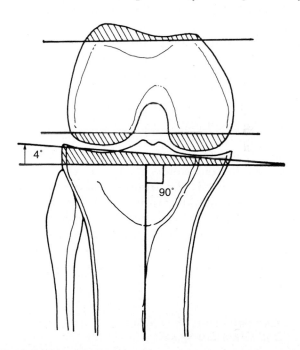

FIGURE 19-27. Bone resection with classic arthroplasty alignment. The tibial plateau is cut perpendicular to its anatomic axis, resulting in more bone resection laterally than medially. To equalize the medial and lateral flexion space, more bone should be resected from the medial posterior femoral condyle. This is achieved by slight external rotation of femoral component.

may be extended proximally within the quad tendon—the standard approach; extended into the muscle close to the tendon; projected otherwise in the mid-aspect of the vastus—a midvastus approach; or extended at the medial margin of the vastus medialis—a subvastus approach. Other variations include (1) the Muller lateral skin incision in combination with a medial capsulotomy, and (2) a lateral incision—lateral capsulotomy generally in combination with a tibial tubercle osteotomy, and generally done for direct access to the lateral stabilizers when managing valgus deformity.

Since approximately 2002 some have been working on minimal incision, small exposure techniques, principally on the medial aspect but also laterally. The term *MIS, for minimal incision surgery,* has been introduced. An analogous approach from the lateral aspect is being developed as well. The goal of all of this work is less soft tissue trauma leading to less discomfort, better initial rehab, and better overall results. It is not clear as of this date whether such techniques are safe, are teachable or transferable, or even whether the final result is any better.

Exposure of the Stiff Knee

The stiff knee, stiff at any point, is much more difficult to expose. Achieving adequate access from the anterior aspect can require extraordinary manipulation of the extensor mechanism. The options include tibial tubercle osteotomy, quadriceps tendon snip, and quite uncommonly today a quad-turndown—modified Coonse-Adams exposure. Another approach is skeletonizing, basically elevating capsular-ligamentous-tendinous tissue as far around and as far proximal and distal as necessary to fold things back and get the knee bent and exposed. The arguments for and against each are voluminous. We very aggressively favor the tibial tubercle osteotomy. It gives the best amount of exposure of the least soft tissue disruption and is associated with the strongest repair. The problems originally noted have largely been overcome.

Gap Balancing, the Flexion, and Extension Spaces

In all cases it is necessary to take care to create essentially equal flexion and extension gaps. The distance from the posterior femoral cut to the proximal tibia approximates the distance of the distal femoral cut surface to the proximal femur when the

tibia is distracted away from the femur and assessed respectively at 90° and 0°. This gap equality is achieved to some degree either by specifically measuring the distances and cutting the bones in the two positions to achieve this, or by using measured resection. Measured resection is accomplished by placing instruments on the distal and posterior femur so that the amounts of bone removed from those aspects of the femoral surface approximate the thickness of the corresponding femoral component surfaces. Pure flexion contracture and pure recurvatum deformity, meaning those without any varus or valgus components, may be viewed as representing a priori inequalities in the flexion versus extension gaps. Viewing the flexion contracture situation as one predisposed to a smaller extension gap as the recurvatum predisposes to a larger extension space.

The knee should be stable in flexion and extension and hyperextension (recurvatum) of the joint should be avoided.

Deformity Balancing

This is another type of balancing that means addressing the *asymmetry* of the soft tissue sleeve as a result of mostly varus and valgus malalignment, but also the presence of flexion contracture. The most common and basic approach is to release those ligamentous, capsular, and tendinous structures that lie on the concave aspect of the deformity, that is the medial side of the varus knee, posteromedial as well if there is flexion contracture. Knees with severe varus deformity need subperiosteal release of the medial collateral ligament from the proximal portion of the tibia. This is required because the medial collateral ligament becomes contracted as the varus alignment becomes more severe. In valgus knees, the iliotibial band, popliteus tendon, and lateral collateral ligament frequently need to be released from the femur. Flexion contractures are corrected by removal of osteophytes from the posterior femoral condyles and release of the posterior joint capsule; occasionally, more distal femoral bone needs removal.

In rare situations the surgeon may elect to tighten the lax, convex side of a deformity. This technique may be indicated in younger patients in whom moving to a higher order of prosthetic constraint—varus or valgus constraint imparted by a highly conforming intercondylar peg, may be undesirable.

Hemostasis

The issue of achieving hemostasis at TKA is handled in a variety of ways. Probably most common is the use of a tourniquet, until components are completely in place. Then, the tourniquet is deflated as the surgeon searches to control the more obvious bleeding points. Some keep the tourniquet inflated until the dressing is wrapped into place. Others let the tourniquet down after bone preparation, search for bleeding points, then reinflate for cementation and closure, or cementation alone. If the surgeon is going to look for bleeding points, and it is our practice and recommendation to do that, *there are at least four locations to check.* The most common moderate bleeding point is at the inferolateral geniculate artery in the posterolateral corner of the knee. This vessel courses between the lateral collateral ligament and the popliteus tendon. Especially with removal of the posterior cruciate ligament for implantation of a PS knee, surgeons are encouraged to inspect the location of the intermediate geniculate at the posterior center. If there has been any lateral patellar release, or significant dissection at the anterolateral fat pad and parapatellar region, then careful examination of the lateral patellar "gutter" is appropriate. A final region is at the medial tibial metaphysis in the case of large medial release for varus deformity. The surgeon can see significant bleeding from injured branches of the inferior medial geniculate vessel.

Cementation

There are many different ways to perform this portion of the surgery and many subtasks and points involved. The surgeon must direct attention to the following elements: (1) definite, adequate pressurization into clean dry cancellous bone; (2) full impaction of the associated component, checking that this is full by seeing that the component is properly down, against the bone surfaces; and (3) clearing of the overflown cement. To accomplish all of this, it is necessary to cleanse and dry the cut surfaces using pulsatile lavage, suction, and sponging. The cement must not be too liquid. Very liquid cement may be injected into the bone, but it then runs away from anything other than a horizontal surface. Also, as the component over the cement is impacted there is less viscosity to create a pressurization at the time of component seating. Similarly, do not use cement that has become too completely cured and cannot intrude into trabecular interstices. Antibiotic impregnated cement is controversial. We use it routinely, and many others do. Most probably do not use it except for revision after infection, for especially long, complicated cases, or because of compromised defense mechanisms in the patient.

Uncemented TKA

Press-fit, uncemented arthroplasty requires accurate bone cuts and achieving initial prosthesis bone fixation. Cuts have to be very accurate; alignment must be nearly perfect and initial stability enhanced to some degree by stems, pegs, or maybe even screws for some designs.

Closure

Wound closure may be considered as "routine"; however, it is crucial. Accurate edge approximation at each level without strangulation and ischemia of tissue is extremely important. The large TKA implant may lie less than a centimeter away from the outer surface of the skin. The chances for retrograde infection due to failure of wound sealing and healing is great.

Computer Navigation

Since approximately 1996, various centers have been using computer assistance to oversee alignment and kinematic features during performance of the total knee operation. This equipment uses high-tech position detection devices that observe using infrared lights on bone and instrument markers. The relative movement of bones and surfaces is immediately detected. Inputting to the computer the locations of those bony features which form the bases of alignment and rotation, the system indicates the relative positions and actual alignment of the components and the respective bones—all at once and essentially instantaneously. Navigation is not currently the standard, but many predict that it will be by the next 5 to 10 years.

Postoperative Rehabilitation

Perhaps the essential features of postoperative rehabilitation are as simple as achieving range of motion and protective as well as functional strength. The real challenge is to get and to keep the knee moving so that the anterior structures do not contract and so the various tissue planes do not get fibrosed to each other and to the components.

REVISION TOTAL KNEE ARTHROPLASTY

The settings of revision TKA include infection, instability, fracture, loosening, poly wear, osteolysis, bone fracture, patellar maltracking, component breakage, and other factors.

The challenges and issues present are all of those mentioned above plus the following:

- Understanding the true cause of failure in the problematic knee
- Difficulties of exposure
- Loss of bone stock, this leading to difficulty with fixation
- Difficulty with fixation
- Difficulty with balancing and stability

Infection

Deep sepsis of total knee arthroplasty is a devastating complication. Preventing infection is an integral part of performing the procedure, while early and appropriate treatment of the established infection is of utmost importance. In recent reports, deep infection complicates 1.3 to 2.9% of total knee arthroplasties.

Causes

Infection occurring in the perioperative period is generally the result of contamination at the time of surgery. Late infection may occur in a previously sterile joint that becomes septic secondary to hematogenous seeding of the arthroplasty. Diabetes mellitus; rheumatoid arthritis and its variant, corticosteroid use; immunosuppressive medications; extreme old age; concurrent infections; prior history of septic arthritis; obesity; and prior knee surgery have all been shown to increase the risk of early and late sepsis of the knee.

Microbiology

The most common organisms isolated from septic arthroplasties have been *Staphylococcus aureus* and *Staphylococcus epidermidis*. Together these microbes are identified in over half of all infected arthroplasties in a wide range of studies. Gram-negative bacilli are involved when arthroplasty infection results from acute wound complications or late hematogenous seeding. Indolent infections presenting 3 to 24 months after surgery are caused by avirulent organisms such as negative staphylococci, viridans streptococci, anaerobic Gram-positive cocci and corynebacteria. Candida organisms that contaminated the wound perioperatively cause rare episodes of indolent prosthetic joint infection. Hematogenous infections of arthroplasties are caused by virulent organisms such as *S. aureus*, β-hemolytic streptococci, and Gram-negative bacilli.

Clinical Presentation

Type I infections occur in the immediate postoperative period. The patient is seen during the first postoperative month, and the diagnosis is evident on the basis of the medical history and physical examination. Systemic signs of infection such as fever, chills, and sweating may be present. Pain is usually continuous, on local examination wound may be erythematous, swollen, fluctuant, and tender. Wound drainage, if present, is usually purulent. Laboratory tests such as white blood cell count (WBC) and erythrocyte sedimentation rate (ESR) are of limited use, since moderate elevation is expected in this time period. C-reactive protein (CRP) normalizes within 3 weeks of surgery, much earlier than ESR and persistent high level of CRP is suggestive but not diagnostic. Clinically, it is difficult to distinguish between sterile and infected hematomas. Culture of drainage fluid has not been reliable. Aspiration is helpful, but if the patient has been on antibiotics within the preceding weeks, a false negative may be obtained. Treatment of the wound is the primary consideration. Tense infusions or hematomas are best surgically evacuated, whether or not infection is present. Infection in this time period is initially treated with surgical debridement, administration of antibiotics, and attempted retention of the components.

Type II infections are also believed to originate at the time of the operation, but because of a small inoculum or the low virulence of the organism the onset of symptoms is delayed. The patient is seen between 6 and 24 months after the index procedure. The hallmark of this type of infection is a gradual deterioration in function and an increase in pain. Type III infections are the least common and are caused by hematogenous spread to a previously asymptomatic arthroplasty, usually 2 or more years after the arthroplasty. Generally there is an acute febrile episode accompanied by sudden rapid deterioration in the function of the knee. The diagnosis can usually be based on history and physical examination. Seeding can occur at the site of a loose prosthesis, a solidly osseo-integrated prosthesis, or a solidly fixed cemented prosthesis. These patients typically have a significant pain-free interval. A type III infection is likely to occur in patients who are immunosuppressed. Other factors that may be associated are dental work, respiratory infection, remote periprosthetic infection, open skin lesions, endoscopy, and contamination of operative sites.

Preoperative Investigations

Plain Radiographs

Plain radiographs should be routinely obtained in evaluating the painful total knee replacement even though they are unremarkable in the majority of cases, particularly in the early period. Occasionally, the patient will have diagnostic changes, such as periostitis, rapidly progressive osteolysis, or endosteal scalloping. The development of a complete radiolucency around a component over a short time is highly suggestive of advanced infection. Subchondral bone resorption and patchy osteoporosis are more subtle, earlier findings present in some infected cases. Periprosthetic osteolysis is the most common finding but is nonspecific. Periosteal new bone formation, with or without loosening of a component, has been considered by some to be pathognomonic of deep infection.

Laboratory Tests

The WBC count is rarely abnormal in patients with suspected total knee infection. In one series, only 28% of infected knees had a WBC greater than 11,000. When a patient does have an abnormal WBC count, the systemic infection is usually clinically obvious.

The ESR and CRP are useful laboratory screening investigations for the diagnosis of a potential infection following total joint replacement. Average ESR of more than 50 has been reported in different series of infected total knee arthroplasty but both false positives and false negatives are seen. False positives can occur because of other inflammatory conditions such as rheumatoid arthritis. The ESR may remain elevated for months after an uncomplicated joint arthroplasty and in early post-operative period. The CRP levels increase from trace amounts to reach maximum values within 48 hours of surgery and then returns to trace amounts in approximately 2 to 3 weeks. Some care must be taken in interpreting the ESR or CRP level before a revision surgery. The physician must determine whether any other factors such as rheumatoid arthritis, a recent operation, neoplasia, collagen vascular disease, infection, or an inflammatory condition are present. *If no such conditions are applicable, an ESR of more than 30 or 35 mm per hour and a C-reactive protein level of more than 10 mg per liter should be considered abnormal and should warrant additional investigations to rule out infection.*

Radionuclide Imaging

Scintigraphy can be of assistance with regard to its potential for the diagnosis of infections following joint replacement. Scintigraphy though is limited by cost of scans, time required, and most importantly its inability to yield consistently acceptable levels of sensitivity and specificity. Often scans are no more accurate than other, less expensive serological investigations. Technetium-99m bone scans are sensitive but not specific. Also persistent increased uptake of Tc-99m adjacent to asymptomatic total knee arthroplasties particularly around the tibial component is expected for up to a year.

Tc scintigraphy has a sensitivity of 95% in detecting TKA infection; its specificity is only 20%. Gallium-67 citrate is a radioisotope that accumulates in areas of inflammation. Gallium scan sensitivity is high and a negative scan can reliably rule out infection; however the positive predictive value is 70 to 75% as gallium may show increased uptake at uninfected sites of bone remodeling. Indium-111-labeled white blood cells are useful for the diagnosis of increased vascularity and white blood cell uptake, and indium-111-labeled WBC scintigraphy has been used to study periprosthetic infection. Other radiolabeled markers like radiolabeled Immunoglobulin G have been investigated and though preliminary results are encouraging, their routine use cannot be advocated till further studies are available. *"Radionuclide scans can be specifically of benefit in equivocal situations in which serological investigations may be falsely elevated and aspirate cultures are unreliable because of the administration of antibiotics."*

Aspiration

Aspiration of the knee is the "standard of care for determining whether there is deep joint infection." It can also identify the bacterial species and antibiotic sensitivity. A synovial fluid WBC of greater than 25,000 or a differential with more than 75% PMNs is suggestive of infection. Also, elevated protein and low glucose are consistent with infections. The most common reason for false negative is the administration of antibiotics before aspiration. If there is any suspicion of infection and the first aspirate is negative, we routinely do repeat weekly aspirations for 3 to 4 weeks.

Management of Established Infection

Several options are available in the management of septic knee arthroplasty. These options include chronic antibiotic suppression, irrigation and debridement with prosthesis retention, arthrodesis, amputation and debridement with reimplantation. A number of factors have to be considered before the treatment option selection. These factors include the time elapsed from index procedure; host factors affecting treatment of infection; soft tissue condition; implant status in terms of fixation, type of organism, and its sensitivity to antibiotics; and, most importantly, the patient's expectations and functional requirements.

Antibiotic Suppression

To sterilize an infected arthroplasty with antibiotics alone is difficult. Long-term suppression with antibiotics alone is rarely indicated. In rare circumstances when medical condition precludes surgery and removal of well-fixed component and the organism has low virulence and is susceptible to an oral antibiotic, oral suppression may be justified. Although this treatment method is rarely indicated, *it is commonly attempted and only prolongs the presence of infection and complicates subsequent treatment attempts.*

Debridement with Prosthetic Retention

This treatment involves removal of all intra-articular infected material and retention of the prosthesis. Suggested treatment criteria include short duration of infection (less than 2 to 3 weeks), susceptible Gram-positive organisms, absence of prolonged drainage of sinus tract, and no prosthetic.

Arthrodesis

Removal of components and surgical arthrodesis is rarely done as first line of management; however it is a potentially beneficial means of managing infected arthroplasties, with low risk of reinfection and reliable pain relief and knee stability. Absence of knee motion and its affect on activities of daily living counterbalance some of its advantages. We consider an arthrodesis generally after failed reimplantation in patients with high functional demand, single joint disease extension mechanism disruption with poor soft tissue envelope.

Amputation

This is reserved as a final option on in the presence of life-threatening systemic sepsis. Earlier attempts at arthrodesis when there is adequate bone stock and a viable soft tissue envelope, rather than repeated attempts at revision in the presence of infection and deceased use of stemmed hinged implants, should lower the incidence of amputation following failed total knee surgery.

Reimplantation

Two-stage exchange arthroplasty involving removal of prosthesis and cement with subsequent arthroplasty at a later date with intervening period of antibiotics is the most commonly used protocol for the treatment of infected total knee arthroplasty. One-stage reimplantations have also been reported in literature; however, most series have small numbers, and the success has not been seen to be corroborated by other groups. We have no personal experience with one-stage revision and believe like most, that two-stage exchanges arthroplasty is still the treatment of choice for infected total knee replacements. Two-stage reimplantation usually implies revision arthroplasty more than 4 to 6 weeks following prosthetic removal. In the first stage, a complete debridement and drainage, including removal of the total-joint prosthesis and acrylic cement, is performed. A 6-week course of antibiotic therapy follows the first stage. At the conclusion of antibiotic therapy, a new knee replacement is inserted as the second stage. The use of modular and custom-designed implants may be necessary to augment any bone loss that may have developed during the active course of the infection.

We have developed an algorithm for assessment and treatment of infection after total knee replacement (Figure 19-28).

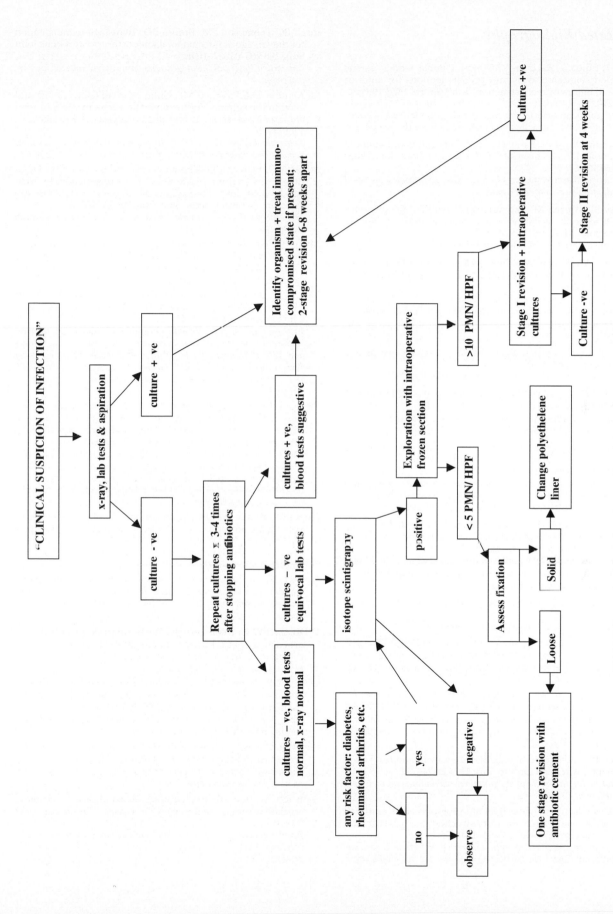

FIGURE 19-28. Algorithm for workup and treatment of suspected TKA infection.

629

Annotated Bibliography

Aglietti P, Buzzi R, Zaccherotti G et al. Patellar tendon versus doubled semitendinosus and gracilis tendons for anterior cruciate ligament reconstruction. Am J Sports Med 1994;22: 211–217.
Article compares 60 patients treated with patellar tendon versus hamstring grafts. There was no difference between the two groups.

Aglietti P, Insall J, Deschamps G et al. The results of treatment of idiopathic osteonecrosis of the knee. J Bone Joint Surg 1983;65B:588.
This article characterizes the clinical course of osteonecrosis based on radiographic area of involvement.

Arnoczky SP, Warren RF. The microvasculature of the meniscus and its response to injury: an experimental study in the dog. Am J Sports Med 1983;11:131–141.
This article forms the basis of meniscal repair.

Barrack RL, Wolfe MW, Waldman DA et al. Resurfacing of the patella in total knee arthroplasty. J Bone Joint Surg 1997; 79A:1121–1131.
A prospective randomized double blind study of eighty nine patients assigned to resurfacing or retention of patella. The prevalence of anterior knee pain was not influenced by whether the patella was resurfaced or not.

Berg EE. Posterior cruciate ligament tibial inlay reconstruction. Arthroscopy 1995;11:69–76.
Inlay technique for PCL reconstruction is described.

Boden BP, Feagin JA Jr. Natural history of the ACL-deficient knee. Sports Med Arthrosc Rev 1997;5:20–28.
The study indicates that incompetence of ACL leads to progressive deterioration of function of the knee.

Boynton MD, Tietjens BR. Long-term follow up of the untreated isolated posterior cruciate ligament-deficient knee. Am J Sports Med 1996;24:306–310.
This study is a retrospective evaluation of 38 patients with isolated PCL deficient knees at 13.4 years after injury. As time from injury increased, articular degeneration on radiographs was seen.

Callaghan JJ, Squire MW, Goetz DD et al. Cemented rotating-platform total knee replacement: a nine- to twelve-year follow-up study. J Bone Joint Surg 2000;82:705–711.
In 119 consecutive TKAs with rotating platform at 9- to 12-year follow-up, no reoperations were required, and no periprosthetic osteolysis and loosening was noted.

Carter TR. Meniscal allograft transplantation. Sports Med Arthrosc Rev 1999;7:51–62.
A review of meniscal transplantation is presented.

DeHaven KE. Meniscus repair. Am J Sports Med 1999;27:242–250.
A review of indications and techniques of meniscus repair.
A review of indications, different techniques for meniscal reapir, patient selection and outcomes.

Font-Rodriguez DE, Scuderi GR, Insall JN. Survivorship of cemented total knee arthroplasty, Clin Orthop 1997;345:79–86.
The surviorship analysis was used to compare the failure rate and overall success of 2629 cemented primary total knee anthroplasties during a 22-year period.

Fulkerson JP. Patellofemoral pain disorders: evaluation and management. J Am Acad Orthop Surg 1994;2:124–132.
Author highlights physical examination, evaluation, and treatment of patellofemoral disorders.

Harner CD, Olson E, Irrgang JJ, et al. Allograft versus autograft anterior cruciate ligament reconstruction: 3- to 5-year outcome. Clin Orthop 1996;324:134–144.
This study compares 64 patients with autograft versus 26 patients with allograft. There was no difference between the two graft sources.

Insall JN, Thompson FM, Brause BD. Two-stage reimplantation for the salvage of infected total knee arthroplasty, J Bone Joint Surg 1983;65A:1087–1098.
This article describes the staged reimplantation of infected knee replacement.

McAlindon TM, LaValley MP, Gulin JP et al. Glucosamine and chondroitin sulphate for treatment of osteoarthritis: a systematic quality assessment and meta-analysis. JAMA 2000;283: 1469–1475.
This meta-analysis showed that glucosamine and chondroitin sulfate demonstrate moderate to large effects on osteoarthritic symptoms.

Miller MD, Harner CD. The anatomic and surgical considerations for posterior cruciate ligament reconstruction. In: Jackson DW, ed. Instr Course Lect 44. Rosemont, IL: American Academy of Orthopaedic Surgeons, 1995:431–440.
The authors discuss anatomy, biomechanics, and current surgical techniques.

Minas T, Peterson L. Advanced techniques in autologue: chondrocyte transplantation, Clin Sports Med 1999;18:13–44.
Patient selection, surgical technique, rehabilitation protocols and results of autologous chondrocyte transplantation discussed.

Naudie D, Bourne RB, Rorabeck CH et al. Survivorship of the high tibial valgus osteotomy: a 10- to 22-year follow up study. Clin Orthop 1999;367:18–27.
In this study 85 patients with minimum 10-year follow up were evaluated. The percentage not requiring TKA was 73% at 5 years and 39% at 15 years. Early failure was associated with age older than 50 years, lateral thrust, previous arthroscopic debridement, range of motion less than 120°, undercorrection, and delayed or nonunion.

Newman JH, Ackroyd CE, Shah NA. Unicompartmental or total knee replacement? Five-year results of prospective, randomized trial of 102 osteoarthritic knees with unicompartmental arthritis. J Bone Joint Surg Br 1998;80B:862–865.
Knees deemed suitable for unicompartmental replacement at the time of surgery were randomized to total or unicompartmental knee replacement. Pain relief was equal in both groups; unicompartmental knee replacement group had better range of motion, less morbidity, and a faster recovery.

Noyes FR, Barber-Westin SD. Treatment of complex injuries involving the posterior cruciate and posterolateral ligaments of the knee. Am J Knee Surg 1996;9:200–214.
The article reviews multiple studies on treatments for PCL and posterolateral injuries of the knee.

Noyes F, Mooar P, Matthews D et al. The symptomatic anterior cruciate deficient knee: part I. J Bone Joint Surg 1983;65A:154–162.
This study presents the natural history of anterior cruciate-deficient knees.

O'Driscoll SW. Current concepts The healing and regeneration of articular cartilage. J Bone Joint Surg 1998;80A:1795–1812.
A general review of the various treatment options available for treating articular cartilage injury.

O'Neill DB. Arthroscopically assisted reconstruction of anterior cruciate ligament: a prospective randomized analysis of three techniques. J Bone Joint Surg 1996;78A:803–813.
No significant difference noted between hamstring autograft, and one and two incision patellar tendon autograft.

Post WR. Clinical evaluation of patients with patellofemoral disorders. Arthroscopy 1999;15:841–851.
Author highlights key components of clinical evaluation and treatment of patellofemoral disorders

Scott RD, Volatile TB. Twelve years' experience with posterior cruciate-retaining total knee arthroplasty. Clin Orthop 1986; 205:100–.
Results of early posterior cruciate retaining design presented with increased range of motion as compared to the early substituting design.

Skyhar MJ, Warren RF, Ortiz GJ et al. The effects of sectioning of the posterior cruciate ligament and the posterolateral complex on the articular contact pressures within the knee. J Bone Joint Surg 1993;75A:694–.

Articular contact pressures in ten cadaveric knees with intact ligaments were measured with the use of film, the measurements were repeated after sequential sectioning of the posterior cruciate ligament and posterolateral complex.

Shelbourne KD, Gray T. Anterior cruciate ligament reconstruct with autogenous patellar tendon autograft followed by accelerated rehabilitation: a two- to nine-year follow-up. Am J Sports Med 1997;25:786–795.

This study describes an accelerated rehabilitation program. The average return to athletic competition was 6.2 months postoperatively.

Shelbourne KD, Patel DV. Management of combined injuries of the anterior cruciate and medial collateral ligaments. J Bone Joint Surg 1995;77A:800–806.

Results of nonsurgical treatment of MCL complex with ACL injuries presented. Authors found that it is possible to treat MCL nonsurgically. The authors also recommended that surgical treatment of ACL should be delayed for 4 to 6 weeks until full knee motion was regained.

Terry GC, LaPrade RF. The posterolateral aspect of the knee: anatomy and surgical approach. Am J Sports Med 1996;24:732–739.

Surgical anatomy of posterolateral corner is meticulously described. The article contains excellent photographs of posterolateral corner of the knee.

Veltri DM, Deng XH, Torzilli PA et al. The role of the cruciate and posterolateral ligaments in stability of knee: a biomechanical study. Am J Sports Med 1995;23:436–443.

Cadaveric study to assess the role of posterolateral and cruciate ligaments in restraining knee motion.

Vince KG, Insall JN, Kelly MA. The total condylar prosthesis: 10- to 12-year results of a cemented knee replacement. J Bone Joint Surg 1989;71B:793–797.

The authors present a long-term evaluation of the original total condylar prosthesis design that sacrificed the posterior cruciate ligament.

20

Stuart L. Weinstein

The Pediatric Foot

PES PLANUS
TARSAL COALITION
CONGENITAL VERTICAL TALUS
CALCANEAL VALGUS

KÖHLER DISEASE
FREIBERG INFARCTION
SEVER DISEASE
METATARSUS ADDUCTUS

CLUBFOOT
IDIOPATHIC TOE-WALKING
TORSIONAL PROBLEMS

Anatomically, the foot can be divided into three sections: the forefoot, midfoot, and hindfoot. The forefoot consists of the metatarsals and phalanges. The cuneiform, cuboid, and navicular bones comprise the midfoot, and the hindfoot consists of the calcaneus and talus. The three foot segments are linked together by strong ligaments; because of this linkage, all foot movements occur concurrently. Supination and pronation are combination movements in the individual foot joints: *supination* refers to the sole pointing inward, and *pronation* refers to sole turning outward (Figure 20-1). Varus (inversion) and valgus (eversion) are motions of a foot segment on a theoretic longitudinal axis (Figure 20-2). When the foot is supinated, the heel goes into varus. When the foot is pronated, the heel goes into valgus (Figure 20-3). Adduction and abduction are motions of the foot segment on a theoretic vertical axis (Figure 20-4).

PES PLANUS

Pes planus is a term describing any condition of the foot in which the longitudinal arch is lowered. It is important to distinguish between physiologic pes planus and pes planus secondary to pathologic conditions.

Physiologic pes planus (hypermobile flatfoot, flexible flatfoot) is characterized by varying degrees of loss of the longitudinal arch of the foot on weight bearing. The foot assumes an apparent pronated posture with abduction of the forefoot and varying degrees of heel valgus (Figure 20-5). The important distinguishing characteristic between physiologic and pathologic pes planus is flexibility. In the physiologic type, the foot remains flexible.

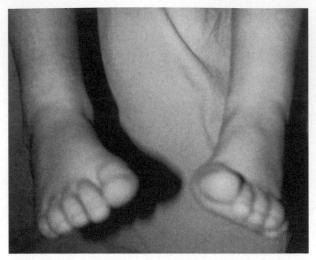

FIGURE 20-1. Foot supination (sole turning inward).

Ninety percent of normal children younger than 2 years have varying degrees of pes planus. This is due to the normal joint hypermobility in this age group and the normal infant fat pad along the medial aspect of the foot (Figure 20-6). In addition, the normal wide-based stance assumed by newly standing or walking children causes the weight-bearing line to fall medial to first or second ray, resulting in the hypermobile foot assuming a pes planus posture.

Between 3 and 5 years of age, the normal longitudinal arch develops in most patients. It is estimated that by age 10 years, only 4% of the population have persistent pes planus.

The normal longitudinal arch of the foot is determined by maintenance of the normal relations between the bones of the foot. These relations are maintained by the supporting ligamentous and capsular structures and can be affected by functional stresses applied to the foot in weight bearing and by muscle contraction. The foot musculature does not maintain the longitudinal arch. Its purpose is to maintain balance, adjust the foot to uneven ground, and propel the body. Biomechanically, when the foot is supinated, the articulations of the midfoot are "locked," and the foot is a rigid structure. When the foot is pronated, however, greater mobility is allowed at the midfoot joints, and maximal motion can occur at the talonavicular and calcaneocuboid joints. The position of heel valgus and forefoot abduction with lowering of the longitudinal arch is often referred to as a *pronated foot,* while in actuality, the forefoot is supinated to varying degrees in relation to the hind foot. Thus, in true physiologic pes planus, as the calcaneus assumes a valgus position, the lateral aspect of the forefoot is in contact only with the ground if the forefoot supinates to some degree in relation to the hindfoot.

The normal weight-bearing pattern includes ground contact with the lateral border of the foot and with the first and fifth metatarsals. In pes planus, as the calcaneus assumes a more valgus position, the talar head loses some of its support and assumes a more vertically oriented position, with

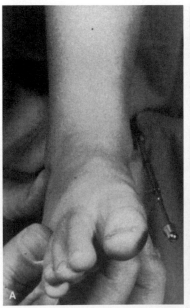
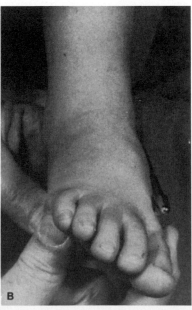

FIGURE 20-2. Forefoot varus (inversion; **A**) and forefoot valgus (eversion; **B**) are motions of a foot segment on a theoretical longitudinal axis.

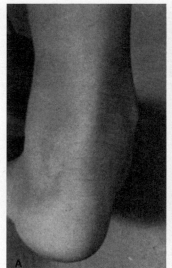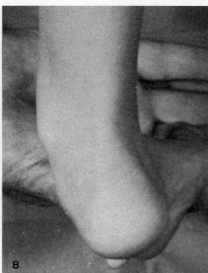

FIGURE 20-3. (A) Heel valgus (eversion) when foot is pronated. **(B)** Heel varus (inversion) when foot is supinated.

subsequent loss of the normal arch (Figure 20-7). Body weight shifts medially, altering the normal weight-bearing pattern and causing increasing ground contact with the medial aspect of the foot. With time, the Achilles tendon may shorten and act as an everter of the foot, accentuating the deformity.

Many theories have been advanced over the years about the cause of physiologic pes planus, most centering around abnormal bone configuration, muscle imbalance, or ligamentous laxity. The origin of persistent physiologic pes planus, however, remains unknown. Many patients have a positive family history of a similar condition or evidence

of generalized ligamentous laxity. Physiologic pes planus may also be associated with obesity. A positive family history should be sought for conditions associated with joint laxity, such as Marfan and Ehlers-Danlos syndromes. Physiologic pes planus is occasionally seen as a residual of the calcaneal valgus foot deformity (discussed later). It is important to obtain a family history of treatment of similar conditions because this may have significant bearing on the patient education necessary in prescribing treatment modalities to the family.

Most children with physiologic pes planus are asymptomatic. They are brought in by their parents

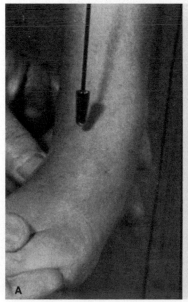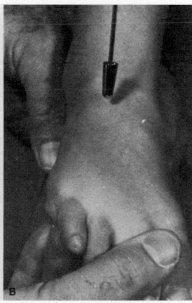

FIGURE 20-4. Forefoot adduction **(A)** and forefoot abduction **(B)** are motions of a foot segment on a theoretic vertical axis.

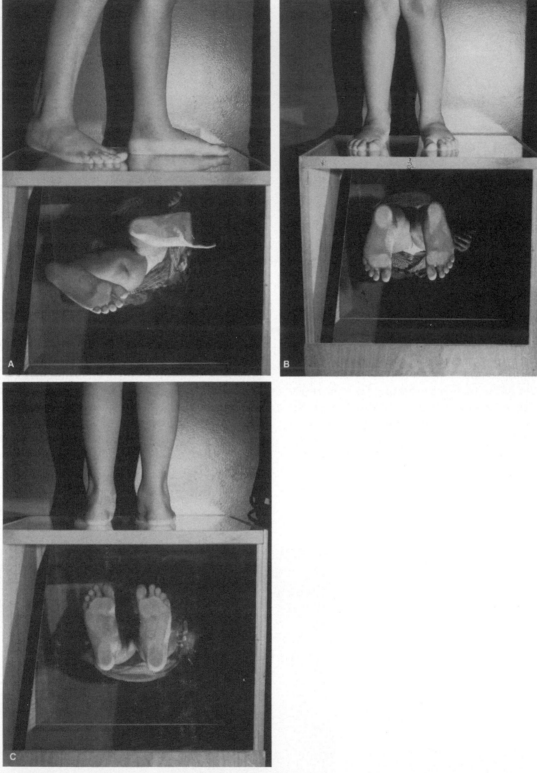

FIGURE 20-5. (A and B) Physiologic pes planus. Note loss of longitudinal arch and apparent pronated posture with abduction of the forefoot. **(C)** Physiologic pes planus. Note heel valgus position with loss of longitudinal arch. **(D)** Physiologic pes planus. With the leg dangling over the examination table in the nonweight-bearing position, the foot assumes a normal appearance to the arch. **(E)** Physiologic pes planus tiptoe test. When the patient stands on tiptoes, normal appearance of the arch is apparent.

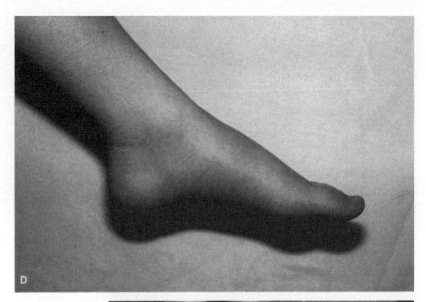

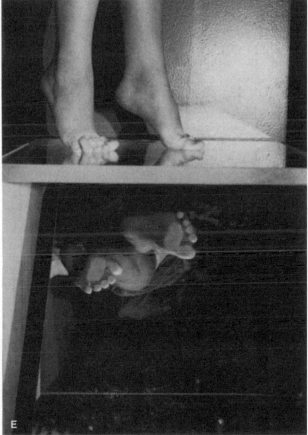

FIGURE 20-5. *(Continued)*

because of the assumption that flatfeet are abnormal and harmful to their child if not treated. Occasionally, some children may complain of symptoms that are referable to foot strain after prolonged activity and generally relieved by rest. Associated leg aches are not uncommon in patients who present with symptomatic pes planus, but because these are present in a large portion of normal people, a cause-and-effect relation is difficult to establish.

Each patient should be thoroughly examined for excessive joint laxity manifested by the ability to hyperextend the metacarpal phalangeal joints,

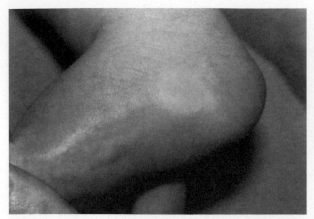

FIGURE 20-6. Four-month-old infant with physiologic pes planus. Note prominence of the medial fat pad contributing to the appearance of pes planus (fat pad is blanched by finger pressure to emphasize its location).

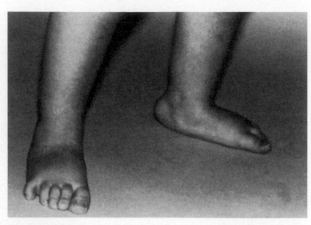

FIGURE 20-8. Hypermobile flatfoot associated with short Achilles tendon. Typical appearance is similar to that of physiologic pes planus.

appose the thumb to the forearm, and hyperextend the elbows and knees. The foot has normal to slightly increased subtalar motion. In weight bearing, varying degrees of loss of the longitudinal medial arch are noted. The heel is in valgus and the forefoot in abduction (see Figure 20-5). With loss of the longitudinal arch on weight bearing, the center of gravity is shifted medially to the second metatarsal or medially to the first metatarsal. The patient may have a toe-in gait in an attempt to shift the weight-bearing axis laterally.

Foot flexibility may be demonstrated in two ways: by examining the feet in the resting position and by the tiptoe test. The patient should be examined with legs dangling over the examination table (see Figure 20-5). In this position, the physiologic pes planus foot assumes a normal contour to the longitudinal arch. In the tiptoe test, the patient's feet are observed when the patient walks on tiptoes (see Figure 20-5). In this position, the normal arch is restored, with the heel going to a neutral or slightly varus position. Muscle strength of the foot should be normal.

It is important to rule out hypermobile flatfoot associated with a short Achilles tendon by history and physical examination (Figure 20-8). This condition, which is often familial, is evidenced by contracture of the gastrocnemius in association with the same clinical features as described previously. This condition is usually symptomatic and associated with long-term disability. These patients can usually correct the deformity by involuntary muscular effort, as demonstrated by the patient restoring the arch by standing on tiptoes.

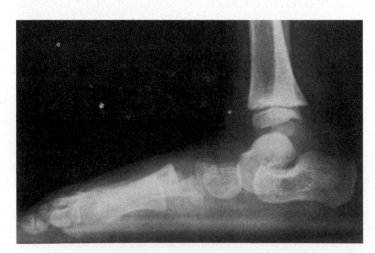

FIGURE 20-7. Physiologic pes planus, standing lateral radiograph. The longitudinal arch is depressed; the talus points directly downward instead of forward in line with the navicular and metatarsals.

In addition, in the nonweight-bearing position, the normal arch is generally present. Contracture of the Achilles tendon is best assessed with the knee in extension and the talonavicular joint locked in inversion so that dorsiflexion is measured only at the ankle. The radiographic features of this condition are characteristic (Figure 20-9). These patients may also show evidence of hypermobility at the midtarsal joints, which allows the heel to touch the floor despite a contracted Achilles tendon. Without treatment, this condition may cause severe disabling pain.

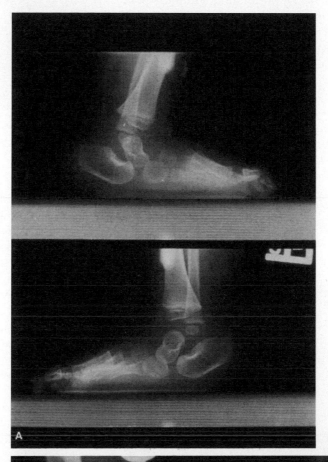

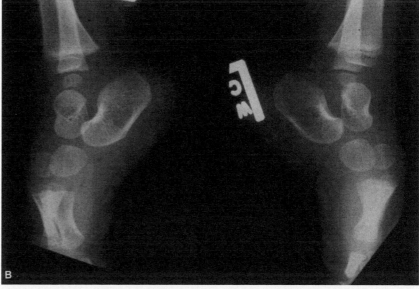

FIGURE 20-9. Hypermobile flatfoot associated with short Achilles tendon. **(A)** Standing lateral radiographs reveal talus in plantar flexion, calcaneus in equinus indicative of contracted Achilles tendon. **(B)** Forced plantar flexion lateral radiograph. The forefoot is collinear with the longitudinal axis of the talus, indicative of passive correctability of this deformity. The patient's condition resolved with Achilles tendon lengthening.

In the child presenting with a complaint of flat-feet, pathologic causes of pes planus must be ruled out. These causes include congenital vertical talus, oblique talus, tarsal coalition, tumor, foreign body reaction, and Köhler disease of the navicular and accessory navicular. Accessory navicular bones are seen in about 12% of the population and are a normal variant. Two patterns are evident. In one pattern, the accessory navicular is a sesamoid bone within the posterior tibial tendon (Figure 20-10). It is anatomically separate from the navicular and usually does not cause symptoms. In the second form, the accessory navicular is in close association with the navicular as an ossification center, causing a change in shape of the navicular. This type may be associated with pain, particularly during adolescence (Figure 20-11). Accessory navicular is not a cause of hypermobile flatfoot, but because both conditions are common, they may present together. Accessory naviculars may be treated symptomatically, but excision may be required if conservative measures fail.

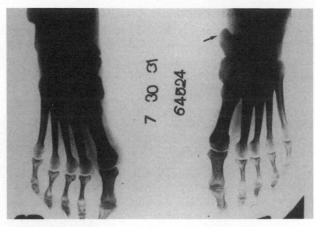

FIGURE 20-11. Accessory navicular. This type of accessory navicular has fused to the primary navicular, altering its shape and leading to prominence of the tuberosity.

The foot with a vertical talus assumes a convex plantar surface that is rigid and has characteristic radiographic findings (Figures 20-12 to 20-14). Neuromuscular causes of pes planus, such as cerebral palsy and muscular dystrophy, can be diagnosed by their typical diagnostic characteristics. The most severe form of physiologic pes planus is referred to as an *oblique talus* because of its radiologic appearance. It has features similar to vertical talus on the standing lateral view, but normal alignment is restored on plantar flexion lateral radiographs. Tarsal coalitions have rigidity of subtalar motion, may be associated with peroneal spastic flatfoot, and are diagnosed radiographically (Figures 20-15 through 20-18). Other causes of pes planus include the so-called skewfoot or Z-foot (see metatarsus adductus) and surgically overcorrected clubfeet.

Radiographs are generally not indicated in the asymptomatic child with a physiologic pes planus. In severe cases, standing anteroposterior (AP) and lateral radiographs should be obtained. On the normal standing AP radiograph, the talocalcaneal angle should be between 15 and 35° (Figure 20-19). Diversion of the AP talocalcaneal angle to greater than 35° is evidence of heel valgus. The midtalar line passing medial to the first metatarsal with the navicular displaced laterally is evidence of forefoot abduction. On the standing lateral radiograph, the normal lateral talocalcaneal angle is between 25 and 50°. The talus first metatarsal angle should be about 0°. On the lateral view, the exact location of loss of longitudinal arch can be determined. This sag may occur at the talonavicular joint, first naviculo-cuneiform joint, and first metatarsocuneiform joint, or combinations thereof. On the standing lateral

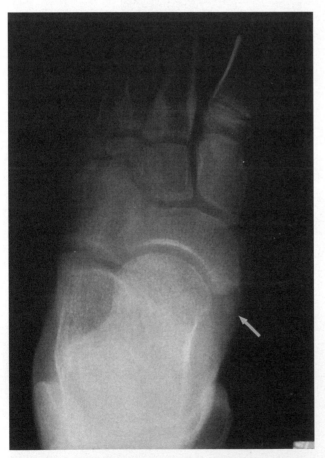

FIGURE 20-10. Accessory navicular. Note the appearance of sesamoid bone within the posterior tibial tendon.

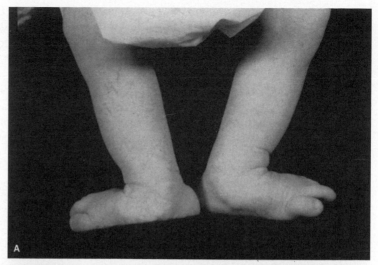

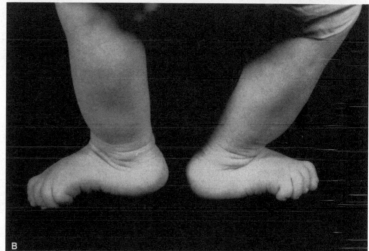

FIGURE 20-12. Congenital vertical talus. Newborn with sacral agenesis and bilateral congenital vertical talus. The heels are in valgus and the forefoot is abducted. The foot has the characteristic rocker-bottom deformity.

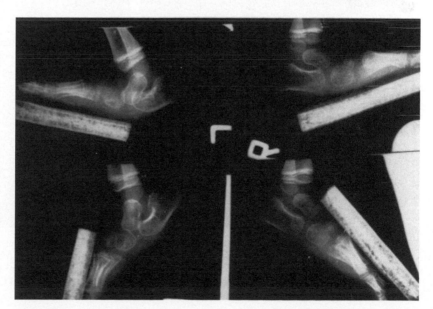

FIGURE 20-13. Congenital vertical talus of left foot. (Hypermobile flatfoot with contracted Achilles tendon on the right foot.) In the simulated weight-bearing views (*upper left and upper right*), both feet have the evidence of a rocker-bottom deformity with dorsiflexion occurring at the midfoot, the hindfoot is in equinus, and the forefoot is in dorsiflexion. The talus is more severely plantar flexed on the left than the right. Both calcanea are in equinus, and on the left foot there is disruption of the calcaneal cuboid joint. On the plantar flexion views (*bottom*), note on the right side the longitudinal axis of the talus is collinear with the forefoot; but on the left (side with congenital vertical talus), the longitudinal axis of the talus is not collinear with the longitudinal axis of the metatarsals, indicative of the rigid nature of the deformity.

radiograph, the talus is more vertically oriented, with the metatarsals and the calcaneus in a more horizontal position than normal because of flattening of the arch (see Figure 20-7).

If the patient presents with a painful flatfoot, oblique views and Harris views (radiograph taken from behind the foot with the x-ray beam at a 45° angle) may be helpful in defining a tarsal coalition or a pathologic process. If tumor, infection, or a

stress fracture is suspected, bone scanning may be helpful. Computed tomography (CT) is indicated if talocalcaneal tarsal coalition is suspected (see Figure 20-18). The diagnosis of physiologic pes planus is one of exclusion.

The natural history of physiologic pes planus is unfortunately clouded by medical and nonmedical mythology. To most parents and many physicians and paramedical personnel, flatfeet are considered

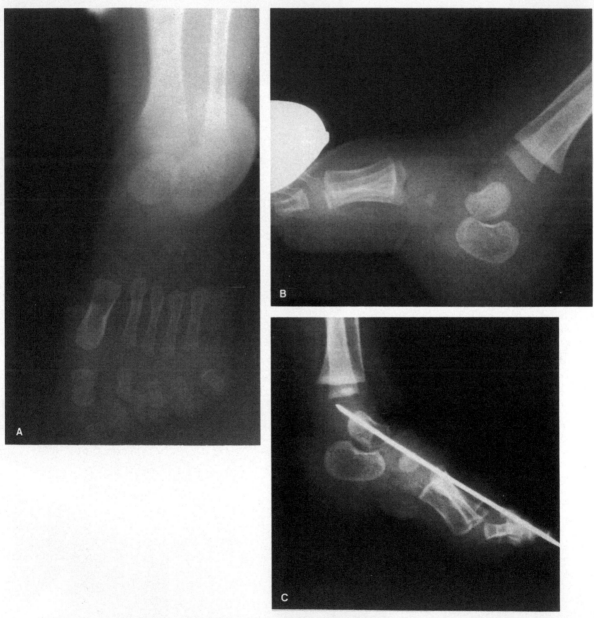

FIGURE 20-14. Congenital vertical talus. **(A)** Standing AP view demonstrates increased angle between talus and calcaneus indicative of the hindfoot valgus. **(B)** Lateral view of plantar flexion indicates failure of realignment of the metatarsals with the long axis of the talus. **(C)** Postsurgical realignment of forefoot, midfoot, and hindfoot. **(D and E)** Standing PA and lateral radiographs 6 years after operation demonstrating restoration of normal anatomic relations.

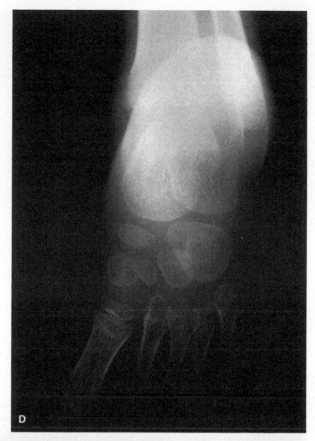

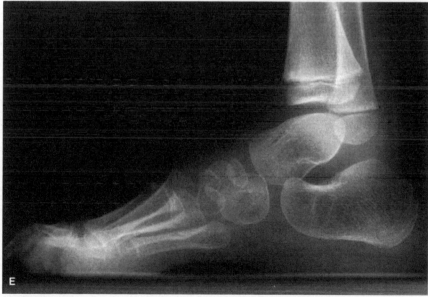

FIGURE 20-14. *(Continued)*

a significant health problem. Unfortunately, good natural history data on this condition are lacking.

Treatments offered in the past have been based on the assumption that patients will have problems in the future if the condition is not treated. In normal children, aged 1 to 3 years, whose parents bring them in for concerns over flatfeet, reassurance and explanation of the cause of pes planus are essential. The parents should be informed about the presence of the normal fat pad, the normal hyperlaxity of

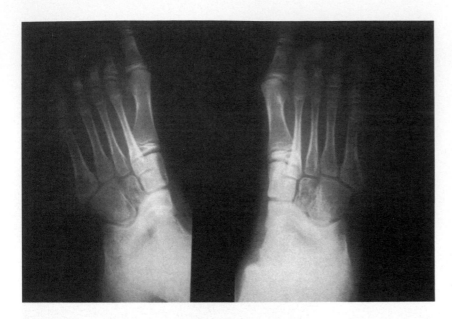

FIGURE 20-15. Calcaneal navicular coalition. Forty-five-degree oblique view demonstrates calcaneal navicular coalitions.

infancy, the often familial nature of the condition. They should also be reassured that, in most children, an arch will develop by 5 years of age. The parents should be informed of the benign natural history of the condition. Appropriate literature should be supplied to the family so they can reassure themselves and other family members who may expect some treatment because of what they have heard from others, what they have read, or treatment they underwent as children. Many parents are under the false assumption that so-called corrective shoes are responsible for the natural development of the longitudinal arch.

The same conservative recommendations apply to all other children with the diagnosis of physiologic pes planus. The educational aspects of the natural

history of the condition cannot be overemphasized. The parents should be instructed that treatment modalities offered in the past were offered without any scientific basis. A recent prospective randomized study of patients with flexible flatfeet treated by corrective shoes and inserts revealed that all patients improved moderately after 3 years of treatment, and no greater improvement was seen in patients who were treated vigorously, even those treated with custom-made inserts. All treatments in the past,

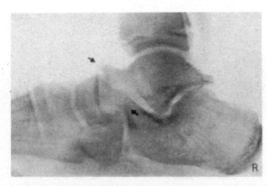

FIGURE 20-16. Calcaneal navicular coalition. In a patient with calcaneal navicular bar, standing lateral radiograph demonstrates prominence of the anterior process of the calcaneus and a spur at the superior talonavicular articulation.

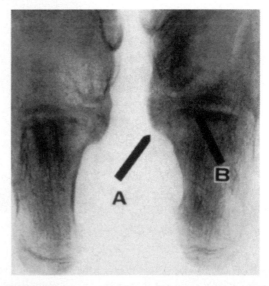

FIGURE 20-17. A talocalcaneal bridge. Harris views of both feet. Note the prominence of the sustentaculum (*arrow A*); talocalcaneal articulation is obliterated in the medial portion (*arrow B*).

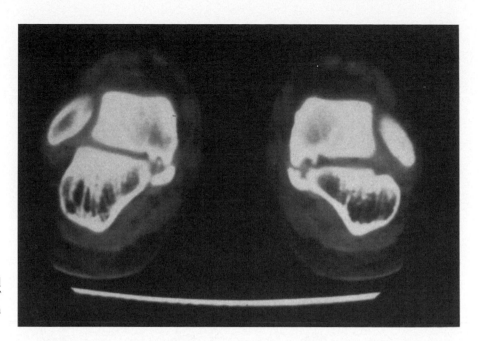

FIGURE 20-18. Talocalcaneal coalition. Frontal section of a CT scan demonstrates tarsal coalition at middle facet joint.

including exercises, varying shoe modifications, and inserts, have been proved to be ineffective.

In a child with a painful flexible flatfoot, the diagnosis must be reassessed and sources of painful flatfeet eliminated. Prophylactic treatment of any type is unwarranted. Treatment for flexible flatfeet is only indicated if the patient presents with pain, usually in the foot or calf, or if the patient has severe excessive shoe wear. The discomfort in the foot and the associated leg aches, which occur in about 15 to 30% of normal people, should be treated symptomatically with acetaminophen, local heat, and massage. If fatigue symptoms or discomfort with increasing activity persists, shoe modifications can be considered. It is important to emphasize that these modifications are not corrective. High-top tennis shoes with a good longitudinal arch can usually be recommended. If symptoms persist, other noncorrective adaptive measures may be tried, such as a medial heel wedge, a long shoe counter, or a navicular pad.

For the more severe symptomatic physiologic pes planus that fails to respond to conservative measures, a more formal shoe orthotic, such as a University of California Biomechanics Lab insert or custom-made insert, may distribute body weight more evenly across the sole of the foot and take the pressure off the prominent talar head. These modalities, however, are expensive, must be changed frequently with foot growth, and have no scientific basis for their use. The use of shoe modification inserts tends to label the child as having a problem.

The use of these devices to appease parents or grandparents should be discouraged.

In young patients with hypermobile flatfoot and a short tendo Achilles, heel cord stretching exercises should be instituted. If symptoms develop or the contracture persists, tendo Achilles lengthening can be considered. The only operative indications in true physiologic pes planus flatfoot are severe malalignment problems causing excessive abnormal shoe wear or pain. Achilles tendon stretching or casting may be of some benefit. Surgical options for these indications are rarely indicated. In the past, these options included soft tissue procedures alone; arthrodeses of the various tarsal joints; osteotomies; and combined osteotomies, arthrodeses, and soft tissue procedures, all with the goal of restoring the normal longitudinal arch, relieving pain, and preserving as much motion as possible. Results of these procedures have been poor.

TARSAL COALITION

The term *tarsal coalition* refers to the union of two or more tarsal bones by fibrous, cartilaginous, or bony tissue. This entity is often called *peroneal spastic flatfoot* because of the high association with contracture of the peroneal tendons. The most common sites of coalition are between the calcaneus and the navicular and between the talus and calcaneus. The most common talocalcaneal coalition is

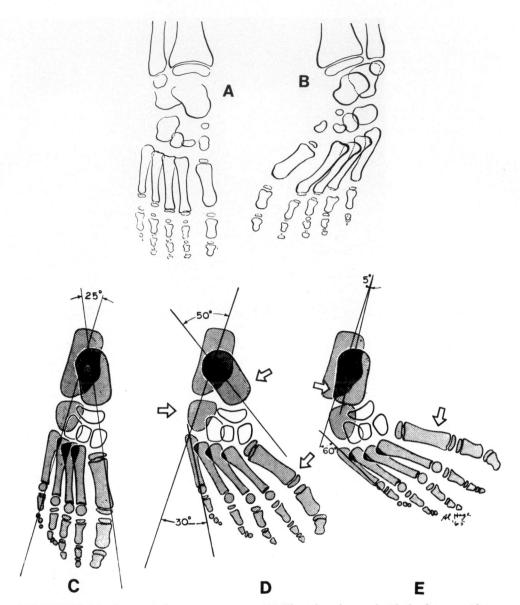

FIGURE 20-19. Congenital metatarsus varus. **(A)** The talus, the scaphoid, the first cuneiform, and the first metatarsal form a straight line. The anterior ends of the talus and the calcaneus are separated. **(B)** The first metatarsal is carried medially and is in line only with the inner cuneiform and the scaphoid, the latter lying lateral to the talar head. The talus and the calcaneus are in the flatfoot position, the anterior ends lying in a divergent relationship. The inversion of the forefoot causes the cuneiforms to overlap and the lateral aspect of the metatarsals to be visualized. The metatarsals normally are bowed dorsalward, and in this view they are wrongly identified as deformed. **(C)** Diagram of radiograph of a normal foot; **(D)** a foot with metatarsus adductus; and **(E)** a clubfoot. Arrows indicate directions and sites of molding during corrective manipulation and plaster-cast application. (Ponseti IV, Becker JR. Congenital metatarsus adductus. J Bone Joint Surg 1966;48A:702)

between the sustentaculum and the talus, with rare coalitions involving the anterior or posterior facet. Other tarsal coalitions are much less common. The coalitions may be complete or partial. When the coalition is fibrous, it is called a *syndesmosis*. When the coalition is cartilaginous, it is referred to as *synchondroses*. A bony union is referred to as a *synostosis*. Tarsal coalition represents the most common nonneuromuscular cause of pathologic pes planus.

The true incidence of tarsal coalition is unknown. It is estimated, however, that less than 1 to 2% of the population is affected. Although tarsal coalitions may be multiple, rarely is there more than one coalition per foot. Bilateralness, however, is common.

Demonstration of coalitions in fetal specimens lends support to the theory of failure of segmentation as the origins of tarsal coalitions (Figure 20-20). This incomplete segmentation of the mesenchymal anlage of the tarsal bones gives rise to the fibrous or cartilaginous coalition, which may ossify later in life. Bilateralness has been reported in up to 70% of calcaneonavicular coalitions and in 20 to 50% of talocalcaneal coalitions. Tarsal coalitions are thought to be an inherited condition, with the most widely accepted pattern being autosomal dominant inheritance with variable penetrance.

Because the true incidence of tarsal coalitions in the population is unknown, the natural history is uncertain. It is apparent that many patients with tarsal coalitions have no symptoms, and many patients with coalitions treated symptomatically can go well into adult life without persistent pain or disability. Symptoms most commonly develop when the coalition begins to ossify. Ossification of the coalition restricts subtalar motion. This alteration in subtalar mechanics leads to increased stress at adjacent joints, particularly the ankle and talonavicular joints. If a coalition remains fibrous (syndesmosis), symptoms may never develop because of the mobility allowed through the syndesmosis.

With increasing ossification of a cartilaginous (synchondrosis) coalition, decreased mobility ensues, increasing the likelihood of the patient developing clinical symptoms. The altered subtalar joint mechanics over time may lead to degenerative joint disease in adjacent joints, causing persistent pain and disability. The limited subtalar motion also causes increased laxity in adjacent joints, particularly the ankle joint, leading to increased incidence of sprains and secondary joint alterations.

The typical patient with tarsal coalition presents during the second decade of life with pain or decreased subtalar motion. Occasionally, the patient complains of a limp, discomfort in the calf region, or nonspecific foot pain. The pain is often localized to the anterior, medial, or lateral aspect of the subtalar joint or to the talonavicular region. The onset of pain is usually insidious or associated with a traumatic event such as a nonresolving ankle sprain. Pain is usually made worse by activities like running and jumping or prolonged standing; it is usually relieved by rest. The symptom onset depends on the nature of the coalition (fibrous, cartilaginous, or bony) and the specific joint involved. Children with the rare talonavicular coalition may present between 2 and 4 years of age. Typically, patients with calcaneonavicular coalitions present between 8 and 12 years of age, and those with talocalcaneal coalitions between 12 and 14 years of age. In any child presenting with a painful rigid foot, tarsal coalition must be ruled out.

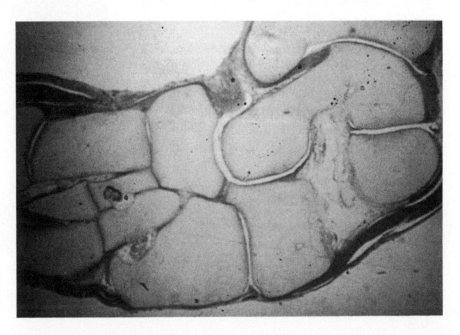

FIGURE 20-20. Tarsal coalition. Fetal specimen demonstrating fibrous tarsal coalition between calcaneus and navicular.

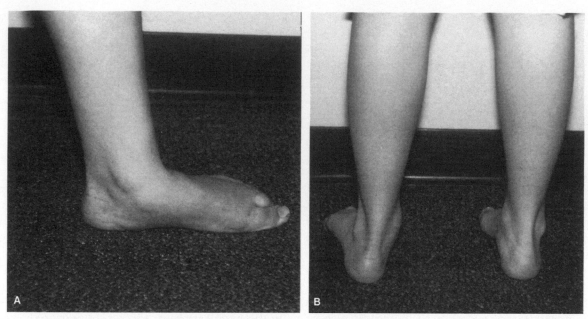

FIGURE 20-21. Tarsal coalition. Note the position of the involved left foot with the forefoot in abduction **(A)** and heel in valgus **(B).** Also note the loss of the longitudinal arch.

Physical examination in patients with tarsal coalition generally reveals decreased hindfoot or midfoot motion, or both. Most commonly, the heel is in valgus and the forefoot in abduction (Figure 20-21). The patient may walk with an antalgic gait, and if symptoms are long-standing and the pain is significant, disuse atrophy may be noted on calf measurements. In about half of cases, contractures of the peroneal muscles is present. This is evidenced by prominence of the peroneal tendons in the lateral aspect of the ankle and foot (Figure 20-22). Attempt at inversion of the deformity causes pain and discomfort along the peroneal region (Figure 20-23). The peroneal tendons are contracted secondary to prolonged positioning of the foot in valgus. True muscle spasms of the peroneal tendons are rare. Increased ankle ligamentous laxity is most commonly seen in patients with long-standing symptoms, particularly those with talocalcaneal coalitions. There may also be varying degrees of loss of the longitudinal arch. Pathologic conditions affecting the subtalar joint, including tumors, rheumatoid arthritis, and traumatic injuries, may mimic the physical findings of tarsal coalition.

When tarsal coalitions are suspected, standing AP, lateral, and 45° medial oblique radiographs should be obtained (see Figure 20-15). The diagnosis of a calcaneonavicular coalition can usually be made on these standard radiographs. The 45° medial oblique radiograph usually demonstrates this coalition. If the coalition is fibrous or cartilaginous, however, it may not be obvious on plain radiographs. Other findings that indicate a possible calcaneonavicular coalition include elongation at the anterior portion of the calcaneus to a point of close proximity to the navicular and irregular, sclerotic

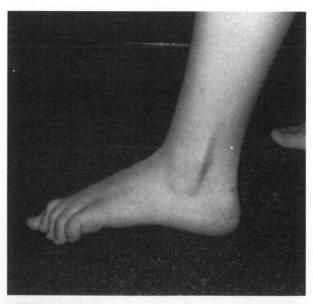

FIGURE 20-22. Tarsal coalition. Note prominence of the perineal tendons on the lateral aspect of the ankle because of prolonged positioning of the hindfoot in valgus and forefoot in abduction.

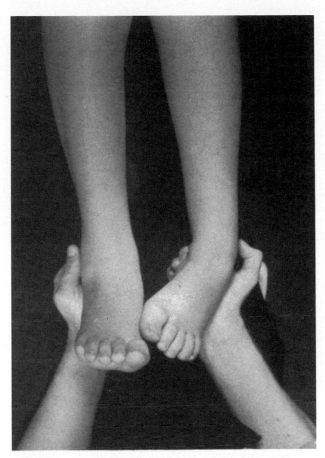

FIGURE 20-23. Tarsal coalition. There is inability to supinate the involved right foot secondary to tarsal coalition with restricted subtalar motion.

margins of the two bones in close approximation (see Figure 20-16).

Before the development of CT scanning, talocalcaneal coalitions were often difficult to diagnose. In suspected talocalcaneal coalitions, Harris views taken from behind the foot at an angle 45° from the horizontal demonstrate the posterior and medial facets of the subtalar joint. Normally, these are parallel, but coalitions may be diagnosed by the loss of the parallel orientation between the two facets, presence of fusion, or irregular or sclerotic surfaces (see Figure 20-17). Other types of tomography also have been used to demonstrate talocalcaneal coalitions; however, CT is the diagnostic method of choice for demonstrating these coalitions. Coronal sections should be obtained to document the coalition (see Figure 20-18). These sections not only document the presence of the coalition but also clearly define its extent. CT scans are most helpful in planning surgical management of this condition.

In patients with talocalcaneal coalitions, abnormal subtalar mechanics may be evident radiographically by secondary adaptive changes. These changes include dorsal beaking or lipping at the head or neck of the talus (see Figure 20-16). This is secondary to stretching of the talonavicular ligaments because of the navicular impinging on the head of the talus. The lateral aspect of the talus may appear broadened, with the undersurface of the talar neck having a concave appearance. There may be apparent narrowing of the posterior talocalcaneal joint space and inability to determine the definition of the middle talocalcaneal articulation.

Radiographs of the ankle joint may demonstrate an apparent ball-and-socket ankle—manifest by convexity of the dome of the talus on both the AP and lateral views. In patients presenting with repeated ankle sprains and radiographic evidence of a ball-and-socket ankle, tarsal coalition should be sought. In these cases, the radiographic changes at the ankle joint are secondary to long-standing ankle instability and adaptive changes of the tibial talar articulation.

Initial management of calcaneonavicular coalitions should be nonoperative because the natural history indicates that many patients have no symptoms, and the literature review of various treatment programs indicates some success with nonoperative treatment. Nonoperative treatment measures are based on immobilizing the subtalar joint. Shoe orthotics, ankle-foot orthoses, nonsteroidal anti-inflammatory agents, and activity restriction may be tried as a first line of treatment. If these fail, a period of cast immobilization with a short-leg walking cast for 3 to 6 weeks should be tried. If symptoms recur or are not alleviated by conservative measures, surgical excision is indicated. The most commonly used surgical technique is wide excision of the bar and interposition of either extensor digitorum brevis tendons or fat. Patients are immobilized in a cast for about 7 to 10 days, followed by range of motion exercise and protected weight bearing. Full weight bearing is allowed in 4 to 6 weeks. The main indication for surgery is pain relief, not restoration of joint motion, although with calcaneonavicular bar excisions, restoration and maintenance of joint motion can be expected if the patient does not have secondary degenerative joint disease changes. If symptoms persist and secondary degenerative joint disease is present in the adjacent joints, triple arthrodesis remains the only option for relief of the patient's symptoms. Success rates of surgery in calcaneonavicular coalitions are best in young patients with cartilaginous bars and no evidence of degenerative joint disease at the talonavicular joint. Talar beaking is not a contraindication for surgery because it does not necessarily represent degenerative changes.

The treatment of talocalcaneal coalitions is somewhat more difficult. Usual treatment should center around nonoperative measures as indicated previously for calcaneonavicular coalitions. If these nonoperative measures fail to provide lasting relief of the patient's symptoms, resection of the coalition with interposition of fat or bone wax should be considered. Specific criteria for resectability of these coalitions are lacking. Long-term series with large numbers of patients are unavailable. Contraindications to resection, however, are an extensive coalition and degenerative joint disease at the adjacent joints. In these circumstances, subtalar fusion or triple arthrodesis should be considered. The most common cause of failure in surgical management of tarsal coalitions is incomplete resection.

CONGENITAL VERTICAL TALUS

Congenital vertical talus is a rare deformity of the foot. It is characterized by a rigid flatfoot deformity, with the plantar aspect of the foot having a convex contour. The heel is in valgus, and the forefoot is abducted (see Figure 20-12). This entity has also been called *congenital convex pes planus, congenital convex pes valgus,* and *congenital flatfoot with talonavicular dislocation.* All these terms are descriptive either of the clinical or radiographic appearance of the foot.

Congenital vertical talus rarely exists alone. It is usually associated with other congenital abnormalities, musculoskeletal defects, or disorders of the central nervous system. There is a high incidence of congenital vertical talus in children with myelomeningocele (10% having congenital vertical talus), congenital hip dysplasia, and several trisomies (13 to 15%, 18%). This entity is more common in boys than girls, and there appears to be a familial tendency. It may be bilateral, but if unilateral, it may be associated with a pathologic condition of the opposite foot, including clubfoot, metatarsus adductus, or calcaneal valgus deformity.

Clinically, the condition can be diagnosed at birth. The involved foot is usually smaller than the opposite side with decreased circumference of the calf. In the newborn, the dorsal aspect of the foot may be in close approximation to the distal aspect of the tibia, similar to the foot position in the calcaneal valgus deformity. Unlike calcaneal valgus, however,

this position is rigid, and the foot cannot be flexed in a plantar direction. The sole of the foot has a convex appearance, the rocker-bottom deformity. The hindfoot is in the equinovalgus position with the Achilles tendon contracted. The forefoot is in the abducted dorsiflexed position. The head of the talus is easily palpable on the plantar medial aspect of the foot at the apex of the foot convexity. The deformity is rigid; it cannot be manipulated into the normal position. The head of the talus is covered dorsolaterally by the displaced navicular. Attempts at manipulation fail to reduce the talonavicular joint. The clinical appearance may mimic a hypermobile flatfoot or calcaneal valgus deformity. In both these conditions, however, normal relations, particularly the talonavicular relation, can be restored by plantar flexion.

AP and simulated standing or standing lateral radiographs should be obtained. Standing or simulated standing lateral radiographs reveal the calcaneus to be in equinus and talus to be vertically oriented parallel to the long axis of the tibia (see Figure 20-13). Because of the extreme plantar flexion of the talus, only the posterior aspect of dome articulates with the distal aspect of the tibia. In children younger than 3 to 5 years of age, the navicular is not ossified, and hence the talonavicular dislocation can only be inferred by noting that the forefoot is displaced dorsally in relation to the talus. Occasionally, a concave depression may be noted on the talar neck induced by the dorsolateral subluxation of the navicular. Once the navicular is ossified, the talonavicular dislocation is easily demonstrated. Radiographs may also demonstrate disruption of the calcaneocuboid joint with dorsolateral displacement of the cuboid. The diagnosis can be confirmed radiographically by a forced plantar flexion lateral view.

In congenital vertical talus, the normal bony relations are not restored on the plantar flexion lateral view. The long axis of the talus is plantar to the cuboid, as opposed to dorsal, and the long axis of the metatarsals cannot be brought into collinear alignment with the long axis of the talus (see Figure 20-13).

Pathoanatomic studies of a few specimens of congenital vertical talus confirm the anatomic distortions evident by the clinical and radiographic presentation. The specimens reported are similar in their clinical features, all demonstrating hindfoot valgus, equinus deformity, and the dorsolateral subluxation of the navicular on the talus. The talus itself may be hypoplastic with a facet joint on the dorsal neck at the point of articulation with the navicular. The sustentaculum talus is hypoplastic and the anterior facet joint absent. The peroneal and posterior tibialis tendons are displaced dorsally, resulting in muscle imbalance. The cause of this condition is unknown.

The natural history of congenital vertical talus depends not only on the foot deformity but also on any associated musculoskeletal or central nervous system disorder. In general, without treatment the ambulatory patient develops significant callosities over the head of the talus. This results in pain and skin breakdown over the talar head. The gait of these children is awkward, and shoeing may be a significant problem.

The treatment of congenital vertical talus depends on whether associated conditions are present. In the isolated deformity, surgical correction is almost always necessary. The foot should be manipulated to try to stretch the dorsolateral soft tissues. The manipulations are followed by casting with a long-leg cast changed at weekly intervals. The purpose of the manipulation and casting is to stretch the dorsolateral constricted soft tissues to minimize surgical complications, particularly skin necrosis. Manipulation and casting should be begun immediately at birth and continued for 6 to 10 weeks. Surgical correction is then performed either as a single or multistage procedure. The surgical correction involves lengthening the contracted dorsolateral structures, reducing the talonavicular or calcaneocuboid (or both) joint subluxations, and correcting of the equinus deformity through a posterior capsulotomy of the ankle and subtalar joint and Achilles tendon lengthening. Reinforcement of the soft tissue structures on the plantar aspect of the navicular by use of the posterior tibial tendon is generally indicated (see Figure 20-14). In older children (over 2.5 years of age), surgical correction is often accompanied by an extra-articular subtalar arthrodesis at the time of surgical correction or as an adjunctive procedure at a later time. Surgical corrections are aimed at restoring normal bony alignment and muscle balance. Complication rates of surgery are high and include aseptic necrosis of the talus, loss of reduction, and stiffness, particularly of the subtalar joint. Success rates are better in children treated surgically when younger than 1 year of age. Tendon transfers may be needed at a later date to restore muscle balance. In the adolescent or adult with untreated or recurrent congenital vertical talus, triple arthrodesis may be the only way to restore normal bony alignment.

CALCANEAL VALGUS

Calcaneal valgus (pes calcaneal valgus, talipes calcaneal valgus, congenital talipes calcaneal valgus) is one of the most common foot deformities seen at birth. The entire foot is held in the dorsiflexed everted position, and in its most severe form, the foot lies adjacent to the anterior border of the tibia (Figure 20-24). Calcaneal valgus is thought to be secondary to intrauterine molding. It is most common in firstborn children and in children of young mothers. It has a female predominance of 1:0.6 and is estimated to occur in 1 of every 1,000 live births.

Clinically, the foot is held in dorsiflexion near the tibia with the forefoot in varying degrees of abduction and the heel in varying degrees of valgus. The peroneal tendons may be subluxated anterior to the lateral malleolus. The soft tissues on the dorsal and lateral aspect of the foot are contracted and restrict plantar flexion and inversion. There may be

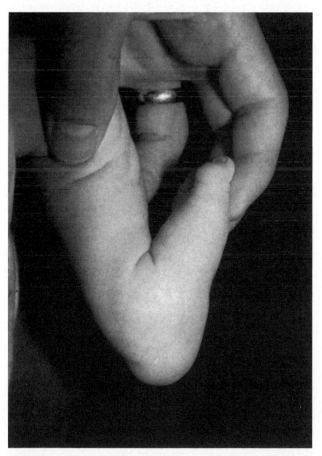

FIGURE 20-24. Calcaneal valgus deformity. There is close approximation of the dorsum of the foot to the anterior aspect of the distal tibia.

a transverse crease just distal to the ankle joint on the dorsal aspect of the foot. The foot can generally be manipulated to neutral or just short of the neutral position and, occasionally in mild cases, just beyond this position (Figure 20-25). The deformity may be accompanied by a mild abduction of the forefoot in varying degrees of heel valgus. There is an occasional association of this deformity with external rotation contractures in the hip and with other conditions thought to be secondary to intrauterine molding deformities (e.g., congenital hip dysplasia and torticollis).

It is important to rule out neuromuscular causes of calcaneal valgus deformity, such as myelomeningocele and arthrogryposis, as well as congenital vertical talus. In congenital vertical talus, the Achilles tendon is contracted, the hindfoot is in equinus, and there is a rocker-bottom deformity. Half the cases of vertical talus are associated with a neuromuscular deformity. All cases of posteromedial bowing of the tibia are associated with a calcaneal valgus deformity of the foot.

Radiographs are not necessary to make the diagnosis of pes calcaneal valgus. The foot can be palpated to show normal alignment with no subluxation at the talonavicular joint. Radiographs are only necessary when the diagnosis is in question.

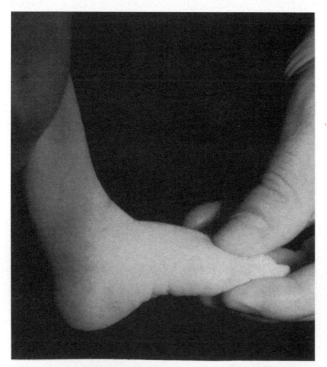

FIGURE 20-25. Calcaneal valgus deformity. The foot can easily be manipulated to or just short of the neutral position.

It is important to stimulate the foot to make certain that the plantar flexors are present.

The natural history of pes calcaneal valgus is one of spontaneous correction. Persistence of some of the deformity may lead to a flexible flatfoot. Casting is rarely necessary. Treatment should be directed at instructing the parents in stretching exercises. The foot should be gently manipulated into plantar flexion and inversion. In general, the deformity is corrected by 2 to 4 months of age. If it is persistent, however, manipulation and casting can be considered.

KÖHLER DISEASE

Köhler disease is an osteochondrosis that affects the tarsal navicular. It is a self-limited condition characterized by pain or swelling in the area of the tarsal navicular in association with certain radiographic features. It occurs in the age range of 4 to 7 years, with 80% of cases occurring in boys. One-fourth to one-third of cases are bilateral.

The cause of Köhler disease is unknown, but it is thought to be related to repetitive trauma and interruption of blood supply to the tarsal navicular. The tarsal navicular is the last bone of the foot to ossify. The appearance of the ossification center varies and is gender related. In girls, the tarsal navicular ossifies between 18 months and 2 years of age. In boys, the ossification occurs between 2.5 and 3 years of age. The normal ossification center has a smooth contour and uniform density. In otherwise normal children who have delay in appearance of the ossification center of the navicular, however, it may appear flat or fragmented with multiple ossification centers of increased density and irregular contour. Several ossification centers may eventually coalesce to form the navicular. Postmortem studies of the navicular in children reveal that the blood supply is tenuous, being supplied by only a single vessel until age 6 years.

Köhler disease is more common in patients (male or female) in whom ossification is delayed. The pathogenesis may be secondary to traumatic interruption of the vasculature to the tarsal navicular at a crucial stage in ossification.

Clinically, children present to the physician with complaints of pain and tenderness to palpation over the tarsal navicular. Localized swelling is occasionally evident. There may be palpable thickening of the soft tissues around the tarsal navicular. Many affected children walk with an antalgic gait and bear weight on the lateral aspect of the foot to avoid pressure over the medial aspect and the tarsal navicular. Active and passive range of motion are normal.

Radiographically, the navicular shows evidence of flattening, sclerosis, and irregular ossification (Figure 20-26). On the standing lateral view, the navicular has a decreased AP diameter with evidence of varying amounts of flattening. Multiple centers of ossification may be present. As mentioned previously, these radiographic features may be a normal variation in as many as one-third of children, particularly those who have late-onset ossification. Therefore, the diagnosis of Köhler disease is made only with the combination of the clinical signs, symptoms, and the radiographic features.

Children with clinical Köhler disease may have similar radiographic changes in the opposite navicular and be totally asymptomatic. In the normal child, the radiographic appearance is assumed to be secondary to coalescence of multiple ossification centers, while in the child with Köhler disease, the radiographic features represent the changes of avascular necrosis, with invasion by granulation tissue, resorption of necrotic trabeculae, and deposition of new bone.

The natural history of Köhler disease is relatively benign. No long-term disabilities have been reported in patients who have Köhler disease despite lack of treatment. In most cases, the navicular assumes a relatively normal appearance within 1 to 3 years after symptom onset.

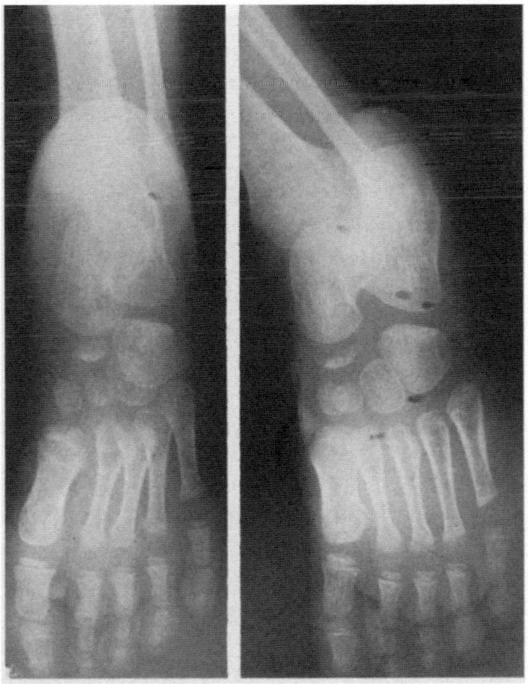

Treatment of the condition is designed to relieve symptoms and not to hasten the reparative process. Treatment for Köhler disease is nonsurgical and depends on the magnitude of symptoms. In patients with mild symptoms, restriction of activities may be all that is necessary. In children with more severe symptoms, a longitudinal arch support can be considered to more evenly distribute the patient's body weight in weight bearing. These measures, in conjunction with avoidance of strenuous activities such as jumping and running, usually relieve symptoms. In patients with more severe symptoms, immobilization in a short-leg cast for 3 to 4 weeks usually provides good relief of symptoms. The patient may need to use crutches with touch weight bearing for a short time but then may bear full weight on the cast as long as symptoms do not recur. Cast treatment should be continued until the patient is asymptomatic. In severe cases, the use of a short-leg walking cast improves the natural history of symptoms dramatically but has no effect on the radiographic course of the disease. Without treatment, most patients have intermittent symptoms for 1 to 3 years that is activity related and relieved by rest.

FIGURE 20-26. Köhler disease or osteochondrosis of the tarsal navicular.

FREIBERG INFARCTION

Freiberg infarction is another type of osteochondrosis. Specifically, it is an aseptic necrosis of the metatarsal head. Three-fourths of cases occur in girls, and the second metatarsal head is the most commonly involved, although the disease may affect the third or fourth metatarsal head. Freiberg disease rarely occurs before the age of 13 or 14 years.

The origin of Freiberg infarction is unknown, but it is thought to be similar to that of osteochondritis dissecans of the knee. The second metatarsal is the longest and the most rigid metatarsal. It is subjected to the greatest amount of stress in walking. Freiberg infarction is sometimes seen with an accompanying stress fracture of the metatarsal.

Clinically, patients present with pain and tenderness around the second metatarsophalangeal joint. They may complain of stiffness and have a limp secondary to the pain. On physical examination, the discomfort is well localized. There may be palpable swelling at the second metatarsophalangeal joint. Pain may be elicited on passive range of motion.

Motion may be limited and painful. The history may be one of exacerbations and remissions, with pain aggravated by activity and relieved by rest.

Radiographically, the second metatarsal head may have a flattened, enlarged appearance with areas of increased sclerosis and fragmentation. The affected metatarsophalangeal joint may be narrowed, and in long-standing disease, secondary degenerative changes may be evident (Figure 20-27).

The natural history of Freiberg infarction is variable. In many cases, the condition is self-limited, with revascularization of the affected metatarsal head. The disease process may leave the metatarsal head deformed. Many patients have no pain or discomfort and good range of motion. In some cases,

however, the disease course involves exacerbations and remissions. Significant deformity may ensue, and secondary degenerative changes may occur at the metatarsophalangeal joint.

The goal of treatment is to obtain healing of the aseptic necrosis. Initial treatment should be symptomatic. Symptomatic treatment includes decreasing activities and using metatarsal pads inserted in the shoe or metatarsal bars on the sole of the shoe. These two measures are designed to allow for weight bearing on the metatarsal neck as opposed to the metatarsal head to decrease the stresses applied to the metatarsal head. In patients who have more acute symptoms, a short-leg walking cast with or without crutches may provide relief. If the joint is free of degenerative changes and symptoms persist, removal of the necrotic fragment alone may provide symptomatic relief. A foot orthosis designed to provide pressure relief over the second metatarsal head may be used on a long-term basis once the acute symptoms have subsided or after surgical removal of the necrotic segment. Mild symptoms may be treated by an orthosis alone.

In patients with long-standing symptoms who fail nonoperative treatment, surgical treatment may be offered. This may include removal of the loose fragment and resection of the base of the proximal phalanx. Alternatively, resection of the metatarsophalangeal joint may be required, with syndactylization of the second and third toe to avoid significant shortening that may follow resection of the metatarsophalangeal joint. This usually provides good relief of symptoms.

SEVER DISEASE

Sever disease, or calcaneal apophysitis, is one of the most common overuse syndromes seen in growing children. It most commonly occurs in the age range of 6 to 12 years and is thought to be due to repeated microtrauma. Most affected children are extremely active. This condition may thus represent chronic strain at the insertion of the tendo Achilles.

Affected children present with activity-related pain over the posterior aspect of the calcaneus. Physical examination reveals tenderness to compression over the calcaneal apophysis. Symptoms may cause discomfort with passive ankle dorsiflexion. The condition must be differentiated from other sources of heel pain in young children (Table 20-1).

In normal children, the calcaneal apophysis appears at an average of 5.6 years of age in girls (range,

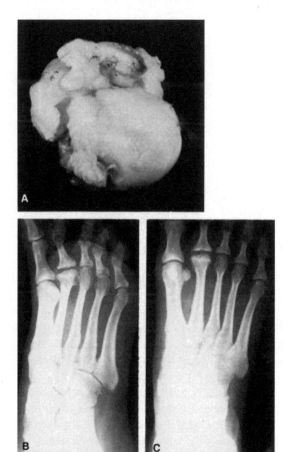

FIGURE 20-27. Freiberg infarction (osteochondrosis of the metatarsal head). **(A)** Frontal view of the resected metatarsal head. The articular cartilage is irregular with areas of loss of articular surface. There are multiple indentations about the head. The capsule about the periphery is thickened, and secondary osteoarthritic spurs are present. A cleft at the margin suggests formation of a loose body by separation. **(B and C)** Radiographs of the second metatarsal head before resection showing sclerosis, irregularity, widening, and spurring with flattening.

TABLE 20-1.
Sources of Heel Pain in Childhood

OVERUSE/OVERGROWTH/TRAUMATIC
Calcaneal apophysitis
Contusion/strain
Stress fracture of calcaneus
Fracture of calcaneus

DEVELOPMENTAL
Tarsal coalition

INFLAMMATORY
Tendinitis (Achilles, patellar, flexor hallux longus)
Plantar fasciitis
Retrocalcaneal bursitis
Periostitis
Os trigonum inflammation

INFECTIOUS
Soft tissue infection
Abscess
Calcaneal osteomyelitis

RHEUMATOLOGIC
Juvenile rheumatoid arthritis
Reiter syndrome
Miscellaneous

TUMORS

BENIGN
Osteoid osteoma
Osteochondroma
Chondroblastoma
Bone cyst (solitary or aneurysmal)

MALIGNANT (RARE)
Leukemia
Metastatic

NEUROLOGIC
Tarsal tunnel syndrome

(Micheli LJ, Ireland ML. Prevention and management of calcaneal apophysitis in children: an overuse syndrome. J Pediatr Orthop 1987;7:34–38)

3 to 8.5 years) and 7.9 years of age in boys (range, 6 to 10 years). In many normal children, the calcaneal apophysis may appear fragmented and then coalesce from two to three separate ossification centers. This normal ossification variant, in combination with symptomatology, is considered diagnostic of Sever disease (Figure 20-28). If patients have bilateral symptoms, radiographs are often not necessary. In unilateral cases, however, radiographs of both feet should be obtained to rule out other causes of

heel pain, such as retrocalcaneal bursitis, stress fractures, infection, rheumatologic conditions, and neoplastic lesions.

Sever disease is a self-limiting condition. In cases of severe symptoms, activity restriction may be necessary. If this alone does not relieve symptoms or if symptoms are acute, a short-leg walking cast may be applied for 3 to 4 weeks. This usually is adequate to curtail symptoms. Longer periods of casting or activity restriction of up to 1 to 3 months may be necessary in some cases. No long-term disability or deformity has been reported from Sever disease.

METATARSUS ADDUCTUS

A wide variety of terms are used to describe this clinical entity, including *metatarsus adductus, metatarsus varus, skew foot, serpentine foot, pes adductus, metatarsus adductovarus, hooked forefoot, metatarsus internus,* and *congenital metatarsus varus.* These terms unfortunately are used inconsistently throughout the medical literature. The two most widely used terms are metatarsus adductus and metatarsus varus, which describe slightly different forefoot variations but are synonymous. In this condition, the forefoot is generally adducted and occasionally inverted (varus) at the tarsometatarsal joint, and the hindfoot is generally neutral to valgus (Figure 20-29; see Figure 20-19). Metatarsus adductus is present at birth but often is overlooked by the family until the child is between 3 months and 1 year of age.

Metatarsus adductus is the most common congenital foot deformity. Its incidence is 1 in 1,000 live births. It has a female predominance of 4:3 and a 5% incidence of the condition in first-degree relatives. There is no known pattern of inheritance, but the risk of a second sibling being affected is 1 in 20. Two-thirds of patients have involvement of both feet. There is a strong association between metatarsus adductus and congenital hip dysplasia and dislocation.

The cause of metatarsus adductus is unknown. It is thought to be secondary to intrauterine molding because 59% of patients are firstborn children. Other etiologic theories include peroneal muscle weakness with overactive anterior tibialis and posterior tibialis; abnormal insertion of the tibialis posterior tendons on the first cuneiform rather than their usual site on the navicular; and posture habits caused by prone, sleeping with the buttocks elevated,

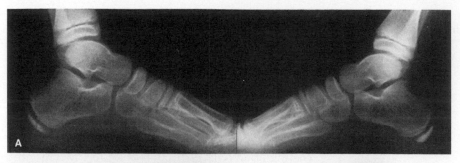

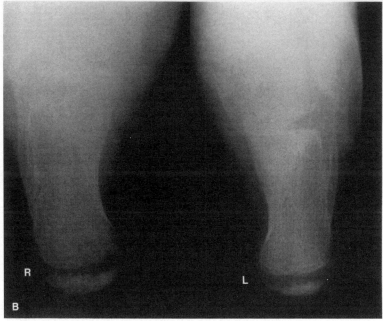

FIGURE 20-28. Severe disease of the calcaneal apophysis. **(A)** Standing lateral radiograph. **(B)** Calcaneal views. Note sclerotic fragmented appearance of the right symptomatic calcaneus as opposed to the sclerotic semifragmented appearance of the asymptomatic left side. (Ponseti IV, Becker JR. Congenital metatarsus adductus. J Bone Joint Surg 1966; 48A:702)

hips and knees in complete flexion, feet adducted and tucked beneath the buttocks, and sitting on the adducted feet. Persistent soft tissue contractures may lead to secondary tarsal changes, making the deformity rigid with time.

Clinically, the deformity is present at birth but usually not noticed by the parents until the child begins to crawl or walk. Occasionally, patients present to a physician in the toddler years when the parents complain of the child in-toeing or having difficulty wearing shoes. On physical examination, all the metatarsals are adducted and the forefoot is occasionally in varus (see Figure 20-29). The heel is in neutral to slight valgus. The great toe is often widely separated from the second toe, and the base of the fifth metatarsal and the cuboid are prominent on the lateral aspect of the foot. The medial border of the foot is concave, and the lateral border is convex. Medial tibial torsion often accompanies metatarsus adductus. The Achilles tendon is not tight, and the foot can be fully dorsiflexed at the ankle joint. The deformity is often accentuated by

overactivity in the abductor hallucis and the short toe flexors.

The deformity is often classified subjectively as mild, moderate, or severe, depending on whether the forefoot can be passively corrected to neutral or to an overcorrected position. Severe deformities are rigid and not passively correctable. The ratio of supple to rigid deformity is about 10:1. The term *serpentine foot* is often used for a rigid adducted forefoot with an accompanying heel valgus.

The heel bisector should pass through the second toe. In a mild deformity, the bisector passes through the third toe; in a moderate deformity, it passes between the third and fourth toes or just the fourth toe; and in a severe deformity, the heel bisector passes between the fourth and fifth toes. The deformity is said to be flexible or passively correctable if the forefoot (second toe) can be passively abducted beyond the heel bisector (see Figure 20-29). Many patients exhibit dynamic hallux varus, whereby the great toe deviates medially during stance phase but the metatarsals are normally aligned.

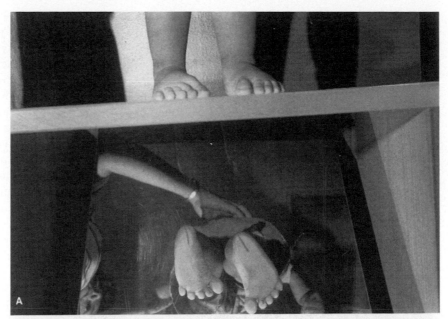

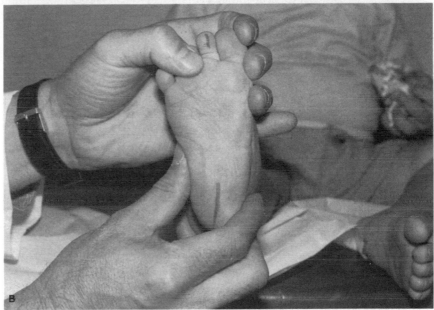

FIGURE 20-29. **(A)** Thirteen-month-old boy with bilateral metatarsus adductus. The left foot is abducted and the right forefoot is adducted and in slight varus. The heel bisector is at the fourth toe on the left foot and between the third and fourth toes on the right foot. **(B)** Note passive correctability of deformity. Forefoot can be passively abducted beyond the heel bisector.

Radiographs are not required to make the diagnosis of metatarsus adductus. Radiographs can, however, document deformity and are used by some to classify the deformity. Radiographs, if taken, should be in the standing position or with the foot resting in a simulated standing position on the radiograph cassette. Radiographs demonstrate sharp medial angulation of the tarsometatarsal joints, with the first metatarsal being more severely adducted than the fifth (see Figure 20-19). Normally, a line drawn through the longitudinal axis of the first metatarsal is parallel or diverges laterally from a line drawn through the longitudinal axis of the talus. In metatarsus adductus, the first metatarsal line falls medial to the talar line. In the weight-bearing or simulated weight-bearing film, the calcaneal line should bisect the cuboid and the base of the fourth metatarsal. In metatarsus adductus, the calcaneal line passes through the lateral portion of the cuboid and through the base of the fifth metatarsal. Heel valgus is evidenced by a greater than 35° AP talocalcaneal angle and by medial and forward displacement of the head of the talus in relation to the anterior portion of the calcaneus. The navicular (generally not seen on radiographs in this age group) is neutral or displaced laterally on the talar head (see Figure 20-19).

The natural history of metatarsus adductus is generally benign. It is estimated that 85 to 90% of cases resolve spontaneously without treatment. In childhood, persistent metatarsus adductus leads to an in-toeing gait and occasional complaints of stumbling or tripping. Adults with uncorrected metatarsus adductus rarely complain of pain but may have hallux valgus and bunions. Shoe wear may be a problem in patients with uncorrected metatarsus adductus. Patients may complain of pain in the lateral foot and in the tarsometatarsal joints. Shoes may irritate this area. It is thus important in infancy to select patients who require treatment.

Treatment decisions for metatarsus adductus are based on the passive correctability of the deformity. In patients in whom the deformity corrects by stimulation of the lateral border of the foot or in those in whom the heel is stabilized, the deformity can be passively corrected or overcorrected, and only observation is necessary. Most cases correct spontaneously. In most large series, if the foot remained passively correctable, the deformity had corrected spontaneously by the age of 3 years. Parents should not be encouraged to do manipulations. Manipulations by parents are generally poorly done and may accentuate heel valgus and only minimally correct forefoot adduction. There is no scientific validity for the use of straight-last or reverse-last shoes in the treatment of metatarsus adductus. Denis Browne splints should not be used because they may accentuate heel valgus.

In patients with rigid, severe, nonpassively correctable metatarsus adductus, manipulation and casting are indicated. Two main components of the deformity, adduction of the metatarsals and varying degrees of valgus of the heel, must be corrected simultaneously. Improper manipulation and casting treatment of metatarsus adductus lead to a pronation deformity of the foot. A flatfoot with residuals of metatarsus adductus and severe heel valgus is a significantly worse problem than the original deformity.

The hindfoot deformity is corrected by supinating the calcaneus underneath the talus. With the calcaneus supinated, the cuneiform, navicular, and cuboid bones are inverted, bringing the bases of the metatarsals in proper alignment with the talus and calcaneus (see Figure 20-19). The metatarsals are then abducted, with counterpressure applied over the cuboid bone. It is important not to pronate the forefoot because a cavus deformity will result. The manipulations of the foot are sustained for several minutes, and this is followed by the application of a thinly padded, well-molded, toe-to-groin plaster cast changed at biweekly intervals until the foot is in the slightly overcorrected position. Complete correction usually requires 3 to 4 long-leg plaster applications. The casting treatment is complete when the lateral aspect of the foot is no longer convex, the heel is in a neutral to slight valgus position, and the forefoot has been completely corrected past neutral. Successful treatment of metatarsus adductus by manipulations and casting in patients older than 8 months of age is not likely, and surgical correction may be necessary.

Surgical correction for metatarsus adductus is indicated only in patients with significant cosmetic or shoe-wearing problems. In patients younger than 2 years of age with rigid metatarsus adductus, first metatarsal cuneiform capsulotomy and release of the abductor hallucis, followed by casting, is usually successful. In older children, corrective bone surgery may be necessary.

CLUBFOOT

Talipes equinovarus is the term most commonly used for clubfeet. *Talipes* is a generic term for any foot deformity that centers around the talus. *Equinus* implies that the foot is flexed in the plantar direction. The term *talipes equinocavovarus* is sometimes used to denote the varying amounts of cavus of the forefoot evident in patients with clubfeet. In the clubfoot, the heel is in varus, and the first metatarsal is in severe plantar flexion, while the fifth metatarsal is normally aligned with the cuboid and calcaneus (Figures 20-30 and 20-31; see Figure 20-19). Cavus is caused by eversion of the forefoot in relation to the hindfoot.

Clubfoot is a complex foot deformity that is readily apparent at birth. All clubfeet are not of the same severity, although all have the basic components of adduction and inversion of the forefoot and midfoot, heel varus, and fixed equinus. The soft tissue changes vary from mild to severe. Clubfoot should best be thought of as a spectrum of deformities. Clubfoot may occur as an isolated disorder or in combination with various syndromes and other associated anomalies, such as arthrogryposis, sacral agenesis, amniotic bands, Larsen syndrome, diastrophic dwarfism, Freeman-Sheldon syndrome, and myelodysplasia.

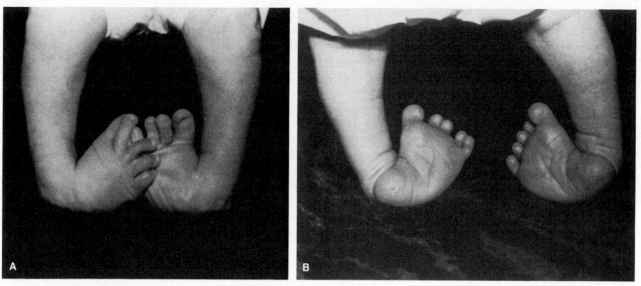

FIGURE 20-30. Severe clubfoot deformity. The heel is in severe varus, and the forefoot is adducted and inverted. The cavus deformity results from the slightly pronated position of the forefoot in relation to the hindfoot.

The incidence of idiopathic clubfoot is estimated to be 1 to 2 per 1,000 live births. It has a male predominance of 2:1 and an incidence of bilateralness estimated to be about 50%. There is an increased

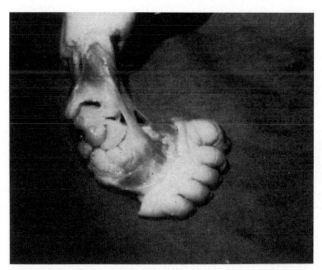

FIGURE 20-31. Clubfoot in a 3-day-old infant. The navicular is medially displaced and articulates only with the medial aspect of the head of the talus. The cuneiforms are seen to the right of the navicular, and the cuboid is underneath it. The calcaneocuboid joint is directed posteromedially. The anterior two-thirds of the os calcis is seen underneath the talus. The tendons of the anterior tibialis extensor hallucis longus and the extensor digitorum longus are medially displaced. (Ponseti IV, Campos J. Observations on pathogenesis and treatment of congenital clubfoot. Corr 1972;84:50–60)

incidence in certain racial and ethnic groups, such as Polynesians, Maoris, and South African blacks, with a much higher incidence if the patient has a positive family history for clubfoot.

The origin of congenital clubfoot in otherwise normal patients remains unknown. Many theories have been advanced, including intrauterine molding defect, blastemic defect of the tarsal cartilage, primary nerve lesion with secondary muscle dysfunction, vascular abnormalities, arrested embryonic development, abnormal tendon insertions, and primary fibrotic contracture. The most widely accepted theory is that of polygenic inheritance modified by environmental factors.

Clinically, the deformity is readily apparent at birth. The child presents with the foot in severe supination with a fixed equinus deformity, heel varus, forefoot and midfoot adduction, and varying amounts of cavus. The involved foot is generally smaller than the opposite side with varying amounts of calf atrophy.

The head of the talus is prominent and easily palpable on the dorsolateral aspect of the foot. Depending on the severity of the cavus deformity, there may be a deep skin crease across the plantar medial aspect of the midfoot. The foot cannot be passively manipulated into the neutral position.

Radiographs are often useful in documenting the deformity. The calcaneus, talus, and cuboid are usually ossified at birth. The navicular does not ossify until about 3 years of age. The normal values of bony relations on standing AP and lateral views of the foot are somewhat variable and age dependent (Figure 20-32).

Radiographs are useful in documenting the deformity (photographs are also useful for this purpose), for follow-up, in assessing the results of nonoperative treatment, and in planning for operative correction of the deformity if necessary. It is best to obtain the initial radiographs in the maximally corrected position. This position varies depending on the flexibility of the individual clubfoot.

In the clubfoot deformity, the talus and calcaneus exhibit parallelism on both the AP and lateral radiographs, indicating hindfoot varus and equinus (see Figure 20-31). The talus first metatarsal angle is negative, indicating adduction of the forefoot. Because of the inversion of the forefoot, the metatarsals appear overlapped. The cuboid is medially displaced on the AP view, indicating the adduction at the midfoot; and on the lateral view, the first metatarsal is in plantar flexion to a greater degree than the fifth metatarsal, indicating cavus deformity.

Pathoanatomically, many specimens of clubfeet have been described, all showing varying degrees of similar abnormalities (see Figure 20-31). In the clubfoot, the talar body is in plantar flexion with the neck angulated medially. The navicular articulates with the medial aspect of the talar neck, and the navicular tuberosity is in close approximation with the medial malleolus. The calcaneus is directly underneath the talus, and the cuboid is medially displaced beneath the navicular. The midfoot is thus adducted and inverted in relation to the talus. The dorsal tendons are medially displaced, and the head of the talus is prominent laterally.

Anatomically, the involved talus is generally smaller than the noninvolved side, with the neck in varying degrees of medial deviation. The navicular is wedge-shaped laterally, with a prominent tuberosity. The calcaneus is small, often with an absent anterior facet. The posterior facet shows varying degrees of hypoplasia and may be linked directly to the middle facet. In unilateral deformities, the foot is always smaller than the noninvolved side, and the calf has varying degrees of atrophy. The tuberosity of the navicular is held in close approximation to the talar neck, the sustentaculum and the medial malleolus by the shortened, thickened tibionavicular ligament, calcaneonavicular ligament, and sheath of the posterior tibial tendon.

Clubfoot deformity, regardless of origin or associated clinical problems, results in a severe handicap unless corrected. The surface area for weight bearing is the lateral aspect of the foot; without treatment, even an otherwise normal patient develops pressure sores and sinuses by the fourth or fifth decade of life (Figure 20-33).

The criteria for successful treatment of a clubfoot deformity vary in the orthopaedic literature. Some judge success only by radiographic criteria, others by function, and others by certain clinical criteria. Thus, the literature on treatment is difficult to compare.

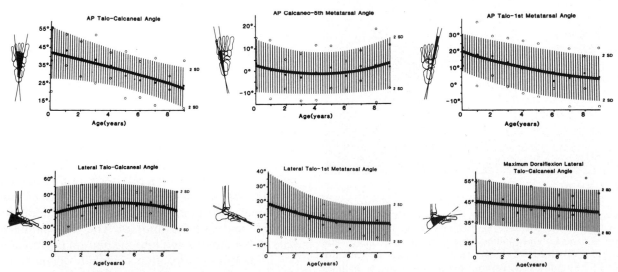

FIGURE 20-32. Normal radiographic values for various foot measurements. (Vanderwilde R, Staheli LT, Chew DE et al. Measurements on radiographs of the foot in normal infants and children. J Bone Joint Surg 1988;70A:407–415)

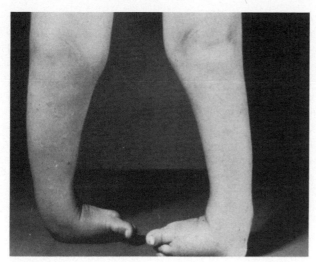

FIGURE 20-33. Four-year-old girl with bilateral untreated clubfeet.

The goal of treatment in clubfoot deformity is to obtain and maintain the foot in plantargrade position. Treatment should be initiated immediately on diagnosis, preferably within the first week of life. Treatment for the newborn with clubfoot is by manipulation and then casting to maintain the correction obtained through manipulation. Corrections begun at a later age may be more difficult owing to ligamentous contracture and joint deformity. Toe-to-groin plaster casts are used to maintain the corrections obtained through manipulation. The equinus deformity is the last deformity corrected to prevent development of a rocker-bottom foot. Casts are changed at weekly intervals, and most deformities are corrected in 5 to 7 casts. Successful treatment rates by casting regimens alone vary in the literature from 85 to 95%. Night splinting is often used for prolonged periods (several years) to maintain correction.

Depending on the initial severity, clubfeet have a natural tendency to recur. The more severe and rigid the initial deformity, the greater the risk of recurrence. Recurrences may be treated by serial manipulations and casting followed by occasional tendon transfers to correct for any muscle imbalance.

The small percentage of deformities that fail to respond to manipulation and casting or that recur may require extensive posterior, medial, and lateral soft tissue releases. The releases are best done at a young age but can be done satisfactorily in children until 5 years of age.

In children older than 3 years of age, lateral column shortening procedures (decancellation of the cuboid or wedge resection of the cuboid in excision of the anterior end of the calcaneus) are often performed in conjunction with posteromedial releases. This is because the greater length of the lateral foot column compared with the medial foot column is thought to be secondary to the medial soft tissue contractures.

The major complications of the extensive posterior, medial, subtalar, and lateral releases performed for residual, resistant, or recurrent clubfoot include skin sloughing on posteromedial aspect of the foot, overcorrection of the deformity, residual forefoot adductus, stiffness, and incomplete correction of the deformity.

Triple arthrodesis may be necessary for recurrent or persistent clubfoot deformity in older children. These procedures are best offered to the patient at 10 to 12 years of age, when foot growth is complete.

IDIOPATHIC TOE-WALKING

This entity is also called *habitual toe-walking, hereditary tendo Achilles contracture,* or *congenital short tendo calcaneus.* Parents notice that the child is walking on the toes either all or most of the time. Idiopathic toe-walking is thought to be an inherited condition because up to 70% of patients have a positive family history. The condition is bilateral and predominantly affects boys (3:1). About 20% of these children have evidence of a learning disability, and an occasional child carries the diagnosis of hyperkinesia with minimal brain dysfunction.

When a child begins to stand and walk, toe-walking is a normal gait variation. Generally, within the first 6 months after walking, the gait may progress from the toe-toe gait or an occasional toe-toe gait to a toe-heel gait and eventually to a heel-toe gait. The mature heel-toe gait pattern is generally established by the time a child is 3 years of age. Careful history of gait development should be obtained in each patient who presents with a chief complaint of toe-walking. Patients with the diagnosis of idiopathic toe-walking have nearly always walked on their toes.

Physical examination includes range of motion of the upper and lower extremities as well as a careful neurologic examination and observation of the patient's gait. Variable amounts of contracture and restriction of ankle dorsiflexion are noted. The amount of contracture or restriction of motion may not be symmetric. These patients have normal sensory examinations and no evidence of muscle weakness. Deep tendon reflexes should be intact without evidence of hyperactivity. The spine should be evaluated for evidence of hair patches, dimpling, hyperpigmentation, or nevi, which are suggestive of spinal dysraphism. There should be minimal or no contracture of the hamstrings, and the patient should have good control of the upper extremities.

The child's gait should be carefully evaluated. Many patients with idiopathic toe-walking can walk on their heels and have a heel-toe gait periodically, but the observed gait pattern usually is toe-toe. Idiopathic toe-walkers with heel cord contractures can generally get their heels down in standing only through knee hyperextension (Figure 20-34).

Idiopathic toe-walking is the diagnosis of exclusion. All conditions that may be associated with an equinus deformity and contracture of the tendo Achilles must be ruled out. Cerebral palsy can be ruled out by the absence of increased deep tendon reflexes, hypertonicity, hamstring contractures, and the lack of posturing abnormalities of the upper extremity during gait. Gait analysis may be of help in

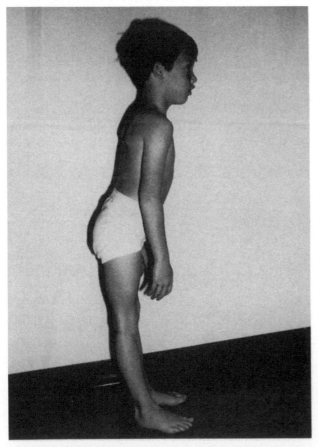

FIGURE 20-34. Three-year-old male idiopathic toe-walker. The heels can be brought to the floor by knee hyperextension.

differentiating the idiopathic toe-walker from the cerebral palsy patient. Other conditions, such as spinal dysraphism, muscular dystrophy, tethered spinal cord, or other central nervous system dysfunctions, must be ruled out. Electromyographs, motor nerve conduction studies, spine films, CT scan of the brain, or MRI may be necessary. Muscle biopsy to rule out muscular dystrophy is also warranted on occasion. Any child with a unilateral deformity, particularly of recent onset, should have an etiologic source sought. A neurologic consultation is often in order.

The typical patient with idiopathic toe-walking has no abnormal findings other than those referable to the equinus deformity with varying degrees of contracture of the Achilles tendon. They have normal sensation, no pain, and no muscle dysfunction.

Treatment of the condition varies according to the age of the patient and the degree of contracture of the Achilles tendon. In patients who are younger than 3 to 4 years of age and have no or minimal contracture of the Achilles tendon, passive range of motion and stretching exercises are indicated. The child's progress should be monitored carefully. If ankle dorsiflexion to at least 10° cannot be restored by this method in 3 to 4 months, serial casts should be applied. If, however, the ankle can be passively dorsiflexed to neutral or beyond, but the child habitually toe-walks, use of a hinged or nonhinged ankle foot orthosis is an option to prevent plantar flexion. These orthoses can be used for a period of weeks to months, depending on the clinical situation. The patient should be continually reevaluated and progress reassessed. In most cases, serial casting in dorsiflexion for 4 to 6 weeks is usually sufficient to resolve the problem. Many patients require postcasting ankle-foot orthoses, passive range of motion, and careful follow-up to ensure that the condition does not recur. In most cases, these noninvasive procedures provide resolution of the problem. For the child who fails to respond to serial casting or is otherwise not a candidate for this procedure, Achilles tendon lengthening provides uniformly good results. Surgical Achilles tendon lengthening is followed by 3 weeks in a nonweight-bearing short-leg cast, then 3 weeks in a weight-bearing short-leg cast. Recurrences after this procedure are rare.

TORSIONAL PROBLEMS

The parents' or grandparents' perception of an abnormal position of the legs of an infant or the way a child walks frequently results in medical consultation.

Unfortunately, these concerns often result in unnecessary, costly treatment.

In the newborn, the proximal femur (femoral head, neck, and trochanter) is usually anteverted about 40° in relation to the transcondylar axis of the distal femur. The intermalleolar axis of the distal tibia in relation to the interplateau axis of the proximal tibia is in about 3° of lateral rotation. During the first year of life, femoral anteversion decreases by about 8° and thereafter decreases by about 1° per year until the adult configuration of about 10 to 15° of anteversion is reached at maturity. Tibial version also increases throughout life until the adult lateral version of 15 to 20° is reached at maturity. Version of more than two standard deviations beyond the mean is referred to as *torsion*.

Any child who is brought in for evaluation because the parents perceive an abnormality should be carefully checked to see whether the child is merely in the normal stages of development or has a torsional problem. The most common torsional problems are femoral antetorsion and medial tibial torsion. The normal values for version vary according to the age of the patient (Figure 20-35). The cause of the torsional problems is unknown but may be due to persistent version or genetic factors. Postnatal sitting and sleeping postures have been implicated as mechanisms that either cause torsional abnormalities or contribute to their lack of resolution, but no conclusive proof exists. Excessive ligament laxity on a genetic basis has been thought by some investigators to contribute to persistent femoral antetorsion in that many children with femoral antetorsion have accompanying physiologic pes planus, genu recurvatum, and excessive lumbar lordosis. The latter two may actually be compensatory measures for femoral antetorsion.

Any child brought in by parents for complaints of in-toeing should have a careful history and physical examination. The history should include the age at which the parents first noted the deformity, how they think it affects the child's function, and any perceived disability because of the deformity. Sleeping and sitting postures should be assessed and a complete history of normal growth and development obtained. The age at onset of walking should be evaluated. Any delay in development of walking beyond 18 months of age may be suggestive of a neuromuscular abnormality such as cerebral palsy. A family history of similar problems should be sought.

Careful physical examination must include a complete neurologic examination and a torsional profile of the patient. The most common abnormalities seen are those of femoral antetorsion, medial tibial torsion, and metatarsus adductus. Other conditions, such as an overactive abductor hallucis, clubfoot deformity, or dynamic in-toeing because of muscle imbalance, must be ruled out.

The parents may complain that the child's problem is worse at the end of the day or when tired, which may indicate failure of compensatory mechanisms. The problem may be of great concern to parents, who often scold the child for walking in a way that is more comfortable because of the child's rotational profile.

The child should be observed walking and running in an unobstructed area. The position of the patella and the feet should be noted. The physician should assess the foot progression angle. The foot progression angle is the axis of the foot as the child walks along an imaginary line of progression. This can be estimated or special paper (footprint paper) can be used to assess the foot progression angle. Negative foot progression angles designate in-toeing; positive foot progression angles designating out-toeing. The normal foot progression angle is usually positive.

Hip rotation should be assessed with the hip in extension in the prone position. The knee is flexed to 90°, and rotation is assessed medially and laterally in relation to the gluteal cleft. The pelvis should be stabilized, and no force should be exerted on the limb. Internal and external rotation are assessed and compared with normal, age-matched values (Figures 20-36 and 20-37).

Tibial rotation is next assessed by use of either the thigh-foot or transmalleolar axis (Figure 20-38). In most cases, the thigh-foot axis is sufficient. Tibial rotation can be assessed in several ways. With the patient in the prone position and the knees flexed to 90°, the thigh-foot axis can easily be assessed and compared with normal, age-matched values. If the patient has a foot deformity, the transmalleolar axis should be used. The transmalleolar axis is assessed by placing the thumb and index finger on the medial and lateral malleoli, respectively, to define the intermalleolar axis; a perpendicular axis is then defined, and the angles between the perpendicular and intermalleolar axis and the long axis of the thigh are assessed. A simpler assessment of the intermalleolar axis is done with the patient sitting with the legs hanging free over the table and the knees at 90°. The thumb and index finger can be placed on the medial and lateral malleoli, respectively, and the intermalleolar axis can be assessed in relation to the tibial tubercle, determining the degree of tibial rotation.

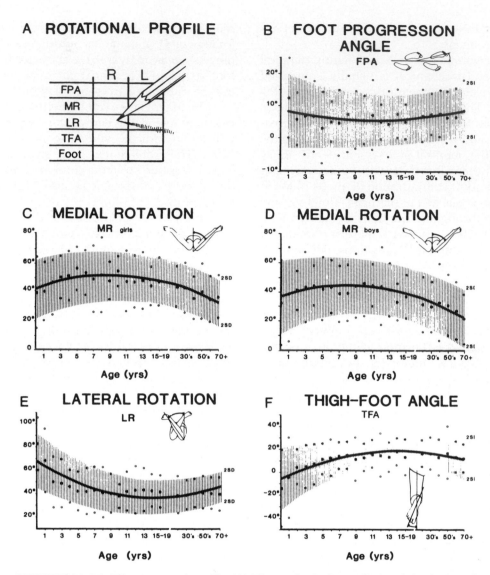

FIGURE 20-35. The rotational profile. **(A)** The method of recording and the degree of measurement for each element of the profile are depicted. This simple chart includes the vital information necessary to establish the diagnosis and to document deformity. **(B through F)** Normal values with the profile based on 1,000 normal limbs are shown. In each figure, the age is listed on the abscissa on a logarithmic scale, and the degrees are shown on the ordinate scale. The mean values are shown in the solid line with a ±2 standard deviation normal range shown in the shaded areas. A gender difference was found from medial rotation, so values are shown independently. (Staheli LT. The lower limb. In: Morrissy RT, ed. Lovell and Winter's Pediatric Orthopedics, 3rd Ed, vol. 2. Philadelphia: JB Lippincott, 1990:742)

The patient's feet should be examined for evidence of metatarsus adductus and residual deformity secondary to previous clubfoot treatment. The cause of the patient's in-toeing gait may be one or more abnormalities in the lower extremity. Occasionally, a rotational profile of the parent may reveal a torsional problem that explains the torsional problem in the child or lack of resolution of the problem in the older child.

Radiographs or special studies are rarely necessary in children with torsional problems. In the infant, congenital hip dysplasia must be ruled out,

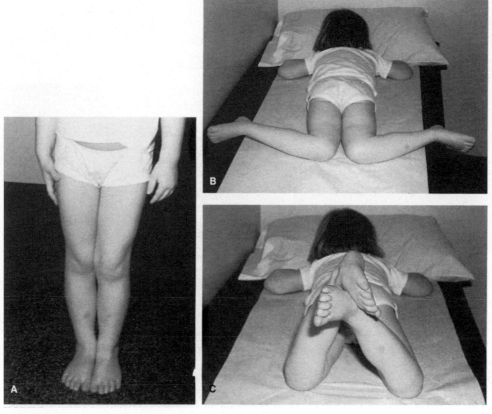

FIGURE 20-36. Femoral antetorsion. **(A)** Four-year-old girl with femoral antetorsion. In the standing view, the patella points inward. In the prone position, excessive femoral antetorsion indicated by internal rotation to about 90° **(B)** and by restricted external rotation **(C).**

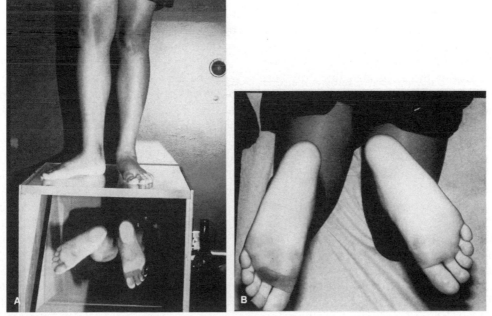

FIGURE 20-37. Lateral tibial torsion. **(A)** Twelve-year-old girl with lateral tibial torsion. **(B)** Unilateral abnormality in the thigh-foot axis is seen.

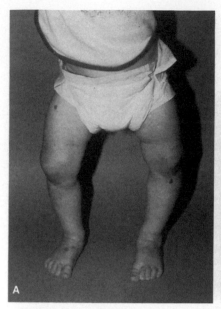
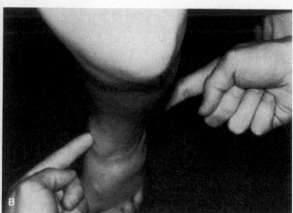

FIGURE 20-38. Medial tibial torsion. **(A)** Eighteen-month-old boy with medial tibial torsion and physiologic bowing. **(B)** Tibial rotation is assessed by visualizing relation of intermalleolar axis in reference to the tibial tubercle with patient sitting with leg over the edge of the examination table.

and if clinical examination warrants, radiographs may be necessary. Determination of version is best done by CT or MRI with cuts through the axis of the femoral neck and the femoral condyles. Torsion of the tibia is easily measured clinically, and hence radiographs or special studies are rarely necessary.

The natural history of torsional problems is one of gradual resolution, and hence treatment of these conditions is rarely necessary. Treatment by devices such as corrective shoes, twister cables, and alteration of sleeping or sitting habits have never been shown to affect the natural history of these conditions and should therefore be avoided. Education of the family regarding the natural history of these conditions is important. The family should be reassured that most torsional problems resolve spontaneously in the course of normal growth. The parents should also be reassured that if there is a positive family history of torsional problems, complete resolution may not occur, but in most cases, no functional disability ensues.

Infants and children before walking age may be brought in by parents for complaints of the feet pointing out. Careful examination of the hips should be done to rule out congenital hip dysplasia. External rotation contractures are normal in the infant and gradually resolve with time. Treatment is never indicated.

In a child who has not reached walking age comes in with the parents complaining of one foot

turning out, a careful hip examination should be performed to rule out any associated congenital hip dysplasia. In general, the out-turned foot is the more normal foot because this condition usually coexists with metatarsus adductus or medial tibial torsion on the opposite side. The natural history should be explained to the parents and observation recommended.

In the prewalking years, the most common cause of in-turning of the lower extremities is metatarsus adductus. Congenital hip dysplasia must, however, be ruled out.

In the walking child between 1 and 3 years of age, the most common cause of in-toeing is medial tibial torsion, which may or may not be accompanied by metatarsus adductus. Reassurance and observation is the treatment of choice.

In the older child, particularly after 3 years of age, medial femoral torsion is a common cause of an in-toeing gait. Natural history studies indicate that medial femoral torsion is not associated with degenerative joint disease over the long term, and hence observation is the only treatment warranted. Radiographs or special studies are not indicated unless there is asymmetry.

Surgical treatment for medial tibial torsion or medial femoral torsion is rarely indicated. Surgical correction can be considered in cases of medial tibial torsion if the child is older than 8 years of age (when spontaneous correction is no longer possible), if the discrepancy is more than three to four standard deviations from the mean, and if the deformity is causing the child significant functional or cosmetic problems. Supramalleolar osteotomy is usually the treatment of choice when surgical correction is contemplated.

Lateral tibial torsion is not an uncommon problem and usually does not resolve with age. Lateral tibial torsion can be considered for correction if it is greater than 30° and causes significant functional or cosmetic deformity to the child (see Figure 20-37).

Medial femoral torsion can be considered for correction if the child is older than 8 years of age and has more than three standard deviations from the mean of torsional deformity (medial rotation greater than 85°, lateral rotation less than 10°, or anteversion greater than 50°). Consideration can be given for correction either at the intertrochanteric level or the supracondylar region; most surgeons prefer the intertrochanteric region. In teenagers, closed intramedullary rotational osteotomy can be considered.

In a certain number of children with severe femoral antetorsion, lateral tibial torsion compensates for the deformity. Surgical treatment should be avoided because the rotational osteotomies would need to be performed in the femur and the tibia, and subsequent patellofemoral malalignment problems could ensue.

Annotated Bibliography

Physiologic Pes Planus

Grogan DP, Gasser SI, Ogden JA. The painful accessory navicular: a clinical and histopathologic study. Foot Ankle 1989; 10:164.
The authors present a review of 22 skeletally immature patients with 39 accessory navicular bones seen during a 4-year period. Twenty-five of the feet were treated surgically after failure of conservative treatment. Symptoms were relieved in all surgically treated patients. Detailed histologic studies of the excised specimens are presented. The changes were consistent with the theory that chronic chondro-osseous tensile failure could occur and that this condition is responsible for the clinical findings.

Harris RI, Beath T. Hypermobile flat-foot with short tendo-achilles. J Bone Joint Surg 1948;30A:116.
This is a classic study of flatfeet in 3,600 Canadian army recruits. The authors found that flexible flatfoot produces disability only when it occurs in combination with a contracted tendo Achilles.

Penneau K, Lutter LD, Winter RD. Pes planus: radiographic changes with foot orthoses and shoes. Foot Ankle 1982;2:299.
This article reports on a radiographic study of 10 children with flexible flatfeet. Radiographs were taken barefoot, with a Thomas heel, with an over-the-counter insert, and with two specially molded plastic foot orthoses. The study showed no difference between the barefoot radiographs and those in which an appliance was used.

Staheli LT, Chew DE, Corbett M. The longitudinal arch: a survey of eight hundred and eighty-two feet in normal children and adults. J Bone Joint Surg 1987;69A:426.
This article reports on a study of 441 normal subjects (1 to 80 years old) that was conducted to determine the configuration of the longitudinal arch. The authors found that flatfeet are usual in infants, common in children, and within the normal range of observations in adults.

Wenger DR, Mauldin D, Speck G et al. Corrective shoes and inserts as treatment for flexible flat foot in infants and children. J Bone Joint Surg 1989;71A:800.
This article reports on a randomized prospective study of 98 patients treated by various "accepted" methods for flexible flatfoot. The authors demonstrated that flexible flatfoot improved naturally over the 3 years of the study and that the degree of improvement was not affected by wearing of a corrective shoe or a shoe with an insert.

Tarsal Coalition

Clarke DM. Multiple tarsal coalitions in the same foot. J Pediatr Orthop 1997;17:777.
The author recommended that CT evaluation of both feet in transaxial and coronal planes be obtained in patients with suspected tarsal coalition. This was based on a study where 6 of 30 children with symptomatic tarsal coalition were found to have multiple coalitions in the same foot, which is a higher percentage than had previously been reported.

Emery KH, Bisset GS III, Johnson ND et al. Tarsal coalition: A blinded comparison of MRI and CT. Pediatric Radiol 1998; 28:612.
Coronal and axial CT and MRI studies were obtained for 40 feet in 20 patients with symptoms suggesting tarsal coalition. The authors concluded that CT is the gold standard and the more cost-effective imaging study for detecting tarsal coalition. MRI is also very good for detecting tarsal coalition, particularly if other causes for ankle or foot pain are being considered.

Gonzalez P, Kumar SJ. Calcaneonavicular coalition treated by resection and interposition of the extensor digitorum brevis muscle. J Bone Joint Surg 1990;72A:71.
The authors present a 2- to 20-year follow-up of 75 calcaneonavicular coalitions treated by resection and interposition of the extensor digitorum brevis muscle. Good or excellent long-term results were reported in 77% of the cases. The best results were reported in patients between 11 and 15 years of age who had a cartilaginous coalition. Talar beaking was not a contraindication to surgery.

Leonard MA. The inheritance of tarsal coalition and its relationship to spastic flat foot. J Bone Joint Surg 1974;56B:520.
The author evaluated 31 index patients with tarsal coalitions and peroneal spastic flatfoot and 90 of their first-degree relatives. Thirty-nine percent of the first-degree relatives were found to have some type of tarsal coalition, but none was ever symptomatic. The study demonstrates that tarsal coalitions are inherited probably as an autosomal dominant disorder and that tarsal coalition is probably not a rare phenomenon.

Mann RA, Beaman DN, Horton GA. Isolated subtalar arthrodesis. Foot Ankle Int 1998;19:511.
Isolated subtalar arthrodesis was performed on 44 feet with hindfoot pathology on which 10 of the feet had a talocalcaneal coalition. The average age at surgery for this subgroup was 26 years. At an average follow-up of 91 months, the AOFAS score was 93 of a possible 100 points, and 88% of the patients were satisfied or very satisfied with their results.

Mosier KM, Asher M. Tarsal coalitions and peroneal spastic flat foot: a review. J Bone Joint Surg 1984;66A:976.
The authors present a superb review of the history, origin, hereditary evidence, incidence, clinical presentations, pathomechanics, radiologic diagnosis, differential diagnosis, and treatment of tarsal coalitions. This article was published before the use of CT scanning

in diagnosis and also before several long-term reviews of treatment. The background information and bibliography on tarsal coalition are superb.

Olney BW, Asher MA. Excision of symptomatic coalition of the middle facet of the talocalcaneal joint. J Bone Joint Surg 1987;69A:539.

The authors report excision of the middle facet of the talocalcaneal joint and autogenous fat grafting in nine patients with 10 symptomatic coalitions. Eight of 10 feet had satisfactory results.

Percy EC, Mann DL. Tarsal coalition: a review of the literature and presentation of 13 cases. Foot Ankle 1988;9:40.

This article adds 13 cases to the world literature. The introductory material surveying the world literature is excellent.

Raikin S, Cooperman DR, Thompson GH. Interposition of the split flexor hallucis longus tendon after resection of a coalition of the middle facet of the talocalcaneal joint. J Bone Joint Surg 1999;81A:11.

Fourteen feet in 10 patients with painful middle facet talocalcaneal coalitions that had failed conservative management underwent resection of the coalition and interposition of a split portion of the flexor hallucis longus tendon. At a mean follow-up of 51 months (range 32 to 60 months), 12 of the feet were rated as excellent and good using the AOFAS rating system. None of the patients had symptoms of functional impairment of the great toe.

Swiontkowski MF, Scranton PE, Hansen S. Tarsal coalitions: long-term results of surgical treatment. J Pediatr Orthop 1983;3:287.

The authors reviewed 40 patients who underwent 57 operations for tarsal coalition. Poor results were correlated with inadequate resection or advanced degenerative joint disease. Talar beaking does not necessarily represent early degenerative joint disease but does represent talonavicular ligament traction spurs, which are not necessarily associated with articular degeneration but are caused by increased stress across the talonavicular joint. This beaking is not a contraindication to bar resection.

Congenital Vertical Talus

Coleman SS, Stelling FH III, Jarrett J. Pathomechanics and treatment of congenital vertical talus. Clin Orthop 1970;70:62.

The authors present a classification of congenital vertical talus, discuss the pathophysiology, and present a surgical method of management. This remains the classic article on the subject.

Kodros SA, Dias LS. Single-stage surgical correction of congenital vertical talus. J Pediatr Orthop 1999;19:42.

A single-stage surgical correction procedure was performed on 41 patients with 55 congenital vertical tali. At follow-up (average 7 years), there were 31 good and 11 fair results. The authors cautioned that underlying diagnoses are common and should be identified to minimize the risk of recurrence.

Ogata K, Shoenecker PL, Sheridan J. Congenital vertical talus and its familial occurrence: an analysis of 36 patients. Clin Orthop 1979;139:128.

The authors report the follow-up of 36 patients with 57 feet with congenital vertical talus. A high incidence of associated congenital hip dislocation, arthrogryposis, congenital hypoplasia of the tibia, and central nervous system abnormalities was noted. Half of the patients with a primary isolated form of congenital vertical talus had a positive family history of foot deformities in first-degree relatives. A method of surgical correction is presented.

Oppenheim W, Smith C, Christie W. Congenital vertical talus. Foot Ankle 1985;5:198.

The authors present a series of 15 congenital vertical tali in 12 patients. They found that the best result was obtained with early subtalar arthrodesis (Grice operation) and plantar K-wire fixations. Attempts to augment push-off power with tendon transfers were unrewarding. Casting alone revealed the worst results. Half of patients had associated abnormalities.

Calcaneal Valgus

Larsen B, Reimann I, Becker-Andersen H. Congenital calcaneovalgus. Acta Orthop Scand 1974;45:145.

In this article, 125 cases of congenital calcaneal valgus are presented. Forty-nine percent were treated with manipulation and taping; 51% were treated with observation alone. The authors demonstrate no significant difference in the outcome between the two groups. The follow-up was between 3 and 11 years, and most feet were normal. Pronation of the feet was often seen when the patients began to walk, and many had slight residual valgus compared with the other side.

Wetzenstein H. The significance of congenital pes calcaneovalgus in the origin of pes palno-valgus in childhood. Acta Orthop Scand 1960;30:64.

The authors reviewed 2,735 consecutive newborns and followed the patients for 2 years. One-hundred and forty-seven of the patients had more than 20° of heel valgus; 333 had 10 to 15°; 759 had 0 to 5°; and 1,496 had 0°. When seen at 2 years of age, 43% of the 147 patients with at least 20° of valgus had flatfeet. Twenty-three percent of the group with normal valgus had flatfeet. The authors conclude that severe calcaneo-valgus is associated with a flatfoot deformity in later life.

Wynne-Davies R. Family studies and the cause of congenital clubfoot: talipes equinovarus, talipes calcaneo-valgus, and metatarsus varus. J Bone Joint Surg 1964;46B:445.

This article deals with family history, associated abnormalities, and causes of clubfoot, metatarsus varus, and calcaneal valgus deformity. This is an excellent review article on the epidemiology and origin of these three foot conditions.

Köhler Disease

Ippolito E, Ricciardi Pollni PT, Falez' F. Köhler's disease of the tarsal navicular: long-term follow-up of 12 cases. J Pediatr Orthop 1984;4:416.

The authors report an average 33-year follow-up of 12 patients with Köhler disease of the tarsal navicular. Complete restoration of normal navicular anatomy averaged 8 months. Treatment did not affect the radiographic course of the disease. All patients reconstituted normal navicular shape, were asymptomatic, and had no evidence of degenerative joint disease.

Karp MG. Köhler's disease of the tarsal scaphoid: an end-result study. J Bone Joint Surg 1937;19:84.

The author reports 45 cases of Köhler disease of the tarsal navicular (39 boys, 6 girls). Treatment had no effect on the radiographic course of the disease. The radiographs of 50 normal children (25 boys, 25 girls) were evaluated for scaphoid development with radiographs taken every 6 months from age 9 months to 4 years. In over half the female patients, a well-developed ossific nucleus of the scaphoid was apparent at 2 years of age; it was apparent by 3.5 years of age in all the patients. More than one-third of the male patients were older than 3.5 years of age before the scaphoid appeared. The average age of appearance of the ossific nucleus for girls is 18 months to 2 years and for boys, 2.5 to 3 years of age. The author also discussed ossification patterns of the scaphoid in relation to time of appearance. The radiographic appearance is unrelated to the duration of symptoms or to treatment. Normal delayed development of the appearance of the ossific nucleus to the scaphoid may simulate a radiographic picture similar to that seen in Köhler disease.

Waugh W. The ossification and vascularization of the tarsal navicular and their relation to Köhler's disease. J Bone Joint Surg 1958;40B:765.

This article reports on an excellent study of the vascular supply to the tarsal navicular and a radiographic study of 52 normal children's feet. Radiographs were taken at 6-month intervals between the ages of 2 and 5 years to assess normal ossification patterns in the navicular. On the basis of the vascular injection studies and the clinical follow-up, the author proposes that Köhler disease of the navicular is caused by compression of the bony nucleus at a critical phase during the growth of a navicular whose appearance is delayed.

Williams GA, Cowell HR. Köhler's disease of the tarsal navicular. Clin Orthop 1981;158:53.
The authors reviewed 20 patients with Köhler disease of the tarsal navicular with an average follow-up of 9.5 years. All patients were asymptomatic and had reconstituted the navicular to the normal radiographic appearance. Short-leg casting significantly affected the morbidity in patients, reducing the symptomatic period from 15 months (untreated patients) to less than 3 months.

Freiberg Infarction

Freiberg AH. The so-called infarction of the second metatarsal bone. J Bone Joint Surg 1926;8:257.
The author, who described the origin of the condition in 1913, discusses Köhler's opinion that the cause of the condition is probably not traumatic. This is a classic paper.

Smillie IS. Freiberg's infarction (Koehler's second disease). J Bone Joint Surg 1955;39B:580.
In this review of 41 cases, female patients predominated. The author proposes a traumatic origin (i.e., stress fracture) for the disease. Treatment options at various disease stages are discussed.

Sever Disease

Liberson A, Lieberson S, Mendes DG et al. Remodeling of the calcaneus apophysis in the growing child. J Pediatr Orthop 1995;4B:74.
The authors used radiographs and CT scans to compare the heels of 36 children with symptoms of calcaneal apophysis and 52 control children. On lateral radiographs, increased density of the calcaneal apophysis was noted in all heels. One or two radiolucent lines (fragmentation) were noted in all of the painful heels but in only 27% of the heels in the control group. CT demonstrated normal increased density with growth.

Micheli LJ, Ireland ML. Prevention and management of calcaneal apophysitis in children: an overuse syndrome. J Pediatr Orthop 1987;7:34.
The authors present an excellent historical review and extensive discussion on the differential diagnosis of heel pain in the child and adolescent. The authors present a large series (85 children, 137 heels) of calcaneal apophysitis (Sever disease) treated by a physical therapy program of lower-extremity stretching, particularly the Achilles tendon, ankle dorsiflexion strengthening, and orthotics. All patients were able to return to their sport of choice 2 months after the diagnosis. The authors proposed that the cause of the condition is an overuse syndrome.

Metatarsus Adductus

Berg EE. A reappraisal of metatarsus adductus and skewfoot. J Bone Joint Surg 1986;68A:1185.
The author describes a radiographic classification in 84 patients with 124 feet with a minimal follow-up of 2 years. The study was devised to determine prospectively whether radiographic evaluation can provide better prognostic information than the usual clinical criteria. The author proposes a four-group classification based on the anteroposterior radiographs: simple metatarsus adductus, complex metatarsus adductus, simple skewfoot, and complex skewfoot. The author reports that all patients with complex skewfoot had flatfoot at follow-up and that there was a strong association with the use of Denis Browne splints and flatfoot deformity at follow-up. Ninety-seven percent of untreated feet responded favorably. The period of cast treatment for patients with complex skewfoot deformity was required twice as long as for those with simple metatarsus adductus, and all had flatfoot at follow-up. This article includes an extensive bibliography.

Bleck EE. Metatarsus adductus: classification relationship to outcomes of treatment. J Pediatr Orthop 1983;3:2.
This was a retrospective study of the results of treatment of 160 children (265 feet) classified by flexibility according to the extent of passive abduction of the forefoot against the stabilized hindfoot with reference to the heel bisector. Results of treatment were statistically significantly better when treatment was begun between the ages of 1 day and 8 months. The only significant predictor of a good outcome was the age of the patient. The recurrence rate was 12%. Severity and flexibility did not appear to affect the treatment outcome. This is an excellent review of the subject with an extensive bibliography.

Farsetti P, Weinstein SL, Ponseti IV. The long-term functional and radiographic outcomes of untreated and non-operatively treated metatarsus adductus. J Bone Joint Surg 1994;76A:257.
Thirty-one patients (45 feet) who had metatarsus adductus were evaluated and followed for an average of 32 years and 6 months. Twelve patients (16 feet) who had a passively correctable deformity (mild or moderate) at the time of the initial presentation had no treatment. Twenty patients (29 feet) who had a partly flexible or rigid deformity (moderate or severe) at the time of the initial presentation were managed with serial manipulation and application of plaster holding casts. (One patient who had a bilateral deformity had no treatment on one side and conservative management on the other). The results were good in all 16 of the untreated feet and in 26 (90%) of the 29 feet that had been conservatively treated. There were no poor results. The passively correctable deformities resolved spontaneously. Radiographs showed an obliquity of the medial cuneiform-metatarsal joint in 21 (68%) of the 31 feet that were examined clinically and radiographically. Similar findings were observed in four of 11 contralateral, normal feet. Hallux valgus was not a common outcome. No patient had operative correction.

Clubfoot

Dietz F, Cooper DM. Treatment of idiopathic clubfoot: a thirty-year follow-up note. J Bone Joint Surg 1995;77:1477.
Forty-five patients who had 71 congenital clubfeet were evaluated at an average age of 34 years (range, 25 to 42 years). With the use of pain and functional limitations as the outcome criteria, 35 (78%) of the 45 patients had an excellent or good outcome compared with 82 (85%) of 97 individuals who did not have congenital deformity of the foot. The technique of treatment led to good long-term results in patients who had clubfoot. The data suggest that a sedentary occupation and avoidance of excessive weight gain may improve the overall long-term result. Excessive weakening of the triceps surae may predispose patients to a poor result. Therefore, it is prudent to avoid overlengthening of this muscle. The outcome could not be predicted from the radiographic result.

Ippolito E, Ponseti IV. Congenital club foot of the human fetus: a histologic study. J Bone Joint Surg 1980;62A:8.
The authors present a superb review of the pathologic anatomy of clubfoot, comparing five clubfeet with three normal control feet in subjects of the same ages. The authors propose a retracting fibrosis as the primary etiologic factor of clubfoot deformity.

Ponseti, IV. Current concepts Review treatment of congenital club foot. J Bone Joint Surg 1992;74:448.
A good general review of the theory behind and the treatment procedure for the correction of clubfoot by a method used at the University of Iowa for over 40 years.

Turco VJ. Resistant congenital clubfoot:—one-stage posteromedial release with internal fixation. J Bone Joint Surg 1979;61A:805.
The author reports modifications of his original technique (most widely used technique with surgical treatment of clubfoot) and end results in 149 feet. The author reports that the best results and fewest complications occurred in patients operated on between 1 and 2 years of age.

Vanderwilde R, Staheli LT, Chew DE et al. Measurements on radiographs of the foot in normal infants and children. J Bone Joint Surg 1988;70A:407.
The authors present a radiographic review of feet of 74 normal infants and children ranging in age from 6 to 127 months. The authors present their results and compare these to results gleaned from the literature in other studies of normal feet.

Wynne-Davies R. Genetic and environmental factors in the etiology of talipes equinovarus. Clin Orthop 1972;84:9.
This review article on the epidemiologic and etiologic theories on idiopathic clubfoot should be read in conjunction with this author's article listed under Calcaneal Valgus.

Idiopathic Toe-Walking

Griffin PTP, Wheelhouse WW, Shiavi R et al. Habitual toe-walkers: clinical and electromyographic gait analysis. J Bone Joint Surg 1977;59A:97.
The authors report a clinical and electromyographic study of six children who are habitual toe-walkers compared to six otherwise normal children walking on their toes. The abnormalities noted on dynamic electromyograms reverted to normal in the habitual toe-walkers after plaster cast treatment.

Hall JE, Salter RB, Bhalla SK. Congenital short tendo-calcaneus. J Bone Joint Surg 1967;49B:695.
This is the first description in the literature of idiopathic toe-walking, which the authors term congenital short tendo-calcaneus. The authors reported on 20 patients with an average follow-up of 3 years (range, 1.5 to 7 years), all treated by Achilles tendon lengthening. All children were otherwise normal. The surgical outcome was good in every patient.

Kalen V, Adler N, Bleck EE. Electromyography of idiopathic toe-walking. J Pediatr Orthop 1986;6:31.
The authors report dynamic electromyograms in 18 patients with idiopathic toe-walking as compared with normal children walking on their toes and cerebral palsy children with equinus deformities. Significant differences in phasic time were demonstrated between cerebral palsy and idiopathic toe-walking patients versus controls,
but no significant differences were noted between idiopathic toe-walkers and the cerebral palsy patients. Because of these gait abnormalities, the authors conclude that idiopathic toe-walking may be due to an unknown nervous system deficiency.

Torsional Problems

Bleck EE. Developmental orthopaedics. III: toddlers Dev Med Child Neurol 1982;24:533.
This excellent review article covers not only torsional abnormalities but also angular deformities of the lower extremity. It includes excellent references.

Hubbard DD, Staheli LT, Chew DE et al. Medial femoral torsion in osteoarthritis. J Pediatr Orthop 1988;8:540.
The authors measured anteversion in 44 hips in 32 patients with idiopathic osteoarthritis of the hip and compared this with measurements in 98 normal adult hips. The differences in the two groups were not significant. The authors did not find medial femoral torsion associated with osteoarthritis of the hip.

Kitaoka HB, Weiner DS, Cook AJ et al. Relationship between femoral anteversion and osteoarthritis of the hip. J Pediatr Orthop 1989;9:396.
In a CT scanning study, the authors demonstrated no difference in anteversion between osteoarthritis subjects and controls with reference to anteversion. They concluded that rotational femoral osteotomies to prevent osteoarthritis are not warranted.

Staheli LT. Torsion-treatment indications. Clin Orthop 1989; 247:61.
The author briefly discusses rotational problems in infants and children and presents the indications and methods of surgical treatment in the rare cases that require operative intervention.

Staheli LT, Corbett M, Wyss C et al. Lower-extremity rotational problems in children: normal values to guide in management. J Bone Joint Surg 1985;67A:39.
The authors present the rotational profile and the normal values for progression angle, medial rotation, lateral rotation, and thigh-foot angle. This is a classic reference article for torsional deformities of the lower extremity.

21

Anand M. Vora,
Gregory P. Guyton

The Adult Ankle and Foot

HALLUX VALGUS

A large proportion of clinical complaints of the foot center on the first metatarsophalangeal (MTP) joint. This articulation alone bears one-third of the weight of the forefoot and helps stabilize the longitudinal arch through the attachment of the plantar aponeurosis into its base. Immediately after the foot hits the ground during ambulation, weight is rapidly transferred from the heel to the metatarsal head region. As a step is taken, the toes are pushed into dorsiflexion. The plantar aponeurosis, which arises from the medial tubercle of the calcaneus and inserts into the base of the proximal phalanx, is pulled over the metatarsal head. In turn, this passively depresses the metatarsal heads and raises the arch (Figure 21-1). This construct is commonly called the "windlass mechanism" after the nautical term for a device for raising a sail by pulling on a rope.

Any disorder of the first metatarsophalangeal joint has the potential to disrupt this critical mechanical function. Weight is then transferred to the lesser metatarsals, and secondary pathology in the remainder of the forefoot can develop. Because of their significant implications for the function of the foot, disorders of the hallux deserve special consideration.

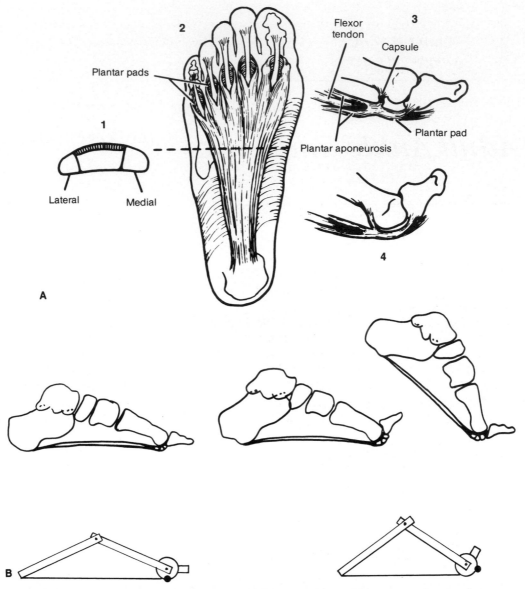

FIGURE 21-1. (A) Plantar aponeurosis. (1) Cross-section. (2) Division of plantar aponeurosis around flexor tendons. (3) Components of the plantar pad and its insertion into the base of the proximal phalanx. (4) Toe in extension with the plantar pad drawn over the metatarsal head. **(B)** The windlass mechanism functions by the passive dorsiflexion of the metatarsophalangeal joints in the last half of the stance phase, which tightens the plantar aponeurosis and mechanically causes the longitudinal arch to rise. This is probably the main stabilizer of the longitudinal arch of the foot. (A from Mann R, Inman VT. Structure and function. In: Du Vries HL. Surgery of the Foot, 2nd Ed. St Louis: CV Mosby, 1965)

The Deformity

Hallux valgus is among the most commonly encountered deformities of the forefoot. It is characterized by lateral deviation of the first toe and, usually, by medial deviation of the first metatarsal. It is commonly known as a bunion deformity after the noticeable prominence on the medial side of the foot. Patients often confuse the medial prominence of hallux valgus with the dorsal osteophyte of hallux rigidus and may refer to both disorders as "bunions."

In most cases, the development of hallux valgus can be directly related to constrictive shoe wear. The disorder was essentially undescribed until the rise of fashionable shoes in France in the 1700s. Numerous surveys of foot deformities in indigenous populations that go unshod demonstrate almost a complete absence of hallux valgus except its relatively rare congenital form. The narrow toe box and raised heel of modern women's shoe wear in particular appear to be the primary culprits in the development of the problem.

Hallux valgus involves lateral deviation of the hallux at the first MTP (Figure 21-2). The toe not only deviates, but it also rotates into pronation. The nail turns to face toward the instep. As these deformities develop, the lateral capsule and the adductor hallucis tendon on the lateral side of the first MTP joint become contracted. The medial capsule becomes attenuated. In the majority of cases, the first metatarsal itself deviates to the medial side, a deformity known as *metatarsus primus varus*. While this happens, the intermetatarsal ligament between the second metatarsal head and lateral sesamoid

remains unchanged in length. The sesamoids therefore retain their original position with regard to the rest of the foot and the first metatarsal head subluxates off of them.

Conservative Management

Once the deformity of hallux valgus is established, there is no conservative maneuver that will restore the normal anatomy. Bunion night splints, toe spacers, and orthotics have all proven unsuccessful. Nevertheless, a large number of patients find relief with simple shoe modifications. In general, shoes should be made of soft material with a minimum of seams over the medial side. The toe box should be wide and accommodative, and the heel should be minimal. If a patient has a significant transfer callus under the second metatarsal head, an orthotic with a metatarsal pad placed immediately behind the painful site may provide relief.

Preoperative Evaluation of a Bunion

Although the simple conservative measures are similar regardless of the specifics of the deformity, a number of factors must be evaluated when choosing a strategy for surgical correction. There are over 100 described operations to correct hallux valgus, and the choice of procedure is critical to a successful outcome.

The only appropriate indications for correction of a bunion deformity are pain at the first MTP joint itself or, occasionally, pain from secondary pathology in the adjacent toes caused by overload and crowding from the hallux. The complication rate in bunion surgery is significant, and there is no role for operations performed only for cosmesis or to allow a return to highly constrictive shoe wear.

As with any surgery contemplated on the foot and ankle, the neurovascular status is important. Patients without palpable dorsalis pedis and tibialis posterior pulses should be evaluated by Doppler exam and, if necessary, referred to a vascular surgeon. Hallux valgus in particular can cause irritation of the dorsomedial cutaneous nerve of the hallux, a sensory nerve on the dorsomedial aspect of the toe. Its status should be assessed carefully.

On clinical examination, the motion of the MTP should be assessed carefully. Almost all bunion procedures result in some loss of motion and the patient should be made aware of this outcome. In many cases, a significant pes planus deformity

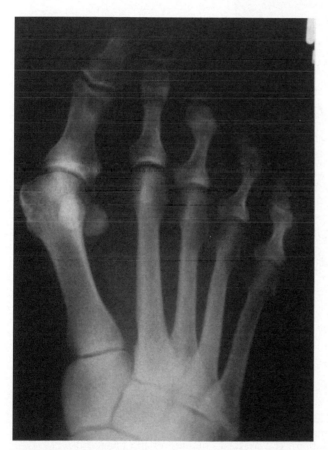

FIGURE 21-2. Radiograph of a hallux valgus deformity. Note the lateral deviation of the proximal phalanx on the metatarsal head, the medial deviation of the metatarsal head, and subluxation of the sesamoids.

would need to be corrected simultaneously with the hallux valgus and the status of the arch should be evaluated. The stability of the first metatarsocuneiform joint should be assessed by stabilizing the lateral forefoot with one hand while dorsiflexing the first ray separately with the other.

Weight-bearing radiographs of the foot are critical in the evaluation of the deformity (Figure 21-3).

The information that should be gleaned from the films includes:

- The intermetatarsal angle formed by the axes of the first and second metatarsals on the AP view.
- The hallux valgus angle formed by the axes of the first metatarsal and the proximal phalanx of the hallux.

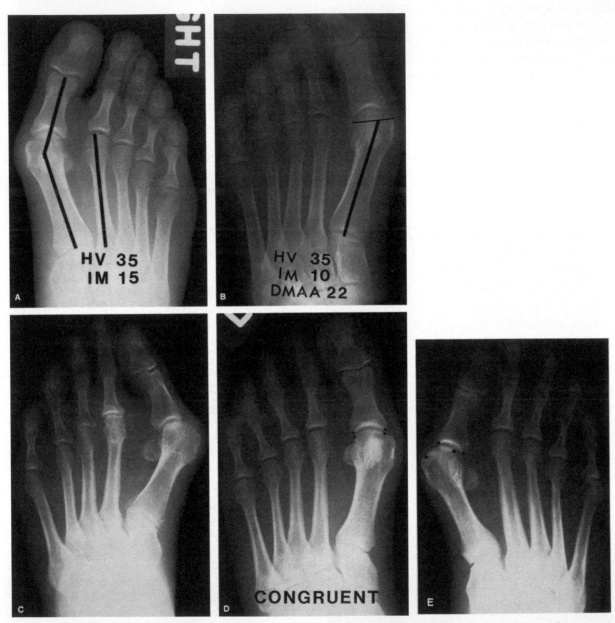

FIGURE 21-3. Radiographic observations of the hallux valgus deformity. **(A)** Hallux valgus angle: normal (less than 15°). Intermetatarsal angle: normal (less than 9°). **(B)** Distal metatarsal articular angle (DMAA): normal (less than 10° lateral deviation). **(C)** Marked obliquity of the metatarsocuneiform joint should alert clinician to possible instability of this joint. **(D)** A congruent joint is one in which there is no lateral subluxation of the proximal phalanx on the articular surface of the metatarsal head. **(E)** The incongruent or subluxated joint has lateral deviation of the proximal phalanx on the metatarsal head.

• The congruity of the joint. In other words, does the articular surface of the proximal phalanx line up with that of the metatarsal head or is it subluxated?
• The distal metatarsal articular angle formed by the alignment of the first metatarsal and the margins of the joint surface of the first MTP.
• The presence or absence of deformity in the hallux itself.
• The presence or absence of arthritis at the first MTP or in the midfoot.
• The presence or absence of instability at the first metatarsocuneiform joint.
• The relative lengths of the first and second metatarsals.

Surgical Procedures

Most cases of hallux valgus severe enough to require surgical correction will involve a widened intermetatarsal angle and an incongruent joint. The magnitude of the intermetatarsal angle is the primary factor that drives the choice of surgical procedure in these cases.

The Distal Soft Tissue Procedure (Modified McBride Procedure)

This procedure was historically used for mild hallux valgus deformities with an intermetatarsal angle of less than 13° (Figure 21-4). It involves releasing the contracted lateral structures (the lateral capsule, the adductor tendon, and the intermetatarsal ligament) and imbricating the attenuated medial capsule. As originally described by McBride, the procedure also included resection of the lateral sesamoid. This component of the procedure was abandoned due to a significant rate of late hallux varus, and the procedure is now known as the "modified" McBride procedure. Although clinically successful for mild deformities, the distal soft tissue procedure performed by itself is less commonly used than the Chevron procedure because of a tendency for some deformity recurrence. Nevertheless, it is always performed in conjunction with a proximal osteotomy or fusion for correction of more severe deformities.

The Chevron Osteotomy

The Chevron osteotomy involves a V-shaped cut in the metatarsal head that allows it to be displaced up to 5 mm laterally (Figure 21-5). The medial capsule is imbricated. Osteonecrosis of the metatarsal head has been reported after the Chevron procedure, and opinion varies as to whether it is safe to perform a concurrent lateral release. In any case, stripping of the lateral side of the metatarsal head must be minimized when performing the procedure.

The Chevron osteotomy is inherently stable and is very well tolerated by patients. Because the amount of displacement of the metatarsal head that can be achieved is limited, the procedure is restricted to correction of less severe deformities with an intermetatarsal angle of less than 13°.

Proximal Osteotomies

More severe hallux valgus deformities with intermetatarsal angles of over 13° require greater correction of the angle of the first metatarsal. This correction can only be achieved by an osteotomy at the proximal end of the bone. Numerous osteotomy techniques have been described, including the curved (crescentic) osteotomy (Figure 21-6), a short oblique (Ludloff) osteotomy, and a V-shaped (proximal Chevron) osteotomy. Long osteotomies involving the diaphysis of the bone have also been described that can essentially accomplish the same goals (the Mitchell osteotomy, the SCARF osteotomy). All have their own technical advantages and pitfalls, and most surgeons become comfortable with one technique. In all cases, the toe is also rebalanced with a distal soft tissue procedure. There is no lower limit to the degree of deformity that can be corrected with a proximal osteotomy, but the intrinsic stability of the distal Chevron makes it the procedure of choice for most deformities of lesser magnitude.

Special Cases

Not all hallux valgus deformities can be neatly categorized by the intermetatarsal angle alone. A number of unique exceptions to the usual surgical strategies must also be accounted for.

Instability of the First Metatarsocuneiform Joint

Some patients will have capsular laxity at the first metatarsocuneiform (MTC) joint that allows the metatarsal to deviate dorsally and medially. This can be detected both clinically and by the presence of subluxation and angular deformity at the first metatarsocuneiform joint on the lateral weight-bearing radiograph (Figure 21-7). The true

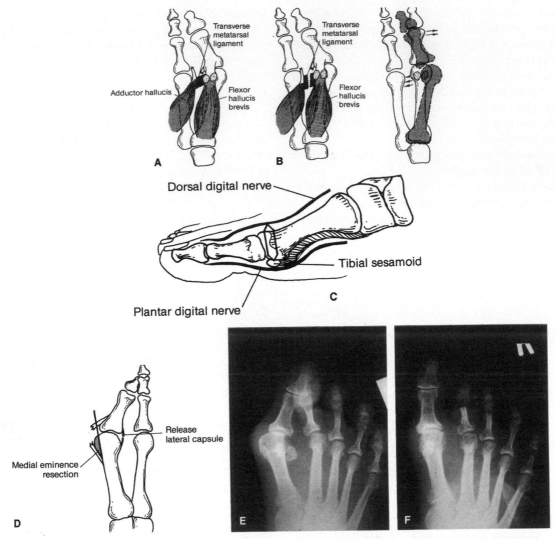

FIGURE 21-4. The distal soft tissue procedure. **(A)** The adductor tendon is released from its insertion into the base of the proximal phalanx and fibular sesamoid. **(B)** The transverse metatarsal ligament is transected and the lateral joint capsule released. **(C)** Through a longitudinal medial incision, a portion of the medial joint capsule is excised. **(D)** The medial eminence is excised in line with the medial aspect of the metatarsal shaft. **(E)** Preoperative radiograph. **(F)** Postoperative radiograph with satisfactory realignment of the metatarsophalangeal joint. (Mann RA, Coughlin MJ. The Video Textbook of Foot and Ankle Surgery. St Louis: Medical Video Productions, 1991)

incidence of this problem continues to be a subject of controversy, but it is felt to represent at least 3 to 5% of cases. If instability at the first MTC exists, the joint must be fused in order to restore the weight-bearing function of the first metatarsal head. The metatarsal is positioned during the fusion to correct the intermetatarsal angle and the toe is rebalanced with a distal soft tissue procedure. This combination of deformity correction, first MTC fusion, and distal soft tissue release is called the Lapidus procedure. The Lapidus procedure can also be used in cases in which the first metatarsocuneiform joint is arthritic.

The Juvenile Bunion

Some patients will present with a hallux valgus deformity that has been present since their adolescence. Typically the first MTP joint is congruent, and the lateral deviation of the hallux is due to the abnormal development of the joint in a deviated position. Although it can be difficult to

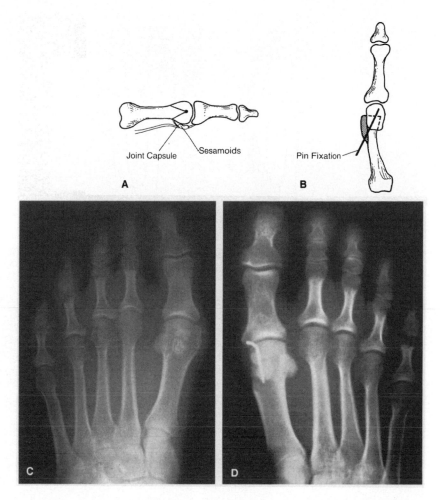

FIGURE 21-5. Chevron procedure. **(A)** The apex of the chevron osteotomy starts in the center of the metatarsal head and is brought proximally. **(B)** The osteotomy site is displaced laterally 20 to 30% of the width of the shaft. Preoperative **(C)** and postoperative **(D)** radiographs demonstrating the Chevron osteotomy. (Mann RA, Coughlin MJ. The Video Textbook of Foot and Ankle Surgery. St Louis: Medical Video Productions, 1991)

assess radiographically, the distal metatarsal articular angle (DMAA) will typically be above 10°. These bunions are not due to shoe wear but rather to a congenital deformity.

An attempt to treat these cases without addressing the deviation of the joint surface may result in creating an incongruent joint out of a congruent one, resulting in stiffness and arthritis. The angle between the joint surface and the metatarsal shaft can be corrected by means of a closing-wedge modification of the Chevron osteotomy. More severe cases require the addition of a proximal procedure as well.

Hallux Valgus Interphalangeus

Occasionally the deviation of the hallux toward the lateral side is due to a deformity at the level of the interphalangeal joint of the hallux itself rather than at the level of the MTP. The MTP joint is congruent in these situations and the phalanx is not deviated. This deformity of the toe can be corrected by a closing-wedge osteotomy of the base of the proximal phalanx, also called the Akin procedure (Figure 21-8).

The Long Second Metatarsal

When a hallux valgus deformity is long standing and the second metatarsal projects significantly more distally than the first, there is a great deal of potential for overload pathology of the second MTP joint. All the osteotomies and fusions involved in hallux valgus correction involve shortening of the first ray at least by the kerf of the saw blade. Because of this, patients who have a long second metatarsal and preoperative transfer pain may also require shortening of the second metatarsal in addition to hallux valgus correction to more fully rebalance the forefoot.

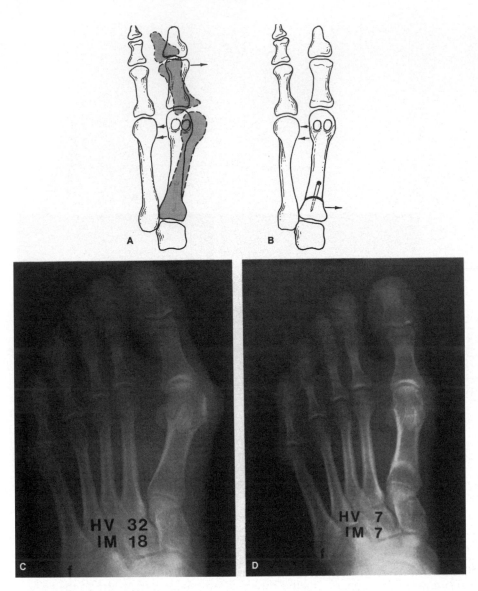

FIGURE 21-6. Distal soft tissue procedure with proximal crescentic metatarsal osteotomy. **(A)** To determine whether an osteotomy is necessary after the soft tissue release has been carried out, the first metatarsal head is pushed laterally. If there is any tendency for the metatarsal head to spring open, an osteotomy should be considered. We add an osteotomy to the distal soft tissue procedure about 85% of the time. **(B)** The osteotomy site is reduced by freeing the soft tissues about the osteotomy and displacing the proximal fragment medially while pushing the meta-tarsal head laterally. Preoperative **(C)** and postoperative **(D)** radiographs demonstrating correction of a moderate hallux valgus deformity with a distal soft tissue procedure and basal metatarsal osteotomy. (Mann RA, Coughlin MJ. The Video Textbook of Foot and Ankle Surgery. St Louis: Medical Video Productions, 1991)

HALLUX RIGIDUS

Primary degenerative arthrosis of the first metatarsophalangeal joint, frequently called *hallux rigidus,* is a common problem. These patients develop a large dorsal osteophytic ridge on the metatarsal head, which results in an impingement of the proximal phalanx to dorsiflexion, limitation of motion, and pain. As the arthritic process advances, the entire joint becomes involved. During normal gait, dorsiflexion occurs at the metatarsophalangeal joint, and if there is an obstruction to the dorsiflexion, then a significant impairment in gait may occur. This is particularly bothersome in patients who engage in athletics. The proliferative bone around the

metatarsal head can also result in significant increased bulk of the joint, which makes wearing shoes difficult.

The patient's main complaint with early stage hallux rigidus is that of pain with dorsiflexion of the metatarsophalangeal joint. This pain is aggravated by increased activities, particularly running and other athletic endeavors. The patient may also complain that, owing to the increased bulk of the joint, wearing shoes is difficult. With advanced hallux rigidus, an arthritic pain pattern of the first metatarsophalangeal joint predominates.

The physical examination frequently demonstrates an abrasion or ulceration over the osteophyte on the dorsal or dorsomedial aspect of the

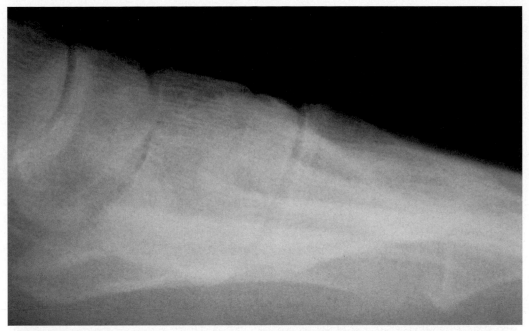

FIGURE 21-7. Subluxation of the first metatarsocuneiform joint demonstrated by plantar joint widening suggestive of joint instability.

metatarsal head. The joint itself is enlarged, there is synovial thickening, and there is significant tenderness around the joint, particularly along the lateral aspect of the metatarsophalangeal joint and over the dorsal ridge (Figure 21-9). There is usually significant restriction of dorsiflexion, and occasionally

the proximal phalanx is held in a position of slight plantar flexion if the deformity is severe. Forced dorsiflexion of the joint causes pain. In advanced presentation, motion may be severely limited. Pain and crepitus is elicited throughout the remaining arc of motion.

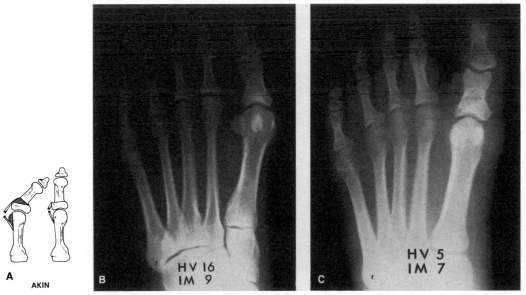

FIGURE 21-8. Akin procedure. **(A)** The medial eminence is excised, and a medially based wedge of bone is removed from the proximal phalanx. Preoperative **(B)** and postoperative **(C)** radiographs demonstrating an Akin procedure.

The radiographs of the patient with hallux rigidus are characteristic, demonstrating degenerative arthritis of the metatarsophalangeal joint on the anteroposterior (AP) view. Besides the narrowing of the joint, significant osteophyte formation is often present along the lateral aspect of the joint. Medially, there rarely is significant osteophyte formation. On the lateral view, there is a dorsal osteophyte of varying degrees. Occasionally, there is an osteophyte on the dorsal aspect of the proximal phalanx as well. In advanced stages, the entire joint space may be compromised. This continuum of disease has been staged as follows:

Grade 1 (mild): joint space is maintained; minimal bony proliferation or spurring on the dorsal aspect of the joint present

Grade 2 (moderate): advanced proliferation of dorsal spurring and more significant joint space narrowing; proximal phalanx may show dorsal spurring; reactive changes about the joint; plantar joint space is preserved

Grade 3 (severe): advanced arthritis stage with significant joint space narrowing and extensive proliferative bone formation; loss of plantar joint space

Management of patients with hallux rigidus involves activity modification, shoe adjustments ensuring adequate room for the metatarsophalangeal joint, and stiffening the shoe by inserting either an orthotic device or a piece of spring steel in the sole to decrease dorsiflexion at the metatarsophalangeal

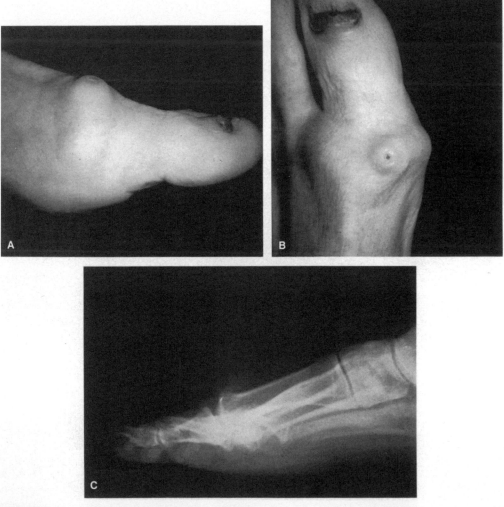

FIGURE 21-9. (**A** and **B**) First metatarsophalangeal joint in a patient with hallux rigidus. Note the increased bulk of the joint and marked osteophyte formation. (**C**) Lateral radiograph of a patient with hallux rigidus, with a large dorsal osteophyte that mechanically blocks dorsiflexion of the proximal phalanx.

joint. Occasionally, nonsteroidal anti-inflammatory medications can be beneficial.

If conservative management fails, then surgical intervention may be indicated if the neurovascular status of the foot is satisfactory. The appropriate operative procedure depends on the amount of arthrosis the patient demonstrates. For early stages of hallux rigidus (grades 1 and 2), a cheilectomy procedure can be effective. Cheilectomy involves resection of the dorsal 20 to 30% of the metatarsal head along with the osteophytes along the lateral side of the metatarsal head. The principle is to relieve the dorsal impingement of the proximal phalanx as dorsiflexion occurs, which usually relieves most of the pain. The procedure only reestablishes about half of normal dorsiflexion but this is usually sufficient to permit the patient to ambulate comfortably and resume most activities.

Arthrodesis of the metatarsophalangeal joint is an excellent procedure for patients who have severe deformity or significant arthroses (grade 3 hallux rigidus). Arthrodesis is also useful for patients who have failed a previous cheilectomy and as a salvage procedure for a failed bunion operation. The optimal positioning of the arthrodesis is 15° of valgus and 10 to 15° of dorsiflexion in relation to the plantar aspect of the foot (or 25 to 30° of dorsiflexion in relation to the first metatarsal shaft, which is inclined in a plantar direction about 20°) (Figure 21-10). After arthrodesis, the patient can be ambulated in a postoperative wooden shoe until the arthrodesis site is solid, which is usually about 10 to 12 weeks after surgery. The main complications of arthrodesis are malalignment of the arthrodesis site and nonunion, although uncommon. If sufficient valgus and dorsiflexion is not placed into the arthrodesis at the time of surgery, excessive wear on the interphalangeal joint occurs—a potential problem.

Occasionally, in an older person whose ambulatory capacity is limited, a Keller procedure can be used for advanced hallux rigidus. In this procedure, the proximal one-third of the proximal phalanx is excised along with the dorsal osteophyte. The problem with this procedure is that it detaches the intrinsic muscles from the base of the phalanx, and as a result, the toe may drift into dorsiflexion or possibly varus or valgus. It is, however, useful in the older patient with marginal circulation.

The use of a Silastic prosthesis to replace the first metatarsophalangeal joint is rarely indicated because stability of the joint is compromised, which may result in a transfer lesion to the adjacent metatarsal head. The active movement of the metatarsophalangeal joint is usually significantly impaired because of the inability to reinsert the intrinsic muscles once the prosthesis has been placed. At times, there is a reaction to the prosthetic materials and a silicon synovitis results. The life expectancy of a prosthesis is rarely more than 5 years. Therefore, it should not be used in any patient who is young and expects to place a great deal of stress on the metatarsophalangeal joint.

DISORDERS OF THE LESSER TOES

Lesser toe deformities are afflictions of the toes other than the great toe. They include mallet toe, hammertoe, and claw toe deformities. Hard and soft corns also occur on the lesser toes. The underlying cause is generally idiopathic or a combination of improper shoe wear. Subtle or overt neuropathy may be contributory. The general patterns of lesser toe deformities are described below:

> Mallet toe: characterized by a fixed flexion deformity of the distal interphalangeal joint, usually involving the second toe but possibly involving the third or fourth toes.
> Hammertoe: characterized by a flexion deformity of the proximal interphalangeal joint, which may be either fixed or flexible. The fixed deformity is one in which the proximal interphalangeal joint cannot be straightened, and a flexible deformity is one in which the proximal interphalangeal joint can be brought back into anatomic alignment.
> Claw toe: characterized by a deformity consisting of the aforementioned mallet toe or hammertoe deformities along with dorsiflexion at the metatarsophalangeal joint. This deformity may involve a single metatarsophalangeal joint or multiple metatarsophalangeal joints. The deformities can be either fixed or flexible.

Symptoms generally arise secondary to irritation from abnormal positioning. Mallet toes usually result in pain on the tip of the toe secondary to pressure from the ground or pain over the distal interphalangeal joint region secondary to pressure against the shoe. With hammertoes, pain occurs over the tip of the toe and over the proximal interphalangeal joint. The patient may develop callus formation beneath the tip of the toe or over the proximal interphalangeal joint region. Claw toes cause pain over the proximal interphalangeal joint

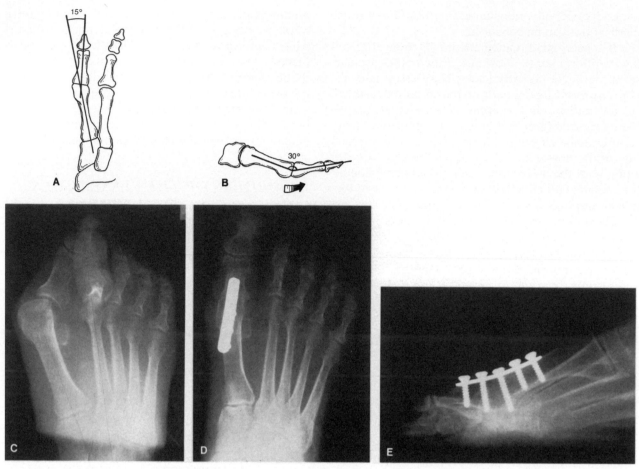

FIGURE 21-10. Arthrodesis of the metatarsophalangeal joint. Proper alignment of the arthrodesed joint is 15° of valgus **(A)** and 30° of dorsiflexion **(B)** in relation to the first metatarsal shaft, which translates to about 10 to 15° of dorsiflexion in relation to the ground. Preoperative **(C)** and postoperative **(D** and **E)** radiographs of an arthrodesis of the first metatarsophalangeal joint using plate fixation. (Mann RA, Coughlin MJ. The Video Textbook of Foot and Ankle Surgery. St Louis: Medical Video Productions, 1991)

region where the toes strike the top of the shoe. If the hyperextension deformity is severe at the metatarsophalangeal joint, progressive dorsiflexion of the proximal phalanx with depression of the metatarsal heads occurs causing plantar metatarsal head prominence. Increased load over the prominence leads to callus formation and pain.

The conservative management of lesser toe deformities consists of adequate padding, offloading with orthotic management, and shoe wear modifications with an adequate shoe box to provide sufficient space for the toes. Orthotic management may be accomplished by simple (i.e., metatarsal pads) or complex (i.e., custom orthotics with offloading bars) means with good results.

The operative treatment of lesser toe deformities can be undertaken when conservative measures fail to provide relief. The goal is to realign the toes at all involved levels to a more anatomic alignment, eliminating prominent sources of irritation. The operative treatment of a mallet toe consists of removing the distal portion of the middle phalanx, which decompresses the distal interphalangeal joint (Figure 21-11). If the deformity is extremely fixed, then a release of the flexor digitorum longus tendon may also be carried out. The operative treatment of a hammertoe consists of excising the distal portion of the proximal phalanx and then holding the toe in correct alignment for about 6 weeks, until a satisfactory fibrous union has occurred (Figure 21-12). Arthrodesis of the proximal interphalangeal joint can be attempted, although the fusion rate is low (about 50%). For this reason, usually a fibrous union is the procedure of choice. Claw toes require correction of the hammer toe or mallet toe deformity as described above as well as addressing the metatarsophalangeal joint

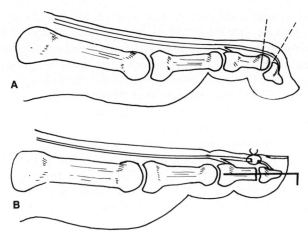

FIGURE 21-11. Mallet toe repair. **(A)** Resection of the condyles of the middle phalanx. **(B)** Intramedullary Kirschner wire fixation. (Mann RA, Coughlin MJ. The Video Textbook of Foot and Ankle Surgery. St Louis Medical Video Productions, 1991)

deformity (Figure 21-13). If the patient has a fixed deformity, then release of the contracted structures on the dorsal aspect of the metatarsophalangeal joint, which consists of both extensor tendons, the joint capsule, and the collateral ligaments, is undertaken to straighten the contracture at the metatarsophalangeal joint. A Girdlestone flexor tendon transfer, in which the flexor digitorum longus tendon is transposed to the dorsal aspect of the proximal phalanx, is carried out to provide increased plantar flexion pull

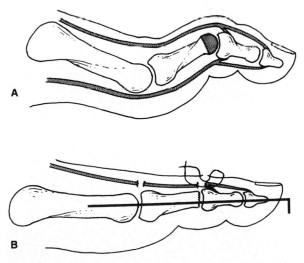

FIGURE 21-12. Fixed hammertoe repair. **(A)** Resection of the condyles of the proximal phalanx. **(B)** Intramedullary Kirschner wire fixation. (Mann RA, Coughlin MJ. The Video Textbook of Foot and Ankle Surgery. St Louis: Medical Video Productions, 1991)

CLAW TOE

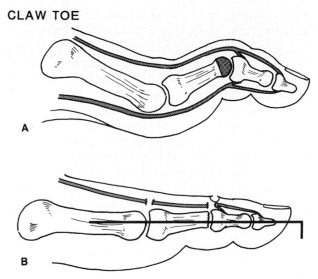

FIGURE 21-13. Fixed claw toe repair. **(A)** Excision of the condyles of the proximal phalanx, metatarsophalangeal joint capsular release, and extensor tenotomy. **(B)** Intramedullary Kirschner wire fixation stabilizes the toe. (Mann RA, Coughlin MJ. The Video Textbook of Foot and Ankle Surgery. St Louis: Medical Video Productions, 1991)

at the metatarsophalangeal joint region. In these cases, pin fixation is often used to maintain satisfactory alignment of the corrected hammertoe and metatarsophalangeal joint until the soft tissues have had a chance to heal. If the deformity is a dynamic one and does not involve any fixed deformity, then a Girdlestone flexor tendon transfer alone may produce a satisfactory clinical result.

DISORDERS OF THE LESSER METATARSOPHALANGEAL JOINTS

Metatarsalgia is a generalized term for pain beneath the metatarsal head region. During normal walking, maximal pressure is applied to the metatarsal region for 50 to 60% of the stance time. As a result, any type of abnormality in this area may cause the patient significant disability. Most commonly, metatarsalgia is secondary to a problem at the metatarsophalangeal joint level. This may be a primary bony problem, joint problem, or less commonly other causative dysfunction may exist. Dysfunction of the metatarsophalangeal joint may be secondary to synovitis associated with inflammatory arthropathy, nonspecific synovitis, plantar plate degeneration, Freiberg infarction, or dysfunction secondary to subluxation or dislocation of the metatarsophalangeal joint. In many patients, metatarsalgia can be treated conservatively by obtaining a shoe of adequate size and then adequately padding the metatarsal area to relieve the areas of maximal pain. At times, however, this conservative management fails, and operative intervention is indicated.

Nonspecific synovitis is a condition in which the patient develops synovial proliferation around the second metatarsophalangeal joint. This usually starts spontaneously, and patients often feel as if they are walking on a painful lump on the bottom of the foot. The physical examination demonstrates generalized synovial thickening around the metatarsophalangeal joint. This is sometimes associated with a hammertoe. This condition often responds to conservative management consisting of adequate shoes and padding and nonsteroidal anti-inflammatory medications. Occasionally, injection of corticosteroid into the joint relieves the condition. If the condition persists, synovectomy of the metatarsophalangeal joint should be considered. At times, this condition results in a patient developing a subluxation of the metatarsophalangeal joint frequently associated with a fixed hammertoe deformity. If symptomatic, this deformity additionally requires correction as discussed previously.

Degeneration of the plantar plate occurs occasionally and is due to cystic changes in the dense plantar plate, which helps to stabilize the metatarsophalangeal joint. It is associated with pain beneath the metatarsal head and often a progressive cocking-up of the metatarsophalangeal joint may develop. Usually, patients do not develop the generalized synovial reaction noted in patients with nonspecific synovitis. The problem can usually be handled conservatively, although occasionally arthroplasty of the metatarsophalangeal joint is indicated.

Subluxations and dislocations of the metatarsophalangeal joint are due to multiple causes, including degeneration of the plantar plate, which permits the extensor tendons to pull the proximal phalanx up into dorsiflexion; chronic pressure of the great toe against the second toe, which may result in a dislocated second metatarsophalangeal joint; nonspecific synovitis; or an undetermined cause. When a severe subluxation or dislocation occurs, the proximal phalanx pushes the metatarsal head into a plantar position (Figure 21-14). As a result, pain and often a large callus develop beneath the metatarsal head. The patient often complains of pain over the dorsal aspect of the toe as well because this strikes the top of the shoe. Under these circumstances, conservative management consists

of a shoe with an adequate toe box to alleviate the pressure on the toe and metatarsal head along with adequate padding to relieve the pressure beneath the metatarsal head. If conservative measures fail, then an operative procedure to reduce the metatarsophalangeal joint may be indicated. These procedures are often successful in alleviating this condition.

Freiberg infarction is an avascular necrosis of unknown origin that occurs in the metatarsal head. This infarction results in collapse of the metatarsophalangeal joint (Figure 21-15). This process is often associated with generalized discomfort around the joint, and the joint may develop a significant synovial reaction or enlargement due to collapse of the bony structures. This condition can often be managed conservatively with adequate shoes and padding, although nonsteroidal anti-inflammatory medications are useful during the acute phases. If the problem significantly limits the patient, arthroplasty may be indicated to remove some of the proliferative bone about the joint.

In inflammatory arthropathy, such as rheumatoid arthritis, psoriatic arthritis, or gout, proliferative synovial tissue develops around the metatarsophalangeal

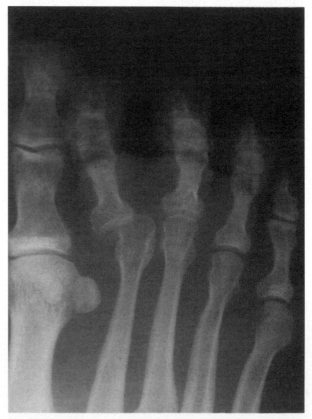

FIGURE 21-14. Subluxation of the second metatarsophalangeal joint in a dorsomedial direction.

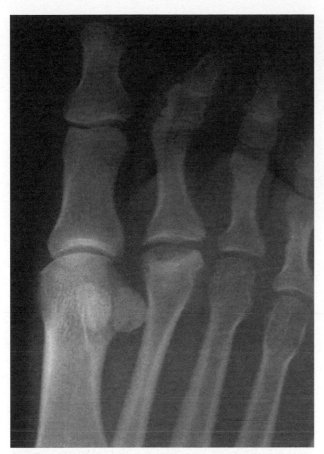

FIGURE 21-15. Radiograph of Freiberg infraction involving the second metatarsal head. This is an avascular necrosis of undetermined cause producing collapse of the metatarsal head.

picture, and over time, the deformities may progress to subluxations and dislocations. This process, particularly in the rheumatoid forefoot, can be helped if synovectomies of the metatarsophalangeal joints are performed before significant capsular destruction has occurred. For advanced rheumatoid forefoot deformity, arthrodesis of the first metatarsophalangeal joint to deformity and lesser metatarsophalangeal joints' decompression by surgical resection of the metatarsal heads is the procedure of choice (Figure 21-17). This procedure allows the fat pad to be drawn back down onto the plantar aspect of the foot and creates a soft cushion for the foot that relieves the metatarsalgia. The lesser toe deformities are corrected by manual osteoclasis and pinning, which corrects the fixed deformities. After this procedure, patients often have increased ambulatory capacity and can wear store-bought shoes.

Pain over the plantar metatarsal head may be due to a prominent fibular condyle, a long metatarsal (Figure 21-18), a so-called Morton foot in which the first metatarsal is short, a hypermobile first ray in which the first metatarsocuneiform joint is of insufficient stability to provide adequate weight bearing, or after trauma in which a metatarsal may be pushed into a plantar or dorsal angulation. Occasionally, after metatarsal surgery to alleviate pressure on one metatarsal, a condition known as a *transfer lesion* may occur. This results in pressure beneath the adjacent metatarsal head due to lack of weight bearing on the previously operated metatarsal. In most of these

joint, which results in an enlargement of the joint as well as a significant inflammatory response by the body. Under these circumstances, placing pressure on the metatarsal head region causes the patient significant discomfort and may make walking extremely difficult. Gout is usually localized to the first metatarsophalangeal joint, whereas rheumatoid and psoriatic arthritis involve multiple metatarsophalangeal joints.

Conservative management of this problem involves placing the patient into an adequate shoe, often extra-depth shoe that has a large toe box with enough room for the patient's forefoot deformities and for an orthotic device to help relieve the stress on the metatarsal heads (Figure 21-16). Gout can often be handled therapeutically, although in some cases with large tophaceous deposits, alteration in shoe wear is necessary.

If the conservative management fails, then a forefoot reconstructive procedure should be considered. The early joint changes begin with a synovitis-type

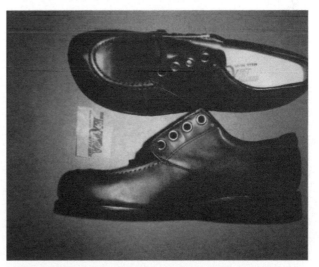

FIGURE 21-16. An extra-depth shoe provides extra room in the toe box as well as extra width to accommodate a deformed foot.

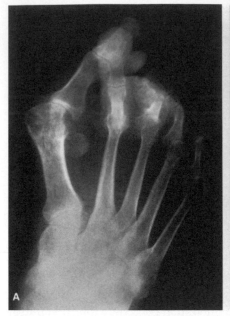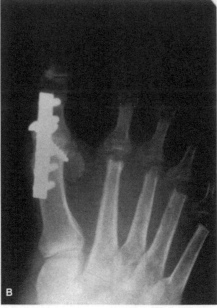

FIGURE 21-17. A rheumatoid foot. (A) Preoperative radiograph of typical rheumatoid changes with a severe hallux valgus deformity and subluxation and dislocation of the lesser metatarsophalangeal joints. (B) Reconstruction using an arthrodesis of the first metatarsophalangeal joint and arthroplasties of the lesser metatarsophalangeal joints.

cases, a callus develops beneath the prominent metatarsal head, which is usually the source of the patient's pain. Conservative treatment involves modifications to provide adequate padding around the area to alleviate the pressure on the involved metatarsal head. If this fails, then a surgical procedure may be indicated either to relieve the prominence or to elevate or shorten the metatarsal and correct any associated joint deformity. One such procedure is the Weil osteotomy, which involves an extra-articular osteotomy of the distal metatarsal allowing decompression and shortening, relieving plantar prominence and joint subluxation.

SOFT TISSUE DISORDERS OF THE FOREFOOT

Forefoot pain due to dermatologic problems can often be a significant cause of discomfort for the patient. The most frequently encountered problems include hard or soft corns, plantar warts, seed corns, or hyperkeratotic skin. A wart is a vascular lesion secondary to a virus and can be differentiated from keratotic skin by carefully trimming the area and observing small punctate bleeders secondary to the fine end arteries, which are present in a wart and not in a keratotic lesion. Treatment includes

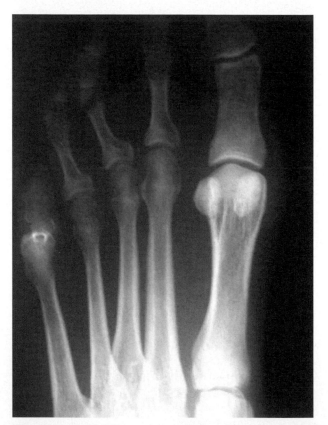

FIGURE 21-18. The presence of a long second metatarsal in the forefoot metatarsal cascade results in excessive pressure beneath metatarsal head, which may predispose to "metatarsalgia" pain.

dermal burning with liquid nitrogen; by using Cantharone, which after multiple applications usually relieves the wart; or occasionally by curettage. Burning the bottom of the foot with electrocautery or surgically excising the wart are not recommended unless other options fail, because they result in a scar on the plantar aspect of the foot, which may become symptomatic.

A seed corn is a small invagination of skin that results in a small keratotic lesion, which at times can be painful. These usually can be managed by trimming the lesion; or if this fails, curettage may alleviate it. Hyperkeratotic skin is observed in some patients and is probably due to a biochemical abnormality that is poorly understood. In these patients, surgical intervention is not indicated; rather, frequent trimming of the hyperkeratotic skin usually is adequate treatment and often can be taught to the patient.

A corn is a keratotic lesion that develops on the skin in response to pressure against the skin by an external force (a shoe). As a general rule, a small bony prominence, termed an *exostosis,* lies beneath the skin, and the shoe covering the foot chafes against this area. Corns are divided into hard and soft corns, depending on their location. A hard corn occurs between the skin and the shoe, whereas a soft corn occurs between one toe and an adjacent toe. In both cases, however, the cause is due to an underlying exostosis. The patient's main complaint is that of buildup of hypertrophic skin over the exostosis. In time, this may become rather large and painful. The conservative management is to trim the lesion and place a soft support around it to alleviate the pressure on the involved area. Usually, a broader, softer shoe helps to accommodate this problem. If conservative management fails, then a surgical procedure may be undertaken that removes the offending prominence.

Other soft tissue problems resulting in forefoot pain include atrophy of the plantar fat pad, synovial cyst arising from the metatarsophalangeal joint, soft tissue tumors such as a lipoma, permanent changes secondary to a crush injury, or a plantar scar secondary to trauma. Atrophy of the plantar fat pad occurs most frequently in older people and can present a significant problem for the patient. Because of loss of adequate padding beneath the metatarsal heads, some callus formation often results, and the metatarsal heads are sensitive to weight bearing. Unfortunately, there is no way to remedy this situation other than to place the patient in a soft-soled shoe with adequate support in the metatarsal area to alleviate the discomfort.

A soft tissue tumor such as a lipoma can also produce metatarsalgia due to its physical prominence. If this fails to respond to conservative management, such as adequate padding and shoe wear, surgical excision may be carried out.

PES PLANUS (FLATFOOT)

Flatfoot is a global term with multiple potential origins. The presence of pes planus itself is not necessarily pathologic. Rather, it is a sign that the underlying cause of the foot deformity should be explored in order to guide treatment. An attempt should be made to differentiate between a congenital versus acquired condition, after which specific diagnoses within each category may be considered. Asymptomatic flexible flatfoot is extremely prevalent, generally requires no treatment, and can be considered a normal variant of foot architecture.

Physical examination demonstrates a diminished longitudinal arch and assessment of alignment reveals excessive hindfoot valgus and forefoot abduction. From behind, the excessive forefoot abduction is demonstrated as the "too many toes" sign, in which an excess of the toes are visualized because of the marked abduction of the forefoot (Figure 21-19). Patients should be thoroughly accessed for motion limitations, particularly of the subtalar joint, which may suggest an underlying coalition. Posterior tibial tendon strength and function should be accessed. When testing the posterior tibial tendon, the foot should begin in a plantarflexed and everted position. The patient should then be asked to invert the foot against the examiner's resistance from this position, eliminating the inversion power of the anterior tibial tendon, which may mask posterior tibial tendon weakness. The ability to perform multiple single heel-rises with initiation of heel inversion confirms intact posterior tibial tendon function (Figure 21-20).

The weight-bearing radiographic findings in the evaluation of a patient with pes planus are present irrespective of the underlying cause. On the lateral radiograph, a line drawn through the long axis of the talus should nearly bisect the navicular and first metatarsal shaft (Figure 21-21). *Mild flatfoot* is indicated by a sag in this line of up to 15°; a sag from 15 to 40° indicates *moderate flatfoot;* and a sag greater than 40° indicates *severe flatfoot.* In the AP radiograph, a line drawn through the long axis of the talus and calcaneus should measure about 15°. An increase in this angle indicates varying degrees of

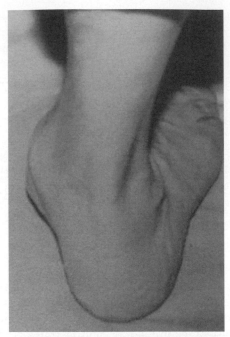

FIGURE 21-19. Clinical examination finding of "too many toes" sign consistent with excessive hindfoot valgus and forefoot abduction resultant from posterior tibial tendon dysfunction.

flatfoot. Observation of the talonavicular joint demonstrates lateral subluxation of the navicular off the head of the talus (Figure 21-21). Associated radiographic findings may suggest the specific underlying cause of the deformity (i.e., midfoot arthrosis, tarsal coalition).

The most common causes of congenital pes planus include asymptomatic flexible pes planus, tarsal coalition (peroneal spastic flatfoot), and residual congenital deformity (i.e., residual clubfoot). Asymptomatic flexible pes planus is a variation of normal foot architecture. This diagnosis generally requires no treatment beyond simple reassurance. Conservative treatment for symptomatic patients involves fitting the foot with a firm shoe that has an extended medial counter to help support the talonavicular joint, a medial heel wedge to help tilt the heel into a neutral position, or a well-molded, semiflexible arch support to further support the longitudinal arch. These treatment modalities suffice in most patients with symptomatic hypermobile flatfoot of congenital origin. If surgery becomes necessary, it is usually in the form of extra-articular osteotomies meant to improve hindfoot alignment (i.e., lateral column lengthening procedures). Rarely, stabilization of the foot with arthrodesis of the joints of the hindfoot may be necessary. The surgeon must always be cautious, however, when carrying out a stabilization procedure of the hindfoot because an excessively flexible foot is being replaced with a rigid foot, and this does not always ensure that the patient will become asymptomatic. In contrast to hypermobile congenital flatfoot, patients with tarsal coalition as a cause of congenital pes planus demonstrate a limitation of tibiotalar, subtalar, or transverse tarsal joint range of motion. This is a condition created by a failure of segmentation of

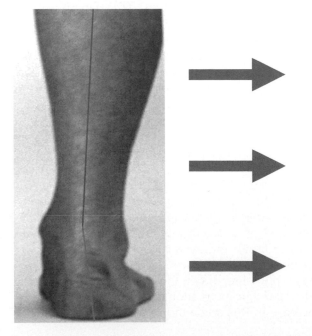

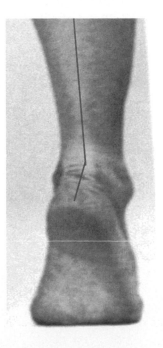

FIGURE 21-20. Clinical examination demonstrating heel inversion with a single heel-rise consistent with intact posterior tibial tendon function.

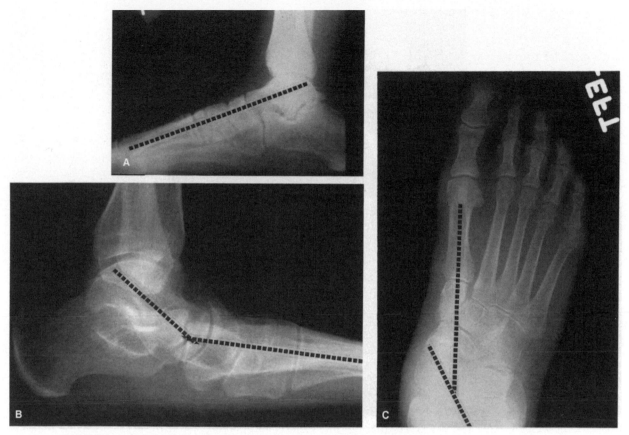

FIGURE 21-21. Radiographs of the flatfoot deformity. **(A)** Normal lateral radiograph demonstrating the relation between the long axis of the talus and first metatarsal. **(B)** In the flatfoot deformity, there is a sagging of the talonavicular joint. **(C)** In the AP view, there should be a straight line relation between the long axis of the talus and first metatarsal. In flatfoot, this line is disrupted, and there is medial deviation of the head of the talus.

the tarsal bones in early development (Figure 21-22). Most often, the talocalcaneal and calcaneonavicular joints are affected. Incidence is reported to be less then 1%, and bilateral coalitions may be present in approximately 50% of those affected. Afflicted individuals notice the condition in adolescence, as the coalition may mature from a cartilaginous to a bony interface and cause symptomatic mechanical irritation. Pain along the peroneal muscles may be present and this is thought to be due to the patient's attempt to compensate and correct the overall hindfoot alignment. It is this latter symptom that lends an alternative name to tarsal coalition: peroneal spastic flatfoot. The acute treatment of a symptomatic coalition is based on relieving the stress at the site of the coalition, generally best performed with immobilization. Patients who have recurrent symptoms despite conservative care may require surgical resection or fusion of the involved areas of the coalition.

The most common causes of acquired pes planus include posterior tibial tendon dysfunction (PTTD) and midfoot arthrosis. These patients can be differentiated from those with congenital flatfoot by history. Patients with acquired flatfoot had at one time a normal architecture of the foot and have since suffered progressive collapse to flatfoot deformity. PTTD is the most common cause of adult acquired flatfoot deformity. The process is initiated by tenosynovitis with progressive inflammation that subsequently causes enlargement and fraying of the tendon, which may progress to frank rupture. As the tendon weakens, the hindfoot demonstrates valgus malalignment secondary to medial column structural laxity. In addition, forefoot abduction occurs.

Four stages of PTTD exist: Stage 1 PTTD demonstrates mild pain along the tendon. The patient retains strength as demonstrated by a preserved ability to perform a single heel-rise. This is the tenosynovitis or tendonitis stage and the patient

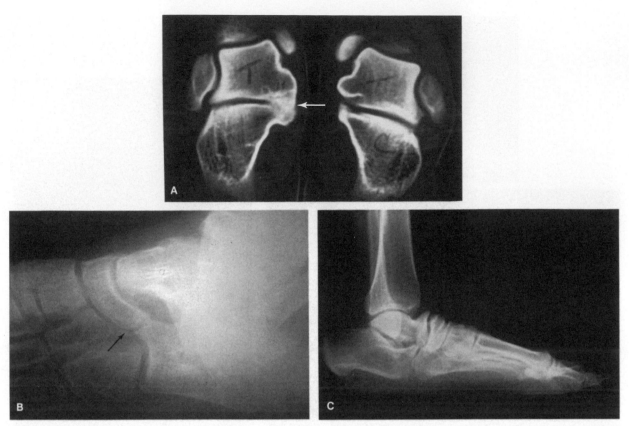

FIGURE 21-22. Tarsal coalitions. **(A)** Talocalcaneal middle facet coalition (*arrow*). **(B)** Calcaneonavicular coalition. **(C)** Changes secondary to a tarsal coalition consist of beaking and irregularity of the talonavicular joint, abnormal appearance of the subtalar joint, and lack of dorsiflexion pitch to the calcaneus.

can generally be managed nonoperatively with a period of immobilization. In no instance should the tendon be injected with corticosteroid, for a number of studies suggest an increased risk of tendon rupture (as high as 25%) with steroid administration. If symptoms persist, a tenosynovectomy of the posterior tibial tendon sheath should be performed to prevent progression of disease. Stage 2 PTTD is characterized by pain along the tendon, inability to perform a single heel-rise or initiate inversion of the heel on heel rise, and postural foot changes (excessive hindfoot valgus or forefoot abduction). The foot does, however, remain supple and motion is retained. This is the "flexible" stage, and the tendon is generally no longer functional. Nonoperative treatment can produce acceptable results with aggressive orthotic management and potentially the long-term use of a solid plastic ankle-foot orthosis, particularly in elderly patients. Many patients, however, improve only with surgical intervention. The most common surgical procedures include posterior tibial tendon debridement, tendon transfer (i.e., flexor digitorum longus [FDL] transfer), and

extra-articular osteotomy procedures to correct bony malalignment (i.e., medial calcaneal slide, lateral column lengthening procedures). Stage 3 PTTD is defined by fixed postural abnormalities secondary to severe chronic malalignment and joint involvement. This is the "rigid" stage and cannot be managed effectively surgically with extra-articular alignment correction or soft tissue procedures alone. If the patient fails nonoperative management, hindfoot arthrodesis is required (selective or triple arthrodesis procedures) to correct the foot to a plantigrade position. Stage 4 PTTD includes the rigid hindfoot changes and additionally involves the tibiotalar joint. If orthotic treatment is ineffective, pantalar fusion (ankle arthrodesis and triple arthrodesis) is required.

Posttraumatic deformity of the hindfoot or midfoot can cause a symptomatic acquired flatfoot deformity. Individuals sustaining a calcaneus or talus fracture may develop hindfoot valgus and collapse of the transverse tarsal joints leading to a flatfoot posture. Primary or posttraumatic midfoot arthrosis may lead to a collapse of the arch and pain (Figure 21-23).

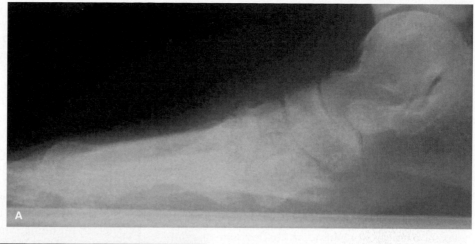

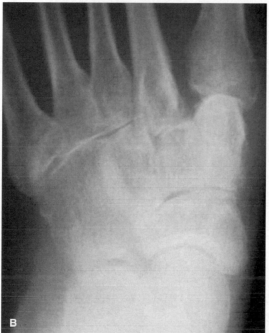

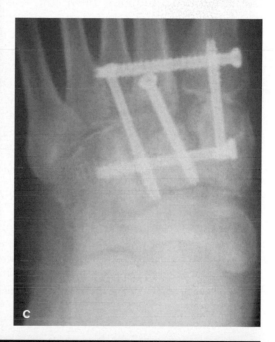

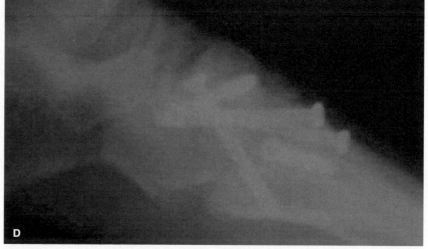

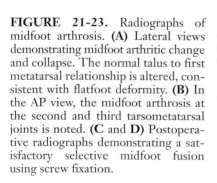

FIGURE 21-23. Radiographs of midfoot arthrosis. **(A)** Lateral views demonstrating midfoot arthritic change and collapse. The normal talus to first metatarsal relationship is altered, consistent with flatfoot deformity. **(B)** In the AP view, the midfoot arthrosis at the second and third tarsometatarsal joints is noted. **(C and D)** Postoperative radiographs demonstrating a satisfactory selective midfoot fusion using screw fixation.

These deformities may be the direct result of the fracture and residual deformity, or it may be secondary to collapse following the development of arthrosis. The treatment for this complication must be individualized given the flexibility and severity of the deformity. Simple arch supports, University of California Berkeley Laboratories (UCBL) inserts, or an ankle-foot orthosis may be sufficient. Surgical stabilization generally involves arthrodesis with interposition of bone graft to lengthen collapsed joints and restore overall foot alignment.

PES CAVUS

A cavus, or high-arched, foot is the opposite of a flat-foot deformity. The foot is often stiff, and the elevated arch does not normalize with weight bearing. The deformity itself may have primarily a hindfoot basis, a forefoot basis, or a combination of both. There should be high index of suspicion for an underlying neuromuscular disorder, although the most common cause is idiopathic. Any new onset presentation should be considered evidence of a possible spinal cord lesion until proven otherwise. The neuromuscular origins associated with a cavus foot include Charcot-Marie-Tooth and polio. Congenital causes (i.e., clubfoot residual) and posttraumatic causes (i.e., compartment syndrome sequelae) may also cause the deformity.

Patients present with pain due to the abnormal distribution of weight and decreased surface area present for weight bearing. The rigid deformity compounds the problem as the foot is unable to absorb the weight-bearing impact. As progressive deformity develops, patients may experience pain on the lateral aspect of the foot, over the fifth metatarsal head, and with severe hindfoot varus secondary ankle instability complaints.

On physical examination, the patient with a cavus deformity demonstrates a high arch while standing, which is associated with a varus deformity of the heel, adduction of the forefoot, and often clawing of the toes. The foot frequently is rigid with restricted motion in all the joints, fixed dorsiflexion contracture of the metatarsophalangeal joints, and fixed hammering of the proximal interphalangeal joints. Muscle testing is essential to determine the cause of the deformity, as most cases are due to hindfoot or forefoot muscle imbalances. This testing allows for localization of deformity and for accurate surgical planning if tendon transfer procedures are being considered. The degree of rigidity of the hindfoot varus can be assessed with the Coleman block test. The heel is placed on a block of wood and the forefoot is allowed to contact the ground, leaving the hindfoot unrestricted. If the hindfoot varus corrects to neutral, the deformity is considered flexible. In a rigid deformity, the hindfoot varus will not correct.

Weight-bearing radiographs of the foot should be obtained to determine the source of the deformity. Primary hindfoot cavus will demonstrate an elevated calcaneal pitch angle with an increased pitch of the calcaneus in relation to the floor of greater than 30°, a normal talometatarsal angle, an elevated longitudinal arch, and forefoot supination (Figure 21-24). Forefoot cavus will demonstrate a normal calcaneal pitch angle, an elevated arch, loss of alignment of the talometatarsal angle, and increased forefoot plantar flexion.

The nonoperative treatment of the cavus foot is usually to provide an accommodative shoe with adequate support and cushioning to help absorb some of the impact of ground contact. If a neurologic disorder

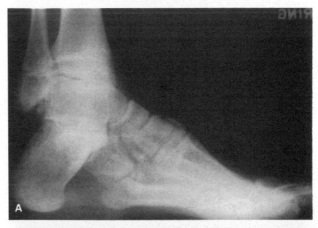

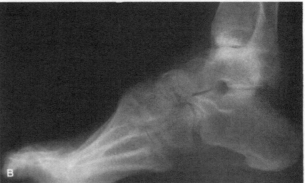

FIGURE 21-24. Radiographs of the cavus foot. **(A)** Marked dorsiflexion pitch of the calcaneus. Normal calcaneal pitch is 20 to 40°. **(B)** Forefoot equinus resulting in a cavus foot. Note the almost normal-appearing pitch to the calcaneus. (Mann RA, Coughlin MJ. The Video Textbook of Foot and Ankle Surgery. St Louis: Medical Video Productions, 1991)

exists, a polypropylene ankle-foot orthosis (AFO) may be necessary to provide stability. Surgical treatment of the cavus foot depends on the precise cause of the problem. The main goals of surgery are to produce a plantigrade foot and, if possible, to lower the longitudinal arch. The type of surgical procedure indicated depends on the specific bony abnormality present and the location of the maximal deformity. Correction should be performed with extra-articular osteotomies with or without tendon transfers at the sites of involvement (i.e., Dwyer calcaneal osteotomy, first metatarsal osteotomy, and plantar fascia release) (Figure 21-25). For patients with severe deformity or with progressive neurologic disease, arthrodesis procedures may be optimal. The goal of all of the surgical procedures is a plantigrade foot, which is stable for weight-bearing.

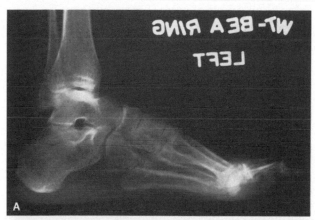
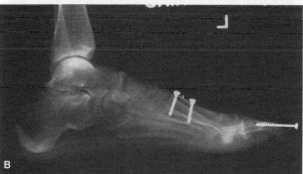

FIGURE 21-25. Operative correction of a cavus foot. **(A)** Preoperative deformity demonstrating the increased dorsiflexion pitch of the calcaneus and mild equinus of the forefoot. **(B)** Postoperative radiograph after a calcaneal osteotomy permitting dorsiflexion of the proximal fragment, dorsiflexion osteotomy of the first metatarsal, release of the plantar fascia, and fusion of the interphalangeal joint of the great toe. The longitudinal arch has been lengthened as a result of this procedure. (Mann RA, Coughlin MJ. The Video Textbook of Foot and Ankle Surgery. St Louis: Medical Video Productions, 1991)

ARTHROSIS OF THE FOOT AND ANKLE

Arthrosis of the foot and ankle may be primary or secondary. Although primary arthrosis of the ankle and subtalar joint is uncommon, it does occur in the talonavicular, tarsometatarsal, and first metatarsophalangeal joints. Why some joints are affected by primary arthroses and others are usually affected after trauma remains an enigma. Because the foot and ankle are weight-bearing structures, joint afflictions may severely limit a person's ability to remain functional. As a general rule, the diagnosis of arthrosis is not difficult to make, and in most cases conservative management can benefit the patient. If conservative management fails, then stabilization of the involved joint may be considered.

Ankle Joint

The ankle joint is rarely afflicted with primary arthrosis, but after an ankle fracture or other various traumas to the ankle joint, degenerative arthritis can occur. The patient complains of pain that is well localized to the ankle joint, and this pain can often lead to a significant degree of disability. After a fracture of the ankle joint, a varus or valgus deformity may result in improper placement of the foot on the ground. The management of the patient with osteoarthritis of the ankle joint is often helped by use of a polypropylene AFO that maintains the ankle joint in a fixed position, relieving the stress across the joint (see Figure 21-26). A rocker-bottom shoe sole permits the patient to roll over the foot, thereby relieving the stress on the ankle joint. If the pain and disability persist, surgical intervention should be considered.

Arthrodesis of the ankle joint remains the gold standard for the treatment of end-stage ankle arthritis. The ankle should be put into neutral position in terms of extension and flexion and into about 5° of valgus (Figure 21-27). The rotation of the foot in relation to the knee joint should be the same as on the uninvolved side. After a successful ankle arthrodesis, patients still maintain some dorsiflexion and plantar flexion motion of the foot, which is mediated through the talonavicular and subtalar joints. Arthrodesis usually results in restoration of function, although most patients cannot participate in running or jumping activities.

Historically, ankle arthroplasty has been a procedure that has not yielded excellent results. Recent

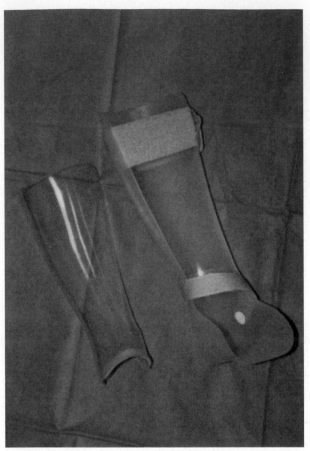

FIGURE 21-26. An ankle-foot orthosis may be used with and without an anterior shell to help contain the foot and ankle.

improvement in design and technique have combined with the significant long-term complications with ankle arthrodesis procedures and have renewed the interest in total ankle arthroplasty. Recent reports of modern implants have demonstrated improved results. The indications for ankle arthroplasty are evolving; the ideal candidate may be an elderly, low demand patient with bilateral disease. Previous infection or neuropathic joint changes are absolute contraindications to this procedure. Obesity, significant articular malalignment, muscle paralysis, instability, severe bone loss, and high demand patients are relative contraindications. The advantage of ankle joint replacement includes preservation of ankle motion, diminishing the risk of adjacent joint arthrosis development as occurs subsequent to ankle arthrodesis and improving functional outcome. The significant risks of soft tissue problems and difficulties with subsequent reconstruction after failure of the implant must be considered before undergoing this procedure.

Hindfoot Joints

Degenerative change of the hindfoot joints (subtalar, talonavicular, and calcaneocuboid joints) can occur as a result of primary osteoarthritis, however, more commonly occur secondary to previous trauma. The subtalar joint, for example, rarely develops primary osteoarthritis but frequently develops posttraumatic arthrosis after an intra-articular calcaneal fracture. These changes result in loss of motion of the subtalar joint and sometimes in a lateral impingement against the fibula. Likewise, the transverse tarsal joints (talonavicular and calcaneocuboid joints) may develop primary arthrosis, or arthrosis may follow trauma to this area. Significant deformity of the talonavicular joint may occur, and the head of the talus tends to drop in a plantar and medial direction. This results in a secondary deformity of the foot in which the calcaneus drifts into valgus and the forefoot into abduction, causing an acquired flatfoot deformity.

Conservative treatment of hindfoot arthrosis includes use of a polypropylene AFO, but in this case, the trim line of the brace can be made to permit 50% ankle joint motion, which gives the patient a smoother gait while providing support to the hindfoot complex. If conservative measures fail, then arthrodesis of the hindfoot joints may be considered. Selective arthrodesis of the talonavicular, calcaneocuboid, or subtalar joints may be effective depending on the clinical circumstances. The hindfoot joints do, however, function as a unit and thus significant compromise of motion may occur even with limited arthrodesis. Selective fusion of the talonavicular joint decreases motion 85%, the subtalar joint 50%, the calcaneocuboid 35%, and any combination thereof (double or triple arthrodesis) nearly 100%. Because of the marginal retention of motion of the hindfoot complex with some selective arthrodesis procedures (i.e., double arthrodesis or talonavicular arthrodesis), a more extensive fusion (i.e., triple arthrodesis) may be the procedure of choice because of the improved union rates with this technique.

When hindfoot arthrodesis is performed, the subtalar joint is placed into about 5° of valgus. If a lateral impingement exists beneath the fibula, this should be excised at the time of the fusion.

After a successful subtalar arthrodesis, patients may resume most activities (Figure 21-28). The transverse tarsal joints (calcaneocuboid and talonavicular joints) should be fused in a neutral position, avoiding excessive pronation or supination.

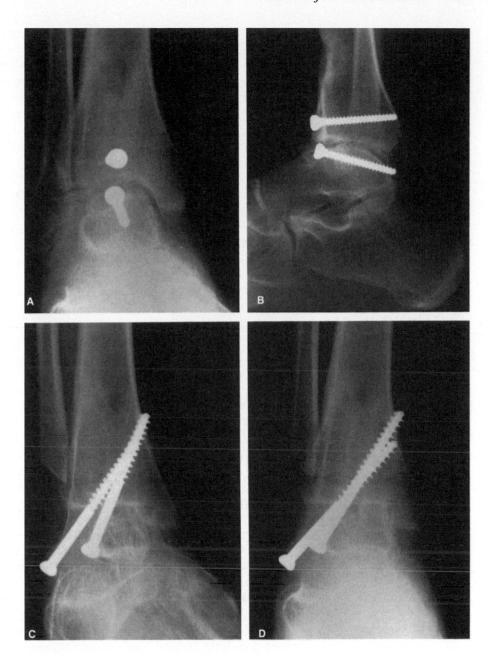

FIGURE 21-27. Ankle fusion. **(A** and **B)** Preoperative radiographs. **(C** and **D)** Postoperative radiographs demonstrating a satisfactory ankle fusion using screw fixation. (Mann RA, Coughlin MJ. The Video Textbook of Foot and Ankle Surgery. St Louis: Medical Video Productions, 1991)

For the talonavicular joint, an isolated arthrodesis produces a satisfactory result in patients older than 50 years of age, but this usually should be combined with a fusion of the calcaneocuboid joint. A triple arthrodesis involves fusion of the subtalar (talocalcaneal), talonavicular, and calcaneocuboid joints. When a triple arthrodesis is carried out, only ankle joint motion is present, and all inversion and eversion function of the foot is lost. Optimal positioning of the subtalar and transverse tarsal joints is necessary to create a plantigrade foot, so that when the foot comes into contact with the ground, there is no abnormal varus or valgus configuration to either the heel or forefoot (Figure 21-29). If the triple arthrodesis is carried out incorrectly, abnormal weight bearing may result. After a successful triple arthrodesis, patients are functional, although there is some added stress to the ankle joint, which can be a problem in some cases. As a general rule, these patients can carry out most functions of daily living, although sports and running are difficult.

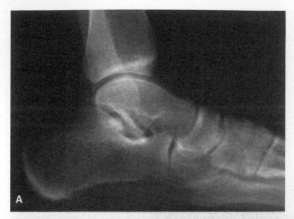

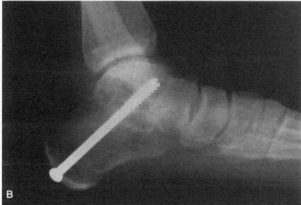

FIGURE 21-28. Subtalar joint arthrodesis. **(A)** Preoperative radiograph of arthrosis of the posterior facet of the subtalar joint. **(B)** Postoperative radiographs demonstrating satisfactory arthrodesis using screw fixation.

Midfoot Arthrosis

Arthrosis of the tarsometatarsal articulation can be primary, or it can be secondary to a Lisfranc fracture dislocation. In both cases, patients note progressive pain and sometimes a progressive abduction deformity of the forefoot, which results in flattening of the longitudinal arch (see Figure 21-23). A prominence often develops, particularly near the first metatarsocuneiform articulation on the plantar medial aspect of the foot. A polypropylene AFO with a trim line cut to permit ankle joint motion and a full-length foot piece often helps provide support. If a large plantar medial prominence is present, however, wearing a brace may be difficult. If conservative management is unsuccessful, arthrodesis to realign the tarsometatarsal articulations can be undertaken.

Arthrodesis of the tarsometatarsal articulation should be carried out to realign the foot, addressing all involved areas of degeneration and deformity.

Often, marked forefoot abduction and dorsiflexion at the tarsometatarsal articulation is present and requires correction. After a successful arthrodesis, the patient has a plantigrade foot and stability of the involved joints. Some patients, however, complain of persistent stiffness in the foot after the fusion, and although they are highly functional, they are encouraged not to engage in high-impact sports.

ANKLE INSTABILITY

Recurrent ankle sprains are a major complaint in young athletic populations. Although the majority of patients who suffer an ankle sprain go on to heal without instability, a small percentage develop chronic laxity of the lateral ankle ligaments. The broad and strong deltoid ligament on the medial side of the ankle is rarely affected. Essentially all cases of lateral ankle ligament laxity involve the anterior talofibular ligament, a thickening of the ankle capsule from the anterior margin of the fibula to the neck of the talus that prevents anterior translation of the talus in the ankle mortise. More severe cases also demonstrate involvement of the stronger calcaneofibular ligament that runs from the tip of the fibula and courses deep to the peroneal tendons to cross the subtalar joint and inserts on the calcaneus. It serves to prevent direct inversion instability both of the ankle and subtalar joint (Figure 21-30).

Bony deformities can predispose patients to develop lateral ankle ligament laxity. When weight bearing, the axis of the calcaneus ordinarily rests in approximately 5 to 7° of valgus compared with the axis of the tibia. This places the line of force lateral to the center of the ankle and does not stress the lateral ankle ligaments. When a varus alignment to the hindfoot is present, however, the lateral ankle ligaments are subject to repetitive loading. The clinical examination of a patient with chronic ankle sprains should include a standing examination from the rear to check hindfoot alignment. Hindfoot varus is most often seen in conjunction with a cavus foot.

In addition to the static ligamentous structures, dynamic support from the peroneal tendons is also important in maintaining ankle stability. The peroneal muscles contract reflexively in response to sudden inversion moments about the subtalar joint and ankle. Because of the peroneal muscle action, many patients with lax ankles on clinical examination do not have a clinical problem with major ankle sprains. In those that do, physical therapy

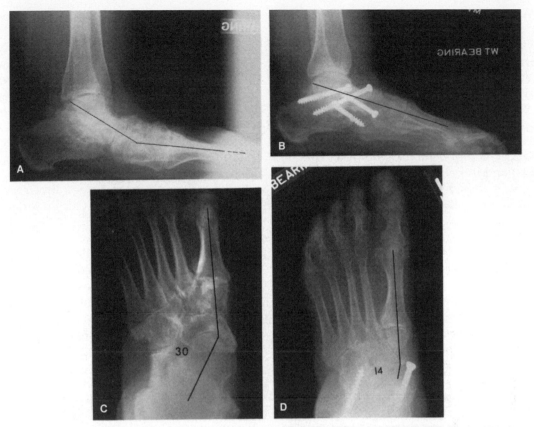

FIGURE 21-29. The triple arthrodesis consists of fusion of the subtalar, talonavicular, and calcaneocuboid joints. Preoperative **(A)** and postoperative **(B)** lateral radiographs demonstrating reestablishment of the longitudinal arch. **(C and D)** AP view demonstrating correction of the abduction deformity of the forefoot. (Mann RA, Coughlin MJ. The Video Textbook of Foot and Ankle Surgery. St Louis: Medical Video Productions, 1991)

aimed at peroneal strengthening and proprioceptive training can be effective in reducing the risk for further major episodes. The mechanism of action is unclear. It takes approximately 50 ms for electrical activity to appear in the peroneal musculature following a sudden unexpected inversion force. Another

70 ms is required for the muscle to develop any significant tension. There is little data to suggest that training can reduce this reaction time. More likely, patients develop more strength in the peroneal tendons and develop motor patterns in which the muscles begin to fire before the foot hits the

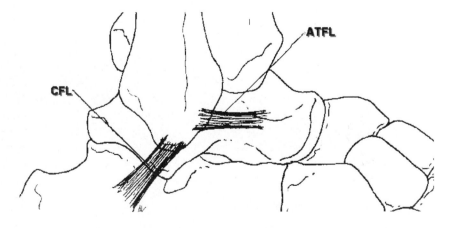

FIGURE 21-30. Schematic diagram depicting course of major lateral ankle ligaments: ATFL (anterior talofibular ligament) and CFL (calcaneofibular ligament). Ligament repair or reconstruction techniques should attempt to recreate ligament isometry.

ground. While this can be effective, some degree of ligament integrity is required to prevent ankle sprains when the foot is going to be subject to sudden unexpected loads as is common in cutting and jumping sports.

The diagnosis of lateral ankle ligament laxity requires both a history of major recurrent ankle sprains and evidence of mechanical laxity on the clinical examination. The ankle should be tested both in direct anterior subluxation (the anterior drawer test) and in inversion (Figure 21-31). Stress radiographs, in which an ankle mortise view is taken while an inversion force is applied, are unreliable. No standards exist to define a threshold of ankle laxity and a large number of false-negative results can be expected because a patient will guard the joint with the peroneal muscles during this awkward test.

The repetitive subluxation events in lateral ankle ligament laxity yield a high rate of associated injuries in other structures about the hindfoot. A high index of suspicion should be maintained in particular for tears of the peroneal tendons and osteochondral lesions of the talus.

Direct repair of the lateral ankle ligaments, usually by imbrication into a small bone trough around the front of the fibula, is known as the Broström procedure. Because it uses the native ligaments and restores the normal anatomy, no limitation of ankle or subtalar motion occurs after the procedure and it is highly effective in restoring stability to the joint. It is the preferred technique for the majority of patients.

Instability may recur after a Broström repair in approximately 15% of cases. One important risk factor for failure is benign joint hypermobility syndrome, a subtle disorder of collagen leading to global ligamentous laxity. It is now regarded by most authorities as synonymous with the mild type III variant of Ehlers-Danlos syndrome. Patients being considered for ligament repair should be evaluated clinically for signs of global ligamentous laxity and for a history of instability problems in other joints.

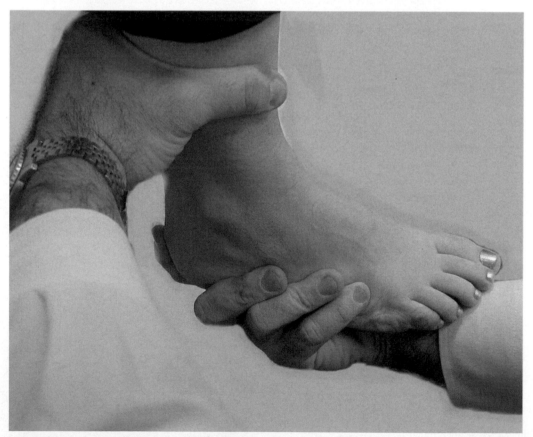

FIGURE 21-31. Anterior drawer physical examination finding in the evaluation of ankle ligament instability. With one hand cupping the heel, an anterior stress is placed on the ankle to elicit the degree of tibiotalar subluxation.

In the case where a previous direct ligament repair has failed or global ligamentous laxity is present, an augmented reconstruction of the lateral ankle ligaments is appropriate. Over 30 procedures have been described to accomplish this using a variety of materials including split or whole peroneus brevis, fascia lata, hamstring tendon, and tendon allograft. All of these augmentation procedures have some potential for causing a pathologic limitation of subtalar motion if the grafts are not placed at the origin and insertion of the anterior talofibular ligament and the calcaneofibular ligament. Whatever graft material is used, the repair should attempt to mimic the normal anatomy as possible.

HEEL PAIN

Pain in the heel pad area may vary from an annoyance to a significantly disabling problem. Heel pain has multiple origins, and it is imperative that a careful history and physical examination be carried out to pinpoint, as precisely as possible, the cause of the pain. In this way, specific treatment can be formulated to relieve the condition. Heel pain can result from disorders of the Achilles tendon, soft tissue disorders near the heel, hindfoot bony injury (i.e. stress fracture), bony prominence irritation, or neurologic disorders about the hindfoot.

Heel pain associated with Achilles tendon disorders is a common problem, particularly with the athlete. Multiple descriptive terms (i.e., tendinitis, tendonitis, tendinosis, tendinopathy, peritendinitis, partial rupture, and so on) have been ascribed to the specific Achilles tendon disorders based on the location of disease and affect on the tendon. These terms are often confusing, occasionally misleading, and many of these disorders often coexist. Perhaps a more simplistic approach is to consider these disorders as a spectrum of disease of the Achilles. The origin, pathogenesis, and natural course of many of these disorders are unknown. Patients generally present with complaints of pain with activities, particularly those sports related. In acute conditions, pain may occur with all activities. In chronic conditions, pain may initially occur only with exertional activities and over time may progress to constant pain, occurring even at rest. Clinical examination may reveal a diffuse selling, crepitation, and tenderness along the tendon in acute disorders. Chronic disorders may present with more subtle and variable findings; often, nodular swelling of the tendon may present suggestive of tendinosis (Figure 21-32). Pain may occur directly over the Achilles tendon proximally, however, it may also occur distally at the heel. If the pain is located at the insertion of the Achilles tendon into the calcaneus, it may be due to some degeneration of the Achilles tendon. In this case, there is thickening of the tendon

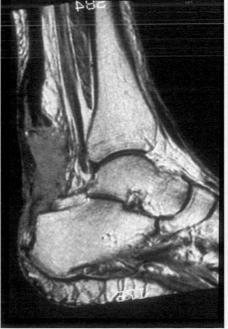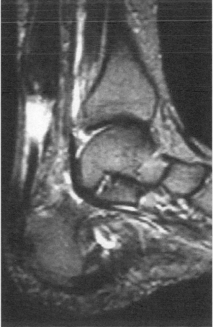

FIGURE 21-32. MRI images of Achilles tendinosis demonstrating intrasubstance tendon degenerative change.

near its insertion, which at times may become large. This can be associated with increased warmth over the area as well. Calcification at the insertion of the Achilles tendon may indicate some degeneration and on rare occasions is a source of pain. At times, pressure from a prominence on the posterosuperior aspect of the calcaneus, known as a *Haglund deformity*, can be the cause of the pain. In the patient with a Haglund deformity, a lateral radiograph of the calcaneus reveals a large posterosuperior prominence on the calcaneus that is responsible for the problem. Initial conservative treatment should be directed toward activity modification, inflammation control, and occasionally immobilization. Corticosteroid use is generally not recommended. If patients fail conservative treatments, surgical intervention may be considered. The procedure of choice depends on the spectrum of disease present and should address all pathology. This may include synovectomy, tendon debridement, tendon repair, tendon augmentation (i.e., tendon transfer [FHL] or Achilles turndown flap), or resection of any bony pathology (i.e., Haglund deformity). The goal of treatment is to return the patient to their desired level of activity without pain.

Soft tissue causes of heel pain include plantar fasciitis and atrophy of the heel pad. Heel pad atrophy is most frequently seen in older patients who develop thinning of the fat pad, which decreases the cushion on the heel. The diagnosis is made by palpation of the heel pad and the observation of lack of adequate fatty tissue. Treatment is conservative with orthotic management for adequate heel cushioning. Plantar fasciitis is the most common cause of inferior heel pain and is very common. It commonly occurs with the first step after a period of rest (e.g., first step in morning) and often improves with activity. This disorder is an inflammatory process and it is postulated that with repeated stress, microtears occur at the bony attachment of the fascia to the calcaneus leading to a chronic inflammatory process. Obesity, repetitive stress in athletics, middle age, and the presence of abnormal foot mechanics (i.e., pes cavus or pes planus) have been associated as risk factors. Although commonly associated with "heel spurs," only 50% of patients with plantar fasciitis have "heel spurs" present radiographically and this finding of itself is not the cause of the patient's subcalcaneal discomfort. Pain is usually located near the tubercle of the calcaneus or just distal to it and palpation along this region reproduces the patient's discomfort. At times, the fasciitis involves the origin of the abductor hallucis muscle, and in these cases, the pain is located along the plantar medial aspect of the heel and is aggravated by palpation of the origin of the muscle. The condition is usually self-limiting and if treatment is begun soon after the onset of symptoms, most patients can expect resolution within 6 weeks. A multitude of treatment options exist and should be exhausted prior to considering surgical intervention. Initial treatment most often consists of Achilles tendon stretching exercises (particularly when limited dorsiflexion is present), oral anti-inflammatory drugs, shoe inserts, and night splints (preventing plantar flexion). For more recalcitrant cases, periodic immobilization may be necessary. Corticosteroid injection at the site of maximal tenderness may be beneficial, but should be used in moderation, rarely exceeding 2 to 3 injections. Extracorporeal shock wave therapy has recently shown benefit in the treatment of refractory fasciitis and should be considered prior to surgical intervention. In rare cases where 6 to 12 months of nonsurgical management has failed to provide relief, surgical intervention, consisting of partial plantar fascia release with or without decompression of the first branch of the lateral plantar nerve and adductor hallucis fascia, should be considered.

Bone-related problems may be the source of heel pain. Occasionally, a stress fracture may involve a calcaneal spur on the plantar aspect of the calcaneus as a cause of heel pain. This occasionally can be demonstrated radiographically, however, often a bone scan is necessary. A bony ridge along the medial or lateral aspect of the insertion of the Achilles tendon may also be a source of heel pain. This bony ridge results in a mechanical problem causing chafing against the counter of the shoe.

The cause of heel pain can be multifactorial, but it is imperative that the clinician accurately diagnoses the origin and directs treatment accordingly. In general, treatment consists of nonsteroidal anti-inflammatory medications, relief of stress over the involved bony prominence, use of a soft orthotic device in the shoe to relieve the heel, cast immobilization, or some combination of these. As a general rule, surgery is not necessary for heel pain. There certainly are exceptions, but the physician should be as conservative as possible in the management of heel pain.

NERVE ENTRAPMENT SYNDROMES

Interdigital Neuroma

Interdigital neuroma is a common cause of pain in the forefoot. The patient may describe a well-localized area of burning pain on the plantar aspect of the foot, which often radiates out toward the tips of the toes. It most frequently involves the third interspace, although it occasionally involves the second interspace. The origin of an interdigital neuroma is not precisely known, although the nerve often becomes thickened secondary to increased hyalinization of the tissues surrounding it and the bursal structures above and below the transverse metatarsal ligament usually enlarge. The pain associated with an interdigital neuroma can be reproduced by squeezing the interspace in a dorsal plantar direction and, when pressure is applied to the interspace, squeezing the foot in a mediolateral direction (Figure 21-33). Conservative management consists of fitting the patient in a wide, soft shoe that also provides metatarsal support. If this fails, excision of the neuroma can be carried out through a dorsal approach to the web space, sectioning the transverse metatarsal ligament and resecting the nerve proximal to the metatarsal head region. This results in a satisfactory response in about 80% of patients.

Tarsal Tunnel Syndrome

Entrapment neuropathy of the posterior tibial nerve with or without involvement of the medial calcaneal nerve can be a neurologic cause of medial ankle and heel pain. The posterior tibial nerve may become compressed within the fibro-osseous tunnel posterior and inferior to the medial malleolus. This may be diagnosed by percussion over the posterior tibial nerve or its terminal branches, which demonstrate a Tinel's sign with radiation toward the heel. The medial calcaneal nerve may be involved at the level of the ankle or at the level of the abductor digiti quinti muscle as the nerve is stretched over the plantar fascia as it passes over it to cross the foot. In these cases, pain is often noted along the plantar medial aspect of the foot, just below the abductor hallucis muscle. Treatment is conservative, with orthotic modifications and measures to decrease the inflammation surrounding the involved nerve. Surgical decompression is performed only in refractory cases, with best results obtained in patients with clearly defined space occupying lesions or masses obstructing the canal.

THE DIABETIC FOOT

Pathology of the foot in diabetes represents a vast public health problem. A typical newly diagnosed patient with diabetes has a roughly 15% chance of developing a foot ulcer over the course of his or her

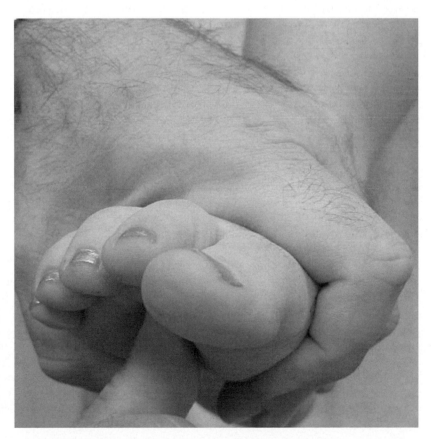

FIGURE 21-33. Clinical examination finding of intradigital neuroma ("Mulder's click"). Reproduction of pain and mechanical subluxation of the thickened nerve and surrounding tissues is produced by squeezing the interspace in a dorsal plantar direction with one hand and applying pressure to the interspace by squeezing the foot in a mediolateral direction with the other hand.

disease. At any given time, roughly 5% of neuropathic diabetics have an ulcer of the foot. Given the increasing trends toward obesity and type II diabetes in Western society, the problem is only likely to become more acute.

Diabetic foot pathology essentially refers to two distinct clinical problems: neuropathic ulceration and the Charcot foot. Both are secondary phenomena to diabetic neuropathy. A recent important prospective study, the Diabetes Control and Complications Trial, demonstrated the arrested progression of diabetic neuropathy with intensive glucose control and close monitoring of glycosylated hemoglobin levels. As a rule, the risk of foot pathology is greatly reduced by diabetics who are successful at long-term diabetic control and can maintain their glycosylated hemoglobin levels under 8%.

Neuropathic Ulceration

Neuropathic ulceration occurs as a consequence of repetitive unrecognized trauma to an insensate foot as a neuropathic patient ambulates. It occurs under load-bearing sites in the foot, most commonly under the metatarsal heads or the heel. A critical level of the loss of sensation appears to be required to lead to ulceration. Semmes-Weinstein monofilaments are short lengths of nylon fishing line of varying thicknesses that can provide a reproducible stimulus to the skin. Ninety percent of patients that are able to feel the Semmes-Weinstein 5.07 monofilament will not develop an ulcer.

Diabetics who have lost more sensation than the critical threshold must maintain a strict regimen of self-care to avoid ulceration. Daily self-examination of the soles of the feet is mandatory. Autonomic neuropathy can lead to a loss of sweat and the resulting cracks and fissures can create portals for infection. The use of a lanolin-rich moisturizer on all dry locations is critical. The single most important measure, however, is the use of appropriate shoe wear. The vast majority of diabetics do not need fully custom shoes. Instead, manufactured accommodative shoes with a wide forefoot and an extra-depth toe box are readily available. These are usually paired with accommodative custom orthotics. The goal of protective diabetic inserts is to accommodate any foot deformities rather than correct them, and no attempt is usually made to significantly reposition the foot. The inserts are usually made of several layers of varying durometer, or hardness. The deeper layers provide a measure of durability while the superficial layers conform to the surface of the foot. Because they are not made of rigid materials, protective orthotics do wear out and compress rapidly. They must typically be replaced several times a year.

Neuropathic ulceration is distinctly different from the vascular gangrene also seen in diabetics with associated atherosclerosis. Vascular gangrene typically strikes distally about the toes and is not purely associated with load-bearing locations in the foot. Numerous studies have demonstrated that poor arterial inflow is not a risk factor for the development of plantar pressure ulcers from weight bearing. Notably, however, a diminished arterial supply can severely affect the ability of those ulcers to heal once they are established.

Other mechanical factors besides the repetitive nature of unrecognized force applied to the neuropathic foot are also at work in developing ulceration. Neuropathic patients will not alter their gait in the presence of any foot deformity. If the patient also has a midfoot or hindfoot collapse from a Charcot arthropathy, these can be severe. Charcot patients have a 350% relative risk of developing ulcerations compared to neuropathic patients without Charcot.

The tight tendo-Achilles complex represents a second important mechanical risk factor. Tight heel cords are prevalent in diabetes because the collagen within the tendon undergoes direct glycosylation with long-standing disease. This leads to abnormal cross-link formation, reduced pliability, and contracture of the motor unit. A tight heel cord paradoxically causes pathology in the forefoot; if the ankle is unable to dorsiflex the heel is brought off the ground earlier in the stance phase of gait. The metatarsal heads are on the ground longer and bear more weight and are therefore highly susceptible to ulceration. Several series have now demonstrated the healing of recalcitrant forefoot ulcers following the release of a heal cord contracture.

Evaluation of an Ulcer

To fully evaluate any diabetic ulcer, it must first be debrided. Superficial calluses must be removed to determine the health of the underlying tissues. Radiographs should be obtained to look for signs of bony erosion indicative of osteomyelitis. These can be deceptive, however, and erosions may not appear for the first several weeks after it develops. If an ulcer clinically probes to bone, there is a 90% chance that osteomyelitis is present based on several studies using histologic diagnosis as the criterion. Osteomyelitis in an adult is a surgical disease; the infected bone must be removed or the ulcer cannot permanently heal.

The presence of cellulitis or a deep abscess is important to diagnose. The only role for MRI in the evaluation of the diabetic foot is to evaluate for the presence of a deep abscess. Bony edema in the diabetic foot, particularly in the presence of Charcot change, makes it extremely difficult to accurately determine the presence of osteomyelitis on MRI criteria, and nuclear medicine studies are more appropriate for this purpose. The overinterpretation of superficial wound culture swabs is another common error. All diabetic ulcers are superficially colonized with a wide variety of organisms including anaerobes. Superficial swabs often differ dramatically from deep, surgically obtained biopsies and treatments based on them may lead to unnecessarily long or risky antibiotic regimens.

The vascular status of the foot is critical in assessing its ability to heal. If the dorsalis pedis and tibialis posterior pulses are not palpable, a Doppler examination is mandated. If there is still suspicion, vascular noninvasive studies are appropriate. The ankle-brachial index (ABI), a ratio of the systolic pressure at the ankle to that in the arm is commonly used. A ratio of 0.4 is a minimally acceptable value, above 0.7 there is little concern. Unfortunately, ABIs can be unreliable in the presence of extensive atherosclerosis. The reduced capacitance of the vascular tree in the leg can falsely elevate the systolic pressure and the ABI reading. Toe pressures represent a simple additional test that can be more informative, but must usually be specifically ordered. A small pressure cuff is placed over the toe and a pressure reading generated. Absolute toe pressures above 40 mm Hg or the presence of pulsatile flow are usually indicative of adequate healing. Transcutaneous oxygen tension within the foot is an excellent means of assessing the vascularity of a foot but is not widely available. If none of these methods can establish the integrity of the arterial blood supply, angiography and referral to a vascular surgeon are required.

The mechanical environment of an ulcer is also important to evaluate. The tightness of the heel cord should be assessed both with the knee extended (gastrocnemius tight) and with the knee flexed (gastrocnemius relaxed). The presence of any varus or valgus deformities in the midfoot or any forefoot deformities should be noted. Bony prominences that would be well-tolerated in a normal individual sometimes lead to disaster for the neuropathic diabetic.

Treatment

Because neuropathic ulcerations are essentially mechanical problems, their treatment is primarily mechanical. Reducing the mechanical stress on the tissues is the primary means of achieving healing. For the forefoot and midfoot, a variety of manufactured pressure-relieving boots and shoes are available. The gold standard in pressure relief, however, continues to be the total contact cast. Most forefoot ulcerations can be healed in 6 to 8 weeks with serial cast treatment and ulcer debridement. Unfortunately, casts and boots do no provide adequate pressure relief for heel ulcerations, and these must be treated with strict non–weight bearing and dressing changes alone.

In some special situations, a variety of wound gels with biologic activity may be appropriate. Becaplermin gel contains recombinant platelet-derived growth factor and may be used in marginally vascularized wounds with atrophic granulation. Copper-containing compounds also provide a stimulatory effect. Mesh embedded with cultured human fibroblasts that secrete an array of growth factors has also been used. Finally, silver-containing gels or slow-release films can be used in the presence of superficial colonization by pseudomonas. It is important to note, however, that all of the biologic adjuvants for wound healing must be used in conjunction with adequate pressure relief.

Hyperbaric oxygen therapy in a chamber has seen mixed support as an adjunctive measure in diabetic ulceration. There is clear support for its use in life- or limb-threatening anaerobic infections following aggressive surgical debridement. For routine neuropathic ulcerations, however, its benefit is unclear. From a practical standpoint the advent of the recombinant wound gels makes them the usual current choice when a biologic adjuvant treatment is desired. There is absolutely no well-controlled evidence that topical normobaric oxygen therapy (placing the foot in an oxygen-filled bag) provides any benefit.

The Charcot Foot

Neuropathic arthropathy was first described by the famous French neurologist Jean-Martin Charcot, who originally described the condition in syphilitics. Typically a dense peripheral neuropathy must be present for approximately 10 to 15 years before the disorder is manifest. Concordantly, the first cases in diabetics were described in the 1930s, approximately 10 years after the availability of insulin extended their lives long enough to develop the complication.

The pathogenesis of neuropathic arthropathy remains obscure. The neurotraumatic hypothesis is the classic model. It holds that accumulated microtrauma to the joint in an insensate limb causes breakdown of the bony architecture. There are, however, well-documented cases of Charcot arthropathy occurring in completely bedridden individuals. In the 1960s, it became clear that Charcot arthropathy is associated with autonomic dysfunction. The neurovascular hypothesis was developed to tie in this observation. It proposed that a loss of the autonomic control of bone blood flow occurs, leading to a "wash out" of bone mineral. There is no causal mechanism to link the increase bone blood flow in Charcot arthropathy to the loss of bone mineral, however. Charcot had originally proposed the neurotrophic hypothesis, theorizing some important "trophic factor" from nerves was critical in maintaining the health of the joints. He may yet prove correct. Evidence from serum markers of bone metabolism indicates a dramatic amount of osteoclastic activity without concordant elevations in osteoblastic activity. A direct link between peripheral nerve and the regulation of osteoclast activity remains to be established.

Eichenholz described three temporal stages of the Charcot joint that remain at least broadly useful for communication, although no clear standards exist to define the precise transitions from one phase to another. Stage I disease represents the acute fracture-like state with dramatic soft-tissue swelling and instability

(Figure 21-34). Stage II represents early coalescence with a stable soft tissue envelope. In stage III, the joint has coalesced and has developed mature calluses and, usually, stability. Classically in the foot the entire process takes approximately 18 months to fully progress to the quiescent stage III, although the time may vary. Approximately 30% of diabetic patients who develop a Charcot foot on one side will eventually suffer the same fate on the contralateral extremity.

The goal of treatment of the Charcot foot is to yield a stable, braceable foot that can be used for ambulation. Any hope of a completely normal foot must be abandoned, and patients must be made aware of this early on. Midfoot Charcot arthropathy accounts for roughly 60% of the cases, and the majority of these can be treated conservatively. During the early stages of the disease, total contact casts are changed at very frequent intervals until the patient's volume status stabilizes. At this point a fully custom clamshell ankle-foot orthosis or Charcot Restrained Orthotic Walker (CROW) is fabricated (Figure 21-35). This device should be used until the foot achieves stability both clinically and radiographically. A portion of patients with midfoot neuropathic arthropathy will go on to develop plantar prominences and ulcers from the collapse of the arch. If the overall degree of collapse is mild and the foot is stable, simple excision of the plantar prominence can be undertaken. In more advanced cases, the arch collapses to the point that it actually reverses, creating a rocker-bottom foot. These cases may require midfoot fusion and reconstruction of the arch to achieve a successful result.

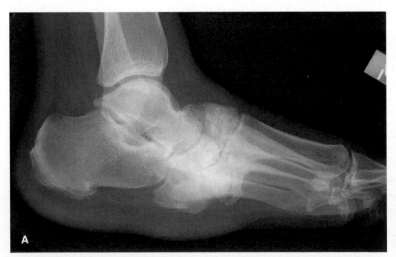
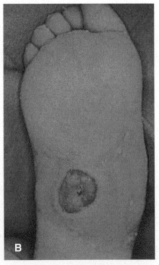

FIGURE 21-34. Diabetic Charcot foot. **(A)** Lateral radiograph demonstrating severe midfoot fracture subluxation with midfoot collapse consistent with rocker-bottom deformity. **(B)** Clinical consequence of ulceration secondary to plantar bony prominence associated with collapse.

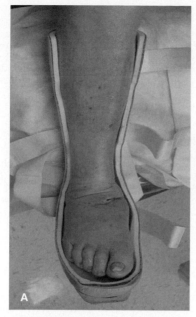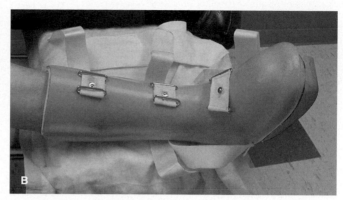

FIGURE 21-35. (A and **B)** Orthotic management of Charcot deformity with a Charcot Restrained Orthotic Walker (CROW) device.

Neuropathic arthropathy of the ankle and hindfoot is less common than in the midfoot but has a much more grim prognosis. This pattern of disease can present in both sporadic forms and after seemingly simple rotational ankle fractures. It often goes on to severe early deformity, ulceration, and osteomyelitis. Although stabilization surgery in the early stages of Charcot arthropathy is usually best avoided, it may be mandatory in the ankle if the patient develops severe early deformity that places the limb at risk. Special fusion techniques including the use of retrograde intramedullary nails are sometimes necessary.

Once a Charcot joint has coalesced, all patients require some form of orthosis. Patients without significant swelling can use a polypropylene molded AFO, but many obese patients find that the degree of day-to-day volume change in the foot requires a less confining brace. A conventional double metal upright AFO attached to the shoe remains an attractive option in this group.

Annotated Bibliography

Mann RA. Biomechanics of the foot and ankle. In: Mann RA, Coughlin MJ, eds. Surgery of the Foot and Ankle, 6th Ed. St. Louis: Mosby-Year Book, 1993:3–43.
This general review article describes the biomechanics of the foot and ankle.

Disorders of the First Metatarsophalangeal Joint

Coughlin MJ. Arthrodesis of the first metatarsophalangeal joint with mini-fragment plate fixation. Orthopaedics 1990; 13:1037.
This article discusses the history of arthrodesis and the indications, surgical technique, results, and complications of this procedure.

Leventen EO. The chevron procedure: etiology and treatment of hallux valgus. Orthopaedics 1990;13:973.
This article discusses the indications, surgical technique, and results of the Chevron procedure.

Mann RA. Decision making in bunion surgery. AAOS Instr Course Lect 1990;39:3.
This article discusses the basic concepts used and presents an algorithm that is helpful in the decision-making process in hallux valgus surgery.

Mann RA. Hallux rigidus. Instr Course Lect 1990; 39:15.
This review article discusses the origin, physical findings, radiographic findings, and treatment of hallux rigidus using various techniques. It emphasizes cheilectomy and arthrodesis as the main surgical procedures.

Mann RA, Coughlin MJ. The great toe. In: The Video Textbook of Foot and Ankle Surgery. St Louis: Medical Video Productions, 1991:145.
This book chapter presents a concise overview of hallux valgus surgery, including the indications, surgical technique, and complications of various surgical procedures.

Mann RA, Coughlin MJ. Hallux valgus: etiology, anatomy, treatment and surgical considerations. Clin Orthop 1981; 157:31.
This article discusses treatment of the hallux valgus deformity using the distal soft tissue procedure. It points out the technical aspects of the procedure, results, and complications.

Mann RA, Rudicel S, Graves S. Repair hallux valgus with a distal soft-tissue procedure and proximal metatarsal osteotomy: a long-term follow-up. J Bone Joint Surg 1992;74A:124.
This is a detailed analysis of the surgical technique, postoperative results, and complications of a review of 109 operative procedures in 75 patients.

Plattner PF, Van Manten JW. Results of Akin type proximal phalangeal osteotomy for correction of hallux valgus deformity. Orthopaedics 1990;13:989.
This article discusses results of the Akin procedure on a series of patients. It points out the indications and complications of this procedure.

Shereff MJ, Bejjani FJ, Kummer FJ. Kinematics of the first metatarsophalangeal joint. J Bone Joint Surg 1986;68A:392.
This article describes the motion of the first metatarsophalangeal joint in terms of its kinematics.

Lesser Toe Deformities

Mann RA, Coughlin MJ. Lesser toe deformities. In: The Video Textbook of Foot and Ankle Surgery. St Louis: Medical Video Productions, 1991:37.
This concise book chapter reviews the various lesser toe deformities. It discusses the definition, evaluation, surgical treatment, and complications of these various deformities.

Metatarsalgia

Mann RA. Intractable plantar keratosis. Instr Course Lect 1984;33:287.
This article reviews the various types of callus formation on the plantar aspect of the foot. It outlines the conservative and operative management of these problems.

Mann RA, Reynolds JC. Interdigital neuroma: a critical clinical analysis. Foot Ankle 1983;3:238.
This article discusses the history, physical findings, and surgical procedure for treatment of the interdigital neuroma. It then analyzes the results of this procedure.

Postural Problems

Mann RA, Coughlin MJ. Postural problems of the foot. In: The Video Textbook of Foot and Ankle Surgery. St Louis: Medical Video Productions, 1991:17.
This book chapter presents an overview of the various types of acquired flatfoot deformities. It points out the physical findings, methods of treatment, and technical aspects of surgery. The chapter further discusses the treatment of the cavus foot.

The Diabetic Foot

Wagner FW. The diabetic foot and amputations of the foot. In: Mann RA, ed. Surgery of the Foot, 5th Ed. St Louis: CV Mosby, 1986:421.
This book chapter presents the problem of the diabetic foot along with a logical approach to treatment. It presents a series of algorithms that enables the clinician to better understand the various modalities of treatment of the diabetic foot.

Arthrosis of the Foot and Ankle

Mann RA, Coughlin MJ. Rheumatoid arthritis and arthrodesis about the foot. In: The Video Textbook of Foot and Ankle Surgery. St Louis: Medical Video Productions, 1991:105.
This chapter describes the surgical treatment of the rheumatoid forefoot, presenting the various types of surgical procedures and postoperative care. It further discusses arthrodesis about the foot, which includes subtalar, talonavicular, and tarsometatarsal arthrodeses. It presents a discussion on triple arthrodesis and double arthrodesis.

Miscellaneous

Baxter DE, Pfeffer GB, Thigpen M. Chronic heel pain: treatment rationale. Orthop Clin North Am 1989;20:563.
This article discusses the various types of heel pain, methods of diagnosis, and conservative and operative management.

Index

Page numbers followed by "f" indicate figures; those followed by "t" indicate tables.

juvenile idiopathic arthritis association, 172, 174
nonarticular, bacterial seeding of joints, 176
olecranon bursitis from, 407
osteomyelitis, 123–140. *See also* Osteomyelitis
  trauma-associated, 125, 176
with total knee arthroplasty, 626–628
  amputation for, 628
  antibiotic suppression for, 628
  arthrodesis for, 628
  aspiration of, 628
  causes of, 626
  clinical presentation of, 626–627
  debridement with prosthetic retention for, 628
  laboratory tests for, 626–627, 629f
  management algorithm for, 628, 629f
  microbiology of, 626
  radiography of, 627
  radionuclide imaging of, 627
  reimplantation for, 628
woven bone association, 11
Infectious arthritis. *See* Septic arthritis
Inferior patella pole-superior patellar ligament junction, chronic tensile stress at, 583
Inflammation
  in acromioclavicular joint, 348, 360
  with bone injury, 58–60
  with calcium pyrophosphate dihydrate deposition disease, 185
  with cartilage injury, 64–65
  with cervical disc disease, 328–329
  with Charcot arthropathy, 228
  with elbow tendonopathies, 410, 412–414
  with foot puncture wound infections, 142
  with gout, 183
  with juvenile rheumatoid arthritis, 337
  in lesser metatarsophalangeal joint disorders, 683–685
  with muscle injury, 69–70, 70t
  with rheumatoid arthritis, 162–163
    of elbow, 409–410
    management of, 164–165, 165f
  with rotator cuff-tear arthropathy, 365, 369
  with septic arthritis, 143, 146
  with systemic lupus erythematosus, 166
  with tendon injury, 67, 68f
Inflammatory bowel disease arthritis, 168, 170
  management of, 171
Inflammatory diseases
  rheumatoid, 151–197. *See also* Rheumatoid diseases; *specific disease*
  woven bone association, 11
Inflammatory enthesitis
  in juvenile idiopathic arthritis, 174
  in spondyloarthropathies, 168, 171
Inflammatory mediators
  of anterior cruciate ligament injury, 601
  of bone injury, 58–60
  release with fractures, 92–93
Infliximab, for rheumatoid arthritis, 434
Infraspinatus musculotendinous unit, in rotator cuff disease, 368, 371

Injury(ies). *See* Trauma; *specific anatomy or injury*
Innervation. *See* Nerve(s)
Innominate osteotomies
  Salter
    for congenital hip dysplasia, 451, 452f
    for Legg-Calvé-Perthes disease, 452f, 463
  triple, for hip dysplasia
    in cerebral palsy, 217
    in pseudochondroplasia, 259
Inorganic matrix
  in bone, 15, 15f
  in connective tissue, 9
Inorganic pyrophosphate (PPi), in calcium pyrophosphate dihydrate deposition disease, 185
Insall-Burstein knee prosthesis, 621
Insertions, of tendons, ligaments, and joint capsules into bone
  direct, 23–24, 23f
  indirect, 23f, 24
Instability. *See* Stability; *specific joint*
Instrumentation
  distraction
    for congenital spinal deformity, 496
    for idiopathic scoliosis, 484, 486, 486f
  for idiopathic scoliosis, 484, 491, 492f–493
  rod. *See* Rod instrumentation
  in spinal fusion
    for cerebral palsy, 213–215, 215f
    for muscular dystrophies, 232
    for myelodysplasia, 224–225
    for spinal muscular atrophy, 230
Insufficiency fractures, 90, 93f
Insulin, bone turnover and, 16
Insulin-like growth factor-I, bone development and, 200
Insurance benefits, gait analysis impact on, 83
Integumentary system. *See* Skin *entries*
Intercondylar notch, in anterior cruciate ligament injury, 601, 603
Intercritical period, of gout inflammation, 183
Interdigital neuroma, in foot, 700–701, 701f
Interdigitation, of muscle cells and tendons, 21, 21f
Interferon, for viral arthritis, 182
Interleukin-1, bone turnover and, 16
Intermediate zone, of articular cartilage, 27, 27f
Intermetatarsal angle, in hallux valgus, 674, 674f, 676
Internal fixation. *See also specific type*
  for fractures
    anatomic reduction with, 107, 109f
    with intramedullary screws, 99, 99f, 106f
    open reduction with. *See* Open reduction and internal fixation
    with plates, 99, 109f
    to promote tissue healing, 57
    with screws, 99, 99f, 106f, 109f
International League of Associations for Rheumatology (ILAR) classification, of juvenile idiopathic arthritis, 172, 174

Interphalangeal (IP) joints
  fractures of, 115
  hallux valgus deformity of, 677, 679f
  in lesser toe disorders, 681–683, 683f
  thumb, in median nerve palsy, 433
Intersection syndrome, of forearm, 410, 412
Intersegmental artery, 46
Inter-segmental forces, in gait analysis, 78, 78f
Interstitial growth, of cartilage, 42, 45f–46f
Interstitial lung disease (ILD), with systemic sclerosis, 188, 189t, 190
Interterritorial matrix, in articular cartilage, 28
Intertransverse process fusion, lumbosacral, for spondylolisthesis, 507–508
Intertrochanteric osteotomy, varus, for hip dysplasia, 530, 530f
Intervertebral (osteo) chondrosis, 156, 157f
Intervertebral disc(s), 31–37
  age-related changes, 32, 34, 36–37
  composition of, 34–37, 34f–35f
    blood supply, 36
    cells, 34, 34f–35f
      connective tissue, 34, 35f
      notochordal, 34, 34f
    matrix, 34–36
    nerve supply, 36
  degeneration of, 32, 34, 330f, 334, 514–515. *See also* Intervertebral disc disease
  elastin in, 8
  function of, 31–32, 55
  infections of, 133, 140–141, 141f
  mycobacterial arthritis involvement, 178
  structure of, 31–34, 33f
    annulus fibrosis, 32–33, 33f
    hyaline cartilage endplate, 32
    nucleus pulposus, 33–34, 33f
    transition zone, 33, 35, 36
Intervertebral disc disease
  cervical, 327–335
    clinical features of, 328–329
    CT scan of, 331
    differential diagnosis of, 328–329, 329t
    diskography of, 331, 333f, 334
    electrodiagnostic studies of, 334
    electromyography of, 334
    incidence of, 328
    local injection for, 334–334
    MRI of, 331, 332f
    myelography of, 328, 331, 331f
    myelopathy with, 329
    pathoanatomy of, 334
    radiculopathy with, 328–329, 330t
      treatment of, 334–335
    radiographic features of, 328–329, 330f, 331
    terms for, 327–328
    treatment of, 334–335, 335f
  as degenerative, 32, 34, 330f, 334, 514–515
  as herniation, 327, 331f, 333f, 334
    in adults, 512–514
    in children, 509